Essentials of Clinical Mycology

Carol A. Kauffman • Peter G. Pappas
Jack D. Sobel • William E. Dismukes
Editors

Essentials of Clinical Mycology

Second Edition

Springer

Editors
Carol A. Kauffman, M.D.
Professor of Internal Medicine
Division of Infectious Diseases
University of Michigan Medical School
Veterans Affairs Ann Arbor Healthcare System
Ann Arbor, MI, USA
ckauff@umich.edu

Jack D. Sobel, M.D.
Professor of Internal Medicine
Division of Infectious Diseases
Detroit Medical Center
Wayne State University School of Medicine
Detroit, MI, USA
JSobel@med.wayne.edu

Peter G. Pappas, M.D.
Professor of Medicine
Division of Infectious Diseases
University of Alabama at Birmingham
School of Medicine
Birmingham, AL, USA
pappas@uab.edu

William E. Dismukes, M.D.
Professor Emeritus of Medicine
Division of Infectious Diseases
University of Alabama at Birmingham
School of Medicine
Birmingham, AL, USA
wed@uab.edu

ISBN 978-1-4899-8227-8 ISBN 978-1-4419-6640-7 (eBook)
DOI 10.1007/978-1-4419-6640-7
Springer New York Dordrecht Heidelberg London

Printed on acid-free paper

Springer is part of Springer Science+Business Media (www.springer.com)

Preface to the Second Edition

Since the publication of the first edition of this book in 2003, the field of clinical mycology has burgeoned. This is in no small measure due to increasing numbers of immunosuppressed hosts. Transplants of both solid organs and stem cells have become commonplace. In addition to patients who classically have been considered to be immune compromised, the expanded use of immune modifiers, such as tumor necrosis factor antagonists and other monoclonal antibodies, has created new populations at risk for fungal infections. Advances in intensive care have allowed survival of desperately ill patients, but also have created another population group at high risk for invasive fungal infections. Our understanding of the epidemiology of fungal infections has expanded with detailed studies on risk factors and effects of various prophylactic regimens in specific at-risk populations and with the use of newer molecular methods.

The treatment of fungal infections has improved markedly in the few short years since the first edition was published. New antifungal agents have been licensed for use, and indications for the use of various antifungal agents have changed. New agents in the echinocandin and azole classes of drugs and the increasing use of lipid formulations of amphotericin B have allowed safer and more effective therapy for severe fungal infections, especially in immunosuppressed patients. The scientific basis of antifungal therapy has been enhanced with new studies on the pharmacodynamics and pharmacokinetics of these agents. Unfortunately, and perhaps not unexpectedly, these positive developments have been tempered by increasing resistance to several classes of antifungal agents.

For each of the medically important fungal diseases, we have attempted to integrate basic aspects of mycology pertinent to an understanding of pathogenesis of infection with an extensive discussion of clinical manifestations, diagnosis, and treatment. Color photographs are used extensively to illustrate the many different manifestations of fungal infections.

The book is organized, as before, into several distinct sections and is extensively indexed to allow easy access to the topics pertinent to patients cared for by busy clinicians. Part I gives a general overview of laboratory aspects of mycology, emphasizing newer molecular techniques that are assuming increasing importance in diagnosis, and of epidemiologic trends in fungal infections. The chapters in Part II give an in-depth review of the antifungal agents available for the treatment of systemic fungal infections. In addition, specific chapters deal with the expanding area of pharmacokinetics and pharmacodynamics, the increasing problem of antifungal resistance, and the use of combination antifungal therapy. Parts III–VI are devoted to individual fungal diseases, and are arranged by diseases caused by yeasts (Part III), moulds (Part IV), dimorphic or endemic fungi (Part V), and other mycoses (Part VI). The final section (Part VII) is devoted to specific immunosuppressed populations who are at high risk for fungal infections.

It is hoped that this text will provide a valuable resource for clinicians who do battle with the medically important fungi in their daily practices, as well as for those who only infrequently are faced with the "odd case" that could possibly be an unusual fungal infection.

C.A.K., P.G.P., J.D.S., W.E.D.

Contents

Contributors

Carlos A. Agudelo M.D.
Department of Internal Medicine, Corporacion para Investigaciones Biologicas, School of Medical Sciences, Universidad Pontificia Bolivriana, Medellin, Colombia
carlosagudelo@yahoo.com

Barbara D. Alexander M.D.
Duke Mycology Research Unit, Division of Infectious Diseases and International Health, Duke University Medical Center, Durham, NC, USA
Alexa011@mcduke.edu

Neil M. Ampel M.D.
Division of Infectious Diseases, Southern Arizona Veterans Affairs Health Care Center, University of Arizona, Tucson, AZ, USA
nampel@email.arizona.edu

David R. Andes M.D.
Department of Medicine, and Medical Microbiology and Immunology, Section of Infectious Diseases, Madison, WI, USA
dra@medicine.wisc.edu

John W. Baddley M.D., MSPH
Division of Infectious Diseases, Birmingham VA Medical Center, University of Alabama at Birmingham School of Medicine, Birmingham, AL, USA
jbaddley@uab.edu

J. Ryan Bariola M.D.
University of Arkansas for Medical Sciences and Central Arkansas Veterans Health Care System, Little Rock, AR, USA
BariolaJeremyR@uams.edu

Robert W. Bradsher Jr M.D.
University of Arkansas for Medical Sciences and Central Arkansas Veterans Health Care System, Little Rock, AR, USA
bradsherrobertw@uams.edu

Mary E. Brandt Ph.D.
Mycotic Diseases Branch, Centers for Disease Control and Prevention, Atlanta, GA, USA
mbb4@cdc.gov

Beatriz Bustamante M.D.
Instituto de Medicina Tropical; "Alexander von Humboldt,"
Universidad Peruana Cayetano Heredia; Departamento de Enfermedades Transmisibles y Dermatológicas, Hospital Nacional
Cayetano Heredia, Lima, Peru
ana.bustamante@upch.pe

Pablo E. Campos M.D., MPH
School of Public Health and Administration, Universidad Peruana
Cayetano Heredia, Lima, Peru
pecampos@upch.pe

Stanley W. Chapman M.D.
School of Medicine, University of Mississippi Medical Center, Jackson, MS, USA
schapman@medicine.umsmed.edu

Tom M. Chiller M.D.
Mycotic Diseases Branch and Division of Foodborne, Bacterial, and Mycotic Diseases, Centers for Disease Control and Prevention, Atlanta, GA, USA
Tchiller@cdc.gov

John D. Cleary Pharm D
Schools of Pharmacy & Medicine, University of Mississippi Medical Center, Jackson, MS, USA
jcleary@medicine.umsmed.edu

Catherine F. Decker M.D.
National Naval Medical Center, Bethesda, MD, USA
catherine.decker@med.navy.mil

William E. Dismukes M.D.
Division of Infectious Diseases, University of Alabama at Birmingham
School of Medicine, Birmingham, AL, USA
wed@uab.edu

Elizabeth Dodds Ashley Pharm D, MHS
School of Medicine and Dentistry, University of Rochester Medical Center, Rochester, NY, USA
Elizabeth_doddsashley@urmc.rochester.edu

Bertrand Dupont M.D.
Maladies Infectieuses, Hopital Necker, Paris, France
bertrand.dupont@nck.aphp.fr

John E. Edwards Jr M.D.
Division of Infectious Diseases, Harbor-UCLA Research and Education Institute, Torrance, CA, USA
jedwards@labiomed.org

Scott G. Filler M.D.
Division of Infectious Diseases, Harbor-UCLA Research and Education Institute, Torrance, CA, USA
sfiller@labiomed.org

Juan C. Gea-Banacloche M.D.
Infectious Diseases Section, Experimental Transplantation and Immunology Branch, National Cancer Institute, National Institutes of Health, Bethesda, MD, USA
banacloj@mail.nih.gov

Angel Gonzalez Ph.D.
Medical and Experimental Mycology Unit, Corporacion para Investigaciones Biologicas, Microbiology School, Universidad de Antioquia, Medellin, Colombia
agonzalezm@cib.org.co

Andreas H. Groll M.D.
Infectious Diseases Research Program, Department of Pediatric Hematology/Oncology and Center for Bone Marrow Transplantation, Children's University Hospital, Muenster, Germany
grollan@ukmuenster.de

Ashraf S. Ibrahim Ph.D.
Division of Infectious Diseases, Harbor-UCLA Research and Education Institute, Torrance, CA, USA
Ibrahim@labiomed.org

Melissa D. Johnson Pharm D, MHS
Division of Infectious Diseases and International Health, Duke University Medical Center, Campbell University School of Pharmacy, Durham, NC, USA
Johns200@mc.duke.edu

Carol A. Kauffman M.D.
Division of Infectious Diseases, University of Michigan Medical School, VA Ann Arbor Healthcare System, Ann Arbor, MI, USA
ckauff@umich.edu

Dimitrios P. Kontoyiannis M.D., Sc D
Department of Internal Medicine, The University of Texas, MD Anderson Cancer Center, Houston TX, USA
dkontoyi@mdanderson.org

Robert A. Larsen M.D.
Department of Internal Medicine, Los Angeles County/USC Medical Center, Los Angeles, CA, USA
rlarsen@usc.edu

Alex J. Lepak M.D.
Department of Medicine, Section of Infectious Diseases, University of Wisconsin, Madison, WI, USA
ajlepak@medicine.wisc.edu

Shawn R. Lockhart Ph.D.
Mycotic Diseases Branch, Centers for Disease Control and Prevention, Atlanta, GA 30333, USA
gyi2@cdc.gov

Olivier Lortholary M.D., Ph.D.
Infectious and Tropical Diseases Departement, Centre d' Infectiologie Necker-Pasteur, Université Paris Descartes, Hôpital Necker Enfants malades, Paris, France
olivier.lortholary@nck.aphp.fr

Kieren A. Marr M.D.
Transplant and Oncology, Infectious Diseases Program, Johns Hopkins University, Baltimore, MD, USA
kmarr4@jhmi.edu

Henry Masur M.D.
Critical Care Medicine, National Institutes of Health, Bethesda, MD, USA
hmasur@nih.gov

Kenrad E. Nelson M.D.
Departments of Epidemiology, Bloomberg School of Public Health,
International Health and Medicine, Johns Hopkins University, Baltimore, MD, USA
kenelson@jhsph.edu

Dionissios Neofytos M.D.
Transplant and Oncology, Infectious Diseases Program,
Johns Hopkins University, Baltimore, MD, USA
dneofyto1@jhmi.edu

Peter G. Pappas M.D.
Division of Infectious Diseases, University of Alabama at Birmingham School of Medicine,
Birmingham, AL, USA
pappas@uab.edu

Benjamin J. Park M.D.
Mycotic Diseases Branch and Division of Foodborne, Bacterial,
and Mycotic Diseases, Centers for Disease Control and Prevention,
Atlanta, GA, USA
Bpark1@cdc.gov

Thomas F. Patterson M.D.
Division of Infectious Diseases, The University of Texas Health Science
Center at San Antonio, San Antonio, TX, USA
patterson@uthscsa.edu

John R. Perfect M.D.
Duke Mycology Research Unit, Division of Infectious Diseases and International Health,
Duke University Medical Center, Durham NC, USA
perfe001@mc.duke.edu

Angela Restrepo M. Ph.D.
Medical and Experimental Mycology Unit, Corporacion para
Investigaciones Biologicas, Medellin, Colombia
angelares@une.net.co

P. David Rogers Pharm D., Ph.D.
University of Tennessee College of Pharmacy, Memphis, TN, USA
drogers@utmem.edu

Dominique Sanglard Ph.D.
Institute of Microbiology, University of Lausanne and
University Hospital Center, Lausanne, Switzerland
Dominique.sanglard@chuv.ch

Wiley A. Schell Ph.D.
Division of Infectious Diseases and International Health, Duke University Medical Center,
Durham NC, USA
wiley.schell@duke.edu

Dominik Schrey M.D.
Infectious Diseases Research Program, Department of Pediatric
Hematology/Oncology and Center for Bone Marrow Transplantation,
Children's University Hospital, Muenster, Germany
Dominik.Schrey@ukmuenster.de

Jack D. Sobel, MD
Division of Infectious Diseases, Wayne State University
School of Medicine, Detroit Medical Center, Detroit, MI, USA
jsobel@med.wayne.edu

Brad Spellberg M.D.
Division of Infectious Diseases, Harbor-UCLA Research and
Education Institute, Torrance, CA, USA
bspellberg@labiomed.org

Khuanchai Supparatpinyo M.D.
Department of Medicine, Chiang Mai University, Chiang Mai, Thailand,
khuanchai@idlhat.org

Harrys A. Torres M.D.
Department of Internal Medicine, The University of Texas,
MD Anderson Cancer Center, Houston, TX, USA
htorres@mdanderson.org

Nongnuch Vanittanakom Ph.D.
Department of Microbiology, Chiang Mai University, Chiang Mai, Thailand,
drnongnuch@gmail.com

Jose A. Vazquez M.D.
Division of Infectious Diseases, Henry Ford Hospital, Wayne State University
School of Medicine, Detroit, MI, USA
jvazque1@hfhs.org

Thomas J. Walsh M.D.
Transplantation-Oncology Infectious Diseases Program, Division of Infectious Diseases,
Weill Cornell Medical College, New York, NY, USA
thomaswalshmd@gmail.com

David W. Warnock Ph.D
Mycotic Diseases Branch and Division of Foodborne, Bacterial,
and Mycotic Diseases, Centers for Disease Control and Prevention, Atlanta, GA, USA
DWarnock@cdc.gov

Part I
Introduction

Laboratory Aspects of Medical Mycology

Mary E. Brandt, Shawn R. Lockhart, and David W. Warnock

Over the course of time, more than 100,000 species of fungi have been recognized and described. However, fewer than 500 of these species have been associated with human disease, and no more than 100 are capable of causing infection in otherwise normal individuals. The remainder are only able to produce disease in hosts that are debilitated or immunocompromised.

What Are Fungi?

Fungi are not plants. Fungi form a separate group of higher organisms, distinct from both plants and animals, which differ from other groups of organisms in several major respects. First, fungal cells are encased within a rigid cell wall, mostly composed of chitin and glucan. These features contrast with the animals, which have no cell walls, and plants, which have cellulose as the major cell wall component.

Second, fungi are heterotrophic. This means that they are lacking in chlorophyll and cannot make their organic food, as plants can, through photosynthesis. Fungi live embedded in a food source or medium, and obtain their nourishment by secreting enzymes for external digestion and by absorbing the nutrients that are released from the medium. The recognition that fungi possess a fundamentally different form of nutrition was one of the characteristics that led to their being placed in a separate kingdom.

Third, fungi are simpler in structure than plants or animals. There is no division of cells into organs or tissues. The basic structural unit of fungi is either a chain of tubular, filament-like cells (termed a hypha) or an independent single cell. Fungal cell differentiation is no less sophisticated than is found in plants or animals, but it is different. Many fungal pathogens of humans and animals change their growth form during the process of tissue invasion. These dimorphic pathogens usually change from a multicellular hyphal form in the natural environment to a budding, single-celled form in tissue.

In most multicellular fungi the vegetative stage consists of a mass of branching hyphae, termed a mycelium. Each individual hypha has a rigid cell wall and increases in length as a result of apical growth. In the more primitive fungi, the hyphae remain aseptate (without cross-walls). In the more advanced groups, however, the hyphae are septate, with more or less frequent cross-walls. Fungi that exist in the form of microscopic multicellular mycelium are often called moulds.

Many fungi that exist in the form of independent single cells propagate by budding out similar cells from their surface. The bud may become detached from the parent cell, or it may remain attached and itself produce another bud. In this way, a chain of cells may be produced. Fungi that do not produce hyphae, but just consist of a loose arrangement of budding cells, are called yeasts. Under certain conditions, continued elongation of the parent cell before it buds results in a chain of elongated cells, termed a pseudohypha.

Fourth, fungi reproduce by means of microscopic propagules called either conidia or spores. Many fungi produce conidia that result from an asexual process. Except for the occasional mutation, these conidia are identical to the parent. Asexual conidia are generally short-lived propagules that are produced in enormous numbers to ensure dispersion to new habitats. Many fungi are also capable of sexual reproduction. Some species are homothallic and able to form sexual structures within individual colonies. Most, however, are heterothallic and do not form their sexual structures unless two different mating strains come into contact. Meiosis then leads to the production of the sexual spores. In some species the sexual spores are borne singly on specialized generative cells and the whole structure is microscopic in size. In other cases, however, the spores are produced in millions in "fruiting bodies" such as mushrooms and puffballs. In current mycological parlance, the sexual stage of a fungus is known as the teleomorph, and the asexual stage is the anamorph.

M.E. Brandt (✉)
Mycotic Diseases Branch, Centers for Disease Control and Prevention, Atlanta, GA, USA
e-mail: mbb4@cdc.gov

C.A. Kauffman et al. (eds.), *Essentials of Clinical Mycology*,
DOI 10.1007/978-1-4419-6640-7_1, © Springer Science+Business Media, LLC 2011

Classification of Fungi

Mycologists are interested in the structure of the reproductive bodies of fungi and the manner in which these are produced because these features form the basis for the classification and naming of fungi. Most recently the kingdom Fungi has been divided into seven lesser groups, termed phyla, based on differences in their reproductive structures, as follows. Three of these phyla contain species that are pathogenic to humans and animals.

Glomeromycota (Formerly Zygomycota)

The phylum name Zygomycota is no longer accepted [1]. In its place, the phylum Glomeromycota and four subphyla have been created pending further resolution of taxonomic questions. In this group of lower fungi, the thallus (vegetative body of a fungus) is aseptate and consists of wide, hyaline (colorless) branched hyphae. The asexual spores, or sporangiospores, are produced inside a closed sac, termed a sporangium, the wall of which ruptures to release them. Sexual reproduction consists of fusion of nuclei from compatible colonies, followed by the formation of a single large zygospore with a thickened wall. Meiosis occurs on germination and haploid mycelium then develops.

The subphylum Mucoromycotina has been proposed to accommodate the order Mucorales, where most human pathogens, such as the genera *Absidia*, *Mucor*, *Rhizomucor*, and *Rhizopus*, are found. The subphylum Entomophthoromycotina includes the genera *Basidiobolus* and *Conidiobolus*, agents of subcutaneous infections.

Ascomycota

In this large group of fungi, the thallus is septate. Asexual reproduction consists of the production of conidia from a generative or conidiogenous cell. In some species the conidiogenous cell is not different from the rest of the mycelium. In others, the conidiogenous cell is contained in a specialized hyphal structure, termed a conidiophore. Sexual reproduction results from fusion of nuclei from compatible colonies. After meiosis, haploid spores, termed ascospores, are produced in a saclike structure, termed an ascus. The Ascomycota show a gradual transition from primitive forms that produce single asci to species that produce large structures, termed ascocarps, containing numerous asci.

This division includes the genus *Ajellomyces*, the main teleomorph of dimorphic systemic fungal pathogens. Anamorphic genera are *Blastomyces*, *Emmonsia*, and *Histoplasma*. The Ascomycota also include the genus *Pseudallescheria*, the teleomorph of some members of the anamorph genus *Scedosporium*. This phylum also includes the ascomycetous yeasts, many of which have an anamorph stage belonging to the genus *Candida*.

Basidiomycota

Most members of this phylum have a septate, filamentous thallus, but some are typical yeasts. Asexual reproduction is variable, with some species producing conidia like those of the Ascomycota, but many others are not known to produce them at all. Sexual reproduction is by fusion of nuclei from compatible colonies, followed by meiosis and production of basidiospores on the outside of a generative cell, termed a basidium. The basidia are often produced in macroscopic structures, termed basidiocarps, and the spores are often forcibly discharged.

Only a few members of this large phylum are of medical importance. The most prominent are the basidiomycetous yeasts with anamorphic stages belonging to the genera *Cryptococcus*, *Malassezia*, and *Trichosporon*. Filamentous basidiomycetes of clinical importance include the genus *Schizophyllum*.

Classification of Anamorphic Fungi

In many fungi asexual reproduction has proved so successful that the sexual stage (the teleomorph) has disappeared or, at least, has not been discovered. Most of these anamorphic fungi are presumed to have (or to have had) a teleomorph that belonged to the phylum Ascomycota; some are presumed to belong to the phylum Basidiomycota. Even in the absence of the teleomorph it is now often possible to assign these fungi to one or other of these phyla on the basis of ultrastructural or molecular genetic characteristics. In the past, however, these anamorphic fungi were termed the Fungi Imperfecti and were divided into several artificial form-classes according to their form of growth and production of asexual reproductive structures. Two form-classes of anamorphic, or "mitosporic," moulds are currently recognized, and continue to offer a useful framework for identification based on morphology.

Hyphomycetes

The mycelium is septate. The conidia are produced directly on the hyphae or on special hyphal branches termed conidiophores. This class contains a large number of anamorphic fungi of medical importance, including the genera *Aspergillus*, *Blastomyces*, *Cladophialophora*, *Fusarium*, *Histoplasma*, *Microsporum*, *Penicillium*, *Phialophora*, *Scedosporium*, and *Trichophyton.*

Coelomycetes

The mycelium is septate. The conidia are produced in elaborate structures that are either spherical with an apical opening (termed pycnidia), or flat and cup-shaped (termed acervuli). Only a few members of this class are of medical importance. These include the genera *Lasiodiplodia* and *Pyrenochaeta*, agents of eumycotic mycetoma.

Nomenclature of Fungi and Fungal Diseases

As Odds has commented, there are few things more frustrating to the clinician than changes in the names of diseases or disease agents, particularly when the diseases concerned are not very common ones [2]. The scientific names of fungi are subject to the International Botanical Code of Nomenclature. In general the correct name for any organism is the earliest (first) name published in line with the requirements of the Code of Nomenclature. To avoid confusion, however, the Code allows for certain exceptions. The most significant of these is when an earlier generic name has been overlooked, a later name is in general use, and a reversion to the earlier name would cause much confusion.

There are two main reasons for renaming. The first is reclassification of a fungus in the light of more detailed investigation of its characteristics. The second is the discovery of the teleomorph (sexual stage) of a previously anamorphic fungus. Many fungi bear two names, one designating their sexual stage and the other their asexual stage. Often there are two names because the anamorphic and teleomorphic stages were described and named at different times without the connection between them being recognized. Both names are valid under the Code of Nomenclature, but that of the teleomorph should take precedence. In practice, however, it is more common (and correct) to refer to a fungus by its asexual designation because this is the stage that is usually obtained in culture.

Unlike the names of fungi, disease names are not subject to strict international control. Their usage tends to reflect local practice. One popular method has been to derive disease names from the generic names of the causal organisms: for example, aspergillosis, candidiasis, sporotrichosis, etc. However, if the fungus changes its name, then the disease name has to be changed as well. For example, moniliasis has become candidiasis or candidosis, and pseudallescheriasis has been variously designated monosporiosis, petriellidiosis, and allescheriasis to match the changing name of the pathogen. In 1992 a subcommittee of the International Society for Human and Animal Mycology recommended that the practice of forming disease names from the names of their causes should be avoided, and that whenever possible individual diseases should be named in the form "pathology A due to (or caused by) fungus B" [3]. This recommendation was not intended to apply to long-established disease names, such as aspergillosis, rather it was intended to offer a more flexible approach to nomenclature.

There is also much to be said for the practice of grouping together mycotic diseases of similar origins under single headings. One of the broadest and most useful of these collective names is the term *phaeohyphomycosis*, which is used to refer to a range of subcutaneous and deep-seated infections caused by brown-pigmented moulds that adopt a septate hyphal form in tissue [4]. The number of organisms implicated as etiologic agents of phaeohyphomycosis has increased from 16 in 1975 to more than 100 at the present time. Often these fungi have been given different names at different times, and the use of the collective disease name has helped to reduce the confusion in the literature.

The term *hyalohyphomycosis* is another collective name that is increasing in usage. This term is used to refer to infections caused by colorless (hyaline) moulds that adopt a septate hyphal form in tissue [5]. To date, more than 70 different organisms have been implicated. The disease name is reserved as a general name for those infections that are caused by less common moulds, such as species of *Fusarium*, that are not the cause of otherwise-named infections, such as aspergillosis.

Laboratory Procedures for the Diagnosis of Fungal Infection

As with other microbial infections, the diagnosis of fungal infection relies upon a combination of clinical observation and laboratory investigation. Superficial and subcutaneous fungal infections often produce characteristic lesions that suggest the diagnosis, but laboratory input can aid the diagnostic process where this is not the case, either because several microorganisms and/or noninfectious processes produce similar clinical pictures, or because the appearance of the lesions has been rendered atypical by previous treatment. In many situations where systemic fungal infection is entertained as a diagnosis, the clinical presentation is nonspecific and can be caused by a wide range of infections, underlying illnesses, or complications of treatment.

The definitive diagnosis of these infections is based almost entirely on the results of laboratory investigation.

The successful laboratory diagnosis of fungal infection depends in major part on the collection of adequate clinical specimens for investigation. Inappropriate collection or storage of specimens can result in a missed diagnosis. Moreover, to ensure that the most appropriate laboratory tests are performed, it is essential for the clinician to indicate that a fungal infection is suspected and to provide sufficient background information. In addition to specifying the source of the specimen, it is important to provide information on any underlying illness, recent travel or previous residence abroad, and the patient's occupation. This information will help the laboratory to anticipate which pathogens are most likely to be involved and permit the selection of the most appropriate test procedures. These differ from one mycotic disease to another, and depend on the site of infection as well as the presenting symptoms and clinical signs. Interpretation of the results of laboratory investigations can sometimes be made with confidence, but at times the findings may not be helpful or even misleading.

Laboratory methods for the diagnosis of fungal infections remain based on three broad approaches: the microscopic detection of the etiologic agent in clinical material; its isolation and identification in culture; and the detection of either a serologic response to the pathogen or some marker of its presence, such as a fungal cell constituent or metabolic product. New diagnostic procedures based on the detection of fungal DNA in clinical material are presently being developed, but have not yet had a significant impact in most clinical laboratories. In the sections that follow, the value and limitations of current diagnostic procedures for fungal infections are reviewed.

Direct Microscopic Examination of Clinical Specimens

In many instances, the tentative or definitive diagnosis of fungal infection can be made by the direct microscopic detection of fungal elements in clinical material. Microscopic examination of skin scrapings or other superficial material can reveal a fungal organism in a matter of minutes. This examination is very helpful to guide treatment decisions, to determine whether an organism recovered later in culture is a contaminant or a pathogen, and to assist the laboratory in selecting the most appropriate culture conditions to recover organisms visualized on direct smear. Because direct microscopic examination is less sensitive than culture, the latter procedure should generally always be performed on clinical materials.

Keratinized tissues require pretreatment to dissolve the material and more readily reveal fungal elements. Skin scrapings and other dermatologic specimens, sputum and other lower respiratory tract specimens, and minced tissue samples can be examined after treatment with warm 10–20% potassium hydroxide (KOH). These samples can then be examined directly, without stain, as a wet preparation (Figs. 1 and 2). Alternatively, a drop of lactophenol cotton blue, methylene blue, or other fungal stain can be mixed with the sample on the microscope slide. Another useful tool is the chemical brightener calcofluor white, a compound that stains the fungal cell wall. The preparation is stained with calcofluor white, with or without KOH, and then read with a fluorescent microscope. The fungal elements appear brightly staining against a dark background.

India ink is useful for negative staining of cerebrospinal fluid (CSF) sediment to reveal encapsulated *Cryptococcus neoformans* cells. Gram staining can be helpful in revealing

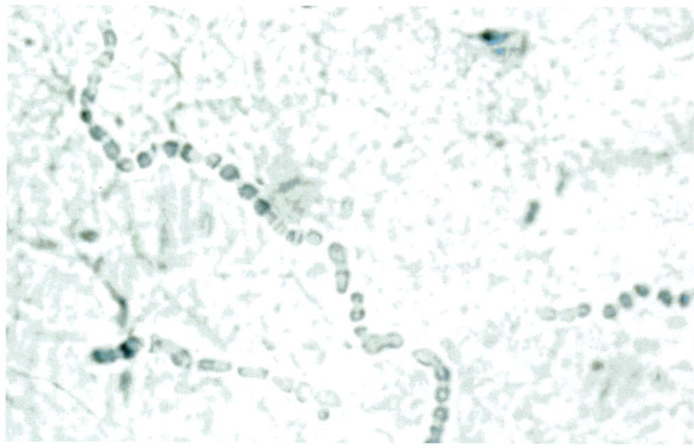

Fig. 1 Unstained potassium hydroxide (*KOH*) preparation of skin scrapings showing the presence of dermatophyte hyphae, which are fragmenting into arthrospores

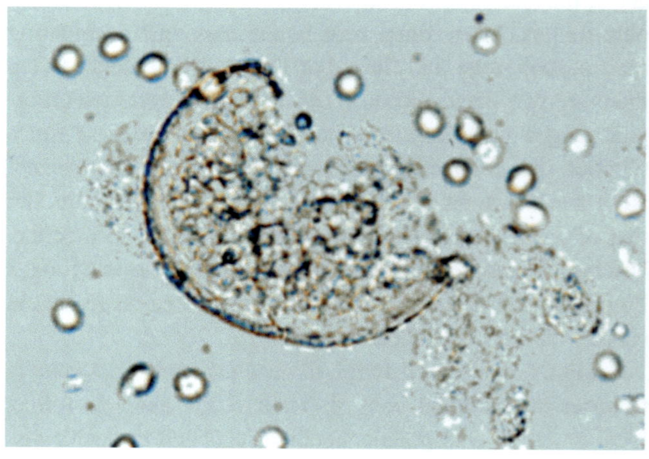

Fig. 2 Unstained potassium hydroxide preparation of purulent material from a soft tissue abscess showing a *Coccidioides immitis* ruptured spherule and released endospores

yeasts in various fluids and secretions. Both Giemsa stain and Wright's stain can be used to detect *Histoplasma capsulatum* in bone marrow preparations or blood smears. The Papanicolaou stain can be used on sputum or other respiratory tract samples to detect fungal elements.

It is necessary to appreciate that both false-positive and false-negative results do occur with direct microscopic examination. The results may vary with the quality and age of the specimen, the extent of the disease process, the nature of the tissue being examined, and the experience of the microscopist.

Histopathologic Examination

Histopathologic examination of tissue sections is one of the most reliable methods of establishing the diagnosis of subcutaneous and systemic fungal infections. However, the ease with which a fungal pathogen can be recognized in tissue is dependent not only on its abundance, but also on the distinctiveness of its appearance. Many fungi stain poorly with hematoxylin and eosin, and this method alone may be insufficient to reveal fungal elements in tissue. There are a number of special stains for detecting and highlighting fungal organisms, and the clinician should request these if a mycotic disease is suspected. Methenamine-silver (Grocott or Gomori) and periodic acid-Schiff (PAS) staining are among the most widely used procedures for specific staining of the fungal cell wall. Mucicarmine can be used to stain the capsule of *C. neoformans*.

It should be appreciated that these staining methods, although useful at revealing the presence of fungal elements in tissue, seldom permit the precise fungal genus involved to be identified. For example, the detection of nonpigmented, branching, septate hyphae is typical of *Aspergillus* infection, but it is also characteristic of a large number of less common organisms, including species of *Fusarium* and *Scedosporium* [6]. Likewise, the detection of small, budding fungal cells seldom permits a specific diagnosis. Tissue-form cells of *H. capsulatum* and *Blastomyces dermatitidis*, for instance, can appear similar, and can be confused with nonencapsulated cells of *C. neoformans*. To overcome this problem, immunohistochemical methods have been developed for identifying various fungal organisms specifically in tissue. Monoclonal antibodies that detect either *Aspergillus* species or members of the order Mucorales are commercially available for use in immunohistochemical procedures (see AbD Serotec, Oxford, UK: www.abdserotec.com), and other antibodies have been evaluated [7, 8]. In the future, it is hoped that monoclonal antibodies specific for *Fusarium* and for *Scedosporium* species will become commercially available.

Culture

Isolation in culture will permit most pathogenic fungi to be identified. Most of these organisms are not fastidious in their nutritional requirements and will grow on the media used for bacterial isolation from clinical material. However, growth on these media can be slow, and development of the structures used in fungal identification can be poor. For these reasons, most laboratories use several different culture media and incubation conditions for recovery of fungal agents. However, a variety of additional incubation conditions and media may be required for growth of particular organisms in culture. The laboratory should be made aware of the particular fungal agent(s) that are suspected in a given sample so that the most appropriate media can be included.

Most laboratories use a medium such as the Emmons modification of Sabouraud's dextrose agar, potato dextrose agar, or potato flakes agar that will recover most common fungi. However, many fastidious organisms, such as yeast-phase *H. capsulatum*, will not grow on these substrates and require the use of richer media, such as brain heart infusion agar. A variety of chromogenic agars that incorporate multiple chemical dyes in a solid medium can be purchased commercially for the detection and preliminary identification of *Candida* spp. (examples are CHROMagar Candida medium [CHROMagar Co., Paris, France]; BBL-ChromAgar Candida (Becton Dickinson); and Albicans ID (bioMerieux, France). The medically important *Candida* spp. appear as different colored colonies due to differential uptake of these chromogenic compounds. For example, on CHROMagar Candida medium after incubation for 48–72 h, *C. albicans* produces green colonies, while *C. tropicalis* produces blue colonies, *C. glabrata* produces dark pink to purple colonies, and *C. parapsilosis* produces cream to pale pink colonies. Chromogenic media can be helpful in detecting the presence of mixed cultures, as well as providing a preliminary species identification. This topic was reviewed by Pincus et al. [9].

Many clinical specimens submitted for fungal culture are contaminated with bacteria, and it is essential to add antibacterial antibiotics to fungal culture media to remove this contamination. Media containing chloramphenicol and gentamicin are commercially available. However, other antimicrobial agents are increasingly being used to suppress growth of bacteria resistant to older agents. If dermatophytes or dimorphic fungi are being isolated, cycloheximide (actidione) should be added to the medium to prevent overgrowth by faster-growing fungi.

The optimum growth temperature for most pathogenic fungi is around 30°C. Material from patients with a suspected superficial infection should be incubated at 25–30°C, because most dermatophytes will not grow at higher temperatures. Material from subcutaneous or deep sites should be incubated at two temperatures, 25–30°C and 37°C. This is because a number of important pathogens, including *H. capsulatum*, *B. dermatitidis* and *Sporothrix schenckii*, are dimorphic and the change in their growth form, depending on the incubation conditions, is useful in identification. At 25–30°C these organisms develop as moulds on Sabouraud's dextrose agar, but at higher temperatures on an enriched medium, such as brain–heart infusion agar, these organisms grow as budding yeasts. Many pathogenic fungi grow slowly in culture and require plates to be held for up to 2 weeks, and in some cases up to 4 weeks, before being discarded as negative. However, some common pathogenic fungi, such as *A. fumigatus* and *C. albicans*, will produce identifiable colonies within 1–3 days. Cultures should be examined at frequent intervals (at least three times weekly) and appropriate subcultures made, particularly from blood-enriched media on which fungi often fail to sporulate.

It is important to appreciate that growth of an organism in culture does not necessarily establish its role as a pathogen. When organisms such as *H. capsulatum* or *Trichophyton rubrum* are isolated, the diagnosis can be established unequivocally. If, however, an opportunistic organism such as *A. fumigatus* or *C. albicans* is recovered, its isolation may have no clinical relevance unless there is additional evidence of its involvement in a pathogenic process. In these cases, culture results should be compared with those of microscopic examination. Isolation of opportunistic fungal pathogens from sterile sites, such as blood or CSF, often provides reliable evidence of deep-seated infection, but their isolation from material such as pus, sputum, or urine must be interpreted with care. Attention should be paid to the amount of fungus isolated and further investigations undertaken.

Many unfamiliar moulds have been reported as occasional causes of lethal systemic infection in immunocompromised patients. No isolate should be dismissed as a contaminant without careful consideration of the clinical condition of the patient, the site of isolation, the method of specimen collection, and the likelihood of contamination. However, it is notable that in a prior study only 24% of 135 unusual moulds isolated from sterile body sites were shown to be responsible for significant clinical disease [10]. In another report, only 245 of 1,209 isolates of *Aspergillus* species collected from hospitalized patients represented cases of clinical aspergillosis [11]. In addition to demonstrating that not every fungal isolate represents a pathogen, these studies also make a case that laboratories should investigate the clinical significance of fungal isolates before indiscriminately identifying to species level every isolate that is recovered from a patient sample.

Although culture often permits the definitive diagnosis of a fungal infection, it has some important limitations. In particular, the failure to recover an organism does not rule out the diagnosis, as this may be due to inadequate specimen collection or improper or delayed transport of specimens. Incorrect isolation procedures and inadequate periods of incubation are other important factors.

Blood Culture

In general, *Candida* species are more readily recovered from blood than are dimorphic fungi and moulds. Isolation rates are higher when the medium is vented and aerated, when multiple samples of blood are collected, and when larger volumes are cultured. The lysis-centrifugation method (Isolator, Wampole Laboratories) remains superior to other systems for recovery of *C. neoformans* and *H. capsulatum* [12], but it is more labor-intensive than other methods, precluding its routine use in some laboratories. With this procedure, 10 mL of blood are collected into a tube containing chemicals that lyse blood cells and inactivate antimicrobial substances present in blood. The tube is centrifuged and the sediment is then inoculated onto appropriate culture media. However, recent improvements in the formulation of blood culture media, together with the development of improved automated blood culture systems, have made the recovery of *Candida* species from standard blood culture bottles generally as effective as that from lysis centrifugation tubes [12], except that in one study use of the specialty Myco/F lytic bottle (Bactec) improved the time to detection of *C. glabrata* [13]. A study comparing the Bactec 9240 and BacT/Alert 3D blood culture systems using simulated *Candida* blood cultures suggests that the BacT performed better than the Bactec in overall growth detection, more rapid growth detection, and fewer false-negative results [14]. An intriguing study suggests that the detection of yeasts in the anaerobic bottle of an aerobic/anaerobic pair incubated in a BACTEC 9240 system was highly predictive for the isolation of *C. glabrata* [15].

Fungal Identification

Most fungi can be identified after growth in culture. Classic phenotypic identification methods for moulds are based on a combination of macroscopic and microscopic morphologic characteristics. Macroscopic characteristics, such as colonial form, surface color and pigmentation, are often helpful in mould identification, but it is essential to examine slide preparations of the culture under a microscope. If well prepared, these will often give sufficient information on the form and arrangement of the conidia and the structures on which they are produced for identification of the fungus to be accomplished. Because identification is usually dependent on visualization of the spore-bearing structures, identification is

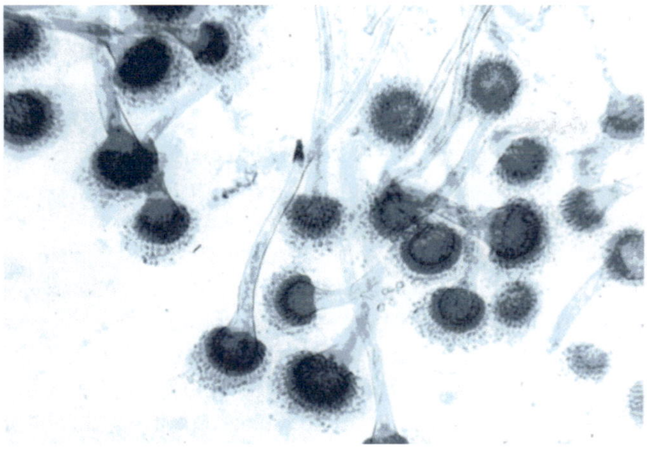

Fig. 3 *Aspergillus fumigatus* conidiophores showing the characteristic pear-shaped vesicles on which are arranged a single layer of spore-producing cells termed phialides

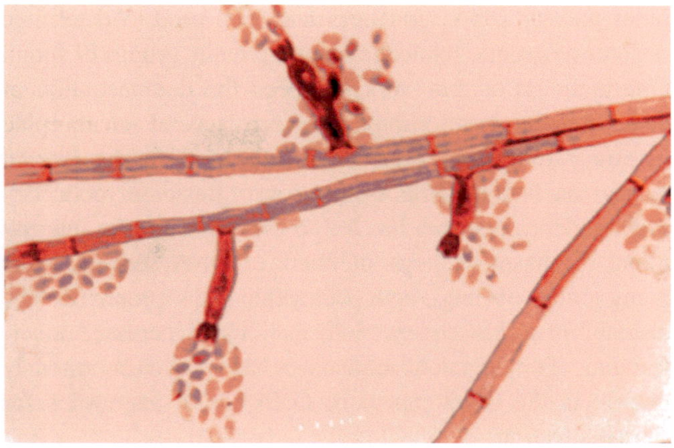

Fig. 4 *Phialophora verrucosa* showing the characteristic small phialides with cup-shaped collarettes from which the conidia are being produced

usually dependent on the ability of the organism to sporulate (Figs. 3 and 4). For "difficult" organisms, much laboratory time can be spent attempting to induce sporulation on various media so that these structures can be studied. Moulds often grow best on rich media, such as Sabouraud's dextrose agar, but overproduction of mycelium often results in loss of sporulation. If a mould isolate fails to produce spores or other recognizable structures after 2 weeks, it should be subcultured to a less-rich medium to encourage sporulation. Media such as cornmeal, oatmeal, malt, and potato-sucrose agars can be used for this purpose. The use of DNA-based identification methods has largely eliminated this requirement.

With some moulds, such as species of *Aspergillus*, the characteristic reproductive structures can be easily identified after a small portion of the growth is removed from the culture plate, mounted in a suitable stain (such as lactofuchsin) on a microscope slide and examined. However, it is sometimes essential to prepare a slide culture in order to identify an isolate. In this technique, a thin square block of a suitable agar is placed on a sterile microscope slide, inoculated with a small amount of the fungal culture, covered with a sterile cover slip, and incubated in a moist environment for up to 2 weeks. The cover slip and agar block are then removed, mounting fluid is added, and a clean cover slip applied to the slide. The fungal growth on the slide is then examined for the presence of spores and other characteristic structures.

Historically, dimorphic fungi such as *H. capsulatum* and *B. dermatitidis* were identified by observing the conversion of mycelial growth at 25°C to yeast-like growth at 37°C. However, development of DNA probe-based tests (Accuprobe; GenProbe Inc., San Diego, CA) has enabled these pathogens to be identified using only a small amount of mycelial material.

Yeasts are usually identified on the basis of their morphologic and biochemical characteristics [9]. Useful morphologic characteristics include the color of the colonies, the size and shape of the cells, the presence of a capsule around the cells, the production of hyphae or pseudohyphae, and the production of chlamydospores. Useful biochemical tests include the assimilation and fermentation of sugars and the assimilation of nitrate and urea. Most yeasts associated with human infections can be identified using one of the numerous commercial identification systems, such as the API 20C, API 32C, Vitek Yeast Biochemical Card, Vitek 2 YST (all BioMerieux), MicroScan Yeast Identification Panel (Dade Behring, West Sacramento, CA) or the Auxacolor (BioRad, Hercules, CA), that are based on the differential assimilation of various carbon compounds. However, it is important to remember that morphologic examination of Dalmau plate cultures on cornmeal agar is essential to avoid confusion between organisms with identical biochemical profiles. A number of simple rapid tests have been devised for the presumptive identification of some of the most important human pathogens. Foremost among these is the serum germ tube test for *C. albicans*, which can be performed in less than 3 h, the urease test for *C. neoformans*, and the rapid trehalose test for *C. glabrata*. Several rapid commercial test panels are also available, most of which are more accurate in the identification of the common rather than unusual yeast pathogens [16].

Molecular Methods for Identification of Fungi

The use of molecular methods to identify organisms relies on the assumption that strains belonging to the same species will demonstrate less genetic variation than organisms that are less closely related [17]. The last decade has seen a massive expansion of research into the phylogenetics of pathogenic fungi [18]. Analysis of aligned ribosomal, mitochondrial, and other nuclear DNA sequences has been used to determine degrees of genetic relatedness among many groups of fungi. One outcome of this work has been the demonstration of close genetic relationships between several anamorphic (asexual) fungi and organisms with teleomorphs (sexual stages) that belong to the Ascomycota or Basidiomycota [19]. Phylogenetics research has led to the deposition in international databases of large numbers of DNA sequences for many groups of fungi, both pathogenic and saprophytic. The availability of this sequence information and increased understanding of phylogenetic relatedness have proven enormously helpful in the development of DNA-based diagnostics for fungal infections.

Portions of the multicopy ribosomal DNA genes are most commonly used as targets in species identification. The internal transcribed spacer (ITS) 1 and ITS2 regions are located between the small and large ribosomal subunits, and the ~600 nucleotide D1/D2 region is part of the large (26 S) ribosomal subunit. These regions have been shown to contain sufficient sequence heterogeneity to provide differences at the species level. Ribosomal genes exist in 50–500 copies per cell, so are detected with better sensitivity than a single-copy gene. In some cases, β tubulin, elongation factor α, calmodulin, or other loci have been used for identification.

Most methods of species identification have exploited the enormous resolving power of the polymerase chain reaction (PCR). With PCR, as little as a few picograms of input DNA can be amplified so that, after 30–40 cycles, the resulting product can be visualized on an agarose gel or detected using chemiluminescence, spectrophotometry, or a laser instrument. Furthermore, amplification occurs in a specific manner that is determined by the temperature selected for the primer annealing step and by the sequence of the complementary primers, the short DNA segments that initiate the PCR elongation step upon binding (annealing) to the input DNA. A variety of methods for amplifying and detecting DNA of interest have been described [20]. Selected methods and studies will be summarized here.

Direct PCR generates a specific DNA product that is visualized on an agarose gel or after capillary electrophoresis. Fungal identification is based on the presence of the fragment, the size of the fragment, or the specific fragment pattern. These methods are very simple to perform, but their sensitivity is directly related to the ability to visualize the fragment(s) and their specificity depends on the uniqueness of the fragment size or pattern for a given species. Misidentification can occur when different species generate fragment(s) of the same size. Different variations of direct PCR have been described. In single-step PCR, the PCR is primed with short oligonucleotides that will amplify only DNA of a particular genus or species, generating a species-specific DNA product or family of products [21]. Nested PCR was originally developed to improve the sensitivity and specificity of first-generation assays. A DNA product of broad specificity is amplified in the first round, and then this product is reacted with species-specific internal primers in a second round of PCR. The product that is generated after the second round is specific for the intended target from the species of interest only [22].

RAPD (randomly amplified polymorphic DNA), also known as AP-PCR (arbitrarily primed PCR), uses random ten-mer oligonucleotide primers to amplify DNA from any region of the genome where the primers can bind. Different species are distinguished by the different patterns of fragments on the gel [23]. This method has found limited utility due to poor interlaboratory reproducibility, but is still helpful in some circumstances. The "rep-PCR" method (Bacterial BarCodes, Athens, GA) involves amplification of repetitive element DNA, which is present in multiple copies throughout the genomes of bacteria and fungi. The resultant rep-PCR pattern is analyzed on a microfluidics chip in an Agilent analyzer. Each unknown DNA generates a pattern of fragments, which are compared to patterns in a library of known species patterns, to identify an unknown DNA by its match to a pattern of a known species in the library. This system has been used for the identification of a number of medically important fungi [24]. The potential utility of this method for fungal identification will be apparent after analysis of a broader panel of species and larger numbers of geographically representative isolates.

PCR-RFLP (PCR restriction fragment length polymorphism) uses restriction enzyme(s) to digest fragment(s) generated by PCR amplification. Species identity is determined by examining the pattern after separation of the fragments using gel electrophoresis. To improve sensitivity and specificity, this has been combined with DNA probe hybridization in a Southern blotting-type format. The first generation of probes were short species-specific DNA fragments labeled with a chemical tag. After restriction enzyme digestion, the amplified DNA is fixed to a membrane and then the membrane is reacted with the labeled probe. Specific binding of a probe to its target is visualized as color development at the position(s) of probe binding. Another modification is PCR-EIA, performed in a microtiter plate, where a universal DNA target is amplified and then challenged with probe(s), each specific for a particular species. Binding of a particular probe to its complementary DNA sequence on the PCR amplicon can be visualized as a change in color in the microtiter well [25]. Other modifications of this approach have included slot blot hybridization, reverse line blot, and reverse hybridization line-probe assays (LiPA) to detect specific binding of probes to DNA targets [26–28]. In reverse line blot assays, up to 43 probes can be used simultaneously. The LiPA is performed on a membrane strip, thus providing flexibility.

Newer generations of probes use fluorescent labels, where complementary binding leads to a release of energy that can be detected by laser-containing instruments. Fluorescence is proportional to the amount of input DNA, so that quantitative results can be provided in "real time" [29]. The newest assays include real-time PCR platforms such as TaqMan [30], FRET or LightCycler systems [31], biprobes, melting curve analysis systems, and molecular beacons. A TaqMan probe consists of a 5′ reporter dye, a 3′ quencher dye, and a 3′ blocking phosphate group. The probe is cleaved by the 5′ endonuclease activity of Taq polymerase, thus releasing the reporter dye fluorescence only when it is hybridized to a complementary target. Fluorescence resonance energy transfer (FRET) assays use two hybridization probes and fluorescence is emitted only if both probes hybridize to the target. Molecular beacons are single-stranded hairpin-shaped oligonucleotide probes, which unfold and release fluorescence when bound to the complementary target. All of these systems have been evaluated in the identification of various fungi, including *Histoplasma*, *Aspergillus*, *Candida*, *Coccidioides*, *Fusarium*, *Penicillium*, and *Paecilomyces* species.

Microarrays are assays where many thousands of probe-to-target sequence binding reactions can be performed on the surface of a tiny microchip, and then rapidly detected and analyzed by computer [32]. Another recent development based on the principle of probe-template binding is the multianalyte profiling (xMAP) system (Luminex Corp., Austin, TX). This assay utilizes a novel flow cytometer and tiny beads color-coded with unique dyes that enable each bead to be distinguished from all other beads in the laser reader. PCR is first performed using universal primers, where the target region of interest is amplified and labeled with biotin. The amplicons are mixed with a series of specific capture probes immobilized each on a different bead. After incubation with streptavidin, the biotin reporter molecule, the beads are analyzed in a laser which distinguishes among the beads and also identifies the bead(s) where a positive biotin-streptavidin reaction has occurred, signifying that the probe has hybridized to a specific amplicon. In this manner, DNA from an unknown organism can be scanned with up to 100 different probes simultaneously in one tube [33].

Isothermal systems represent another strategy for identifying fungal DNA. These methods do not require a thermal cycler, as the entire assay is conducted at a single temperature. These systems include nucleic acid sequence-based amplification (NASBA), loop-mediated isothermal amplification (LAMP), and rolling circle amplification (RCA). NASBA uses three enzymes to produce a cDNA product from single-stranded RNA. LAMP uses six specific primers to form multiple stem-loop structures when primers anneal to alternate inverted repeats of the gene target. RCA is based on the rolling replication of short ssDNA circles.

The peptide nucleic acid fluorescent in situ hybridization assay (PNA-FISH) is commercially available for the detection and identification of *Candida* DNA in smears directly from blood culture bottles [34]. PNA molecules are synthetic DNA mimics which allow hybridization with high specificity. The commercially available Yeast Traffic Light PNA FISH (AdvanDx, Woburn, MA) contains three probes: *C. albicans*/*C. parapsilosis* (green fluorescence), *C. glabrata*/*C. krusei* (red fluorescence), and *C. tropicalis* (yellow fluorescence). The color is read with a fluorescent microscope.

DNA sequencing offers a method for identifying organisms that fail to sporulate or are otherwise refractory to conventional identification methods. The Clinical and Laboratory Standards Institute [www.clsi.org] has recently issued guidelines establishing interpretive criteria for identification of fungi using DNA target sequencing [35]. With most fungal isolates, the ITS region(s) and the D1/D2 or D2 ribosomal regions are the most commonly sequenced loci. In a few cases, ITS sequencing does not provide sufficient resolution, so that protein-coding regions such as β tubulin, elongation factor α, or RPB2 (the second largest RNA polymerase subunit) are used for species identification. Pyrosequencing, which is performed on a short taxonomically significant region of 20 or so nucleotides, has also been reported as a more rapid and economical alternative to full-length sequencing for yeast identification [36].

The reliability of the molecular identification is, of course, directly related to the reliability of the database with which comparisons are made. Identification of unknown fungal isolates can be made by comparing a partial DNA sequence of that organism with sequences in a central database such as GenBank, operated by the National Library of Medicine [www.ncbi.nlm.nih.gov/ BLAST], or the CBS database operated by the Centraalbureau voor Schimmelcultures in the Netherlands [www.cbs.knaw.nl]. GenBank contains thousands of DNA sequences from medically important as well as saprophytic fungi. Any investigator can submit a new DNA sequence to GenBank for no cost, thus continually expanding the number of sequences in the database. An extensive GenBank database of D1D2 large ribosomal subunit sequences exists for ascomycetous and basidiomycetous yeasts. Many ITS sequencing studies are also contributing to an expansion of that database as well [20, 35]. The main disadvantage of the GenBank database is the lack of curatorial control. Incorrect entries are not challenged, and phylogenetic changes in genus/species names are not always made. The more restricted CBS databases contain sequences from isolates whose identification has been well validated phenotypically and taxonomically. The MicroSeq D2 LSU fungal sequencing system (Applied Biosystems) is a commercially available fungal identification system which provides reagents for sequencing the ~300 nucleotide D2 region of the large ribosomal subunit, identification and analysis software, and a library of fungal sequences. Another commercial system, SmartGene IDNS (SmartGene, Lausanne, Switzerland; www.smartgene.com) offers a system where proofreading of DNA sequences, sequence alignment, interpretation, phylogenetic tree, and report creation are integrated into a set of web-based modules.

Many techniques have been described in the literature for the DNA-based identification of fungal isolates. In general, these procedures have not been validated using large representative populations of the species of interest. Furthermore, only a few of these methods are commercially available and most require expertise usually found only in research laboratories. Their interlaboratory reproducibility is also generally unknown. In time, we will develop more knowledge and understanding of these tools as we continue to employ them with a wider range of fungi. Each clinical laboratory will decide how to integrate molecular methods into their standard identification practices [37]. These decisions will be made based on workflow, specimen volume, turnaround time, and cost. However, it is important to note that, as has been stated earlier, many fungal isolates recovered from clinical samples do not represent significant disease. The identification of fungal pathogens requires input from both the clinician and the laboratorian for the diagnostic process to be successful and productive.

Molecular Subtyping of Fungi

Molecular subtyping is the process of assessing the genetic relatedness of a group of isolates of the same species. Molecular subtyping may be performed in the context of an epidemiologic investigation where particular isolates are being assessed as the potential source of an outbreak. In a broader sense, molecular subtyping data can also be used to determine the relationship between colonization and infection, to trace the emergence of drug-resistant strains in a population, or to address questions regarding the role of relapse versus reinfection in recurrent disease. In a global sense, molecular subtyping data can be used to trace the spread of virulent clones throughout a particular geographic region or around the world.

Various methods can be used for fungal subtyping. In general, phenotype-based methods have proved irreproducible and are no longer used for this purpose. Furthermore, *C. albicans* and related species have been shown to undergo high-frequency switching among a number of phenotypes, thus altering a number of phenotypic traits with each activation–deactivation of the switch phenotype.

Strain typing methods for pathogenic fungi are now based on procedures that measure genetic relatedness. To be successful, DNA fingerprinting methods should meet several criteria: they should not be affected by changes in the environment, and they should provide, as much as possible, an effective measure of genetic distance between any two isolates in the population. In addition, typing methods should assess DNA sequences that are fairly stable over time, i.e., do not undergo recombination, gene exchange, or genomic switching events at high frequencies. The ability to store data electronically and to retrieve data rapidly is also helpful as it enables results of different studies to be compared over time and among different investigators [38].

In interpreting subtyping data, it is important to understand that every genome contains segments that evolve at different rates. Thus it is important to assess the resolution of the subtyping probe, i.e., which "speed" of the molecular clock is being measured by the chosen probe. It is also important to decide the epidemiologic question being asked prior to choosing molecular subtyping probes. This is important because different probes may be more or less useful for different circumstances. For example, a study examining serial patient isolates collected over a period of years may require a distinction to be made between bands that change as a result of microevolution (undergo recombination at extremely high frequency) and bands that change less rapidly. Thus when any two isolates are examined, it can be determined whether band changes are due to microevolution within a single isolate, or due to the appearance of a second unrelated fungal strain. The ideal subtyping probe for this type of study may be different from that chosen for an analysis of a hospital outbreak, where isolates collected at one point in time are to be studied.

A number of methods briefly described here have historically been used for subtyping, but have largely been supplanted by direct DNA sequencing-based techniques [39]. Multilocus enzyme electrophoresis (MEE) was one of the first methods used to assess the presence of cellular isoenzymes or allozymes. The enzyme activities are directly related to the alleles of the genes coding for these enzymes, so that by comparing allelic differences within a series of isolates their genetic relatedness can be directly assessed. RFLP analysis (see previous section) was another early method used to assess genetic relatedness. The classical RFLP method suffers from a lack of sensitivity for strain discrimination, which was improved somewhat by transferring the DNA to a membrane and hybridizing with a labeled DNA probe. The resolution of single-copy probes, which generate one or two bands per sample, is usually not sufficient for most epidemiologic studies. Southern blotting has also been applied using complex or repetitive element probes, which are DNA fragments containing sequences that are dispersed throughout the genome of the organism. Repetitive element probes have been described for *A. fumigatus*, *C. albicans*, *C. glabrata*, *C. parapsilosis*, *C. tropicalis*, and *C. dubliniensis* [38]. These probes provide fingerprints of sufficient complexity so that genetic variability can be analyzed at multiple levels. The fingerprint patterns contain bands that arise as a result of microevolution (most variable), as well as bands of moderate variability and low or no variability. Repeat sequences have also been used to develop probes for *C. neoformans* [40] and *Aspergillus flavus* [41]. This method suffers from a lack of portability and ease of result exchange, and has been largely replaced with direct DNA sequencing.

Electrophoretic karyotyping, or separation of fungal chromosomes using pulsed-field gel electrophoresis, has also been used to fingerprint a number of *Candida* spp., as well as *C. neoformans*, *A. nidulans*, *H. capsulatum*, and *C. immitis* [38]. Karyotyping appears to be able to discriminate among unrelated strains. However, the phenomenon of high-frequency switching in *C. albicans* may make karyotyping unsuitable for studying moderately related isolates.

RAPD analysis has also been used in DNA fingerprinting of many organisms including *C. albicans*, *C. glabrata*, *C. parapsilosis*, *C. tropicalis*, *C. lusitaniae*, *A. fumigatus*, *A. flavus*, *C. neoformans*, *B. dermatitidis*, and *H. capsulatum* [38]. One reason for its popularity is that no prior information about the genome of the organism is required. However, a number of problems have been identified in obtaining intra- and interlaboratory reproducibility of this method [42]. Longer repetitive sequences such as the minisatellite M13 (from the phage M13), T3B (from the transfer RNA sequence), and TELO1 (from telomeric sequences) have also been used as fingerprinting primers. They can demonstrate reliable discrimination among strains under carefully controlled conditions.

Amplified fragment length polymorphism (AFLP) cuts genomic DNA with two enzymes, ligates synthetic DNA fragments to these ends, and then amplifies these ligated fragments in a PCR reaction. The result is a complex banding pattern of 50–500 base pair fragments [43]. This method has been used for typing of a number of fungal loci, with high discriminatory power.

The most recently developed methods employ direct sequencing to analyze the relationship among various DNA fragments. Multilocus sequence typing (MLST) is a method in which the DNA sequences of six to eight polymorphic fragments of "housekeeping" genes are directly obtained and compared to one another. The results can be expressed as individual sequences (genotypes) at each locus, or as diploid sequence types (DSTs), unique combinations of the genotypes in each isolate. The use of MLST does require prior knowledge of the relevant housekeeping gene sequences. MLST data for a number of fungal taxa have been stored on a central database and are available through the internet (www.mlst.net). New genotypes and DSTs can be contributed by investigators around the world, and can thus add to the information about the genetic and population structure of the fungal species for which MLST is useful. MLST has demonstrated typing results comparable to those obtained with older methods with *C. albicans* [44] and other medically important organisms [45], and has been used to demonstrate strain replacement and microvariation in *C. albicans* [46]. MLST methods are generally useful for typing most of the pathogenic *Candida* species except *C. parapsilosis*, which does not demonstrate sufficient sequence diversity.

Microsatellites, or short tandem repeats, are stretches of tandemly repeated mono- to hexanucleotide sequences dispersed throughout the genome. They have a high level of polymorphism due to expansion and contraction of the number of repeat elements during each cycle of DNA replication. Microsatellite polymorphisms are manifested as allelic length differences due to the different number of repeated units present in the alleles. Microsatellites are analyzed by amplifying the polymorphic loci directly using fluorescently-labeled primers, and then either measuring the fragment sizes directly using a laser, or obtaining the full DNA sequence of the target product. When a number of methods were compared for their ability to type the highly genetically variable species *A. fumigatus*, microsatellite typing showed the highest discriminatory power [43, 47]. A variation of microsatellite typing that has been used with several fungal species is inter-simple-sequence-repeat (ISSR) PCR typing. This method involves amplification of DNA fragments that are located between two closely adjacent microsatellite sequences. The resulting PCR products are labeled with fluorescent tags and are sized when separated in a capillary. This method has been used to type 84 isolates of *Scedosporium prolificans* collected worldwide [48].

Retrotransposon-like insertion context (RISC) typing has also been used for *A. fumigatus* [49] as an alternative to Southern blotting. This method employs retrotransposon-like sequences as amplification targets. An adapter is ligated to cohesive ends generated by restriction enzyme digestion of genomic DNA. The flanking sequences of the retrotransposon elements are then amplified using an outward oriented, fluorescently labeled internal primer targeting the 5′ long terminal repeat of the *Afut* 1 element. Fluorescent amplification products can be analyzed using capillary electrophoresis.

Serologic Testing

Serologic testing often provides the most rapid means of diagnosing a fungal infection. The majority of tests are based on the detection of antibodies to specific fungal pathogens, although tests for fungal antigens are now becoming more widely available. At their best, individual serologic tests can be diagnostic, e.g., tests for antigenemia in cryptococcosis and histoplasmosis. In general, however, the results of serologic testing are seldom more than suggestive or supportive of a fungal diagnosis. These tests must be interpreted with caution and considered alongside the results of other clinical and laboratory investigations.

Tests for antibodies have proved useful in diagnosing endemic fungal infections, such as histoplasmosis and coccidioidomycosis in immunocompetent persons. In these individuals, the interval between exposure and the development of symptoms (2–6 weeks) is usually sufficient for a humoral response to develop. Tests for fungal antibodies are most helpful when paired serum specimens (acute and convalescent) are obtained, so that it can be determined whether titers are rising or falling. Tests for detection of antibodies are much less useful in immunocompromised persons, many of whom are incapable of mounting a detectable humoral response to infection.

In this situation, tests for detecting fungal antigens can be helpful. Antigen detection is an established procedure for the diagnosis of cryptococcosis and histoplasmosis, and similar tests have been developed for aspergillosis and candidiasis. Antigen detection methods are complicated by several important factors. First, antigen is often released in minute amounts from fungal cells necessitating the use of highly sensitive test procedures to detect low amounts of antigen circulating in serum. Second, fungal antigen is often cleared very rapidly from the circulation, necessitating frequent collection of samples [50]. Third, antigen is often bound to circulating IgG, even in immunocompromised individuals, and therefore steps must be taken to dissociate these complexes before antigen can be detected [51].

Numerous methods are available for the detection of antibodies in persons with fungal diseases. Immunodiffusion (ID) is a simple, specific and inexpensive method, but it is insensitive and this reduces its usefulness as a screening test. Complement fixation (CF) is more sensitive, but more difficult to perform and interpret than ID. However, CF remains an important test for a number of fungal diseases, including histoplasmosis and coccidioidomycosis. Latex agglutination (LA) is a simple but insensitive method that can be used for detection of antibodies or antigens. It has proved most useful for detection of the polysaccharide capsular antigens of *C. neoformans* that are released in large amounts in most patients with cryptococcosis. More sensitive procedures, such as enzyme-linked immunosorbent assay (ELISA), have also been developed and evaluated for the diagnosis of a number of fungal diseases.

Serologic testing is a valuable adjunct to the diagnosis of histoplasmosis. At this time the CF and ID tests are the principal methods used to detect antibodies in individuals with this disease [52, 53]. The principal antigen used in both these tests is histoplasmin, a soluble filtrate of *H. capsulatum* mycelial cultures. The CF test is more sensitive, but less specific than ID. Approximately 95% of patients with histoplasmosis are positive by CF, but 25% of these are positive only at titers of 1:8 or 1:16. CF titers of at least 1:32 or rising titers in serial samples are considered to be strong presumptive evidence of infection. Because low titers of CF antibodies can persist for years following acute histoplasmosis, and because cross-reactions can occur in patients with other fungal infections, care must be taken to exclude these diseases if the clinical signs and symptoms are not typical of histoplasmosis. The ID test is more specific, but less sensitive than CF and can be used to assess the significance of weakly positive CF results. Using histoplasmin as antigen, two major precipitin bands can be detected with the ID test. The M band can be detected in up to 75% of patients with acute histoplasmosis, but may also be found in nearly all individuals with a past infection. The H band is specific for active disease, but only occurs in 10–20% of proven cases. Attempts to improve the serologic diagnosis of histoplasmosis by replacing the CF test with more sensitive procedures, such as ELISA, have largely proved unsuccessful, due to the presence of cross-reactive moieties associated with the H and M antigens.

Antigen detection has proved a more useful method for the rapid diagnosis of histoplasmosis in patients presenting with acute disease, as well as in those with disseminated infection [52]. In acute disease, antigen can be detected within the first month after exposure before antibodies appear. The most popular test is a quantitative enzyme immunoassay (MiraVista Diagnostics, Indianapolis, IN) [54], but similar assays are offered by several other vendors. *Histoplasma* polysaccharide antigen has been detected in serum, urine, CSF, and bronchoalveolar lavage fluid. The test has proved particularly successful in detecting antigen in urine from HIV-infected individuals with disseminated histoplasmosis. Antigen usually disappears with effective treatment, and its reappearance can be used to diagnose relapse [52]. Care should be taken in interpreting results obtained from different laboratories [55]. In addition, false-positive reactions have been reported in patients with blastomycosis, paracoccidioidomycosis, coccidioidomycosis, and penicilliosis [56, 57].

Serologic testing is also invaluable in the diagnosis and management of patients with coccidioidomycosis [58]. In the immunodiffusion tube precipitin (IDTP) test, heated coccidioidin (a filtrate of autolysed *C. immitis/C. posadasii* mycelial cultures) is used as antigen to detect IgM antibodies to *Coccidioides* spp. These can be found within 1–3 weeks after the onset of symptoms, but disappear within a few months of self-limited disease [59]. The sensitivity of the IDTP test is improved by concentration of serum prior to performing the test. Several commercial LA tests are available for the detection of IgM antibodies. These also utilize heated coccidioidin as antigen, are simpler and faster to perform, and are more sensitive than the IDTP test in detecting early infection. However, LA has a false-positive rate of at least 6%, and the results should be confirmed using the ID method.

In the CF test, a heat-labile protein antigen derived from coccidioidin is used to measure IgG antibodies against

Coccidioides species [59]. These antibodies do not appear until 4–12 weeks after infection, but may persist for long periods in patients with chronic pulmonary or disseminated disease, thus providing useful diagnostic information. Low CF titers of 1:2 to 1:4 are usually indicative of early, residual, or meningeal disease, but are sometimes found in individuals without coccidioidomycosis. Titers of >1:16 or rising titers of CF antibodies are consistent with spread of disease beyond the respiratory tract. More than 60% of patients with disseminated coccidioidomycosis have CF titers of >1:32. However, titer alone should not be used as the basis for diagnosis of dissemination, but should be considered alongside the results of other clinical and laboratory investigations.

A commercially available enzyme immunoassay (Premier *Coccidioides* EIA; Meridian Bioscience Inc., Cincinnati, OH) measures IgM and IgG antibodies, and displays acceptable sensitivity and specificity.

Antigen assays are now commercially available for the diagnosis of coccidioidomycosis [60] and blastomycosis [61] (MiraVista Diagnostics). Urine, serum, and bronchial lavage fluid can be tested. These assays display good sensitivity, but cross-reactivity has been reported with samples from patients with histoplasmosis, paracoccidioidomycosis, and penicilliosis.

Tests for *Aspergillus* antibodies have been extensively evaluated for the rapid diagnosis of invasive aspergillosis, but their role remains uncertain. Tests for detection of antibodies include ID, indirect hemagglutination, and ELISA. The ID test is simple to perform and has proved valuable for the diagnosis of aspergilloma and allergic bronchopulmonary aspergillosis in immunocompetent individuals [53]. Tests for *Aspergillus* antibodies have, however, seldom been helpful in diagnosis of invasive or disseminated infection in immunocompromised patients.

Tests for the detection of *Aspergillus* antigens in blood and other body fluids offer a rapid means of diagnosing aspergillosis in these individuals. Low concentrations of galactomannan, a major cell wall component of *Aspergillus* species, have been detected in serum, urine, and bronchoalveolar lavage fluid from infected patients. However, galactomannan is rapidly cleared from the blood, and tests for its detection are helpful in management only if performed on a regular basis. Antigen testing is now included within the consensus definitions for diagnosing aspergillosis in immunocompromised patients with cancer and hematopoietic stem cell transplant (HSCT) recipients [62].

A commercial sandwich ELISA (Platelia *Aspergillus*; BioRad Laboratories, Hercules, CA) for measuring *Aspergillus* cell wall galactomannan antigen levels in serum was approved by the US Food and Drug Administration (FDA) in 2006. As clinical experience with this ELISA has increased, it has become clear that results obtained depend on a number of factors, including the stage of the disease at the time of testing and the use of antifungal drugs as treatment or prophylaxis [62]. The latter factor has been shown to significantly reduce levels of circulating galactomannan. Published results have also depended on several test parameters, including the cut-off value used, and whether two consecutive positive test results were required for significance.

The Platelia *Aspergillus* ELISA results are reported as a ratio between the optical density of the patient's sample and that of a control with a low but detectable amount of galactomannan. The optimal cut-off value to maximize test sensitivity and specificity has been the subject of debate since this test first became available. Until recently, a ratio of >1.5 was considered to be positive, and a ratio <1.0 to be negative. More recent studies have used a cut-off ratio of 0.5:1.0, and the FDA approved a value of 0.5. This greatly increases the sensitivity of the test, albeit at some loss of specificity [63].

Although the Platelia *Aspergillus* ELISA is a promising tool for the early diagnosis of aspergillosis, false-positive results have been reported for 75% of pediatric HSCT recipients [64], and for 20% of lung transplant recipients [65]. Among the causes of these false-positive results have been the administration of piperacillin-tazobactam and other beta-lactam antibiotics, neonatal gastrointestinal colonization with *Bifidobacterium*, and enteral feeding with a liquid nutrient that contained soybean protein [62, 66].

Tests for *Candida* antibodies have been extensively evaluated but remain of limited usefulness in the diagnosis of invasive forms of candidiasis. These tests are complicated by false-positive results in patients with mucosal colonization or superficial infection, and by false-negative results in immunocompromised individuals. Antigen detection tests have also been extensively evaluated for the rapid diagnosis of invasive forms of candidiasis. Numerous circulating antigens have been studied as potential targets, including mannan (a heat-stable cell wall component), enolase, proteinase, and other immunodominant antigens [67]. Test formats that have been investigated include LA, ELISA, and dot immunoassay.

Several commercial LA tests have been developed for detection of mannan, but these have been found to be relatively insensitive. More recently, a sandwich ELISA (Platelia *Candida* Antigen; Bio-Rad Laboratories) has been marketed in Europe. By combining the results of the Platelia *Candida* Antigen ELISA with those of a commercial ELISA for detection of antimannan antibodies (Platelia *Candida* Antibody; Bio-Rad Laboratories), mannan antigen and/or antimannan antibodies have been found in 69% of patients with invasive candidiasis by the time the first positive blood culture was obtained [68]. Non-neutropenic surgical patients present first with positive antibody tests, while hematologic patients present with antigenemia.

The LA test for *C. neoformans* capsular polysaccharide antigen in serum and CSF is invaluable in the diagnosis of meningeal and disseminated forms of cryptococcosis [53]. The test is sensitive and specific, giving positive results with CSF specimens from well over 90% of infected patients. In general, CSF and serum antigen titers are higher in persons with acquired immunodeficiency syndrome (AIDS) than in other immunocompromised individuals. High or rising titers indicate progression of infection, while falling titers indicate regression of disease and response to treatment. Occasional false-positive results have been caused by infection with organisms, such as *Trichosporon asahii* (*T. beigelii*), that share cross-reacting antigens with *C. neoformans*, or by non-specific interference from rheumatoid factor, which can be eliminated by prior treatment of the sample with pronase. False-negative results can occur if the organism load is low, or if the organisms are not well-encapsulated. False-negative results have also been reported with the LA test owing to a prozone effect, but this can be corrected by dilution of the sample.

In general, tests for antibodies to *C. neoformans* are of little diagnostic usefulness. However, they can be of value for assessing prognosis. Antibodies may be detected during the early stages of the disease or in patients with localized infection, but they are rapidly eliminated by the large amounts of capsular antigen released during evolution of the infection. Antibodies may subsequently reappear after successful treatment.

β-D-Glucan Testing

(1–3)-β-D-glucan is a cell wall component of many fungi, including *Aspergillus* and *Candida* spp., but is not found in *Cryptococcus* species or zygomycetes. It can be detected in serum during fungal infection by using a chromogenic variant of the limulus amoebocyte lysate assay [69]. In 2006, the FDA approved the Fungitell assay (Associates of Cape Cod, Inc., East Falmouth, MA) for the presumptive diagnosis of invasive fungal infections, and β-D-glucan testing is now included within the consensus definitions for diagnosing these infections in immunocompromised patients with cancer and HSCT recipients [70]. Although a positive test result for the presence of (1–3)-β-D-glucan does not identify the etiologic agent, the Fungitell assay can be used as a screening method for invasive fungal infection, allowing the earlier initiation of antifungal treatment. However, false-positive reactions have been reported in patients with bacterial infections, in those who have recently received albumin or immunoglobulin products, and among those exposed to other sources of glucan, such as are found in cotton bandages, hemodialysis membranes and filters. The test also requires endotoxin-free dedicated glassware to reduce laboratory contamination [66].

Molecular Diagnostics

DNA-based assays for the detection of pathogenic fungi in clinical samples are now beginning to be marketed in some countries. This section will not attempt to list exhaustively all studies on this topic, but will sample the current published literature. Brief descriptions of the methods can be found in the section on Fungal Identification. Assays have been described for the detection of fungal DNA from nearly all body sites, but particularly blood (serum, plasma, and whole blood), respiratory fluids, CSF, ophthalmic materials, and dermatologic samples. Most molecular diagnostic assays are PCR-based, to take advantage of the increase in sensitivity offered by the many-fold amplification of PCR targets as well as the specificity offered through appropriate primer/probe design. The LightCycler SeptiFast (Roche Molecular Systems) was the first commercial in vitro diagnostic assay for PCR-based detection of fungal pathogens in whole blood [71]. The MYC Assay (Myconostica, Manchester, UK) is currently undergoing evaluation as a molecular beacon assay to detect *Aspergillus* and *Pneumocystis* in respiratory samples (www.myconostica.co.uk).

The most active area of research is in the development of assays to detect and identify *Candida* and *Aspergillus* species in blood. Generally, these tests are intended for prospective monitoring of immunosuppressed patients at risk for fungal diseases, particularly hepatosplenic candidiasis or invasive forms of aspergillosis, and for the early detection of these difficult-to-diagnose diseases so that appropriate therapy can be initiated.

A recent review describes platforms and strategies for detection of *Aspergillus* DNA in blood [72]. In one of the earliest papers on this topic, Einsele et al. described a PCR designed to amplify a fungal-specific 18S ribosomal sequence from blood and then to identify the fungal pathogen using species-specific hybridization [73]. Since then, numerous papers have been published on this subject, using Southern blotting, PCR-EIA, nested PCR, and real-time PCR formats to detect *Aspergillus* DNA in bronchial lavage fluids, whole blood, plasma, or serum samples. A meta-analysis of 16 studies describing the use of PCR tests for the diagnosis of invasive aspergillosis was recently published [74], and results from more than 10,000 blood, serum, or plasma samples from 1,618 patients at risk were evaluated. These authors concluded that a single PCR-negative test is sufficient to exclude a diagnosis of proven or probable invasive aspergillosis according to the European Organization for Research and Treatment of Cancer-Mycoses Study Group (EORTC-MSG) definitions; however, two positive tests are required to confirm the diagnosis due to a requirement for higher specificity. They comment that future studies should distinguish between the use of the test to screen for the presence or absence of invasive aspergillosis in high-risk patients as compared to use of the test to confirm the disease in symptomatic patients. The use of two different PCR targets might be appropriate for the latter purpose. They also found a need for standardizing the PCR methodology, including the nature of the sample, volume tested, DNA extraction methods, choice of target gene, detection of PCR products, and use of appropriate controls.

PCR detection of *Candida* species in blood has been investigated in many studies, due in part to the recognition that blood cultures are positive in fewer than half the cases of invasive candidiasis. Methods used have included PCR-RFLP, Southern blot hybridization, PCR-EIA, microarrays, LightCycler FRET, TaqMan, molecular beacons, biprobes and melt curve analysis, and Luminex [20]. Most studies have reported high sensitivity and specificity, although the fungal load in blood is low (as low as <1 cfu/mL in some cases). Several groups have reported that *Candida* DNA was detected more readily in serum and plasma than in whole blood, but there is no current consensus on the most appropriate clinical sample for *Candida* diagnostics.

A number of publications describe the use of PCR to detect fungal pathogens in maxillary sinus tissue, nails, corneal tissue, vitreous fluids, and other ophthalmic samples [75]. In one representative study, nested PCR was used for detection and identification of *C. albicans*, *A. fumigatus*, and *F. solani* [76]. The authors noted that one patient sample was PCR positive but culture negative, suggesting that molecular testing may permit a diagnosis to be made even when organisms cannot be grown from the sample. A nested PCR has been described that detects DNA from *Trichophyton* and *Microsporum* species in human and veterinary dermatologic samples [77]. DNA could be detected even in the presence of contaminating bacterial organisms. DNA from various *Malassezia* species could be detected in dressings applied to skin lesions of affected patients [78].

Historically, diagnosis of fungal infections using fresh or paraffin-embedded tissue has been complicated by several problems. Fungi can be extremely difficult to distinguish from one another in tissue, contributing to misdiagnosis [6]. Many organisms demonstrate atypical morphology in tissue. Many fungi, particularly mucormycetes (formerly zygomycetes) cannot be reliably cultured from tissue. Finally in many cases fungal culture is never ordered, so that histopathologic findings cannot be extended or confirmed. A number of PCR-based approaches and in situ hybridization assays have been developed to address these problems and to identify DNA recovered from tissue blocks. In the former category, a panfungal PCR targeting the ITS-1 region combined with DNA sequencing [79], a seminested PCR with sequencing [80], and PCR combined with Southern blot analysis [81] have been described. In the second category, in situ hybridization using probes directed against fungal ribosomal DNA has been used for the identification of fungi in tissue sections from five skin biopsies [82]. In situ hybridization is not helpful unless fungal organisms can be visualized using conventional histopathologic staining. Varying degrees of success have been reported in the recovery of DNA from formalin-fixed tissues. The formalin fixation step has been reported to cause degradation of amplifiable DNA as a result of DNA cross-linking. In cases where DNA cannot be recovered, immunohistochemical staining of tissue may be helpful (see Histopathologic Examination).

Molecular diagnostics offer great hope for the rapid detection and identification of difficult-to-culture organisms, for detection of antifungal drug resistance, and for rapid diagnosis directly from host tissues and fluids. At this time, many research laboratories offer "in-house" procedures for molecular identification of fungal isolates from culture plates, from tissue, or from body fluids. Their sensitivity, specificity, predictive value, and clinical relevance have not always been rigorously investigated. It is to be hoped that in the future the relevance of these assays will be demonstrated and that they will be introduced to a broader audience in the clinical microbiology laboratory community.

Antifungal Drug Susceptibility Testing

As with antibacterial compounds, tests designed to ascertain the minimum amount of drug needed to inhibit the growth of fungal strains in culture (minimum inhibitory concentration or MIC) are often assumed to be the most dependable means of determining the relative effectiveness of different antifungal agents and of detecting the development of drug-resistant strains. In addition, it is often assumed that the clinical outcome of treatment can be predicted from the results of in vitro testing of a patient's isolate against a panel of potentially useful agents. Such an approach to the selection of antifungal agents has become more reasonable with the development of a reliable and reproducible reference procedure for in vitro testing of fungal species against antifungal agents and the demonstration of correlations with clinical outcome, at least for some forms of candidiasis. However, the pitfalls of assuming a correlation between the results of susceptibility testing of other antifungal drugs and organisms in vitro and outcome in vivo should not be underestimated. With an increase in drug resistance demonstrated among such diverse fungi as *C. glabrata*, *A. fumigatus*, *A. terreus*, *C. neoformans*, and *S. apiospermum* [83–87], and the expanded range of antifungal agents, it is clear that the need for meaningful methods of in vitro testing of both new and established agents is increasing.

Starting in the mid-1980s there was a movement to establish a standardized methodology for antifungal susceptibility testing, and to this end the CLSI (formerly the National

Committee for Clinical Laboratory Standards [NCCLS]) formed a Subcommittee on Antifungal Susceptibility Testing. The first publication of a standardized methodology for antifungal susceptibility testing occurred in 1997 when the NCCLS published an approved reference method (document M27-A) for the in vitro testing of five antifungal agents (amphotericin B, flucytosine, fluconazole, itraconazole, and ketoconazole) against *Candida* species and *C. neoformans* by the broth macrodilution and microdilution methodologies [88]. Although imperfect, this first document facilitated the establishment of interpretive breakpoints for fluconazole and itraconazole against *Candida* spp., specified a defined test medium (RPMI-1640 broth buffered to pH 7.0 with MOPS), and recommended an inoculum standardized by spectrophotometric reading to around 1,000 cells/mL. Two expanded editions of this document have now been published. The third document in this series is M27-A3 [89]. This document provides quality control (QC) limits at 24 and 48 h for amphotericin B, flucytosine, fluconazole, itraconazole, voriconazole, posaconazole, ravuconazole, ketoconazole, anidulafungin, micafungin, and caspofungin against an expanded set of QC strains [90].

The M27-A reference series has permitted much greater standardization of the in vitro testing of antifungal agents; however, several problems remain unresolved. These include the poor performance of the recommended culture medium in tests with some organisms and with amphotericin B, the method of end point determination, and the proper interpretation of trailing growth in tests with azole agents [91].

The defined culture medium described in the CLSI reference procedure (RPMI-1640 broth buffered to pH 7.0 with MOPS) has proven less than ideal for the testing of some *Candida* species and *C. neoformans*. Increasing the glucose concentration of the medium from 0.2% to 2% results in better growth of most isolates of *Candida* species, making the visual determination of end points easier without significantly altering the observed MICs of amphotericin B, flucytosine, fluconazole, or ketoconazole [92, 93]. Another modification that appears to be helpful is the use of yeast nitrogen base medium in tests with *C. neoformans* [94]. Although not specifically recommended, both of these modifications have been noted in Supplement M27-S3 [95].

It has become evident that the use of the M27-A method to test *Candida* species against amphotericin B results in a restricted range of MICs. Given these results, there has been concern that the reference procedure might not detect resistance to amphotericin B. The difference in amphotericin B MICs between susceptible and resistant strains is more pronounced when antibiotic medium 3 (AM3) is used instead of standard RPMI-1640 medium [96]. However, complete separation of resistant from susceptible isolates has not been achieved by using AM3 medium. In addition, AM3 is a nonstandardized medium and lot-to-lot variation is a limiting factor to its use [97]. It is recommended that laboratories that use this alternative medium introduce strains of *Candida* species with known amphotericin B MICs as controls.

The M27-A procedure relies upon the visual determination of MIC end points. However, the recommended end points differ for different antifungal agents. For amphotericin B, the end point is defined as the lowest concentration at which there is complete inhibition of growth. The end point for azoles and echinocandins for both macro- and microdilution testing has been defined as the point at which there is a prominent reduction in growth. For macrodilution testing, prominent reduction in growth has been shown to correspond to an 80% reduction in growth relative to that observed in the growth control. However, when the microdilution format is utilized and read with a spectrophotometer, the specified prominent visual reduction in growth best corresponds to a 50% spectrophotometric growth inhibition end point [98, 99].

The M27-A3 document recommends 24-h readings for caspofungin, micafungin, and anidulafungin, 24- or 48-h readings for fluconazole and amphotericin B, and 48-h readings for voriconazole, itraconazole, posaconazole, and flucytosine. An investigation of 11,000 clinical isolates of *Candida* species using the CLSI broth microdilution methodology to compare 24- and 48-h test results for fluconazole showed 93.8% categorical agreement with only 0.1% very major errors. The essential agreement, two $\log_2$ dilutions, was 99.6% [100]. The lowest categorical agreement was for *C. glabrata* and was predominantly the result of isolates that were susceptible at 24 h but susceptible-dose dependent at 48 h [100]. When the initial dosing and outcome data set used to establish the 48-h breakpoints for fluconazole was reevaluated using the 24-h readings, the clinical outcome and pharmacodynamic data strongly supported the early reading [101]. Again, the exceptions were those species with MIC distributions at the higher end of the range, such as *C. glabrata*.

Readings taken at 24 h may be more relevant for some isolates. Isolates for which the earlier reading is important show a dramatic rise in drug MIC between 24 and 48 h due to "trailing" growth. The term *trailing* has been used to describe the reduced but persistent growth which some isolates of *Candida* species (primarily *C. albicans* and *C. tropicalis*) exhibit over an extended range of azole drug concentrations, making interpretation of the MIC end point difficult [102, 103]. Estimated as occurring in about 5% of isolates [104], this trailing growth can be so great as to make an isolate that appears to be susceptible after 24 h appear completely resistant at 48 h. Two independent in vivo investigations of this phenomenon that employed murine models of disseminated candidiasis [103, 104] have shown that trailing isolates should be classed as susceptible rather than resistant. This concept has been corroborated by the clinical demonstration that most episodes of oropharyngeal candidiasis due to trailing isolates respond to low doses of fluconazole, used to treat typical susceptible isolates [102].

The inclusion of a colorimetric indicator into the culture medium has been found to produce much clearer visual end points in tests with azole antifungal agents and to generate MICs that are in close agreement with those obtained using the standard broth dilution procedures [105, 106]. Commercial colorimetric microdilution plate panels for the in vitro testing of antifungal agents are now available for diagnostic use in the United States. Comparisons of the Sensititre YeastOne Colorimetric Antifungal Panel (Trek Diagnostics Systems Inc., Westlake, OH), which incorporates alamar blue as the colorimetric indicator, with the M27-A reference procedure have demonstrated good agreement between the methods [107–111]. In addition to clearer end points, other benefits include reduced incubation times and storage of the panels for up to 2 years at room temperature. There are also some data showing a good correlation between Sensititre YeastOne and the M38-A reference procedure [112].

Interpretive guidelines (breakpoints) have been determined for fluconazole, itraconazole, voriconazole, caspofungin, anidulafungin, micafungin, and flucytosine against all *Candida* species [113–115]. Initial breakpoints for fluconazole and itraconazole were based largely on studies of mucosal candidiasis and there were very little clinical outcome data for isolates with elevated MIC values to fluconazole [113]. Subsequently, a reanalysis of the breakpoints incorporating additional clinical trial data and pharmacodynamic analysis, as well as consideration of mechanisms of resistance, reaffirmed the original breakpoints [116]. Breakpoints for voriconazole were developed in 2006 and were based largely on outcome data from six phase III clinical trials with 1,681 *Candida* isolates from nonneutropenic patients with candidemia [115]. The relevance of these breakpoints in other clinical settings remains to be established.

Interpretive criteria for echinocandin antifungal agents were published in 2008 [114]. Because of a lack of clinical isolates with elevated MIC values to the echinocandins, a single "susceptible only" breakpoint was assigned for caspofungin, anidulafungin, and micafungin at ≤2 μg/mL. A lower breakpoint would encompass almost all isolates of *C. albicans, C. glabrata* and *C. tropicalis*, but the higher breakpoint was chosen to avoid bisecting the distribution of *C. parapsilosis* MIC values.

Following the principles established for testing *Candida* species and *C. neoformans*, the CLSI subcommittee on antifungal susceptibility testing has developed an approved reference procedure (document M38-A) for broth microdilution susceptibility testing of conidium-forming filamentous fungi [117]. The essential features of this method include the use of a broth microdilution format, a defined test medium (RPMI-1640 broth buffered to pH 7.0 with MOPS), an inoculum standardized by spectrophotometric reading to around 10,000 colony-forming units per milliliter, and visual determination of the MIC end point after incubation at 35°C for 24–72 h. This procedure was developed using isolates of *Aspergillus* species, *Fusarium* spp., *S. apiospermum*, and *S. schenckii*. The methods of inoculum preparation, choice of inoculum size, time of reading, and end point selection have all been evaluated in a series of multicenter investigations [118, 119]. Nongerminated conidia are used because, at least with *Aspergillus* species, similar results have been obtained for germinated and nongerminated conidia [120, 121]. Quality control guidelines have been established for amphotericin B, itraconazole, voriconazole, and posaconazole [122].

Although the M27-A reference procedure served as the starting point for the M38 document, there are several significant differences between the two methods. The inoculum is about ten times higher than for yeasts and requires a different method of preparation. Because of the differences in the size and light-scattering properties of the spores produced by these fungi, the M38-A document specifies different optical densities for each genus. Careful preparation of the inoculum is essential, since a concentration outside the specified range will result in an altered MIC to most antifungal agents [123].

The end point definition is another point where the M38 and M27 procedures differ. In M27, azoles and echinocandins are read at a partial inhibition end point (defined as the lowest drug concentration producing a prominent reduction in growth). In the M38-A2 standard it is recommended that reading the end point at 100% inhibition (no growth) better detects resistance of *Aspergillus* species to itraconazole and the newer triazoles [121, 124]. For the echinocandins it is recommended that the minimum effective concentration (MEC) be used to define breakpoints. The MEC is the lowest concentration of drug that leads to growth of small, rounded, compact hyphal forms as compared to the control well.

The development of the M27 and M38 reference procedures for in vitro testing has provided an essential standard against which possible alternative methods can be evaluated. Microdilution procedures are time-consuming and labor-intensive, and there is a need for simpler and more economical methods of antifungal susceptibility testing for routine clinical use. Among the simpler methods that are now being evaluated are the agar disk diffusion tests and the Etest.

The most recent set of standards from CLSI is M44-A, a reference method for antifungal disk diffusion susceptibility testing [125]. Disk diffusion is already widely used in clinical laboratories for testing bacteria, so this document provides a simple, rapid, and cost-effective method for susceptibility testing of fungi. Mueller-Hinton agar, which may already be available in some clinical laboratories, supplemented with 2% glucose and methylene blue dye, is the recommended testing medium. Quality control limits for fluconazole and voriconazole have been developed [126, 127]. Criteria have been established for fluconazole against *Candida* species by comparing inhibition zone diameters to MICs generated by the M27-A broth microdilution method and by testing against isolates with known resistance mechanisms [128, 129]. One advantage of the disk diffusion assay is that the zone diameters are read at 24 h. However, reading the prominent reduction in growth is highly subjective and can lead to susceptible isolates being categorized as resistant [130]. Otherwise, there is very good agreement between broth microdilution and disk diffusion for fluconazole [130], and even though there are no approved criteria at this writing, for voriconazole as well [131]. Standards for disk diffusion susceptibility testing of moulds are currently under consideration [132].

The Etest (AB Biodisk, Solna, Sweden) is a patented commercial method for the quantitative determination of MICs. It is set up in a manner similar to a disk diffusion test, but the disk is replaced with a calibrated plastic strip impregnated with a continuous concentration gradient of the antimicrobial agent. Following incubation, the MIC is determined from the point of intersection of the growth inhibition zone with the calibrated strip. Both nonuniform growth of the fungal lawn and the presence of a trailing growth edge can make end point determination difficult. However, with experience and standardized procedures, the correlation between the Etest and the M27-A reference procedure has been acceptable for most *Candida* species and the azole and echinocandin antifungal agents [111, 133–135]. For many moulds, including *Aspergillus* species, good correlations with amphotericin B, posaconazole and itraconazole Etest and MICs by the M38 method have been reported [136–139]. The Etest has proved useful for the determination of amphotericin B MICs and represents one of the more reliable ways to detect resistant isolates [140–142]. QC Etest limits for the two M27 QC isolates against amphotericin B, flucytosine, fluconazole, itraconazole, and ketoconazole have been proposed [133].

Currently, there are only three commercially available systems that are FDA approved for in vitro susceptibility testing of fluconazole. These are the Sensititre YeastOne System (Trek Diagnostics, Cleveland, OH), Etest (AB BIODISK, Solna Sweden) and the VITEK2 system (bioMerieux, Hazelwood, MO). The VITEK2 is a fully automated and standardized spectrophotometric system, already in use for bacteriology in many clinical laboratories, that computes MIC values from closed cards containing dehydrated drug. In a multicenter evaluation of 426 *Candida* isolates, the overall agreement with broth microdilution read at 24 and 48 h was 97.9% and 93.1%, respectively. Categorical agreement with the 24-h read was 97.2% but dropped to 88.3% at 48 h. This was mainly attributable to trailing growth of *C. glabrata* isolates. The mean time of incubation for the VITEK2 cards was 13 h, greatly reducing the time needed for an accurate result [143]. Cards with voriconazole, flucytosine, and amphotericin B also show strong categorical agreement with broth microdilution [144].

The European Union Committee on Antimicrobial Susceptibility Testing (EUCAST) has developed a similar but slightly modified set of standards for susceptibility testing of yeasts that result in essentially the same MIC values as the CLSI methodology [145, 146]. Quality control strains and quality control ranges for amphotericin B, flucytosine, fluconazole, itraconazole, posaconazole, and voriconazole have been established [147]. The EUCAST methodology has some notable differences from the CLSI method. Both use RPMI 1640 as the growth medium, but the EUCAST methodology adjusts the glucose concentration to 2%, which has been shown to enhance the growth of most yeasts without significantly impacting the MIC value [148]. The inoculum used in the EUCAST methodology is 50 times that dictated by CLSI. Finally, all MIC values are determined by measuring absorbance using a plate reader, and they are determined after 24 h of incubation [145, 149]. For these reasons, the CLSI breakpoints cannot be applied to isolates whose MIC values were determined by the EUCAST methodology [150].

For fluconazole, the MICs generated by the EUCAST method and by the CLSI method are essentially the same up to 2 μg/mL, but above this level the CLSI generated MIC values are twofold higher [150]. The result is that there are two sets of breakpoints for fluconazole depending upon the standards on which the testing was based [113, 145]. It must be borne in mind that the EUCAST breakpoints currently only include the species *C. albicans*, *C. tropicalis*, and *C. parapsilosis*, do not include a susceptible dose-dependent category, and the pharmacodynamic analyses used to evaluate the breakpoints were based on doses of 400 and 800 mg [145]. That being said, when 475 *Candida* isolates were tested by the two methodologies simultaneously and the respective breakpoints were applied, there were only eight major discrepancies. Three isolates that were resistant by the EUCAST method were susceptible by the CLSI method, and five isolates that were susceptible by the EUCAST method were resistant by the CLSI method [150]. The latter five isolates all had a trailing growth phenotype and all were susceptible by the CLSI methodology when MIC values were determined at 24 h. Breakpoints for voriconazole have been established for C. *albicans*, *C. tropicalis*, and *C. parapsilosis*. Like the fluconazole breakpoints, the EUCAST voriconazole breakpoints are much lower than the CLSI breakpoints and there is no susceptible dose-dependent category [151, 152].

The EUCAST group has also established a standardized methodology for the determination of microbroth MIC values to moulds [153]. This is essentially the same as that used for yeasts, with the exceptions that the inoculum is calculated by counting spores under a hemocytometer, the MIC end points are determined visually, and MEC values are determined for the echinocandins. No interpretive criteria have been established for any species of mould.

As Rex et al. have commented [91], the ability to generate an MIC is of little value without the corresponding ability to interpret its clinical meaning. However, this process is far from straightforward for a number of reasons. First, MICs are not a physical measurement. Second, host factors play a critical role in determining clinical outcome. Third, susceptibility in vitro does not uniformly predict therapeutic success in vivo. Fourth, resistance in vitro will often, but not always, correlate with treatment failure [113]. After compiling clinical correlation data for both bacteria and fungi, Rex and Pfaller devised what they called the "90-60 rule" [154]. The 90-60 rule made the observation that infections due to isolates which are susceptible in vitro respond to appropriate therapy approximately 90% of the time while infections due to isolates which are resistant in vitro (or which are treated with inappropriate therapy) respond to treatment approximately 60% of the time. In this way, susceptibility testing is seen only as a portion of the process in determining proper therapy for a patient and may be better described as a process for identification of antimicrobial therapy which is less likely to succeed [154].

Although antifungal susceptibility testing has come a long way in the last 20 years there are still some major gaps to be filled. There is no standardized methodology for testing dimorphic fungi in either the yeast or mould form. There are no breakpoints for any drugs against *Cryptococcus* species or any of the moulds. A more critical evaluation of current breakpoints, including their correlation with therapeutic outcome and species-specific breakpoints, is needed. Susceptibility testing is often helpful for isolates of *Candida* species (especially for species other than *C. albicans*) from deep sites, and may help physicians with step-down therapy now that the antifungal armamentarium has expanded. Testing of oropharyngeal isolates of *Candida* species from patients who have failed to respond to standard azole treatment can help to distinguish failures due to drug resistance from other causes. At this point in time, for moulds, species identification will have a larger impact on choice of therapy than in vitro susceptibility testing. However, testing for a resistant isolate following a prolonged nonresponse to therapy may help the clinician determine the proper course of therapy. Given these limitations, antifungal susceptibility testing has now become a useful clinical tool. It is not, however, an infallible guide to the treatment of fungal infections.

References

1. Hibbett DS, Binder M, Bischoff JF, et al. A higher – level phylogenetic classification of the fungi. Mycol Res 2007;111: 509–47
2. Odds FC. The fungal kingdom: essentials of mycology. In: Kibbler CC, Mackenzie DWR, Odds FC, eds. Principles and Practice of Clinical Mycology. Chichester: Wiley, 1996:1–6.
3. Odds FC, Arai T, Disalvo AF, et al. Nomenclature of fungal diseases: a report and recommendations from a sub-committee of the International Society for Human and Animal Mycology (ISHAM). J Med Vet Mycol 1992;30:1–10
4. Ajello L. Phaeohyphomycosis: definition and etiology. In: Proceedings of the Third International Conference on the Mycoses. Scientific Publication 304. Washington, DC: Pan American Health Organization, 1975:126–133
5. Ajello L. Hyalohyphomycosis and phaeohyphomycosis: two global disease entities of public health importance. Eur J Epidemiol 1986;2:243–51
6. Sangoi AR, Rogers WM, Longacre TA, Montoya JG, Baron EJ, Banaei N. Challenges and pitfalls of morphologic identification of fungal infections in histologic and cytologic specimens. Am J Clin Pathol 2009;33:364–75
7. Jensen HE, Salonen J, Ekfors TO. The use of immunohistochemistry to improve sensitivity and specificity in the diagnosis of systemic mycoses in patients with hematological malignancies. J Pathol 1997;181:100–5
8. Schuetz AN, Cohen C. *Aspergillus* immunohistochemistry of culture-proven fungal tissue isolates shows high cross-reactivity. Appl Immunohistochem Mol Morphol 2009;17:524–9
9. Pincus DH, Orenga S, Hotelier S. Yeast identification-past, present, and future methods. Med Mycol 2007;45:97–121
10. Rees JR, RW Pinner, RA Hajjeh, ME Brandt, AL Reingold. The epidemiological features of invasive mycotic infections in the San Francisco Bay area 1992–1993: results of population-based active surveillance. Clin Infect Dis 1998;27:1138–47
11. Perfect JR, Cox GM, Lee JY, et al. The impact of culture isolation of *Aspergillus* species: a hospital-based survey of aspergillosis. Clin Infect Dis 2001;33:1924–33
12. Vetter E, Torgerson C, Feuker A, et al. Comparison of the BACTEC Myco/F lytic bottle to the Isolator tube, BACTEC Plus Aerobic F/bottle, and BACTEC Anaerobic Lytic/10 bottle and comparison of the BACTEC Plus Aerobic F/bottle to the Isolator tube for recovery of bacteria, mycobacteria, and fungi from blood. J Clin Microbiol 2001;39:4380–6
13. Kirby JE, Delaney M, Qian Q, Gold HS. Optimal use of Myco/F lytic and standard BACTEC blood culture bottles for detection of yeast and mycobacteria. Arch Pathol Lab Med 2009; 133:93–6
14. Horvath LL, George BJ, Murray CK, Harrison LS, Hospenthal DR. Direct comparison of the BACTEC 9240 and BacT/ALERT 3D automated blood culture systems for *Candida* growth detection. J Clin Microbiol 2004;42:115–8
15. Foster N, Symes C, Barton R, Hobson R. Rapid identification of *Candida glabrata* in *Candida* bloodstream infections. J Med Microbiol 2007;56(Part 12):1639–43
16. Espinel-Ingroff A, Stockman L, Roberts G, et al. Comparison of RapID Yeast Plus system with API 20C system for identification of common, new, and emerging yeast pathogens. J Clin Microbiol 1998;36:1443–5
17. Taylor JW, Jacobson DJ, Kroken S, et al. Phylogenetic species recognition and species concepts in fungi. Fungal Genet Biol 2000;31:21–32
18. Guarro J, Gené J, Stchigel AM. Developments in fungal taxonomy. Clin Microbiol Rev 1999;12:454–500

19. Gené J, Guillamon JM, Guarro J, Pujol J, Ulfig K. Molecular characterization, relatedness, and antifungal susceptibility of the basidiomycetous *Hormographiella* species and *Coprinus cinereus* from clinical and environmental sources. Antonie Leeuwenhoek Int J Genet 1996;70:49–57
20. Balajee SA, Sigler L, Brandt ME. DNA and the classical way: identification of medically important molds in the 21st century. Med Mycol 2007;45:475–90
21. Abliz P, Fukushima K, Takizawa K, Nieda N, Miyaji M, Nishimura K. Rapid identification of the genus *Fonsecaea* by PCR with specific oligonucleotide primers. J Clin Microbiol 2004;42:404–7
22. Zhao J, Kong F, Li R, Wang X, Wan Z, Wang D. Identification of *Aspergillus fumigatus* and related species by nested PCR targeting ribosomal DNA internal transcribed spacer regions. J Clin Microbiol 2001;39:2261–6
23. Berg DE, Akopyants NS, Kersulyte D. Fingerprinting microbial genomes using the RAPD or AP-PCR method. Methods Mol Cell Biol 1994;5:13–24
24. Hansen D, Healy M, Reece K, Smith C, Woods GL. Repetitive-sequence-based PCR using the DiversiLab system for identification of *Aspergillus* species. J Clin Microbiol 2008;46:1835–9
25. Elie CM, Lott TJ, Burns BM, Reiss E, Morrison CJ. Rapid identification of *Candida* species using species-specific DNA probes. J Clin Microbiol 1998;36:3260–5
26. Kong F, Gilbert GL. Multiplex PCR-based reverse line blot hybridization assay (mPCR/RLB)-a practical epidemiological and diagnostic tool. Nat Protoc 2006;1:2668–80
27. Loeffler J, Hebart H, Magga S, et al. Identification of rare *Candida* species and other yeasts by polymerase chain reaction and slot blot hybridization. Diagn Microbiol Infect Dis 2000;38:207–12
28. Martin C, Roberts D, van der Weide M, et al. Development of a PCR-based line probe assay for identification of fungal pathogens. J Clin Microbiol 2000;38:3735–42
29. Espy MJ, Uhl JR, Sloan LM, et al. Real-time PCR in clinical microbiology: applications for routine laboratory testing. Clin Microbiol Rev 2006;19:165–256
30. Guiver M, Levi K, Oppenheim BA. Rapid identification of *Candida* species by TaqMan PCR. J Clin Pathol 2001;54:362–6
31. Loeffler J, Henke N, Hebart H, et al. Quantification of fungal DNA by using fluorescence resonance energy transfer and the light cycler system. J Clin Microbiol 2000;38:586–90
32. Huang A, Li JW, Shen ZQ, Wang XW, Jin M. High-throughput identification of clinical pathogenic fungi by hybridization to an oligonucleotide microarray. J Clin Microbiol 2006;44:3299–305
33. Landlinger C, Preuner S, Willinger B, et al. Species-specific identification of a wide range of clinically relevant fungal pathogens by use of Luminex xMAP technology. J Clin Microbiol 2009;47:1063–73
34. Shepard JR, Addison RM, Alexander BD, et al. Multicenter evaluation of the *Candida albicans/Candida glabrata* peptide nucleic acid fluorescent in situ hybridization method for simultaneous dual-color identification of *C. albicans* and *C. glabrata* directly from blood culture bottles. J Clin Microbiol 2008;46:50–5
35. Petti CA, Bosshard PP, Brandt ME, et al. MM18-A: Interpretive Criteria for Identification of Bacteria and Fungi by DNA Target Sequencing: Approved Guideline. Wayne: Clinical and Laboratory Standards Institute, 2008
36. Borman AM, Linton CJ, Miles SJ, Johnson EM. Molecular identification of pathogenic fungi. J Antimicrob Chemother 2008;61(Suppl 1):i7–12
37. Pounder JI, Simmons KE, Barton CA, Hohmann SL, Brandt ME, Petti CA. Discovering potential pathogens among fungi identified as nonsporulating molds. J Clin Microbiol 2007;45:568–71
38. Soll DR. The ins and outs of DNA fingerprinting the infectious fungi. Clin Microbiol Rev 2000;13:332–70
39. Gil-Lamaignere C, Roilides E, Hacker J, Muller F-MC. Molecular typing for fungi-a critical review of the possibilities and limitations of currently and future methods. Clin Microbiol Infect 2003;9:172–85
40. Spitzer ED, SG Spitzer. Use of a dispersed repetitive DNA element to distinguish clinical isolates of *Cryptococcus neoformans*. J Clin Microbiol 1992;30:1094–7
41. McAlpin CE, Mannarelli B. Construction and characterization of a DNA probe for distinguishing strains of *Aspergillus flavus*. Appl Environ Microbiol 1995;61:1068–72
42. Meunier J-R, Grimont PAD. Factors affecting reproducibility of random amplified polymorphic DNA fingerprinting. Res Microbiol 1993;144:373–9
43. de Valk HA, Klaassen CHW, Meis JFGM. Molecular typing of *Aspergillus* species. Mycoses 2008;51:463–76
44. Robles JC, Koreen L, Park S, Perlin DS. Multilocus sequence typing is a reliable alternative method to DNA fingerprinting for discriminating among strains of *Candida albicans*. J Clin Microbiol 2004;42:2480–8
45. Odds FC, Jacobsen MD. Multilocus sequence typing of pathogenic *Candida* species. Eukaryot Cell 2008;7:1075–84
46. Odds FC, Davidson AD, Jacobsen MD, et al. *Candida albicans* strain maintenance, replacement, and microvariation demonstrated by multilocus sequence typing. J Clin Microbiol 2006;44:3647–58
47. Vanhee LM, Symoens F, Jacobsen MD, Nelis HJ, Coenye T. Comparison of multiple typing methods for *Aspergillus fumigatus*. Clin Microbiol Infect 2009;15:643–50
48. Sole M, Cano J, Rodriguez-Tudela JL, et al. Molecular typing of clinical and environmental isolates of *Scedosporium prolificans* by inter-simple-sequence-repeat polymerase chain reaction. Med Mycol 2003;41:293–300
49. de Ruiter MT, de Valk HA, Meis JFGM, Klassen CHW. Retrotransposon insertion-site context (RISC) typing: a novel typing method for *Aspergillus fumigatus* and a convenient PCR alternative to restriction fragment length polymorphism analysis. J Microbiol Meth 2007;70:528–34
50. Jones JM. Kinetics of antibody responses to cell wall mannan and a major cytoplasmic antigen of *Candida albicans* in rabbits and humans. J Lab Clin Med 1980;96:845–60
51. Reiss E, Stockman L, Kuykendall RS, Smith SJ. Dissociation of mannan-serum complexes and detection of *Candida albicans* mannan by enzyme immunoassay variations. Clin Chem 1982;28:306–10
52. Wheat LJ. Improvements in diagnosis of histoplasmosis. Expert Opin Biol Ther 2006;6:1207–21
53. Lindsley MD, Warnock, DW, Morrison, CJ. Serological and molecular diagnosis of fungal infection. In: Rose NR, Hamilton RG, Detrick B, eds. Manual of Clinical Laboratory Immunology, 7th edn. Washington, DC: ASM Press, 2006:569–605
54. Connolly PA, Durkin MM, LeMonte AM, Hackett EJ, Wheat LJ. Detection of *Histoplasma* antigen by quantitative enzyme immunoassay. Clin Vac Immunol 2007;14:1587–91
55. McKinsey DS, McKinsey JP, Northcutt N, Sarria JC. Interlaboratory discrepancy of antigenuria results in 2 patients with AIDS and histoplasmosis. Diagn Microbiol Infect Dis 2009;63:111–4
56. Wheat J, Wheat H, Connally P, et al. Cross-reactivity in *Histoplasma capsulatum* variety *capsulatum* antigen assays of urine samples from patients with endemic mycoses. Clin Infect Dis 1997;24:1169–71
57. Kuberski T, Myers R, Wheat LJ, Kubal BM, Bruckner D, Pegues D. Diagnosis of coccdioidomycosis by antigen detection using cross-reaction with *Histoplasma* antigen. Clin Infect Dis 2007;44:e50–4
58. Einstein HE, Johnson RE. Coccidioidomycosis: new aspects of epidemiology and therapy. Clin Infect Dis 1993;16:349–56

59. Pappagiannis D, Zimmer BL. Serology of coccidioidomycosis. Clin Microbiol Rev 1990;3:247–68
60. Durkin M, Connolly P, Kuberski T, et al. Diagnosis of coccidioidomycosis with use of the *Coccidioides* antigen enzyme immunoassay. Clin Infect Dis 2008;47:69–73
61. Durkin M, Witt J, LeMonte A, Wheat B, Connolly, P. Antigen assay with the potential to aid in diagnosis of blastomycosis. J Clin Microbiol 2004;42:4873–75
62. Maertens J, Theunissen K, Lodewyck T. Advances in the serological diagnosis of invasive *Aspergillus* infections in patients with hematological disorders. Mycoses 2007;50(Suppl 1):2–17
63. Marr KA, Balajee SA, McLaughlin L, Tabouret M, Bentsen C, Walsh TJ. Detection of galactomannan antigenemia by enzyme immunoassay for the diagnosis of invasive aspergillosis: variables that affect performance. J Infect Dis 2004;190:641–9
64. Herbrecht R, Letscher-Bru V, Oprea C, et al. *Aspergillus* galactomannan detection in the diagnosis of invasive aspergillosis in cancer patients. J Clin Oncol 2002;20:1898–906
65. Husain S, Kwak EJ, Obman A, et al. Prospective assessment of Platelia *Aspergillus* galactomannan antigen for the diagnosis of invasive aspergillosis in lung transplant recipients. Am J Transplant 2004;4:796–802
66. Balajee SA, Magill SS, Brandt ME. The role of molecular methods in the identification of fungal infections. Curr Fung Infect Rep 2007;1:65–71
67. Ponton J, Moragues MD, Quindos G. Non-culture-based diagnostics. In: Calderone RA, ed. Candida and Candidiasis. Washington, DC: ASM Press, 2002:395–425
68. Yera H, Sendid B, Francois N, Camus D, Poulain D. Contribution of serological tests and blood culture to the early diagnosis of systemic candidiasis. Eur J Clin Microbiol Infect Dis 2001; 20:864–70
69. Odabasi Z, Mattiuzzi G, Estey E, et al. Beta-D-glucan as a diagnostic adjunct for invasive fungal infections: validation, cutoff development, and performance in patients with acute myelogenous leukemia and myelodysplastic syndrome. Clin Infect Dis 2004; 39:199–205
70. De Pauw B, W. T., Donnelly JP, et al. Revised definitions of invasive fungal disease from the European Organization for Research and Treatment of Cancer/Invasive Fungal Infections Cooperative Group and the National Institute of Allergy and Infectious Diseases Mycoses Study Group (EORTC/MSG) Consensus Group. Clin Infect Dis 2008;46:1813–21
71. Mancini N, Clerici D, Diotti R, et al. Molecular diagnosis of sepsis in neutropenic patients with hematological malignancies. J Med Microbiol 2008;57:601–4
72. White PL, Barton R, Guiver M, et al. A consensus on fungal polymerase chain reaction diagnosis?: a United Kingdom-Ireland evaluation of polymerase reaction methods for detection of systemic fungal infections. J Mol Diagn 2006;8:376–84
73. Einsele H, Hebart H, Roller G, et al. Detection and identification of fungal pathogens in blood by using molecular probes. J Clin Microbiol 1997;35:1353–60
74. Mengoli C, Cruciani M, Barnes RA, Loeffler J, Donnelly JP. Use of PCR for diagnosis of invasive aspergillosis: systematic review and meta-analysis. Lancet Infect Dis 2009;9:89–96
75. Okhravi N, Adamson P, Lightman S. Use of PCR in endophthalmitis. Ocul Immunol Inflamm 2000;8:189–200
76. Jaeger EEM, Carroll NM, Choudhury S, et al. Rapid detection and identification of *Candida*, *Aspergillus*, and *Fusarium* species in ocular samples using nested PCR. J Clin Microbiol 2000;38:2902–8
77. Turin L, Riva F, Galbiati G, Cainelli T. Fast, simple and highly sensitive double-rounded polymerase chain reaction assay to detect medically relevant fungi in dermatological specimens. Eur J Clin Invest 2000;30:511–8
78. Sugita T, Suto H, Unno T, et al. Molecular analysis of *Malassezia* microflora on the skin of atopic dermatitis patients and healthy subjects. J Clin Microbiol 2001;39:3486–90
79. Lau A, Chen S, Sorrell T, et al. Development and clinical application of a panfungal PCR assay to detect and identify fungal DNA in tissue specimens. J Clin Microbiol 2007;45:380–5
80. Rickerts V, Mousset S, Lambrecht E, et al. Comparison of histopathological analysis, culture, and polymerase chain reaction assays to detect invasive mold infections from biopsy specimens. Clin Infect Dis 2007;44:1078–83
81. Paterson PJ, Seaton S, McHugh TD, et al. Validation and clinical application of molecular methods for the identification of molds in tissue. Clin Infect Dis 2006;42:51–6
82. Abbott JJ, Hamacher KL, Ahmed I. *In situ* hybridization in cutaneous deep fungal infections: a valuable diagnostic adjunct to fungal morphology and tissue cultures. J Cutan Pathol 2006; 33:426–32
83. Pfaller MA, Messer SA, Hollis RJ, Boyken L, Tendolkar S, Kroeger J, Diekema DJ. Variation in susceptibility of bloodstream isolates of *Candida glabrata* to fluconazole according to patient age and geographic location in the United States, 2001–2007. J Clin Microbiol 2009;47:3185–90
84. Denning DW, Venkateswarlu K, Oakley KL, et al. Itraconazole resistance in *Aspergillus fumigatus*. Antimicrob Agents Chemother 1997;41:1364–8
85. Perfect JR, Cox GM. Drug resistance in *Cryptococcus neoformans*. Drug Resist Updat 1999;2:259–69
86. Sutton DA, Sanche SE, Revankar SG, Fothergill AW, Rinaldi MG. In vitro amphotericin B resistance in clinical isolates of *Aspergillus terreus*, with a head-to-head comparison to voriconazole. J Clin Microbiol 1999;37:2343–5
87. Walsh TJ, Peter J, McGough DA, Fothergill AW, Rinaldi MG, Pizzo PA. Activities of amphotericin B and antifungal azoles alone and in combination against *Pseudallescheria boydii*. Antimicrob Agents Chemother 1995;39:1361–4
88. National Committee for Clinical Laboratory Standards. Reference method for broth dilution antifungal susceptibility testing of yeasts. Approved standard. Document M27-A. Wayne: National Committee for Clinical Laboratory Standards, 1997
89. Clinical Laboratory Standards Institute. Reference method for broth dilution antifungal susceptibility testing of yeasts; approved standard-third edition. Document M27-A3. Wayne. Clinical and Laboratory Standards Institute, 2008
90. Barry AL, Pfaller MA, Brown SD, et al. Quality control limits for broth microdilution susceptibility tests of ten antifungal agents. J Clin Microbiol 2000;38:3457–9
91. Rex JH, Pfaller MA, Walsh TJ, et al. Antifungal susceptibility testing: practical aspects and current challenges. Clin Microbiol Rev 2001;14:643–58
92. Cuenca Estrella M, Diaz-Guerra TM, Mellado E, Rodriguez-Tudela JL. Influence of glucose supplementation and inoculum size on growth kinetics and antifungal susceptibility testing of *Candida* spp. J Clin Microbiol 2001;39:525–32
93. Rodriguez-Tudela JL, Martinez-Suarez JV. Defining conditions for microbroth antifungal susceptibility tests: influence of RPMI and RPMI-2% glucose on the selection of endpoint criteria. J Antimicrob Chemother 1995;35:739–49
94. Sanati H, Messer SA, Pfaller M, et al. Multi-center evaluation of broth microdilution method for susceptibility testing of *Cryptococcus neoformans* against fluconazole. J Clin Microbiol 1996;34:1280–2
95. Clinical Laboratory Standards Institute. Reference method for broth dilution antifungal susceptibility testing of yeasts; third informational supplement. CLSI document M27-S3. Wayne: Clinical and Laboratory Standards Institute, 2008
96. Rex JH, Cooper CR, Merz WG, Galgiani JN, Anaissie EJ. Detection of amphotericin B-resistant *Candida* isolates in a broth-based system. Antimicrob Agents Chemother 1995;39:906–9

97. Lozano-Chiu M, Nelson PW, Lancaster M, Pfaller MA, Rex JH. Lot-to-lot variability of antibiotic medium 3 used for testing susceptibility of *Candida* isolates to amphotericin B. J Clin Microbiol 1997;35:270–2
98. Odds FC, Vranckx L, Woestenborghs F. Antifungal susceptibility testing of yeasts: evaluation of technical variables for test automation. Antimicrob Agents Chemother 1995;39:2051–60
99. Pfaller MA, Messer SA, Coffmann S. Comparison of visual and spectrophotometric methods of MIC endpoint determinations by using broth microdilution methods to test five antifungal agents, including the new triazole, D0870. J Clin Microbiol 1995;33:1094–7
100. Pfaller MA, Boyken LB, Hollis RJ, et al. Validation of 24-hour fluconazole MIC readings versus the CLSI 48-hour broth microdilution reference method: results from a global *Candida* antifungal surveillance program. J Clin Microbiol 2008;46:3585–90
101. Ostrosky-Zeichner L, Rex JH, Pfaller MA, et al. Rationale for reading fluconazole MICs at 24 hours rather than 48 hours when testing *Candida* spp. by the CLSI M27-A2 standard method. Antimicrob Agents Chemother 2008;52:4175–7
102. Revankar SG, Kirkpatrick WR, McAtee RK, et al. Interpretation of trailing endpoints in antifungal susceptibility testing by the National Committee for Clinical Laboratory Standards method. J Clin Microbiol 1998;36:153–6
103. Rex JH, Nelson PW, Paetznick VL, Lozano-Chiu M, Espinel-Ingroff A, Anaissie EJ. Optimizing the correlation between results of testing in vitro and therapeutic outcome in vivo for fluconazole by testing critical isolates in a murine model of invasive candidiasis. Antimicrob Agents Chemother 1998;42:129–34
104. Arthington-Skaggs BA, Warnock DW, Morrison CJ. Quantitation of *Candida albicans* ergosterol content improves the correlation between in vitro antifungal susceptibility test results and in vivo outcome after fluconazole treatment in a murine model of invasive candidiasis. Antimicrob Agents Chemother 2000;44:2081–5
105. Pfaller MA, Vu Q, Lancaster M, et al. Multisite reproducibility of colorimetric broth microdilution method for antifungal susceptibility testing of yeast isolates. J Clin Microbiol 1994;32:1625–8
106. To WK, Fothergill AW, Rinaldi MG. Comparative evaluation of macrodilution and alamar colorimetric microdilution broth methods for antifungal susceptibility testing of yeast isolates. J Clin Microbiol 1995;33:2660–4
107. Davey KG, Szekely A, Johnson EM, Warnock DW. Comparison of a new commercial colorimetric microdilution method with a standard method for in-vitro susceptibility testing of *Candida* spp. and *Cryptococcus neoformans*. J Antimicrob Chemother 1998;42:439–44
108. Espinel-Ingroff A, Pfaller M, Messer SA, et al. Multicenter comparison of the Sensititre YeastOne Colorimetric Antifungal Panel with the National Committee for Clinical Laboratory Standards M27-A reference method for testing clinical isolates of common and emerging *Candida* spp., *Cryptococcus* spp., and other yeasts and yeast-like organisms. J Clin Microbiol 1999;37:591–5
109. Pfaller MA, Messer SA, Hollis RJ, et al. Multisite reproducibility of MIC results by the Sensititre YeastOne colorimetric antifungal susceptibility panel. Diagn Microbiol Infect Dis 1998;31:543–7
110. Pfaller MA, Chaturvedi V, Diekema DJ, et al. Clinical evaluation of the Sensititre YeastOne colorimetric antifungal panel for antifungal susceptibility testing of the echinocandins anidulafungin, caspofungin, and micafungin. J Clin Microbiol 2008;46:2155–9
111. Alexander BD, Byrne TC, Smith KL, et al. Comparative evaluation of Etest and Sensititre YeastOne panels against the Clinical and Laboratory Standards Institute M27-A2 reference broth microdilution method for testing *Candida* susceptibility to seven antifungal agents. J Clin Microbiol 2007;45:698–706
112. Martín-Mazuelos E, Pemán J, Valverde A, Chaves M, Serrano MC, Cantón E. J. Comparision of the Sensititre Yeast One colorimetric antifungal panel and E-test with the NCCLS M38-A methods to determine the activity of amphotericin B and itraconazole against clinical isolates of *Aspergillus* of Antimicrob Chemother 2003;52:365–70
113. Rex JH, Pfaller MA, Galgiani JN, et al. Development of interpretive breakpoints for antifungal susceptibility testing: conceptual framework and analysis of in vitro – in vivo correlation data for fluconazole, itraconazole, and *Candida* infections. Clin Infect Dis 1997; 24:235–47.
114. Pfaller MA, Diekema DJ, Ostrosky-Zeichner L, et al. Correlation of MIC with outcome for *Candida* species tested against caspofungin, anidulafungin, and micafungin: analysis and proposal for interpretive MIC breakpoints. J Clin Microbiol 2008;46:2620–9
115. Pfaller MA, Diekema DJ, Rex JH, et al. Correlation of MIC with outcome for *Candida* species tested against voriconazole: analysis and proposal for interpretive breakpoints. J Clin Microbiol 2006;44:819–26
116. Pfaller MA, Diekema DJ, Sheehan DJ. Interpretive breakpoints for fluconazole and *Candida* revisited: a blueprint for the future of antifungal susceptibility testing. Clin Microbiol Rev 2006; 19:435–47
117. National Committee for Clinical Laboratory Standards. Reference method for broth dilution antifungal susceptibility testing of filamentous fungi. Approved standard. Document M38-A. Wayne: National Committee for Clinical Laboratory Standards, 2002
118. Espinel-Ingroff A, Dawson K, Pfaller M, et al. Comparative and collaborative evaluation of standardization of antifungal susceptibility testing for filamentous fungi. Antimicrob Agents Chemother 1995;39:314–9
119. Espinel-Ingroff A, Bartlett M, Bowden R, et al. Multicenter evaluation of proposed standardized procedure for antifungal susceptibility testing of filamentous fungi. J Clin Microbiol 1997; 35:139–43
120. Manavathu EK, Cutright J, Chandrasekar PH. Comparative study of susceptibilities of germinated and ungerminated conidia of *Aspergillus fumigatus* to various antifungal agents. J Clin Microbiol 1999;37:858–61
121. Espinel-Ingroff A, Bartlett M, Chaturvedi V, et al. Optimal susceptibility testing conditions for detection of azole resistance in *Aspergillus* spp.: NCCLS collaborative evaluation. Antimicrob Agents Chemother 2001;45:1828–35
122. Espinel-Ingroff A, Fothergill A, Ghannoum M, et al. Quality control and reference guidelines for CLSI broth microdilution susceptibility method (M 38-A document) for amphotericin B, itraconazole, posaconazole, and voriconazole. J Clin Microbiol 2005;43:5243–6
123. Gehrt A, Peter J, Pizzo PA, Walsh TJ. Effect of increasing inoculum sizes of pathogenic filamentous fungi on MICs of antifungal agents by broth microdilution method. J Clin Microbiol 1995; 33:1302–7
124. Denning DW, Radford SA, Oakley KL, Hall L, Johnson EM, Warnock DW. Correlation between in vitro susceptibility testing to itraconazole and in-vivo outcome of *Aspergillus fumigatus* infection. J Antimicrob Chemother 1997;40:401–14
125. National Committee for Clinical Laboratory Standards. Method for antifungal disk diffusion susceptibility testing of yeasts: approved guideline. NCCLS document M44-A. Wayne: National Committee for Clinical Laboratory Standards, 2004
126. Barry A, Bille J, Brown S, et al. Quality control limits for fluconazole disk susceptibility tests on Mueller-Hinton agar with glucose and methylene blue. J Clin Microbiol 2003;41:3410–2
127. Pfaller MA, Barry A, Bille J, et al. Quality control limits for voriconazole disk susceptibility tests on Mueller-Hinton agar with glucose and methylene blue. J Clin Microbiol 2004;42:1716–8
128. Barry AL, Pfaller MA, Rennie RP, Fuchs PC, Brown SD. Precision and accuracy of fluconazole susceptibility testing by broth microdilution, Etest, and disk diffusion methods. Antimicrob Agents Chemother 2002;46:1781–4

129. Matar MJ, Ostrosky-Zeichner L, Paetznick VL, Rodriguez JR, Chen E, Rex JH. Correlation between E-test, disk diffusion, and microdilution methods for antifungal susceptibility testing of fluconazole and voriconazole. Antimicrob Agents Chemother 2003;47:1647–51
130. Pfaller MA, Hazen KC, Messer SA, et al. Comparison of results of fluconazole disk diffusion testing for *Candida* species with results from a central reference laboratory in the ARTEMIS global antifungal surveillance program. J Clin Microbiol 2004; 42:3607–12
131. Pfaller MA, Boyken L, Messer SA, Tendolkar S, Hollis RJ, Diekema DJ. Comparison of results of voriconazole disk diffusion testing for *Candida* species with results from a central reference laboratory in the ARTEMIS global antifungal surveillance program. J Clin Microbiol 2005;43:5208–13
132. Espinel-Ingroff A, Arthington-Skaggs B, Iqbal N, et al. Multicenter evaluation of a new disk agar diffusion method for susceptibility testing of filamentous fungi with voriconazole, posaconazole, itraconazole, amphotericin B, and caspofungin. J Clin Microbiol 2007;45:1811–20
133. Pfaller MA, Messer SA, Bolmstrom A, Odds FC, Rex JH. Multisite reproducibility of the E test method for antifungal susceptibility of yeast isolates. J Clin Microbiol 1996;34:1691–3
134. Pfaller MA, Messer SA, Mills K, Bolmström A, Jones RN. Evaluation of Etest method for determining caspofungin (MK-0991) susceptibilities of 726 clinical isolates of *Candida* species. J Clin Microbiol 2001;39:4387–9
135. Warnock DW, Johnson EM, Rogers TRF. Multi-centre evaluation of the Etest method for antifungal drug susceptibility testing of *Candida* spp. and *Cryptococcus neoformans*. J Antimicrob Chemother 1998;42:321–31
136. Pfaller MA, Messer SA, Mills K, Bolmstrom A. In vitro susceptibility testing of filamentous fungi: comparison of Etest and reference microdilution methods for determining itraconazole MICs. J Clin Microbiol 2000;38:3359–61
137. Szekely A, Johnson EM, Warnock DW. Comparison of E-test and broth microdilution methods for antifungal drug susceptibility testing of molds. J Clin Microbiol 1999;37:1480–3
138. Espinel-Ingroff A. Comparison of the E-test with the NCCLS M38-P method for antifungal susceptibility testing of common and emerging pathogenic filamentous fungi. J Clin Microbiol 2001;39:1360–7
139. Espinel-Ingroff A. Comparison of three commercial assays and a modified disk diffusion assay with two broth microdilution reference assays for testing zygomycetes, *Aspergillus* spp., *Candida* spp., and *Cryptococcus neoformans* with posaconazole and amphotericin B. J Clin Microbiol 2006;44:3616–22
140. Clancy CJ, Nguyen MH. Correlation between in vitro susceptibility determined by E test and response to therapy with amphotericin B: results from a multicenter prospective study of candidemia. Antimicrob Agents Chemother 1999;43:1289–90
141. Peyron F, Favel A, Michel-Nguyen A, Gilly M, Regli P, Bolmstrom A. Improved detection of amphotericin B-resistant isolates of *Candida lusitaniae* by Etest. J Clin Microbiol 2001;39:339–42
142. Wanger A, Mills K, Nelson PW, Rex JH. Comparison of Etest and National Committee for Clinical Laboratory Standards broth macrodilution method for antifungal susceptibility testing: enhanced ability to detect amphotericin B-resistant *Candida* isolates. Antimicrob Agents Chemother 1995;39:2520–2
143. Pfaller MA, Diekema DJ, Procop GW, Rinaldi MG. Multicenter comparison of the VITEK 2 yeast susceptibility test with the CLSI broth microdilution reference method for testing fluconazole against *Candida* spp. J Clin Microbiol 2007;45:796–802
144. Pfaller MA, Diekema DJ, Procop GW, Rinaldi MG. Multicenter comparison of the VITEK 2 antifungal susceptibility test with the CLSI broth microdilution reference method for testing amphotericin B, flucytosine, and voriconazole against *Candida* spp. J Clin Microbiol 2007;45:3522–8
145. Subcommittee on Antifungal Susceptibility Testing (AFST) of the ESCMID European Committee for Antimicrobial Susceptibility Testing (EUCAST). EUCAST definitive document EDef 7.1: method for the determination of broth dilution MICs of antifungal agents for fermentative yeasts. Clin Microbiol Infect 2008; 14:398–405
146. Espinel-Ingroff A, Barchiesi F, Cuenca-Estrella M, et al. International and multicenter comparison of EUCAST and CLSI M27-A2 broth microdilution methods for testing susceptibilities of *Candida* spp. to fluconazole, itraconazole, posaconazole, and voriconazole. J Clin Microbiol 2005;43:3884–9
147. Cuenca-Estrella M, Arendrup MC, et al. Multicentre determination of quality control strains and quality control ranges for antifungal susceptibility testing of yeasts and filamentous fungi using the methods of the Antifungal Susceptibility Testing Subcommittee of the European Committee on Antimicrobial Susceptibility Testing (AFST-EUCAST). Clin Microbiol Infect 2007;13: 1018–22
148. Rodriguez-Tudela JL, Martinez-Suarez JV. Improved medium for fluconazole susceptibility testing of *Candida albicans*. Antimicrob Agents Chemother 1995;38:45–8
149. Cuenca-Estrella M, Moore CB, Barchiesi F, et al. Multicenter evaluation of the reproducibility of the proposed antifungal susceptibility testing method for fermentative yeasts of the Antifungal Susceptibility Testing Subcommittee of the European Committee on Antimicrobial Susceptibility Testing (AFST-EUCAST). Clin Microbiol Infect 2003;9:467–74
150. Rodriguez-Tudela JL, Donnelly JP, Pfaller MA, et al. Statistical analyses of correlation between fluconazole MICs for *Candida* spp. assessed by standard methods set forth by the European Committee on Antimicrobial Susceptibility Testing (E.Dis. 7.1) and CLSI (M27-A2). J Clin Microbiol 2007;45:109–11
151. European Committee on Antimicrobial Susceptibility Testing-Subcommittee on Antifungal Susceptibility Testing (EUCAST-AFST). EUCAST technical note on fluconazole. Clin Microbiol Infect 2008;14:193–5
152. Subcommittee on Antifungal Susceptibility Testing of the ESCMID European Committee for Antimicrobial Susceptibility Testing. EUCAST Technical Note on voriconazole. Clin Microbiol Infect 2008;14:985–7
153. Subcommittee on Antifungal Susceptibility Testing of the ESCMID European Committee for Antimicrobial Susceptibility Testing. EUCAST Technical Note on the method for the determination of broth dilution minimum inhibitory concentrations of antifungal agents for conidia-forming moulds. Clin Microbiol Infect 2008;14:982–4
154. Rex JH, Pfaller MA. Has antifungal susceptibility testing come of age? Clin Infect Dis 2002;35:982–9

Epidemiology of Systemic Fungal Diseases: An Overview

Benjamin J. Park, Tom M. Chiller, Mary E. Brandt, and David W. Warnock

The epidemiology of systemic fungal diseases has evolved rapidly over the past 2 decades. Advances in medical treatment have led to improved survival in the general population, but these advances have also led to larger numbers of individuals (including those who have indwelling catheters, who are in intensive care, who have received various immunosuppressive therapies, and who are undergoing organ or stem cell transplantation) being at risk for fungal infection. The global human immunodeficiency virus (HIV) pandemic has led to unprecedented numbers of opportunistic fungal infections, including candidiasis, cryptococcosis, histoplasmosis, and penicilliosis. While the numbers have dropped dramatically in developed nations [1–4], many countries in sub-Saharan Africa [5–7] and parts of Asia [8–10] remain highly affected by these and other fungal diseases. Migration patterns, land use, and climate factors are thought to have contributed to a marked increase in the incidence of coccidioidomycosis [11] in the endemic areas of the southwestern USA and in the emergence of *Cryptococcus gattii* infections [12, 13] in British Columbia, Canada, and the Pacific northwestern USA.

This chapter will focus on public health aspects of systemic fungal diseases. It will discuss principles of epidemiology, risk factors, and prevention of infection by using specific fungal diseases as examples of broader public health principles. Major public health issues will be discussed, including potential strategies for minimizing morbidity and mortality related to fungal diseases.

Cycle of Disease Prevention

Prevention of disease is the ultimate goal of public health. Prevention measures may include limiting risk factors, developing educational campaigns, and administering vaccination programs, but can also include improved methods for early diagnosis or improved treatment strategies to prevent disease sequelae. Once measures are identified it is important to act to reduce disease and disease-related morbidity and mortality.

In order to achieve the ultimate goal of prevention, public health activities need to encompass a wide array of interrelated issues, including understanding disease occurrence or incidence (the number of new cases of a disease during a period of time), performing surveillance to identify disease, investigating outbreaks to determine the source and stop disease transmission, defining risk factors for disease, and ultimately implementing prevention strategies. Some in public health refer to these activities as the cycle of disease control and prevention (Fig. 1).

As depicted in Fig. 1, activities of public health are related and lead from one to another. For example, surveillance can determine the incidence of disease in a given population. Surveillance may also help identify outbreaks of disease and may lead to further epidemiologic investigation. These activities are useful to identify risk factors or prevention measures, as well as to guide applied research projects so that epidemiologic findings can be better understood. Applied research may in turn identify useful prevention tools, such as new vaccine candidates.

Finally, an important role of public health is to measure the effect of prevention measures and to determine how to improve the effectiveness of any prevention effort. This is performed through continued surveillance for the disease, thus beginning the cycle anew.

Surveillance

Public health surveillance is defined as the ongoing, systematic collection, analysis, interpretation, and dissemination of data regarding a health-related event for use in public health action to reduce morbidity and mortality and to improve health [14, 15]. It is one of the most vital functions of public health agencies. Surveillance data are used to measure the burden and trends of diseases, to detect new pathogens, and

B.J. Park (✉)
Mycotic Diseases Branch and Division of Foodborne, Bacterial, and Mycotic Diseases, Centers for Disease Control and Prevention, Atlanta, GA, USA
e-mail: Bpark1@cdc.gov

C.A. Kauffman et al. (eds.), *Essentials of Clinical Mycology*,
DOI 10.1007/978-1-4419-6640-7_2, © Springer Science+Business Media, LLC 2011

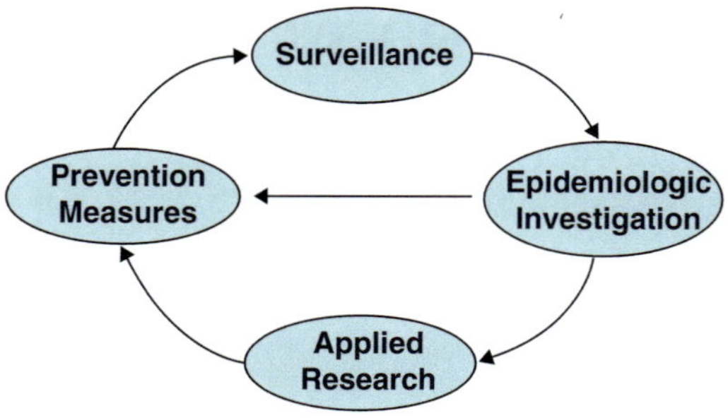

Fig. 1 The cycle of disease control and prevention

to evaluate quality of care [15]. It is also essential to determine the effectiveness of interventions such as prevention guidelines and vaccination programs. Various epidemiologic surveillance systems (to be distinguished from microbiologic surveillance) have been used to examine systemic fungal diseases [3, 7, 16–25].

Surveillance systems can vary by the population under surveillance (population-based surveillance vs sentinel surveillance), or by the method of data collection (active vs passive surveillance).

Population-Based Surveillance

Population-based surveillance is a type of surveillance performed within a well-defined catchment area where data on the population are accessible. This catchment area is often a geographic location, such as a city, county, state, or province, because a reliable population can be derived from census data. In population-based surveillance programs, all cases of the disease under surveillance in the catchment area are identified. However, only cases occurring among residents of the catchment area are counted toward the incidence calculation because the denominator (population as defined by census) only includes residents of that geographic area. Incidence can then be calculated as the number of new cases occurring in the population during a defined time period, divided by the total population (i.e., cases of disease per 100,000 residents of the surveillance area per year).

Population-based surveillance programs for a number of systemic fungal diseases have now been conducted in a number of different countries worldwide. For example, the Centers for Disease Control and Prevention (CDC) conducted population-based surveillance for *Candida* bloodstream infections (candidemia) at different sites in the USA during 1992–1994, and again during 1998–2000. These studies were conducted in metropolitan San Francisco and Atlanta (1992–1994) [26], Baltimore City/County, and the state of Connecticut (1998–2000) [20] and showed that the annual incidence of candidemia was 8–10 cases per 100,000 population [20, 26]. Another population-based surveillance conducted in the state of Iowa between 1998 and 2001 demonstrated an annual incidence of candidemia of 6 cases per 100,000 population [27]. Population-based surveillance has also been conducted in a number of European countries, where the annual incidence of candidemia has been lower, generally between 1.8 and 4.9 cases per 100,000 persons [16, 28–31].

Population-based surveillance has the advantage of providing the most representative description of the epidemiology of a disease in the area under surveillance, because large numbers of individuals may be included and because cases are detected in a multitude of settings, from small outpatient clinics to large tertiary-care centers. For example, in the population-based surveillance of candidemia in Connecticut and Baltimore, a total of 4.7 million persons were under surveillance in 47 hospitals [20]. However, performing such wide-scale surveillance often requires considerable expense and is difficult to sustain for long periods of time.

Another type of population-based surveillance is one in which the catchment area is not defined by geography, but by a common cohort (group) of persons. In such cohort studies, adequate follow-up is essential to determine the presence or absence of infection and therefore inclusion as a case of disease or as a noncase. Cohort studies, as opposed to geographically defined populations, are advantageous when only subsets of the general population are at risk for a certain infection. For example, a cohort study conducted among persons with HIV in Uganda during 1995–1999 determined an annual incidence of cryptococcosis of 4.0% [5].

Recently, a cohort strategy was used to determine incidence of fungal diseases in a transplant population. CDC, in partnership with academic transplant centers across the USA, conducted surveillance for invasive fungal infections among stem cell and organ transplant recipients between 2001 and 2006 [32]. This network of tertiary care transplant centers was appropriate for surveillance of this patient population because these procedures are generally only performed at these types of institutions. Data from this large network are more broadly representative of systemic fungal diseases following transplantation performed in the USA than studies from individual centers.

Sentinel Surveillance

Another important type of surveillance is sentinel surveillance. This is usually conducted at selected sites (often medical centers), rather than in the entire population of a geographic area. Sentinel surveillance is generally easier to perform and less costly than population-based surveillance, and as a result, is performed more frequently. Although it is not possible to estimate the total burden of disease in a population with this form of surveillance, it can be helpful for diseases such as candidemia for which the at-risk population is captured.

Since candidemia is primarily a healthcare-associated infection, hospitals are good sites for sentinel surveillance, since hospital-based denominators such as hospital admissions and patient-days can be used. As a result, numerous sentinel surveillance studies for candidemia have been performed. Published incidence rates for candidemia have ranged from 2.0 cases per 10,000 hospital admissions in France during 1997–1999 [33] to 24.9 cases per 10,000 admissions in Brazil during 2003–2004 [17]. Explanations for these differences in incidence rates by geographic region are not obvious, but may be related to differences in the prevalence of particular risk factors in the population. Such factors likely include differences in antibacterial or antifungal agent use, differences in patient demographics, including race and sociodemographic factors, infection control practices, or medical care, such as frequency of central venous catheter utilization or abdominal surgery.

One particular benefit of performing surveillance over time is to be able to determine trends in incidence. In the examples we have noted earlier, studies conducted over time cannot only determine if the incidence of candidemia in general is changing, but can also detect changes in the incidence of individual pathogens. Some surveillance data from intensive care units in the USA have suggested that although the species distribution has shifted from predominantly *Candida albicans* in the 1980s to an increase in the proportion of non-*albicans* species during the 1990s, it was a decrease in the incidence of *C. albicans* that led to this shift [24]. Some reports from Europe have demonstrated stable incidence rates of both *C. albicans* and non-*albicans* candidemia [34], while others have actually demonstrated an increase in candidemia incidence overall [30, 31].

It is important to distinguish surveillance from disease registries, which are collections of cases. Registries can be useful sources of information about clinical details of cases, particularly for rare diseases, such as mucormycosis [35], or even for diseases occurring in special hosts, such as transplant recipients [36, 37]. However, for the purposes of public health surveillance, registries are of limited value. They do not provide information on incidence because meaningful and appropriate denominator data do not exist. Registries are also subject to ascertainment bias, in which selected participation or case finding can lead to biased data. As a result, registries may not be representative of broader populations and probably should not be interpreted as such.

Active Surveillance

Active surveillance is a surveillance method whereby data collection is initiated by the investigator or public health authority. In these systems, one or more components of the surveillance, such as case finding and detection, are performed consistently and periodically throughout the length of the surveillance period. An example of active surveillance is a system whereby microbiology laboratory records are reviewed and audited periodically to detect new cases of a disease. Clinical information about the cases may then be collected and recorded to describe the epidemiology.

Active surveillance for fungal diseases is expensive and often difficult to conduct, but it results in more complete and accurate information because virtually all cases of the disease in question are being counted. It has enabled accurate population-based incidence rates to be determined for several invasive fungal infections, including *Candida* bloodstream infections and cryptococcosis [3, 16, 17, 19, 20, 23, 26]. It has also permitted a more representative description of the epidemiology of these diseases.

One difficulty with performing active surveillance is the amount of resources required to sustain this effort for prolonged periods. Dedicated staff are generally needed to perform case finding and confirmation, as well as to recover clinical data. Isolates are often submitted to a central laboratory, which may perform species confirmation and antimicrobial susceptibility testing. Because of the resources required, surveillance may not be conducted continuously in order to measure trends in incidence. One strategy to overcome this is to repeat surveillance at periodic intervals in the same population. Active, population-based surveillance for candidemia is currently ongoing in Atlanta and Baltimore, where population-based surveillance was performed previously [20, 26]. These data will describe the changing epidemiology of candidemia in these populations and ascertain whether changes in incidence of antifungal susceptibility or species distribution have occurred.

Passive Surveillance

Passive surveillance systems are provider-initiated: the data are reported to public health authorities without being actively requested. The vast majority of public health surveillance is passive. The advantage of passive surveillance systems is their low cost, as fewer resources are required. However, the quality and completeness of the data are not as high as that collected through active systems.

An example of a passive surveillance system for a fungal disease is the notifiable disease surveillance system for coccidioidomycosis. In the endemic states of the southwest USA, cases of coccidioidomycosis are reported by providers or laboratories to state health departments. Data submitted generally include basic demographic data only. Total case counts are then submitted to CDC, which compiles and reports state, regional, and national data in the Morbidity and Mortality Weekly Report (available at www.cdc.gov/mmwr.pdf).

These data show that the incidence of coccidioidomycosis has been increasing steadily, especially in the endemic states of Arizona and California [38, 39]. In Arizona, coccidioidomycosis is now the third-most-common infection reported to the state health department with an annual incidence of 91 per 100,000 population in 2006 [40]. In California, in 2006, the overall incidence in the state was 8 per 100,000 population, but in the highly endemic area of Kern County, the incidence was 150 per 100,000 population [39].

Passive surveillance data, while easier to collect, are often limited in scope. Clinical and demographic data, which would require more active methods to capture, are often sparse. In addition, case counts may not be complete, as the public health authority is not actively collecting cases or performing audits to ensure that all cases have been reported.

Issues with Surveillance

Case Definitions

In order to perform reliable surveillance for a disease, standard case definitions must be applied. Case definitions may vary depending on their purpose. For example, a definition used for surveillance purposes may not need to be as strict as a definition used for enrollment criteria in a clinical trial.

One example of this is the case definition used for invasive mould infections. Although consensus case definitions have been developed for clinical trial enrollment of immunocompromised patients with cancer and hematopoietic stem cell transplant recipients, [41, 42] these definitions are complicated and are therefore cumbersome for surveillance purposes.

Establishing accurate incidence estimates of invasive mould infections, such as aspergillosis and zygomycosis, remains a major challenge. CDC performed active population-based surveillance for mould infections as a part of a broader laboratory-based fungal surveillance conducted in San Francisco in 1992–1993 [23]. However, for case detection this study relied on laboratory reports of positive fungal cultures [23]. This case definition may not have been accurate: A positive mould culture has a poor positive predictive value because it fails to distinguish between colonization and infection. Furthermore, not all mould infections result in a positive culture result. Indeed, patients who are diagnosed with an invasive mould infection often have this diagnosis reached by a combination of approaches including culture, histopathology, and increasingly, antigenic markers, such as galactomannan. When future surveillance studies in the general population are performed, simpler and more reliable surveillance case definitions for mould infections will need to be developed.

Case definitions can be complicated, but public health authorities have sometimes been successful in simplifying these definitions for surveillance purposes. Prior to 2007, the serologic component of the case definition for coccidioidomycosis required a documented rise in IgG titer for a case to count as a reportable infection. After consulting with experts in the disease and considering the relative cost and benefit of a simplified definition, the Council of State and Territorial Epidemiologists in 2007 agreed to modify the case definition to include persons with a single positive serologic test result as adequate for definition of a case for surveillance purposes [43]. This simplified surveillance case definition may result in an increase in reported cases, but is likely to provide a better total estimate of the burden of disease, and this will be helpful for public health purposes.

Administrative data, such as International Classification of Diseases (ICD) codes, have also been used for fungal surveillance. These data are often used as the case definitions for surveillance. However, since administrative data are usually coded by personnel who are trained for reimbursement purposes, these criteria have been shown to have poor predictive value for fungal diseases, such as aspergillosis, when used as a case definition [44]. Their sensitivity for screening for fungal diseases is considerably more useful.

Burden of Disease

Understanding the actual burden of a disease as it relates to other diseases is one of the major challenges for public health. In most cases, surveillance systems do not accurately estimate the total burden of disease in a population. Often this occurs because there are many steps between the actual reporting of a case of disease and its occurrence in a population. To begin with, a person must have symptoms of disease; these must rise to the level of concern to initiate a visit to a clinician for evaluation. The clinician must then collect an appropriate sample and submit it to a capable laboratory. The laboratory must identify the causative organism by an appropriate methodology. Lastly, the case must be reported to public health authorities by the defined method used for surveillance. These steps, when taken together, constitute what can be described as the burden of illness pyramid (Fig. 2a) [45]. The shape of the pyramid varies for every disease and situation (Fig. 2b). For example, for a disease such as a viral hemorrhagic fever, it is likely that nearly all of the cases in a population will be

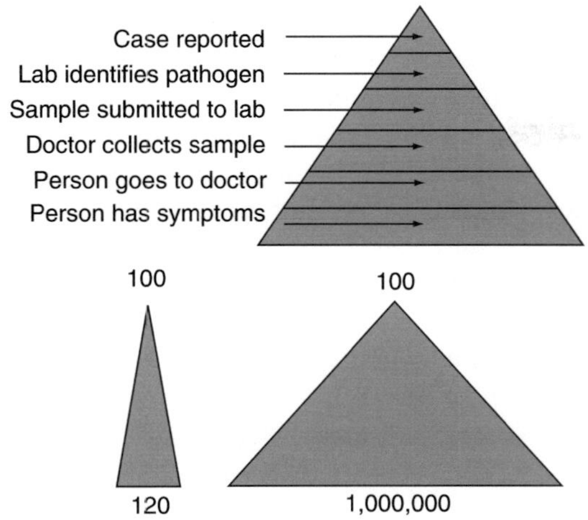

Fig. 2 (**a**) and (**b**) Pyramid of surveillance

Table 1 Estimated cryptococcal meningitis (CM) cases and deaths among 10 UN AIDS global regions by using published incidence rates from studies conducted in those regions (Adapted from [51])

Region	Estimated yearly CM cases (range), in 1,000 s	Estimated deaths (range), in 1,000 s
Sub-Saharan Africa	720 (144.0–1,296.0)	504.0 (100.8–907.2)
East Asia	13.6(2.7–24.5)	1.2 (0.2–2.2)
Oceania	0.1 (0.0–0.1)	0.009 (0.0–0.009)
South and Southeast Asia	120 (24.0–216.0)	66.0 (13.2–118.8)
Eastern Europe, Central Asia	27.2 (5.4–49.0)	15.0 (3.0–27.0)
Western and Central Europe	0.5 (0.1–1.0)	0.045 (0.009–0.09)
North Africa, Middle East	6.5 (1.3–11.6)	3.6 (0.7–6.4)
North America	7.8 (1.6–14.0)	0.7 (0.1–1.3)
Caribbean	7.8 (1.6–14.1)	4.3 (0.9–7.8)
Latin America	54.4 (10.9–97.9)	29.9 (6.0–53.8)
Global	957.9 (371.7–1,544)	624.7 (125.0–1,124.9)

detected; but for a disease such as salmonellosis, studies have demonstrated that only 1 in 38.6 cases are reported to public health authorities [46].

Because surveillance may not estimate the entire burden of a disease, it is helpful to estimate the incidence using burden of disease calculations. Burden of disease estimates allow for comparison with other disease burdens and help public health authorities determine disease priorities and resource allocation. CDC and the World Health Organization have conducted numerous studies to measure the burden due to specific diseases throughout the world [47–50].

One of the most striking estimates recently was the global burden of cryptococcal meningitis, including yearly cases and deaths, in persons with HIV infection [51]. According to the estimate, approximately 958,000 cases of cryptococcal meningitis occur each year (range, 371,700–1,544,000) (Table 1). The region with the greatest number of cases was sub-Saharan Africa, with 720,000 cases per year, followed by South and Southeast Asia, with 120,000 cases per year. Western and Central Europe (500 cases) and Oceania (100 cases) had the fewest number of estimated cases. In addition, an estimated 625,000 deaths were estimated to occur globally, with most deaths in sub-Saharan Africa, with over 500,000 deaths per year.

Similar burden of disease estimates have not been developed for other systemic fungal diseases. Such estimates would allow public health agencies to place particular diseases in the context of other diseases. In the case of cryptococcosis, the recent burden estimates showed that the disease is one of the leading causes of infection-related mortality in sub-Saharan Africa [51] and the most common cause of meningitis in that part of world. It is estimated to cause more deaths in this region than diseases such as tuberculosis, which are more common in the population (Fig. 3) [50].

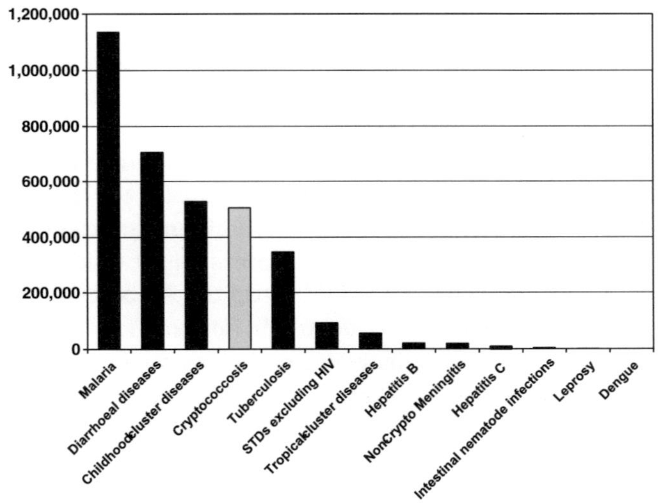

Fig. 3 Comparison of deaths in sub-Saharan Africa due to human immunodeficiency virus (HIV)-related cryptococcosis and common infectious diseases, excluding HIV, as estimated by WHO [51]

Reducing the Public Health Burden of Systemic Fungal Diseases

The ultimate goal of public health is to reduce morbidity and mortality related to a disease, either through reduction of the number of cases of a disease or by improving the outcomes associated with the infection. Prevention of some fungal infections may be performed by identifying outbreaks and eliminating the transmission of disease. Fungal outbreaks may be associated with hospital construction [52, 53], point-sources from the community [54–56], and even novel medical devices [57, 58]. An adequate understanding of the mechanisms of transmission of these infections has important implications for prevention strategies, ranging from the need for specific containment and environmental control measures to the consideration of antifungal drug prophylaxis.

Environmental Control Measures

The ubiquitous occurrence of many opportunistic moulds in the environment and the ecology of others, such as the endemic pathogens *Histoplasma capsulatum* and *Coccidioides* species, make it difficult to prevent exposure. Environmental control measures designed to protect high-risk patients from exposure to moulds at home or in the hospital are difficult. Housing these individuals in rooms supplied with HEPA-filtered air has helped to prevent the acquisition of *Aspergillus* infection within the hospital. The CDC, in collaboration with the Hospital Infection Control Practices Advisory Committee (HICPAC), has published guidelines that describe many of these environmental measures for preventing aspergillosis in the hospital environment (available at: http://www.cdc.gov/ncidod/dhqp/hicpac_pubs.html).

In the case of *Candida* bloodstream infections, evidence from outbreak investigations has implicated carriage of organisms on the hands of healthcare providers as a cause of transmission of some *Candida* species in hospitals. Guidelines have been developed by the CDC and the Association for Professionals in Infection Control and Epidemiology (http://www.cdc.gov/ncidod/dhqp/hicpac_pubs.html) to enforce rigorous hand washing before and between all patient contacts, especially when dealing with high-risk patients.

Guidelines have also been developed for protection against some community-acquired infections in special risk groups. Examples include prevention of histoplasmosis among workers (http://www.cdc.gov/niosh/docs/2005-109/) and prevention of opportunistic fungal infections in persons with AIDS, developed in collaboration with the Infectious Diseases Society of America (IDSA) (http://www.cdc.gov/mmwr/preview/mmwrhtml/rr5108a1.htm).

Improving the Diagnosis of Fungal Infections

Although improved diagnostics may not prevent disease, simpler and easier diagnosis may lead to increased numbers of patients being treated for fungal infections, and this may in turn reduce the morbidity and mortality related to these diseases. Improved diagnostic tools would be beneficial in the diagnosis and early management of many systemic fungal infections.

The detection of cryptococcosis in resource-poor countries is a major concern and an area in which improved diagnostic capabilities could dramatically benefit patients. Currently, in many of the countries with the highest burden of this infection (e.g., sub-Saharan Africa and South and Southeast Asia) laboratory capacity is not uniformly capable of reliably detecting *Cryptococcus*. Many clinical laboratories in these countries are small and poorly equipped and may be staffed by persons with minimal training. Improving capacity for diagnosis, as well as development of simple diagnostic technologies, such as lateral flow assays for antigen detection, may be increasingly important in these areas.

Improved diagnostic practices are also being encouraged for coccidioidomycosis. Although the incidence of disease currently reported from the southwestern USA through passive surveillance is quite high, there is evidence that the actual burden is much higher. Only 2–13% of individuals with compatible respiratory illnesses are tested for *Coccidioides* antibodies, [59] despite prospective studies showing that 8–29% of cases of community acquired pneumonias in endemic regions may be caused by this organism [59–61]. To lessen this diagnostic gap, public health authorities are encouraging increased testing for coccidioidomycosis among persons in endemic areas presenting to clinical providers with community-acquired pneumonia.

Vaccination

Vaccination is the ultimate tool for prevention and control of disease. Unfortunately, few vaccines are being developed for fungal diseases. For coccidioidomycosis, a vaccine may be an attractive option because natural infection almost always confers lifelong immunity to reinfection [62]. Over the last decade, the Valley Fever Vaccine Project, a consortium of researchers coordinated by the California State University, Bakersfield campus, has identified candidate vaccines for further development. Despite an economic analysis published in 2001 which suggested that a vaccine would have substantial public health benefit [63] funding for research has been inconsistent. Nonetheless, numerous candidate vaccines have been developed [62, 64–66], and phase I or phase II trials may be possible in the near future.

Encouraging Improved Therapeutics

Just as improved diagnostics may help to reduce the morbidity and mortality related to disease, so can improved therapeutics. Clinical trials are being conducted for infections such as aspergillosis and candidiasis. Similar efforts for diseases such as coccidioidomycosis and histoplasmosis, which have been given less attention, have been advocated by public health authorities.

Until prevention efforts such as a vaccine are available, prevention of coccidioidomycosis will prove to be challenging. The infective dose for *Coccidioides* is very low, and although dust-generating activities such as digging have been associated with outbreaks, the vast majority of cases that occur in the endemic area are sporadic. Because of this, public health officials are also focusing on strategies to reduce the morbidity and mortality of this disease. One potential intervention that has only been studied retrospectively is the utility of antifungal treatment for primary infection [67]. While studies have shown that the majority of cases resolve eventually without treatment, many persons may be ill for months and consequently may be absent from work or school [11]. It is not known if treatment of primary infection can reduce symptoms or quicken improvement, or if it can help to prevent disseminated disease, which is uniformly fatal when untreated. Further study should determine if rapid diagnosis and treatment of primary pulmonary infection can reduce the complications of infection, and which groups of patients, if any, benefit the most.

Another situation that warrants further study is the best approach to treatment of cryptococcosis in resource-limited areas. Although current IDSA guidelines recommend treatment of cryptococcal meningitis with amphotericin B and flucytosine [68], these medications are not available or are cost-prohibitive to use in many countries in sub-Saharan Africa. Additionally, the complex medical infrastructure required for the management of these patients (which includes frequent lumbar punctures to manage intracranial pressure and monitoring of renal function for those on amphotericin B) is often not available. Therefore, creative treatment and sustainable management solutions will need to be developed. One promising strategy is the use of fluconazole at high doses for treatment. Recent data have shown that fluconazole at dosages of up to 1,200 mg daily is safe and effective [69]. Additionally, combination therapy with fluconazole and amphotericin B is safe and may be effective [70].

In areas in which amphotericin B and/or flucytosine are not available, these treatment strategies may be considered. Public health officials should work with ministries of health to determine the most cost-effective strategies for prevention of cryptococcal disease given the numerous competing resources for HIV/AIDS care and treatment. This situation also offers an example of the interrelated nature of the cycle of disease prevention. Surveillance can offer an estimate of the burden of fungal infection in this patient population; such burden estimates can then be used to inform public health officials so that appropriate employment of health resources can be made.

Prophylaxis

The investment in organ and stem cell transplantation is large and increasing. Public health efforts are not only aimed at maintaining the safety and quality of transplanted tissues and organs, but also focus on reducing risk of infection after transplantation has occurred. Invasive fungal infections remain one of the leading causes of infection-related morbidity and mortality. In stem cell transplant populations, antifungal prophylaxis, in particular with fluconazole [71–73] and posaconazole [74, 75], has been shown to be effective at reducing systemic fungal infections. Of the few clinical trials that have been performed among organ transplant recipients, fluconazole and itraconazole have demonstrated efficacy in preventing fungal infections in liver transplant recipients [76–78]. Prophylaxis with trimethoprim-sulfamethoxazole for prevention of *Pneumocystis jiroveci* infection is standard of care for organ transplant recipients.

Candidemia is one of the most common health care-associated infections. The burden of candidemia among neonates and infants is particularly high, with an incidence as high as 160 cases per 100,000 population among black infants in Baltimore [20]. Clinical trials of fluconazole prophylaxis for the prevention of candidiasis have demonstrated efficacy, particularly among very-low-birth-weight neonates, against this disease [79–82]. Antifungal prophylaxis is not widely practiced in these infants, partly due to concerns for the emergence of resistant *Candida* species [83]. Recommendations for prophylaxis focus on those whose birth weight is <1,000 g and who are cared for in units that have high rates of invasive candidiasis.

Primary prophylaxis to prevent cryptococcosis in high-risk HIV patients merits further clinical study. Prophylaxis trials among HIV-infected persons performed in the 1990s in developed countries (USA, Europe, and Australia) using either fluconazole or itraconazole showed a reduction of risk for development of cryptococcal infection, but without an overall survival benefit [84–86]. As a result, primary prophylaxis was never recommended as a prevention strategy. However, these studies were all performed in developed countries in optimized clinical conditions where the incidence and attributable mortality from cryptococcal disease among the cohorts was low, relative to the current reality in resource-limited countries in which cryptococcosis has a higher incidence and higher case-fatality rate. In developing countries, trials may be more likely to achieve statistical significance in demonstrating a benefit for primary prophylaxis in selected HIV-infected populations.

Two studies have been performed recently in Thailand with differing results. The first study involved 129 HIV-infected patients with CD4 counts <300 cells/μL who received either itraconazole prophylaxis or placebo; this study did not show a survival benefit from receiving antifungal medication, but no patients in the itraconazole arm developed cryptococcosis [87]. Another small study, which randomized 90 HIV-infected patients with CD4 <100 cells/μL to either fluconazole, 400 mg each week, or placebo, did suggest a survival benefit [88]. Overall, 3 of 44 (6.8%) patients on the fluconazole arm developed cryptococcal disease, compared with 7 of 46 (15.2%) in the placebo arm, although this outcome was not statistically different [88]. To date, no randomized trials to evaluate prophylaxis have been published from sub-Saharan Africa.

Empirical and Pre-Emptive Therapy

Empirical therapy consists of identifying persons at high risk for development of an invasive fungal infection by recognition of clinical signs and symptoms that are consistent with early fungal disease, and then initiating antifungal therapy. Empirical approaches have been studied extensively in high-risk neutropenic patients; amphotericin B deoxycholate, liposomal formulations of amphotericin B, voriconazole, itraconazole, and caspofungin are recommended as options for treatment of persistently febrile neutropenic patients by IDSA guidelines [89].

In contrast to empirical therapy, a pre-emptive therapy strategy is one in which patients with evidence of fungal infection are identified early in the course of disease, allowing early initiation of antifungal therapy. These strategies have been extensively studied in invasive aspergillosis. High levels of antigenic markers, such as galactomannan, have been shown to be helpful to identify persons who may benefit from early initiation of antifungal therapy, and certain radiographic findings on high-resolution chest computed tomography scans have been shown to be early predictors of worse disease in many cases [90–93]. Prospective studies have shown value in a pre-emptive approach to treatment of patients with prolonged neutropenia [90, 94].

Pre-emptive treatment may also be valuable in cryptococcal meningitis. Most patients with cryptococcal meningitis in sub-Saharan Africa present very late in the course of disease, often with very low CD4 counts and with signs of advanced cryptococcal infection; survival rates are extremely poor [5, 7, 95]. Pre-emptive treatment may be beneficial among asymptomatic or mildly symptomatic persons with a positive serum cryptococcal antigen test. Studies using prospective or retrospective serum antigen screening have reported a prevalence of cryptococcal antigenemia of 6–18% [96–100]. Antigenemia has also been shown to precede clinical disease and independently predict poor outcomes. In a study from Uganda, antigenemia preceded clinical symptoms of cryptococcosis by a median of 22 days (range, 5–234), with 11% of individuals demonstrating positivity for greater than 100 days [5]. Another study found that asymptomatic cryptococcal antigenemia was associated with a higher risk of death (RR 6.6, 95% CI 1.9–23.6), and had a population-attributable risk for mortality similar to that of active tuberculosis [98].

Identifying antigenemic persons with few or no symptoms would allow for early antifungal treatment using an oral agent, such as fluconazole, which is widely available and inexpensive. In a Cambodian study, 10 persons with asymptomatic antigenemia were treated with fluconazole, 200 mg daily for 12 weeks [100]. When evaluated after completion of therapy, none had developed cryptococcal meningitis. Early treatment may also help to prevent immune reconstitution inflammatory syndrome (IRIS), which may contribute substantially to early mortality among persons initiating antiretroviral medication.

Disclaimer: The findings and conclusions in this presentation/report are those of the author(s) and do not necessarily represent the official position of the Centers for Disease Control and Prevention.

This information is distributed solely for the purpose of predissemination peer review under applicable information quality guidelines. It has not been formally disseminated by the Centers for Disease Control and Prevention. It does not represent and should not be construed to represent any agency determination or policy.

References

1. Dromer F, Mathoulin-Pelissier S, Fontanet A, et al. Epidemiology of HIV-associated cryptococcosis in France (1985–2001): comparison of the pre- and post-HAART eras. AIDS 2004;18:555-62.
2. Kaplan JE, Hanson D, Dworkin MS, et al. Epidemiology of human immunodeficiency virus-associated opportunistic infections in the United States in the era of highly active antiretroviral therapy. Clin Infect Dis 2000;30(Suppl 1):S5-14.
3. Mirza SA, Phelan M, Rimland D, et al. The changing epidemiology of cryptococcosis: an update from population-based active surveillance in 2 large metropolitan areas, 1992-2000. Clin Infect Dis 2003;36:789-94.
4. van Elden LJ, Walenkamp AM, Lipovsky MM, et al. Declining number of patients with cryptococcosis in the Netherlands in the era of highly active antiretroviral therapy. AIDS 2000;14:2787-8.
5. French N, Gray K, Watera C, et al. Cryptococcal infection in a cohort of HIV-1-infected Ugandan adults. AIDS 2002;16:1031-8.
6. Mbanya DN, Zebaze R, Minkoulou EM, Binam F, Koulla S, Obounou A. Clinical and epidemiologic trends in HIV/AIDS patients in a hospital setting of Yaounde, Cameroon: a 6-year perspective. Int J Infect Dis 2002;6:134-8.
7. McCarthy KM, Morgan J, Wannemuehler KA, et al. Population-based surveillance for cryptococcosis in an antiretroviral-naive South African province with a high HIV seroprevalence. AIDS 2006;20:2199-206.
8. Klotz SA, Nguyen HC, Van Pham T, Nguyen LT, Ngo DT, Vu SN. Clinical features of HIV/AIDS patients presenting to an inner city clinic in Ho Chi Minh City, Vietnam. Int J STD AIDS 2007;18:482-5.

9. Kong BN, Harwell JI, Suos P, et al. Opportunistic infections and HIV clinical disease stage among patients presenting for care in Phnom Penh, Cambodia. Southeast Asian J Trop Med Public Health 2007;38:62-8.
10. Kumarasamy N, Solomon S, Flanigan TP, Hemalatha R, Thyagarajan SP, Mayer KH. Natural history of human immunodeficiency virus disease in southern India. Clin Infect Dis 2003;36:79-85.
11. Park BJ, Sigel K, Vaz V, et al. An epidemic of coccidioidomycosis in Arizona associated with climatic changes, 1998-2001. J Infect Dis 2005;191:1981-7.
12. Chambers C, MacDougall L, Li M, Galanis E. Tourism and specific risk areas for *Cryptococcus gattii*, Vancouver Island, Canada. Emerg Infect Dis 2008;14:1781-3.
13. MacDougall L, Kidd SE, Galanis E, et al. Spread of *Cryptococcus gattii* in British Columbia, Canada, and detection in the Pacific Northwest, USA. Emerg Infect Dis 2007;13(1):42-50.
14. Centers for Disease Control and Prevention. Guidelines for evaluating surveillance systems. MMWR – Morb Mortal Wkly Rep 1988;37(Suppl 5):1-18.
15. German RR, Lee LM, Horan JM, et al. Updated guidelines for evaluating public health surveillance systems: recommendations from the Guidelines Working Group. MMWR Recomm Rep 2001;50:1-35.
16. Almirante B, Rodriguez D, Park BJ, et al. Epidemiology and predictors of mortality in cases of *Candida* bloodstream infection: results from population-based surveillance, Barcelona, Spain, from 2002 to 2003. J Clin Microbiol 2005;43:1829-35.
17. Colombo AL, Nucci M, Park BJ, et al. Epidemiology of candidemia in Brazil: a nationwide sentinel surveillance of candidemia in eleven medical centers. J Clin Microbiol 2006;44: 2816-23.
18. Hajjeh RA, Brandt ME, Pinner RW. Emergence of cryptococcal disease: epidemiologic perspectives 100 years after its discovery. Epidemiol Rev 1995;17:303-20.
19. Hajjeh RA, Conn LA, Stephens DS, et al. Cryptococcosis: population-based multistate active surveillance and risk factors in human immunodeficiency virus-infected persons. Cryptococcal Active Surveillance Group. J Infect Dis 1999;179:449-54.
20. Hajjeh RA, Sofair AN, Harrison LH, et al. Incidence of bloodstream infections due to *Candida* species and in vitro susceptibilities of isolates collected from 1998 to 2000 in a population-based active surveillance program. J Clin Microbiol 2004;42:1519-27.
21. Pfaller MA, Diekema DJ, Gibbs DL, et al. Results from the ARTEMIS DISK global antifungal surveillance study, 1997-2007: 10.5-year analysis of susceptibilities of noncandidal yeast species to fluconazole and voriconazole determined by CLSI standardized disk diffusion testing. J Clin Microbiol 2009;47:117-23.
22. Pfaller MA, Messer SA, Boyken L, et al. Global trends in the antifungal susceptibility of *Cryptococcus neoformans* (1990 to 2004). J Clin Microbiol 2005;43:2163-7.
23. Rees JR, Pinner RW, Hajjeh RA, Brandt ME, Reingold AL. The epidemiological features of invasive mycotic infections in the San Francisco Bay area, 1992-1993: results of population-based laboratory active surveillance. Clin Infect Dis 1998;27: 1138-47.
24. Trick WE, Fridkin SK, Edwards JR, Hajjeh RA, Gaynes RP, National Nosocomial Infections Surveillance System H. Secular trend of hospital-acquired candidemia among intensive care unit patients in the United States during 1989-1999. Clin Infect Dis 2002;35:627-30.
25. Viscoli C, Girmenia C, Marinus A, et al. Candidemia in cancer patients: a prospective, multicenter surveillance study by the Invasive Fungal Infection Group (IFIG) of the European Organization for Research and Treatment of Cancer (EORTC). Clin Infect Dis 1999;28:1071-9.
26. Kao AS, Brandt ME, Pruitt WR, et al. The epidemiology of candidemia in two United States cities: results of a population-based active surveillance. Clin Infect Dis 1999;29:1164-70.
27. Diekema DJ, Messer SA, Brueggemann AB, et al. Epidemiology of candidemia: 3-year results from the emerging infections and the epidemiology of Iowa organisms study. J Clin Microbiol 2002;40:1298-302.
28. Asmundsdottir LR, Erlendsdottir H, Gottfredsson M. Increasing incidence of candidemia: results from a 20-year nationwide study in Iceland. J Clin Microbiol 2002;40:3489-92.
29. Laupland KB, Gregson DB, Church DL, Ross T, Elsayed S. Invasive *Candida* species infections: a 5 year population-based assessment. J Antimicrob Chemother 2005;56:532-7.
30. Poikonen E, Lyytikainen O, Anttila VJ, Ruutu P. Candidemia in Finland, 1995-1999. Emerg Infect Dis 2003;9:985-90.
31. Sandven P, Bevanger L, Digranes A, et al. Candidemia in Norway (1991 to 2003): results from a nationwide study. J Clin Microbiol 2006;44:1977-81.
32. Morgan J, Wannemuehler KA, Marr KA, et al. Incidence of invasive aspergillosis following hematopoietic stem cell and solid organ transplantation: interim results of a prospective multicenter surveillance program. Med Mycol 2005;43(Suppl 1):S49-58.
33. Tortorano AM, Peman J, Bernhardt H, et al. Epidemiology of candidaemia in Europe: results of 28-month European Confederation of Medical Mycology (ECMM) hospital-based surveillance study. Eur J Clin Microbiol Infect Dis 2004;23:317-22.
34. Marchetti O, Bille J, Fluckiger U, et al. Epidemiology of candidemia in Swiss tertiary care hospitals: secular trends, 1991-2000. Clin Infect Dis 2004;38:311-20.
35. Roden MM, Zaoutis TE, Buchanan WL, et al. Epidemiology and outcome of zygomycosis: a review of 929 reported cases. Clin Infect Dis 2005;41:634-53.
36. Horn DL, Fishman JA, Steinbach WJ, et al. Presentation of the PATH alliance registry for prospective data collection and analysis of the epidemiology, therapy, and outcomes of invasive fungal infections. Diagn Microbiol Infect Dis 2007;59:407-14.
37. Neofytos D, Horn D, Anaissie E, et al. Epidemiology and outcome of invasive fungal infection in adult hematopoietic stem cell transplant recipients: analysis of Multicenter Prospective Antifungal Therapy (PATH) Alliance registry. Clin Infect Dis 2009;48:265-73.
38. Centers for Disease Control and Prevention. Increase in Coccidioi domycosis – Arizona, 1998-2001. MMWR – Morb Mortal Wkly Rep 2003;52:109-12.
39. Centers for Disease Control and Prevention. Increase in Coccidioi domycosis – California, 2000-2007. MMWR – Morb Mortal Wkly Rep 2009;58:105-9.
40. Sunenshine RH, Anderson S, Erhart L, et al. Public health surveillance for coccidioidomycosis in Arizona. Ann NY Acad Sci 2007;1111:96-102.
41. Ascioglu S, Rex JH, de Pauw B, et al. Defining opportunistic invasive fungal infections in immunocompromised patients with cancer and hematopoietic stem cell transplants: an international consensus. Clin Infect Dis 2002;34:7-14.
42. De Pauw B, Walsh TJ, Donnelly JP, et al. Revised definitions of invasive fungal disease from the European Organization for Research and Treatment of Cancer/Invasive Fungal Infections Cooperative Group and the National Institute of Allergy and Infectious Diseases Mycoses Study Group (EORTC/MSG) Consensus Group. Clin Infect Dis 2008;46:1813-21.
43. *Coccidioides* (*Coccidioides* spp., Valley fever) 2008 case definition: Centers for Disease Control and Prevention, 2008. (Accessed December 1, 2009, at http://www.cdc.gov/ncphi/disss/nndss/casedef/coccidioid2008.htm.)
44. Chang DC, Burwell LA, Lyon GM, et al. Comparison of the use of administrative data and an active system for surveillance of invasive aspergillosis. Infect Control Hosp Epidemiol 2008;29:25-30.

45. Hardnett FP, Hoekstra RM, Kennedy M, Charles L, Angulo FJ, Emerging Infections Program FoodNet Working Group. Epidemiologic issues in study design and data analysis related to FoodNet activities. Clin Infect Dis 2004;38(Suppl 3):S121-6.
46. Voetsch AC, Van Gilder TJ, Angulo FJ, et al. FoodNet estimate of the burden of illness caused by nontyphoidal Salmonella infections in the United States. Clin Infect Dis 2004;38(Suppl 3): S127-34.
47. Mead PS, Slutsker L, Dietz V, et al. Food-related illness and death in the United States. Emerg Infect Dis 1999;5:607-25.
48. Crump JA, Luby SP, Mintz ED. The global burden of typhoid fever. Bull World Health Organ 2004;82:346-53.
49. Crump JA, Youssef FG, Luby SP, et al. Estimating the incidence of typhoid fever and other febrile illnesses in developing countries. Emerg Infect Dis 2003;9:539-44.
50. Revised Global Burden of Disease (GBD) 2002 Estimates: World Health Organization, 2002. (Accessed December 1, 2009, at http://www.who.int/healthinfo/bodgbd2002revised/en/index.html.)
51. Park BJ, Wannemuehler KA, Marston BJ, Govender N, Pappas PG, Chiller TM. Estimation of the current global burden of cryptococcal meningitis among persons living with HIV/AIDS. AIDS 2009;23:525-30.
52. Panackal AA, Dahlman A, Keil KT, et al. Outbreak of invasive aspergillosis among renal transplant recipients. Transplantation 2003;75:1050-3.
53. Vonberg RP, Gastmeier P. Nosocomial aspergillosis in outbreak settings. J Hosp Infect 2006;63:246-54.
54. Chamany S, Mirza SA, Fleming JW, et al. A large histoplasmosis outbreak among high school students in Indiana, 2001. Pediatr Infect Dis J 2004;23:909-14.
55. Huhn GD, Austin C, Carr M, et al. Two outbreaks of occupationally acquired histoplasmosis: more than workers at risk. Environ Health Perspect 2005;113:585-9.
56. Kauffman CA. Endemic mycoses: blastomycosis, histoplasmosis, and sporotrichosis. Infect Dis Clin North Am 2006;20:645-62.
57. Chang DC, Grant GB, O'Donnell K, et al. Multistate outbreak of *Fusarium* keratitis associated with use of a contact lens solution. JAMA 2006;296:953-63.
58. Grant GB, Fridkin S, Chang DC, Park BJ. Postrecall surveillance following a multistate *Fusarium* keratitis outbreak, 2004 through 2006. JAMA 2007;298:2867-8.
59. Chang DC, Anderson S, Wannemuehler K, et al. Testing for coccidioidomycosis among patients with community-acquired pneumonia. Emerg Infect Dis 2008;14:1053-9.
60. Kim MM, Blair JE, Carey EJ, Wu Q, Smilack JD. Coccidioidal pneumonia, Phoenix, Arizona, USA, 2000-2004. Emerg Infect Dis 2009;15:397-401.
61. Valdivia L, Nix D, Wright M, et al. Coccidioidomycosis as a common cause of community-acquired pneumonia. Emerg Infect Dis 2006;12:958-62.
62. Cox RA, Magee DM. Coccidioidomycosis: host response and vaccine development. Clin Microbiol Rev 2004;17:804-39.
63. Barnato AE, Sanders GD, Owens DK. Cost-effectiveness of a potential vaccine for *Coccidioides immitis*. Emerg Infect Dis 2001;7:797-806.
64. Capilla J, Clemons KV, Liu M, Levine HB, Stevens DA. *Saccharomyces cerevisiae* as a vaccine against coccidioidomycosis. Vaccine 2009;27:3662-8.
65. Tarcha EJ, Basrur V, Hung CY, Gardner MJ, Cole GT. Multivalent recombinant protein vaccine against coccidioidomycosis. Infect Immun 2006;74:5802-13.
66. Xue J, Chen X, Selby D, Hung CY, Yu JJ, Cole GT. A genetically engineered live attenuated vaccine of *Coccidioides posadasii* protects BALB/c mice against coccidioidomycosis. Infect Immun 2009;77:3196-208.
67. Ampel NM, Giblin A, Mourani JP, Galgiani JN. Factors and outcomes associated with the decision to treat primary pulmonary coccidioidomycosis. Clin Infect Dis 2009;48:172-8.
68. Perfect JR, Dismukes WE, Dromer F, et al. Clinical practice guidelines for the management of cryptococcal disease: 2010 update by the Infectious Diseases Society of America. Clin Infect Dis 2010;50:291-322.
69. Longley N, Muzoora C, Taseera K, et al. Dose response effect of high-dose fluconazole for HIV-associated cryptococcal meningitis in Southwestern Uganda. Clin Infect Dis 2008;47:1556-61.
70. Pappas PG, Chetchotisakd P, Larsen RA, et al. A phase II randomized trial of amphotericin B alone or combined with fluconazole in the treatment of HIV-associated cryptococcal meningitis. Clin Infect Dis 2009;48:1775-83.
71. Goodman JL, Winston DJ, Greenfield RA, et al. A controlled trial of fluconazole to prevent fungal infections in patients undergoing bone marrow transplantation. N Engl J Med 1992;326:845-51.
72. Marr KA, Seidel K, Slavin MA, et al. Prolonged fluconazole prophylaxis is associated with persistent protection against candidiasis-related death in allogeneic marrow transplant recipients: long-term follow-up of a randomized, placebo-controlled trial. Blood 2000;96:2055-61.
73. Slavin MA, Osborne B, Adams R, et al. Efficacy and safety of fluconazole prophylaxis for fungal infections after marrow transplantation – a prospective, randomized, double-blind study. J Infect Dis 1995;171:1545-52.
74. Cornely OA, Maertens J, Winston DJ, et al. Posaconazole vs. fluconazole or itraconazole prophylaxis in patients with neutropenia. N Engl J Med 2007;356:348-59.
75. Ullmann AJ, Lipton JH, Vesole DH, et al. Posaconazole or fluconazole for prophylaxis in severe graft-versus-host disease. N Engl J Med 2007;356:335-47.
76. Winston DJ, Pakrasi A, Busuttil RW. Prophylactic fluconazole in liver transplant recipients. A randomized, double-blind, placebo-controlled trial. Ann Intern Med 1999;131:729-37.
77. Lumbreras C, Cuervas-Mons V, Jara P, et al. Randomized trial of fluconazole versus nystatin for the prophylaxis of *Candida* infection following liver transplantation. J Infect Dis 1996;174:583-8.
78. Sharpe MD, Ghent C, Grant D, Horbay GL, McDougal J, David Colby W. Efficacy and safety of itraconazole prophylaxis for fungal infections after orthotopic liver transplantation: a prospective, randomized, double-blind study. Transplantation 2003;76:977-83.
79. Kaufman D. Fluconazole prophylaxis decreases the combined outcome of invasive *Candida* infections or mortality in preterm infants. Pediatrics 2008;122:1158-9.
80. Kaufman D, Boyle R, Hazen KC, Patrie JT, Robinson M, Donowitz LG. Fluconazole prophylaxis against fungal colonization and infection in preterm infants. N Engl J Med 2001;345:1660-6.
81. Kaufman D, Boyle R, Hazen KC, Patrie JT, Robinson M, Grossman LB. Twice weekly fluconazole prophylaxis for prevention of invasive *Candida* infection in high-risk infants of <1000 grams birth weight. J Pediatr 2005;147:172-9.
82. Kicklighter SD, Springer SC, Cox T, Hulsey TC, Turner RB. Fluconazole for prophylaxis against candidal rectal colonization in the very low birth weight infant. Pediatrics 2001;107:293-8.
83. Burwell LA, Kaufman D, Blakely J, Stoll BJ, Fridkin SK. Antifungal prophylaxis to prevent neonatal candidiasis: a survey of perinatal physician practices. Pediatrics 2006;118:e1019-26.
84. McKinsey DS, Wheat LJ, Cloud GA, et al. Itraconazole prophylaxis for fungal infections in patients with advanced human immunodeficiency virus infection: randomized, placebo-controlled, double-blind study. National Institute of Allergy and Infectious Diseases Mycoses Study Group. Clin Infect Dis 1999;28:1049-56.
85. Powderly WG, Finkelstein D, Feinberg J, et al. A randomized trial comparing fluconazole with clotrimazole troches for the

prevention of fungal infections in patients with advanced human immunodeficiency virus infection. NIAID AIDS Clinical Trials Group. N Engl J Med 1995;332:700-5.
86. Smith DE, Bell J, Johnson M, et al. A randomized, double-blind, placebo-controlled study of itraconazole capsules for the prevention of deep fungal infections in immunodeficient patients with HIV infection. HIV Med 2001;2:78-83.
87. Chariyalertsak S, Supparatpinyo K, Sirisanthana T, Nelson KE. A controlled trial of itraconazole as primary prophylaxis for systemic fungal infections in patients with advanced human immunodeficiency virus infection in Thailand. Clin Infect Dis 2002; 34:277-84.
88. Chetchotisakd P, Sungkanuparph S, Thinkhamrop B, Mootsikapun P, Boonyaprawit P. A multicentre, randomized, double-blind, placebo-controlled trial of primary cryptococcal meningitis prophylaxis in HIV-infected patients with severe immune deficiency. HIV Med 2004;5:140-3.
89. Walsh TJ, Anaissie EJ, Denning DW, et al. Treatment of aspergillosis: clinical practice guidelines of the Infectious Diseases Society of America. Clin Infect Dis 2008;46:327-60.
90. Maertens J, Theunissen K, Verhoef G, et al. Galactomannan and computed tomography-based preemptive antifungal therapy in neutropenic patients at high risk for invasive fungal infection: a prospective feasibility study. Clin Infect Dis 2005;41:1242-50.
91. Maertens J, Van Eldere J, Verhaegen J, Verbeken E, Verschakelen J, Boogaerts M. Use of circulating galactomannan screening for early diagnosis of invasive aspergillosis in allogeneic stem cell transplant recipients. J Infect Dis 2002;186:1297-306.
92. Maertens J, Verhaegen J, Lagrou K, Van Eldere J, Boogaerts M. Screening for circulating galactomannan as a noninvasive diagnostic tool for invasive aspergillosis in prolonged neutropenic patients and stem cell transplantation recipients: a prospective validation. Blood 2001;97:1604-10.
93. Segal BH, Almyroudis NG, Battiwalla M, et al. Prevention and early treatment of invasive fungal infection in patients with cancer and neutropenia and in stem cell transplant recipients in the era of newer broad-spectrum antifungal agents and diagnostic adjuncts. Clin Infect Dis 2007;44:402-9.
94. Cordonnier C, Pautas C, Maury S, et al. Empirical versus preemptive antifungal therapy for high-risk, febrile, neutropenic patients: a randomized, controlled trial. Clin Infect Dis 2009;48: 1042-51.
95. Hovette P, Soko TO, Raphenon G, Camara P, Burgel PR, Garraud O. Cryptococcal meningitis in AIDS patients: an emerging opportunistic infection in Senegal. Trans R Soc Trop Med Hyg 1999; 93:368.
96. Desmet P, Kayembe KD, De Vroey C. The value of cryptococcal serum antigen screening among HIV-positive/AIDS patients in Kinshasa, Zaire. AIDS 1989;3:77-8.
97. Lara-Peredo O, Cuevas LE, French N, Bailey JW, Smith DH. Cryptococcal infection in an HIV-positive Ugandan population. J Infect 2000;41:195.
98. Liechty CA, Solberg P, Were W, et al. Asymptomatic serum cryptococcal antigenemia and early mortality during antiretroviral therapy in rural Uganda. Trop Med Int Health 2007;12:929-35.
99. Tassie JM, Pepper L, Fogg C, et al. Systematic screening of cryptococcal antigenemia in HIV-positive adults in Uganda: JAIDS 2003;33:411-2.
100. Micol R, Lortholary O, Sar B, et al. Prevalence, determinants of positivity, and clinical utility of cryptococcal antigenemia in Cambodian HIV-infected patients. JAIDS 2007;45:555-9.

Part II
Systemic Antifungal Drugs

Amphotericin B

Stanley W. Chapman, John D. Cleary, and P. David Rogers

Amphotericin B (AmB) has been the cornerstone of antifungal therapy for almost 50 years. Discovered in the late 1950s, it was approved for human use as an antifungal agent in 1960. Initial formulations of AmB were plagued with impurities. Allergic responses, presumably secondary to these impurities, and endotoxin-like infusion-related reactions were common. Although improvements in purification and fermentation over the last 30 years have enhanced tolerability, infusion-related reactions and renal dysfunction are still commonplace with the use of the deoxycholate solubilized formulation. Formulations using a lipid carrier have significantly improved tolerability. Safety aside, AmB remains the most effective, broad-spectrum, fungicidal agent with the greatest experience for the treatment of systemic mycoses. Both intrinsic and acquired resistance are limited. The treatment failures seen with AmB are multifaceted. These can be attributed to delays in diagnosis of invasive mycoses, the immune compromised state of the patient being treated, the unique pharmacokinetic/pharmacodynamic properties of the different formulations, and dose limitations related to toxicity. In an effort to enhance antifungal efficacy and reduce toxicity, AmB has been combined with other antifungals and new nonlipid formulations are being evaluated.

Alternative formulations of AmB have been devised in an effort to improve the therapeutic index of this agent. A water-soluble methyl ester preparation showed promise; unfortunately, several patients developed leukoencephalopathy in clinical trials and the product was abandoned [1]. Nanoparticle science has led to investigation of novel orally absorbed AmB and intravenous products [2, 3]. In addition, highly purified AmB and biosynthesis of deoxyamphotericins have been reported in the literature [4]. Nebulized AmB lipid formuations are currently being investigated for prophylaxis in lung transplant receipients [5].

J.D. Cleary (✉)
Schools of Pharmacy & Medicine, University of Mississippi Medical Center, Jackson, MS, USA
e-mail: jcleary@medicine.umsmed.edu

This chapter discusses FDA-approved AmB deoxycholate (AmB-d) and the lipid preparations of amphotericin B separately. Where appropriate, we compare and contrast these different formulations with an emphasis on unique pharmacologic properties or clinically relevant differences in toxicity or outcome that favor one preparation over another.

Amphotericin B Deoxycholate

Chemistry

AmB is one of several polyene antifungals produced by the soil actinomycete *Streptomyces nodosus*. The AmB molecule is a heptaene macrolide consisting of seven conjugated double bonds within the main ring, a connecting mycosamine through a glycoside side chain, and a connecting free carboxyl group (Fig. 1). AmB is relatively insoluble in water and derives its name from its amphoteric property to form methanol soluble salts under both basic and acidic conditions [6]. AmB is available as an intravenous preparation formulated by combination with sodium deoxycholate (AmB-d), which results in formation of a micellar dispersion upon reconstitution in 5% dextrose in water [6].

Mechanisms of Action

The primary antifungal activity of AmB is mediated by its preferential binding to fungal cell membrane ergosterol. This interaction results in the formation of pores consisting of eight AmB molecules in the membrane, allowing leakage of cellular components, such as potassium, that ultimately leads to cell death [7]. Although AmB has a greater affinity for the fungal ergosterol, it still has some affinity for binding to the cholesterol of mammalian cell membranes. The latter probably plays an important role in its associated toxicity [8].

C.A. Kauffman et al. (eds.), *Essentials of Clinical Mycology*,
DOI 10.1007/978-1-4419-6640-7_3, © Springer Science+Business Media, LLC 2011

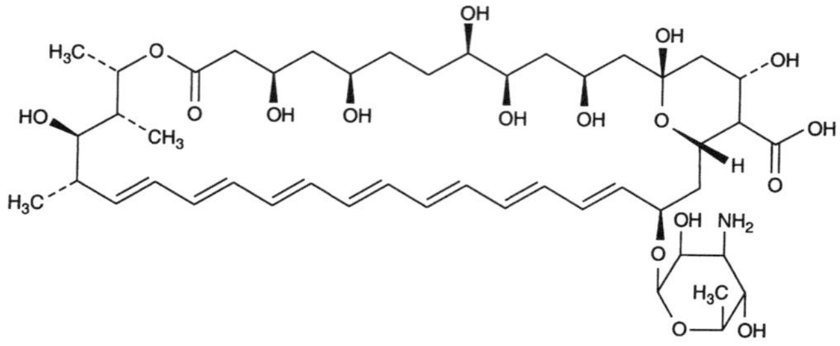

Fig. 1 Amphotericin B polyene structure. The molecular formula of the drug is $C_{47}H_{73}NO_{17}$; the molecular weight is 924.10

There is also evidence suggesting that cell death may be due in part to the oxidizing properties of the drug that results in the production of reactive oxygen species and lipid peroxidation of fungal cell membranes [7]. In support of oxidative cell injury, Sokol-Anderson and colleagues have shown that AmB-mediated lysis of *Candida albicans* protoplasts and whole cells is reduced, independent of potassium leakage, in the absence of oxygen and in the presence of exogenous catalase and superoxide dismutase [9]. The presence of seven conjugated double bonds in the chemical structure of AmB renders it prone to auto-oxidation [9], leading some investigators to speculate that AmB may also act as an antioxidant, although clinical data to support this hypothesis are lacking. Finally, AmB also has been shown to inhibit the respiration of actively metabolizing *Aspergillus fumigatus* [10].

AmB may indirectly modulate antifungal efficacy by its ability to alter immune function. The immunomodulatory effects of AmB have been found to be diverse, and research results are contradictory. The reported differences in AmB-induced immunomodulation may be the result of a number of factors, including antifungal concentration, the in vitro conditions, and the animal model used. AmB has been shown to act as an immunoadjuvant by stimulating cell proliferation and cell-mediated immunity in murine models [11]. AmB has also been shown to enhance the phagocytic, tumoricidal, and antibacterial activity of macrophages along with increasing colony-stimulating factor concentrations in mice [12]. AmB induces production of multiple inflammatory cytokines (i.e., IL-1β, TNF-α, and IL-1RA) and increases nitric oxide synthesis in vitro while increasing immune modulators (i.e., IL-12 and IFN-γ) in mice [13–15].

In contrast, AmB has been shown to inhibit chemotactic responsiveness, phagocytic capacity, and killing by human neutrophils [16]. Inhibition of both spontaneous and antigen-induced transformation, as well as antibody-dependent cellular toxicity of human lymphocytes, has been reported with AmB [17]. It has also been reported to diminish human peripheral blood mononuclear cell along with T-cell responses to phytohemagglutinin [18] and to impair NK cell activity [17].

Taken collectively, these data suggest that AmB exerts its direct antifungal activity through three mechanisms of action: pore formation, oxidative damage, and inhibition of metabolic activity. While the direct antifungal activity of AmB has been extensively validated, the in vivo role of its immunomodulatory properties has not been sufficiently defined.

Spectrum of Activity

AmB is active against most of the common yeasts, moulds, and dimorphic fungi causing human infection including: *Candida* species, *Cryptococcus neoformans*, *Blastomyces dermatitidis*, *Histoplasma capsulatum*, *Coccidioides* species, *Paracoccidioides brasiliensis*, *Sporothrix schenckii*, *Aspergillus* species, and the zygomycetes. This polyene also has some degree of activity against the protozoa *Leishmania brasiliensis*, *Trypanosoma* species, and *Naegleria fowleri* [6].

Relatively few organisms manifest intrinsic resistance to AmB. *Scedosporium apiospermum* (*Pseudallescheria boydii*), *Candida lusitaniae*, *Candida guilliermondii*, *Scopulariopsis* species, *Aspergillus terreus* and *Fusarium* species generally are considered intrinsically resistant to AmB [19]. Acquired resistance to AmB, whether through selective laboratory techniques or after clinical usage, appears to be uncommon. Recently, however, resistant isolates of *C. albicans*, *C. glabrata*, *C. tropicalis*, and *C. neoformans* have been isolated from patients with AIDS [20–23].

Studies of resistant clinical isolates of *C. albicans* and *C. neoformans* suggest that resistance occurs through alterations of the genes encoding $\alpha^{8,7}$-isomerase or $\alpha^{5,6}$-desaturase within the sterol biosynthesis pathway. These isolates accumulate alternative sterols, allowing the organism to evade the activity of AmB [21, 22, 24]. Others have suggested that resistance to AmB in yeasts may occur through increased catalase activity, impairing AmB-induced oxidative damage [24, 25].

Susceptibility Testing

The recent efforts of the Clinical Laboratory Standards Institute (CLSI) have been instrumental in the development of standardized methodology for antifungal susceptibility testing for yeasts and moulds [26–28]. Despite these improvements, the routine use of susceptibility testing of clinical isolates to AmB is not recommended. Susceptibility testing of clinical isolates may be helpful for patients who are failing therapy. For example, clinical failure using AmB-d to treat serious candidal and cryptococcal infections has been associated with minimum inhibitory concentrations (MICs) of >1.0 μg/mL [20, 29].

It should be noted, however, that clinical failure in AmB-treated patients is not necessarily indicative of fungal resistance, but is often related to the underlying immunodeficiency of the patient. Susceptibility testing may also be clinically useful in guiding treatment of rare pathogens for which resistance is likely or unpredictable. Interpretive break points that correlate in vitro activity with clinical outcomes are limited for moulds.

Pharmacology and Pharmacokinetics

Polyenes are poorly absorbed through mammalian membranes (less than 5%), hence the requirement of an intravenous formulation for the treatment of systemic mycoses. Following an intravenous infusion, AmB-d is bound primarily to lipoproteins, cholesterol, and erythrocytes. Peak serum concentrations of approximately 1–3 μg/mL are achieved during the first hour following a 4- to 6-h AmB-d infusion at a dose of 0.6 mg/kg. Serum concentrations rapidly fall to a prolonged plateau phase with measured concentrations of 0.2–0.5 μg/mL. Following an initial half-life of 24–48 h, there is a terminal elimination half-life of approximately 15 days. This terminal elimination phase most likely represents the slow release of AmB from the tissues (Table 1).

AmB-d is distributed to many tissues, including the lungs, spleen, liver, and kidneys [30]. The volume of distribution is 4 L/kg and appears to follow a three-compartment model of distribution. AmB-d, however, does not distribute into adipose tissue, supporting the premise that dosage should be based on lean body mass. Unfortunately, the measurement of lean body mass is not always practical. Hence dosing of AmB-d in obese patients should be based on calculated ideal body weight. AmB-d is bound extensively in tissues and can be detected in the liver, spleen, and kidney for months after treatment has been terminated [31]. Despite this extensive and prolonged tissue binding, the relationship of serum versus tissue concentration and clinical efficacy or toxicity has not been clearly established.

AmB-d concentrations in peritoneal, pleural, and synovial fluids are less than half of the simultaneous serum concentrations [32]. Concentrations in the vitreous body in noninflamed eyes are not measurable. Although clinical efficacy of AmB-d has been repeatedly documented for the treatment of central nervous system fungal infections, such as cryptococcal meningitis, cerebrospinal fluid levels are low, usually less than 5% even in the presence of inflamed meninges. This enhanced clinical efficacy may reflect higher levels of AmB-d in the meninges as compared to the cerebrospinal fluid, as has been documented in animal models of meningitis [6].

Despite almost 50 years of clinical experience, little is known about the metabolism of AmB-d. No metabolites have yet been identified. Less than 5% of the administered dose is excreted in the urine and bile. Serum concentrations, as such, are not changed and accumulation of AmB-d does not occur in patients with hepatic or renal failure. Likewise, hemodialysis or peritoneal dialysis does not influence serum concentrations [6, 33–35].

Several pharmacokinetic parameters of AmB-d are different in children than in adults [36, 37]. For instance, children have a smaller volume of distribution and a larger clearance compared to adults. When equivalent weight-based doses of AmB-d are administered, peak serum concentrations in children are approximately one-half of those obtained in adults. The increased clearance of AmB-d in children may, in part, explain the clinical finding that higher doses are better tolerated in children as compared to adults. Cerebrospinal fluid concentrations of AmB-d treated neonates are higher than those noted in adults.

Pharmacodynamics

Pharmacodynamics involves the integration of several pharmacologic measurements made in vitro (e.g., susceptibility studies, time-kill studies, dynamic models, viability, postantifungal effect [PAFE], etc.) and in vivo (drug concentrations, toxicity, efficacy, etc.). For antibacterial agents. several variables have been assigned quantitative limits that are predictive of therapeutic success and include the time that the serum drug concentration exceeds MIC [$T >$ MIC]; the ratio of maximum serum drug concentration to MIC [C_{max}:MIC]; and the ratio of the area under the concentration–time curve during a 24-h dosing period to MIC [AUC_{0-24}:MIC] [38]. These parameters have proven useful in classifying antibiotics as either concentration-dependent or time-dependent in their bactericidal activity and have also been instrumental in selecting the optimal antibacterial treatment regimens.

Pharmacodynamic parameters are less clearly defined for the antifungal drugs. AmB has traditionally been portrayed as a concentration-dependent antifungal agent. Concentration-dependence is characterized by a long PAFE and therapeutic success when the C_{max}:MIC ratio is high. Determination of C_{max}:MIC ratios of AmB and their relationship to clinical outcome in human infections is incomplete. Additional studies are required to evaluate the predictive value and clinical usefulness of these pharmacodynamic parameters in optimizing therapy of human infections.

Initial studies evaluating AmB pharmacodynamic models in vitro and in vivo have been contradictory. For example, the PAFE of AmB-d for *Candida* species was prolonged when studied in vivo. In a study of neutropenic mice infected with *Candida*, the antifungal effects of AmB-d were observed for 23–30 h [39]. In contrast, several in vitro studies have shown

Table 1 Characteristics of amphotericin B formulations

Category	Amphotericin B [AmB-d; Fungizone®]	Amphotericin B Lipid Complex [ABLC™; Abelcet]	Amphotericin B Colloidal Dispersion [ABCD; Amphotec®]	Liposomal Amphotericin B [L-amB; AmBisome®]
Primary Reference	[31, 92]	Package Insert	Package Insert	Package Insert
FDA Approved Indication	Life threatening fungal infections Visceral leishmaniasis	Refractory/ intolerant to AmB	Invasive aspergillosis in patients refractory/ intolerant to AmB	Empirical therapy in neutropenic fever Refractory/ intolerant to AmB Visceral leishmaniasis
Formulation	Micelle	Ribbons/Sheets	Lipid Disk	Unilamellar Vesicles
Sterol	None	None	Cholesterol Sulfate	Cholesterol Sulfate (5)+
Phospholipid	None	DMPC & DMPG(7:3)+	None	EPC & DSPG(10:4)+
Size (nm)	<10	1600-11000	122(±48)	80-120
Stability	1 week at 2-8°C or 24 hrs at 27°C	15 hrs at 2-8°C or 6 hrs at 27°C	24 hrs at 2-8°C	24 hours at 2-8°C
Dosage & Rate	0.3-1.0 mg/kg/d over 1-6hrs	5.0 mg/kg/d at 2.5 mg/kg/hr	3.0-6.0 mg/kg/day over 2 hrs	3.0-5.0 mg/kg/d over 2 hrs
Lethal Dose 50%	3.3 mg/kg	10-25 mg/kg	68 mg/kg	175 mg/kg
Pharmacokinetic Parameters				
Dose	0.5 mg/kg	5.0 mg/kg x 7d	5.0 mg/kg x 7d	5 mg/kg x 7d
Serum Concentrations				
Peak	1.2 ug/mL	1.7 ug/mL	3.1 ug/mL	83.0 ug/mL
Trough	0.5 ug/mL	0.7 ug/mL		4.0 ug/mL
Half-life (Beta)	91.1 hrs	173.4 hrs	28.5 hrs	6.8 hrs
Area Under the Curve	14 ug/mL·hr	17 ug/mL·hr	43.0 ug/mL·hr	555 ug/mL·hr
Volume of Distribution	3-5.0 L/kg	131.0 L/kg	4.3 L/kg	0.10 L/kg
Protein Binding (%)	<10%	ND	ND	ND
Adipose^	0.12(ND)	ND	ND	ND
Brain^	1.02(0.3)	1.6 (ND)	ND	0.56 (0.1)
CSF/Serum (%)	2-4 (40-90 in neonates)	9.7	ND	ND
Heart^	1.73(0.4)	5 (ND)	ND	4.3 (0.1)
Kidney^	10.4-18.9(0.8-1.5)	6.9(ND)	ND	22.8 (0.3)
Liver^	45.9-93.2(26.2-27.5)	196(ND)	ND	175.7 (18.3)
Lung^	5.29-12.9(3.1-3.2)	222(ND)	ND	16.8 (0.6)
Pancreas^	7.6(0.2)	ND	ND	ND
Spleen^	28.7-59.3(1-5.2)	290(ND)	ND	201.5
Clearance	38.0 mL/hr/kg	436.0 mL/hr/kg	0.117 mL/hr/kg	11.0 mL/hr/kg
Urine (%)	2-5% in 24 hours			
Feces (%)	ND			

EPC - Egg phosphatidylcholine; +- Molar ratio of each component, respectively.
DSPG - Distearolyphosphatidyglycerol; ^-Amount in tissue (ug/g) then in parenthesis (%) of total dose.
DMPC - Dimyristoyl phosphatidycholine
DMPG - Dimyristoyl phosphatidyglycerol
ND - Not Determined

a shorter duration of antifungal effect (0–10.6 h) depending on the MIC and the length of drug exposure [40, 41]. The longer PAFE noted in vivo might be due to the immunomodulatory properties and/or the slow release of AmB-d from tissue. Also confounding pharmacodynamic studies on drug concentration at the site of infection, the MIC of the organism, and the density of organisms at the site of infection impact the composite sum of these factors. Data on these important parameters affecting antifungal pharmacodynamics and clinical outcome have not been adequately defined.

A few studies have attempted to define clinically relevant pharmacodynamic parameters of AmB-d that affect clinical outcome. Drutz and colleagues reported improved clinical outcomes when AmB-d serum concentrations were maintained greater than twice the fungal MIC [42]. Animal models of infection have further demonstrated that high peaks relative to the MIC are correlated with improved survival and decreased fungal burden, as defined by CFU per gram of tissue in a variety of organs [39, 43]. When studied in a neutropenic mouse model of infection, a serum C_{max}: MIC ratio of 10:1 was associated with the greatest decrease in kidney fungal burden. Additionally, using nonlinear regression, a strong relationship was also found for the length of time the serum concentration remained above the MIC. This latter pharmacodynamic property is characteristic of a non-concentration-dependent, that is time-dependent antifungal agent [39, 43]. A reasonable hypothesis in reconciling these results involves the enhanced tissue binding of AmB-d. Specifically, the enhanced tissue storage and long elimination rates of AmB-d confound traditional dynamic estimates, and the release of free drug from tissue sites is difficult to discriminate from the residual effects of inhibitory antifungal concentrations.

Adverse Effects

The utility of AmB-d is hindered by significant toxicity. Although AmB-d has a greater affinity for ergosterol, its affinity for cholesterol in the mammalian cell membrane likely plays a role in its toxicity [8]. The resulting nonselective disruption of mammalian cells is believed to be the underlying cause of most of the adverse effects associated with this drug [44–46].

It is clinically useful to classify AmB-d-associated reactions as infusion-related, dose-related, or idiosyncratic reactions. Infusion-related reactions include a symptom complex of fever, chills, nausea, vomiting, headache, and hypotension. Infusion-related fever and chills are observed in over half the patients receiving AmB-d. Our clinical experience is that patients having severe infusion reactions often have undiagnosed adrenal insufficiency (especially those with disseminated histoplasmosis); consequently, adrenal function should be evaluated in these individuals. These infusion-related effects are believed to be due to the production of proinflammatory mediators by monocytes and macrophages in response to AmB-d [46–48]. AmB-d has been shown to up-regulate a number of genes encoding pro-inflammatory proteins such as IL-1α, IL-1β, TNFα, IL-8, MIP-1α, MIP-1β, and MCP-1 [14, 47, 48]. Production of these respective gene products, along with release of PGE_2 from endothelial cells, likely mediates the infusion-related toxicity. The patient-to-patient variability of AmB-d infusion-related toxicity may correlate with quantitative differences in cytokine production in vivo. Other adverse effects that may be related to the cytokine mechanism include thrombophlebitis, nausea, vomiting, headaches, myalgias, and arthralgias.

Less frequently, cardiac arrhythmias have been reported. Arrhythmias may occur when high concentrations are rapidly infused, especially in patients with heart disease, patients with renal failure, and those receiving an accidental drug overdosage [49]. Caution is also recommended for patients receiving the drug by a central venous catheter.

Dose-related reactions occur with longer courses of treatment and are related to total dose. AmB-induced nephrotoxicity includes decreased glomerular filtration, decreased renal blood flow, and renal tubular acidosis. Secondary consequences, such as hypokalemia and hypomagnesemia are common. Additionally, normochromic, normocytic anemia is frequently observed, likely in response to decreased erythropoietin production [50]. Calcium deposits have been found in the renal tubule lumen, tubule cells, and interstitium upon histopathologic examination of renal tissue specimens obtained from patients treated with AmB-d [51, 52]. Reversible renal impairment occurs within 2 weeks of therapy in more than 80% of AmB-d treated patients [53]. Onset of nephrotoxicity may occur before laboratory or clinical signs and symptoms are evident. With the onset of nephrotoxicity, the action taken ranges from AmB-d discontinuation or dosage reduction, stopping concurrent nephrotoxic drugs, changing to an alternate day infusion schedule, or pretreating patients with normal saline. There are no clinical trials that identify the optimal therapeutic option.

The mechanism of AmB-d-induced nephrotoxicity is multifaceted. Animal studies have demonstrated the vasoconstrictive properties of AmB-d, particularly with regard to the afferent arteriole [54]. Increased tubule permeability has also been demonstrated [55]. Other studies suggest that AmB-d inhibits sodium-potassium ATPases and affects proton exchange, which could contribute to renal tubular acidosis. Conversely, damage to the medullary thick ascending limb was ameliorated by ouabain in a rat kidney model, suggesting an alternative role for this pump in AmB-d-induced nephrotoxicity. Others have suggested a role for AmB-d-induced release of prostaglandins and leukotrienes as well as oxidative injury in this process [52].

The tubuloglomerular feedback mechanism normally involved in renal homeostasis also plays a prominent role in the pathogenesis of AmB-d-induced nephrotoxicity [56]. This feedback process is believed to be activated by transport of sodium chloride across the macula densa cells into the distal nephron, resulting in constriction of the afferent arteriole, possibly mediated by adenosine, and subsequent impairment of glomerular filtration [51]. Dehydration and sodium depletion accentuate this response and exacerbate AmB-d related renal failure. Sodium loading with intravenous administration of 500–1,000 mL of normal saline prior to initiation of AmB-d, when tolerated by the patient, is recommended in order to decrease the likelihood of renal toxicity [57].

Idiosyncratic reactions are rare, unpredictable, and include anaphylaxis, liver failure, hypertension, and respiratory failure.

Drug Interactions

Corticosteroids and nonsteroidal antiinflammatory drugs (NSAIDs) are the agents most frequently used to prevent infusion-related toxicities [58]. Controversy exists concerning the risk:benefit ratio of corticosteroids for prevention of infusion-related reactions. Clinical experience overwhelmingly supports the therapeutic benefit of administering hydrocortisone to patients suffering infusion-related reactions. However, circumstantial evidence suggests that administration of this immunosuppressant could be detrimental to the therapeutic success of AmB-d [59, 60]. Although further investigation of this therapeutic issue is required, it seems prudent to limit the dose and duration of corticosteroids by a therapeutic taper once infusion-related reactions are ameliorated. Likewise, routine use of NSAIDs for premedication should be avoided owing to their potential to enhance AmB-d related renal insufficiency. Intravenous meperidine has proven useful in abrogating infusion-related rigors [61].

Enhanced nephrotoxicity associated with AmB-d administration has been observed with cyclosporine or tacrolimus, diuretics, NSAIDs, pentamidine [62], and other nephrotoxic agents, such as aminoglycosides or radio-opaque dyes. Diligent monitoring of renal function is warranted in patients treated concurrently with these nephrotoxic agents.

A variety of other therapeutic agents may result in AmB-d associated adverse events that require diligent monitoring. Pulmonary leukostasis and respiratory failure associated with concomitant leukocyte transfusions or indium-labeled leukocyte scanning can be life-threatening [63, 64]. However, the incidence of this reaction has markedly decreased with less frequent use of leukocyte infusions. Skeletal muscle relaxants and neuromuscular blocking agents have been reported to enhance curariform effects related to hypokalemia. AmB-d-induced hypokalemia can also enhance the cardiac effects of digitalis glycosides. In these cases, patients suffered cardiac dysfunction that would be difficult to differentiate from the direct effects of AmB-d on the myocardial tissue [46]. Amiloride has been suggested for concomitant administration to decrease the hypokalemia in patients receiving digitalis glycosides. However, the effect is difficult to predict and requires further study. Cyclophosphamide and doxorubicin appear to penetrate cells more effectively when administered with AmB-d and this results in enhanced toxicity [65].

Drug interactions also encompass incompatibilities of pharmaceuticals in solution. AmB-d, and the AmB lipid formulations are incompatible in solutions with high saline content, including lactated Ringer's or normal (0.9%) sodium chloride. In addition, the infusion of AmB formulations concomitantly with other antiinfectives (amikacin, ampicillin, aztreonam, carbenicillin, clindamycin, cotrimoxazole, fluconazole, gentamicin, linezolid, nitrofurantoin, penicillin G, and piperacillin) may induce precipitation of either agent.

Combination Therapy

One approach to improving the activity and/or toxicity profile of AmB-d is its administration in combination with another antifungal or pharmacologic agent. Animal data and anecdotal experience suggest that colony-stimulating factors, rifampin, or tetracyclines may be effective adjuvants [66, 67]. A more traditional approach would be to use another antifungal in combination with AmB-d. While many in vitro studies of antifungal combinations with AmB-d have been performed, the results of these have not been consistent. For example, pretreatment with an imidazole prior to the administration of AmB-d has been reported to be antagonistic [68]. Other studies, however, have documented additive or synergistic activity when triazoles were combined with AmB-d [69]. Owing to these differing results, the routine use of an azole with AmB-d has not been recommended. However, one randomized blinded clinical trial showed no antagonism and actually improvement in clearing candidemia when fluconazole was combined with AmB-d [70]. In contrast to studies with the azoles, the clinical benefit of using AmB-d in combination with flucytosine for the treatment of cryptococcal meningitis has been clearly documented in both AIDS and non-AIDS patients [71–73]. In addition, smaller cohorts of patients with candidemia and other serious candidal infections have been treated successfully with AmB-d combined with flucytosine. Unfortunately, clinical studies evaluating the efficacy of other antifungal combinations are relatively few [74].

Administration

There are no well-controlled trials that delineate the optimal dosing regimen for AmB-d. The daily dose has traditionally ranged from 0.3 mg/kg up to 1.5 mg/kg depending on the specific mycosis and severity of disease. The duration of therapy for most systemic fungal infections has varied from 4 to 12 weeks, although courses of many months have been reported. The availability of the triazoles, however, has resulted in AmB-d being used for shorter treatment courses, usually until clinical improvement is evident, before step-down therapy is initiated with a less toxic azole.

Specific administration and dosing recommendations are as variable as the number of institutions that utilize this antifungal polyene. Selection of dosing regimens, including premedications, is often based on clinicians' concerns for toxicity, rather than achievement of efficacy. Dosing recommendations that have been approved by the Food and Drug Administration are outlined in Table 1. Specific recommendations for the administration of AmB-d, based on the authors' clinical experiences, are outlined in Table 2.

The practice of administering a 1 mg test dose of AmB prior to the initial dose, while recommended by the manufacturer, is controversial among clinicians [75]. The dose is administered as 1 mg AmB-d in 50 mL of D5W administered over 30–60 min. In most instances, however, the test dose is given as part of the initial dose, which in turn is then given in full if no adverse effects are observed. The test dose is designed to identify patients who will experience immediate type hypersensitivity reactions or pronounced infusion-related reactions. While evidence supporting this practice is sparse, many experienced clinicians continue to use this approach. Others argue that immediate type hypersensitivity would be observed with the test dose, whereas the AmB-d concentration provided by a test dose would be insufficient to produce the proinflammatory response responsible for fever and chills. Also of concern is the potential delay in therapy that may occur with the use of an initial test dose [75]. The authors do not recommend a test dose.

A second controversy centers around the length of infusions, e.g., short versus long. Several studies have explored toxicity and tolerability of standard infusion times (4–6 h) versus more rapid infusions of 2–4 h and even less than an hour [76]. The results of these studies indicate that rapid infusion times are equally well tolerated and have similar rates of adverse events as compared to infusions given over 4–6 h. Due to the risk of cardiac arrhythmias, rapid infusions should not be used in patients with renal failure, heart disease, and history of cardiac arrhythmias, and in those receiving AmB-d through a central venous catheter [77, 78]. A recent study reported less toxicity, including nephrotoxicity, in febrile neutropenic patients treated with continuous-infusion AmB-d when compared to

Table 2 Amphotericin B infusion protocol

Administration and dosing

Dilute amphotericin B in D5W, the final concentration not exceeding 0.1 mg/mL. Infuse the dose over 2–4 h. Record temperature, pulse rate, and blood pressure every 30 min for 4 h. If patient develops significant chills, fever, respiratory distress, or hypotension, administer adjunctive medication prior to next infusion. Consult an Infectious Diseases clinician for any questions concerning maximum daily dose, total dose, and duration of therapy

Adjunctive medications

1. Heparin 1,000 units may diminish thrombophlebitis for peripheral lines. Please observe the contraindications to the use of heparin; thrombocytopenia, increased risk of hemorrhage, and concomitant anticoagulation
2. Administration of 250 mL of normal saline prior to amphotericin B may help decrease renal dysfunction
3. Acetaminophen administered 30 min prior to amphotericin B infusion may ameliorate the fever
4. Hydrocortisone 0.7 mg/kg (Solu-Cortef) can be added to the amphotericin B infusion. Hydrocortisone is given to decrease the infusion-related reactions. This should only be used for significant fever (>2.0°F elevation from baseline), and chills with infusions and should be discontinued as soon as possible (3–5 days). It is not necessary to add hydrocortisone if the patient is receiving supraphysiologic doses of corticosteroids
5. Meperidine hydrochloride 25–50 mg parenterally in adults may be utilized to prevent or ameliorate chills

Monitoring

1. At least twice weekly for the first 4 weeks, then weekly: hematocrit, reticulocyte count, magnesium, potassium, BUN, creatinine, bicarbonate, urinalysis. The GFR may fall 40% before stabilizing in these patients. Discontinue for 2–5 days if renal function continues to deteriorate and reinstate after improvement. Hematocrit frequently falls from 22% to 35% of baseline
2. Monitor closely for hypokalemia and hypomagnesemia

Caveats and patients requiring closer monitoring

1. Electrolytes: Addition of an electrolyte to the amphotericin B solution causes the colloid to aggregate and probably gives a suboptimal therapeutic effect. This includes IV piggyback medications containing electrolytes
2. Filtering: The colloidal solution is partially retained by 0.22-μm pore membrane filter, so do not use filters
3. The infusion bottle need not be light-shielded
4. Patients with adrenal insufficiency tolerate infusions poorly. Treatment with corticosteroids improves patient tolerance
5. Patients should not receive granulocyte transfusions
6. Patients with anuria or previous cardiac history may have an increased risk of arrhythmias and slower infusion rates are recommended

patients treated with 4-h infusions [79]. However, clinical experience with continuous infusion of AmB-d is limited, and there is concern about achieving adequate serum concentrations for maximum efficacy of AmB. Until safety and efficacy are better documented, continuous infusion cannot be recommended at this time.

Other routes of administration for AmB-d are used when therapeutic goals are not or cannot be achieved with intravenous dosing [6, 69]. Topical preparations (3% lotion, creams, or ointments, 10-mg lozenges or oral suspension, 100 mg/mL) may be compounded as needed for the treatment of superficial or cutaneous yeast infections. Intrathecal or intraventricular routes have been used in refractory cases of fungal meningitis, most frequently coccidioidal meningitis [6, 69, 80]. Intrathecal administration is problematic due to the poor distribution and the development of arachnoiditis at the injection site. Intraventricular administration is preferred. Long-term administration should be performed using a subcutaneous Ommaya or Rickham reservoir. AmB-d should be mixed with sterile water to a final concentration of 250 μg/mL. Initial dosing (10–25 μg) can be escalated slowly up to a dose of 250 μg/day to as high as 500 μg/day day, depending on the mycosis being treated and patient's tolerance of this therapy. This route of administration is often limited by local reactions (radicular pain, headache, vomiting, and arachnoiditis). More severe neurologic complications include ventricular hemorrhage and bacterial superinfection [80].

Ocular administration of AmB-d is frequently used for the treatment of fungal eye infections [6, 81]. Topical ophthalmic application (0.25–1.5% solution) or subconjunctival injection (100–200 μg/0.5 mL) is appropriate for most superficial infections. However, little medication penetrates into the vitreous body, and intravitreal injection of 5–10 μg/0.1 mL is often used for vitritis [81].

The therapeutic benefit and optimal dose of nonparenteral routes of administration are not well established, and local inflammatory responses specific to the sites of administration are common and are frequently dose limiting [6, 69]. Intraperitoneal administration for the treatment of peritoneal dialysis-associated *Candida* infections can be achieved by administering AmB-d within the dialysate or intraperitoneally, but this is extremely irritating and is no longer recommended [82]. Intraarticular doses (5–15 mg) administered for fungal arthritis are rarely indicated. Bladder instillation/irrigation with an AmB-d solution (50 mg/L) by continuous infusion through a triple-lumen catheter for 5 days has been used for candidal cystitis and candiduria [83] AmB-d (10 mg) in 5 ml has been administered twice a day via nebulization for prevention of pulmonary aspergillosis in neutropenic patients [84, 85]. Specific adverse reactions with aerosolized AmB-d include dyguesia, gastrointestinal distress, dyspnea, and cough. Less frequently, intracavitary irrigation has been used for treatment of pulmonary aspergilloma.

Use in Pregnancy

AmB is the antifungal agent with which there has been the most experience in pregnancy [86, 87]. Both the deoxycholate and lipid-based formulations are assigned to risk category B by their manufacturers. While the pharmacokinetics of AmB in pregnancy have not been studied, the drug appears to cross the placenta and enter the fetal circulation [85]. Among case reports of AmB use in pregnancy, azotemia was the most common maternal adverse drug reaction reported, followed by anemia, hypokalemia, acute nephrotoxicity, fever, chills, headache, nausea, and vomiting. Individual cases of possible fetal toxicity include transient acidosis with azotemia, anemia, transient maculopapular rash, and respiratory failure requiring mechanical ventilation. Only a single case of congenital malformation (microcephaly with a pilonidal dimple) has been associated with AmB-d [86]. To date there have been no reports of animal teratogenesis attributed to AmB [86, 87].

Lipid Preparations of Amphotericin B

Three lipid-based products are currently available in the United States: AmB colloidal dispersion (ABCD), liposomal AmB (L-AmB), and AmB lipid complex (ABLC) (Fig. 2). In addition to these commercial formulations, lipid-based preparations have been admixed by individual institutions by combining AmB deoxycholate and 20% lipid emulsion [88, 89]. While AmB lipid emulsion is attractive from the standpoint of cost, several concerns have been raised, encompassing the stability of the emulsion, the need for filtration, and the possibility of fat overload syndrome. One pharmaceutical company pursued development of this formulation for several years, but a stable suspension was not achieved. Administration of this formulation is, therefore, not recommended [90].

Chemistry

The commercial lipid formulations are distinct as regards their phospholipid content, particle size and shape, electrostatic charge, and bilayer rigidity [91]. Liposomal AmB is formulated as a unilamellar spherical vesicle with a single lipid bilayer comprised of hydrogenated phosphatidylcholine, cholesterol, and distearoyl phosphatidylglycerol in a 2:1:0.8 ratio. Amphotericin is located on the inside and outside of the vesicle. L-AmB has the smallest particle size. ABCD was developed by complexing AmB with cholesteryl sulfate in a 1:1 molar ratio. These complexes form tetramers

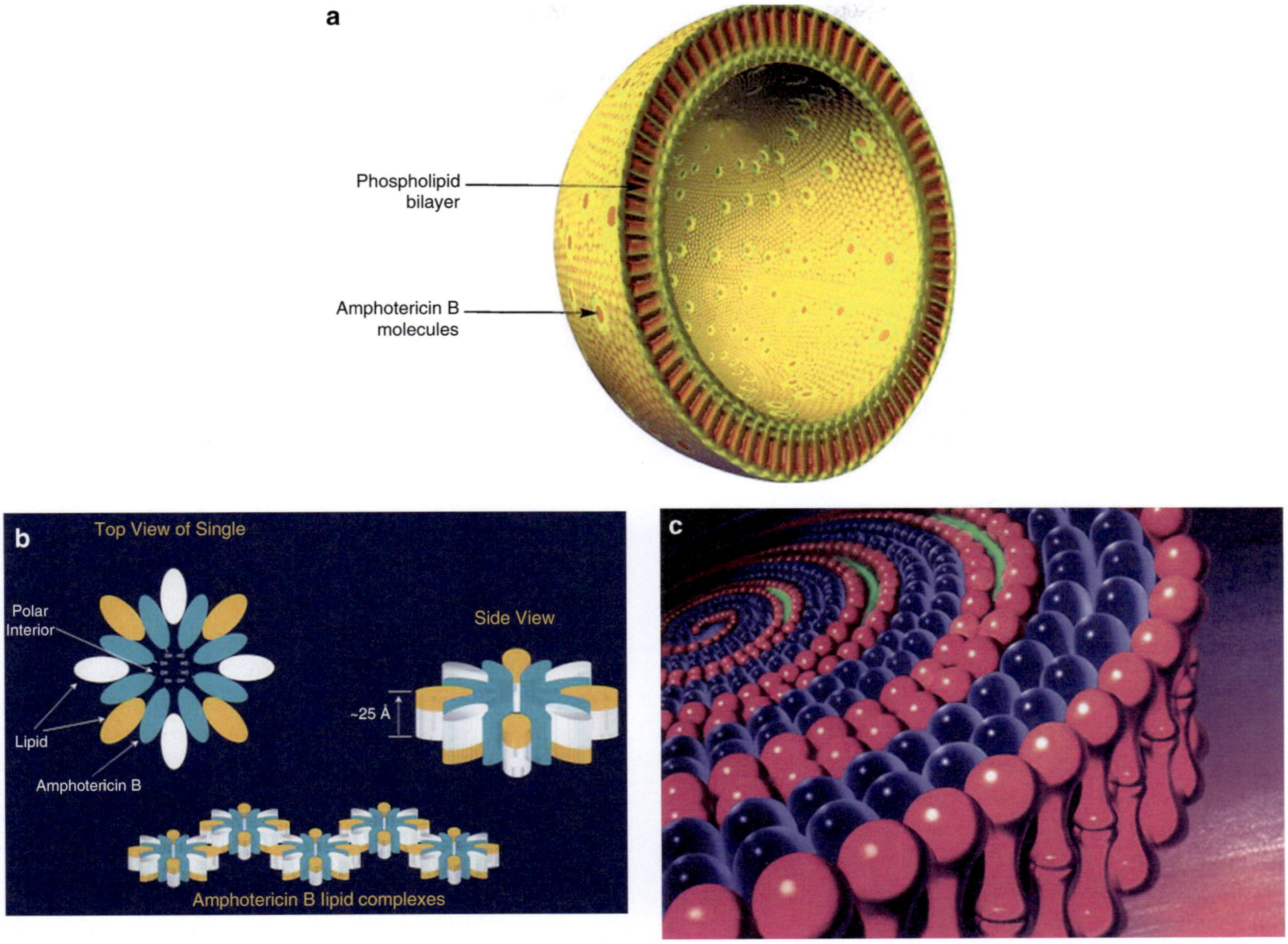

Fig. 2 Amphotericin B lipid-based formulations represented in artistic drawings: (**a**) liposomal amphotericin B; (**b**) amphotericin B lipid complex; (**c**) amphotericin B colloidal dispersion

that have a hydrophobic and a hydrophilic portion. The tetramers aggregate to form disk-like structures that are larger in size than L-AmB. ABLC consists of nonliposomal AmB-complexed ribbon structures and was originally derived from multilaminar liposomes prepared by mixing two phospholipids, dimyristoyl phosphatidylcholine (DMPC) and dimyristoyl phosphatidylglycerol (DMPG) in a 7:3 molar ratio. ABLC is much larger than the other two formulations [91–93] (Table 1).

Proposed Mechanisms for Enhanced Therapeutic Index

Although the lipid formulations have been shown to have an improved therapeutic index as compared to AmB-d, the mechanism(s) by which this occurs has not been adequately defined. Several mechanisms have been proposed. The unifying concept in all of these proposals involves the ability of lipid formulations to prevent binding to the kidney and the selective distribution of lipid-bound AmB to other tissues [91].

The first mechanism involves the rapid endocytic uptake of lipid-associated AmB by macrophages in tissues, often at the sites of infection. Following this targeted delivery, AmB is then slowly released into the tissues and the circulation. In addition to this selective tissue targeting, macrophage uptake of AmB also limits the amount of free drug, and presumably also LDL-bound drug, in the circulation capable of binding to human cells. The second mechanism involves the selective transfer of AmB from the lipid carrier to the fungal cell membrane. In this instance, AmB has a stronger affinity for the lipid carrier than for the cholesterol in mammalian cells. On the other hand, the affinity of AmB for ergosterol in the fungal cell is stronger than its affinity for either the lipid carrier or cholesterol. A third mechanism proposes that the lipid-based formulations are less nephrotoxic by limiting the amount of free drug in the blood and by preventing AmB binding to circulating LDL. Free AmB and LDL-bound AmB are considered to be more nephrotoxic than either HDL or other lipid-bound AmB. The fourth mechanism proposes that the lipid-based formulations elicit reduced cytokines, such as TNF-α or IL-1 from human cells as compared with AmB-d. These proinflammatory cytokines are putative mediators for infusion-related reactions and nephrotoxicity. This fourth hypothesis is supported primarily by in vitro data. The final purported mechanism involves the action of extracellular phospholipases produced by yeasts and moulds in releasing the lipid-bound AmB at the site of infection. As such, more AmB is released in the infected tissues. The phospholipid carrier of ABLC is especially susceptible to these fungal phospholipases.

Therapeutic Indications

In general, all three lipid formulations are indicated for the treatment of systemic fungal infection in patients refractory to or intolerant of therapy with AmB-d (Table 1) [91, 93]. L-AmB has also been approved for the empiric therapy of presumed fungal infection in febrile neutropenic patients [94]. In routine clinical practice, however, lipid formulations are frequently used as primary therapy for patients with baseline renal insufficiency and in patients at high risk for renal failure, including transplant recipients and patients receiving concurrent treatment with other nephrotoxic agents. Lipid preparations, however, should not be used as primary therapy for dialysis-dependent patients unless they fail therapy with AmB-d. Some authors consider the lipid formulations, due to their high concentrations in the liver and spleen, to be ideal for the treatment of patients with chronic disseminated candidiasis [95]. Finally, many infectious disease physicians consider lipid formulations of AmB to be superior to AmB-d for the treatment of patients with aggressive mould infections, such as invasive aspergillosis and zygomycosis. The data supporting this use are anecdotal, and comparative trials documenting the superiority of lipid formulations for these infections are lacking at present.

Pharmacology and Pharmacokinetics

The lipid agents' biochemical/biophysical properties have a profound effect on the pharmacology of these lipid formulations (Table 1). For example, L-AmB is not as readily taken up by macrophages, and L-AmB achieves higher serum concentrations and a greater area under the curve (AUC) in blood compared to AmB-d or the other lipid preparations. On the other hand, the larger lipid formulation, ABLC, is more readily taken up by the tissues and has the greatest volume of distribution. Comparative data on the pharmacokinetic parameters of the lipid formulations, either compared to each other or to AmB-d, are limited. However, profound differences in some of the parameters have been documented and have led to unique therapeutic options (Table 1) [92, 96]. In amimals, ABLC lung penetration far exceeds (70- to 375-fold) the penetration by other formulations [97]. This tissue saturation also results in increased drug clearance from the serum. Whether any of these pharmacologic differences significantly affect clinical outcome or toxicity has not been studied adequately.

Pharmacodynamics

Owing to a variety of confounding variables, the pharmacodynamic information obtained with AmB-d cannot be directly extrapolated to the lipid formulations. In general, studies utilizing AmB lipid formulations have revealed a poor correlation between pharmacodynamic parameters and outcome [43]. Measurement of free AmB has been hypothesized to potentially resolve these discrepancies. However, the ability to accurately measure or predict free AmB is difficult [95].

As mentioned earlier, L-AmB achieves serum concentrations many-fold higher than the other lipid formulations of AmB, leading to a tremendously increased AUC versus time curve that in turn impacts all pharmacodynamic calculations. Using traditional calculations, L-AmB would not be predicted to be an effective therapy for central nervous system infections. To the contrary, L-AmB proved effective in animal studies [43] and a clinical trial of patients with AIDS-associated cryptococcal meningitis [98]. Although cerebrospinal fluid levels were low or undetectable, brain tissue concentrations exceeded expectations and, in the animal studies, were higher than those found with either AmB-d or the other lipid formulations. Brain tissue concentrations in patients receiving L-AmB were not as high as those documented in the animal studies [43, 98].

After 7 days of parenteral treatment of rabbits, mean AmB concentrations in inflamed eyes were significantly higher in the aqueous humor for L-AmB (0.73 μg/mL) compared with ABLC (0.03 μg/mL) and AmB-d (0.13 μg/mL). Levels in the vitreous body were also higher for L-AmB (0.47 μg/mL) than for ABLC (0.27 μg/mL) and AmB-d (0.16 μg/mL). Little, if any AmB-d can be detected in noninflamed eyes [99, 100].

Disproportionate distribution into the reticuloendothelial system has been observed for two lipid formulations, ABLC and L-AmB. As a result, very high tissue concentrations of these agents are detected in the liver and spleen relative to serum. These high tissue concentrations have been hypothesized to be a therapeutic advantage for these agents in treating patients with chronic disseminated candidiasis [95]. In support of this theory, clearance of *C. albicans* from the liver was superior in mice treated with L-AmB (1.5 mg/kg) compared to mice treated with AmB-d at equal doses [101]. In contrast, clearance of yeasts from lung was not enhanced in L-AmB-treated mice, but high concentrations of ABLC were detected in lung tissue, suggesting that this fomulation may be optimal for the treatment of pulmonary mycoses.

Adverse Events

All three lipid-based preparations currently available in the United States exhibit less nephrotoxicity than AmB-d [91, 102]. However, infusion-related toxicities similar to AmB-d are still observed [103, 104]. Several studies have demonstrated significantly fewer infusion-related adverse events associated with L-AmB when compared with AmB-d or with ABLC [91, 94, 102].

Although uncommon, acute respiratory events have been associated with administration of AmB and are typically characterized by tachypnea, dyspnea, and wheezing. Recently, there have also been reports of chest discomfort and altered pulmonary function associated with the lipid-based preparations of AmB [105, 106]. In fact, a triad of symptoms including: (1) chest pain, dyspnea, and hypoxia; (2) severe abdominal, flank, and leg pain; and (3) flushing and urticaria, has been reported with L-AmB [107]. These reactions appear in approximately 20% of patients, start within 5 min of infusion, and respond to antihistamines (diphenydramine).

The mechanisms causing these "uncommon" reactions are unclear, but may be related to the ability of AmB to elicit chemokine production from monocytes [14, 48]. The ability of IL-8 to recruit neutrophils could then mediate the pulmonary toxicity occasionally observed during administration of this agent. The lipid formulations of AmB deliver higher amounts of drug to the pulmonary tissue [105]. Thus, it is conceivable that enhanced pulmonary neutrophil recruitment in response to elevated local concentrations of IL-8 could lead to pulmonary leukostasis and thereby explain in part the pulmonary toxicity associated with AmB preparations. Indeed, studies in animal models have demonstrated that AmB pulmonary toxicity involves neutrophil recruitment to the lungs [108, 109]. Another possibility is that the lipid component of these preparations may itself contribute to these physiologic effects. Irrespective of the cause of the pulmonary toxicity, it seems prudent to administer the initial dose of any of the AmB lipid formulations under close observation and to reduce the rate of infusion in instances in which these effects are observed [105, 106].

Other adverse events reported with the lipid preparations include headache, hypotension, hypertension, diarrhea, nausea, vomiting, and rashes. Laboratory abnormalities reported include hypokalemia, hypomagnesemia, hypocalcemia, elevated liver function tests, and thrombocytopenia [91]. Regarding frequency of infusion-related adverse events of available AmB preparations, data suggest the following rank order by greatest to least frequency: AmB-d > ABCD > ABLC > L-AmB.

Comparative Trials

Comparative trials between lipid AmB preparations and AmB-d are enlightening. Empiric therapy for febrile neutropenic patients has received the most attention. In two different studies, ABCD (4 mg/kg/day) and L-AmB (3 mg/kg/day) were each compared to standard therapy with AmB-d (0.6–0.8 mg/kg/day) [94, 104]. In both studies, patients treated with the lipid preparations had a more rapid defervescence and lower death rate, although in neither study were these clinical differences statistically significant. In contrast, patients receiving either of the lipid preparations had statistically superior outcomes compared to patients treated with AmB-d for (1) the time to onset and rates of renal dysfunction; (2) rates of infusion-related reactions; and (3) prevention of breakthrough invasive fungal infections [94, 104]. Another study of therapy for febrile neutropenic patients compared two different doses of L-AmB (3 mg/kg/day and 5 mg/kg/day) to ABLC (5 mg/kg/day). Clinical outcomes were equivalent for all patient groups, except that the rates of renal dysfunction were significantly less for both doses of L-AmB compared to the ABLC formulation [102].

Comparative studies of the different AmB formulations in the treatment of documented infections have been primarily nonblinded and limited in number. ABCD (0.5–8 mg/kg/day), L-AmB (4 mg/kg/day) and ABLC (1.2–5 mg/kg/day) have been compared with AmB-d (0.1–1.5 mg/kg/day) for the treatment of invasive aspergillosis [103, 110] and cryptococcal meningitis [98, 111]. Patients with proven or probable aspergillosis who received ABCD experienced higher response rates (50%) compared to a historical control group treated with AmB-d [103]. However, in a randomized, double-blind trial, ABCD showed equal but no better efficacy than AmB-d as therapy for invasive aspergillosis (52% vs 51%) [110]. In two open label, randomized trials comparing a lipid formulation for the treatment of AIDS-associated cryptococcal meningitis, the clinical and microbiologic responses rates favored the lipid preparations [98, 111]. Of note, in these studies, significantly lower rates of nephrotoxicity were observed in patients treated with the lipid formulations.

A randomized, blinded treatment trial compared AmB-d, 0.7 mg/kg daily, with L-AmB, 3 mg/kg daily, for AIDS patients who had moderately severe to severe disseminated histoplasmosis. L-AmB was found to be superior in regard to efficacy and time to defervescence and there were fewer adverse reactions in the L-AmB arm [112].

Administration and Dosage

The approved daily dose and rate of administration are different for each lipid formulation. Other than for ABCD, the maximal daily dose that can be safely administered in humans has not been adequately defined. More interestingly, the equivalent doses of the individual lipid formulations that compare to the recommended dose of AmB-d for a particular fungal infection has not been established.

The recommended initial dose of L-AmB is 3 mg/kg/day for empiric therapy and 3–5 mg/kg/day for documented systemic fungal infections. The drug is usually infused over 2 h, but the infusion time can be decreased to 1 h if tolerated. The currently approved daily dose of ABLC is 5 mg/kg, and this is infused at a rate of 2.5 mg/kg/h. Daily doses of L-AmB and ABLC have been titrated considerably higher than the recommended daily doses and appear to be well tolerated in selected patients with refractory diseases. Treatment with ABCD should be initiated with a daily dose of 3–4 mg/kg. The dose can then be escalated to 6 mg/kg/day based on patient tolerance and clinical response. The recommended maximal daily dose is 7.5 mg/kg. Infusion-related toxicities with ABCD become more severe with doses of 8 mg/kg or greater.

Costs

A major consideration regarding the lipid-based formulations of AmB is their high cost in comparison to AmB-d. Data indicate that the lipid formulations range from 10- to 50-fold higher in acquisition cost per dose [113]. These agents are less nephrotoxic than AmB-d, and their overall therapeutic:toxic ratio is clearly improved over that of the parent drug. However, superiority in clinical efficacy has been definitively established in head-to-head comparative trials only in the case of disseminated histoplasmosis. Consequently, well-done pharmacoeconomic studies are needed to justify the higher cost of the lipid formulations.

References

1. Schmitt HJ. New methods of delivery of amphotericin B. Clin Infect Dis. 1993;17 Suppl 2:S501–6.
2. Wasan EK, Bartlett K, Gershkovich P, et al. Development and characterization of oral lipid-based amphotericin B formulations with enhanced drug solubility, stability and antifungal activity in rats infected with *Aspergillus fumigatus* or *Candida albicans*. Int J Pharm. 2009;372:76–84.
3. Fukui H, Koike T, Saheki A, Sonoke S, Tomii Y, Seki J. Evaluation of the efficacy and toxicity of amphotericin B incorporated in lipid nano-sphere (LNS). Int J Pharm. 2003;263:51–60.
4. Cleary JD, Chapman SW, Swiatlo E, Kramer R. High purity amphotericin B. J Antimicrob Chemother. 2007;60(6):1331–40.
5. Monforte V, Ussetti P, López R, et al. Nebulized liposomal amphotericin B prophylaxis for *Aspergillus* infection in lung transplantation: pharmacokinetics and safety. J Heart Lung Transpl. 2009;28:170–5.
6. Gallis HA, Drew RH, Pickard WW. Amphotericin B: 30 years of clinical experience. Rev Infect Dis. 1990;12:308–29.
7. Brajtburg J, Powderly WG, Kobayashi GS, Medoff G. Amphotericin B: current understanding of mechanisms of action. Antimicrob Agents Chemother. 1990;34:183–8.
8. Abu-Salah KM. Amphotericin B: An update. Br J Biomed Sci. 1996;53:122–33.
9. Sokol-Anderson ML, Brajtburg J, Medoff G. Amphotericin B-induced oxidative damage and killing of *Candida albicans*. J Infect Dis. 1986;154:76–83.
10. Sandhu DK. Effect of amphotericin B on the metabolism of *Aspergillus fumigatus*. Mycopathologia. 1979;68:23–9.
11. Bistoni F, Vecchiarelli A, Mazzolla R, Puccetti P, Marconi P, Garaci E. Immunoadjuvant activity of amphotericin B as displayed in mice infected with *Candida albicans*. Antimicrob Agents Chemother. 1985;27:625–31.
12. Lin H, Medoff G, Kobayashi GS. Effects of amphotericin B on macrophages and their precursor cells. Antimicrob Agents Chemother. 1977;11:154–60.
13. Mozaffarian N, Berman JW, Casadevall A. Enhancement of nitric oxide synthesis by macrophages represents an additional mechanism of action for amphotericin B. Antimicrob Agents Chemother. 1997;41:1825–9.
14. Rogers PD, Jenkins JK, Chapman SW, Ndebele K, Chapman BA, Cleary JD. Amphotericin B activation of human genes encoding for cytokines. J Infect Dis. 1998;178:1726–33.
15. Cenci E, Mencacci A, Del Sero G, Bistoni F, Romani L. Induction of protective Th1 responses to *Candida albicans* by antifungal therapy alone or in combination with an interleukin-4 antagonist. J Infect Dis. 1997;176:217–26.
16. Marmer DJ, Fields BT, France GL, Steele RW. Ketoconazole, amphotericin B, and amphotericin B methyl ester: Comparative in vitro and in vivo toxicological effects on neutrophil function. Antimicrob Agents Chemother. 1981;20:660–5.
17. Nair MPN, Schwartz SA. Immunomodulatory effects of amphotericin-B on cellular cytotoxicity of normal human lymphocytes. Cell Immunol. 1982;70:287–300.
18. Stewart SJ, Spagnuolo PJ, Ellner JJ. Generation of suppressor T lymphocytes and monocytes by amphotericin B. J Immunol. 1981;127:135–9.
19. Speeleveld E, Gordts B, Van Landuyt HW, De Vroey C, Raes-Wuytack C. Susceptibility of clinical isolates of *Fusarium* to antifungal drugs. Mycoses. 1996;39:37–40.
20. Powderly WG, Keath EJ, Sokol-Anderson M, Robinson K, Kitzd, Little JR. Amphotericin B resistant *Cryptococcus neoformans* in a patient with AIDS. Infect Dis Clin Pract. 1992;1:314–6.

21. Le TP, Tuazoncu CU, Levine M, Borum M, Rollhauser C. Resistance to fluconazole and amphotericin B in patients with AIDS who are being treated for candidal esophagitis. Clin Infect Dis. 1996;23:649–50.
22. Kelly SL, Lamb DC, Kelly DE, et al. Resistance to fluconazole and cross resistance to amphotericin B in *Candida albicans* from AIDS patients caused by defective sterol delta 5, 6-desaturation. FEBS Lett. 1997;400:80–2.
23. Lass-Flörl C. The changing face of epidemiology of invasive fungal disease in Europe. Mycoses. 2009;52:197–205.
24. Georgopapadakou NH, Walsh TJ. Antifungal agents: chemotherapeutic targets and immunologic stratagies. Antimicrob Agents Chemother. 1996;40:279–91.
25. Ghannoum MA, Rice LB. Antifungal agents: mode of action, mechanisms of resistance, and correlation of these mechanisms with bacterial resistance. Clin Microbiol Rev. 1999;12:501–17.
26. Park BJ, Arthington-Skaggs BA, Hajjeh RA, et al. Evaluation of amphotericin B interpretive breakpoints for *Candida* bloodstream isolates by correlation with therapeutic outcome. Antimicrob Agents Chemother. 2006;50:1287–92.
27. Clinical Laboratory Standards Institute. Reference method for broth dilution antifungal susceptibility testing of yeasts; approved standard-third edition. Document M27-A3. Wayne: Clinical and Laboratory Standards Institute, 2008
28. Clinical Laboratory Standards Institute. Reference method for broth dilution antifungal susceptibility testing of filamentous fungi. Approved standard CLSI document M38-A. Wayne: Clinical Laboratory Standards Institute, 2001.
29. Larsen RA, Bauer M, Brouwer AE, et al. In vitro-clinical correlations for amphotericin B susceptibility in AIDS-associated cryptococcal meningitis. Antimicrob Agents Chemother. 2007;51:343–5.
30. Collette N, van der Auwera P, Lopez AP, Heymans C, Meunier F. Tissue concentrations and bioactivity of amphotericin B in cancer patients treated with amphotericin B-deoxycholate. Antimicrob Agents Chemother. 1989;33:362–8.
31. Christiansen KJ, Bernard EM, Gold JWM, Armstrong D. Distribution and activity of amphotericin B in humans. J Infect Dis. 1985;152:1037–43.
32. van der Voort PH, Boerma EC, Yska JP. Serum and intraperitoneal levels of amphotericin B and flucytosine during intravenous treatment of criticly ill patients with *Candida* peritonitis. J Antimicrob Chemother. 2007;59:952–6.
33. Atkinson Jr AJ, Bennett JE. Amphotericin B pharmacokinetics in humans. Antimicrob Agents Chemother. 1978;13:271–6.
34. Daneshmend TK, Warnock DW. Clinical pharmacokinetics of systemic antifungal drugs. Clin Pharmacokinet. 1983;8:17–42.
35. Gussak HM, Rahman S, Bastani B. Administration and clearance of amphotericin B during high-efficiency or high-efficiency/high-flux dialysis. Am J Kidney Dis. 2001;37:E45.
36. Starke JR, Mason Jr EO, Kramer WG, Kaplan SL. Pharmacokinetics of amphotericin B in infants and children. J Infect Dis. 1987;155:766–74.
37. Benson JM, Nahata MC. Pharmacokinetics of amphotericin B in children. Antimicrob Agents Chemother. 1989;33:1989–93.
38. Gunderson BW, Ross GH, Ibrahim KH, Rotschafer JC. What do we really know about antibiotic pharmacodynamics? Pharmacotherapy. 2001;21:302S–18.
39. Andes D, Stamsted T, Conklin R. Pharmacodynamics of amphotericin B in a neutropenic-mouse disseminated-candidiasis model. Antimicrob Agents Chemother. 2001;45(3):922–6.
40. Turnidge JD, Gudmondsson S, Vogelman B, Craig WA. The post-antibiotic effect of antifungal agents against common pathogenic yeast. J Antimicrob Chemother. 1994;34:83–92.
41. Ernst E, Klepser ME, Pfaller MA. Post-antifungal effects of echinocandin, azole, and polyene antifungal agents against *Candida albicans* and *Cryptococcus neoformans*. Antimicrob Agents Chemother. 2000;44:1108–11.
42. Drutz DJ, Spickard A, Rogers DE, Koenig MG. Treatment of disseminated mycotic infections. A new approach to amphotericin B therapy. Am J Med. 1968;5:405–18.
43. Groll AH, Giri N, Petraitis V, et al. Comparative efficacy and distribution of lipid formulations of amphotericin B in experimental *Candida albicans* infection of the central nervous system. J Infect Dis. 2000;182:274–82.
44. Andreoli TE. On the anatomy of amphotericin B-cholesterol pores in lipid bilayer membranes. Kidney Int. 1973;4:337–45.
45. Hsuchen CC, Feingold DS. Selective membrane toxicity of the polyene antibiotics: studies on natural membranes. Antimicrob Agents Chemother. 1973;4:316–9.
46. Cleary JD, Chapman SW, Nolan RL. Pharmacologic modulation of interleukin-1 expression by amphotericin B-stimulated human mononuclear cells. Antimicrob Agents Chemother. 1992;36:977–81.
47. Rogers PD, Stiles JK, Chapman SW, Cleary JD. Amphotericin B induces expression of genes encoding chemokines and cell adhesion molecules in the human monocytic cell line THP-1. J Infect Dis. 2000;182:1280–3.
48. Rogers PD, Perason MM, Cleary JD, Chapman SW, Sullivan DC. Differential expression of genes encoding for immunodulatory proteins in response to amphotericin B in the human monocytic cell line THP-1 identified by cDNA array analysis. J Antimicrob Chemother. 2002;50:811–7.
49. Cleary JD, Hayman J, Sherwood J, Lasala GP, Piazza-Hepp T. Amphotericin B overdose in pediatric patients with associated cardiac arrest. Ann Pharmacother. 1993;27:715–8.
50. Lin AC, Goldwasser E, Bernard EM, Chapman SW. Amphotericin B blunts erythropoietin response to anemia. J Infect Dis. 1990;161:348–51.
51. Sabra R, Branch RA. Amphotericin B nephrotoxicity. Drug Saf. 1990;5:94–108.
52. Carlson MA, Condon RE. Nephrotoxicity of amphotericin B. J Am Coll Surg. 1994;179:361–81.
53. Butler WT, Bennett JE, Alling DW, Wertlake PT, Utz JP, Hill G. Nephrotoxicity of amphotericin B. Early and late effects in 81 patients. Ann Intern Med. 1964;61:175–87.
54. Sawaya BP, Weihprech TH, Campbell WR, et al. Direct basal vasoconstriction as a possible cause for amphotericin B nephrotoxicity in rats. J Clin Inves. 1991;87:2097–107.
55. Cheng JT, Witty RT, Robinson RR, Yarger WE. Amphotericin B nephrotoxicity: increased renal resistance and tubule permeability. Kidney Int. 1982;22:626–33.
56. Branch RA, Jackson EK, Jacqz E, et al. Amphotericin B nephrotoxicity in humans decreased by sodium supplements with coadministration of ticarcillin or intravenous saline. Klin Wochenschr. 1987;65:500–6.
57. Branch RA. Prevention of amphotericin B-induced renal impairment: a review of the use of sodium supplementation. Arch Intern Med. 1988;148:2389–94.
58. Goodwin SD, Cleary JD, Walawander CA, Taylor JW, Grasela TH. Pretreatment regimens for adverse events related to infusion of amphotericin B. Clin Infect Dis. 1995;20:755–61.
59. North RJ. The action of cortisone acetate on cell-mediated immunity to infection: Suppression of host cell proliferation and alteration of cellular composition of infective foci. J Exp Med. 1971;134:1485–500.
60. Snyder DS, Unanue ER. Corticosteroids inhibit murine macrophage Ia expression and interleukin 1 production. J Immunol. 1982;129:1803–5.
61. Burks LC, Aisner J, Fortner CL, Wiernik PH. Meperidine for the treatment of shaking chills and fever. Arch Intern Med. 1980;140:483–4.

62. Antoniskis D, Larsen RA. Acute, rapidly progressive renal failure with simultaneous use of amphotericin B and pentamidine. Antimicrob Agents Chemother. 1990;34:470–2.
63. Wright DG, Robichaud KJ, Pizzo PA, Deisseroth AB. Lethal pulmonary reactions associated with the combination use of amphotericin B and leukcocyte transfusions. N Engl J Med. 1981;304:1185–9.
64. Dutcher JP, Kendall J, Norris D, Schiffer C, Aisner J, Wiernik PH. Granulocyte transfusion therapy and amphotericin B adverse reactions. Am J Hematol. 1989;31:102–8.
65. Present CA, Klahr C, Santala R. Amphotericin B induction of sensitivity to adriamycin, 1, 3-bis (2-chloroethyl)-1 nitrosourea (BCNU) plus cyclophosphamide in human neoplasia. Ann Intern Med. 1977;86:47–9.
66. Medoff G. Controversial areas in antifungal chemotherapy: short-course and combination therapy with amphotericin B. Rev Infect Dis. 1987;9:403–7.
67. Stevens DA. Combination immunotherapy and antifungal chemotherapy. Clin Infect Dis. 1998;26:1266–9.
68. Sugar AM. Use of amphotericin B with azoles with antifungal drugs: what are we doing? Antimicrob Agents Chemother. 1995;39:1907–12.
69. Peacock Jr JE, Herrington DA, Cruz JM. Amphotericin B therapy: past, present, future. Infect Dis Clin Pract. 1993;2:81–93.
70. Rex JH, Pappas PG, Karchmer AW, et al. A randomized and blinded multicenter trial of high-dose fluconazole plus placebo versus fluconazole plus amphotericin B as therapy for candidemia and its consequences in nonneutropenic subjects. Clin Infect Dis. 2003;36:1221–8.
71. Bennett JE, Dismukes WE, Duma RJ, et al. A comparison of amphotericin B alone and combined with flucytosine in the treatment of cryptococcal meningitis. N Engl J Med. 1979;301:126–31.
72. Dismukes WE, Cloud G, Gallis HA, et al. Treatment of cryptococcal meningitis with combination amphotericin B and flucytosine for four as compared with six weeks. N Engl J Med. 1987;317:334–41.
73. Van der Horst CM, Saag MS, Cloud GA, et al. Treatment of cryptococcal meningitis associated with the acquired immunodeficiency syndrome. N Engl J Med. 1997;337:15–21.
74. Lewis RE, Kontoyiannis P. Rationale for combination antifungal therapy. Pharmacotherapy. 2001;21:149S–64.
75. Griswold MW, Briceland LL, Stein DS. Is amphotericin B test dosing needed? Ann Pharmacother. 1998;32:475–7.
76. Cleary JD, Weisdorf D, Fletcher CV. Effect of infusion rate on amphotericin B-associated febrile reactions. Drug Intell Clin Pharm. 1988;22:769–72.
77. Craven PC, Gremillion DH. Risk factors for ventricular fibrillation during rapid amphotericin B infusion. Antimicrob Agents Chemother. 1985;27:868–71.
78. Bowler WA, Weiss PJ, Hill HE, et al. Risk of ventricular dysrythmias during one hour infusions of amphotericin B in patients with preserved renal function. Antimicrob Agents Chemother. 1992;36:2542–3.
79. Eriksson U, Seifert B, Schaffner A. Comparison of effects of amphotericin B deoxycholate infused over 4 or 24 hours: randomized controlled trial. Br Med J. 2001;322:579–82.
80. Wen DY, Bottini AG, Hall WA, Haines SJ. Infections in neurologic surgery. The intraventricular use of antibiotics. Neurosurg Clin N Am. 1992;3:343–54.
81. Lesar TS, Fiscella RG. Antimicrobial drug delivery to the eye. Drug Intell Clin Pharm. 1985;19:642–54.
82. Piraino B, Bailie GR, Bernardini J, et al. ISPD guidelines/recommendations. Peritoneal dialysis-related infections recommendations: 2005 update. Perit Dial Int. 2005;25:107–31.
83. Fan-Havard P, Odonovan C, Smith SM, Oh J, Bamberger M, Eng RHK. Oral fluconazole versus amphotericin B bladder irrigation for treatment of candidal funguria. Clin Infect Dis. 1995; 21:960–5.
84. O'Riordan T, Faris M. Inhaled antimicrobial therapy. Respir Care Clin N Am. 1999;5:617–31.
85. Diot P, Dequin PF, Rivoire B, et al. Aerosols and anti-infectious agents. J Aerosol Med. 2001;14:55–64.
86. King CT, Rogers PD, Cleary JD, Chapman SW. Antifungal therapy during pregnancy. Clin Infect Dis. 1998;27:1151–60.
87. Sobel JD. Use of antifungal drugs in pregnancy: a focus on safety. Drug Saf. 2000;23:77–85.
88. Caillot D, Casasnovas O, Solary E, et al. Efficacy and tolerance of an amphotericin B lipid (Intralipid) emulsion in the treatment of candidemia in neutropenic patients. J Antimicrob Chemother. 1993;31:161–9.
89. Ayestaran A, Lopez RM, Montoro JB, et al. Pharmacokinetics of conventional formulation versus fat emulsion formulation of amphotericin B in a group of patients with neutropenia. Antimicrob Agents Chemother. 1996;40:609–12.
90. Cleary JD. Amphotericin B formulated in a lipid emulsion. Ann Pharmacother. 1996;30:409–12.
91. Slain D. Lipid-based amphotericin B for the treatment of fungal infections. Pharmacotherapy. 1999;19:306–23.
92. Janknergt R, de Marie S, Bakker-Woudenberg IAJM, Crommelin DJA. Liposomal and lipid formulations of amphotericin B: clinical pharmacokinetics. Clin Pharmacokinet. 1992;23: 279–91.
93. Robinson RF, Nahata MC. A comparative review of conventional and lipid formulations of amphotericin B. J Clin Pharm Ther. 1999;24:249–57.
94. Walsh TJ, Finberg RW, Arndt C, et al. Liposomal amphotericin B for empirical therapy in patients with persistent fever and neutropenia. N Engl J Med. 1999;340:764–71.
95. Walsh TJ, Whitcomb P, Piscitelli S, et al. Safety, tolerance, and pharmacokinetics of amphotericin B lipid complex in children with hepatosplenic candidiasis. Antimicrob Agents Chemother. 1997;41:1944–8.
96. Villani R, Regazzi MB, Maserati R, Viale P, Alberici F, Giacchino R. Clinical and pharmacokinetic evaluation of a new lipid-based delivery system of amphotericin B in AIDS patients. Arzneimittelforschung. 1996;46:445–9.
97. Groll AH, Lyman CA, Petraitis V, Petraitiene R, Armstrong D, Mickiene D, et al. Compartmentalized intrapulmonary pharmacokinetics of amphotericin B and its lipid formulations. Antimicrob Agents Chemother. 2006;50:3418–23.
98. Leenders C, Reiss P, Portegies P, et al. Liposomal amphotericin B (AmBisome) compared with amphotericin B both followed by oral fluconazole in the treatment of AIDS-associated cryptococcal meningitis. AIDS. 1997;11:1463–71.
99. Goldblum D, Rohrer K, Frueh BE, Theurillat R, Thormann W, Zimmerli S. Corneal concentrations following systemic administration of amphotericin B and its lipid preparations in a rabbit model. Ophthalmic Res. 2004;36:172–6.
100. Goldblum D, Rohrer K, Frueh BE, Theurillat R, Thormann W, Zimmerli S. Ocular distribution of intravenously administered lipid formulations of amphotericin B in a rabbit model. Antimicrob Agents Chemother. 2002;46:3719–23.
101. Kretschmar M, Nichterlein T, Hannak D, Hof H. Effects of amphotericin B incorporated into liposomes and in lipid suspensions in the treatment of murine candidiasis. Arzneimittelforschung. 1996;46:711–5.
102. Wingard JR, White MH, Anaissie E, Raffalli J, Goodman J, Arrieta AL Amph/ ABLC Collaborative Study Group. a randomized, double-blind comparative trial evaluating the safety of

liposomal amphotericin B versus amphotericin B lipid complex in the empirical treatment of febrile neutropenia. Clin Infect Dis. 2000;31:1155–63.
103. White MH, Anaissie EJ, Kusne S, et al. Amphotericin B colloidal dispersion vs. amphotericin B as therapy for invasive aspergillosis. Clin Infect Dis. 1997;24:635–42.
104. White MH, Bowden RA, Sandler ES, et al. Randomized, double-blind clinical trial of amphotericin B colloidal dispersion vs. amphotericin B in the empirical treatment of fever and neutropenia. Clin Infect Dis. 1998;27:296–302.
105. Johnson MD, Drew RH, Perfect JR. Chest discomfort associated with liposomal amphotericin B: report of three cases and review of the literature. Pharmacotherapy. 1998;18:1053–61.
106. Collazos J, Martinez E, Mayo J, Ibarra S. Pulmonary reactions during treatment with amphotericin B: review of published cases and guidelines for management. Clin Infect Dis. 2001;33:E75–82.
107. Roden MM, Nelson LD, Knudsen TA, et al. Triad of acute infusion-related reactions associated with liposomal amphotericin B: analysis of clinical and epidemiological characteristics. Clin Infect Dis. 2003;36:1213–20.
108. McDonnell TJ, Chang SW, Westcott JY, Voelkel NF. Role of oxidants, eicosanoids, and neutrophils in amphotericin B lung injury in rats. J Appl Physiol. 1988;65:2195–206.
109. Hardie WD, Wheeler AP, Wright PW, Swindell BB, Bernard GR. Effect of cyclooxygenase inhibition on amphotericin B-induced lung injury in awake sheep. J Infect Dis. 1992;166:134–8.
110. Bowden R, Chandrasekar P, White MH, et al. A double-blind, randomized, controlled trial of amphotericin B colloidal dispersion for treatment of invasive aspergillosis in immunocompromised patients. Clin Infect Dis. 2002;35:359–66.
111. Sharkey PK, Graybill JR, Johnson ES, et al. Amphotericin B lipid complex compared with amphotericin B in the treatment of cryptococcal meningitis in patients with AIDS. Clin Infect Dis. 1996;22:329–30.
112. Johnson PC, Wheat LJ, Cloud GA, Goldman M, Lancaster D, Bamberger DM, et al. Safety and efficacy of liposomal amphotericin B compared with conventional amphotericin B for induction therapy of histoplasmosis in patients with AIDS. Ann Intern Med. 2002;137:105–9.
113. Rex JH, Walsh TJ. Editorial response: estimating the true cost of amphotericin B. Clin Infect Dis. 1999;29:1408–10.

Flucytosine

Robert A. Larsen

Flucytosine (5-fluorocytosine; 5-flucytosine; 5-FC) is one of the oldest antifungal agents in use [1]. It was initially synthesized in 1957, but was not discovered to possess significant antifungal properties until 1964, when activity against *Cryptococcus neoformans* and *Candida* species was shown [2]. Human clinical trials were initiated in the late 1960s for both cryptococcal meningitis and disseminated candidiasis [3, 4]. The rapid emergence of flucytosine resistance was observed, particularly among *C. neoformans* isolates, limiting its utility as single-agent therapy [5–7]. Presently, flucytosine is utilized as single-agent therapy in only a limited number of settings, including urinary candidiasis and chromoblastomycosis [8]. The seminal studies of combination therapy of flucytosine with amphotericin B for patients with cryptococcal meningitis were the first to firmly establish a role for combination antifungal therapy for a well-defined invasive fungal infection [9, 10].

Mechanism of Action

Flucytosine is taken up by fungal cells by a unique fungal-specific cytosine permease. Two important and independent pathways for fungal cell injury occur: one leading to protein synthesis inhibition and the other resulting in DNA synthesis inhibition. Flucytosine is converted by intracellular deamination to 5-fluorouracil and ultimately processed into 5-fluorouridine triphosphate, which is incorporated into fungal RNA. This results in miscoding during translation from RNA into amino acid sequencing, causing structural abnormalities during protein synthesis [11, 12]. The second mechanism of action is characterized by the conversion of 5-fluorouracil to 5-fluorodeoxyuridine monophosphate, which inhibits thymidylate synthetase and subsequently DNA biosynthesis [13].

R.A. Larsen (✉)
Department of Internal Medicine, Los Angeles County/USC Medical Center, Los Angeles, CA, USA
e-mail: rlarsen@usc.edu

Resistance to flucytosine may arise from mutations that affect the production of three key enzymes (uridine monophosphate pyrophosphorylase, cytosine permease, and cytosine deaminase) or through increased production of pyrimidines [14].

Pharmacology

Both intravenous and oral formulations of flucytosine have been developed and are in clinical use. However, in the USA, only the oral formulation of flucytosine is available and comes as 250- and 500-mg capsules. Following oral administration, 78–89% of the drug is absorbed, with peak concentrations achieved in approximately 2 h [15]. Food, antacids, and renal insufficiency can impair absorption. Over 90% of the drug is eliminated by urinary excretion unchanged [16]. As such, impaired renal function leads to drug accumulation and dramatically alters the serum half-life from approximately 4 h in those with normal renal function (range 2.4–4.8 h) to over 85 h in those with severe renal impairment [17]. Consequently, the daily dose must be adjusted for patients with renal dysfunction [18]. Hemodialysis, hemofiltration, and peritoneal dialysis reduce plasma flucytosine levels [19]. Flucytosine demonstrates only limited protein binding (approximately 3–4%). The penetration of flucytosine into cerebrospinal, peritoneal, and synovial fluids is approximately 75% of simultaneous plasma concentrations [11].

Following oral administration of 2 g of flucytosine in subjects with normal renal function, peak serum levels reach 30–40 mcg/mL. Repeated dosing every 6 h results in peak concentrations of 70–80 mcg/mL. Serum concentrations of greater than 100 mcg/mL are associated with increased toxicity and can rapidly be achieved in the setting of renal failure, particularly that caused by concomitant amphotericin B administration [18, 20]. For these reasons, it is important to monitor renal function closely among all patients receiving flucytosine and adjust dosing for changes in renal function. A nomogram for flucytosine dosing is shown in Table 1.

C.A. Kauffman et al. (eds.), *Essentials of Clinical Mycology*,
DOI 10.1007/978-1-4419-6640-7_4,

Table 1 Dose adjustment of flucytosine with renal insufficiency

Renal function (mL/min)	Oral dosing
>40	25 mg/kg every 6 h
20–39	25 mg/kg every 12 h
10–19	25 mg/kg every 24 h
<10	25 mg/kg after dialysis and monitor peak levels

Modified from Stamm et al. [18]

Estimate of renal function can be made by the Cockroft-Gualt Equation:

$$eCc_r = \frac{(140 - \text{age}) \times \text{mass (in kg)} \times [0.85 \text{ if female}]}{72 \times \text{serum creatinine (in mg/dL)}}$$

This formula expects weight to be measured in kilograms and creatinine to be measured in milligrams per deciliter (mg/dL), as is standard in the USA. The resulting value is multiplied by a constant of 0.85 if the patient is female

For creatinine in µmol/L:

$$eCc_r = \frac{(140 - \text{age}) \times \text{mass (in kg)} \times \text{constant}}{\text{serum creatinine (in µmol/L)}}$$

Where constant is 1.23 for men and 1.04 for women

Dosage and Administration

The current standard daily dose of flucytosine is 100 mg/kg daily given in four divided doses in persons with normal renal function. Doses ranging between 50 and 150 mg/kg daily have been utilized successfully among patients with established fungal infection, but the 150 mg/kg daily dose is often associated with serious side effects [10, 18, 20].

Early studies among patients with cryptococcal meningitis used flucytosine doses of 150 mg/kg daily, but in these studies, serum levels were monitored carefully and adjustments in dosing were made based on these determinations. Recent studies have employed lower-dose regimens of flucytosine (100 mg/kg daily) for shorter periods (2–4 weeks) and have relied less on monitoring serum levels [21–26].

Serum flucytosine levels are not universally available, and delays in obtaining test results often reduce or limit the clinical impact of the information. When available, flucytosine levels can be a helpful adjunct to monitoring therapy and preventing hematologic toxicities. Frequent monitoring of white blood cell and platelet counts can be used as a means of monitoring toxicity if flucytosine levels are not available; the dosage should be decreased at the first sign of a decrease in white blood cell or platelet counts. Alternatively, flucytosine serum levels can be reasonably predicted based upon population pharmacokinetic studies [27]. When monitored, serum levels should be maintained between 50 and 70 mcg/mL although lower levels may be effective [14].

Clinical Indications

Flucytosine is indicated for patients with cryptococcosis, various forms of candidiasis, and chromoblastomycosis. Development of drug resistance is more common in patients treated with flucytosine alone. The most common use of flucytosine is in the management of serious infections caused by *C. neoformans* [28, 29]. In this setting, flucytosine is usually combined with amphotericin B [9, 10, 22, 26, 30, 31] or fluconazole [21, 25, 32], and occasionally with itraconazole [33–36]. Combinations of an azole or amphotericin B with flucytosine have generally been shown to result in more rapid culture conversion of the cerebrospinal fluid from positive to negative and to improved clinical outcomes when compared to single-agent therapy.

Flucytosine can be employed as a single agent or in combination with amphotericin B against organisms responsible for chromoblastomycosis, e.g., *Fonsecaea* and *Cladosporium* species, with moderate success [37–39]. Evaluation of in vitro activity of flucytosine against over 8,500 clinical isolates of *Candida* species showed that primary resistance to flucytosine was very uncommon among all species with the exception of *C. krusei* (only 5% susceptible) [40]. Even though most *Candida* species are susceptible to flucytosine, most invasive *Candida* infections are not treated with flucytosine alone. However, combination therapy with flucytosine and amphotericin B has been used successfully for several forms of invasive candidiasis [41–44]. Given the availability of effective alternative agents, such as the azoles and the echinocandins, flucytosine as part of combination therapy with amphotericin B is an increasingly uncommon approach to serious *Candida* infections. However, recent guidelines recommend flucytosine in combination with amphotericin B for selected patients with central nervous system candidiasis, *Candida* endocarditis, and *Candida* endophthalmitis [45]. In addition, flucytosine is sometimes used as a single agent to treat urinary candidiasis [45].

Aspergillus species may respond to the combination of amphotericin B and flucytosine, but the benefit of adding flucytosine is not well established [46–49]. *Histoplasma capsulatum*, *Coccidioides* species, *Blastomyces dermatitidis*, *Sporothrix schenckii*, and *Scedosporium apiospermum* are not susceptible to flucytosine and therefore this drug has no role in these fungal infections. Although *Penicillium marneffei* is inhibited in vitro by flucytosine [50], the therapeutic utility of flucytosine for penicilliosis is not established.

Adverse Effects

The most common adverse effects associated with flucytosine use are gastrointestinal complaints of nausea, vomiting, and diarrhea. These events are rarely serious, and can often be ameliorated by taking the oral medication over 15–30 min. Hepatic toxicities, including elevated transaminase and alkaline phosphatase levels, have been reported in 0–25% of subjects taking flucytosine. Rarely, hyperbilirubinemia occurs with flucytosine administration, but bilirubin levels usually decline once the drug is stopped [51]. Clinically significant hepatitis is rare, but deaths have been attributed to flucytosine-induced hepatic disease. The gastrointestinal and hepatic side effects have not been demonstrated to be dose dependent [52]. Although the mechanism of gastrointestinal toxicity is not well established, it is postulated to result from 5-fluorouracil accumulation from intestinal microflora metabolism of flucytosine [53, 54].

Serious adverse effects usually arise from bone marrow injury [18, 20]. Thrombocytopenia, granulocytopenia, and anemia may arise at any time during the course of therapy, particularly if flucytosine drug levels accumulate because of decreased renal clearance associated with concomitant amphotericin B administration. Bone marrow toxicity has been observed in 60% of subjects with flucytosine serum levels greater than 100 mcg/mL, whereas only 12% developed bone marrow toxicity when serum levels were less than 100 mcg/mL [20]. Although flucytosine-induced blood dyscrasias are usually reversible on discontinuation of drug, fatal bone marrow suppression has been reported. Prior radiation therapy appears to exacerbate the potential for bone marrow toxicity.

Therapeutic monitoring of serum flucytosine levels followed by adjustment of flucytosine dose may reduce the frequency of severe bone marrow toxicity. A complete blood and platelet count provides a good indication of flucytosine toxicity when serum levels are unavailable. Flucytosine may be safely employed in settings with limited ability to monitor drug levels through very careful observation of renal function and white blood cell and platelet counts; dosage adjustments must be made if renal function changes or white blood cell or platelet counts fall.

Cytosine arabinoside has been reported to inactivate flucytosine [55]. No other significant drug–drug interactions are known.

Precautions

Flucytosine should be used with care during pregnancy. Teratogenic effects have been observed in rats and rabbits (spinal fusion, cleft lip and palate, and micrognathia); thus, this agent is assigned pregnancy category C by the US Food and Drug Administration. On occasion, flucytosine has been given during pregnancy with success [56, 57]. Flucytosine has not been approved for use in children, but there has been considerable experience in this age group, particularly for treatment of central nervous system and urinary infections due to *Candida* species [58, 59]. Nursing mothers should avoid flucytosine as it may be excreted in breast milk.

References

1. Utz JP. Flucytosine. N Engl J Med. 1972;286:777–8.
2. Grunberg E, Titsworth E, Bennett M. Chemotherapeutic activity of 5-flourocytosine. Antimicrob Agents Chemother. 1964;3:566–8.
3. Tassel D, Madoff MA. Treatment of *Candida* species and *Cryptococcus* meningitis with 5-fluorocytosine: a new antifungal agent. JAMA. 1968;206:830–2.
4. Utz JP, Tynes BS, Shadomy HJ, Duma RJ, Kannan MM, Mason N. 5-fluorocytosine in human cryptococcosis. Antimicrob Agents Chemother. 1968;8:344–6.
5. Normark S, Schönebeck J. In vitro studies of 5-flucytosine resistance in *Candida albicans* and *Torulopsis glabrata*. Antimicrob Agents Chemother. 1972;2:114–21.
6. Block ER, Jennings AE, Bennett JE. 5-fluorocytosine resistance in *Cryptococcus neoformans*. Antimicrob Agents Chemother. 1973;3:649–56.
7. Hospenthal DR, Bennett JE. Flucytosine monotherapy for cryptococcosis. Clin Infect Dis. 1998;27:260–4.
8. Graybill JR, Craven PC. Antifungal agents used in systemic mycoses. activity and therapeutic use. Drugs. 1983;25:41–62.
9. Bennett JE, Dismukes WE, Duma RJ, et al. A comparison of amphotericin B alone and combined with flucytosine in the treatment of cryptococcal meningitis. N Engl J Med. 1979;301:126–31.
10. Dismukes WE, Cloud G, Gallis HA, et al. Treatment of cryptococcal meningitis with combination amphotericin B and flucytosine for four as compared with six weeks. N Engl J Med. 1987;317:334–41.
11. Bennett JE. Flucytosine. Ann Intern Med. 1977;86:319–21.
12. Diasio RB, Bennett JE, Myers CE. Mode of action of 5–fluorocytosine. Biochem Pharmacol. 1978;27:703–7.
13. Waldorf R, Polak A. Mechanisms of action of 5-fluorocytosine. Antimicrob Agents Chemother. 1983;23:79–85.
14. Francis P, Walsh TJ. Evolving role of flucytosine in immunocompromised patients: new insights into safety, pharmacokinetics, and antifungal therapy. Clin Infect Dis. 1992;15:1003–18.
15. Cutler RE, Blair AD, Kelly MR. Flucytosine kinetics in subjects with normal and impaired renal function. Clin Pharmacol Ther. 1978;24:333–42.
16. Schönebeck J, Polak A, Fernex M, Scholer HJ. Pharmacokinetic studies on the oral antimycotic agent 5-fluorocytosine in individuals with normal and impaired kidney function. Chemotherapy. 1973; 18:321–36.
17. Daneshmend TK, Warnock DW. Clinical pharmacokinetics of systemic antifungal drugs. Clin Pharmacokinet. 1983;8:17–42.
18. Stamm AM, Diasio RB, Dismukes WE, et al. Toxicity of amphotericin B plus flucytosine in 194 patients with cryptococcal meningitis. Am J Med. 1987;83:236–42.
19. Lau AH, Kronfol NO. Elimination of flucytosine by continuous hemofiltration. Am J Nephrol. 1995;15:327–31.
20. Kauffman CA, Frame PT. Bone marrow toxicity associated with 5-fluorocytosine therapy. Antimicrob Agents Chemother. 1977; 11:244–7.
21. Larsen RA, Bozzette SA, Jones BE, et al. Fluconazole combined with flucytosine for treatment of cryptococcal meningitis in patients with AIDS. Clin Infect Dis. 1994;19:741–5.
22. van der Horst CM, Saag MS, Cloud GA, et al. Treatment of cryptococcal meningitis associated with the acquired immunodeficiency syndrome. N Engl J Med. 1997;337:15–21.

23. Brouwer AE, Rajanuwong A, Chierakul W, et al. Combination antifungal therapies for HIV-associated cryptococcal meningitis: a randomised trial. Lancet. 2004;363:1764–7.
24. Brouwer AE, van Kan HJ, Johnson E, et al. Oral versus intravenous flucytosine in patients with human immunodeficiency virus-associated cryptococcal meningitis. Antimicrob Agents Chemother. 2007;51:1038–42.
25. Milefchik E, Leal MA, Haubrich R, et al. Fluconazole alone or combined with flucytosine for the treatment of AIDS-associated cryptococcal meningitis. Med Mycol. 2008;46:393–5.
26. Bicanic T, Wood R, Meintjes G, et al. High-dose amphotericin B with flucytosine for the treatment of cryptococcal meningitis in HIV-infected patients: a randomized trial. Clin Infect Dis. 2008;47:123–30.
27. Vermes A, Mathot RAA, ven der Sijs IH, Dankert J, Guchelaar HJ. Population pharmacokinetics of flucytosine: comparison and validation of three models using STS, NPEM, and NONMEM. Therapeutic Drug Monitor. 2000;22:676–87.
28. Pappas PG, Perfect JR, Cloud GA, et al. Cryptococcosis in human immunodeficiency virus-negative patients in the era of effective azole therapy. Clin Infect Dis. 2001;33:690–9.
29. Perfect JR, Dismukes WE, Dromer F, et al. Clinical practice guidelines for the management of cryptococcal disease: 2010 update by the Infectious Diseases Society of America. Clin Infect Dis. 2010;50:291–322.
30. Larsen RA, Leal MA, Chan LS. Fluconazole compared to amphotericin B plus flucytosine for cryptococcal meningitis in AIDS: a randomized trial. Ann Intern Med. 1990;113:183–7.
31. de Gans J, Portegies P, Tiessens G, et al. Itraconazole compared with amphotericin B plus flucytosine in AIDS patients with cryptococcal meningitis. AIDS. 1992;6:185–90.
32. Mayanja-Kizza H, Oishi K, Mitarai S, et al. Combination therapy with fluconazole and flucytosine for cryptococcal meningitis in Ugandan patients with AIDS. Clin Infect Dis. 1998;26:1362–6.
33. Chotmongkol V, Jitpimolmard S. Treatment of cryptococcal meningitis with combination itraconazole and flucytosine. J Med Assoc Thailand. 1994;77:253–6.
34. Chotmongkol V, Jitpimolmard S. Treatment of cryptococcal meningitis with triple combination of amphotericin B, flucytosine and itraconazole. Southeast Asian J Trop Med Pub Health. 1995; 26:381–3.
35. Chotmongkol V, Sukeepaisarncharoen W, Thavornpitak Y. Comparison of amphotericin B, flucytosine and itraconazole with amphotericin B and flucytosine in the treatment of cryptococcal meningitis in AIDS. J Med Assoc Thailand. 1997;80:416–25.
36. Riantawan P, Ponglertnapakorn P. Clinical efficacy of itraconazole with initial flucytosine in AIDS-related cryptococcal meningitis: a preliminary study. J Med Assoc Thailand. 1996;79:429–33.
37. Lopes CF, Alvarenga RJ, Cispalpino EO, Resende MA, Oliveira LG. Six years experience in treatment of chromomycosis with 5-fluorocytosine. Int J Dermatol. 1978;17:414–8.
38. Silber JG, Gombert ME, Green KM, Shalita AR. Treatment of chromomycosis with ketoconazole and 5-fluorocytosine. J Am Acad Dermatol. 1983;8:236–8.
39. Restrepo A. Treatment of tropical mycoses. J Am Acad Dermatol. 1994;31:S91–S102.
40. Pfaller MA, Messer SA, Boyken L, Huynh H, Hollis RJ, Diekema DJ. In vitro activities of 5-fluorocytosine against 8, 803 clinical isolates of Candida spp global assessment of primary resistance using National Committee for Clinical Laboratory Standards susceptibility testing methods. Antimicrob Agents Chemother. 2002;46:3518–21.
41. Record CO, Skinner JM, Sleight P, Speller DC. *Candida* endocarditis treated with 5-fluorocytosine. Brit Med J. 1971;1:262–4.
42. Smego Jr RA, Perfect JR, Durack DT. Combined therapy with amphotericin B and 5-fluorocytosine for *Candida* meningitis. Rev Infect Dis. 1984;6:791–801.
43. Kujath P, Lerch K, Kochendorfer P, Boos C. Comparative study of the efficacy of fluconazole versus amphotericin B/flucytosine in surgical patients with systemic mycoses. Infection. 1993;21:376–82.
44. Abele-Horn M, Kopp A, Sternberg U, et al. A randomized study comparing fluconazole with amphotericin B/5-flucytosine for the treatment of systemic *Candida* infections in intensive care patients. Infection. 1996;24:426–32.
45. Pappas PG, Kauffman CA, Andes D, et al. Clinical practice guidelines for the management of candidiasis. 2009 update by the Infectious Diseases Society of America. Clin Infect Dis. 2009;48:503–35.
46. Denning DW, Stevens DA. Antifungal and surgical treatment of invasive aspergillosis: review of 2,121 published cases. Rev Infect Dis. 1990;12:1147–201 [erratum appears in Rev Infect Dis 13:345, 1991].
47. Pogliani E, Clini E. Association therapy as a prognostic factor in deep fungal infection complicating oncohaematological diseases. Supportive Care Cancer. 1994;2:385–8.
48. Denning DW, Marinus A, Cohen J, et al. An EORTC multicentre prospective survey of invasive aspergillosis in haematological patients: diagnosis and therapeutic outcome. EORTC Invasive Fungal Infections Cooperative Group. J Infect. 1998;37:173–80.
49. Yu VL, Wagner GE, Shadomy S. Sino-orbital aspergillosis treated with combination antifungal therapy. Successful therapy after failure with amphotericin B and surgery. JAMA. 1980;244:814–5.
50. Supparatpinyo K, Nelson KE, Merz WG, et al. Response to antifungal therapy by human immunodeficiency virus-infected patients with disseminated *Penicillium marneffei* infections and in vitro susceptibilities of isolates from clinical specimens. Antimicrob Agents Chemother. 1993;37:2407–11.
51. Scholer HJ. Flucytosine. In: Speller DCE, editor. Antifungal Chemotherapy. Chichester: Wiley; 1980. p. 35–106.
52. Vermes A, van der Sijs IH, Guchelaar J. Flucytosine: correlation between toxicity and pharmacokinetic parameters. Chemotherapy. 2000;46:86–94.
53. Harris BE, Manning WB, Federle TW, Diasio RB. Conversion of 5-fluorocytosine to 5-fluorouracil by human intestinal microflora. Antimicrob Agents Chemother. 1986;29:44–8.
54. Malet-Marino MC, Martino R, de Forni M, Andremont A, Hartman O, Armand JP. Flucytosine conversion to fluorouracil in humans: does a correlation with gut flora status exist? Infection. 1991;19:178–80.
55. Holt RJ. Clinical problems with 5-fluorocytosine. Mykosen. 1978;21:363–9.
56. Ely EW, Peacock Jr JE, Haponik EF, Washburn RG. Cryptococcal pneumonia complicating pregnancy. Medicine (Baltimore). 1998;77:153–67.
57. Chen CP, Wang KG. Cryptococcal meningitis in pregnancy. Am J Perinatol. 1996;13:35–6.
58. Stamos JK, Rowley AH. Candidemia in a pediatric population. Clin Infect Dis. 1995;20:571–5.
59. Rowen JL, Tate JM. Management of neonatal candidiasis. Neonatal Candidiasis Study Group. Pediat Infect Dis J. 1998;17:1007–11.

Azoles

David R. Andes and William E. Dismukes

The introduction of the azole class of antifungal drugs with the licensing of miconazole in 1979 marked the beginning of a new era in therapy for systemic fungal diseases. Although miconazole, an intravenous formulation associated with significant toxicity, is no longer commercially available, it set the stage for the development and subsequent licensing of three oral azole drugs: ketoconazole, fluconazole, and itraconazole [1]. For many systemic mycoses, these drugs have been effective and safe alternatives to the older antifungal drugs – amphotericin B, a member of the polyene class and for years the so-called "gold standard" of therapy, and flucytosine, a fluorinated pyrimidine. Ketoconazole, introduced in 1981, fluconazole (1990), and itraconazole (1992) have been attractive agents because of their excellent spectrum of activity against *Candida* species and endemic fungi and their overall efficacy, safety, and ease of oral administration. However, these drugs for the most part lack significant activity against mould pathogens, an important group of emerging opportunistic fungi. Consequently, the past several years have witnessed the development of an exciting group of second-generation triazole drugs, which possess an expanded spectrum of activity, especially against various moulds and resistant *Candida* species. Voriconazole, approved in 2002, is the first of these to become commercially available; posaconazole was most recently licensed – in 2006 [2, 3]. Our purpose in this chapter is to compare and contrast the pharmacologic properties of the older oral azoles and the newer triazoles and to provide perspective on the clinical indications for these agents. Since ketoconazole is the oldest azole and now the least used, our comments about ketoconazole will be limited.

D.R. Andes (✉)
Department of Medicine, and Medical Microbiology and Immunology, Section of Infectious Diseases, Madison, WI, USA
e-mail: dra@medicine.wisc.edu

Chemistry

Chemical structures for the commercially useful (fluconazole, itraconazole, voriconazole, and posaconazole) azole drugs are shown in Fig. 1. The antifungal zoles are classified chemically as imidazoles or triazoles based on the number of nitrogen atoms (two or three, respectively) in the azole ring [4]. Voriconazole, a second-generation triazole, was developed via systematic chemical manipulation of fluconazole to produce a compound with enhanced potency and spectrum of activity. Voriconazole's structure is similar to fluconazole, but one triazole ring is replaced with a fluorinated pyrimidine, and an α-methyl group is added to the propanol backbone. These modifications increase voriconazole's affinity for the target enzyme in *Aspergillus fumigatus* by 10-fold over that of fluconazole. Posaconazole is chemically similar to itraconazole. The structures of both azoles contain extended piperazine-phenyl-triazole side-chains, but posaconazole is composed of a furan ring with fluorine substituted for chlorine.

These azole drugs can also be distinguished by their relative molecular size and aqueous solubility. Fluconazole is unique among the antifungal azoles owing to its relatively small molecular size and high aqueous solubility. Itraconazole, voriconazole, and posaconazole are less soluble or insoluble in water at physiologic pH, thereby reducing their oral bioavailability and complicating the development of a suitable parenteral dosage form. Different approaches have been taken to assure efficient and safe delivery of these lipophilic compounds into the systemic circulation. As one example, the oral solution and parenteral formulations of itraconazole have incorporated the azole in a carrier complex of hydroxypropyl-β-cyclodextrin, a large ring of substituted glucose molecules with a hydrophilic outer surface and a cylindrical hydrophobic inner core [5–8]. A similar formulation was developed for the parenteral formulation of voriconazole [2]. The manufacturers of posaconazole are also conducting investigations with a parenteral cyclodextrin formulation.

C.A. Kauffman et al. (eds.), *Essentials of Clinical Mycology*,
DOI 10.1007/978-1-4419-6640-7_5,

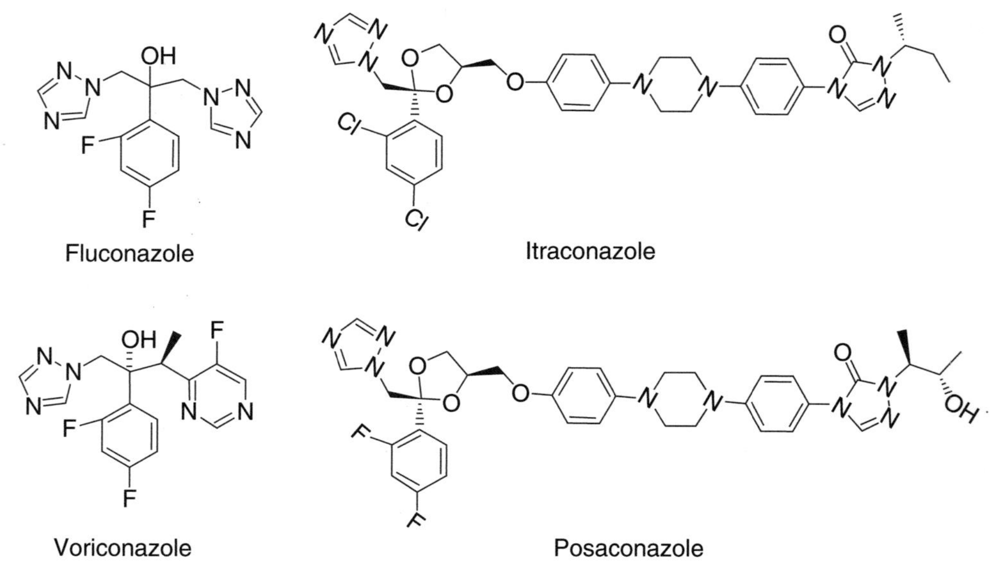

Fig. 1 Structures of azole antifungal agents

Mechanism of Action

The primary antifungal effect of the azoles occurs via inhibition of a fungal cytochrome P-450 enzyme involved in the synthesis of ergosterol, the major sterol in the fungal cell membrane [1, 9–11]. On a molecular level, binding of the free azole nitrogen with the heme moiety of fungal C-14α demethylase inhibits demethylation of lanosterol, thereby depriving the cell of ergosterol and allowing accumulation of various 14α methylsterols. The net result is a disruption of normal structure and function of the cell membrane and, ultimately, the inhibition of cell growth and morphogenesis. More recent experiments with newer azoles have concluded the antifungal activities of the triazole derivatives are due to the inhibition of 14α demethylase exclusively [12, 13].

Azoles are generally recognized as fungistatic agents at clinically achievable concentrations. However, recent in vitro studies with itraconazole and voriconazole demonstrated fungicidal activity against conidial suspensions of *Aspergillus fumigatus* and several other *Aspergillus* species at concentrations below those attained with recommended dosages [14].

Formulations and Dosing

Fluconazole is formulated as an oral tablet (50, 100, 150, or 200 mg), a powder for oral suspension (10 mg/mL, 50 mg/5 mL, 40 mg/mL, 200 mg/5 mL), and as an intravenous formulation (400 mg/200 mL, 200 mg/100 mL). The recommended regimen for invasive candidiasis is a loading dose 800 mg (12 mg/kg) followed by 400 mg (6 mg/kg) daily [15]. A dosage of 400 mg daily is recommended for antifungal prophylaxis in neutropenic patients. Lower dosages can be administered for treatment of noninvasive infections. A single 150-mg dose is effective for treatment of vulvovaginal candidiasis. Fluconazole dosages of 100–200 mg daily are recommended for treatment of oropharyngeal candidiasis. Dosages of 200–400 mg daily should be administered for esophageal candidiasis. For suppression of mucosal candidiasis in patients with recurrent disease, fluconazole 200 mg 3×/week is recommended. Treatment and suppression of cryptococcosis requires dosages of 200–800 mg daily, depending on the severity of the infection. Fluconazole can be safely administered to infants and children [16]. Fluconazole is cleared more rapidly in children than adults and higher weight-based dosages are required to produce therapeutic exposures. For treatment of systemic candidiasis in children, a dosage of 6–12 mg/kg daily is recommended. A lower daily dose (3 mg/kg) can be administered for mucosal candidiasis, but a loading dose of 6 mg/kg should be given. For treatment of cryptococcal meningitis in children, fluconazole can be administered as a 12 mg/kg IV loading dosage, followed by 6 mg/kg daily.

Available preparations of itraconazole include a 100-mg capsule and an oral solution (10 mg/mL complexed with 400 mg hydroxypropyl-β-cyclodextrin/mL). Itraconazole has also been formulated for intravenous administration, but this product is available in only a few countries. For treatment of invasive fungal infections, including aspergillosis, blastomycosis, and histoplasmosis, loading doses are recommended to more rapidly achieve steady-state serum concentrations. Loading doses can be administered by the intravenous route (200 mg IV twice daily for four doses) or oral route (200 mg three times daily for 3 days). The dose can then be decreased to 200 mg once or twice daily. Loading dosages are not considered necessary for less severe infections, including mucosal candidiasis and onychomycosis. The itraconazole oral solution should be administered as swish and swallow for esophageal candidiasis (200 mg daily) and oropharyngeal candidiasis (100–200 mg daily). The approved regimens for onychomycosis include daily itraconazole (200 mg daily for 12 weeks) or pulse therapy (200 mg twice daily for 1 week, then off drug for 3 weeks, repeated for 12 weeks). Itraconazole is not approved for pediatric patients. However, the itraconazole oral solution has been studied in infants and children for the treatment of mucosal candidiasis and as antifungal prophylaxis at dosages of 5 mg/kg daily, 2.5 mg/kg daily, and 2.5 mg/kg twice daily [17, 18]. Limited studies in infants and younger children suggest that intravenous itraconazole can be administered based upon weight as well. A single 2.5 mg/kg dosage was well tolerated in young children and resulted in serum itraconazole levels similar to adults [19].

Voriconazole is formulated as an oral tablet (50 or 200 mg), a powder for oral suspension (40 mg/mL), and a solution complexed with sulfobutyl-ether β-cyclodextrin (SEBCD) for intravenous administration (10 mg/mL voriconazole, 160 mg/mL SEBCD). The recommended intravenous regimen includes a 6 mg/kg loading for two doses followed by 4 mg/kg BID. The recommended oral dosing regimen also involves a loading period (400 mg BID for two doses) followed by 200 mg BID. If the patient is not responding to therapy, the oral dosing regimen can be increased to 300 mg BID. The oral dose may be smaller than the intravenously administered dosages on a weight basis. Some experts recommend increasing the oral dosage based on weight (4 mg/kg) rounded up to convenient pill sizes. However, weight-based oral dosing has not been extensively examined. Patients 12 years of age or older should receive adult doses of voriconazole. In contrast, younger children require higher weight-based dosages of voriconazole to achieve the same serum concentrations as adults [20, 21]. A pediatric dosage of 7 mg/kg administered every 12 h results in similar voriconazole serum concentrations as an adult dosage of 4 mg/kg given every 12 h and is the currently recommended regimen for this group [22]. Study of voriconazole in newborn infants is limited.

Posaconazole is currently available only as an immediate-release oral suspension containing polysorbate 80 as an emulsifying agent. The suspension is cherry-flavored and contains 40 mg of posaconazole per milliliter. Due to saturable absorption, loading doses are not advised, and doses should be divided into two to four daily doses. The recommended dose of posaconazole is 800 mg daily for treatment of fungal infection and 600 mg daily for prophylaxis of fungal infection. Posaconazole is FDA approved for prophylaxis in adolescents 13 years or older who are at risk for invasive fungal infection due to severe immunocompromise. In these studies, adolescents received posaconazole doses identical to adults (200 mg TID) [23, 24]. Ongoing pharmacokinetic studies are attempting to determine appropriate dosing in the younger pediatric population.

Pharmacokinetics

The major pharmacokinetic parameters of the antifungal azoles are presented in Table 1. The bioavailability of fluconazole is near 90% and is not significantly impacted by administration of food or gastric acidity [25–27]. Itraconazole is highly lipophilic and poorly soluble in aqueous solutions at neutral pH. The bioavailability of itraconazole is dependent upon the formulation. Absorption of the capsule formulation is only 55% [28]. An acidic gastric environment enhances solubility of the capsule formulation and optimizes absorption. Conversely, itraconazole absorption is reduced when coadministered with medications which suppress gastric acidity, such as proton pump inhibitors or histamine-2 blockers. This effect can be reversed by administering an acidic beverage, e.g., Coca-Cola, with the itraconazole capsules to healthy individuals [29]. Food also positively impacts itraconazole bioavailability [27, 30]. The development of an oral solution with hydroxypropyl-β-cyclodextrin as a carrier molecule for itraconazole has improved the bioavailability of itraconazole to nearly 80% by enhancing the solubility of the lipophilic molecule [6, 7, 31]. Food and gastric acidity do not enhance absorption of the solution formulation.

The bioavailability of voriconazole is >90% in healthy volunteers and is optimal in the fasted state, approximately 1 h before or after a meal [28, 32]. Unlike itraconazole capsules, gastric acid does not impact absorption of voriconazole. In contrast, the presence of food, especially a high-fat meal, significantly increases absorption of posaconazole [33–35]. Similar to itraconazole, absorption of posaconazole is reduced by coadministration of drugs that raise the gastric pH [36–38].

Peak plasma concentrations of azoles are typically reached within 2–3 h after administration. With fluconazole, peak concentrations are proportional to the dose administered [1, 39]. Posaconazole exhibits dose-limited (saturable) absorption [28, 40]. In contrast, peak serum levels of voriconazole and itraconazole increase disproportionately with larger doses, suggesting the presence of saturable first-pass metabolism [41–46]. For example, increasing the voriconazole by two-fold results in an approximately three-fold increase in Cmax and AUC [46]. Initiation of therapy with the parenteral formulation and the administration of a loading regimen helps to assure rapid attainment of therapeutic concentrations for each of the triazoles, with the exception of posaconazole [1, 2, 47].

Table 1 Pharmacokinetic parameters of antifungal azoles

Parameter	Fluconazole	Itraconazole	Voriconazole	Posaconazole
Bioavailability (%)	>90	55–>90[a]	>90	8–47[b]
Effect of food	No effect	Decreases capsule Increases solution	Decreases	Increases
Peak concentration (μg/mL)				
At steady state:	3.86–4.96	2.9 [1.9][c]	3.0	NA
IV (dosage)	(100 mg daily)	(200 mg bid × 2, then 200 mg daily × 5)	(3 mg/kg bid)	
Oral (dosage)	4.1–8.1 (400 mg × 1)	2.0–2.3 [2.1–2.6][c](200 mg bid)	1.9 (200 mg bid)	1.1 (200 mg bid)
Volume of distribution (L/kg)	0.7–1	10.7	4.6	7–15
Tissue penetration (% simultaneous serum)				
CSF	50–94	<1	42–67	NA
Protein binding (%)	11–12	99.8 [99.5][c]	58	>98
Elimination half-life (h)	22–31	38–64[d] [27–56][c]	6[d]	24
% Unchanged drug in urine	80	<1	<5	<1

CSF cerebrospinal fluid, *NA* data not available

[a] Oral bioavailability is dependent on dosage form. Higher values represent data from commercially available oral solution when given to healthy volunteers

[b] Human data not currently available. Values represent data from animal studies. Absolute oral bioavailability is not known due to absence of parenteral dosage form. Value represents bioavailability relative to oral solution

[c] Values in brackets are parameters for hydroxyitraconazole

[d] Dose-dependent elimination has been reported. Values may be higher or lower depending on dosage

Once absorbed into the systemic circulation, the portion of an azole drug not bound to plasma proteins distributes readily to body tissues and fluids. Fluconazole is estimated to be 11–13% protein-bound in the serum of healthy volunteers [48]. Fluconazole penetrates most tissues, including the liver, spleen, lung, brain, muscle, and eye [42, 49, 50]. Therapeutic concentrations have been measured in all body fluids sampled, including the brain parenchyma and the cerebrospinal fluid (CSF), achieving concentrations near those observed in serum. Fluconazole also accumulates in the compartments of the inflamed and noninflamed eye. Fluconazole is the sole triazole that is excreted in active form into the urine. In healthy volunteers, urinary fluconazole concentrations are approximately 10-fold higher than serum concentrations [51, 52]. Significant and prolonged vaginal penetration has also been noted and is the basis for dosing as infrequently as every 72 h for treatment of vaginal candidiasis. A single-dose fluconazole (150 mg) produces peak concentrations in vaginal secretions similar to plasma and concentrations remain above 1 μg/g for 72 h [53].

Itraconazole is 99.8% bound to plasma protein; therefore, levels of itraconazole in body fluids, such as CSF, are relatively low in relation to plasma levels (2–5%) [5]. Itraconazole accumulation in the vitreous is also limited [54]. Itraconazole has a large volume of distribution (11 L/kg), and drug has been demonstrated to accumulate in tissues, such as lung, kidney, muscle, bone, and the gastrointestinal tract [42]. Similar to fluconazole, high levels of itraconazole are found in the female genital tract [55]. In addition, concentrations of itraconazole in keratinous tissues are exceptionally high (up to 19-fold higher than plasma), thereby allowing intermittent or pulse therapy for infections localized to the skin and nails [41, 44, 56].

Voriconazole is 58% protein bound in the serum with a volume of distribution of 4.6 L/kg. Several studies demonstrate extensive voriconazole tissue penetration to extravascular tissues, including the CNS and compartments of the eye [28, 57, 58]. Voriconazole assay in the CSF of patients receiving therapy for CNS fungal infection demonstrated concentrations of more than 40% of concentrations measured in serum. A similar study in a cohort with ocular fungal infections reported voriconazole concentrations in the vitreous humor and aqueous humor that were 38% and 53% of those observed in plasma, respectively [59].

Protein binding for posaconazole is similar to itraconazole (>98%). Although posaconazole CSF levels in a rabbit model of cryptococcal meningitis were undetectable (<0.05 μg/mL), posaconazole was as effective as fluconazole in treatment of meningitis, suggesting that CSF posaconazole levels may not predict drug efficacy for treatment of meningitis [60]. An open-label trial of posaconazole therapy of refractory central nervous system fungal infections also demonstrated efficacy [61]. These data suggest that posaconazole achieves therapeutic CNS concentrations. Vitreal penetration observations suggest posaconazole achieves concentrations (21%) that are lower than those described for voriconazole (38%) and fluconazole (28–75%), but higher than that reported for itraconazole (10%) [28, 59].

Fluconazole is the sole triazole that does not undergo extensive metabolism, but is eliminated largely as unchanged drug in the urine. The elimination half-life of fluconazole is approximately 30 h. Clearance declines with increasing degrees of renal impairment, and dosages of this agent should be reduced accordingly. For patients with a creatinine clearance of 10–60 mL/min, the fluconazole dosage should be decreased by 50%. Adjustments are not necessary for loading dosages or single-dose fluconazole [62]. Standard hemodialysis and some forms of continuous hemofiltration remove significant amounts of fluconazole from plasma, [63–66] and it is recommended that fluconazole be administered following hemodialysis. Conversely, in a case study of a patient on continuous arteriovenous hemodiafiltration (CAVHD), fluconazole administered without dosage adjustment resulted in pharmacokinetic parameters similar to patients with normal renal function [67]. Fluconazole does not require dose reduction for patients with hepatic impairment.

Itraconazole and voriconazole undergo extensive hepatic metabolism via cytochrome P-450 enzymes and are eliminated in urine or bile as inactive metabolites [1, 41, 42, 45, 68–70]. Itraconazole is metabolized, primarily by the CYP450 isoenzyme 3A4, to at least three metabolites: hydroxyitraconazole, keto-itraconazole, and *N*-desalkyl-itraconazole. Itraconazole is unique because one of these metabolites, hydroxyitraconazole, exhibits antifungal activity similar to or greater than the parent compound [41]. Elimination of itraconazole and hydroxyitraconazole follow saturable pharmacokinetics, and the half-life is greater than 24 h [34]. The metabolites are recovered in the feces (54%) and urine (35%) [42]. All excreted metabolites in the urine are not microbiologically active [71]. Renal elimination is not a major route for itraconazole clearance, and the dosing regimen of itraconazole does not need to be adjusted for renal insufficiency. However, the major route of elimination of a hydroxypropyl-β-cyclodextrin vehicle is glomerular filtration, and higher levels are found in patients with reduced renal function (creatinine clearance of <19 mL/min). Therefore, the intravenous formulation of itraconazole is not recommended for patients with creatinine clearance of <30 mL/min and should be used with caution in those with creatinine clearance of 30–80 mL/min. However, the itraconazole oral solution can be used in patients with renal insufficiency because the hydroxypropyl-β-cyclodextrin carrier is degraded by amylases in the gastrointestinal tract and is thus not systemically absorbed (<3%) [7]. Itraconazole is not dialyzable by either hemodialysis or continuous ambulatory peritoneal dialysis (CAPD) [72]. Hepatic metabolism of itraconazole is necessary for elimination. Studies examining the use of itraconazole in patients with liver disease are limited; however, elevated serum itraconazole concentrations are expected in patients with hepatic impairment and dose reduction is recommended [41, 42].

Voriconazole is hepatically metabolized by CYP450 isoenzymes CYP2C9, CYP2C19, and CYP3A4 via N-oxidation, with CYP2C19 as the major metabolic enzyme [73]. Recent investigations with voriconazole [74] indicate clearance may be reduced significantly in patients with impaired hepatic function; therefore, dosage reduction is warranted in patients with mild-to-moderate cirrhosis of the liver (Child-Pugh Classes A and B). The elimination half-life of voriconazole is short (6.5 h) compared to the other triazoles. However, metabolism of voriconazole is saturable within the range of clinically effective dosages, and plasma clearance of these agents is significantly reduced (elimination half-life is prolonged) as doses approach 400 mg. Renal elimination of the parent compound is minimal, and no adjustments of oral voriconazole are required for decreased renal function. However, in using the intravenous formulation one must consider the renally cleared cyclodextrin vehicle, and use of the intravenous formulation is not recommended in patients with reduced renal function (CrCl<50 mL/min). The oral formulation does not contain the cyclodextrin vehicle and is safe in patients with renal insufficiency. Voriconazole is not readily dialyzable, with <1% found in the dialysate of patients receiving peritoneal dialysis [75]. Voriconazole has been administered without dosage adjustments to patients undergoing continuous venovenous hemodiafiltration, peritoneal dialysis, and hemodialysis [75, 76].

Posaconazole undergoes minimal metabolism (15%) and is primarily excreted unchanged into the feces [77]. Studies in rodents indicate that posaconazole undergoes significant enterohepatic circulation and is eliminated almost entirely in bile and feces [69]. Dosing adjustments are not required in patients with renal dysfunction, and posaconazole is not removed by hemodialysis [78]. Posaconazole has not been studied extensively in patients with hepatic insufficiency and should be used with caution in these patient populations.

Therapeutic Drug Monitoring

Numerous studies have demonstrated wide patient-to-patient variability in serum concentrations for three of the triazole drugs: itraconazole, voriconazole, and posaconazole. A growing body of evidence suggests a relationship between serum concentrations and either treatment efficacy or adverse effects [79]. This combination of pharmacologic factors warrants consideration of therapeutic drug monitoring.

Both healthy volunteer and population pharmacokinetic studies have demonstrated large kinetic variability for itraconazole and posaconazole that is related predominantly to erratic absorption [80–82]. For the capsule formulation of itraconazole and for posaconazole, absorption is impacted by gastric acidity and drugs that control gastric pH. In addition, food has a significant influence on absorption of all three triazoles in the monitoring category. Much of the intersubject variability in voriconazole serum concentrations has been linked to allelic polymorphisms in the gene encoding the primary metabolic enzyme for voriconazole (CYP2C19) [73, 83]. Patients with polymorphisms conferring poor voriconazole metabolism have higher drug concentrations and are at increased risk for toxicity [21, 84–86]. Conversely, low serum voriconazole levels are observed in patients with polymorphisms resulting in extensive metabolism, and these lower concentrations have been associated with treatment failure [84]. Intersubject variability in voriconazole exposure is more pronounced in certain patient cohorts, suggesting that variables other than CYP2C19 metabolizer status may impact voriconazole drug exposure [85].

Numerous studies have demonstrated a strong relationship between triazole serum concentration and treatment efficacy [87–90]. The itraconazole serum concentration-efficacy relationship has been studied in a variety of disease states, including candidiasis, aspergillosis, cryptococcosis, and coccidioidomycosis. The utility of monitoring has been examined using two treatment strategies, including prophylaxis to prevent the development of an invasive fungal infection, as well as treatment of documented fungal infections. Interpretation of itraconazole serum concentrations is dependent upon the assay method. Serum levels can be measured by either high-performance liquid chromatography (HPLC), which is able to differentiate the active metabolite of itraconazole, hydroxyitraconazole, from itraconazole or bioassays which are not able to make this distinction. The bioassay values are typically 10-fold higher than HPLC values due to the additional activity of the metabolite [91, 92].

The largest study experience with itraconazole therapeutic drug monitoring has been in the setting of antifungal prophylaxis [93–96]. Two independent studies demonstrated that achieving an itraconazole trough concentration greater than 0.25–0.50 μg/mL favored prevention of breakthrough fungal infections [93, 94]. Among the cohort with concentrations below this value, 50% of patients developed an invasive fungal infection while only 30% of those with concentrations above this value developed fungal infections. A third study demonstrated a survival advantage in patients with breakthrough fungal infections associated with higher (>0.5 compared to 0.12 μg/mL) itraconazole trough concentrations [96].

Examination of the role for itraconazole serum concentration montoring in the setting of treatment of documented fungal infections is smaller; however, the relationships are similar. In a group of 21 patients with invasive aspergillosis, the mean itraconazole trough concentration (based upon microbiologic assay) in responders was 6.5 μg/mL compared to only 4.2 μg/mL in nonresponders [88, 91]. The same serum concentration-efficacy relationship was observed in a cohort of 39 patients with nonmeningeal coccidioidomycosis [90]. In another study, investigators examined the impact of itraconazole trough concentrations (determined by HPLC) on treatment outcome in 25 patients with HIV and cryptococcal meningitis. Treatment success was observed in 100% of patients with trough concentrations >1 μg/mL. In contrast, only a partial clinical response was achieved in 66% of those patients with concentrations <1 μg/mL [89]. The largest database used to investigate the relationship between itraconazole serum levels and efficacy was composed of 250 patients with oral candidiasis [97]. The analysis examined the impact of both itraconazole trough concentration (by HPLC) and *Candida* in vitro susceptibility on outcome. The trough concentrations associated with the highest success rate (83%) were >0.5 μg/mL, while only 76% of patients with trough concentrations <0.5 μg/mL responded to therapy. The significantly lower value observed for noninvasive fungal infections suggests that lower exposures may be sufficient for treatment of *Candida* noninvasive infection.

More recently, clinical studies demonstrating the utility of monitoring voriconazole and posaconazole serum concentrations have emerged. Reports from patients receiving voriconazole therapy for invasive aspergillosis demonstrated favorable outcome associated with trough concentrations greater than 1–2 μg/mL [98, 99]. Studies of monitoring in patients receiving voriconazole prophylaxis suggest that serum trough concentrations as low as 0.5 μg/mL may be sufficient [100]. For posaconazole, monitoring was undertaken in an open-label trial for treatment of refractory aspergillosis. In this patient cohort, a statistically and clinically meaningful relationship between posaconazole serum concentration and treatment outcome was observed. Efficacy was greatest in patients with steady-state concentrations >1.25 μg/mL and intermediate in those with concentrations above 0.5 μg/mL [81]. In a randomized trial of antifungal prophylaxis for allogeneic hematopoietic stem cell transplant recipients with GVHD, only five patients receiving posaconazole developed an invasive fungal infection. However, these patients were found to have lower median plasma posaconazole concentrations (Cmax 699 ng/mL, Cav 611 ng/mL) compared to the 241 patients who did not develop infection (Cmax 1,360 ng/ml, Cav 922 ng/mL). With only a small subset of patients diagnosed with an infection, a statistically significant relationship between serum drug level and infection could not be established [101].

Drug Interactions

Clinical use of the antifungal azoles is problematic in some patients because of the potential for interactions with coadministered drugs [32, 66, 102–113]. Thus a patient's concomitant medications should be carefully reviewed for potential drug interactions prior to start and discontinuation of triazole therapy. These interactions can be broadly categorized in two major types: those that result in decreased or, less commonly, increased serum concentrations of the azoles, and those interactions in which the azoles produce increased plasma concentrations and/or clinical effect of another agent. Because several of the interactions pose sufficient risk, coadministration is not recommended. Specific interactions reported with individual azoles are provided in Table 2.

The most commonly encountered interaction is due to a CYP450 interaction resulting in an increase in the concentration of the coadministered medication [105, 114]. Each of the triazoles is a substrate for one or more of the CYP450 isoenzymes; however, the individual triazoles vary in their affinity for the various enzymes [115]. This interaction includes fluconazole and posaconazole, which are not significantly metabolized by the CYP450 enzymes but are substrates for the inhibition of CYP450 isoenzymes. Fluconazole is an inhibitor of CYP3A4, CYP2C9, and CYP2C19 [103]. The following drugs should not be administered with fluconazole due to risk of QT prolongation: astemizole, bepridil, cisapride, levomethadyl, mesoridazine, pimozide, ranolazine, terfenadine, thioridazine, or ziprasidone. Fluconazole also increases serum levels of ergot alkaloids, and concomitant use is contraindicated due to risk of toxicity.

Itraconazole is both a substrate and an inhibitor of the CYP450 enzymes, specifically CYP3A4 and CYP2C9 [103]. Itraconazole is the most potent triazole inhibitor of CYP3A4. Coadministration of itraconazole with cisapride, dofetilide, pimozide, terfenadine, levacetylmethadol, or quinidine results in elevated concentrations of these drugs and is contraindicated due to risk of QT prolongation, torsades de pointes, and ventricular arrhythmia [116, 117]. Lovastatin, simvastatin, oral midazolam, triazolam, and ergot alkaloid clearance are also markedly reduced, and coadministration is contraindicated [118]. Itraconazole may expose patients to higher levels of vinca alkaloids, and concomitant use of itraconazole and vincristine in patients with leukemia or lymphoma was associated with increased risk of neurotoxicity, including severe myalgias, arthralgias, paralysis, and paralytic ileus [119, 120].

Voriconazole is both a substrate and an inhibitor of the CYP450 enzymes, specifically CYP2C19, CYP2C9, and CYP3A4 [70, 114, 121]. Similar to the other triazoles, coadministration of voriconazole with astemizole, cisapride, pimozide, quinidine, or terfenadine is contraindicated due to risk of QT prolongation and torsades de pointes. Voriconazole can also substantially increase serum levels of ergot alkaloids, and concomitant use is not recommended.

Although posaconazole is not extensively metabolized by CYP450 enzyme system, it is an inhibitor of the CYP450 3A4 isoenzyme and has the capacity for drug-drug interactions through this mechanism. Posaconazole is not a major substrate or inhibitor of other isoenzymes, including CYP2C8/9, CYP1A2, CYP2D6, or CYP2E1 [122]. In patients taking posaconazole, contraindicated drugs include astemizole, cisapride, dihydroergotamine, ergoloid mesylates, ergonovine, ergotamine, halofantrine, methylergonovine, methysergide, pimozide, quinidine, and terfenadine.

Other CYP450 interactions due to this class of interactions are common but can often be managed by monitoring and dose adjustment of the coadministered medication. For example, interaction with the calcineurin inhibitors in the transplant population is common to all of the triazoles to some degree. Similarly, interaction with warfarin requires enhanced monitoring of the degree of anticoagulation when administered with the azole class of drugs.

Drug interactions that result in decreased concentrations of the azole occur via two primary mechanisms. In the first type, solubilization and subsequent absorption of weakly basic, highly lipophilic azoles is impaired by agents that decrease gastric acidity. The agents affected are ketoconazole, itraconazole capsules, and posaconazole. In situations where ketoconazole, itraconazole capsules, or posaconazole is used in patients receiving antisecretory therapy, administration of the azole with an acidic beverage, e.g., Classic Coca-Cola® or Pepsi®, is recommended [29, 36, 123].

The second mechanism by which serum concentrations of the azole are reduced is via induction or inhibition of azole metabolism by agents that impact hepatic cytochrome P-450 activity [103, 105, 114]. All azoles are affected, although clinical significance of these interactions is least with fluconazole since hepatic metabolism plays only a minor role in clearance of this drug. In contrast, the impact on other agents is substantial and therapeutic failures are possible in patients receiving the other azoles with enzyme-inducing agents [105, 124–129]. Whenever possible, concomitant therapy with azoles and these inducing agents, including phenytoin, carbamezapine, and rifampin, should be avoided [130].

Another mechanism, via which antifungal azoles may increase plasma concentrations and/or the effect of coadministered agents, involves inhibition of P-glycoprotein, an ATP-dependent plasma membrane transporter involved in intestinal absorption, brain penetration, and renal secretion of a number of chemically diverse agents [131]. Of the available azoles, itraconazole, ketoconazole, and posaconazole have the highest potential to interact with P-glycoprotein. Inhibition of this transporter is thought to be the primary mechanism by which itraconazole enhances the neurotoxicity of vincristine [119, 120, 132, 133] and decreases renal clearance (increases serum concentration) of digoxin [115, 134, 135]. Further investigation is necessary to determine the extent to which the newer triazole derivatives interact with P-glycoprotein.

Table 2 Drug interactions involving antifungal azoles

Effect of interaction	Fluconazole	Itraconazole	Voriconazole	Posaconazole
Decreased absorption of azoles		Antacids- aluminum carbonate (basic), aluminum hydroxide, aluminum phosphate, calcium, dihydroxyaluminum aminoacetate, dihydroxyaluminum sodium carbonate, magaldrate, magnesium carbonate, magnesium hydroxide, magnesium trisilicate, sodium bicarbonate H2-blockers-cimetidine, famotidine, nizatidine, ranitidine, roxatidine Proton pump inhibitors-esomeprazole, lansoprazole, omeprazole, pantoprazole, rabeprazole		H2-blockers-cimetidine Proton pump inhibitors-esomeprazole, lansoprazole, omeprazole, pantoprazole, rabeprazole
Decreased plasma concentration of azole due to metabolism	Antibiotics- rifampin, rifapentine	Antibiotics-isoniazid, rifabutin, rifampin, rifapentine Antiepileptics-carbamazepine, fosphenytoin, phenytoin Antiretrovirals-darunavir, didanosine, efavirenz, etravirine, nevirapine Barbiturates-phenobarbital	Antibiotics- rifabutin, rifampin, rifapentine Antiepileptics-carbamazepine, fosphenytoin, phenytoin Antiretrovirals-amprenavir, darunavir, delavirdine, efavirenz, nevirapine, ritonavir, tipranavir Barbiturates-alfuzosin, aprobarbital, butabarbital, eterobarb, heptabarbital, hexobarbital, mephobarbital, pentobarbital, phenobarbital, secobarbital	Antibiotics-rifabutin, rifampin, rifapentine Antiepileptics-phenytoin
Increased plasma concentration of azole due to coadministered drug		Antibiotics-clarithromycin Antiretrovirals-amprenavir, darunavir, fosamprenavir, lopinavir, ritonavir	Antiretrovirals-delavirdine, etravirine, fosamprenavir, nelfinavir, nevirapine, saquinavir, tipranavir Oral contraceptives- ethinyl estradiol, norethindrone Proton pump inhibitor – omeprazole	
Increased plasma concentration of coadministered drug	Aldosterone antagonists-eplerenone Anesthetics-enflurane, halothane, isoflurane Antianginal-ranolazine Antiarrhythmics-acecainide, ajmaline, amiodarone, aprindine, azimilide, bretylium, disopyramide, flecainide, hydroquinidine, ibutilide, lorcainide, pirmenol, prajmaline, procainamide, propafenone quinidine, sematilide, sotalol, tedisamil	Aldosterone antagonists-eplerenone Alpha-adrenergic blocker-alfuzosin Antianginal- ranolazine Antiarrhythmics-digoxin, disopyramide, dofetilide, quinidine Antibiotics-clarithromycin, erythromycin, telithromycin, trimetrexate Anticholingergic-oxybutynin	Alpha-adrenergic blockers-alfuzosin Antianginal-ranolazine Antiarrhythmics-quinidine Antibiotics-clarithromycin, erythromycin, rifabutin Anticoagulants-acenocoumarol, dicumarol, phenprocoumon, warfarin	Antiarrhythmics-quinidine Antibiotics- rifabutin Antiepileptics-phenytoin Antimalarials-halofantrine Antipsychotics-pimozide Antiretrovirals-etravirine Antihistamine-astemizole(off market), terfenadine (off market)

Antibiotics-clarithromycin, erythromycin, gemifloxacin, levofloxacin, nitrofurantoin, rifabutin, spiramycin, sulfamethoxazole, telithromycin, trimethoprim, trimetrexate(?) Anticoagulants- acenocoumarol, anisindione, dicumarol, phenindione, phenprocoumon, warfarin Antidepressants-amitriptyline, amoxapine, desipramine, dibenzepin, doxepin, fluoxetine, imipramine, nortriptyline, trimipramine Antiemetic-dolasetron, droperidol, prochlorperazine Antiepileptics-carbamazepine, fosphenytoin, phenytoin Antihistamines- astemizole, terfenadine Antimalarials-chloroquine, halofantrine, mefloquine Antineoplastic agents-arsenic trioxide, ixabepilone, tretinoin Antiprotozoal-pentamidine Antipsychotics-amisulpride, chlorpromazine, haloperidol, mesoridazine, pimozide, quetiapine, risperidone, sertindole, sultopride, thioridazine, trifluoperazine, ziprasidone, zotepine Antiretrovirals-atevirdine, etravirine, nevirapine, tipranavir, zidovudine Antiviral-foscarnet Benzodiazepines-alprazolam, midazolam, triazolam Calcium channel blockers-amlodipine, bepridil, felodipine, isradipine, lidoflazine, nicardipine, nifedipine	Anticoagulants- acenocoumarol, anisindione, dicumarol, phenindione, phenprocoumon, warfarin Antidepressants-buspirone, trazodone Antidiarrheal agents-loperamide Antiemetic-aprepitant Antihistamines-astemizole, terfenadine Antimalarials-halofantrine Antineoplastic agents-bexarotene, busulfan, docetaxel, erlotinib, gefitinib, imatinib, ixabepilone, lapatinib, nilotinib, sunitinib, vinblastine, vincamine, vincristine, vincristine liposome, vindesine, vinorelbine Antiparasitic-praziquantel Antipsychotics-aripiprazole, pimozide, quetiapine, risperidone Antiretrovirals- amprenavir, darunavir, etravirine, fosamprenavir, indinavir, maraviroc, saquinavir Benzodiazepines- alprazolam, diazepam, midazolam, triazolam Calcium channel blockers-amlodipine, felodipine, isradipine, nicardipine, nifedipine, nimodipine, verapamil Calcimimetic-cinacalcet Calcitriol analog- paricalcitol Corticosteroids- betamethasone, budesonide, corticotropin, cosyntropin, deflazacort, dexamethasone, fludrocortisone, fluocortolone, hydrocortisone, methylprednisolone, paramethasone, prednisolone, prednisone, triamcinolone Endothelin receptor antagonists-ambrisentan, bosentan Ergot alkaloids- dihydroergotamine, ergoloid mesylates, ergonovine, ergotamine, methylergonovine, methysergide Glucose lowering agents-repaglinide Immunosuppressants-cyclosporine, sirolimus, tacrolimus, temsirolimus Lipid-lowering agents- atorvastatin, cerivastatin, lovastatin, rosuvastatin, simvistatin Muscarinic receptor antagonist-darifenacin	Antiepileptics-fosphenytoin, phenytoin Antineoplastic agents-erlotinib, imatinib, ixabepilone, lapatinib, nilotinib, vinblastine, vincristine, vincristine liposome, vinorelbine, sunitinib, temsirolimus, tretinoin Antipsychotics-pimozide Antiretrovirals-amprenavir, atazanavir, delavirdine, efavirenz, etravirine, fosamprenavir, maraviroc, nelfinavir, nevirapine, saquinavir, tipranavir Antihistamines- astemizole, terfenadine Benzodiazepines-alprazolam, midazolam, triazolam Calcium channel blockers-amlodipine, diltiazem, felodipine, lercanidipine, nifedipine, nisoldipine, nitrendipine, verapamil Calcimimetic-cinacalcet Calcitriol analog-paricalcitol Ergot alkaloids-dihydroergotamine, ergoloid mesylates, ergonovine, ergotamine, methylergonovine, methysergide Proton pump inhibitors-esomeprazole, omeprazole Immunosuppressants-cyclosporine, sirolimus, tacrolimus Opiods- alfentanil, methadone	Antiarrhythmics-quinidine Antibiotics- rifabutin Antiepileptics-phenytoin Antimalarials-halofantrine Antipsychotics-pimozide Antiretrovirals-etravirine Antihistamine-astemizole(off market), terfenadine (off market) Benzodiazepines-midazolam Calcium channel blockers-amlodipine, diltiazem, felodipine, lercanidipine, nifedipine, nisoldipine, nitrendipine, verapamil Ergot alkaloids-dihydroergotamine, ergoloid mesylates, ergonovine, ergotamine, methylergonovine, methysergide Immunosuppressants-cyclosporine, sirolimus, tacrolimus Serotonic receptor antagonists-cisapride (off market) Statins-atorvastatin, lovastatin, simvistatin

(continued)

Table 2 (continued)

Effect of interaction	Fluconazole	Itraconazole	Voriconazole	Posaconazole
	Corticosteroids-prednisone COX2-inhibitors-celecoxib, valdecoxib Endothelin receptor antagonist-bosentan Ergot alkaloids- dihydroergotamine, ergoloid mesylates, ergonovine, ergotamine, methylergonovine, methysergide Immunosuppressants-cyclosporine, sirolimus, tacrolimus Lipid-lowering agents- atorvastatin, cerivastatin, fluvastatin, lovastatin, probucol, rosuvastatin, simvistatin Melatonin receptor agonists- ramelteon Opiods- alfentanil, fentanyl, levomethadyl, methadone Oral contraceptives- ethinyl estradiol, etonogestrel, levonorgestrel, mestranol, norelgestromin, norethindrone, norgestrel Peptides-octreotide, vasopressin Sedatives-chloral hydrate Serotonic receptor antagonists-cisapride Sulfonylureas-glimepiride, glipizide, glyburide, tolbutamide Triptans-eletriptan, zolmitriptan	Opiods- alfentanil, fentanyl, levomethadyl, mifepristone Oral contraceptives and hormonal replacement-estrogens, estradiol, estriol, estrone, estropipate, eszopiclone Phosphodiesterase inhibitors- cilostazol, sildenafil, tadalafil, vardenafil Serotonic receptor antagonists-cisapride Stimulants-modafinil Triptans- almotriptan, eletriptan Vasopressin receptor antagonists-conivaptan	Oral contraceptives- ethinyl estradiol, norethindrone Serotonic receptor antagonists-cisapride Statins-atorvastatin, cerivastatin, lovastatin, simvistatin Sulfonylureas-glipizide, glyburide, tolbutamide Triptans-eletriptan	Vinca alkaloids-vinblastine, vincristine, vincristine liposome, vinorelbine

Spectrum of Activity

As a class, the azoles possess a broad spectrum of activity that includes most of the fungal pathogens associated with systemic infections (Table 3) [60, 136–162].

Among the *Candida* species, drugs are most active against *C. albicans*, *C. parapsilosis*, *C. tropicalis*, *C. lusitaniae*, and *C. dubliniensis* [163]. With the exception of voriconazole, the triazoles are generally not active against *C. krusei*. Although fluconazole activity has also been demonstrated against some strains of *C. glabrata*, MICs are higher and resistance is common [137, 157, 163]. Few *C. glabrata* isolates that exhibit resistance to fluconazole remain susceptible to second-generation triazoles [164–166].

The entire triazole class also exhibits in vitro activity against *Cryptococcus neoformans* [60, 145, 163, 167–169]. Against the dimorphic fungi, the older azoles ketoconazole and itraconazole have better activity than fluconazole [156]. Voriconazole and posaconazole, the new triazoles, are also quite active against this group of organisms [155, 160].

Fluconazole is the sole triazole that exhibits poor activity against the common moulds or filamentous organisms and only moderate activity against dimorphic fungi. The second-generation triazoles exhibit significantly enhanced in vitro activity against *Aspergillus* species and variable activity against *Scedosporium* species, *Fusarium* species, and the dematiaceous fungi [138, 152, 154, 162, 170–174]. Voriconazole is not active in vitro against Zygomycetes, whereas posaconazole does show promising activity against some Zygomycetes, especially *Rhizopus* species [146, 147, 150, 152, 153].

In vitro Susceptibility Testing

Until recently, in vitro antifungal susceptibility testing has been considered to be of limited clinical value due to lack of a reproducible in vitro susceptibility testing procedure and the apparent poor correlation between in vitro test results and outcomes [175, 176]. In 1997, the National Committee for Clinical Laboratory Standards (NCCLS) published reference guidelines (M27-A Method) for conducting in vitro susceptibility testing of *Candida* species and *Cryptococcus neoformans*. These guidelines have recently been updated to the essentially identical M27-A2 methodology [177]. In addition to specifying conditions for performing the tests, the guidelines also provide antifungal concentration breakpoints for interpreting results of tests with fluconazole, itraconazole, and voriconazole. Breakpoints have not yet been determined for posaconazole.

The information utilized in the development of these guidelines includes MIC distribution data as well as pharmacokinetic and pharmacodynamic studies from animal models and patients [97]. Animal data using a murine candidiasis model have shown that treatment outcomes for triazole antifungals are associated with a drug concentration relative to the MIC or AUC/MIC ratio of 25 [178–180]. Clinical studies with fluconazole from 1,295 patients with either oropharyngeal candidiasis or invasive candidiasis provided a dataset allowing pharmacodynamic analysis. Considering the fluconazole dose and the *Candida* species MICs, the AUC/MIC associated with efficacy was similarly near a value of 25. Analysis supported the following MIC breakpoints for fluconazole and *Candida* species: susceptible (S), ≤8 μg/mL; susceptible dose-dependent (SDD), 16–32 μg/mL; and resistant (R), ≥64 μg/mL. The dose-dependent category was determined using a higher dosage of fluconazole. A significantly lower clinical success rate was seen for patients with resistant isolates (42%) compared to those with susceptible (85%) or susceptible dose-dependent isolates (67%). Based on this dataset, isolates of *Candida* species with an MIC <8 μg/mL are considered susceptible to fluconazole and isolates with a MIC >32 μg/mL are considered resistant. Fluconazole MICs of 16–32 μg/mL are reported as susceptible dose-dependent (S-DD), implying that positive outcomes are more likely with higher dosages. Several published clinical observations in both mucosal and invasive candidiasis have corroborated these reports [181, 182].

A similar approach was taken for development of breakpoints for itraconazole, although the data available for analysis were more limited. Clinical studies evaluated in this process included data for 316 HIV-infected patients with oropharyngeal candidiasis enrolled in four trials investigating the efficacy of itraconazole oral solution. Outcome relative to itraconazole MIC was investigated [97]. The combined data supported the following MIC breakpoints for itraconazole and *Candida* species: susceptible (S), ≤0.125 μg/mL; susceptible dose-dependent (SDD), 0.25–5 μg/mL; and resistant (R), ≥1 μg/mL. The dose-dependent category was based upon therapeutic drug monitoring and an itraconazole plasma concentration cutoff of 0.5 μg/mL. For isolates with MICs 0.25–0.5 μg/mL, 76% of patients with itraconazole levels of >0.5 μg/mL responded to therapy while only 50% of those with serum concentrations of <0.5 μg/mL received benefit. However, for isolates with MICs≤0.125 μg/mL, success rates were achieved in approximately 80% of patients regardless of itraconazole plasma concentrations.

More recently these principles have been applied for the development of *Candida* species breakpoints for voriconazole. Outcomes from 249 patients enrolled in six phase III voriconazole trials were correlated with the MICs of infecting

Table 3 Spectrum of activity of antifungal azoles against selected pathogenic fungi

	Fluconazole	Itraconazole	Voriconazole	Posaconazole
	MIC 90% [a] (μg/mL)	MIC 90%[a] (μg/mL)	MIC 90%[a] (μg/mL)	MIC 90%[a] (μg/mL)
Candida spp.				
C. albicans	0.5–2 ++	0.12–0.25 ++	0.015–0.06 ++	0.03–0.06 ++
C. glabrata	32–> 128 –/+	2–8 –/+	1–2 –/+	2–4 –/+
C. parapsilosis	2–4 ++	0.25–0.5 ++	0.06–0.12 ++	0.12–0.25 ++
C. tropicalis	2–4 ++	0.5 ++	0.12–0.25 ++	0.25 ++
C. dubliniensis	0.5–32 +	0.25–0.5 ++	0.03 ++	0.06–0.12 ++
C. krusei	64–> 128 –	1 –/+	0.5–1 ++	0.5–1 ++
C. lusitaniae	2–4 ++	0.25–2 ++	0.015–0.06 ++	0.12–0.25 ++
C. guilliermondii	8–32 +	4 –/+	0.25–0.5 ++	0.5–1 +
C. famata	16 –/+	1 –/+	0.12 ++	1 +
C. rugosa			0.12	0.25 +
C. neoformans	8 ++	0.5 ++	0.12 ++	0.5 ++
B. dermatitidis	4–32 +	0.25–2 ++	0.25 ++	0.12 ++
H. capsulatum	2–32 +	0.06–1 ++	0.25–1 ++	0.25–2 ++
Coccidioides spp.	2–64 +	0.25–1 ++	0.25–0.5 ++	0.25–1 ++
S. schenckii	>64 –	0.5–4 ++	4–16 –	1–2 +
P. brasiliensis		0.06 ++		0.12 ++
Aspergillus				
A. fumigatus	–	0.5–2 +	0.25–0.5 ++	0.5 ++
A. flavus	–	0.5–1 +	1 ++	0.5 ++
A. niger	–	0.5–2 +	1–2 ++	0.5–1 ++
A. versicolor	–	2 +	1 ++	1 ++
A. terreus	–	0.25–0.5 +	0.25–1 ++	0.25 ++
A. nidulans	–	0.25–0.5 +	8–>8 –	
Fusarium spp.	>64 –	>8–>16 –	>8–>64 +	8–32 +
Rhizopus spp.	>64 –	1–32 –/+	8–>64 –	1–8 +
Mucor spp.	>64 –	>8–32 –	8–>64 –	2–16 +
Rhizomucor spp.	>64 –	0.02–0.25 –/+	16–>64 –	0.016–0.25 ++
Absidia spp.	>64 –	0.25–0.5 +	>8–>64 –	0.12–0.25 ++
Cunninghamella spp.	>64 –	0.12–2 +	>64 –/+	0.03–1 +
Apophysomyces spp.	>64 –	0.03–8 –/+	2 +	0.03–4 +
Paecilomyces spp.	16–>64 –	4–>8 –	0.25 +	2 +
Cladophialophora spp.	16–64 –	0.12–16 –/+		0.25 +
Fonsecaea pedrosoi	16–64 –	0.25 +1–4 +	2 +	
Pseudallescheria spp.	4–64 –	1–4 +		1–2 +
Scedosporium spp.				
S. apiospermum	16–>16 –	2-32-/+	0.25–5 +	1–2 +
S. prolificans	>16 –	>16–>32 –	4–	32+
Penicillium spp.	–	2 +	1–2 +	0.016–1 ++
Bipolaris spp.	–	0.25 +		0.12 ++
Exophilia spp.	–	0.5–1 +		0.5 ++
Phialophora spp.	–			
Wangiella spp.	–	0.12 +		
Alternaria spp.	–	1 +		0.25 ++
Dactylaria sp.	–	0.5 +		
Trichoderma sp.	–	>8 –		

+, Moderate activity in vitro; ++, excellent activity in vitro, –, no clinical useful activity, –/+, minimal activity in vitro

[a]MIC 90% = MIC at which 90% of isolates were inhibited

Candida isolates [183]. The data supported the following MIC breakpoints for voriconazole and *Candida* species: susceptible (S), ≤1 μg/mL; susceptible dose–dependent (SDD), 2 μg/mL; and resistant (R), ≥4 μg/mL. When correlated with clinical outcome, isolates with MICs of >2 μg/mL were associated with lower clinical success than isolates with MIC <1 μg/mL (43% vs 74%).

Standards for performing susceptibility tests with filamentous fungi have also been approved (NCCLS document M38-P), but studies to determine the correlation with clinical outcomes are ongoing. For a more detailed discussion of in vitro susceptibility testing of fungi, see Chap. 1.

Drug Resistance

Two types of resistance to azoles have been described. Primary or "intrinsic" resistance results from the natural interaction between an organism and the antifungal agent and is independent of previous drug exposure [184]. The most notable example of intrinsic resistance involving azoles is the universal resistance to fluconazole among isolates of *C. krusei*. Since primary resistance is usually predictable and based on fungal species, it rarely presents a problem in patient management if clinicians are aware of the differences in susceptibility to the azoles for the organism(s) causing the infection. The more problematic clinical issue related to secondary resistance is the selection of resistant organisms during azole therapy. The development of resistance can involve selection of a less susceptible species or the emergence of a resistant clone within a fungal species. For example, the emergence of *C. krusei* or *C. glabrata* during fluconazole prophylaxis or therapy for *C. albicans* is now a well-recognized example of the former in patients receiving antifungal prophylaxis [185–187]. The second phenomenon is currently less common, but was more frequent in the pre-HAART era in HIV-infected patients and continues to be seen occasionally in other immunosuppressed patients after organ transplantation or chemotherapy [187–196]. Increases in the frequency of isolation of resistant *Candida* species have been attributed to both host immune deficits and the extensive use of triazoles in a specific institution or local geographic region. Clinicians should be aware of location-specific resistance frequencies when selecting empirical antifungal therapy.

Extensive laboratory investigation with *Candida* species has revealed several mechanisms to explain the azole resistance phenotype [197–206]. Common mechanisms include alteration or overexpression of the fungal target enzyme (C-14α demethylase) of azole drugs, extrusion of drug from fungal cells, and reduction or loss of function of Δ5,6 desaturase, thereby preventing intracellular accumulation of toxic 14-methoxysterols. Of these mechanisms, extrusion of the azole via activation of energy-dependent drug-efflux pumps is thought to the most common and clinically relevant. Two families of multidrug efflux pumps have been identified in clinical isolates: the major facilitators, which are encoded by the MDR1 gene, and the ATP-binding cassette transporters (ABC), which are expressed by CDR1 and CDR2 genes in *Candida* species. All azoles are substrates for ABC efflux pumps, but current data suggest that only fluconazole is a substrate for the major facilitator transport.

With few exceptions, resistance to one drug in the azole class is predictive of reduced susceptibility to the other drugs in the class. A study of 157 fluconazole-resistant (MIC >64 μg/mL) *Candida* isolates showed that 71% were also resistant to itraconazole (MIC >1 μg/mL) as well [165, 166]. More recently, Pfaller et al. examined azole susceptibility of over 13,000 *Candida* strains and identified a strong correlation between fluconazole resistance and voriconazole resistance ($r=0.93$). Although MICs for voriconazole were 16- to 32-fold lower than those for fluconazole, [166] fluconazole MICs of <32 μg/mL correlated well with susceptibility to voriconazole and has been proposed as a surrogate marker for voriconazole susceptibility. This trend in cross-resistance is present for all *Candida* species and azoles with the exception of *C. krusei*. The majority of fluconazole-resistant *C. krusei* strains remain susceptible to voriconazole (98%).

Acquired resistance to itraconazole has been reported in *Aspergillus fumigatus* isolates from patients receiving prolonged azole treatment. The most frequently described mechanisms of resistance for *A. fumigatus* include various point mutations in CYP51A, the gene encoding 14-alpha demethylase [207–210]. Upregulation of efflux pumps (MDR3, MDR4 and atrF) has also been shown to play a role in itraconazole resistance in vitro [211, 212]. More recently *Aspergillus* infections in Europe (up to 10%) with primary resistance to all second-generation triazoles have been reported. It is hypothesized that resistance developed in the environment associated with agricultural antifungal use [213, 214]. The significance of these observations in other geographic regions remains unclear.

Adverse Effects

The clinical attractiveness of the antifungal azoles is due in part to their low potential for serious adverse effects (Table 4), especially compared with polyene agents (nystatin and amphotericin B). The most common patient complaints about azole drugs are directed at the GI tract and consist primarily of anorexia, nausea, vomiting, diarrhea, and abdominal pain [215]. These side effects appear most common with itraconazole [216].

Table 4 Adverse effects of currently available antifungal azoles

	Fluconazole	Itraconazole	Voriconazole	Posaconazole
Gastrointestinal tract	Anorexia, nausea, vomiting	Anorexia, nausea, vomiting	Anorexia, nausea, vomiting	Anorexia, nausea, vomiting
Skin	Rash	Rash	Rash, photosensitivity	Rash
Liver	Hepatitis[a]	Hepatitis[a]	Hepatitis[a]	?
Cardiac	QT prolongation	QT prolongation	QT prolongation	QT prolongation
Other	Alopecia, teratogenicity	Hypokalemia, pedal edema, hypertension, heart failure, teratogenicity	Visual disturbances, encephalopathy teratogenicity	

[a]Usually asymptomatic elevations of transaminases, but liver failure can occur

Fortunately, rates of discontinuation due to GI side effects range from only 1–6% when daily dosages are 400 mg or lower [86, 217]. Another shared adverse effect is the potential of antifungal azoles to cause disturbances in hepatic function [99, 218]. All available azoles may reversibly increase transaminase levels; therefore, baseline and periodic monitoring of hepatic enzymes is warranted in any patient receiving an azole for more than a few days [1, 219]. Rare instances of severe, and sometimes fatal, hepatic failure associated with ketoconazole, fluconazole, itraconazole, and voriconazole indicate practitioners should be more vigilant in monitoring hepatic function in patients receiving these agents [220]. A third common side effect of the azoles is development of a generalized erythematous rash, with or without pruritus [221]. More severe cutaneous reactions, such as Stevens-Johnson syndrome and toxic epidermal necrolysis, have been associated with voriconazole and fluconazole, typically in patients with serious underlying disease who are also receiving other medications. Voriconazole has also been associated with photosensitivity-induced erythema/desquamation of exposed skin and blistering of lips. Therefore, patients should be instructed to avoid strong, direct sunlight while receiving voriconazole. Rarely, cardiac events, including prolongation of the QT interval, have been reported, usually in the setting of another interacting drug [116, 117, 222]. Finally, the triazole class should be avoided in pregnant and nursing mothers due to the risk of teratogenicity. Case reports have linked fluconazole exposure during pregnancy to congenital birth defects [223]. Reports of infants included description of craniofacial, skeletal, and cardiac anomalies following fluconazole administration to mothers being treated for coccidioidomycosis. Similar findings have been reported with the other triazoles in animal studies. The triazole class is an FDA pregnancy category C and should not be given to a pregnant woman unless the potential benefit justifies the risk.

In addition to these common, shared adverse effects, each of the commercially available azoles is associated with unique reactions that merit physician awareness. Most notable among these are: endocrine disturbances secondary to ketoconazole, reversible alopecia with fluconazole, negative inotropic effects leading rarely to congestive heart failure associated with itraconazole, and reversible neurologic symptoms ascribed to high serum concentrations of voriconazole [221, 224–227]. All of these effects are dose-related and are usually reversible after discontinuation of the azole. For most practitioners, the most likely unique azole-specific side effect that will be encountered in clinical practice is visual disturbance with voriconazole [2]. Approximately 30% of subjects receiving this azole experience altered visual perception, blurred vision, and/or photopsia. Fortunately, these effects are mild, transient, and appear to be fully reversible after discontinuation of therapy. Onset is commonly within 30 min after administration, and duration is typically 30 min or less [221]. Patients receiving voriconazole should be warned about these visual effects and the potential hazards of driving or operating equipment. The mechanism of this voriconazole-associated visual disturbance is unknown; no permanent sequelae have been reported.

Clinical Indications

Candidiasis

For an in-depth discussion of the treatment approaches, including use of azole drugs, for the various *Candida* syndromes, see Chap. 11, Candidiasis.

The advent of the AIDS epidemic in the early 1980s brought new focus to the management of oropharyngeal candidiasis (OPC). Physicians quickly recognized that many patients with OPC failed therapy with topical agents, including nystatin swish and swallow, clotrimazole troches, and oral amphotericin B [228, 229]. Consequently, much attention shifted to evaluation of the efficacy and safety of oral azoles, especially fluconazole and itraconazole, for treatment of OPC.

Numerous treatment trials have investigated the efficacy of fluconazole for treatment of these infections. Fluconazole has been shown to be effective for treatment of mucosal candidiasis in HIV-infected patients in randomized studies. A comparative trial involving 334 HIV-positive patients with oral candidiasis observed similar efficacy for fluconazole (100 mg daily for 14 days) and clotrimazole (10 mg 5 times daily). Clinical success rates of >90% were documented for both treatment groups, but fluconazole was more successful in mycologic eradication (65% vs 48%) and provided longer relief of symptoms [229]. Another study compared fluconazole (3 mg/kg PO daily) to combination therapy with itraconazole (3 mg/kg PO daily) and flucytosine (100 mg/kg PO daily) for treatment of esophageal candidiasis in 85 HIV-infected patients [230]. This double-blind, placebo-controlled trial found fluconazole to be as effective as combination therapy [230].

Additional studies have shown that the clinical responses of OPC are excellent for all of the triazoles [17, 228, 231–233]. Several multicenter, randomized trials have compared the efficacy of fluconazole and itraconazole oral solution for the treatment of oral and esophageal candidiasis in immunosuppressed patients [233–235]. For the most part, itraconazole does not offer significant advantage over fluconazole for uncomplicated disease, but has been shown to be useful in fluconazole-refractory cases [232, 236]. Among itraconazole trials, higher success rates have been observed for the itraconazole oral solution than itraconazole capsules [233, 234, 237, 238].

In the mid 1990s, concerns developed about the emergence of *Candida* species, particularly *C. albicans*, that were resistant to the azole drugs, especially fluconazole, in patients with low CD4 cell counts (<100/μL) and those receiving prolonged courses of azoles [191–193]. In such patients with recurrent or fluconazole-resistant OPC, alternative treatment strategies have evolved, including high-dose fluconazole (400–800 mg daily); switching to another azole, e.g., itraconazole oral solution, [236] voriconazole, [239] or posaconazole [231]; or switching to another class of drug, e.g., a polyene or an echinocandin. The most commonly recommended alternative is itraconazole solution. To date, the incidence of fluconazole-resistant *Candida* species causing OPC appears to have leveled off in the 5% range. Fluconazole is approved by the FDA for treatment of oral and esophageal candidiasis. The current 2009 Infectious Diseases Society of America (IDSA) guidelines recommend fluconazole as first-line therapy for treatment of esophageal candidiasis and moderate-to-severe cases of OPC [15]. For patients with recurrent disease requiring suppressive therapy, fluconazole (200 mg 3×/week) is the regimen of choice. Fluconazole is also recommended for treatment of chronic mucocutaneous candidiasis.

Esophageal candidiasis, regardless of the host, cannot be successfully treated with a topical agent, such as nystatin or clotrimazole. The efficacy of each of the available triazoles has been examined in randomized trials and has demonstrated equivalent efficacy. The drug of initial choice for esophageal candidiasis remains fluconazole based on the rationale used in OPC drug choice. The recommended doses are fluconazole tablet or suspension, 100–400 mg/day for 14–21 days [234, 240, 241]. Itraconazole solution, voriconazole, and posaconazole are typically reserved for fluconazole refractory disease [242–244]. For example, in a open-label trial enrolling 100 HIV-infected patients with OPC or esophageal candidiasis refractory to previous azole therapy, posaconazole (400 mg twice daily for 3 months) was successful in 86% of patients [242]. In those few patients who fail azole therapy, treatment with intravenous amphotericin B or an echinocandin is warranted.

Topical azole drugs, such as clotrimazole or miconazole, or nonazole topical agents, such as nystatin or boric acid, have long been associated with high rates of success as therapy for *Candida* vaginitis, especially in immunocompetent patients with infrequent episodes. However, these topical agents are messy, inconvenient to use, and not always effective. Increasingly, women are utilizing short-course, oral azole therapy for treatment of *Candida* vaginitis. Oral fluconazole and itraconazole are both highly effective [245–247]. The 2009 IDSA guidelines recommend either oral fluconazole or topical agents as first-line agents for treatment of uncomplicated vaginal candidiasis in nonpregnant women [15]. Single-dose fluconazole (150 mg) has been shown effective for >80% of patients with uncomplicated vaginal candidiasis. Comparable efficacy has also been demonstrated for itraconazole. A meta-analysis examined comparative trials of the efficacy and safety of itraconazole and fluconazole for the treatment of uncomplicated acute vaginal and vulvovaginal candidiasis. Data from six randomized trials, including a total of 1,092 nonpregnant women, found no difference in clinical or mycologic cure or adverse events [248].

For complicated vulvovaginal candidiasis, based on severity of symptoms or in an immunocompromised host, a regimen of fluconazole, 150 mg every 72 h for three doses, has been shown to be superior to single-dose therapy [249]. A multiple-dose regimen is also recommended for patients infected with *C. glabrata.* For patients with recurring disease (>4 episodes in 1 year), 10–14 days of induction therapy with a topical or oral azole, followed by fluconazole 150 mg weekly for 6–12 months has been shown to be effective [250]. A placebo-controlled, randomized trial examined the efficacy of fluconazole, 150 mg weekly, for preventing relapse in 387 patients with recurrent vaginal candidiasis. Significantly more patients receiving weekly fluconazole remained disease-free at 6, 9, and 12 months (91%, 73%, and 43%) compared to placebo-treated patients (36%, 28%, and 22%). Weekly fluconazole therapy was safe and did not appear to promote emergence of less susceptible *Candida* species.

Asymptomatic colonization of the bladder by *Candida* species in a patient with an indwelling Foley catheter is common but rarely requires treatment [251]. In such a patient, treatment will not typically eradicate *Candida* from the bladder as long as the catheter remains in place. Within a few days after stopping therapy, the urine will again become colonized with *Candida* [252]. For those occasional patients who have symptomatic *Candida* cystitis and no indwelling catheter, fluconazole is the azole of choice and an effective therapy, owing to the high concentration of active drug in the urine [253, 254] (Table 1). Most recent guidelines recommend treatment of asymptomatic candiduria in patients at high risk for developing invasive infection, including neutropenic patients, low-birth-weight neonates, and patients undergoing urologic procedures [15].

Candida onychomycosis, a less frequent occurrence than dermatophyte onychomycosis and frequently associated with *Candida* paronychia, is most effectively treated with an oral azole, either itraconazole or fluconazole. Most patients are treated with itraconazole, utilizing a so-called "pulse regimen," 1 week per month for 3 months or a daily regimen for 3 months [56, 255, 256]. Fluconazole is also administered in a variant of the itraconazole pulse regimen [257, 258]. Both drugs are associated with remission rates in the 60% range and both are well tolerated. Griseofulvin, frequently used in the past to treat dermatophyte onychomycosis, is not active in vitro against *Candida* species.

Among the various forms of systemic or invasive candidiasis, the syndrome of candidemia is the most common and lends itself to comparative clinical trials for evaluation of management strategies. In several trials, amphotericin B and fluconazole were the two comparators. Three of the trials were randomized multicenter studies in nonneutropenic patients; among these, two were nonblinded [259, 260] and one was blinded [261]. The fourth study was a prospective observational trial in nonneutropenic patients, [262] and the fifth study was a matched cohort trial in cancer patients (including a few patients with neutropenia) [263].

Several important findings emerged from these trials. First, in all trials fluconazole was associated with less toxicity than amphotericin B, irrespective of the different doses of study drugs. Second, the success rates were comparable in the two randomized trials that used similar doses of fluconazole, 400 mg/day, and amphotericin B, 0.5–0.6 mg/day [259, 260] and in the matched cohort study [263]. Third, significant differences were observed in two measures of outcome only in the blinded trial, which compared combination amphotericin B and high-dose fluconazole, 800 mg/day, to high-dose fluconazole alone, with success rates of 69% and 56%, respectively, and persistent candidemia rates of 6% and 17%, respectively [261]. The 6% rate of persistent candidemia for the combination treatment arm was lower than the rates of persistent candidemia for all treatment arms in the prior studies. Also of note in this study, the baseline APACHE II scores were higher in the fluconazole alone treatment group. While the mortality rates in both treatment groups were similar, the toxicity rate was significantly higher in the combination treatment arm. Fourth, in this same study, the combination of amphotericin B and fluconazole was not microbiologically antagonistic compared to fluconazole alone. Fifth, in all studies, removal of vascular catheters reduced time to clearance of the candidemia [264].

The collective results of these five trials establish that fluconazole and amphotericin B are equally effective therapies for candidemia, especially in nonneutropenic patients, and fluconazole is better tolerated and less toxic than amphotericin B. Combination fluconazole and amphotericin B may have a role in selected patients with candidemia, e.g., critically ill and neutropenic patients.

Fluconazole has been compared to the echinocandin anidulafungin for treatment of invasive candidiasis. Anidulafungin was found to be at least as effective as fluconazole for treatment of invasive candidiasis [265]. Success rates after 10 days of therapy were 76% for anidulafungin (200 mg IV on day 1, then 100 mg IV daily) and 60% for fluconazole (800 mg IV on day 1, then 400 mg IV daily). At 6-week follow-up, success rates (fluconazole 44%, anidulafungin 56%) and mortality rates (fluconazole 31%, anidulafungin 23%) did not differ significantly between the two groups. The efficacy of other FDA-approved echinocandins, caspofungin and micafungin, have also been demonstrated efficacious in treatment of candidemia, but were not compared to a triazole regimen.

Voriconazole has also been studied in the setting of candidemia [266]. In a randomized, multicenter trial, voriconazole was compared to a regimen of amphotericin B followed by fluconazole for treatment of invasive candidiasis. Twelve weeks after the end of therapy, successful clinical outcome was observed for 41% of patients in each group, and voriconazole met noninferiority criteria. Median time to blood culture negativity and mortality were also similar between the two study groups.

Fluconazole (400 mg daily oral or IV) is recommended by the 2009 IDSA treatment guidelines as an initial therapy option for invasive candidiasis with the exception of patients who are critically ill, neutropenic, or at risk for fluconazole-resistant isolates due to recent azole exposure [15]. Patients in these high-risk cohorts should receive an echinocandin or an amphotericin B formulation as initial therapy. The basis for these recommendations includes lack of study in neutropenic patients, theoretical concern about use of an inhibitory compared to a fungicidal drug in severe illness, and reduced activity against *Candida* species, such as *C. glabrata* and *C. krusei*, which has been observed in some cohorts following fluconazole prophylaxis. Fluconazole is also commonly used to transition to oral therapy following initial echinocandin or amphotericin therapy if the isolate is susceptible and the patient is clinically stable. The role of voriconazole for candidemia has not been clearly defined but appears to be limited to step-down therapy for the small subset of *C. glabrata* that are resistant to fluconazole but susceptible to voriconazole or for *C. krusei*. Itraconazole and posaconazole have not been similarly studied and at this time appear to have a limited role for invasive candidiasis.

Fluconazole and voriconazole have been used successfully for other forms of systemic or invasive candidiasis, including endophthalmitis, peritonitis, bone/joint disease, hepatosplenic disease, renal parenchymal disease, and endocarditis.

Cryptococcosis

Azole drugs have greatly impacted the management of cryptococcosis over the past several years. While amphotericin B and flucytosine remain key drugs for this disease, fluconazole and, to a lesser extent, itraconazole, have a definite role, especially in the management of AIDS-associated cryptococcosis. Cryptococcal meningitis is the most common form of fungal meningitis in both normal and immunocompromised hosts. Moreover, fluconazole is the most attractive of the available azoles for therapy of fungal meningitis because of its excellent penetration into the CSF (Table1). Although the measurable concentrations in CSF of itraconazole are low, this drug does show moderate efficacy in treatment of cryptococcal meningitis [89, 267].

Fluconazole and itraconazole have been used as treatment approaches for different clinical manifestations of cryptococcosis; however, most of the experience has been in therapy of cryptococcal meningitis. Many authorities agree that optimal primary therapy consists of two parts: an induction regimen for 2–3 weeks with combination amphotericin B and flucytosine, followed by a consolidation regimen for 8–10 weeks with an azole, preferably fluconazole [268]. The definitive study in AIDS patients of this treatment approach showed the following: (1) after 2 weeks of induction therapy, CSF cultures were negative in 60% of patients who received the combination regimen versus 51% of patients who received amphotericin B alone ($p=0.06$); (2) at the conclusion of the 10-week induction/consolidation treatment regimen, clinical responses were similar – 68% in the fluconazole-treated patients and 70% in the itraconazole-treated patients; (3) CSF cultures were negative in 72% of patients in the fluconazole group, and 60% of the itraconazole group [269]. Although this important study was performed in AIDS patients, the results have been extrapolated to the management of cryptococcal meningitis in non-AIDS patients.

Fluconazole has also been explored in primary therapy of cryptococcal meningitis in a randomized comparison with amphotericin B [270]. Microbiologic success was not significantly different for patients receiving fluconazole (34%) and those treated with amphotericin B (40%). However, the mortality rate within the first 2 weeks was higher in the fluconazole treatment group (15% vs 8%). In addition, the median length of time for CSF clearance was longer in patients receiving fluconazole (64 vs 42 days). Considering the trend of increased risk of early death and increased time for CSF sterilization in fluconazole-treated patients, amphotericin B is recommended for most serious infections.

More recently, the combination of fluconazole and amphotericin B therapy has been investigated for induction therapy in HIV-associated cryptococcal meningitis [271]. Patients were randomized to amphotericin B (0.7 mg/kg), amphotericin B plus fluconazole (400 mg/day), or amphotericin B and high-dose fluconazole (800 mg/day). The combinations were found to be safe and antagonism was not observed. The high-dose combination was more effective at the early treatment end point (14 days), and a difference in favor of this combination was similarly observed at later study periods (42 and 72 days). The results are encouraging and suggest a possible role for the combination of amphotericin B and high-dose fluconazole. This induction regimen may be particularly useful in developing countries where flucytosine and toxicity monitoring availability are limited.

The potential role of voriconazole in the treatment of refractory cryptococcosis has been limited to open-label, salvage trials [272]. Of the 18 patients in one trial with refractory cryptococcosis, 39% responded to voriconazole treatment. Study with posaconazole has been limited to animal model investigation.

Another important indication for fluconazole relates to maintenance therapy in AIDS patients with cryptococcal meningitis. Once primary therapy is completed and successful, maintenance therapy is required to prevent relapse, which occurs in approximately 15% of patients [273]. Two large randomized trials demonstrated the efficacy of fluconazole in this setting. An initial trial compared oral fluconazole, 200 mg daily, to intravenous amphotericin B, 1 mg/kg/week. The relapse rate in the fluconazole-treated group was only 2% versus 18% in the amphotericin B–treated group [274]. A subsequent trial compared two azoles, fluconazole, 200 mg daily, versus itraconazole, 200 mg daily. Again fluconazole was superior, showing a 4% relapse rate compared with a 23% relapse rate in the itraconazole group [275]. Accordingly, fluconazole is the recommended maintenance therapy in AIDS patients who have successfully completed primary therapy for cryptococcal meningitis [268]. Recent evidence supports discontinuation of maintenance therapy in patients who have no symptoms of cryptococcosis and have achieved immune reconstitution with HAART therapy [276].

Azole therapy, especially fluconazole, has also been utilized for nonmeningeal forms of cryptococcosis, including pulmonary disease, bone disease, skin disease, and isolated cryptococcemia, in AIDS and non-AIDS patients [89, 277, 278]. For a more detailed discussion about azole therapy of cryptococcosis, the reader is referred to the 2010 IDSA consensus guidelines [268]. These guidelines recommend fluconazole for treatment of mild-to-moderate pulmonary disease (200–400 mg daily for 6–12 months). For HIV-positive patients and other immunocompromised patients, fluconazole may also be administered for life-long suppression or for the duration of immunosuppression at a dose of 200–400 mg daily.

Endemic Mycoses (Blastomycosis, Coccidioidomycosis, Histoplasmosis, Penicilliosis, Paracoccidioidomycosis, and Sporotrichosis)

The endemic mycoses, as a rule, tend to be indolent illnesses. However, each can cause life-threatening meningitis and disseminated disease. In addition, these same endemic mycoses are opportunistic in nature and associated with more serious disease in immunocompromised hosts, such as HIV/AIDS patients, transplant recipients, and those receiving corticosteroid therapy. Since the introduction of ketoconazole in 1981, the older oral antifungal azoles have played an important role in the therapy of the endemic mycoses. For those patients with serious life-threatening endemic fungal diseases, amphotericin B formulation is usually given as an initial therapy; after the patient is stabilized, an azole drug is usually employed. Here, data on azole treatment of each mycosis are summarized briefly.

Both ketoconazole and itraconazole are highly effective in the majority of patients with blastomycosis. Early on, several studies established the efficacy (70–100%) and relative safety of ketoconazole [279, 280]. Subsequently, a large open-label study demonstrated similar efficacy (90–95% of patients) with itraconazole and fewer adverse events compared with ketoconazole. The dose of itraconazole is lower, 200–400 mg daily, compared to ketoconazole, 400–800 mg daily. Fluconazole is less active in vitro against *Blastomyces dermatitidis*. Several open-label trials have investigated the utility of fluconazole for treatment of blastomycosis. While the results demonstrated efficacy, the rate of response was lower than that observed in similar studies with itraconazole and higher daily doses of fluconazole (400–800 mg/day) were required for efficacy [281, 282]. Voriconazole, the newest triazole, is active in vitro [156] and in animals, but use of this drug has been limited to case series. However, reported successes from these observations were encouraging and suggest a potential role for voriconazole in patients intolerant of itraconazole [283]. The 2008 IDSA guidelines recommend amphotericin B and itraconazole as first-line agents for treatment of blastomycosis, depending on the severity of the infection [284]. This change was not made as requested on first edit [280, 284].

Over the years, coccidioidomycosis has been considered one of the most difficult to treat systemic mycoses. Formerly, intravenous amphotericin B was the mainstay of therapy. Nowadays, itraconazole and fluconazole are the principal antifungal drugs for this disease, owing in large part to their efficacy, ease of administration by either the oral or intravenous routes, and relatively low toxicity profiles [285–289] when compared to amphotericin B.

A large, comparative trial of itraconazole and fluconazole in patients with progressive, nonmeningeal coccidioidomycosis confirmed the efficacy of these drugs [219]. Cure or improvement was achieved in 63% (61/97) of itraconazole recipients and in 50% (47/94) of fluconazole recipients (absolute difference, 13%, 95% CI, –2 to 28). In addition, itraconazole tended to be more effective in patients with coccidioidal skeletal disease. Both drugs were well tolerated. Serious adverse events occurred in 6% of itraconazole patients and 8% of fluconazole patients. While initial studies with oral ketoconazole demonstrated moderate efficacy, the high daily doses (400–800 mg) to achieve efficacy were poorly tolerated [290, 291]. In addition, ketoconazole, because of its poor penetration into CSF, is not recommended for coccidioidal meningitis [292]. Voriconazole has good in vitro activity against *C. immitis* [156] and good penetration into CSF, but there is minimal clinical experience with this newer triazole drug in coccidioidomycosis. However, the utility of posaconazole for treatment of chronic coccidioidomycosis has been recently explored in two open-label trials [293, 294]. One trial enrolled 20 patients with nonmeningeal disseminated or chronic pulmonary coccidioidomycosis to receive 400 or 800 mg of posaconazole daily [294]. At 24 weeks, 85% of patients received benefit, and the drug was well tolerated with a median duration of therapy of 173 days. A similar trial investigated the utility of posaconazole (400 mg BID) in a small group of patients with chronic pulmonary or disseminated coccidioidomycosis refractory to conventional therapy [293]. After 1 month of therapy, 73% of patients experienced a partial or complete clinical response. IDSA consensus guidelines emphasize the important role of the antifungal azoles in the management of coccidioidomycosis and indicate that both itraconazole and fluconazole provide attractive options as initial therapy for most patients with this disease [295–297]. Fluconazole is the treatment of choice for patients with coccidioidal meningitis and must be continued for life in most patients [288, 296, 297].

Azole drugs have also significantly altered the approach to therapy of histoplasmosis. Formerly, amphotericin B was the treatment of choice for this disease, with clinical response rates ranging from 57% to 100% in patients with chronic pulmonary disease and 71–88% in patients with disseminated disease. However, amphotericin B was poorly tolerated. Ketoconazole was the first azole drug to prove effective in patients with both forms of histoplasmosis, but relapse rates were high and drug-associated toxicity was problematic [298, 299]. Later studies with itraconazole established this azole as the treatment of choice, initially in non-HIV-infected patients and subsequently in AIDS patients with disseminated histoplasmosis [279, 300–304]. Itraconazole is clearly more effective than ketoconazole in AIDS-associated histoplasmosis. Utilizing a regimen of a loading dose of 600 mg daily for 3 days, followed by a daily dose of 400 mg, itraconazole was effective in 85% (50 of 59) of patients with AIDS-associated indolent disseminated disease [303]. In a second study, maintenance therapy with itraconazole, 200 mg daily, prevented relapse of histoplasmosis in 85% of AIDS patients [304]. Fluconazole is a less effective therapy for histoplasmosis than either ketoconazole or itraconazole, [305, 306] as is the case with blastomycosis and coccidioidomycosis. Voriconazole and posaconazole show good in vitro activity against *H. capsulatum*, [156] but limited data from human studies are available. Small numbers of patients with pulmonary or disseminated histoplasmosis refractory or intolerant to conventional therapy have been treated with either posaconazole, 800 mg daily, or voriconazole, 200 mg twice daily, as salvage therapy [283, 307]. Most patients were intolerant of amphotericin B due to elevated creatinine or electrolyte disturbance. Both new triazoles were well tolerated, and treatment success was observed in the majority of patients.

Consensus 2007 guidelines by the IDSA indicate that itraconazole remains the first choice of therapy for the majority of non-AIDS patients with chronic indolent forms of histoplasmosis; ketoconazole is an acceptable alternative and less expensive [308]. For most AIDS patients with disseminated histoplasmosis, itraconazole is the drug of choice for both primary and maintenance therapy. For patients with serious life-threatening pulmonary or disseminated histoplasmosis, a lipid formulation of amphotericin B is the preferred initial treatment.

The therapy of paracoccidioidomycosis, which is highly endemic in selected areas of Mexico and Central and South America, has also benefited from the advent of azole drugs. For years, sulfonamides and amphotericin B were the mainstays of treatment for this chronic, multiorgan mycosis. Studies with ketoconazole, 200–400 mg daily, showed high efficacy rates, 85–95%, but prolonged duration of therapy was required [298, 309]. Subsequent studies with itraconazole, 50–100 mg daily, showed even higher efficacy rates, 90–95%, with duration of therapy in the 6-month range [302, 310]. Both drugs, at the doses employed, are generally well tolerated. Limited data suggest that fluconazole might be effective [287].

In vitro activity of voriconazole against *P. brasiliensis* has been shown, but limited clinical experience in humans has been reported. One open-label randomized comparative study of 53 patients found voriconazole as effective as itraconazole. Complete or partial response was observed in 87% of patients receiving voriconazole 200 mg twice daily and 94% of those treated with itraconazole 100 mg twice daily [311]. Authorities agree that itraconazole is the azole drug of choice for paracoccidioidomycosis on the basis of its superior efficacy, low daily dose, low frequency of adverse events, and relatively short duration of therapy [312].

Itraconazole has replaced saturated solution of potassium iodide (SSKI) as the drug of choice for lymphocutaneous sporotrichosis [313]. Several open-label trials have shown superior efficacy of itraconazole, 100–200 mg daily for 3–6 months with response rates ranging from 80% to 100% in various disease forms, and fewer side effects of this azole compared with SSKI [314–316]. Previous experiences with ketoconazole as treatment for sporotrichosis were disappointing [299, 317]. Similarly, fluconazole at high doses, 400–800 mg daily, was only moderately effective [287, 318]. Itraconazole is recommended in the 2007 IDSA guidelines for treatment of sprorotrichosis [319]. For cutaneous and lymphocutaneous disease, therapy with 200 mg daily should be given for at least 2–4 weeks after all lesions have resolved, which is usually for a total of 3–6 months. Higher doses (200 mg twice daily) can be used if the patient does not respond to lower doses. For patients with osteoarticular and pulmonary sporotrichosis, the higher dose itraconazole, 200 mg twice daily, is recommended for at least 12 months. Although itraconazole has become the treatment of choice for most patients with sporotrichosis, primary therapy with amphotericin B should be initiated in those rare patients with disseminated or severe pulmonary sporotrichosis [313].

Finally, recent studies have demonstrated the efficacy of azole therapy, namely itraconazole, for patients with disseminated penicilliosis. This opportunistic mycosis, which is endemic in Southeast Asia, especially northern Thailand, has been a significant cause of morbidity and mortality in HIV/AIDS patients in that geographic area. While both amphotericin B and itraconazole have been utilized as primary therapy of penicilliosis in these patients, data indicate that combination therapy with amphotericin B and itraconazole is more effective primary therapy than either drug alone [320]. After completion of successful primary therapy, maintenance therapy is required and itraconazole (200 mg/day), the drug of choice, is associated with a very low rate of relapse [321]. Moreover, in Thailand, where the incidences of penicilliosis, cryptococcosis and histoplasmosis are high, primary prophylaxis with itraconazole is significantly effective [322].

No large clinical trials have evaluated ketoconazole and fluconazole as therapy or prevention of penicilliosis. An open-label salvage trial of voriconazole was conducted in 11 HIV-positive patients with systemic *Penicillium marneffei* infections [272, 323]. Two patients discontinued therapy prematurely due to adverse events. Of the 9 remaining patients, 8 patients received benefit from voriconazole, including 5 patients who responded completely to therapy. This relatively high response rate suggests that the role of voriconazole in treatment of refractory *P. marneffei* infections should be further explored.

Mould Diseases

Moulds have emerged as an important group of pathogens in compromised hosts, especially heart and lung transplant recipients, AIDS patients, and patients with neutropenia secondary to chemotherapy or bone marrow transplantation. Whereas *Aspergillus* species remain the most common opportunistic mould organisms, other opportunistic moulds are increasingly recognized, including *Fusarium* species, *Scedosporium apiospermum*, the asexual form of *Pseudallescheria boydii*, *Scedosporium prolificans*, Zygomycetes, and dematiaceous fungi such as *Alternaria* species, *Bipolaris* species, and *Cladophialophora* species. Among the older azoles, only itraconazole exhibits moderately good in vitro activity against *Aspergillus* species, *F. solani*, *S. apiospermum*, and some dematiaceous fungi (Table 3). By contrast, the newer triazoles have more promising in vitro activity against these same mould organisms. Of note, neither itraconazole nor voriconazole show significant activity against Zygomycetes. However, posaconazole has activity against several Zygomycetes.

Invasive aspergillosis is notoriously refractory to treatment, especially in the face of persistent immunocompromise, such as persistent neutropenia or prolonged high-dose corticosteroid therapy. Until fairly recently, the standard therapy for invasive aspergillosis has been amphotericin B deoxycholate, although responses are suboptimal (less than 40%) [324] and toxicity is common at the doses required for efficacy. Less toxic treatment approaches were developed including lipid formulations of amphotericin B and itraconazole (both oral and intravenous formulations) without significant improvement in outcome. Several studies have evaluated itraconazole therapy of invasive aspergillosis and reported cure/improvement rates ranging from 39% to 63% [325–327]. However, several problems with itraconazole are encountered, including patient intolerance of the drug, inadequate absorption of the oral capsules, and significant itraconazole–drug interactions. The current IDSA guidelines recommend itraconazole as salvage therapy in patients refractory to or intolerant of voriconazole and amphotericin B formulations [324]. In addition, some authorities have advocated itraconazole as a consolidation regimen following initial therapy with amphotericin B.

Current first-line therapy is based on results of a randomized multicenter trial that compared voriconazole versus amphotericin B as primary therapy of invasive aspergillosis [328]. Successful outcomes (complete or partial responses) were noted in 53% of the voriconazole group and 32% of the amphotericin B group (absolute difference 21%, 95% CI, 10.4–32.9). The survival rate was also higher in the voriconazole group, 71% versus 58%, and voriconazole-treated patients had significantly fewer severe drug-related adverse events. An earlier open, noncomparative multicenter trial of voriconazole therapy for invasive aspergillosis in immunocompromised patients showed similarly good outcomes [329]. Taken together, the results of these two studies were extremely encouraging and suggest that voriconazole should replace amphotericin B as the "gold standard" therapy for invasive aspergillosis. The recently published IDSA guidelines recommend voriconazole as the first-line choice for the primary treatment of invasive aspergillosis [324].

Fewer data are available examining the utility of posaconazole for invasive aspergillosis; however, the results are promising. Two open-label salvage trials in patients with invasive aspergillosis observed response rates of 40–42% in patients failing other antifungal therapy [81, 330]; however, posaconazole has not been directly compared to other agents as primary therapy for aspergillosis. Based on available trial data, posaconazole was approved by the EMEA as salvage therapy for patients with invasive aspergillosis who are refractory to amphotericin B or itraconazole.

Another promising approach to treatment of invasive aspergillosis is to combine a new triazole and an echinocandin. Numerous in vitro and in animal models demonstrate enhanced efficacy with a variety of antifungal combinations [331, 332]. Several case–control studies suggest the utility of the combination concept. A retrospective review of 47 patients who had failed amphotericin B as primary therapy of aspergillosis examined the response to salvage therapy with either voriconazole alone or voriconazole and caspofungin in combination [333]. Kaplan-Meier analysis identified higher overall survival rates 3 months after diagnosis in patients who had received combination therapy with voriconazole and caspofungin. A prospective, randomized clinical trial of a combination of voriconazole and anidulafungin is underway.

With regard to azole therapy of non-*Aspergillus* mould diseases, experience until recently has been primarily with itraconazole. This older triazole has mainly been used to treat phaeohyphomycosis [334, 335] and scedosporiosis [336]. However, no large trials have been performed, reports consist of only one to a few cases, and only moderate success has been observed. Given the promising in vitro activity of voriconazole against many non-*Aspergillus* moulds, this new triazole has been given to a number of patients on a compassionate basis, and encouraging results have been noted. One multicenter, open-label trial examined the efficacy of voriconazole in the treatment of 273 patients with emerging or refractory fungal infections [272]. Of the 11 patients with fusariosis, 5 patients had complete or partial response. Of the 10 patients with scedosporiosis, 3 patients received benefit from voriconazole. A second salvage trial in pediatric patients with these emerging mould infections suggested similar efficacy [20]. These results are encouraging considering that patients with fusariosis and scedosporiosis generally respond poorly to treatment with amphotericin B and the diseases are associated with high mortality rates. However, among *Scedosporium* species, activity appears limited to *S. apiospermum*, with reduced activity against *S. prolificans*, for which there are very limited treatment options. These findings led to FDA approval of voriconazole for the treatment of *Scedosporium* species and *Fusarium* species in patients with intolerance of other antifungal therapy or refractory disease.

Posaconazole has also been examined in open-label series for emerging mould infections. In a retrospective analysis of three open-label trials for fusariosis, 21 patients refractory to or intolerant of at least 7 days of conventional therapy received posaconazole as salvage therapy [337]; 48% of patients experienced a complete or partial response. Two additional open-label trials studied posaconazole in patients with zygomycosis, refractory to or intolerant of conventional therapy with remarkable success rates of 60% and 80%, respectively [338, 339]. Posaconazole has joined amphotericin B as the sole treatment option for the Zygomycetes group of fungi.

Febrile Neutropenia

Both itraconazole and voriconazole have been evaluated as empirical therapy in persistently febrile neutropenic patients, a population at high risk for invasive mould diseases. Both triazoles were compared to polyene therapy and found to be similarly effective. In the itraconazole open-label trial against amphotericin B there were no differences in breakthrough fungal infections or mortality rates. However, itraconazole was associated with fewer adverse effects than amphotericin B [340]. Voriconazole was compared to liposomal amphotericin B [341]. The composite success rates were 26% for the voriconazole-treated patients and 31% for the liposomal amphotericin B–treated patients (95% CI for difference in percentages –10.6% to 1.6%). Voriconazole patients experienced fewer breakthrough invasive fungal infections, fewer infusion-related reactions, and less nephrotoxicity. These results led the investigators to conclude that voriconazole is a suitable alternative to amphotericin B formulations for empirical antifungal therapy in persistently neutropenic patients.

Prophylaxis and Empirical Therapy

Azole drugs have been used extensively as prophylaxis in various non-AIDS patient population groups at risk for systemic fungal diseases. These groups include neutropenic patients, bone marrow transplant recipients, selected solid organ (e.g., liver and lung) transplant recipients, and intensive care unit patients.

Fluconazole is recommended by the IDSA for antifungal prophylaxis in bone marrow transplant recipients with neutropenia and patients with chemotherapy-induced neutropenia [15]. The efficacy of fluconazole for prophylaxis of invasive fungal infection in patients undergoing bone marrow transplantation was established in a randomized, double-blind placebo-controlled trial of 300 patients [342]. Patients treated with fluconazole, 400 mg daily, for 75 days after transplantation developed fewer systemic fungal infections (7%) compared to placebo-treated patients (18%). In addition, a mortality benefit was found for fluconazole-treated patients at 110 days, with 52 deaths in the placebo arm compared to 31 deaths in the fluconazole treatment arm.

Other comparative investigations have examined the efficacy of fluconazole or amphotericin B for prevention of fungal infection in patients with hematologic malignancies and neutropenia [343–345]. One randomized trial compared fluconazole (400 mg daily) and amphotericin B (0.5 mg/kg IV 3×/week) antifungal prophylaxis in 71 patients with acute leukemia undergoing remission induction chemotherapy [345]. Proven, probable, or possible fungal infections were diagnosed in 31% of amphotericin B–treated patients and 17% of fluconazole-treated patients. Amphotericin B was tolerated poorly and was more frequently discontinued (42% vs 20%).

Similar studies have investigated the role of itraconazole in these populations. Efficacy was demonstrated in one double-blind randomized, placebo-controlled trial of itraconazole capsules, 100 mg BID, in neutropenic patients with hematologic malignancy or undergoing autologous bone marrow transplantation. The incidence of fungal infection was reduced from 15% in patients receiving placebo to 6% in those administered itraconazole therapy [346]. In a similar patient cohort, the efficacy of itraconazole oral solution, 2.5 mg/kg BID, was confirmed in a randomized, double-blind, placebo-controlled trial [347]. Itraconazole prophylaxis resulted in a reduced rate of proven or suspected deep fungal infection (24% compared to 33%) and fewer episodes of candidemia (0.5% vs 4%). In addition, data from an open-label trial suggested itraconazole prophylaxis may be associated with a decreased mortality rate due to invasive fungal infection in neutropenic patients [348].

The efficacy and safety of fluconazole and itraconazole have also been compared in several trials for prevention of fungal infection in neutropenic patients. A meta-analysis was performed on a subset of five randomized, controlled, comparative trials in this patient population [349]. Although fluconazole prophylaxis resulted in significantly more documented or suspected fungal infections (OR = 1.62), itraconazole was more frequently discontinued due to adverse drug event (OR = 0.27). The study concluded that itraconazole was more effective as antifungal prophylaxis, but fluconazole was much better tolerated.

Fluconazole has been compared to posaconazole for antifungal prophylaxis in two multicenter, randomized trials [23, 24]. Posaconazole was compared to prophylaxis with either fluconazole or itraconazole in 602 neutropenic patients undergoing chemotherapy for acute myelogenous leukemia or myelodysplastic syndrome. Significantly fewer invasive fungal infections were diagnosed in patients receiving posaconazole (2%) compared to those receiving either fluconazole or itraconazole (8%) [23]. Kaplan-Meier analysis also identified significant survival benefit for patients receiving posaconazole. In another large trial in 600 hematopoietic stem cell transplant recipients with severe graft-versus-host disease, prophylaxis with posaconazole was compared to fluconazole [24]. Posaconazole was established as noninferior based on analysis of the primary end point, occurrence of invasive fungal infection (posaconazole 5.3%, fluconazole 9%). A mortality benefit was not observed. Both studies found posaconazole significantly more successful in preventing invasive aspergillosis and similar to fluconazole in preventing candidiasis.

A consensus has not been reached regarding administration of antifungal prophylaxis in ICU patients. The current 2009 IDSA candidiasis guidelines recommend fluconazole for antifungal prophylaxis for high-risk patients only in those adult ICUs reporting a high incidence of invasive candidiasis [15]. Several studies, including two meta-analyses and a multicenter, randomized trial have examined the role of fluconazole prophylaxis in this patient cohort [350–353]. One meta-analysis included four randomized, double-blind trials composed of a total of 626 patients in surgical ICUs. Fluconazole (100–400 mg daily) treatment was found to significantly decrease the rate of fungal infections compared to placebo (OR = 0.44) [350]. However, a significant survival benefit was not identified (OR=0.87). The low rate of candidemia (2.2%) observed in the studies was not impacted by fluconazole administration. A second meta-analysis included trials comparing ketoconazole or fluconazole to placebo [351]. Data from 1226 patients enrolled in nine trials (seven double-blind) were analyzed. Azole prophylaxis was associated with a decreased rate of candidemia (RR = 0.3), lower mortality from candidiasis (RR = 0.25), and lower overall mortality (RR = 0.6).

A recent large, multicenter, randomized trial investigated the efficacy of fluconazole empirical treatment, rather than prophylaxis, in ICU patients with fever despite administration of broad-spectrum antibiotics [352]. Documented invasive candidiasis occurred in 5% of the patients receiving fluconazole (800 mg daily for 14 days) and 9% of placebo recipients. The sum of studies suggests a benefit in a select group of high-risk patients. The optimal strategy to define this group has not yet been identified and remains an area of intense study.

Prophylaxis studies have been undertaken in the preterm neonatal population. Fluconazole has been shown effective and is recommended by the IDSA for antifungal prophylaxis in preterm neonates (<1,000 g) in nurseries with high rates of invasive candidiasis. A multicenter, randomized trial examined the impact of fluconazole for prevention of fungal colonization and infection in 322 preterm neonates weighing less than 1,500 g at birth [354]. Fluconazole was administered every third day for 2 weeks, then every other day until day 30 and decreased the rate of invasive fungal infection. A mortality benefit was not observed.

Another high-risk population for which azole prophylaxis has been considered is certain solid organ transplant recipients, including those with liver, pancreas, and small bowel transplants. The effectiveness of fluconazole and itraconazole oral solution for antifungal prophylaxis was compared in a randomized, controlled trial of 188 liver transplant recipients [355]. The rates of proven invasive fungal infection were similar between patients treated with fluconazole 400 mg daily (3%) and those receiving itraconazole 200 mg BID (7%). The mortality rate was similar in both patient groups (fluconazole 8%, itraconazole 12%), with only one patient dying from fungal infection. The utility of routine use of prophylaxis in this subset of solid organ transplant recipients remains unclear.

Dermatophytosis

Both itraconazole and fluconazole have been examined for treatment of fungal infections of the skin and nails. Itraconazole has been considered superior to fluconazole for most dermatophyte infections and equivalent to or slightly inferior to the allylamine, terbinafine. In open-label studies, itraconazole 100–200 mg daily for approximately 3–6 months achieved clinical response rates of 64–80% and 60–73% in patients with dermatophyte onychomycosis of the fingernails and toenails, respectively [256, 356]. Another open-label dose-ranging comparison trial found itraconazole 200 mg daily to be more effective than 100 mg daily dosing, presumably due to achievement of over five-fold higher itraconazole concentrations in the nails [357].

Itraconazole is lipophilic and keratophilic, with pharmacokinetics ideal for pulse dose therapy. When given in high doses, itraconazole concentrates in the nail bed and remains active for months. Pulse itraconazole therapy (400 mg daily for 1 week per month for 3–4 consecutive months) successfully treated 85–93% of patients with onychomycosis enrolled in open trials [255, 358]. A double-blind, multicenter, randomized trial by Haru et al. of 129 patients with confirmed dermatophyte onychomycosis compared itraconazole pulse therapy (400 mg daily 1 week per month for 3 months) to continuous itraconazole therapy (200 mg daily for 3 months) [359]. Although the clinical response rates favored pulse itraconazole therapy (81%) over continuous therapy (69%) at 12 month follow-up, statistical superiority was not established. Mycologic cure rates were similar between the groups (69% for pulse therapy versus 66% for continuous therapy). The pulse dose therapy regimen is at least as effective as continuous therapy and has the added benefits of decreased systemic drug exposure and lower treatment cost.

Of four trials comparing the efficacy of itraconazole to terbinafine for the treatment of onychomycosis, three of the trials demonstrated superiority of terbinafine. In a multicenter double-blind trial, itraconazole 200 mg daily for 12 weeks was significantly less effective than terbinafine 250 mg daily for the treatment of toenail onychomycosis, with a lower mycologic cure rate (63% vs 81%) [360]. Similar results have been found in additional randomized comparisons [361]. Taken together, these studies demonstrate the superiority of terbinafine in treatment of onychomycosis and suggest itraconazole as a safe and effective alternative.

Open-label studies demonstrated the utility of both fluconazole and itraconazole daily for the treatment of cutanteous dermatophytosis such as tinea pedis, tinea cruris, and tinea corporis, with clinical response rates of 70–96% [362–365]. Trials comparing the two azoles have not been undertaken. However, double-blind, randomized trials comparing itraconazole with terbinafine for treating dermatophytosis have established the superiority of terbinafine based on significantly higher clinical and mycologic cure rates [366].

References

1. Como JA, Dismukes WE. Oral azole drugs as systemic antifungal therapy. N Engl J Med. 1994;330:263–72.
2. Johnson LB, Kauffman CA. Voriconazole: a new triazole antifungal agent. Clin Infect Dis. 2003;36:630–7.
3. Nagappan V, Deresinski S. Reviews of anti-infective agents: posaconazole: a broad-spectrum triazole antifungal agent. Clin Infect Dis. 2007;45:1610–7.
4. Saag MS, Dismukes WE. Azole antifungal agents: emphasis on new triazoles. Antimicrob Agents Chemother. 1988;32:1–8.
5. Willems L, van der Geest R, de Beule K. Itraconazole oral solution and intravenous formulations: a review of pharmacokinetics and pharmacodynamics. J Clin Pharm Ther. 2001;26:159–69.
6. Hostetler JS, Hanson LH, Stevens DA. Effect of cyclodextrin on the pharmacology of antifungal oral azoles. Antimicrob Agents Chemother. 1992;36:477–80.
7. Stevens DA. Itraconazole in cyclodextrin solution. Pharmacotherapy. 1999;19:603–11.
8. Szente L, Szejtli J. Highly soluble cyclodextrin derivatives: chemistry, properties, and trends in development. Adv Drug Deliv Rev. 1999;36:17–28.
9. Vanden Bossche H. Biochemical targets for antifungal azole derivatives: hypothesis on the mode of action. Curr Top Med Mycol. 1985;1:313–51.
10. Munayyer HK, Mann PA, Chau AS, et al. Posaconazole is a potent inhibitor of sterol 14alpha-demethylation in yeasts and molds. Antimicrob Agents Chemother. 2004;48:3690–6.
11. Heimark L, Shipkova P, Greene J, et al. Mechanism of azole antifungal activity as determined by liquid chromatographic/mass spectrometric monitoring of ergosterol biosynthesis. J Mass Spectrom. 2002;37:265–9.
12. Sanati H, Belanger P, Fratti R, Ghannoum M. A new triazole, voriconazole (UK-109, 496), blocks sterol biosynthesis in *Candida albicans* and *Candida krusei*. Antimicrob Agents Chemother. 1997;41:2492–6.
13. Hitchcock CA, Dickinson K, Brown SB, Evans EG, Adams DJ. Interaction of azole antifungal antibiotics with cytochrome P-450-dependent 14 alpha-sterol demethylase purified from *Candida albicans*. Biochem J. 1990;266:475–80.
14. Manavathu EK, Cutright JL, Chandrasekar PH. Organism-dependent fungicidal activities of azoles. Antimicrob Agents Chemother. 1998;42:3018–21.
15. Pappas PG, Kauffman CA, Andes D, et al. Clinical practice guidelines for the management of candidiasis: 2009 update by the Infectious Diseases Society of America. Clin Infect Dis. 2009; 48:503–35.
16. Presterl E, Graninger W. Efficacy and safety of fluconazole in the treatment of systemic fungal infections in pediatric patients. Multicentre Study Group. Eur J Clin Microbiol Infect Dis. 1994;13:347–51.
17. Groll AH, Wood L, Roden M, et al. Safety, pharmacokinetics, and pharmacodynamics of cyclodextrin itraconazole in pediatric patients with oropharyngeal candidiasis. Antimicrob Agents Chemother. 2002;46:2554–63.
18. de Repentigny L, Ratelle J, Leclerc JM, et al. Repeated-dose pharmacokinetics of an oral solution of itraconazole in infants and children. Antimicrob Agents Chemother. 1998;42: 404–8.
19. Abdel-Rahman SM, Jacobs RF, Massarella J, et al. Single-dose pharmacokinetics of intravenous itraconazole and hydroxypropyl-beta-cyclodextrin in infants, children, and adolescents. Antimicrob Agents Chemother. 2007;51:2668–73.
20. Walsh TJ, Lutsar I, Driscoll T, et al. Voriconazole in the treatment of aspergillosis, scedosporiosis and other invasive fungal infections in children. Pediatr Infect Dis J. 2002;21:240–8.
21. Walsh TJ, Karlsson MO, Driscoll T, et al. Pharmacokinetics and safety of intravenous voriconazole in children after single- or multiple-dose administration. Antimicrob Agents Chemother. 2004;48:2166–72.
22. Groll AH, Roilides E, Walsh TJ. Pediatric pharmacology of antifungal agents. Curr Fungal Infect Rep. 2008;2:49–56.

23. Cornely OA, Maertens J, Winston DJ, et al. Posaconazole vs. fluconazole or itraconazole prophylaxis in patients with neutropenia. N Engl J Med. 2007;356:348–59.
24. Ullmann AJ, Lipton JH, Vesole DH, et al. Posaconazole or fluconazole for prophylaxis in severe graft-versus-host disease. N Engl J Med. 2007;356:335–47.
25. Thorpe JE, Baker N, Bromet-Petit M. Effect of oral antacid administration on the pharmacokinetics of oral fluconazole. Antimicrob Agents Chemother. 1990;34:2032–3.
26. Lazar JD, Wilner KD. Drug interactions with fluconazole. Rev Infect Dis. 1990;12 Suppl 3:S327–33.
27. Zimmermann T, Yeates RA, Laufen H, Pfaff G, Wildfeuer A. Influence of concomitant food intake on the oral absorption of two triazole antifungal agents, itraconazole and fluconazole. Eur J Clin Pharmacol. 1994;46:147–50.
28. Dodds Ashley ES, Lewis R, Lewis JS, Martin C, Andes D. Pharmacology of systemic antifungal agents. Clin Infect Dis. 2006;43(S1):S28–39.
29. Lange D, Pavao JH, Wu J, Klausner M. Effect of a cola beverage on the bioavailability of itraconazole in the presence of H2 blockers. J Clin Pharmacol. 1997;37:535–40.
30. Van Peer A, Woestenborghs R, Heykants J, Gasparini R, Gauwenbergh G. The effects of food and dose on the oral systemic availability of itraconazole in healthy subjects. Eur J Clin Pharmacol. 1989;36:423–6.
31. Prentice AG, Glasmacher A. Making sense of itraconazole pharmacokinetics. J Antimicrob Chemother. 2005;56 Suppl 1:i17–22.
32. Purkins L, Wood N, Kleinermans D, Greenhalgh K, Nichols D. Effect of food on the pharmacokinetics of multiple-dose oral voriconazole. Br J Clin Pharmacol. 2003;56 Suppl 1:17–23.
33. Courtney R, Wexler D, Radwanski E, Lim J, Laughlin M. Effect of food on the relative bioavailability of two oral formulations of posaconazole in healthy adults. Br J Clin Pharmacol. 2004;57: 218–22.
34. Barone JA, Koh JG, Bierman RH, et al. Food interaction and steady-state pharmacokinetics of itraconazole capsules in healthy male volunteers. Antimicrob Agents Chemother. 1993;37:778–84.
35. Barone JA, Moskovitz BL, Guarnieri J, et al. Food interaction and steady-state pharmacokinetics of itraconazole oral solution in healthy volunteers. Pharmacotherapy. 1998;18:295–301.
36. Krishna G, Moton A, Ma L, Medlock MM, McLeod J. Pharmacokinetics and absorption of posaconazole oral suspension under various gastric conditions in healthy volunteers. Antimicrob Agents Chemother. 2009;53:958–66.
37. Courtney R, Radwanski E, Lim J, Laughlin M. Pharmacokinetics of posaconazole coadministered with antacid in fasting or nonfasting healthy men. Antimicrob Agents Chemother. 2004;48:804–8.
38. Alffenaar JW, van Assen S, van der Werf TS, Kosterink JG, Uges DR. Omeprazole significantly reduces posaconazole serum trough level. Clin Infect Dis. 2009;48:839.
39. Ezzet F, Wexler D, Courtney R, Krishna G, Lim J, Laughlin M. Oral bioavailability of posaconazole in fasted healthy subjects: comparison between three regimens and basis for clinical dosage recommendations. Clin Pharmacokinet. 2005;44:211–20.
40. Courtney R, Pai S, Laughlin M, Lim J, Batra V. Pharmacokinetics, safety, and tolerability of oral posaconazole administered in single and multiple doses in healthy adults. Antimicrob Agents Chemother. 2003;47:2788–95.
41. Haria M, Bryson HM, Goa KL. Itraconazole. A reappraisal of its pharmacological properties and therapeutic use in the management of superficial fungal infections. Drugs. 1996;51:585–620.
42. Grant SM, Clissold SP. Itraconazole. A review of its pharmacodynamic and pharmacokinetic properties, and therapeutic use in superficial and systemic mycoses. Drugs. 1989;37:310–44.
43. Heykants J, Van Peer A, Lavrijsen K, Meuldermans W, Woestenborghs R, Cauwenbergh G. Pharmacokinetics of oral antifungals and their clinical implications. Br J Clin Pract Suppl. 1990;71:50–6.
44. Heykants J, Van Peer A, Van de Velde V, et al. The clinical pharmacokinetics of itraconazole: an overview. Mycoses. 1989; 32 Suppl 1:67–87.
45. Purkins L, Wood N, Greenhalgh K, Eve MD, Oliver SD, Nichols D. The pharmacokinetics and safety of intravenous voriconazole - a novel wide-spectrum antifungal agent. Br J Clin Pharmacol. 2003;56 Suppl 1:2–9.
46. Purkins L, Wood N, Ghahramani P, Greenhalgh K, Allen MJ, Kleinermans D. Pharmacokinetics and safety of voriconazole following intravenous- to oral-dose escalation regimens. Antimicrob Agents Chemother. 2002;46:2546–53.
47. Poirier JM, Hardy S, Isnard F, Tilleul P, Weissenburger J, Cheymol G. Plasma itraconazole concentrations in patients with neutropenia: advantages of a divided daily dosage regimen. Ther Drug Monit. 1997;19:525–9.
48. Debruyne D. Clinical pharmacokinetics of fluconazole in superficial and systemic mycoses. Clin Pharmacokinet. 1997;3 3:52–77.
49. Thaler F, Bernard B, Tod M, et al. Fluconazole penetration in cerebral parenchyma in humans at steady state. Antimicrob Agents Chemother. 1995;39:1154–6.
50. Walsh TJ, Foulds G, Pizzo PA. Pharmacokinetics and tissue penetration of fluconazole in rabbits. Antimicrob Agents Chemother. 1989;33:467–9.
51. Foulds G, Wajszczuk C, Weidler DJ, Garg DJ, Gibson P. Steady state parenteral kinetics of fluconazole in man. Ann NY Acad Sci. 1988;544:427–30.
52. Shiba K, Saito A, Miyahara T. Safety and pharmacokinetics of single oral and intravenous doses of fluconazole in healthy subjects. Clin Ther. 1990;12:206–15.
53. Houang ET, Chappatte O, Byrne D, Macrae PV, Thorpe JE. Fluconazole levels in plasma and vaginal secretions of patients after a 150-milligram single oral dose and rate of eradication of infection in vaginal candidiasis. Antimicrob Agents Chemother. 1990;34:909–10.
54. Savani DV, Perfect JR, Cobo LM, Durack DT. Penetration of new azole compounds into the eye and efficacy in experimental Candida endophthalmitis. Antimicrob Agents Chemother. 1987;31: 6–10.
55. Larosa E, Cauwenbergh G, Cilli P, Woestenborghs R, Heykants J. Itraconazole pharmacokinetics in the female genital tract: plasma and tissue levels in patients undergoing hysterectomy after a single dose of 200 mg itraconazole. Eur J Obstet Gynecol Reprod Biol. 1986;23:85–9.
56. De Doncker P, Decroix J, Pierard GE, et al. Antifungal pulse therapy for onychomycosis. A pharmacokinetic and pharmacodynamic investigation of monthly cycles of 1-week pulse therapy with itraconazole. Arch Dermatol. 1996;132:34–41.
57. Lutsar I, Roffey S, Troke P. Voriconazole concentrations in the cerebrospinal fluid and brain tissue of guinea pigs and immunocompromised patients. Clin Infect Dis. 2003;37:728–32.
58. Thiel MA, Zinkernagel AS, Burhenne J, Kaufmann C, Haefeli WE. Voriconazole concentration in human aqueous humor and plasma during topical or combined topical and systemic administration for fungal keratitis. Antimicrob Agents Chemother. 2007;51:239–44.
59. Hariprasad SM, Mieler WF, Holz ER, et al. Determination of vitreous, aqueous, and plasma concentration of orally administered voriconazole in humans. Arch Ophthalmol. 2004;122:42–7.
60. Perfect JR, Cox GM, Dodge RK, Schell WA. In vitro and in vivo efficacies of the azole SCH56592 against *Cryptococcus neoformans*. Antimicrob Agents Chemother. 1996;40:1910–3.
61. Pitisuttithum P, Negroni R, Graybill JR, et al. Activity of posaconazole in the treatment of central nervous system fungal infections. J Antimicrob Chemother. 2005;56:745–55.

62. Cousin L, Berre ML, Launay-Vacher V, Izzedine H, Deray G. Dosing guidelines for fluconazole in patients with renal failure. Nephrol Dial Transplant. 2003;18:2227–31.
63. Valtonen M, Tiula E, Neuvonen PJ. Effect of continuous venovenous haemofiltration and haemodiafiltration on the elimination of fluconazole in patients with acute renal failure. J Antimicrob Chemother. 1997;40:695–700.
64. Muhl E. Antimycotic drugs under continuous renal replacement therapy. Mycoses. 2005;48 Suppl 1:56–60.
65. Muhl E, Martens T, Iven H, Rob P, Bruch HP. Influence of continuous veno-venous haemodiafiltration and continuous veno-venous haemofiltration on the pharmacokinetics of fluconazole. Eur J Clin Pharmacol. 2000;56:671–8.
66. Grant SM, Clissold SP. Fluconazole. A review of its pharmacodynamic and pharmacokinetic properties, and therapeutic potential in superficial and systemic mycoses. Drugs. 1990;39:877–916.
67. Nicolau DP, Crowe H, Nightingale CH, Quintiliani R. Effect of continuous arteriovenous hemodiafiltration on the pharmacokinetics of fluconazole. Pharmacotherapy. 1994;14:502–5.
68. Weiss J, Ten Hoevel MM, Burhenne J, et al. CYP2C19 genotype is a major factor contributing to the highly variable pharmacokinetics of voriconazole. J Clin Pharmacol. 2009;49:196–204.
69. Hoffman HL, Ernst EJ, Klepser ME. Novel triazole antifungal agents. Expert Opin Investig Drugs. 2000;9:593–605.
70. Sabo JA, Abdel-Rahman SM. Voriconazole: a new triazole antifungal. Ann Pharmacother. 2000;34:1032–43.
71. Hardin TC, Graybill JR, Fetchick R, Woestenborghs R, Rinaldi MG, Kuhn JG. Pharmacokinetics of itraconazole following oral administration to normal volunteers. Antimicrob Agents Chemother. 1988;32:1310–3.
72. Boelaert J, Schurgers M, Matthys E, et al. Itraconazole pharmacokinetics in patients with renal dysfunction. Antimicrob Agents Chemother. 1988;32:1595–7.
73. Theuretzbacher U, Ihle F, Derendorf H. Pharmacokinetic/pharmacodynamic profile of voriconazole. Clin Pharmacokinet. 2006; 45:649–63.
74. Alffenaar JW, de Vos T, Uges DR, Daenen SM. High voriconazole trough levels in relation to hepatic function: how to adjust the dosage? Br J Clin Pharmacol. 2009;67:262–3.
75. Peng LW, Lien YH. Pharmacokinetics of single, oral-dose voriconazole in peritoneal dialysis patients. Am J Kidney Dis. 2005;45: 162–6.
76. Fuhrmann V, Schenk P, Jaeger W, et al. Pharmacokinetics of voriconazole during continuous venovenous haemodiafiltration. J Antimicrob Chemother. 2007;60:1085–90.
77. Krieter P, Flannery B, Musick T, Gohdes M, Martinho M, Courtney R. Disposition of posaconazole following single-dose oral administration in healthy subjects. Antimicrob Agents Chemother. 2004;48:3543–51.
78. Courtney R, Sansone A, Smith W, et al. Posaconazole pharmacokinetics, safety, and tolerability in subjects with varying degrees of chronic renal disease. J Clin Pharmacol. 2005;45:185–92.
79. Andes D, Pascual A, Marchetti O. Antifungal therapeutic drug monitoring: established and emerging indications. Antimicrob Agents Chemother. 2009;53:24–34.
80. Krishna G, Sansone-Parsons A, Martinho M, Kantesaria B, Pedicone L. Posaconazole plasma concentrations in juvenile patients with invasive fungal infection. Antimicrob Agents Chemother. 2007;51:812–8.
81. Walsh TJ, Raad I, Patterson TF, et al. Treatment of invasive aspergillosis with posaconazole in patients who are refractory to or intolerant of conventional therapy: an externally controlled trial. Clin Infect Dis. 2007;44:2–12.
82. Gubbins PO, Krishna G, Sansone-Parsons A, et al. Pharmacokinetics and safety of oral posaconazole in neutropenic stem cell transplant recipients. Antimicrob Agents Chemother. 2006;50:1993–9.
83. Desta Z, Zhao X, Shin JG, Flockhart DA. Clinical significance of the cytochrome P450 2C19 genetic polymorphism. Clin Pharmacokinet. 2002;41:913–58.
84. Smith J, Safdar N, Knasinski V, et al. Voriconazole therapeutic drug monitoring. Antimicrob Agents Chemother. 2006;50:1570–2.
85. Trifilio S, Ortiz R, Pennick G, et al. Voriconazole therapeutic drug monitoring in allogeneic hematopoietic stem cell transplant recipients. Bone Marrow Transplant. 2005;35:509–13.
86. Boyd AE, Modi S, Howard SJ, Moore CB, Keevil BG, Denning DW. Adverse reactions to voriconazole. Clin Infect Dis. 2004; 39:1241–4.
87. Berenguer J, Ali NM, Allende MC, et al. Itraconazole for experimental pulmonary aspergillosis: comparison with amphotericin B, interaction with cyclosporin A, and correlation between therapeutic response and itraconazole concentrations in plasma. Antimicrob Agents Chemother. 1994;38:1303–8.
88. Denning DW, Tucker RM, Hanson LH, Stevens DA. Treatment of invasive aspergillosis with itraconazole. Am J Med. 1989;86: 791–800.
89. Denning DW, Tucker RM, Hanson LH, Hamilton JR, Stevens DA. Itraconazole therapy for cryptococcal meningitis and cryptococcosis. Arch Intern Med. 1989;149:2301–8.
90. Tucker RM, Denning DW, Arathoon EG, Rinaldi MG, Stevens DA. Itraconazole therapy for nonmeningeal coccidioidomycosis: clinical and laboratory observations. J Am Acad Dermatol. 1990; 23:593–601.
91. Warnock DW, Turner A, Burke J. Comparison of high performance liquid chromatographic and microbiological methods for determination of itraconazole. J Antimicrob Chemother. 1988;21:93–100.
92. Odds FC, Dupont B, Rinaldi MG, Stevens DA, Warnock DW, Woestenborghs R. Bioassays for itraconazole blood levels: an interlaboratory collaborative study. J Antimicrob Chemother. 1999;43:723–7.
93. Boogaerts MA, Verhoef GE, Zachee P, Demuynck H, Verbist L, De Beule K. Antifungal prophylaxis with itraconazole in prolonged neutropenia: correlation with plasma levels. Mycoses. 1989;32 Suppl 1:103–8.
94. Tricot G, Joosten E, Boogaerts MA, Vande Pitte J, Cauwenbergh G. Ketoconazole vs. itraconazole for antifungal prophylaxis in patients with severe granulocytopenia: preliminary results of two nonrandomized studies. Rev Infect Dis. 1987;9 Suppl 1:S94–9.
95. Glasmacher A, Hahn C, Molitor E, Marklein G, Sauerbruch T, Schmidt-Wolf IG. Itraconazole trough concentrations in antifungal prophylaxis with six different dosing regimens using hydroxypropyl-beta-cyclodextrin oral solution or coated-pellet capsules. Mycoses. 1999;42:591–600.
96. Glasmacher A, Hahn C, Leutner C, et al. Breakthrough invasive fungal infections in neutropenic patients after prophylaxis with itraconazole. Mycoses. 1999;42:443–51.
97. Rex JH, Pfaller MA, Galgiani JN, et al. Development of interpretive breakpoints for antifungal susceptibility testing: conceptual framework and analysis of in vitro-in vivo correlation data for fluconazole, itraconazole, and *Candida* infections. Subcommittee on Antifungal Susceptibility Testing of the National Committee for Clinical Laboratory Standards. Clin Infect Dis. 1997;24:235–47.
98. Smith J, Andes D. Therapeutic drug monitoring of antifungals: pharmacokinetic and pharmacodynamic considerations. Ther Drug Monit. 2008;30:167–72.
99. Pascual A, Calandra T, Bolay S, Buclin T, Bille J, Marchetti O. Voriconazole therapeutic drug monitoring in patients with invasive mycoses improves efficacy and safety outcomes. Clin Infect Dis. 2008;46:201–11.
100. Trifilio S, Singhal S, Williams S, et al. Breakthrough fungal infections after allogeneic hematopoietic stem cell transplantation in patients on prophylactic voriconazole. Bone Marrow Transplant. 2007;40:451–6.

101. Krishna G, Martinho M, Chandrasekar P, Ullmann AJ, Patino H. Pharmacokinetics of oral posaconazole in allogeneic hematopoietic stem cell transplant recipients with graft-versus-host disease. Pharmacotherapy. 2007;27:1627–36.
102. Wood N, Tan K, Purkins L, et al. Effect of omeprazole on the steady-state pharmacokinetics of voriconazole. Br J Clin Pharmacol. 2003;56 Suppl 1:56–61.
103. Brüggemann RJM, Alffenaar JC, Blijlevens NMA, et al. Pharmacokinetic drug interactions of azoles. Curr Fungal Infect Rep. 2008;2:20–7.
104. Bruggemann RJ, Alffenaar JW, Blijlevens NM, et al. Clinical relevance of the pharmacokinetic interactions of azole antifungal drugs with other coadministered agents. Clin Infect Dis. 2009;48:1441–58.
105. Lomaestro BM, Piatek MA. Update on drug interactions with azole antifungal agents. Ann Pharmacother. 1998;32:915–28.
106. Piscitelli SC, Gallicano KD. Interactions among drugs for HIV and opportunistic infections. N Engl J Med. 2001;344:984–96.
107. Kuypers DR, Claes K, Evenepoel P, Vanrenterghem Y. Clinically relevant drug interaction between voriconazole and tacrolimus in a primary renal allograft recipient. Transplantation. 2006;81: 1750–2.
108. Marty FM, Lowry CM, Cutler CS, et al. Voriconazole and sirolimus coadministration after allogeneic hematopoietic stem cell transplantation. Biol Blood Marrow Transplant. 2006;12:552–9.
109. Purkins L, Wood N, Kleinermans D, Nichols D. Voriconazole potentiates warfarin-induced prothrombin time prolongation. Br J Clin Pharmacol. 2003;56 Suppl 1:24–9.
110. Purkins L, Wood N, Ghahramani P, Love ER, Eve MD, Fielding A. Coadministration of voriconazole and phenytoin: pharmacokinetic interaction, safety, and toleration. Br J Clin Pharmacol. 2003;56 Suppl 1:37–44.
111. Romero AJ, Le Pogamp P, Nilsson LG, Wood N. Effect of voriconazole on the pharmacokinetics of cyclosporine in renal transplant patients. Clin Pharmacol Ther. 2002;71:226–34.
112. Saari TI, Laine K, Leino K, Valtonen M, Neuvonen PJ, Olkkola KT. Effect of voriconazole on the pharmacokinetics and pharmacodynamics of intravenous and oral midazolam. Clin Pharmacol Ther. 2006;79:362–70.
113. Saari TI, Laine K, Bertilsson L, Neuvonen PJ, Olkkola KT. Voriconazole and fluconazole increase the exposure to oral diazepam. Eur J Clin Pharmacol. 2007;63:941–9.
114. Nivoix Y, Leveque D, Herbrecht R, Koffel JC, Beretz L, Ubeaud-Sequier G. The enzymatic basis of drug-drug interactions with systemic triazole antifungals. Clin Pharmacokinet. 2008;47: 779–92.
115. Albengres E, Le Louet H, Tillement JP. Systemic antifungal agents. Drug interactions of clinical significance. Drug Saf. 1998;18:83–97.
116. Crane JK, Shih HT. Syncope and cardiac arrhythmia due to an interaction between itraconazole and terfenadine. Am J Med. 1993;95:445–6.
117. Pohjola-Sintonen S, Viitasalo M, Toivonene L, Neuvonen P. Torsades de pointes after terfenadine-itraconazole interaction. BMJ (Clin Res Ed). 1993;306:186.
118. Olkkola KT, Backman JT, Neuvonen PJ. Midazolam should be avoided in patients receiving the systemic antimycotics ketoconazole or itraconazole. Clin Pharmacol Ther. 1994;55: 481–5.
119. Bermudez M, Fuster JL, Llinares E, Galera A, Gonzalez C. Itraconazole-related increased vincristine neurotoxicity: case report and review of literature. J Pediatr Hematol Oncol. 2005; 27:389–92.
120. Takahashi N, Kameoka Y, Yamanaka Y, et al. Itraconazole oral solution enhanced vincristine neurotoxicity in five patients with malignant lymphoma. Intern Med. 2008;47:651–3.
121. Jeong S, Nguyen PD, Desta Z. Comprehensive in vitro analysis of voriconazole inhibition of eight cytochrome P450 (CYP) enzymes: major effect on CYPs 2B6, 2C9, 2C19, and 3A. Antimicrob Agents Chemother. 2009;53:541–51.
122. Wexler D, Courtney R, Richards W, Banfield C, Lim J, Laughlin M. Effect of posaconazole on cytochrome P450 enzymes: a randomized, open-label, two-way crossover study. Eur J Pharm Sci. 2004;21:645–53.
123. Johnson MD, Hamilton CD, Drew RH, Sanders LL, Pennick GJ, Perfect JR. A randomized comparative study to determine the effect of omeprazole on the peak serum concentration of itraconazole oral solution. J Antimicrob Chemother. 2003;51:453–7.
124. Krishna G, Parsons A, Kantesaria B, Mant T. Evaluation of the pharmacokinetics of posaconazole and rifabutin following coadministration to healthy men. Curr Med Res Opin. 2007; 23:545–52.
125. Krishna G, Sansone-Parsons A, Kantesaria B. Drug interaction assessment following concomitant administration of posaconazole and phenytoin in healthy men. Curr Med Res Opin. 2007;23:1415–22.
126. Zilly W, Breimer DD, Richter E. Pharmacokinetic interactions with rifampicin. Clin Pharmacokinet. 1977;2:61–70.
127. Jaruratanasirikul S, Sriwiriyajan S. Effect of rifampicin on the pharmacokinetics of itraconazole in normal volunteers and AIDS patients. Eur J Clin Pharmacol. 1998;54:155–8.
128. Drayton J, Dickinson G, Rinaldi MG. Coadministration of rifampin and itraconazole leads to undetectable levels of serum itraconazole. Clin Infect Dis. 1994;18:266.
129. Ducharme MP, Slaughter RL, Warbasse LH, et al. Itraconazole and hydroxyitraconazole serum concentrations are reduced more than tenfold by phenytoin. Clin Pharmacol Ther. 1995;58: 617–24.
130. Tucker RM, Denning DW, Hanson LH, et al. Interaction of azoles with rifampin, phenytoin, and carbamazepine: in vitro and clinical observations. Clin Infect Dis. 1992;14:165–74.
131. Venkatakrishnan K, von Moltke LL, Greenblatt DJ. Effects of the antifungal agents on oxidative drug metabolism: clinical relevance. Clin Pharmacokinet. 2000;38:111–80.
132. Miyama T, Takanaga H, Matsuo H, et al. P-glycoprotein-mediated transport of itraconazole across the blood-brain barrier. Antimicrob Agents Chemother. 1998;42:1738–44.
133. Bohme A, Ganser A, Hoelzer D. Aggravation of vincristine-induced neurotoxicity by itraconazole in the treatment of adult ALL. Ann Hematol. 1995;71:311–2.
134. Kauffman CA, Bagnasco FA. Digoxin toxicity associated with itraconazole therapy. Clin Infect Dis. 1992;15:886–7.
135. Rex J. Itraconazole-digoxin interaction. Ann Intern Med. 1992; 116:525.
136. Pfaller MA, Messer SA, Hollis RJ, et al. In vitro susceptibilities of *Candida* bloodstream isolates to the new triazole antifungal agents BMS-207147, Sch 56592, and voriconazole. Antimicrob Agents Chemother. 1998;42:3242–4.
137. Pfaller MA, Diekema DJ, Gibbs DL, et al. Results from the ARTEMIS DISK Global Antifungal Surveillance study, 1997 to 2005: an 8.5-year analysis of susceptibilities of *Candida* species and other yeast species to fluconazole and voriconazole determined by CLSI standardized disk diffusion testing. J Clin Microbiol. 2007;45:1735–45.
138. Pfaller MA, Messer SA, Hollis RJ, Jones RN. Antifungal activities of posaconazole, ravuconazole, and voriconazole compared to those of itraconazole and amphotericin B against 239 clinical isolates of *Aspergillus* spp. and other filamentous fungi: report from SENTRY Antimicrobial Surveillance Program, 2000. Antimicrob Agents Chemother. 2002;46:1032–7.
139. Ostrosky-Zeichner L, Rex JH, Pappas PG, et al. Antifungal susceptibility survey of 2,000 bloodstream Candida isolates in the

United States. Antimicrob Agents Chemother. 2003;47: 3149–54.
140. Marco F, Pfaller MA, Messer S, Jones RN. In vitro activities of voriconazole (UK-109, 496) and four other antifungal agents against 394 clinical isolates of *Candida* spp. Antimicrob Agents Chemother. 1998;42:161–3.
141. Cuenca-Estrella M, Ruiz-Diez B, Martinez-Suarez JV, Monzon A, Rodriguez-Tudela JL. Comparative in-vitro activity of voriconazole (UK-109, 496) and six other antifungal agents against clinical isolates of *Scedosporium prolificans* and *Scedosporium apiospermum*. J Antimicrob Chemother. 1999;43:149–51.
142. Ramos G, Cuenca-Estrella M, Monzon A, Rodriguez-Tudela JL. In-vitro comparative activity of UR-9825, itraconazole and fluconazole against clinical isolates of *Candida* spp. J Antimicrob Chemother. 1999;44:283–6.
143. Gomez-Lopez A, Garcia-Effron G, Mellado E, Monzon A, Rodriguez-Tudela JL, Cuenca-Estrella M. In vitro activities of three licensed antifungal agents against spanish clinical isolates of *Aspergillus* spp. Antimicrob Agents Chemother. 2003;47: 3085–8.
144. Cuenca-Estrella M, Rodriguez D, Almirante B, et al. In vitro susceptibilities of bloodstream isolates of Candida species to six antifungal agents: results from a population-based active surveillance programme, Barcelona, Spain, 2002–2003. J Antimicrob Chemother. 2005;55:194–9.
145. De Bedout C, Ordonez N, Gomez BL, et al. In vitro antifungal susceptibility of clinical isolates of Cryptococcus neoformans var. neoformans and C. neoformans var. gattii. Rev Iberoam Micol. 1999;16:36–9.
146. Espinel-Ingroff A, Johnson E, Hockey H, Troke P. Activities of voriconazole, itraconazole and amphotericin B *in vitro* against 590 moulds from 323 patients in the voriconazole Phase III clinical studies. J Antimicrob Chemother. 2008;61:616–20.
147. Sun QN, Fothergill AW, McCarthy DI, Rinaldi MG, Graybill JR. In vitro activities of posaconazole, itraconazole, voriconazole, amphotericin B, and fluconazole against 37 clinical isolates of zygomycetes. Antimicrob Agents Chemother. 2002;46:1581–2.
148. McGinnis MR, Nordoff N, Li RK, Pasarell L, Warnock DW. *Sporothrix schenckii* sensitivity to voriconazole, itraconazole and amphotericin B. Med Mycol. 2001;39:369–71.
149. Alvarado-Ramirez E, Torres-Rodriguez JM. In vitro susceptibility of *Sporothrix schenckii* to six antifungal agents determined using three different methods. Antimicrob Agents Chemother. 2007;51:2420–3.
150. Dannaoui E, Meletiadis J, Mouton JW, Meis JF, Verweij PE. In vitro susceptibilities of zygomycetes to conventional and new antifungals. J Antimicrob Chemother. 2003;51:45–52.
151. Paphitou NI, Ostrosky-Zeichner L, Paetznick VL, Rodriguez JR, Chen E, Rex JH. In vitro antifungal susceptibilities of *Trichosporon* species. Antimicrob Agents Chemother. 2002;46:1144–6.
152. Sabatelli F, Patel R, Mann PA, et al. In vitro activities of posaconazole, fluconazole, itraconazole, voriconazole, and amphotericin B against a large collection of clinically important molds and yeasts. Antimicrob Agents Chemother. 2006;50:2009–15.
153. Almyroudis NG, Sutton DA, Fothergill AW, Rinaldi MG, Kusne S. In vitro susceptibilities of 217 clinical isolates of zygomycetes to conventional and new antifungal agents. Antimicrob Agents Chemother. 2007;51:2587–90.
154. Meletiadis J, Meis JF, Mouton JW, Rodriquez-Tudela JL, Donnelly JP, Verweij PE. In vitro activities of new and conventional antifungal agents against clinical *Scedosporium* isolates. Antimicrob Agents Chemother. 2002;46:62–8.
155. Gonzalez GM, Fothergill AW, Sutton DA, Rinaldi MG, Loebenberg D. In vitro activities of new and established triazoles against opportunistic filamentous and dimorphic fungi. Med Mycol. 2005;43:281–4.
156. Li RK, Ciblak MA, Nordoff N, Pasarell L, Warnock DW, McGinnis MR. In vitro activities of voriconazole, itraconazole, and amphotericin B against *Blastomyces dermatitidis*, *Coccidioides immitis*, and *Histoplasma capsulatum*. Antimicrob Agents Chemother. 2000;44:1734–6.
157. Pfaller MA, Messer SA, Hollis RJ, Jones RN, Diekema DJ. In vitro activities of ravuconazole and voriconazole compared with those of four approved systemic antifungal agents against 6, 970 clinical isolates of *Candida* spp. Antimicrob Agents Chemother. 2002;46:1723–7.
158. Espinel-Ingroff A. In vitro fungicidal activities of voriconazole, itraconazole, and amphotericin B against opportunistic moniliaceous and dematiaceous fungi. J Clin Microbiol. 2001;39:954–8.
159. Gonzalez GM, Sutton DA, Thompson E, Tijerina R, Rinaldi MG. In vitro activities of approved and investigational antifungal agents against 44 clinical isolates of basidiomycetous fungi. Antimicrob Agents Chemother. 2001;45:633–5.
160. Espinel-Ingroff A. In vitro activity of the new triazole voriconazole (UK-109, 496) against opportunistic filamentous and dimorphic fungi and common and emerging yeast pathogens. J Clin Microbiol. 1998;36:198–202.
161. Fernandez-Torres B, Vazquez-Veiga H, Llovo X, Pereiro Jr M, Guarro J. In vitro susceptibility to itraconazole, clotrimazole, ketoconazole and terbinafine of 100 isolates of *Trichophyton rubrum*. Chemotherapy. 2000;46:390–4.
162. Carrillo AJ, Guarro J. In vitro activities of four novel triazoles against *Scedosporium* spp. Antimicrob Agents Chemother. 2001;45:2151–3.
163. Pfaller MA, Messer SA, Boyken L, et al. In vitro activities of voriconazole, posaconazole, and fluconazole against 4,169 clinical isolates of *Candida* spp. and *Cryptococcus neoformans* collected during 2001 and 2002 in the ARTEMIS global antifungal surveillance program. Diagn Microbiol Infect Dis. 2004;48:201–5.
164. Panackal AA, Gribskov JL, Staab JF, Kirby KA, Rinaldi M, Marr KA. Clinical significance of azole antifungal drug cross-resistance in *Candida glabrata*. J Clin Microbiol. 2006;44:1740–3.
165. Pfaller MA, Diekema DJ, Messer SA, Hollis RJ, Jones RN. In vitro activities of caspofungin compared with those of fluconazole and itraconazole against 3,959 clinical isolates of *Candida* spp., including 157 fluconazole-resistant isolates. Antimicrob Agents Chemother. 2003;47:1068–71.
166. Pfaller MA, Messer SA, Boyken L, et al. Use of fluconazole as a surrogate marker to predict susceptibility and resistance to voriconazole among 13, 338 clinical isolates of *Candida* spp. Tested by clinical and laboratory standards institute-recommended broth microdilution methods. J Clin Microbiol. 2007;45:70–5.
167. Pfaller MA, Zhang J, Messer SA, et al. In vitro activities of voriconazole, fluconazole, and itraconazole against 566 clinical isolates of *Cryptococcus neoformans* from the United States and Africa. Antimicrob Agents Chemother. 1999;43:169–71.
168. Pfaller MA, Messer SA, Boyken L, et al. Global trends in the antifungal susceptibility of *Cryptococcus neoformans* (1990 to 2004). J Clin Microbiol. 2005;43:2163–7.
169. Gomez-Lopez A, Zaragoza O, Dos Anjos Martins M, Melhem MC, Rodriguez-Tudela JL, Cuenca-Estrella M. In vitro susceptibility of *Cryptococcus gattii* clinical isolates. Clin Microbiol Infect. 2008;14:727–30.
170. Te Dorsthorst DT, Verweij PE, Meis JF, Punt NC, Mouton JW. In vitro interactions between amphotericin B, itraconazole, and flucytosine against 21 clinical *Aspergillus* isolates determined by two drug interaction models. Antimicrob Agents Chemother. 2004;48:2007–13.
171. Espinel-Ingroff A. Comparison of in vitro activities of the new triazole SCH56592 and the echinocandins MK-0991 (L-743, 872) and LY303366 against opportunistic filamentous and dimorphic fungi and yeasts. J Clin Microbiol. 1998;36:2950–6.

172. Diekema DJ, Messer SA, Hollis RJ, Jones RN, Pfaller MA. Activities of caspofungin, itraconazole, posaconazole, ravuconazole, voriconazole, and amphotericin B against 448 recent clinical isolates of filamentous fungi. J Clin Microbiol. 2003;41:3623–6.
173. Cacciapuoti A, Loebenberg D, Corcoran E, et al. In vitro and in vivo activities of SCH 56592 (posaconazole), a new triazole antifungal agent, against *Aspergillus* and *Candida*. Antimicrob Agents Chemother. 2000;44:2017–22.
174. Alastruey-Izquierdo A, Cuenca-Estrella M, Monzon A, Mellado E, Rodriguez-Tudela JL. Antifungal susceptibility profile of clinical *Fusarium* spp. isolates identified by molecular methods. J Antimicrob Chemother. 2008;61:805–9.
175. Anaissie EJ, Karyotakis NC, Hachem R, Dignani MC, Rex JH, Paetznick V. Correlation between in vitro and in vivo activity of antifungal agents against *Candida* species. J Infect Dis. 1994;170:384–9.
176. Graybill JR, Montalbo E, Kirkpatrick WR, Luther MF, Revankar SG, Patterson TF. Fluconazole versus *Candida albicans*: a complex relationship. Antimicrob Agents Chemother. 1998;42:2938–42.
177. NCCLS. Clinical Laboratory Standards Institute. In: Reference method for broth dilution antifungal susceptibility testing Document M27-A2. 2nd ed. Wayne: National Committee for Clinical Laboratory Standards; 2002.
178. Andes D, van Ogtrop M. Characterization and quantitation of the pharmacodynamics of fluconazole in a neutropenic murine disseminated candidiasis infection model. Antimicrob Agents Chemother. 1999;43:2116–20.
179. Andes D. In vivo pharmacodynamics of antifungal drugs in treatment of candidiasis. Antimicrob Agents Chemother. 2003;47:1179–86.
180. Andes D, Marchillo K, Stamstad T, Conklin R. In vivo pharmacokinetics and pharmacodynamics of a new triazole, voriconazole, in a murine candidiasis model. Antimicrob Agents Chemother. 2003;47:3165–9.
181. Baddley JW, Patel M, Bhavnani SM, Moser SA, Andes DR. Association of fluconazole pharmacodynamics with mortality in patients with candidemia. Antimicrob Agents Chemother. 2008;52:3022–8.
182. Rex JH, Pfaller MA, Barry AL, Nelson PW, Webb CD. Antifungal susceptibility testing of isolates from a randomized, multicenter trial of fluconazole versus amphotericin B as treatment of nonneutropenic patients with candidemia. NIAID Mycoses Study Group and the Candidemia Study Group. Antimicrob Agents Chemother. 1995;39:40–4.
183. Pfaller MA, Diekema DJ, Rex JH, et al. Correlation of MIC with outcome for *Candida* species tested against voriconazole: analysis and proposal for interpretive breakpoints. J Clin Microbiol. 2006;44:819–26.
184. White TC, Marr KA, Bowden RA. Clinical, cellular, and molecular factors that contribute to antifungal drug resistance. Clin Microbiol Rev. 1998;11:382–402.
185. Wingard JR. Infections due to resistant *Candida species* in patients with cancer who are receiving chemotherapy. Clin Infect Dis. 1994;19 Suppl 1:S49–53.
186. Wingard JR, Merz WG, Rinaldi MG, Johnson TR, Karp JE, Saral R. Increase in *Candida krusei* infection among patients with bone marrow transplantation and neutropenia treated prophylactically with fluconazole. N Engl J Med. 1991;325:1274–7.
187. Wingard JR, Merz WG, Rinaldi MG, Miller CB, Karp JE, Saral R. Association of *Torulopsis glabrata* infections with fluconazole prophylaxis in neutropenic bone marrow transplant patients. Antimicrob Agents Chemother. 1993;37:1847–9.
188. Baily GG, Perry FM, Denning DW, Mandal BK. Fluconazole-resistant candidosis in an HIV cohort. AIDS (London, England). 1994;8:787–92.
189. Redding S, Smith J, Farinacci G, et al. Resistance of *Candida albicans* to fluconazole during treatment of oropharyngeal candidiasis in a patient with AIDS: documentation by in vitro susceptibility testing and DNA subtype analysis. Clin Infect Dis. 1994;18:240–2.
190. Ruhnke M, Eigler A, Tennagen I, Geiseler B, Engelmann E, Trautmann M. Emergence of fluconazole-resistant strains of *Candida albicans* in patients with recurrent oropharyngeal candidosis and human immunodeficiency virus infection. J Clin Microbiol. 1994;32:2092–8.
191. Maenza JR, Merz WG, Romagnoli MJ, Keruly JC, Moore RD, Gallant JE. Infection due to fluconazole-resistant *Candida* in patients with AIDS: prevalence and microbiology. Clin Infect Dis. 1997;24:28–34.
192. Maenza JR, Keruly JC, Moore RD, Chaisson RE, Merz WG, Gallant JE. Risk factors for fluconazole-resistant candidiasis in human immunodeficiency virus-infected patients. J Infect Dis. 1996;173:219–25.
193. Revankar SG, Kirkpatrick WR, McAtee RK, et al. Detection and significance of fluconazole resistance in oropharyngeal candidiasis in human immunodeficiency virus-infected patients. J Infect Dis. 1996;174:821–7.
194. Martins MD, Lozano-Chiu M, Rex JH. Point prevalence of oropharyngeal carriage of fluconazole-resistant *Candida* in human immunodeficiency virus-infected patients. Clin Infect Dis. 1997;25:843–6.
195. He X, Tiballi RN, Zarins LT, Bradley SF, Sangeorzan JA, Kauffman CA. Azole resistance in oropharyngeal *Candida albicans* strains isolated from patients infected with human immunodeficiency virus. Antimicrob Agents Chemother. 1994;38:2495–7.
196. Abi-Said D, Anaissie E, Uzun O, Raad I, Pinzcowski H, Vartivarian S. The epidemiology of hematogenous candidiasis caused by different *Candida* species. Clin Infect Dis. 1997;24:1122–8.
197. Sanglard D, Kuchler K, Ischer F, Pagani JL, Monod M, Bille J. Mechanisms of resistance to azole antifungal agents in *Candida albicans* isolates from AIDS patients involve specific multidrug transporters. Antimicrob Agents Chemother. 1995;39:2378–86.
198. White TC, Holleman S, Dy F, Mirels LF, Stevens DA. Resistance mechanisms in clinical isolates of *Candida albicans*. Antimicrob Agents Chemother. 2002;46:1704–13.
199. Sanglard D, Ischer F, Koymans L, Bille J. Amino acid substitutions in the cytochrome P-450 lanosterol 14alpha-demethylase (CYP51A1) from azole-resistant *Candida albicans* clinical isolates contribute to resistance to azole antifungal agents. Antimicrob Agents Chemother. 1998;42:241–53.
200. Sanglard D, Ischer F, Monod M, Bille J. Cloning of *Candida albicans* genes conferring resistance to azole antifungal agents: characterization of CDR2, a new multidrug ABC transporter gene. Microbiology (Reading, England). 1997;143(Pt 2):405–16.
201. Sanglard D, Ischer F, Monod M, Bille J. Susceptibilities of *Candida albicans* multidrug transporter mutants to various antifungal agents and other metabolic inhibitors. Antimicrob Agents Chemother. 1996;40:2300–5.
202. Sanglard D, Ischer F, Bille J. Role of ATP-binding-cassette transporter genes in high-frequency acquisition of resistance to azole antifungals in Candida glabrata. Antimicrob Agents Chemother. 2001;45:1174–83.
203. Sanglard D. Clinical relevance of mechanisms of antifungal drug resistance in yeasts. Enferm Infecc Microbiol Clín. 2002;20:462–9. quiz 70, 79.
204. Sanglard D, Ischer F, Parkinson T, Falconer D, Bille J. *Candida albicans* mutations in the ergosterol biosynthetic pathway and resistance to several antifungal agents. Antimicrob Agents Chemother. 2003;47:2404–12.
205. Chau AS, Gurnani M, Hawkinson R, Laverdiere M, Cacciapuoti A, McNicholas PM. Inactivation of sterol Delta5, 6-desaturase

attenuates virulence in Candida albicans. Antimicrob Agents Chemother. 2005;49:3646–51.
206. Marr KA, Lyons CN, Rustad TR, Bowden RA, White TC. Rapid, transient fluconazole resistance in *Candida albicans* is associated with increased mRNA levels of *CDR*. Antimicrob Agents Chemother. 1998;42:2584–9.
207. Chen J, Li H, Li R, Bu D, Wan Z. Mutations in the cyp51A gene and susceptibility to itraconazole in *Aspergillus fumigatus* serially isolated from a patient with lung aspergilloma. J Antimicrob Chemother. 2005;55:31–7.
208. Howard SJ, Webster I, Moore CB, et al. Multi-azole resistance in *Aspergillus fumigatus*. Int J Antimicrob Agents. 2006;28:450–3.
209. Mellado E, Garcia-Effron G, Alcazar-Fuoli L, Cuenca-Estrella M, Rodriguez-Tudela JL. Substitutions at methionine 220 in the 14alpha-sterol demethylase (Cyp51A) of *Aspergillus fumigatus* are responsible for resistance in vitro to azole antifungal drugs. Antimicrob Agents Chemother. 2004;48:2747–50.
210. Diaz-Guerra TM, Mellado E, Cuenca-Estrella M, Rodriguez-Tudela JL. A point mutation in the 14alpha-sterol demethylase gene cyp51A contributes to itraconazole resistance in *Aspergillus fumigatus*. Antimicrob Agents Chemother. 2003;47:1120–4.
211. Nascimento AM, Goldman GH, Park S, et al. Multiple resistance mechanisms among *Aspergillus fumigatus* mutants with high-level resistance to itraconazole. Antimicrob Agents Chemother. 2003;47:1719–26.
212. Slaven JW, Anderson MJ, Sanglard D, et al. Increased expression of a novel *Aspergillus fumigatus* ABC transporter gene, atrF, in the presence of itraconazole in an itraconazole resistant clinical isolate. Fungal Genet Biol. 2002;36:199–206.
213. Snelders E, van der Lee HA, Kuijpers J, et al. Emergence of azole resistance in Aspergillus fumigatus and spread of a single resistance mechanism. PLoS Med. 2008;5:e219.
214. Snelders E, Huis In 't Veld RA, Rijs AJ, Kema GH, Melchers WJ, Verweij PE. Possible environmental origin of resistance of Aspergillus fumigatus to medical triazoles. Appl Environ Microbiol. 2009;75:4053–7.
215. Van Cauteren H, Lampo A, Vandenberghe J, et al. Toxicological profile and safety evaluation of antifungal azole derivatives. Mycoses. 1989;32 Suppl 1:60–6.
216. Tucker RM, Haq Y, Denning DW, Stevens DA. Adverse events associated with itraconazole in 189 patients on chronic therapy. J Antimicrob Chemother. 1990;26:561–6.
217. Eiden C, Peyriere H, Cociglio M, et al. Adverse effects of voriconazole: analysis of the French Pharmacovigilance Database. Ann Pharmacother. 2007;41:755–63.
218. Gearhart MO. Worsening of liver function with fluconazole and review of azole antifungal hepatotoxicity. Ann Pharmacother. 1994;28:1177–81.
219. Galgiani JN, Catanzaro A, Cloud GA, et al. Comparison of oral fluconazole and itraconazole for progressive, nonmeningeal coccidioidomycosis. A randomized, double-blind trial. Mycoses Study Group. Ann Intern Med. 2000;133:676–86.
220. Scherpbier HJ, Hilhorst MI, Kuijpers TW. Liver failure in a child receiving highly active antiretroviral therapy and voriconazole. Clin Infect Dis. 2003;37:828–30.
221. Hoffman HL, Rathbun RC. Review of the safety and efficacy of voriconazole. Expert Opin Investig Drugs. 2002;11:409–29.
222. Tran HT. Torsades de pointes induced by nonantiarrhythmic drugs. Conn Med. 1994;58:291–5.
223. Pursley TJ, Blomquist IK, Abraham J, Andersen HF, Bartley JA. Fluconazole-induced congenital anomalies in three infants. Clin Infect Dis. 1996;22:336–40.
224. Weinroth SE, Tuazon CU. Alopecia associated with fluconazole treatment. Ann Intern Med. 1993;119:637.
225. Pappas PG, Kauffman CA, Perfect J, et al. Alopecia associated with fluconazole therapy. Ann Intern Med. 1995;123:354–7.
226. Ahmad SR, Singer SJ, Leissa BG. Congestive heart failure associated with itraconazole. Lancet. 2001;357:1766–7.
227. Stevens DA, Diaz M, Negroni R, et al. Safety evaluation of chronic fluconazole therapy. Fluconazole Pan-American Study Group. Chemotherapy. 1997;43:371–7.
228. Koletar SL, Russell JA, Fass RJ, Plouffe JF. Comparison of oral fluconazole and clotrimazole troches as treatment for oral candidiasis in patients infected with human immunodeficiency virus. Antimicrob Agents Chemother. 1990;34:2267–8.
229. Pons V, Greenspan D, Debruin M. Therapy for oropharyngeal candidiasis in HIV-infected patients: a randomized, prospective multicenter study of oral fluconazole versus clotrimazole troches. The Multicenter Study Group. J Acquir Immune Defic Syndr. 1993;6:1311–6.
230. Barbaro G, Barbarini G, Di Lorenzo G. Fluconazole vs itraconazole-flucytosine association in the treatment of esophageal candidiasis in AIDS patients. A double-blind, multicenter placebo-controlled study. The Candida Esophagitis Multicenter Italian Study (CEMIS) Group. Chest. 1996;110:1507–14.
231. Skiest DJ, Vazquez JA, Anstead GM, et al. Posaconazole for the treatment of azole-refractory oropharyngeal and esophageal candidiasis in subjects with HIV infection. Clin Infect Dis. 2007;44:607–14.
232. Phillips P, Zemcov J, Mahmood W, Montaner JS, Craib K, Clarke AM. Itraconazole cyclodextrin solution for fluconazole-refractory oropharyngeal candidiasis in AIDS: correlation of clinical response with in vitro susceptibility. AIDS (London, England). 1996;10:1369–76.
233. Graybill JR, Vazquez J, Darouiche RO, et al. Randomized trial of itraconazole oral solution for oropharyngeal candidiasis in HIV/AIDS patients. Am J Med. 1998;104:33–9.
234. Wilcox CM, Darouiche RO, Laine L, Moskovitz BL, Mallegol I, Wu J. A randomized, double-blind comparison of itraconazole oral solution and fluconazole tablets in the treatment of esophageal candidiasis. J Infect Dis. 1997;176:227–32.
235. Phillips P, De Beule K, Frechette G, et al. A double-blind comparison of itraconazole oral solution and fluconazole capsules for the treatment of oropharyngeal candidiasis in patients with AIDS. Clin Infect Dis. 1998;26:1368–73.
236. Saag MS, Fessel WJ, Kauffman CA, et al. Treatment of fluconazole-refractory oropharyngeal candidiasis with itraconazole oral solution in HIV-positive patients. AIDS Res Hum Retroviruses. 1999;15:1413–7.
237. Cartledge JD, Midgely J, Gazzard BG. Itraconazole solution: higher serum drug concentrations and better clinical response rates than the capsule formulation in acquired immunodeficiency syndrome patients with candidosis. J Clin Pathol. 1997;50:477–80.
238. Cartledge JD, Midgley J, Youle M, Gazzard BG. Itraconazole cyclodextrin solution–effective treatment for HIV-related candidosis unresponsive to other azole therapy. J Antimicrob Chemother. 1994;33:1071–3.
239. Hegener P, Troke PF, Fatkenheuer G, Diehl V, Ruhnke M. Treatment of fluconazole-resistant candidiasis with voriconazole in patients with AIDS. AIDS (London, England). 1998;12:2227–8.
240. Barbaro G, Barbarini G, Calderon W, Grisorio B, Alcini P, Di Lorenzo G. Fluconazole versus itraconazole for *Candida* esophagitis in acquired immunodeficiency syndrome. Gastroenterology. 1996;111:1169–77.
241. Laine L, Dretler RH, Conteas CN, et al. Fluconazole compared with ketoconazole for the treatment of *Candida* esophagitis in AIDS. A randomized trial. Ann Intern Med. 1992;117:655–60.
242. Vazquez JA, Skiest DJ, Tissot-Dupont H, Lennox JL, Boparai N, Isaacs R. Safety and efficacy of posaconazole in the long-term treatment of azole-refractory oropharyngeal and esophageal candidiasis in patients with HIV infection. HIV Clin Trials. 2007; 8:86–97.

243. Ally R, Schurmann D, Kreisel W, et al. A randomized, double-blind, double-dummy, multicenter trial of voriconazole and fluconazole in the treatment of esophageal candidiasis in immunocompromised patients. Clin Infect Dis. 2001;33:1447–54.
244. Smith DE, Midgley J, Allan M, Connolly GM, Gazzard BG. Itraconazole versus ketaconazole in the treatment of oral and oesophageal candidosis in patients infected with HIV. AIDS (London, England). 1991;5:1367–71.
245. Sobel JD, Brooker D, Stein GE, et al. Single oral dose fluconazole compared with conventional clotrimazole topical therapy of *Candida* vaginitis. Fluconazole Vaginitis Study Group. Am J Obstet Gynecol. 1995;172:1263–8.
246. Brammer KW, Feczko JM. Single-dose oral fluconazole in the treatment of vaginal candidosis. Ann NY Acad Sci. 1988;544:561–3.
247. Stein GE, Mummaw N. Placebo-controlled trial of itraconazole for treatment of acute vaginal candidiasis. Antimicrob Agents Chemother. 1993;37:89–92.
248. Pitsouni E, Iavazzo C, Falagas ME. Itraconazole vs fluconazole for the treatment of uncomplicated acute vaginal and vulvovaginal candidiasis in nonpregnant women: a metaanalysis of randomized controlled trials. Am J Obstet Gynecol. 2008;198:153–60.
249. Sobel JD, Kapernick PS, Zervos M, et al. Treatment of complicated *Candida* vaginitis: comparison of single and sequential doses of fluconazole. Am J Obstet Gynecol. 2001;185:363–9.
250. Sobel JD, Wiesenfeld HC, Martens M, et al. Maintenance fluconazole therapy for recurrent vulvovaginal candidiasis. N Engl J Med. 2004;351:876–83.
251. Kauffman CA, Vazquez JA, Sobel JD, et al. Prospective multicenter surveillance study of funguria in hospitalized patients. The National Institute for Allergy and Infectious Diseases (NIAID) Mycoses Study Group. Clin Infect Dis. 2000;30:14–8.
252. Sobel JD, Kauffman CA, McKinsey D, et al. Candiduria: a randomized, double-blind study of treatment with fluconazole and placebo. The National Institute of Allergy and Infectious Diseases (NIAID) Mycoses Study Group. Clin Infect Dis. 2000;30:19–24.
253. Jacobs LG, Skidmore EA, Freeman K, Lipschultz D, Fox N. Oral fluconazole compared with bladder irrigation with amphotericin B for treatment of fungal urinary tract infections in elderly patients. Clin Infect Dis. 1996;22:30–5.
254. Fan-Havard P, O'Donovan C, Smith SM, Oh J, Bamberger M, Eng RH. Oral fluconazole versus amphotericin B bladder irrigation for treatment of candidal funguria. Clin Infect Dis. 1995;21:960–5.
255. De Doncker P, Van Lint J, Dockx P, Roseeuw D. Pulse therapy with one-week itraconazole monthly for three or four months in the treatment of onychomycosis. Cutis. 1995;56:180–3.
256. Walsoe I, Stangerup M, Svejgaard E. Itraconazole in onychomycosis. Open and double-blind studies. Acta Derm Venereol. 1990;70:137–40.
257. Arca E, Tastan HB, Akar A, Kurumlu Z, Gur AR. An open, randomized, comparative study of oral fluconazole, itraconazole and terbinafine therapy in onychomycosis. J Dermatol Treat. 2002;13:3–9.
258. Scher RK, Breneman D, Rich P, et al. Once-weekly fluconazole (150, 300, or 450 mg) in the treatment of distal subungual onychomycosis of the toenail. J Am Acad Dermatol. 1998;38: S77–86.
259. Rex JH, Bennett JE, Sugar AM, et al. A randomized trial comparing fluconazole with amphotericin B for the treatment of candidemia in patients without neutropenia. Candidemia Study Group and the National Institute. N Engl J Med. 1994;331:1325–30.
260. Phillips P, Shafran S, Garber G, et al. Multicenter randomized trial of fluconazole versus amphotericin B for treatment of candidemia in non-neutropenic patients. Canadian Candidemia Study Group. Eur J Clin Microbiol Infect Dis. 1997;16:337–45.
261. Rex JH, Pappas PG, Karchmer AW, et al. A randomized and blinded multicenter trial of high-dose fluconazole plus placebo versus fluconazole plus amphotericin B as therapy for candidemia and its consequences in nonneutropenic subjects. Clin Infect Dis. 2003;36:1221–8.
262. Nguyen MH, Peacock Jr JE, Tanner DC, et al. Therapeutic approaches in patients with candidemia. Evaluation in a multicenter, prospective, observational study. Arch Intern Med. 1995;155:2429–35.
263. Anaissie EJ, Vartivarian SE, Abi-Said D, et al. Fluconazole versus amphotericin B in the treatment of hematogenous candidiasis: a matched cohort study. Am J Med. 1996;101:170–6.
264. Rex JH, Bennett JE, Sugar AM, et al. Intravascular catheter exchange and duration of candidemia. NIAID Mycoses Study Group and the Candidemia Study Group. Clin Infect Dis. 1995;21:994–6.
265. Reboli AC, Rotstein C, Pappas PG, et al. Anidulafungin versus fluconazole for invasive candidiasis. N Engl J Med. 2007;356: 2472–82.
266. Kullberg BJ, Sobel JD, Ruhnke M, et al. Voriconazole versus a regimen of amphotericin B followed by fluconazole for candidaemia in non-neutropenic patients: a randomised non-inferiority trial. Lancet. 2005;366:1435–42.
267. de Gans J, Portegies P, Tiessens G, et al. Itraconazole compared with amphotericin B plus flucytosine in AIDS patients with cryptococcal meningitis. AIDS (London, England). 1992;6:185–90.
268. Perfect JR, Dismukes WE, Dromer F, et al. Clinical Practice guidelines for the management of cryptococcal disease: 2010 update by the Infectious Diseases Society of America. Clin Infect Dis. 2010;50:291–322.
269. van der Horst CM, Saag MS, Cloud GA, et al. Treatment of cryptococcal meningitis associated with the acquired immunodeficiency syndrome. National Institute of Allergy and Infectious Diseases Mycoses Study Group and AIDS Clinical Trials Group. N Engl J Med. 1997;337:15–21.
270. Saag MS, Powderly WG, Cloud GA, et al. Comparison of amphotericin B with fluconazole in the treatment of acute AIDS-associated cryptococcal meningitis. The NIAID Mycoses Study Group and the AIDS Clinical Trials Group. N Engl J Med. 1992;326:83–9.
271. Pappas PG, Chetchotisakd P, Larsen RA, et al. A phase II randomized trial of amphotericin B alone or combined with fluconazole in the treatment of HIV-associated cryptococcal meningitis. Clin Infect Dis. 2009;48:1775–83.
272. Perfect JR, Marr KA, Walsh TJ, et al. Voriconazole treatment for less-common, emerging, or refractory fungal infections. Clin Infect Dis. 2003;36:1122–31.
273. Bozzette SA, Larsen RA, Chiu J, et al. A placebo-controlled trial of maintenance therapy with fluconazole after treatment of cryptococcal meningitis in the acquired immunodeficiency syndrome. California Collaborative Treatment Group. N Engl J Med. 1991;324:580–4.
274. Powderly WG, Saag MS, Cloud GA, et al. A controlled trial of fluconazole or amphotericin B to prevent relapse of cryptococcal meningitis in patients with the acquired immunodeficiency syndrome. The NIAID AIDS Clinical Trials Group and Mycoses Study Group. N Engl J Med. 1992;326:793–8.
275. Saag MS, Cloud GA, Graybill JR, et al. A comparison of itraconazole versus fluconazole as maintenance therapy for AIDS-associated cryptococcal meningitis. National Institute of Allergy and Infectious Diseases Mycoses Study Group. Clin Infect Dis. 1999;28:291–6.
276. Kaplan JE, Benson C, Holmes KK, et al. Guidelines for prevention and treatment of opportunistic infections in HIV-infected adults and adolescents. Recommendations from CDC, the National Institutes of Health, and the HIV Medicine Association of the Infectious Diseases Society of America. MMWR 2009;58:1–206.

277. Yamaguchi H, Ikemoto H, Watanabe K, Ito A, Hara K, Kohno S. Fluconazole monotherapy for cryptococcosis in non-AIDS patients. Eur J Clin Microbiol Infect Dis. 1996;15:787–92.
278. Pappas PG, Perfect JR, Cloud GA, et al. Cryptococcosis in human immunodeficiency virus-negative patients in the era of effective azole therapy. Clin Infect Dis. 2001;33:690–9.
279. Dismukes WE, Bradsher Jr RW, Cloud GC, et al. Itraconazole therapy for blastomycosis and histoplasmosis. NIAID Mycoses Study Group. Am J Med. 1992;93:489–97.
280. Chapman SW, Bradsher Jr RW, Campbell Jr GD, Pappas PG, Kauffman CA. Practice guidelines for the management of patients with blastomycosis. Infectious Diseases Society of America. Clin Infect Dis. 2000;30:679–83.
281. Pappas PG, Bradsher RW, Kauffman CA, et al. Treatment of blastomycosis with higher doses of fluconazole. The National Institute of Allergy and Infectious Diseases Mycoses Study Group. Clin Infect Dis. 1997;25:200–5.
282. Pappas PG, Bradsher RW, Chapman SW, et al. Treatment of blastomycosis with fluconazole: a pilot study. The National Institute of Allergy and Infectious Diseases Mycoses Study Group. Clin Infect Dis. 1995;20:267–71.
283. Freifeld A, Proia L, Andes D, et al. Voriconazole use for endemic fungal infections. Antimicrob Agents Chemother. 2009;53:1648–51.
284. Chapman SW, Dismukes WE, Proia LA, et al. Clinical practice guidelines for the management of blastomycosis: 2008 update by the Infectious Diseases Society of America. Clin Infect Dis. 2008;46:1801–12.
285. Graybill JR, Stevens DA, Galgiani JN, Dismukes WE, Cloud GA. Itraconazole treatment of coccidioidomycosis. NAIAD Mycoses Study Group. Am J Med. 1990;89:282–90.
286. Tucker RM, Denning DW, Dupont B, Stevens DA. Itraconazole therapy for chronic coccidioidal meningitis. Ann Intern Med. 1990;112:108–12.
287. Diaz M, Negroni R, Montero-Gei F, et al. A Pan-American 5-year study of fluconazole therapy for deep mycoses in the immunocompetent host. Pan-American Study Group. Clin Infect Dis. 1992;14 Suppl 1:S68–76.
288. Galgiani JN, Catanzaro A, Cloud GA, et al. Fluconazole therapy for coccidioidal meningitis. The NIAID-Mycoses Study Group. Ann Intern Med. 1993;119:28–35.
289. Catanzaro A, Galgiani JN, Levine BE, et al. Fluconazole in the treatment of chronic pulmonary and nonmeningeal disseminated coccidioidomycosis. NIAID Mycoses Study Group. Am J Med. 1995;98:249–56.
290. DeFelice R, Galgiani JN, Campbell SC, et al. Ketoconazole treatment of nonprimary coccidioidomycosis. Evaluation of 60 patients during three years of study. Am J Med. 1982;72:681–7.
291. Galgiani JN, Stevens DA, Graybill JR, Dismukes WE, Cloud GA. Ketoconazole therapy of progressive coccidioidomycosis. Comparison of 400- and 800-mg doses and observations at higher doses. Am J Med. 1988;84:603–10.
292. Graybill JR, Stevens DA, Galgiani JN, et al. Ketoconazole treatment of coccidioidal meningitis. Ann NY Acad Sci. 1988;544:488–96.
293. Stevens DA, Rendon A, Gaona-Flores V, et al. Posaconazole therapy for chronic refractory coccidioidomycosis. Chest. 2007;132:952–8.
294. Catanzaro A, Cloud GA, Stevens DA, et al. Safety, tolerance, and efficacy of posaconazole therapy in patients with nonmeningeal disseminated or chronic pulmonary coccidioidomycosis. Clin Infect Dis. 2007;45:562–8.
295. Galgiani JN, Ampel NM, Blair JE, et al. Coccidioidomycosis. Clin Infect Dis. 2005;41:1217–23.
296. Dewsnup DH, Galgiani JN, Graybill JR, et al. Is it ever safe to stop azole therapy for *Coccidioides immitis* meningitis? Ann Intern Med. 1996;124:305–10.
297. Galgiani JN, Ampel NM, Blair JE, et al. Coccidioidomycosis. Clin Infect Dis. 2005;41:1217–23.
298. Negroni R, Robles AM, Arechavala A, Tuculet MA, Galimberti R. Ketoconazole in the treatment of paracoccidioidomycosis and histoplasmosis. Rev Infect Dis. 1980;2:643–9.
299. Dismukes WE, Stamm AM, Graybill JR, et al. Treatment of systemic mycoses with ketoconazole: emphasis on toxicity and clinical response in 52 patients. National Institute of Allergy and Infectious Diseases collaborative antifungal study. Ann Intern Med. 1983;98:13–20.
300. Negroni R, Taborda A, Robies AM, Archevala A. Itraconazole in the treatment of histoplasmosis associated with AIDS. Mycoses. 1992;35:281–7.
301. Negroni R, Robles AM, Arechavala A, Taborda A. Itraconazole in human histoplasmosis. Mycoses. 1989;32:123–30.
302. Negroni R, Palmieri O, Koren F, Tiraboschi IN, Galimberti RL. Oral treatment of paracoccidioidomycosis and histoplasmosis with itraconazole in humans. Rev Infect Dis. 1987;9 Suppl 1:S47–50.
303. Wheat J, Hafner R, Korzun AH, et al. Itraconazole treatment of disseminated histoplasmosis in patients with the acquired immunodeficiency syndrome. AIDS Clinical Trial Group. Am J Med. 1995;98:336–42.
304. Wheat J, Hafner R, Wulfsohn M, et al. Prevention of relapse of histoplasmosis with itraconazole in patients with the acquired immunodeficiency syndrome. Ann Intern Med. 1993;118:610–6.
305. Wheat J, MaWhinney S, Hafner R, et al. Treatment of histoplasmosis with fluconazole in patients with acquired immunodeficiency syndrome. National Institute of Allergy and Infectious Diseases Acquired Immunodeficiency Syndrome Clinical Trials Group and Mycoses Study Group. Am J Med. 1997;103:223–32.
306. McKinsey DS, Kauffman CA, Pappas PG, et al. Fluconazole therapy for histoplasmosis. The National Institute of Allergy and Infectious Diseases Mycoses Study Group. Clin Infect Dis. 1996;23:996–1001.
307. Restrepo A, Tobon A, Clark B, et al. Salvage treatment of histoplasmosis with posaconazole. J Infect. 2007;54:319–27.
308. Wheat LJ, Freifeld AG, Kleiman MB, et al. Clinical practice guidelines for the management of patients with histoplasmosis: 2007 update by the Infectious Diseases Society of America. Clin Infect Dis. 2007;45:807–25.
309. Restrepo A, Gomez I, Cano LE, et al. Treatment of paracoccidioidomycosis with ketoconazole: a three-year experience. Am J Med. 1983;74:48–52.
310. Naranjo MS, Trujillo M, Munera MI, Restrepo P, Gomez I, Restrepo A. Treatment of paracoccidioidomycosis with itraconazole. J Med Vet Mycol. 1990;28:67–76.
311. Queiroz-Telles F, Goldani LZ, Schlamm HT, Goodrich JM, Espinel-Ingroff A, Shikanai-Yasuda MA. An open-label comparative pilot study of oral voriconazole and itraconazole for long-term treatment of paracoccidioidomycosis. Clin Infect Dis. 2007;45:1462–9.
312. Restrepo A. Treatment of tropical mycoses. J Am Acad Dermatol. 1994;31:S91–102.
313. Kauffman CA, Hajjeh R, Chapman SW. Practice guidelines for the management of patients with sporotrichosis. For the Mycoses Study Group. Infectious Diseases Society of America. Clin Infect Dis. 2000;30:684–7.
314. Winn RE, Anderson J, Piper J, Aronson NE, Pluss J. Systemic sporotrichosis treated with itraconazole. Clin Infect Dis. 1993;17:210–7.
315. Restrepo A, Robledo J, Gomez I, Tabares AM, Gutierrez R. Itraconazole therapy in lymphangitic and cutaneous sporotrichosis. Arch Dermatol. 1986;122:413–7.

316. Sharkey-Mathis PK, Kauffman CA, Graybill JR, et al. Treatment of sporotrichosis with itraconazole. NIAID Mycoses Study Group. Am J Med. 1993;95:279–85.
317. Calhoun DL, Waskin H, White MP, et al. Treatment of systemic sporotrichosis with ketoconazole. Rev Infect Dis. 1991;13:47–51.
318. Kauffman CA, Pappas PG, McKinsey DS, et al. Treatment of lymphocutaneous and visceral sporotrichosis with fluconazole. Clin Infect Dis. 1996;22:46–50.
319. Kauffman CA, Bustamante B, Chapman SW, Pappas PG. Clinical practice guidelines for the management of sporotrichosis: 2007 update by the Infectious Diseases Society of America. Clin Infect Dis. 2007;45:1255–65.
320. Sirisanthana T, Supparatpinyo K, Perriens J, Nelson KE. Amphotericin B and itraconazole for treatment of disseminated *Penicillium marneffei* infection in human immunodeficiency virus-infected patients. Clin Infect Dis. 1998;26:1107–10.
321. Supparatpinyo K, Perriens J, Nelson KE, Sirisanthana T. A controlled trial of itraconazole to prevent relapse of *Penicillium marneffei* infection in patients infected with the human immunodeficiency virus. N Engl J Med. 1998;339:1739–43.
322. Chariyalertsak S, Supparatpinyo K, Sirisanthana T, Nelson KE. A controlled trial of itraconazole as primary prophylaxis for systemic fungal infections in patients with advanced human immunodeficiency virus infection in Thailand. Clin Infect Dis. 2002;34:277–84.
323. Supparatpinyo K, Schlamm HT. Voriconazole as therapy for systemic *Penicillium marneffei* infections in AIDS patients. Am J Trop Med Hyg. 2007;77:350–3.
324. Walsh TJ, Anaissie EJ, Denning DW, et al. Treatment of aspergillosis: clinical practice guidelines of the Infectious Diseases Society of America. Clin Infect Dis. 2008;46:327–60.
325. Dupont B. Itraconazole therapy in aspergillosis: study in 49 patients. J Am Acad Dermatol. 1990;23:607–14.
326. Denning DW, Lee JY, Hostetler JS, et al. NIAID Mycoses Study Group multicenter trial of oral itraconazole therapy for invasive Aspergillosis. Am J Med. 1994;97:135–44.
327. Stevens DA, Lee JY. Analysis of compassionate use itraconazole therapy for invasive aspergillosis by the NIAID Mycoses Study Group criteria. Arch Intern Med. 1997;157:1857–62.
328. Herbrecht R, Denning DW, Patterson TF, et al. Voriconazole versus amphotericin B for primary therapy of invasive aspergillosis. N Engl J Med. 2002;347:408–15.
329. Denning DW, Ribaud P, Milpied N, et al. Efficacy and safety of voriconazole in the treatment of acute invasive aspergillosis. Clin Infect Dis. 2002;34:563–71.
330. Raad II, Hanna HA, Boktour M, et al. Novel antifungal agents as salvage therapy for invasive aspergillosis in patients with hematologic malignancies: posaconazole compared with high-dose lipid formulations of amphotericin B alone or in combination with caspofungin. Leukemia. 2008;22:496–503.
331. Kirkpatrick WR, Perea S, Coco BJ, Patterson TF. Efficacy of caspofungin alone and in combination with voriconazole in a Guinea pig model of invasive aspergillosis. Antimicrob Agents Chemother. 2002;46:2564–8.
332. Perea S, Gonzalez G, Fothergill AW, Kirkpatrick WR, Rinaldi MG, Patterson TF. In vitro interaction of caspofungin acetate with voriconazole against clinical isolates of *Aspergillus* spp. Antimicrob Agents Chemother. 2002;46:3039–41.
333. Marr KA, Boeckh M, Carter RA, Kim HW, Corey L. Combination antifungal therapy for invasive aspergillosis. Clin Infect Dis. 2004;39:797–802.
334. Sharkey PK, Graybill JR, Rinaldi MG, et al. Itraconazole treatment of phaeohyphomycosis. J Am Acad Dermatol. 1990;23:577–86.
335. Whittle DI, Kominos S. Use of itraconazole for treating subcutaneous phaeohyphomycosis caused by Exophiala jeanselmei. Clin Infect Dis. 1995;21:1068.
336. Goldberg SL, Geha DJ, Marshall WF, Inwards DJ, Hoagland HC. Successful treatment of simultaneous pulmonary *Pseudallescheria boydii* and *Aspergillus terreus* infection with oral itraconazole. Clin Infect Dis. 1993;16:803–5.
337. Raad II, Hachem RY, Herbrecht R, et al. Posaconazole as salvage treatment for invasive fusariosis in patients with underlying hematologic malignancy and other conditions. Clin Infect Dis. 2006;42:1398–403.
338. Greenberg RN, Mullane K, van Burik JA, et al. Posaconazole as salvage therapy for zygomycosis. Antimicrob Agents Chemother. 2006;50:126–33.
339. van Burik JA, Hare RS, Solomon HF, Corrado ML, Kontoyiannis DP. Posaconazole is effective as salvage therapy in zygomycosis: a retrospective summary of 91 cases. Clin Infect Dis. 2006; 42:e61–5.
340. Boogaerts M, Winston DJ, Bow EJ, et al. Intravenous and oral itraconazole versus intravenous amphotericin B deoxycholate as empirical antifungal therapy for persistent fever in neutropenic patients with cancer who are receiving broad-spectrum antibacterial therapy. A randomized, controlled trial. Ann Intern Med. 2001;135:412–22.
341. Walsh TJ, Pappas P, Winston DJ, et al. Voriconazole compared with liposomal amphotericin B for empirical antifungal therapy in patients with neutropenia and persistent fever. N Engl J Med. 2002;346:225–34.
342. Slavin MA, Osborne B, Adams R, et al. Efficacy and safety of fluconazole prophylaxis for fungal infections after marrow transplantation – a prospective, randomized, double-blind study. J Infect Dis. 1995;171:1545–52.
343. Rozenberg-Arska M, Dekker AW, Branger J, Verhoef J. A randomized study to compare oral fluconazole to amphotericin B in the prevention of fungal infections in patients with acute leukaemia. J Antimicrob Chemother. 1991;27:369–76.
344. Menichetti F, Del Favero A, Martino P, et al. Preventing fungal infection in neutropenic patients with acute leukemia: fluconazole compared with oral amphotericin B. Ann Intern Med. 1994;120:913–8.
345. Bodey GP, Anaissie EJ, Elting LS, Estey E, O'Brien S, Kantarjian H. Antifungal prophylaxis during remission induction therapy for acute leukemia fluconazole versus intravenous amphotericin B. Cancer. 1994;73:2099–106.
346. Nucci M, Biasoli I, Akiti T, et al. A double-blind, randomized, placebo-controlled trial of itraconazole capsules as antifungal prophylaxis for neutropenic patients. Clin Infect Dis. 2000;30:300–5.
347. Menichetti F, Del Favero A, Martino P, et al. Itraconazole oral solution as prophylaxis for fungal infections in neutropenic patients with hematologic malignancies: a randomized, placebo-controlled, double-blind, multicenter trial. GIMEMA Infection Program. Gruppo Italiano Malattie Ematologiche dell' Adulto. Clin Infect Dis. 1999;28:250–5.
348. Glasmacher A, Molitor E, Hahn C, et al. Antifungal prophylaxis with itraconazole in neutropenic patients with acute leukaemia. Leukemia. 1998;12:1338–43.
349. Vardakas KZ, Michalopoulos A, Falagas ME. Fluconazole versus itraconazole for antifungal prophylaxis in neutropenic patients with haematological malignancies: a meta-analysis of randomised-controlled trials. Br J Haematol. 2005;131:22–8.
350. Shorr AF, Chung K, Jackson WL, Waterman PE, Kollef MH. Fluconazole prophylaxis in critically ill surgical patients: a meta-analysis. Crit Care Med. 2005;33:1928–35. quiz 36.
351. Cruciani M, de Lalla F, Mengoli C. Prophylaxis of *Candida* infections in adult trauma and surgical intensive care patients: a systematic review and meta-analysis. Intens Care Med. 2005;31:1479–87.
352. Schuster MG, Edwards Jr JE, Sobel JD, et al. Empirical fluconazole versus placebo for intensive care unit patients: A randomized trial. Ann Intern Med. 2008;149:83–90.

353. Eggimann P, Francioli P, Bille J, et al. Fluconazole prophylaxis prevents intra-abdominal candidiasis in high-risk surgical patients. Crit Care Med. 1999;27:1066–72.
354. Manzoni P, Stolfi I, Pugni L, et al. A multicenter, randomized trial of prophylactic fluconazole in preterm neonates. N Engl J Med. 2007;356:2483–95.
355. Winston DJ, Busuttil RW. Randomized controlled trial of oral itraconazole solution versus intravenous/oral fluconazole for prevention of fungal infections in liver transplant recipients. Transplantation. 2002;74:688–95.
356. Hay RJ, Clayton YM, Moore MK, Midgely G. An evaluation of itraconazole in the management of onychomycosis. Br J Dermatol. 1988;119:359–66.
357. Willemsen M, De Doncker P, Willems J, et al. Posttreatment itraconazole levels in the nail. New implications for treatment in onychomycosis. J Am Acad Dermatol. 1992;26:731–5.
358. Haneke E, Abeck D, Ring J. Safety and efficacy of intermittent therapy with itraconazole in finger- and toenail onychomycosis: a multicentre trial. Mycoses. 1998;41:521–7.
359. Havu V, Brandt H, Heikkila H, et al. A double-blind, randomized study comparing itraconazole pulse therapy with continuous dosing for the treatment of toe-nail onychomycosis. Br J Dermatol. 1997;136:230–4.
360. Brautigam M. Terbinafine versus itraconazole: a controlled clinical comparison in onychomycosis of the toenails. J Am Acad Dermatol. 1998;38:S53–6.
361. De Backer M, De Vroey C, Lesaffre E, Scheys I, De Keyser P. Twelve weeks of continuous oral therapy for toenail onychomycosis caused by dermatophytes: a double-blind comparative trial of terbinafine 250 mg/day versus itraconazole 200 mg/day. J Am Acad Dermatol. 1998;38:S57–63.
362. Montero-Gei F, Perera A. Therapy with fluconazole for tinea corporis, tinea cruris, and tinea pedis. Clin Infect Dis. 1992;14 Suppl 1:S77–81.
363. Katsambas A, Antoniou C, Frangouli E, et al. Itraconazole in the treatment of tinea corporis and tinea cruris. Clin Exp Dermatol. 1993;18:322–5.
364. Degreef H, Marien K, De Veylder H, Duprez K, Borghys A, Verhoeve L. Itraconazole in the treatment of dermatophytoses: a comparison of two daily dosages. Rev Infect Dis. 1987;9 Suppl 1:S104–8.
365. Legendre R, Esola-Macre J. Itraconazole in the treatment of tinea capitis. J Am Acad Dermatol. 1990;23:559–60.
366. De Keyser P, De Backer M, Massart DL, Westelinck KJ. Two-week oral treatment of tinea pedis, comparing terbinafine (250 mg/day) with itraconazole (100 mg/day): a double-blind, multicentre study. Br J Dermatol. 1994;130 Suppl 43:22–5.

Echinocandins

Andreas H. Groll, Dominik Schrey, and Thomas J. Walsh

Ever since the discovery that penicillin inhibits bacterial cell wall synthesis, developing equivalent agents to target the fungal cell wall has been a focus of antifungal drug development. Because the cell wall is essential to the vitality of fungal organisms and because its components are absent in the mammalian host, the fungal cell wall represents an ideal target for antifungal compounds. With considerable variation among different species, the gross macromolecular components of the cell wall of most fungi include chitin, alpha- or beta-linked glucans, and a variety of mannoproteins. The dynamics of the fungal cell wall are closely coordinated with cell growth and cell division, and the predominant function of the cell wall is to control the internal turgor of the cell. Disruption of the cell wall structure leads to osmotic instability and may ultimately result in the lysis of the fungal cell. The echinocandins are antifungal agents whose actions are directed against the major constituents of the fungal cell wall.

The echinocandins are a class of semisynthetic amphiphilic lipopeptides that are composed of a cyclic hexapeptide core linked to a variably configured N-acyl lipid side chain. The first compound of this class undergoing major preclinical evaluation was cilofungin (LY 121019), a semisynthetic echinocandin B derivative with activity limited against *Candida* spp. However, clinical development was abandoned in early stages due to toxicity concerns associated with the intravenous polyethylene glycol formulation vehicle [1–3].

Over the past decade, second generation semisynthetic echinocandins with extended antifungal spectrum against *Candida* and *Aspergillus* spp., excellent safety profiles, and favorable pharmacokinetic characteristics have been developed. These include anidulafungin (Ecalta™ and Eraxis™), caspofungin (Cancidas™), and micafungin (Mycamine™) (Fig. 1). With individual exceptions, current data indicate that these agents are not fundamentally different with respect to spectrum, pharmacodynamics, pharmacokinetics, safety, and antifungal efficacy (Table 1).

Mechanism of Action

The echinocandins act by noncompetitive inhibition of the synthesis of (1→3)-β-D-glucan, a polysaccharide in the cell wall of many pathogenic fungi (Fig. 2). Together with chitin, the rope-like glucan fibrils are responsible for the strength and shape of the cell wall. They are important in maintaining the osmotic integrity of the fungal cell and play a key role in cell division and cell growth [1–3]. The proposed molecular target of the echinocandins, glucan synthase, is a heteromeric enzyme complex composed of at least one large integral membrane protein encoded by the *FKS* genes that bind the substrate (UDP-glucose), and one small regulatory subunit, Rho1p, a GTP-binding protein; other, yet unidentified components may also be involved [11]. Additional immunomodulatory effects through unmasking of (1→3)-β-D-glucan and induction of proinflammatory cytokine release from host immune cells have been described recently and may be important to explain the observed in vivo efficacy of echinocandins against moulds that are typically resistant in vitro [12].

The echinocandins demonstrate a species-dependent mode of action. Whole cell in vitro assays reveal fungicidal activity against most *Candida* spp. but not against *Aspergillus* spp. [13, 14]. Examination of exposed *Aspergillus* organisms shows a dose-dependent formation of microcolonies with progressively truncated, swollen hyphal elements that appear to be cell wall deficient, but are able to regain their cell walls upon subculture in the absence of drug [15–17]. Vital fluorescence staining of *Aspergillus fumigatus* exposed to caspofungin or micafungin revealed a differential killing effect on apical and subapical branching cells with little reduction in vital staining of subapical cells, suggesting that only cells at the active centers for new cell wall synthesis within *A. fumigatus* hyphae are killed [14, 17]. These observations indicate differences in functional target sensitivity, the implications of which are not yet understood.

A.H. Groll (✉)
Infectious Diseases Research Program, Department of Pediatric Hematology/Oncology and Center for Bone Marrow Transplantation, Children's University Hospital, Muenster, Germany
e-mail: grollan@ukmuenster.de

C.A. Kauffman et al. (eds.), *Essentials of Clinical Mycology*,
DOI 10.1007/978-1-4419-6640-7_6, © Springer Science+Business Media, LLC 2011

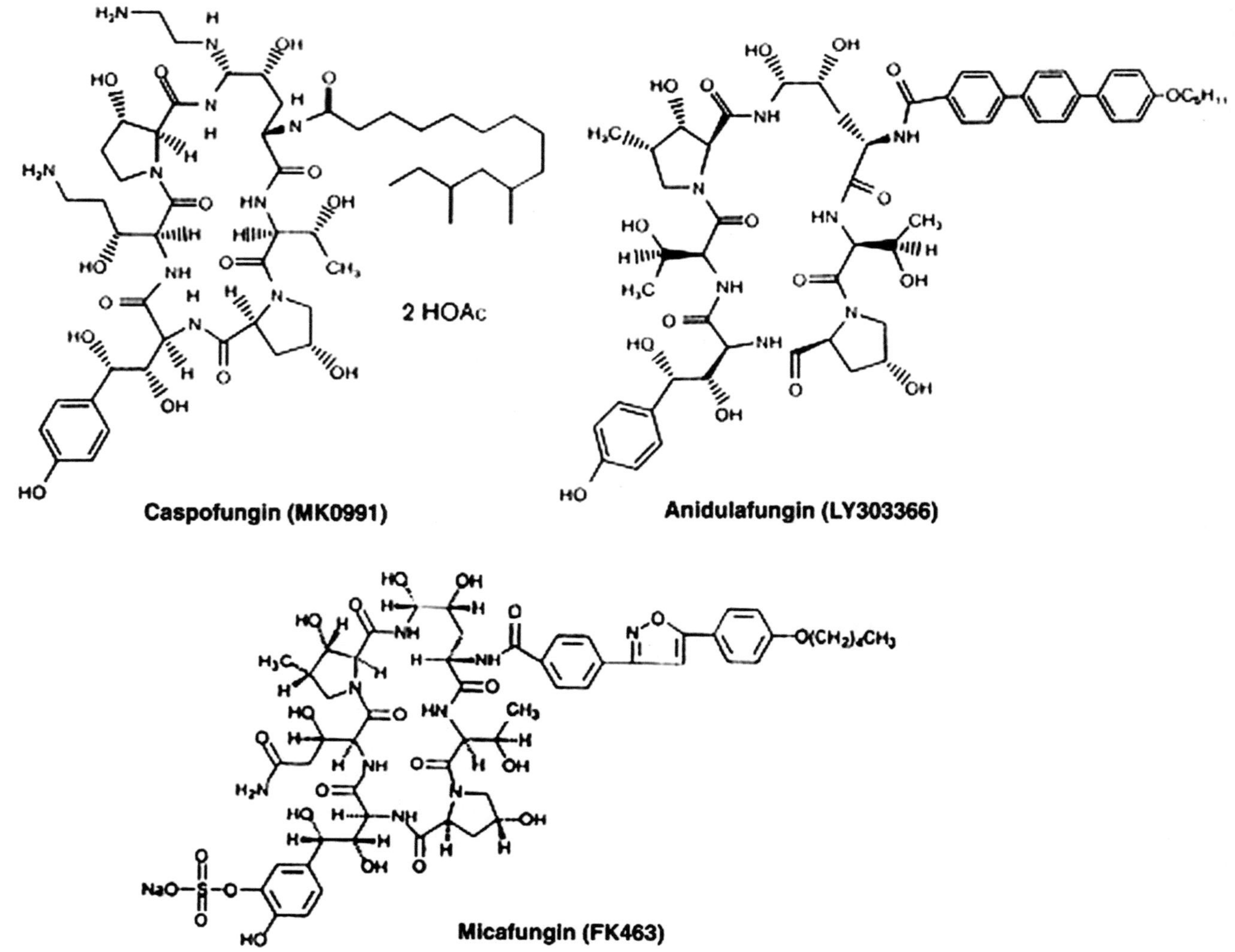

Fig. 1 Structural formulas of anidulafungin, caspofungin, and micafungin. The echinocandins are composed of a cyclic hexapeptide core that is attached to an individually configurated acyl side chain

Table 1 Principal pharmacokinetic properties of anidulafungin, caspofungin, and micafungin

	Anbidulafungin	Caspofungin	Micafungin
Formulation	IV	IV	IV
Dose-linearity	yes	yes	yes
Oral bioavailability [%]	n/a	n/a	n/a
Protein binding [%]	84	97	99
Volume of distribution [L/kg]	0.7–0.9	n/a	0.24
Elimination half-life [h]	24–26	9–11	11–17
Substrate/inhibitor of CYP450	no	Poor substrate/weak inhibitor	Poor substrate/weak inhibitor
Metabolism	Via chemical degradation to inactive metabolites	Via peptide hydrolysis and N-acetylation	Via arylsulfatase and catechol-O-methyltransferase
Elimination	Primarily in feces (10% unchanged); 1% in urine	35% in feces, 41% in urine (1.4% unchanged)	40% in feces, < 15% in urine (<1% unchanged)
Dosage adjustment in renal impairment	No adjustment needed	No adjustment needed	No adjustment needed
Dosage adjustment in hepatic impairment	No adjustment needed	Child-Pugh <7: No adjustment; 7–9: 35 mg maintenance; >9: No data	Child-Pugh ≤ 9: No adjustment; > 9: No data

Data compiled from Refs. [4–10]
n/a, not applicable

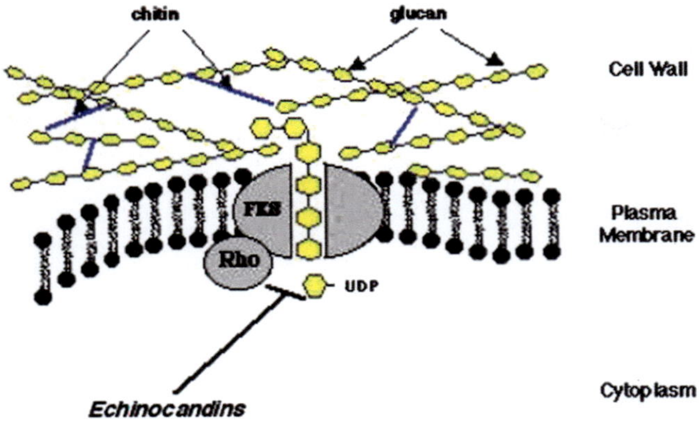

Fig. 2 Schematic of the proposed mechanism of action of echinocandin lipopeptides. Echinocandins inhibit the synthesis of cell wall 1,3-beta glucan at the level of the cell membrane. FKS is the proposed catalytic subunit, and RHO the proposed regulatory subunit of the glucan synthase complex (Modified from Kurtz and Douglas 1997 [11], by permission of the publisher)

Antifungal Activity and Resistance

The echinocandins have potent and broad spectrum in vitro activity against clinically relevant *Candida* spp. with somewhat higher minimum inhibitory concentration (MIC) values for *Candida parapsilosis*, *Candida guilliermondii*, and *Candida famata* (Table 2). They have shown activity against *Saccharomyces cerevisiae* but virtually no in vitro activity against *Cryptococcus neoformans* and *Trichosporon asahii*. The echinocandins also have broad spectrum activity against *Aspergillus* spp. They have variable activity against dematiaceous and endemic moulds, and are considered inactive in vitro against most hyalohyphomycetes and the zygomycetes. Efficacy against invasive infections by *Candida* and *Aspergillus* spp has been demonstrated in various experimental models in immunocompetent and immunocompromised animals. Of note, all echinocandins have shown preventive and therapeutic activity in animal models of *Pneumocystis* pneumonia [13, 18–27].

As expected from their mechanism of action, the echinocandins show no cross-resistance to amphotericin and fluconazole-resistant *Candida* and *Aspergillus* isolates. Primary resistance to echinocandins in otherwise susceptible fungal species remains rare [18, 28]. While results from resistance-induction studies demonstrate an overall low potential for induced resistance in *Candida* spp. [13], development of secondary echinocandin resistance has been reported in patients [29–35]. Of note, resistance to one agent appears to be generally associated with cross-resistance to other echinocandins [36, 37]. Development of secondary resistance to *Aspergillus* spp. is conceivable based on laboratory experiments [36], but has not been observed yet in patients.

Most mutations in *Candida* and *Aspergillus* spp. conferring resistance have been mapped to two "hot-spot" regions of the *FKS1* gene [11, 36–40]. Recent findings indicate that a naturally occurring substitution in *FKS1* from the *C. parapsilosis* group accounts for the reduced susceptibility phenotype of these organisms [41]. *FKS1* sequences also appear to represent determinants of intrinsic echinocandin resistance in *Fusarium* and *Scedosporium* species [42]. In contrast, the primary resistance of *C. neoformans* to echinocandins appears to be unrelated to (1→3)-β-D-glucan synthase resistance [43].

The observation of a paradoxical effect of caspofungin and other amine-substituted echinocandins against some *C. albicans* isolates at supra-MIC concentrations has been linked to upregulation of *FKS1*, *MKC1*, *GSL2* and *GSC1* gene expression [44, 45], but also to the derepression or activation of resistance mechanism that do not involve (1→3)-β-D-glucan synthesis [46, 47] and may include high affinity uptake transporters [48], efflux pumps [49], and mechanisms involved in remodeling or maintenance of cell wall components [38, 44, 45, 50]. In animals, a paradoxical effect could not be reproducibly demonstrated [51, 52], and, similar to the realm of antibacterial chemotherapy, there has been no signal in patients treated with high doses of echinocandin compounds. That these in vitro paradoxical effects tend to occur at echinocandin concentrations greatly exceeding those that are safely achieved in plasma may explain the absence of an in vivo correlate.

Antimicrobial Interactions

In vitro studies using checkerboard methodologies, time kill and metabolic assays have consistently shown no antagonism in vitro between echinocandins and other antifungal agents; however, indifference, additivity, and synergy have been noted when tested against *Aspergillus* spp., *C. albicans* and non-*albicans Candida* spp. [13, 53–65]. In vivo, beneficial effects of combinations of echinocandins with triazoles or amphotericin B have been shown in animal models of disseminated and pulmonary aspergillosis [66–70], experimental invasive candidiasis [57, 71, 72], disseminated coccidioidomycosis [73], and disseminated *R. oryzae* zygomycosis [74].

When tested in combination with human phagocytes against *C. albicans*, all echinocandins had variably enhancing effects on phagocytosis, oxidative burst, and intracellular killing of the organism [75, 76]. Enhancing effects on these functions were also seen against *A. fumigatus* [77–79]. Echinocandins have also been shown to decrease the adherence of *C. albicans* to plastic coated with extracellular matrix proteins [80], to decrease the ability of *C. albicans* to subsequently

Table 2 In vitro susceptibilities of 5.346 clinical isolates of *Candida* spp. to anidulafungin, caspofungin, and micafungin

Organism	No. of isolates	Antifungal agent	MIC 90% [ug/mL]	MIC Range [ug/mL]
C. albicans	2,857	Anidulafungin	0.06	0.007–1.0
		Caspofungin	0.06	0.007–0.5
		Micafungin	0.03	0.007–1.0
C. parapsilosis	771	Anidulafungin	2	0.03–4.0
		Caspofungin	1	0.015–4.0
		Micafungin	2	0.015–2.0
C. glabrata	747	Anidulafungin	0.12	0.015–4.0
		Caspofungin	0.06	0.015–≥8.0
		Micafungin	0.015	0.007–1.0
C. tropicalis	625	Anidulafungin	0.06	0.007–2.0
		Caspofungin	0.06	0.007–≥8.0
		Micafungin	0.06	0.007–1.0
C. krusei	136	Anidulafungin	0.06	0.015–0.5
		Caspofungin	0.25	0.015–1.0
		Micafungin	0.12	0.015–0.25
C. guilliermondii	61	Anidulafungin	2	0.12–4.0
		Caspofungin	1	0.03–≥8.0
		Micafungin	1	0.015–2.0
C. lusitaniae	58	Anidulafungin	0.5	0.06–1.0
		Caspofungin	0.5	0.03–1.0
		Micafungin	0.25	0.03–1.0
C. kefyr	37	Anidulafungin	0.12	0.015–0.12
		Caspofungin	0.015	0.007–0.03
		Micafungin	0.06	0.015–0.06
C. famata	24	Anidulafungin	2	0.015–2.0
		Caspofungin	1	0.015–2.0
		Micafungin	1	0.015–2.0
Candida spp.	30	Anidulafungin	1	0.007–≥8.0
		Caspofungin	0.25	0.015–0.5
		Micafungin	0.5	0.015–0.5
Total	5,346	Anidulafungin	2	0.007–≥8.0
		Caspofungin	0.25	0.007–≥8.0
		Micafungin	1	0.007–2.0

Table modified from Ref. [18]

form biofilms [81], and, in contrast to antifungal triazoles and conventional but not lipid-associated amphtericin B, to exert potent antifungal activity against sessile *C. albicans* and *C. parapsilosis* within biofilms [81–83].

Pharmacodynamics

Time kill studies in *Candida* spp. have demonstrated strain- and species-dependent, both concentration- and time-dependent fungicidal activity and rate of kill at concentrations above the MIC for all three compounds. In addition, prolonged post-antifungal effects between 5 and 12 h at concentrations above the MIC have been demonstrated [84–90].

In persistently neutropenic rabbit models, anidulafungin showed highly predictable concentration-effect relationships in experimental disseminated candidiasis; however, no concentration-effect relationships were observed in experimental pulmonary aspergillosis despite full exploration of the dosage range [91]. Pharmacodynamic studies in murine kidney target models of disseminated candidiasis indicated that the Cmax/MIC and AUC/MIC are strongly predictive of antifungal efficacy [92–94] and that free drug exposures associated with efficacy are similar across *Candida* spp and similar across agents [93, 94]. In a murine model of invasive pulmonary aspergillosis, the Cmax/MEC ratio appeared to be the parameter most closely associated with efficacy [95].

In patients, pharmacokinetic/pharmacodynamic (PK/PD) correlations of all echinocandins have been explored using clinical data from Phase II and III clinical studies in patients with esophageal and oropharyngeal candidiasis. These studies consistently demonstrated dose response and PK/PD relationships that allowed for the definition of pharmacokinetic target values for exposure, average plasma levels, and plasma trough levels, that were well exceeded at the the dosages investigated in pivotal clinical trials in patients with invasive *Candida* infections. However, the analysis of isolates of patients enrolled in four clinical trials of caspofungin for esophageal and invasive candidiasis revealed no relationship of MIC to outcome for the entire data set, the different types of candidiasis, or specific *Candida* spp. [96]. Similar data were obtained for anidulafungin and micafungin [97]. This observation may be explained by the high efficacy of the dosages used in these studies and the absence of *Candida* isolates with elevated MICs in the clinical trial data sets.

In Vitro Susceptibility Testing

The European Committee on Antimicrobial Susceptibility Testing (EUCAST) and the Clinical and Laboratory Standards Institute (CLSI) have developed standardized methods based on broth dilution for the susceptibility testing of yeasts, that, despite methodological differences, generate overall similar results [98–100] (Table 2). Recently, the CLSI proposed a value of ≤ 2 μg/mL as a tentative susceptibility breakpoint for anidulafungin, caspofungin, and micafungin for *Candida* spp. on the basis of mechanisms of resistance, an epidemiological MIC population distribution, parameters associated with success in pharmacodynamic models, and results of clinical efficacy studies [97, 98]. Whether current susceptibility testing methods and breakpoints reliably identify isolates with resistance mechanisms associated with treatment failures, is not clear: In a recent study using a collection of blinded *FKS* hot spot mutant and wild type isolates, the CLSI breakpoint of ≤ 2 μg/mL resulted in 89.2% being classified as anidulafungin susceptible, 60.7% as caspofungin susceptible, and 92.9% as micafungin susceptible [101].

Anidulafungin

Pharmacokinetics and Metabolism

In healthy volunteers, after intravenous dosages of 35–100 mg, anidulafungin demonstrated linear pharmacokinetics with mean peak plasma levels ranging from 1.71 to 3.82 μg/mL, and mean $AUC_{0-\infty}$ values from 37.46 to 104.81 μg•h/mL. The mean volume of distribution was between 0.72 and 0.90 L/kg, and the terminal half-life was approximately 40 h (Table 3) [23]. Population based analysis of concentration data from 225 patients with serious fungal diseases collected during four phase II/III clinical studies revealed no relevant differences in pharmacokinetics as compared to healthy subjects [102].

Anidulafungin is not metabolized by the liver but slowly degraded chemically to inactive products. Mass balance studies showed that anidulafungin is eliminated in the feces predominantly as degradation products, with only a small fraction (10%) eliminated as unchanged drug; fecal elimination likely occurs via biliary excretion. Only negligible renal involvement in the drug's elimination was observed [4]. In laboratory animals, tissue concentrations at trough after multiple dosing were highest in lung and liver, followed by spleen and kidney. Measurable concentrations in brain tissue were noted only at the higher end of the dosage range. No relevant inter-species differences were observed [5, 91].

The pharmacokinetics of anidulafungin are not altered in subjects with mild, moderate and severe (creatinine clearance of <30 mL/min) renal impairment, nor in end-stage renal disease or during hemodialysis; likewise, hepatic impairment does not cause clinically relevant changes in the pharmacokinetics [103].

In pediatric patients, in a sequential cohort, age-stratified, dose-escalation study, concentrations and AUC were similar across patients, and, in contrast to caspofungin and micafungin, weight adjusted clearance rates were consistent

Table 3 Single-dose anidulafungin pharmacokinetics in pediatric and adult patients

	Pediatric patients (2–17 years)		Adults	
Dosage	0.75 mg/kg	1.5 mg/kg	50 mg	100 mg
Cmax (μg/mL)	4.02	6.09	2.51	3.82
AUC 0–24 h (μg·h/mL)	48.0	89.7	53.3	104.8
T ½ beta (h)	20.8	19.5	39.3[a]	42.3[a]
CL (L/h/kg)	0.0175	0.0191	n/a	n/a
VDss (L/kg)	0.45	0.49	0.72	0.78

Pharmacokinetic parameters are expressed as mean values. Data were obtained in groups of six pediatric patients with compromised immunity and neutropenia per age group and dosage level, and compared to those obtained in 26 adult healthy volunteers (Modified from Refs. [102, 104])

n/a, not available

[a]T½ gamma

across age (Table 3). Pharmacokinetic parameters following 0.75 or 1.5 mg/kg/day were similar to those observed in adult patients receiving 50 or 100 mg/day, respectively [104]. No data have yet been published for neonates.

Clinical Efficacy

The clinical efficacy of anidulafungin against *Candida* infections has been demonstrated in phase II and phase III studies in immunocompromised patients with esophageal candidiasis and in patients with candidemia or other forms of invasive candidiasis [105–108]. Anidulafungin had equivalent efficacy to fluconazole in a randomized, double-blind phase III international multicenter study in mostly HIV-infected patients with esophageal candidiasis [106]. Patients received intravenous anidulafungin (100 mg on day 1, followed by 50 mg daily) or oral fluconazole (200 mg on day 1, followed by 100 mg daily) for 7 days beyond resolution of symptoms (range, 14–21 days). At the end of therapy, the rate of endoscopic success for anidulafungin (242 [97.2%] of 249 treated patients) was found to be statistically noninferior to that for fluconazole (252 [98.8%] of 255 treated patients).

In a non-comparative dose-ranging study, 123 patients with invasive candidiasis, including candidemia, were randomized to one of three intravenous once daily regimens of 50, 75, or 100 mg of anidulafungin. Non-*albicans Candida* species accounted for approximately one-half of all isolates. Treatment continued for 2 weeks beyond resolution or improvement of signs and symptoms. The primary endpoint was clinical and microbiological success in the evaluable population at 2 weeks after end of therapy. Among the 68 patients evaluable for efficacy, success rates at end of therapy were 84%, 90%, and 89%, respectively [105]. This study was followed by a randomized, double blind phase III study that compared anidulafungin,100 mg daily, to fluconazole,400 mg daily, for treatment of invasive candidiasis in a total of 245 mostly non-neutropenic patients [107]. Patients were stratified for neutropenia and APACHE II scores (> or ≤ 20) and, in either arm, could switch to oral fluconazole after at least 10 days of intravenous therapy. The primary efficacy endpoint was global response (clinical and microbiological success) in the modified intent-to-treat (MITT) population at end of intravenous therapy. Of 261 enrolled patients, 245 had received at least one dose of study drug and were proved to have candidiasis. Overall, 89% had candidemia, and 97% were not neutropenic. The groups were well matched; the mean APACHE II score was 15 and 14.4. *C. albicans* was the species isolated in 62% of patients. Clinical and microbiological success was superior for anidulafungin, when compared with fluconazole, at the end of therapy (74% vs 57%, $p = .02$) and at 2 weeks after the end of therapy (65% vs 49%, $p = .02$). A trend toward increased survival was noted in the anidulafungin group (77% vs 69%; $P = .13$).

Safety and Tolerance

In initial dose-optimization studies in healthy volunteers receiving daily maintenance doses of 70–130 mg for 9 days following a loading dose of up to 260 mg on day one, anidulafungin was well tolerated without encountering dose limiting toxicities [23].

Anidulafungin was overall well tolerated. In the dose-ranging trial in patients with invasive *Candida* infections, review of adverse events and laboratory data indicated no dose response for safety parameters. Adverse events considered to be related to treatment were reported by <5% of patients in each dosage group. The most common events, irrespective of relationship to treatment, were hypotension, vomiting, constipation, nausea and pyrexia [105]. In the two randomized, comparative trials, the safety profile of anidulafungin was similar to that of fluconazole. Type and frequency of adverse events were comparable with <5% of patients discontinuing the randomized study drug because of drug-related adverse events [106, 107].

Of note, infusion-related reactions have been reported with anidulafungin. In the pivotal invasive candidiasis study, these included flushing (2.3%), pruritus (2.3%), rash (1.5%), and urticaria (0.8%). Other treatment-related adverse reactions that occurred in <5% of patients in the pivotal study included hypokalemia, diarrhea, increased hepatic enzymes and bilirubin [107]. In individual patients, cases of hepatic dysfunction, hepatitis, or worsening hepatic failure have been reported. Exacerbation of infusion-related reactions by coadministration of anesthetics has been noted in a study in rats; the clinical relevance of this is unknown [109, 110].

Drug Interactions

In vitro studies showed that anidulafungin is not a clinically relevant substrate, inducer, or inhibitor of important human cytochrome P450 isoforms at safely achievable concentrations, and it is not an inhibitor of P-glycoprotein [4]. Formal interaction studies demonstrated that no dosage adjustment of either drug is warranted when anidulafungin is coadministered with cyclosporine A, tacrolimus, voriconazole, liposomal amphotericin B, or rifampin [109–113]. In a large population-based pharmacokinetic analysis, there was no evidence that the presence of rifampin or metabolic substrates, inhibitors, or inducers of cytochrome p450 influenced the clearance of anidulafungin [4].

Approval Status and Dosing Recommendations

Anidulafungin is licensed in USA in patients ≥ 18 years of age for esophageal candidiasis, candidemia, and other forms of invasive *Candida* infections, including intra-abdominal abscesses and peritonitis, in non-neutropenic patients [110]. In Europe, anidulafungin is licensed for treatment of candidemia in adult non-neutropenic patients [109]. The recommended dosage is 100 mg daily after a loading dose of 200 mg for invasive candidiasis and 50 mg daily after a loading dose of 10 mg for esophageal candidiasis. No dosage adjustment is needed in subjects with mild, moderate or severe renal impairment, those undergoing hemodialysis and in patients with mild, moderate or severe hepatic impairment (Child-Pugh class A, B and C).

Safety and antifungal efficacy of anidulafungin in pediatric patients has not been established, but is actively being studied. Anidulafungin has been shown to cross the placental barrier and may be embryotoxic in rats. Adequate data in pregnant and lactating women do not exist, and the compound should only be used if the potential benefit justifies the risk to the fetus [109, 110].

Caspofungin

Pharmacokinetics and Metabolism

Administration of single dosages of 5–100 mg of caspofungin to healthy volunteers demonstrated linear pharmacokinetics with a beta half-life of 9–10 h and an average plasma clearance of 10–12 mL/min (Table 4). At higher dosages, an additional, longer gamma half-life of 40–50 h was evident. Multiple dose studies at dosages of 15, 35, and 70 mg daily for 2 or 3 weeks revealed dose-dependent accumulation of drug in plasma of up to 50%. A loading dose of 70 mg, followed by 50 mg daily, maintained plasma concentrations above 1 μg/mL from day 1 onward; this is above the reported MIC values for most susceptible fungi [117]. Investigation of higher dosages revealed constant pharmacokinetics after single doses of 150 and 210 mg and following 14-days of 100 mg, respectively [25].

Tissue distribution, particularly to the liver through specific uptake transporters, is the predominant mechanism influencing clearance of caspofungin: Mass balance studies demonstrate that approximately 92% of the administered radioactivity distributes to tissues at 36–48 h [6, 48, 118, 119]. Tissue distribution studies in mice revealed preferential exposure of liver, kidney, and large intestine, whereas exposure for small intestine, lung and spleen was equivalent to that for plasma. Organs with a lower level of exposure included the heart, thigh, and brain [120]. Excretion of caspofungin in humans is slow, with 41% and 35% of the dosed radioactivity being recovered in urine and feces, respectively, over 27 days. Caspofungin is slowly metabolized by peptide hydrolysis and N-acetylation; only a small fraction of caspofungin (~1.4% of dose) is excreted unchanged in urine [6, 7, 118–120].

Dosage adjustment is not necessary for patients with impaired renal function and end-stage renal insufficiency. While patients with mild hepatic insufficiency do not require a dosage adjustment, a dosage of 35 mg daily after the initial 70 mg loading dose is recommended for patients with moderate hepatic insufficiency (Child-Pugh score 7–9) due to an average increase of 76% in AUC. No clinical experience exists in patients with severe hepatic insufficiency (Child-Pugh score >9). Dosage adjustment based on weight, age, gender, serum albumin concentration or on the basis of race is not required [21, 25, 121].

Table 4 Single-dose caspofungin pharmacokinetics in pediatric and adult patients

	Premature neonates	Infants and toddlers (3–24 months)	Children (2–11 years)	Adolescents (12–17 years)	Adults
Dosage	25 mg/m²	50 mg/m²	50 mg/m²	50 mg/m²	50 mg
AUC 0–24 h (μg·h/mL)	n/a	120	96.4	77.6	70.6
C1 (μg/mL)	10.2	17.46	13.9	8.95	7.67
C24 (ug/mL)	2.3	1.34	1.09	1.26	1.35
T ½ beta (h)	n/a	7.79	7.6	10.51	11.7
CL (mL/min/m²)	n/a	6.05	7.78	6.3	6.07

Least square means are reported for AUC, C1 (Cmax), and C24 (Cmin), and harmonic means for t ½ beta. Data were obtained in groups of 6–10 pediatric patients and compared to those obtained in 32 adult patients with mucosal candidiasis

Compiled from Refs. [8, 114–116]

n/a, data not available from the publication

In pediatric patients 2–17 years old, 50 mg/m²/day provided similar or slightly higher exposure relative to adults dosed with 50 mg daily [8] and was selected for further study. While this dosage was also found to be appropriate in infants 3 months to 2 years of age [114], limited data indicate that a dosage of 25 mg/m² daily is indicated to achieve comparable exposures in premature neonates (Table 4) [115].

Clinical Efficacy

The clinical efficacy of caspofungin has been investigated for oropharyngeal and esophageal candidiasis, invasive candidiasis, invasive aspergillosis, and for empiric treatment of persistently febrile neutropenic patients. In a multicenter, randomized, double blind study comparing caspofungin (50 mg daily) and fluconazole (200 mg daily) for treatment of esophageal candidiasis in 177 mostly HIV-infected patients, response rates as assessed by the combined response of symptom resolution and significant endoscopic improvement 5–7 days after discontinuation of treatment were similar for both cohorts (81% vs 85%) [116]. These favorable data were supported by two further, randomized, double-blind, multicenter trials that compared caspofungin with conventional amphotericin B (0.5 mg/kg/day) [122, 123] and a retrospective case series of patients with esophageal candidiasis resistant to fluconazole [124].

The efficacy of caspofungin as primary treatment of invasive *Candida* infections has been investigated in a multicenter, randomized, double-blind phase III clinical trial comparing caspofungin, 50 mg daily after a loading dose of 70 mg, to amphotericin B deoxycholate,0.6–1 mg/kg daily. Patients were treated for 14 days after the last positive culture, but could be switched to fluconazole after 10 days of intravenous therapy. Success required both symptom resolution and microbiological clearance. At study entry, 13% of patients were neutropenic; the majority had candidemia (83%). The predominant organism was *C. albicans* (45%). Among patients receiving at least one dose of study drug, 73% (80/109) of the caspofungin cohort and 61.7% (71/115) of the amphotericin B cohort were classified as therapeutic success at the end of intravenous therapy. There was no difference in relapse or survival at 6–8 weeks follow up [125].

The clinical usefulness of caspofungin for treatment of patients with invasive candidiasis is further corroborated by a randomized, double-blind phase III trial comparing micafungin 100 mg daily and micafungin 150 mg daily with the standard dosage of caspofungin, 50 mg daily, in a total of 595 adults. This study showed similar success rates at the end of therapy (76%, 71%, and 72%, respectively) and no significant differences in time to culture negativity, mortality, relapses and emerging infections [126]. In a more recent randomized phase III trial, high-dose caspofungin, 150 mg daily, was compared to treatment with the standard dose of 50 mg daily in a total of 204 patients. No safety concerns were found for the higher dose of caspofungin; however, no significant benefit in regards to clinical response or mortality was found [127]. Among 48 patients with non-fungemic invasive candidiasis and chronic disseminated candidiasis who received caspofungin primary or salvage monotherapy at the standard dosage had an overall success rate at the end of therapy of 81% [128]. A review of 27 neutropenic patients showed a favorable response in 17 of 27 patients (63%) [129].

The clinical efficacy of caspofungin, 50 mg daily after a loading dose of 70 mg, against invasive aspergillosis has been studied in a multicenter, open-label, noncomparative phase II trial in patients with definite or probable invasive aspergillosis refractory to or intolerant of standard therapies [130]. A total of 83 patients received caspofungin for a mean duration of 28 days (range, 1–162 days). The majority had hematological malignancies or had undergone bone marrow transplantation, and most had refractory *Aspergillus* infections. Complete or partial responses at end of therapy were achieved in 44.6% of patients receiving at least one dose of caspofungin; in patients receiving the drug for≥7 days, a favorable response was seen in 56%.

Caspofungin has also been explored as first line treatment of invasive aspergillosis in two phase II pilot trials initiated by the EORTC Infectious Diseases Group. In 61 mostly neutropenic patients with hematological malignancies or undergoing autologous stem cell transplantation, 20 (31%) patients had a complete and partial response at end of treatment, and 9 (15%) achieved stabilization. The 12-week survival rate was 53% (32/60) [131]. Among 24 eligible allogeneic stem cell transplant recipients, of whom 12 were neutropenic at baseline, 10 (44%) had a complete or partial response at end of treatment, and one (4%) had stable disease. Survival at day 84 was 48% [132].

Retrospective series suggest a potential usefulness of combination therapies of caspofungin with either voriconazole [133] or amphotericin B [134]. In a multicenter, prospective noncomparative study of caspofungin combined with other antifungal agents, including 53 adults with invasive aspergillosis refractory or intolerant to prior therapy, the overall success rate at end of therapy was 55%. Success in patients with >7 days of combination therapy was 66% (27/41) [135]. In a prospective, randomized open pilot study in 30 patients with proven or probable invasive aspergillosis, combination of liposomal amphotericin B 3 mg/kg daily and caspofungin was tested against monotherapy with high-dose amphotericin B 10 mg/kg daily; while complete or partial response rates were higher in the combination group, survival rates at 12 weeks after inclusion were 100% and 80%, respectively [136]. Finally, in a single center retrospective observational study including 41 patients with biopsy-proven rhino-orbital-cerebral mucormycosis identified over 12 years, treatment with polyene-caspofungin therapy had superior success compared with patients treated with polyene monotherapy. In multivariate analysis, only receipt of combination therapy was significantly associated with improved outcomes [137].

In a randomized, double-blind, multinational trial of empirical antifungal therapy in febrile neutropenic patients, the overall success rate of caspofungin treatment was non-inferior to that with liposomal amphotericin B 3 mg/kg daily [138]. However, among patients with baseline fungal infections, a higher proportion of those treated with caspofungin had a successful outcome (51.9% vs 25.9%, $P=0.04$). Similarly, the proportion of patients who survived at least 7 days after therapy was greater in the caspofungin group (92.6% vs 89.2%, $P=0.05$) and premature study discontinuation occurred less often in the caspofungin group (10.3% vs 14.5%, $P=0.03$). Randomized data also indicate that caspofungin may provide similar protection as itraconazole against invasive fungal infections when given as prophylaxis in patients undergoing remission induction chemotherapy for acute myelogenous leukemia or myelodysplastic syndrome [139].

For children, efficacy data have been collected for caspofungin, 50 mg/m^2 daily adfter a loading dose of 70 mg/m^2, in the setting of fever and neutropenia and in patients with documented infections. As compared to liposomal amphotericin B, 3 mg/kg daily, caspofungin was equaly effective as empirical therapy but better tolerated [140]. Among 48 pediatric patients with proven or probable invasive fungal infections, success at end of therapy was achieved in 5 of 10 patients with invasive aspergillosis, and 30 of 37 with invasive candidiasis [141]. Limited data support the use of caspofungin for treatment of neonatal candidemia [142–144]. Among 36 neonates, most of whom were premature, with candidemia refractory to therapy with amphotericin B, treatment with caspofungin at 2 mg/kg daily (mean: 23 mg/m^2), 35 (97%) had a successful outcome [144].

Safety and Tolerance

Caspofungin is generally well tolerated: In the seven randomized, comparative clinical trials discussed in detail earlier, less than 5% of patients discontinued the drug prematurely due to drug-related clinical adverse experiences [116, 122–128, 138]. Exploration of higher dosages of up to 210 mg daily in healthy volunteers [25] and of up to 150 mg daily in patients with invasive candidiasis [127] revealed no new or increased rates of adverse events.

The most commonly reported drug-related clinical adverse experiences occurring in $\geq$5% of 228 patients in 3 active control studies included fever, phlebitis, nausea, and headache [145, 146]. Symptoms such as rash, facial swelling, pruritus, or sensation of warmth, potentially mediated through endogenous histamine release [147], have been reported in isolated cases [148]. Laboratory abnormalities occurring in $\geq$5% of patients were increased liver enzymes, decreased serum potassium, decreased hemoglobin, and decreased white blood cell count [145, 146]. A similar incidence and pattern of adverse events has been observed larger surveys outside the setting of clinical trials [149, 150].

Caspofungin appears to be well-tolerated in pediatric patients: In a phase I/II dose-finding study in 39 children and adolescents, none of the patients developed a serious drug-related adverse event nor was therapy discontinued for toxicity [114]. A similarly favorable safety profile has also been reported in immunocompromised pediatric patients who received the compound within pharmacokinetic dose finding trials, as empirical therapy, or for treatment of invasive infections [151] and in neonates with refractory invasive candidiasis [144]. As caspofungin solution contains sucrose, patients with rare hereditary problems of fructose intolerance or sucrase–isomaltase insufficiency should not receive this agent.

Because of transient elevations of hepatic transaminases in single-dose interaction studies, the concomitant use of caspofungin with cyclosporine is not recommended by the manufacturer [145, 146]. However, retrospective analyses [152, 153] did not show evidence of a toxicodynamic interaction of caspofungin and cyclosporine.

Drug Interactions

Caspofungin is not a substrate of P-glycoprotein and is a poor substrate of cytochrome P-450 enzymes and a weak cytochrome P-450 enzyme inhibitor [7]. No pharmacokinetic interactions were observed in healthy volunteers between caspofungin and itraconazole, amphotericin B deoxycholate, mycophenolate mofetil, and nelfinavir [21, 25, 154], and no clinically relevant interactions have been found between tacrolimus or cyclosporine A and caspofungin. In vitro, caspofungin significantly inhibited the metabolism of cytarabine, a substrate of CYP3A4; no in vivo interaction studies have been conducted as to determine the clinical relevance of this finding [155].

Coadministration of inducers of drug clearance and/or mixed inducer/inhibitors, namely efavirenz, nevirapine, phenytoin, rifampin, dexamethasone, and carbamazepine with caspofungin may result in clinically meaningful reductions in caspofungin concentrations. The manufacturer recommends an increase in the dosage of caspofungin to 70 mg daily in patients on concurrent therapy with these drugs [21, 25, 145, 146].

Results from regression analyses indicate that pediatric patients will have similar reductions with inducers as seen in adults. If caspofungin is co-administered with the listed inducers of drug clearance, a dose of 70 mg/m² daily (maximum daily dose of 70 mg) should be considered [145, 146].

Approval Status and Dosing Recommendations

In USA, caspofungin is licensed in adults and pediatric patients 3 months and older for treatment of esophageal candidiasis, candidemia, certain forms of invasive *Candida* infections, including intra-abdominal abscesses, peritonitis and pleural space infections. It is recommenrded as second line therapy of proven or probable invasive aspergillosis and for empirical antifungal therapy in granulocytopenic patients with persistent fever [145]. In Europe, the compound is approved in adult and pediatric patients of all ages for treatment of invasive candidiasis, second line treatment of invasive aspergillosis, and for empirical therapy for presumed fungal infections in neutropenic patients [146].

The recommended dose regimen for adults consists of a single 70-mg loading dose on day 1, followed by 50 mg daily thereafter, administered over 1 h. The regimen approved in pediatric patients 3 months to 17 years is 50 mg/m² daily after a 70 mg/m² loading dose (maximum daily dose 70 mg). The preliminary dosage in infants < 3 months and in premature neonates is 25 mg/m² daily. No dosage adjustment is required in patients with renal insufficiency. In patients with mild hepatic insufficiency (Child-Pugh category A), no adjustments are needed; in patients with moderate hepatic insufficiency (Child-Pugh category B), decreasing the maintenance dose to 35 mg/day is recommeded after the loading dose of 70 mg. No recommendations exist for patients with severe hepatic insufficiency (Child-Pugh category C).

Caspofungin has been shown to cross the placental barrier and to be embryotoxic in rats and rabbits. Adequate data in pregnant and lactating women do not exist, and the compound should only be used if the potential benefit justifies the risk to the fetus [145, 146].

Micafungin

Pharmacokinetics and Metabolism

Micafungin exhibits linear plasma pharmacokinetics with doses ranging from 12.5 to 200 mg. There is no evidence of systemic accumulation with repeated administration, and steady state is generally reached within 4–5 days [156–158]. Following a standard single therapeutic dose of 100 mg, the mean peak plasma level was 8.8 μg/mL, the $AUC_{0-\infty}$ 125.9 μg.h/mL, half-life 14.6 h, and total clearance 9.8 mL/h/kg, respectively [159] (Table 5).

In plasma, the drug is highly (>99%) bound primarily to albumin and is rapidly distributed into tissues [22]. Tissue concentrations in animals were highest in the lung, liver, spleen, and kidney. Micafungin was undetectable in CSF, but brain tissue concentrations exceeded MIC_{90} values in a dose dependent manner [9, 22]. Micafungin is metabolized in the liver and excreted in inactive form into bile and urine. In healthy volunteers, during washout, less than 1% of drug was found in the urine in unchanged form [22]. Even though micafungin is a substrate for CYP3A in vitro, hydroxylation by CYP3A is not a major pathway for micafungin metabolism in vivo [22].

Renal dysfunction (creatinine clearance < 30 mL/min) or hemodialysis have no relevant impact on the pharmacokinetics of micafungin [159]. In subjects with moderate hepatic dysfunction, weight-normalized clearance was not altered [9]. In living donor liver recipients, no significant differences were observed in the disposition of micafungin [162], and no differences in disposition were noted in elderly patients aged 66–78 years [22].

In febrile neutropenic pediatric patients 2–17 years of age dosed from 0.5 to 4 mg/kg, micafungin pharmacokinetics were linear and overall similar to those observed in adults. However, in patients 2–8 years old, clearance was approximately 1.35 times that of patients > 9 years of age. Exposures following a dose of 1 and 2 mg/kg corresponded to those following 50 and 100 mg in adults, respectively

Table 5 Single-dose micafungin pharmacokinetics in pediatric and adult patients

	Premature neonates	Pediatric patients (2–17 years)		Adults	
Dosage	3 mg/kg	1 mg/kg	2 mg/kg	50 mg	100 mg
Cmax (μg/mL)	9.3	10.8	15.3	3.6	7.1
AUC 0–24 h (μg·h/mL)	69.0	40.3	83.0	33.9	59.9
T ½ beta (h)	8.2	12.5	13.2	12.5	13.0
CL (L/h/kg)	0.039	0.021	0.020	0.017[a]	0.018[a]
VDss (L/kg)	0.44	0.33	0.31	0.31[a]	0.32[a]

Pharmacokinetic parameters are expressed as mean values. Data were obtained in groups of 6–15 pediatric patients or neonates, and compared to those obtained in cohorts of 8–9 adult patients with hematopoietic stem cell transplantation (Modified from Refs [22, 160, 161, 163])

[a] Weight normalization calculated by assuming an average body weight of 70 kg

(Table 5) [160, 163] and were selected for the further pediatric development. Current pharmacokinetic data in premature neonates indicate a considerably higher clerance rate than in other pediatric age groups and adults and the potential need for larger doses in these infants [161, 164–166].

Clinical Efficacy

The antifungal efficacy and the dose-response relationship of micafungin against human *Candida* infections were investigated in a series of phase II and III clinical trials in mostly HIV-infected patients with esophageal candidiasis [167–169]. In a randomized, double-blind clinical trial including a total of 245 patients ≥ 18 years with HIV-infection and esophageal candidiasis, the endoscopic cure rate was dose-dependent with 68.8%, 77.4%, and 89.8%, respectively, following 50, 100, and 150 mg of micafungin. The endoscopic cure rate for 100 and 150 mg of micafungin combined (83.5%) was comparable to that of fluconazole (86.7%) [169]. In a further randomized, double-blind comparative trial conducted in a total of 523 patients ≥ 16 years with esophageal candidiasis, micafungin (150 mg) was as effective as fluconazole (200 mg daily) with endoscopic cure rates of 87.7% versus 88.0%, and recurrence rates at 4-weeks post-treatment were not different [169].

The efficacy of micafungin as first line therapy of invasive *Candida* infections has been established through two large randomized, double-blind phase III clinical trials [126, 170]. The first trial compared micafungin 100 mg daily to liposomal amphotericin B 3 mg/kg daily in a total of 531 adult patients. Treatment success was defined as clinical response combined with mycological response at end of therapy. Candidemia constituted approximately 85% of the cases, and non-*albicans* infections comprised approximately 60% of cases. Most patients (88%) were non-neutropenic. The overall success rate in both treatment arms was similar – 74% of those receiving micafungin and 70% in those receiving liposomal amphotericin B, and there was no difference in survival [170]. The second trial compared micafungin 100 mg daily and micafungin 150 mg daily to the standard dosage of caspofungin, 50 mg daily, in a total of 595 mostly non-neutropenic (92%) adults with candidemia and other forms of invasive candidiasis. At the end of blinded intravenous therapy, treatment was considered successful for 76.4% of patients in the micafungin 100 mg group, 71.4% in the micafungin 150 mg group, and 72.3% in the caspofungin group. There were no significant differences in time to culture negativity, mortality, relapses and emerging infections among the study arms [126]. The clinical efficacy of micafungin against invasive candidiasis is further supported by an open label, non-comparative trial in 126 patients with new or refractory candidemia who received the drug alone or in combination with another agent. Complete or partial responses were observed in 83.3% patients overall without apparent species-related differences [171].

A multi-national, non-comparative open-label clinical trial investigated micafungin for proven or probable invasive aspergillosis alone or in combination with another systemic antifungal agent in 225 patients. A favorable response rate at the end of therapy was seen in 35.6%. Of those treated only with micafungin, favorable responses were seen in 6/12 of the primary and 9/22 of the salvage therapy group. Most patients were treated with one or two other drugs as well as micafungin, and the overall response rate for those patients was 34% [172]. In the subgroup of 98 hematopoietic stem cell transplant recipients, a partial or complete response was seen in 3 of 8 patients who were treated with micafungin alone [173].

Micafungin was also compared with fluconazole for prophylaxis against invasive fungal infections during neutropenia in patients undergoing hematopoietic stem cell transplantation. In a randomized, double-blind, multi-institutional, phase III trial involving 882 adult and pediatric patients, patients received either 50 mg of micafungin (1 mg/kg for <50 kg body weight) or 400 mg of fluconazole (8 mg/kg for <50 kg) daily. Success was defined as the absence of suspected, proven, or probable invasive fungal infection (IFI) through the end of therapy and as the absence of proven or probable IFI through the end of the 4-week period after treatment. The overall efficacy of micafungin was superior to that of fluconazole as antifungal prophylaxis (80.0% vs. 73.5%, $p = .03$), thus demonstrating efficacy of micafungin for antifungal prophylaxis in neutropenic patients [174] A further, smaller randomized trial in 106 adult HSCT patients compared prophylaxis with micafungin 150 mg to fluconazole 400 mg. Success, defined the same as noted above, was 94% in the micafungin-treated patients ans 88% in the fluconazole recipients [175].

In pediatric patients, efficacy data from substudies of two large randomized comparative trials have been reported [174, 176]. In patients undergoing stem cell transplantation, prophylaxis with micafungin was as effective as prophylaxis with fluconazole without signals for differences in comparison to the entire study population [174]. Similar observations were made in 98 pediatric patients with invasive candidiasis or candidemia, 57 of whom were <2 years old and 19 who were premature neonates. Treatment success was observed for 35/48 (72.9%) patients treated with micafungin and 38/50 (76.0%) patients treated with liposomal amphotericin B. Efficacy findings were independent of neutropenia status, age, and whether the patient was premature at birth [176].

Safety and Tolerance

In dose-ranging studies in immunocompromised adult patients, micafungin was well tolerated during chronic dosing at dosages up to 200 mg or 8 mg/kg daily without reaching a maximum tolerated dose [156, 168, 177]. A pooled analysis from 17 clinical efficacy and safety studies with micafungin, including 3,028 mostly immunocompromised patients who received at least one single dose of micafungin, has been reported. The mean age of patients was 41.4 years with 296 (9.8%) children <16 years and 387 (12.8%) older patients ≥ 65 years. The median micafungin daily dose was 100 mg for adult patients and 1.5 mg/kg for children. The mean duration of exposure was 18 and 29 days, respectively. The most frequently reported treatment-related adverse events (≥ 2%) were nausea, vomiting, phlebitis, hypokalemia, fever, and diarrhea. Increases in liver enzymes occurred in about 2% of patients (2.0%) [178]. In the pivotal comparative studies, micafungin had a similar safety profile compared to fluconazole and caspofungin and was better tolerated than liposomal amphotericin B; less than 5% of patients discontinued treatment with micafungin related to adverse events [126, 168, 170, 174].

Clinical trials in pediatric patients revealed no differences in safety as compared to adults [163, 174, 176]. In premature neonates, micafungin has been tolerated without limiting toxicity or higher rates of adverse events at multiple doses of up to 15 mg/kg daily [165, 166].

Because of the observation of foci of altered hepatocytes and hepatocellular tumors after long-term exposure studies in rats, the European Summary of Product Characteristics recommends careful monitoring of liver function values during micafungin treatment and early discontinuation in the presence of significant and persistent elevation of liver transaminases, and also recommends a careful risk/benefit evaluation, particularly in patients having severe liver function impairment, chronic liver diseases or receiving concomitant hepatotoxic therapy [179]. The clinical relevance of these observed preclinical findings, however, is unknown.

Drug Interactions

Studies using human liver microsomes revealed neither inhibition nor stimulation of CYP1A2, CYP2D6, CYP2E1, CYP2C9, and CYP2C19 but inhibition of CYP3A4 in a manner comparable to fluconazole [180–182]. However, studies in healthy volunteers revealed no drug interaction between micafungin and mycophenolate mofetil, cyclosporine, tacrolimus, prednisolone, sirolimus, nifedipine, fluconazole, ritonavir, rifampicin, itraconazole, voriconazole and amphotericin B. In these studies, no evidence of altered pharmacokinetics of micafungin was observed. Exposure (AUC) of itraconazole, sirolimus, and nifedipine was slightly increased in the presence of micafungin. Patients receiving sirolimus, nifedipine or itraconazole in combination with micafungin should be monitored for toxicity due to these agents and the dosage of sirolimus, nifedipine or itraconazole should be reduced, if necessary [10, 179, 183–185].

Approval Status and Dosing Recommendations

In USA, micafungin is licensed in adults for treatment of esophageal candidiasis, candidemia, acute disseminated candidiasis, *Candida* peritonitis and abscesses, and as prophylaxis against *Candida* infections in patients undergoing hematopoietic stem cell transplantation [183]. In Europe, micafungin is approved for treatment of esophageal candidiasis in patients ≥ 16 years of age for whom intravenous therapy is appropriate, for treatment of invasive candidiasis in all age groups, and for prophylaxis of *Candida* infection in patients undergoing allogeneic hematopoietic stem cell transplantation or patients who are expected to have neutropenia for >10 days [179].

The recommended dosage regimens approved by both the FDA and the EMEA for adults is 150 mg for esophageal candidiasis,100 mg for invasive candidiasis, and 50 mg for prophylaxis of *Candida* infections, administered once daily over 1 h. The corresponding regimens approved by the EMEA in pediatric patients ≤ 40 kg of body weight are 3, 2, and 1 mg/kg, respectively. In patients with invasive candidiasis, the option of dose escalation to 200 mg or 4 mg/kg, respectively, in patients with persistent clinical or microbiological findings is offered [179, 183].

No dosage adjustments are required based on race, gender, in patients with renal insufficiency, or in patients with mild to moderate hepatic insufficiency (Child-Pugh category A and B). No recommendations exist for patients with severe hepatic insufficiency (Child-Pugh category C).

Micafungin has been shown to cross the placental barrier and to be embryotoxic in laboratory animals. Adequate data in pregnant and lactating women do not exist, and the compound should only be used if the potential benefit justifies the risk to the fetus [179, 183].

References

1. Hector RF. Compounds active against cell walls of medically important fungi. Clin Microbiol Rev. 1993;6:1–21.
2. Debono M, Gordee RS. Antibiotics that inhibit fungal cell wall development. Ann Rev Microbiol. 1994;48:471–97.

3. Groll AH, Piscitelli SC, Walsh TJ. Clinical pharmacology of systemic antifungal agents: a comprehensive review of agents in clinical use, current investigational compounds, and putative targets for antifungal drug development. Adv Pharmacol. 1998;44:343–500.
4. Damle BD, Dowell JA, Walsky RL, Weber GL, Stogniew M, Inskeep PB. In vitro and in vivo studies to characterize the clearance mechanism and potential cytochrome P450 interactions of anidulafungin. Antimicrob Agents Chemother. 2009;53:1149–56.
5. Damle B, Stogniew M, Dowell J. Pharmacokinetics and tissue distribution of anidulafungin in rats. Antimicrob Agents Chemother. 2008;52:2673–6.
6. Hajdu R, Thompson R, Sundelof JG, et al. Preliminary animal pharmacokinetics of the parenteral antifungal agent MK-0991 (L-743, 872). Antimicrob Agents Chemother. 1997;41:2339–44.
7. Stone JA, Xu X, Winchell GA, et al. Disposition of caspofungin: role of distribution in determining pharmacokinetics in plasma. Antimicrob Agents Chemother. 2004;48:815–23.
8. Walsh TJ, Adamson PC, Seibel NL, et al. Pharmacokinetics, safety, and tolerability of caspofungin in children and adolescents. Antimicrob Agents Chemother. 2005;49:4536–45.
9. Niwa T, Yokota Y, Tokunaga A, et al. Tissue distribution after intravenous dosing of micafungin, an antifungal drug, to rats. Biol Pharm Bull. 2004;27:1154–6.
10. Hebert MF, Townsend RW, Austin S, et al. Concomitant cyclosporine and micafungin pharmacokinetics in healthy volunteers. J Clin Pharmacol. 2005;45:954–60.
11. Kurtz MB, Douglas CM. Lipopeptide inhibitors of fungal glucan synthase. J Med Vet Mycol. 1997;35:79–86.
12. Leventakos K, Ben Ami R, Lewis RE, Kontoyiannis DP. Immunomodulating effects of antifungal therapy. Curr Fungal Infect Rep. 2009;3:43–50.
13. Bartizal K, Gill CJ, Abruzzo GK, et al. In vitro preclinical evaluation studies with the echinocandin antifungal MK-0991 (L-743, 872). Antimicrob Agents Chemother. 1997;41:2326–32.
14. Watabe E, Nakai T, Matsumoto S, Ikeda F, Hatano K. Killing activity of micafungin against *Aspergillus fumigatus* hyphae assessed by specific fluorescent staining for cell viability. Antimicrob Agents Chemother. 2003;47:1995–8.
15. Kurtz MB, Heath IB, Marrinan J, Dreikorn S, Onishi J, Douglas CM. Morphological effects of lipopeptides against *Aspergillus fumigatus* correlate with activities against (1, 3)-beta-D-glucan synthase. Antimicrob Agents Chemother. 1994;38:1480–9.
16. Oakley KL, Moore CB, Denning DW. In vitro activity of the echinocandin antifungal agent LY303, 366 in comparison with itraconazole and amphotericin B against *Aspergillus* spp. Antimicrob Agents Chemother. 1998;42:2726–30.
17. Bowman JC, Hicks PS, Kurtz MB, et al. The antifungal echinocandin caspofungin acetate kills growing cells of *Aspergillus fumigatus* in vitro. Antimicrob Agents Chemother. 2002;46:3001–12.
18. Pfaller MA, Boyken L, Hollis RJ, et al. In vitro susceptibility of invasive isolates of *Candida* spp. to anidulafungin, caspofungin, and micafungin: six years of global surveillance. J Clin Microbiol. 2008;46:150–6.
19. Espinel-Ingroff A. Comparison of in vitro activities of the new triazole SCH56592 and the echinocandins MK-0991 (L-743, 872) and LY303366 against opportunistic filamentous and dimorphic fungi and yeasts. J Clin Microbiol. 1998;36:2950–6.
20. Tawara S, Ikeda F, Maki K, et al. In vitro activities of a new lipopeptide antifungal agent, FK463, against a variety of clinically important fungi. Antimicrob Agents Chemother. 2000;44:57–62.
21. Groll AH, Walsh J. Caspofungin: Pharmacology, safety, and therapeutic potential in superficial and invasive fungal infections. Exp Opin Invest Drugs. 2001;10:1545–58.
22. Groll AH, Stergiopoulou T, Roilides E, Walsh TJ. Micafungin: pharmacology, experimental therapeutics and clinical applications. Expert Opin Invest Drugs. 2005;14:489–509.
23. Vazquez JA, Sobel JD. Anidulafungin: a novel echinocandin. Clin Infect Dis. 2006;43:215–22.
24. Wiederhold NP, Lewis JS. The echinocandin micafungin: a review of the pharmacology, spectrum of activity, clinical efficacy and safety. Expert Opin Pharmacother. 2007;8:1155–66.
25. Hope WW, Shoham S, Walsh TJ. The pharmacology and clinical use of caspofungin. Expert Opin Drug Metab Toxicol. 2007;3:263–74.
26. Estes KE, Penzak SR, Calis KA, Walsh TJ. Pharmacology and antifungal properties of anidulafungin, a new echinocandin. Pharmacotherapy. 2009;29:17–30.
27. Pfaller MA, Boyken L, Hollis RJ, et al. In vitro susceptibility of clinical isolates of *Aspergillus* spp. to anidulafungin, caspofungin, and micafungin: A head-to-head comparison using the CLSI M38-A2 broth microdilution method. J Clin Microbiol. 2009;47:3323–5.
28. Eschertzhuber S, Velik-Salchner C, Hoermann C, Hoefer D, Lass-Florl C. Caspofungin-resistant *Aspergillus flavus* after heart transplantation and mechanical circulatory support: a case report. Transplant Infect Dis. 2008;10:190–2.
29. Hernandez S, Lopez-Ribot JL, Najvar LK, McCarthy DI, Bocanegra R, Graybill JR. Caspofungin resistance in *Candida albicans*: correlating clinical outcome with laboratory susceptibility testing of three isogenic isolates serially obtained from a patient with progressive *Candida* esophagitis. Antimicrob Agents Chemother. 2004;48:1382–3.
30. Moudgal V, Little T, Boikov D, Vazquez JA. Multiechinocandin- and multiazole-resistant *Candida parapsilosis* isolates serially obtained during therapy for prosthetic valve endocarditis. Antimicrob Agents Chemother. 2005;49:767–9.
31. Laverdière M, Lalonde RG, Baril JG, Sheppard DC, Park S, Perlin DS. Progressive loss of echinocandin activity following prolonged use for treatment of *Candida albicans* oesophagitis. J Antimicrob Chemother. 2006;57:705–8.
32. Krogh-Madsen M, Arendrup MC, Heslet L, Knudsen JD. Amphotericin B and caspofungin resistance in *Candida glabrata* isolates recovered from a critically ill patient. Clin Infect Dis. 2006;42:938–44.
33. Thompson 3rd GR, Wiederhold NP, Vallor AC, Villareal NC, Lewis JS, Patterson TF. Development of caspofungin resistance following prolonged therapy for invasive candidiasis secondary to *Candida glabrata* infection. Antimicrob Agents Chemother. 2008;52: 3783–5.
34. Garcia-Effron G, Kontoyiannis DP, Lewis RE, Perlin DS. Caspofungin-resistant *Candida tropicalis* strains causing breakthrough fungemia in patients at high risk for hematologic malignancies. Antimicrob Agents Chemother. 2008;52:4181–3.
35. Cleary JD, Garcia-Effron G, Chapman SW, Perlin DS. Reduced *Candida glabrata* susceptibility secondary to an FKS1 mutation developed during candidemia treatment. Antimicrob Agents Chemother. 2008;52:2263–5.
36. Perlin DS. Resistance to echinocandin-class antifungal drugs. Drug Resist Update. 2007;10:121–30.
37. Espinel-Ingroff A. Mechanisms of resistance to antifungal agents: Yeasts and filamentous fungi. Rev Iberoam Micol. 2008;25:101–6.
38. Gardiner RE, Souteropoulos P, Park S, Perlin DS. Characterization of *Aspergillus fumigatus* mutants with reduced susceptibility to caspofungin. Med Mycol. 2005;43 Suppl 1:S299–305.
39. Park S, Kelly R, Kahn JN, et al. Specific substitutions in the echinocandin target Fks1p account for reduced susceptibility of rare laboratory and clinical *Candida* spp. isolates. Antimicrob Agents Chemother. 2005;49:3264–73.
40. Rocha EM, Garcia-Effron G, Park S, Perlin DS. A Ser678Pro substitution in *FKS1P* confers resistance to echinocandin drugs in *Aspergillus fumigatus*. Antimicrob Agents Chemother. 2007;51:4174–6.
41. Garcia-Effron G, Katiyar SK, Park S, Edlind TD, Perlin DS. A naturally occurring proline-to-alanine amino acid change in *FKS1p* in *Candida parapsilosis, Candida orthopsilosis,* and *Candida*

metapsilosis accounts for reduced echinocandin susceptibility. Antimicrob Agents Chemother. 2008;52:2305–12.

42. Katiyar SK, Edlind TD. Role for *FKS1* in the intrinsic echinocandin resistance of *Fusarium solani* as evidenced by hybrid expression in *Saccharomyces cerevisiae*. Antimicrob Agents Chemother. 2009;53:1772–8.
43. Maligie MA, Selitrennikoff CP. *Cryptococcus neoformans* resistance to echinocandins: (1, 3)beta-glucan synthase activity is sensitive to echinocandins. Antimicrob Agents Chemother. 2005;49:2851–6.
44. Wiederhold NP, Kontoyiannis DP, Prince RA, Lewis RE. Attenuation of the activity of caspofungin at high concentrations against *Candida albicans*: possible role of cell wall integrity and calcineurin pathways. Antimicrob Agents Chemother. 2005;49:5146–8.
45. Wiederhold NP. Paradoxical echinocandin activity: a limited in vitro phenomenon? Med Mycol. 2009;47 Suppl 1:S369–75.
46. Stevens DA, Espiritu M, Parmar R. Paradoxical effect of caspofungin: reduced activity against *Candida albicans* at high drug concentrations. Antimicrob Agents Chemother. 2004;48:3407–11.
47. Stevens DA, White TC, Perlin DS, Selitrennikoff CP. Studies of the paradoxical effect of caspofungin at high drug concentrations. Diagn Microbiol Infect Dis. 2005;51:173–8.
48. Paderu P, Park S, Perlin DS. Caspofungin uptake is mediated by a high-affinity transporter in *Candida albicans*. Antimicrob Agents Chemother. 2004;48:3845–9.
49. Schuetzer-Muehlbauer M, Willinger B, Krapf G, Enzinger S, Presterl E, Kuchler K. The *Candida albicans* Cdr2p ATP-binding cassette (ABC) transporter confers resistance to caspofungin. Mol Microbiol. 2003;48:225–35.
50. Liu TT, Lee RE, Barker KS, Lee RE, Wei L, Homayouni R, et al. Genome-wide expression profiling of the response to azole, polyene, echinocandin, and pyrimidine antifungal agents in *Candida albicans*. Antimicrob Agents Chemother. 2005;49:2226–36.
51. Clemons KV, Espiritu M, Parmar R, Stevens DA. Assessment of the paradoxical effect of caspofungin in therapy of candidiasis. Antimicrob Agents Chemother. 2006;50:1293–7.
52. Lewis RE, Albert ND, Kontoyiannis DP. Comparison of the dose-dependent activity and paradoxical effect of caspofungin and micafungin in a neutropenic murine model of invasive pulmonary aspergillosis. J Antimicrob Chemother. 2008;61:1140–4.
53. Arikan S, Lozano-Chiu M, Paetznick V, Rex JH. In vitro synergy of caspofungin and amphotericin B against *Aspergillus* and *Fusarium*. Antimicrob Agents Chemother. 2002;46:245–7.
54. Stevens DA. Drug interaction studies of a glucan synthase inhibitor (LY 303366) and a chitin synthase inhibitor (Nikkomycin Z) for inhibition and killing of fungal pathogens. Antimicrob Agents Chemother. 2000;44:2547–8.
55. Perea S, Gonzalez G, Fothergill AW, Kirkpatrick WR, Rinaldi MG, Patterson TF. In vitro interaction of caspofungin acetate with voriconazole against clinical isolates of *Aspergillus* spp. Antimicrob Agents Chemother. 2002;46:3039–41.
56. Roling EE, Klepser ME, Wasson A, Lewis RE, Ernst EJ, Pfaller MA. Antifungal activities of fluconazole, caspofungin (MK0991), and anidulafungin (LY 303366) alone and in combination against *Candida* spp. and *Crytococcus neoformans* via time-kill methods. Diagn Microbiol Infect Dis. 2002;43:13–7.
57. Hossain MA, Reyes GH, Long LA, Mukherjee PK, Ghannoum MA. Efficacy of caspofungin combined with amphotericin B against azole-resistant *Candida albicans*. J Antimicrob Chemother. 2003;51:1427–9.
58. Manavathu EK, Alangaden GJ, Chandrasekar PH. Differential activity of triazoles in two-drug combinations with the echinocandin caspofungin against *Aspergillus fumigatus*. J Antimicrob Chemother. 2003;51:1423–5.
59. O'Shaughnessy EM, Meletiadis J, Stergiopoulou T, Demchok JP, Walsh TJ. Antifungal interactions within the triple combination of amphotericin B, caspofungin and voriconazole against *Aspergillus* species. J Antimicrob Chemother. 2006;58:1168–76.
60. Barchiesi F, Spreghini E, Fothergill AW, et al. Caspofungin in combination with amphotericin B against *Candida glabrata*. Antimicrob Agents Chemother. 2005;49:2546–9.
61. Cuenca-Estrella M, Gomez-Lopez A, Garcia-Effron G, et al. Combined activity in vitro of caspofungin, amphotericin B, and azole agents against itraconazole-resistant clinical isolates of *Aspergillus fumigatus*. Antimicrob Agents Chemother. 2005;49:1232–5.
62. Oliveira ER, Fothergill AW, Kirkpatrick WR, Coco BJ, Patterson TF, Redding SW. In vitro interaction of posaconazole and caspofungin against clinical isolates of *Candida glabrata*. Antimicrob Agents Chemother. 2005;49:3544–5.
63. Ganesan LT, Manavathu EK, Cutright JL, Alangaden GJ, Chandrasekar PH. In-vitro activity of nikkomycin Z alone and in combination with polyenes, triazoles or echinocandins against *Aspergillus fumigatus*. Clin Microbiol Infect. 2004;10:961–6.
64. Heyn K, Tredup A, Salvenmoser S, Muller FM. Effect of voriconazole combined with micafungin against *Candida, Aspergillus,* and *Scedosporium* spp. and *Fusarium solani*. Antimicrob Agents Chemother. 2005;49:5157–9.
65. Philip A, Odabasi Z, Rodriguez J, et al. In vitro synergy testing of anidulafungin with itraconazole, voriconazole, and amphotericin B against *Aspergillus* spp. and *Fusarium* spp. Antimicrob Agents Chemother. 2005;49:3572–4.
66. Kirkpatrick WR, Perea S, Coco BJ, Patterson TF. Efficacy of caspofungin alone and in combination with voriconazole in a guinea pig model of invasive aspergillosis. Antimicrob Agents Chemother. 2002;46:2564–8.
67. Petraitis V, Petraitiene R, Sarafandi AA, et al. Combination therapy in treatment of experimental pulmonary aspergillosis: synergistic interaction between an antifungal triazole and an echinocandin. J Infect Dis. 2003;187:1834–43.
68. Graybill JR, Bocanegra R, Gonzalez GM, Najvar LK. Combination antifungal therapy of murine aspergillosis: liposomal amphotericin B and micafungin. J Antimicrob Chemother. 2003;52:656–62.
69. MacCallum DM, Whyte JA, Odds FC. Efficacy of caspofungin and voriconazole combinations in experimental aspergillosis. Antimicrob Agents Chemother. 2005;49:3697–701.
70. Sionov E, Mendlovic S, Segal E. Efficacy of amphotericin B or amphotericin B-intralipid in combination with caspofungin against experimental aspergillosis. J Infect. 2006;53:131–9.
71. Barchiesi F, Spreghini E, Tomassetti S, Arzeni D, Giannini D, Scalise G. Comparison of the fungicidal activities of caspofungin and amphotericin B against *Candida glabrata*. Antimicrob Agents Chemother. 2005;49:4989–92.
72. Olson JA, Adler-Moore JP, Smith PJ, Proffitt RT. Treatment of *Candida glabrata* infection in immunosuppressed mice by using a combination of liposomal amphotericin B with caspofungin or micafungin. Antimicrob Agents Chemother. 2005;49:4895–902.
73. González GM, González G, Najvar LK, Graybill JR. Therapeutic efficacy of caspofungin alone and in combination with amphotericin B deoxycholate for coccidioidomycosis in a mouse model. J Antimicrob Chemother. 2007;60:1341–6.
74. Spellberg B, Fu Y, Edwards Jr JE, Ibrahim AS. Combination therapy with amphotericin B lipid complex and caspofungin acetate of disseminated zygomycosis in diabetic ketoacidotic mice. Antimicrob Agents Chemother. 2005;49:830–2.
75. Frank U, Greiner M, Engels I, Daschner FD. Effects of caspofungin (MK-0991) and anidulafungin (LY303366) on phagocytosis, oxidative burst and killing of *Candida albicans* by human phagocytes. Eur J Clin Microbiol Infect Dis. 2004;23:729–31.
76. Gil-Lamaignere C, Salvenmoser S, Hess R, Muller FM. Micafungin enhances neutrophil fungicidal functions against *Candida* pseudohyphae. Antimicrob Agents Chemother. 2004;48:2730–2.

77. Brummer E, Chauhan SD, Stevens DA. Collaboration of human phagocytes with LY 303366 for antifungal activity against *Aspergillus fumigatus*. J Antimicrob Chemother. 1999;43:491–6.
78. Chiller T, Farrokhshad K, Brummer E, Stevens DA. The interaction of human monocytes, monocyte-derived macrophages, and polymorphonuclear neutrophils with caspofungin (MK-0991), an echinocandin, for antifungal activity against *Aspergillus fumigatus*. Diagn Microbiol Infect Dis. 2001;39:99–103.
79. Choi JH, Brummer E, Stevens DA. Combined action of micafungin, a new echinocandin, and human phagocytes for antifungal activity against *Aspergillus fumigatus*. Microbes Infect. 2004;6:383–9.
80. Soustre J, Rodier MH, Imbert-Bouyer S, Daniault G, Imbert C. Caspofungin modulates in vitro adherence of *Candida albicans* to plastic coated with extracellular matrix proteins. J Antimicrob Chemother. 2004;53:522–5.
81. Kuhn DM, George T, Chandra J, Mukherjee PK, Ghannoum MA. Antifungal susceptibility of *Candida* biofilms: unique efficacy of amphotericin B lipid formulations and echinocandins. Antimicrob Agents Chemother. 2002;46:1773–80.
82. Bachmann SP, VandeWalle K, Ramage G, Patterson TF, Wickes BL, Graybill JR, et al. In vitro activity of caspofungin against *Candida albicans* biofilms. Antimicrob Agents Chemother. 2002;46:3591–6.
83. Ramage G, VandeWalle K, Bachmann SP, Wickes BL, Lopez-Ribot JL. In vitro pharmacodynamic properties of three antifungal agents against preformed *Candida albicans* biofilms determined by time-kill studies. Antimicrob Agents Chemother. 2002;46: 3634–6.
84. Ernst ME, Klepser ME, Wolfe EJ, Pfaller MA. Antifungal dynamics of LY 303366, an investigational echinocandin B analog, against *Candida* spp. Diagn Microbiol Infect Dis. 1996;26:125–31.
85. Ernst EJ, Klepser ME, Ernst ME, Messer SA, Pfaller MA. In vitro pharmacodynamic properties of MK-0991 determined by time-kill methods. Diagn Microbiol Infect Dis. 1999;33:75–80.
86. Ernst EJ, Roling EE, Petzold CR, Keele DJ, Klepser ME. In vitro activity of micafungin (FK-463) against *Candida* spp.: microdilution, time-kill, and postantifungal-effect studies. Antimicrob Agents Chemother. 2002;46:3846–53.
87. Petraitis V, Petraitiene R, Groll AH, et al. Comparative antifungal activity of the echinocandin micafungin against disseminated candidiasis and invasive pulmonary aspergillosis in persistently neutropenic rabbits. Antimicrob Agents Chemother. 2002;46:1857–69.
88. Manavathu EK, Ramesh MS, Baskaran I, Ganesan LT, Chandrasekar PH. A comparative study of the post-antifungal effect (PAFE) of amphotericin B, triazoles and echinocandins on *Aspergillus fumigatus* and *Candida albicans*. J Antimicrob Chemother. 2004;53:386–9.
89. Clancy CJ, Huang H, Cheng S, Derendorf H, Nguyen MH. Characterizing the effects of caspofungin on *Candida albicans*, *Candida parapsilosis*, and *Candida glabrata* isolates by simultaneous time-kill and postantifungal-effect experiments. Antimicrob Agents Chemother. 2006;50:2569–72.
90. Nguyen KT, Ta P, Hoang BT, et al. Anidulafungin is fungicidal and exerts a variety of postantifungal effects against *Candida albicans, C. glabrata, C. parapsilosis,* and *C. krusei* isolates. Antimicrob Agents Chemother. 2009;53:3347–52.
91. Groll AH, Mickiene D, Petraitiene R, et al. Pharmacokinetic and pharmacodynamic modeling of anidulafungin (LY303366): Reappraisal of its efficacy in neutropenic animal models of opportunistic mycoses using optimal plasma sampling. Antimicrob Agents Chemother. 2001;45:2845–55.
92. Louie A, Deziel M, Liu W, Drusano MF, Gumbo T, Drusano GL. Pharmacodynamics of caspofungin in a murine model of systemic candidiasis: importance of persistence of caspofungin in tissues to understanding drug activity. Antimicrob Agents Chemother. 2005;49:5058–68.
93. Andes D, Diekema DJ, Pfaller MA, Prince RA, Marchillo K, Ashbeck J, et al. In vivo pharmacodynamic characterization of anidulafungin in a neutropenic murine candidiasis model. Antimicrob Agents Chemother. 2008;52:539–50.
94. Andes DR, Diekema DJ, Pfaller MA, Marchillo K, Bohrmueller J. In vivo pharmacodynamic target investigation for micafungin against *Candida albicans* and *C. glabrata* in a neutropenic murine candidiasis model. Antimicrob Agents Chemother. 2008;52:3497–503.
95. Wiederhold NP, Kontoyiannis DP, Chi J, Prince RA, Tam VH, Lewis RE. Pharmacodynamics of caspofungin in a murine model of invasive pulmonary aspergillosis: Evidence of concentration-dependent activity. J Infect Dis. 2004;190:1464–71.
96. Kartsonis N, Killar J, Mixson L, et al. Caspofungin susceptibility testing of isolates from patients with esophageal candidiasis or invasive candidiasis: relationship of MIC to treatment outcome. Antimicrob Agents Chemother. 2005;49:3616–23.
97. Pfaller MA, Diekema DJ, Ostrosky-Zeichner L, et al. Correlation of MIC with outcome for *Candida* species tested against caspofungin, anidulafungin, and micafungin: analysis and proposal for interpretive MIC breakpoints. J Clin Microbiol. 2008;46:2620–9.
98. Clinical and Laboratory Standards Institute (CLSI). Reference method for broth dilution antifungal susceptibility testing of yeasts; Approved standard – third edition; CLSI document M27-A3(28). 2008. Clinical and laboratory Standards Institute, Pennsylvania, USA.
99. Rodriguez-Tudela JL, Arendrup MC, Barchiesi F, et al. EUCAST definitive document EDef 7.1: method for the determination of broth dilution MICs of antifungal agents for fermentative yeasts. ClinMicrobiol Infect. 2008;14:398–405.
100. Rodriguez-Tudela JL, Donnelly JP, Pfaller MA, et al. Statistical analyses of correlation between fluconazole MICs for *Candida* spp. assessed by standard methods set forth by the European Committee on Antimicrobial Susceptibility Testing (E.Dis. 7.1) and CLSI (M27-A2). J ClinMicrobiol. 2007;45:109–11.
101. Arendrup MC, Garcia-Effron G, Lass-Flörl C, et al. Susceptibility testing of *Candida* species to echinocandins: comparison of EUCAST EDef 7.1, CLSI M27-A3, Etest, disk diffusion and agar-dilution using RPMI and IsoSensitest medium. Antimicrob Agents Chemother. 2010;54:426–39.
102. Dowell JA, Knebel W, Ludden T, Stogniew M, Krause D, Henkel T. Population pharmacokinetic analysis of anidulafungin, an echinocandin antifungal. J Clin Pharmacol. 2004;44:590–8.
103. Dowell JA, Stogniew M, Krause D, Damle B. Anidulafungin does not require dosage adjustment in subjects with varying degrees of hepatic or renal impairment. J Clin Pharmacol. 2007;47:461–70.
104. Benjamin Jr DK, Driscoll T, Seibel NL, et al. Safety and pharmacokinetics of intravenous anidulafungin in children with neutropenia at high risk for invasive fungal infections. Antimicrob Agents Chemother. 2006;50:632–8.
105. Krause DS, Reinhardt J, Vazquez JA, et al. Phase 2, randomized, dose-ranging study evaluating the safety and efficacy of anidulafungin in invasive candidiasis and candidemia. Antimicrob Agents Chemother. 2004;48:2021–4.
106. Krause DS, Simjee AE, van Rensburg C, et al. A randomized, double-blind trial of anidulafungin versus fluconazole for the treatment of esophageal candidiasis. Clin Infect Dis. 2004;39:770–5.
107. Reboli AC, Rotstein C, Pappas PG, et al. Anidulafungin versus fluconazole for invasive candidiasis. N Engl J Med. 2007;356: 2472–82.
108. Vazquez JA, Schranz JA, Clark K, Goldstein BP, Reboli A, Fichtenbaum C. A phase 2, open-label study of the safety and efficacy of intravenous anidulafungin as a treatment for azole-refractory mucosal candidiasis. J Acquir Immune Defic Syndr. 2008;48:304–9.

109. Ecalta™ Summary of Product Characteristics. European Medicines Agency. 2009. http://www.emea.europa.eu/humandocs/Humans/EPAR/ecalta/ecalta.htm. Accessed 23 July 2009.
110. Eraxis™ U.S. Prescribers Information. U.S. Food and Drug Administration. 2006. http://www.accessdata.fda.gov/scripts/cder/drugsatfda/index.cfm?fuseaction = Search.Label_ApprovalHistory. Accessed 17 Feb 2006.
111. Dowell JA, Stogniew M, Krause D, Henkel T, Weston IE. Assessment of the safety and pharmacokinetics of anidulafungin when administered with cyclosporine. J Clin Pharmacol. 2005;45:227–33.
112. Dowell JA, Schranz J, Baruch A, Foster G. Safety and pharmacokinetics of coadministered voriconazole and anidulafungin. J Clin Pharmacol. 2005;45:1373–82.
113. Dowell JA, Stogniew M, Krause D, Henkel T, Damle B. Lack of pharmacokinetic interaction between anidulafungin and tacrolimus. J Clin Pharmacol. 2007;47:305–14.
114. Neely M, Jafri HS, Seibel N, et al. Pharmacokinetics and safety of caspofungin in older infants and toddlers. Antimicrob Agents Chemother. 2009;53:1450–6.
115. Sáez-Llorens X, Macias M, Maiya P, et al. Pharmacokinetics and safety of caspofungin in neonates and infants less than 3 months of age. Antimicrob Agents Chemother. 2009;53:869–75.
116. Villanueva A, Gotuzzo E, Arathoon EG, et al. A randomized double-blind study of caspofungin versus fluconazole for the treatment of esophageal candidiasis. Am J Med. 2002;113:294–9.
117. Stone JA, Holland SD, Wickersham PJ, et al. Single- and multiple-dose pharmacokinetics of caspofungin in healthy men. Antimicrob Agents Chemother. 2002;46:739–45.
118. Sandhu P, Lee W, Xu X, et al. Hepatic uptake of the novel antifungal agent caspofungin. Drug Metab Dispos. 2005;33:676–82.
119. Sandhu P, Xu X, Bondiskey PJ, et al. Disposition of caspofungin, a novel antifungal agent, in mice, rats, rabbits, and monkeys. Antimicrob Agents Chemother. 2004;48:1272–80.
120. Balani SK, Xu X, Arison BH, et al. Metabolites of caspofungin acetate, a potent antifungal agent, in human plasma and urine. Drug Metab Dispos. 2000;28:1274–8.
121. Mistry GC, Migoya E, Deutsch PJ, et al. Single- and multiple-dose administration of caspofungin in patients with hepatic insufficiency: Implications for safety and dosing recommendations. J Clin Pharmacol. 2007;47:951–61.
122. Villanueva A, Arathoon EG, Gotuzzo E, Berman RS, DiNubile MJ, Sable CA. A randomized double-blind study of caspofungin versus amphotericin for the treatment of candidal esophagitis. Clin Infect Dis. 2001;33:1529–35.
123. Arathoon EG, Gotuzzo E, Noriega LM, Berman RS, DiNubile MJ, Sable CA. Randomized, double-blind, multicenter study of caspofungin versus amphotericin B for treatment of oropharyngeal and esophageal candidiasis. Antimicrob Agents Chemother. 2002;46:451–7.
124. Kartsonis N, DiNubile MJ, Bartizal K, Hicks PS, Ryan D, Sable CA. Efficacy of caspofungin in the treatment of esophageal candidiasis resistant to fluconazole. J Acquir Immune Defic Syndr. 2002;3:183–7.
125. Mora-Durate J, Betts R, Rotstein C, et al. Comparison of caspofungin and amphotericin B for invasive candidiasis. N Engl J Med. 2002;347:2020–9.
126. Pappas PG, Rotstein CM, Betts RF, et al. Micafungin versus caspofungin for treatment of candidemia and other forms of invasive candidiasis. Clin Infect Dis. 2007;45:883–93.
127. Betts RF, Nucci M, Talwar D, et al. A multicenter, double-blind trial of a high-dose caspofungin treatment regimen versus a standard caspofungin treatment regimen for adult patients with invasive candidiasis. Clin Infect Dis. 2009;48:1676–84.
128. Cornely OA, Lasso M, Betts R, et al. Caspofungin for the treatment of less common forms of invasive candidiasis. J Antimicrob Chemother. 2007;60:363–9.
129. Betts R, Glasmacher A, Maertens J, et al. Efficacy of caspofungin against invasive *Candida* or invasive *Aspergillus* infections in neutropenic patients. Cancer. 2006;106:466–73.
130. Maertens J, Raad I, Petrikkos G, et al. Efficacy and safety of caspofungin for treatment of invasive aspergillosis in patients refractory to or intolerant of conventional antifungal therapy. Clin Infect Dis. 2004;39:1563–71.
131. Viscoli C, Herbrecht R, Akan H, et al. An EORTC Phase II study of caspofungin as first-line therapy of invasive aspergillosis in haematological patients. J Antimicrob Chemother. 2009;64:1274–81.
132. Herbrecht R, Maertens J, Biala L, et al. Caspofungin as first line therapy of invasive aspergillosis in allogeneic hematopoietic stem cell transplant recipients: A study of the EORTC Infectious Diseases Group. Program and Abstracts of the 49th Interscience Conference on Antimicrobial Agents and Chemotherapy. American Society for Microbiology, Washington, DC: abst. M-2168, p. 674 (2009).
133. Marr KA, Boeckh M, Carter RA, Kim HW, Corey L. Combination antifungal therapy for invasive aspergillosis. Clin Infect Dis. 2004;39:797–802.
134. Kontoyiannis DP, Hachem R, Lewis RE, et al. Efficacy and toxicity of caspofungin in combination with liposomal amphotericin B as primary or salvage treatment of invasive aspergillosis in patients with hematologic malignancies. Cancer. 2003;98:292–9.
135. Maertens J, Glasmacher A, Herbrecht R, et al. Multicenter, noncomparative study of caspofungin in combination with other antifungals as salvage therapy in adults with invasive aspergillosis. Cancer. 2006;107:2888–97.
136. Caillot D, Thiébaut A, Herbrecht R, et al. Liposomal amphotericin B in combination with caspofungin for invasive aspergillosis in patients with hematologic malignancies: a randomized pilot study (Combistrat trial). Cancer. 2007;110:2740–6.
137. Reed C, Bryant R, Ibrahim AS, et al. Combination polyene-caspofungin treatment of rhino-orbital-cerebral mucormycosis. Clin Infect Dis. 2008;47:364–71.
138. Walsh TJ, Teppler H, Donowitz GR, et al. Caspofungin versus liposomal amphotericin B for empirical antifungal therapy in patients with persistent fever and neutropenia. N Engl J Med. 2004;351:1391–402.
139. Mattiuzzi GN, Alvarado G, Giles FJ, et al. Open-label, randomized comparison of itraconazole versus caspofungin for prophylaxis in patients with hematologic malignancies. Antimicrob Agents Chemother. 2006;50:143–7.
140. Maertens JA, Madero-Lopez L, Reilly AF, et al. A randomized, double-blind, multicenter study of caspofungin versus liposomal amphotericin B for empirical antifungal therapy in pediatric patients with persistent fever and neutropenia. Pediatr Infect Dis J. 2010;29(5):415–20.
141. Zaoutis TE, Jafri HS, Huang LM, et al. A prospective, multicenter study of caspofungin for the treatment of documented *Candida* or *Aspergillus* infections in pediatric patients. Pediatrics. 2009;123:877–84.
142. Odio CM, Araya R, Pinto LE, et al. Caspofungin therapy of neonates with invasive candidiasis. Pediatr Infect Dis J. 2004;23:1093–7.
143. Natarajan G, Lulic-Botica M, Rongkavilit C, Pappas A, Bedard M. Experience with caspofungin in the treatment of persistent fungemia in neonates. J Perinatol. 2005;25:770–7.
144. Odio CM, Castro CE, Vasques S, Lazo J, Herrera ML. Caspofungin therapy for neonates with invasive candidiasis cared for at intensive care units. In Program and Abstracts of the 47th Interscience Conference on Antimicrobial Agents and Chemotherapy. American Society for Microbiology, Washington, DC: abst. G-976, p. 270 (2007).

145. Cancidas™ U.S. Prescribers Information. U.S. Food and Drug Administration. 2009. http://www.accessdata.fda.gov/scripts/cder/drugsatfda/index.cfm?fuseaction = Search.Label_ApprovalHistory. Accessed 26 June 2009.
146. Cancidas™ Summary of Product Characteristics. European Medicines Agency. 2009. http://www.emea.europa.eu/humandocs/Humans/EPAR/cancidas/cancidas.htm. Accessed 23 July 2009.
147. Cleary JD, Schwartz M, Rogers PD, de Mestral J, Chapman SW. Effects of amphotericin B and caspofungin on histamine expression. Pharmacotherapy. 2003;23:966–73.
148. Sable CA, Nguyen BY, Chodakewitz JA, DiNubile MJ. Safety and tolerability of caspofungin acetate in the treatment of fungal infections. Transpl Infect Dis. 2002;4:25–30.
149. Glasmacher A, Cornely OA, Orlopp K, et al. Caspofungin treatment in severely ill, immunocompromised patients: a case-documentation study of 118 patients. J Antimicrob Chemother. 2006;57:127–34.
150. Groll AH, Attarbaschi A, Schuster FR, et al. Treatment with caspofungin in immunocompromised paediatric patients: a multicentre survey. J Antimicrob Chemother. 2006;57:527–35.
151. Zaoutis T, Lehrnbecher T, Groll AH, et al. Safety experience with caspofungin in pediatric patients. Pediatr Infect Dis J. 2009;28:1132–5.
152. Marr KA, Hachem R, Papanicolaou G, et al. Retrospective study of the hepatic safety profile of patients concomitantly treated with caspofungin and cyclosporin A. Transpl Infect Dis. 2004;6: 110–6.
153. Sanz-Rodriguez C, Lopez-Duarte M, Jurado M, et al. Safety of the concomitant use of caspofungin and cyclosporin A in patients with invasive fungal infections. Bone Marrow Transplant. 2004;34:13–20.
154. Stone JA, Migoya EM, Hickey L, et al. Potential for interactions between caspofungin and nelfinavir or rifampin. Antimicrob Agents Chemother. 2004;48:4306–14.
155. Colburn DE, Giles FJ, Oladovich D, Smith JA. In vitro evaluation of cytochrome P450-mediated drug interactions between cytarabine, idarubicin, itraconazole and caspofungin. Hematology. 2004;9:217–21.
156. Hiemenz J, Cagnoni P, Simpson D, et al. Pharmacokinetic and maximum tolerated dose study of micafungin in combination with fluconazole versus fluconazole alone for prophylaxis of fungal infections in adult patients undergoing a bone marrow or peripheral stem cell transplant. Antimicrob Agents Chemother. 2005;49:1331–6.
157. Tabata K, Katashima M, Kawamura A, Kaibara A, Tanigawara Y. Population pharmacokinetic analysis of micafungin in Japanese patients with fungal infections. Drug Metab Pharmacokinet. 2006;21:324–31.
158. Gumbo T, Hiemenz J, Ma L, Keirns JJ, Buell DN, Drusano GL. Population pharmacokinetics of micafungin in adult patients. Diagn Microbiol Infect Dis. 2008;60:329–31.
159. Hebert MF, Smith HE, Marbury TC, et al. Pharmacokinetics of micafungin in healthy volunteers, volunteers with moderate liver disease, and volunteers with renal dysfunction. J Clin Pharmacol. 2005;45:1145–52.
160. Hope WW, Seibel NL, Schwartz CL, et al. Population pharmacokinetics of micafungin in pediatric patients and implications for antifungal dosing. Antimicrob Agents Chemother. 2007;51:3714–9.
161. Hope WW, Mickiene D, Petraitis V, et al. The pharmacokinetics and pharmacodynamics of micafungin in experimental hematogenous *Candida* meningoencephalitis: implications for echinocandin therapy in neonates. J Infect Dis. 2008;197:163–71.
162. Kishino S, Ohno K, Shimamura T, Furukawatodo H. Optimal prophylactic dosage and disposition of micafungin in living donor liver recipients. Clin Transplant. 2004;18:676–80.
163. Seibel NL, Schwartz C, Arrieta A, et al. Safety, tolerability, and pharmacokinetics of micafungin (FK463) in febrile neutropenic pediatric patients. Antimicrob Agents Chemother. 2005;49:3317–24.
164. Heresi GP, Gerstmann DR, Reed MD, et al. The pharmacokinetics and safety of micafungin, a novel echinocandin, in premature infants. Pediatr Infect Dis J. 2006;25:1110–5.
165. Benjamin Jr DK, Smith PB, Arrieta A, et al. Safety and pharmacokinetics of repeat-dose micafungin in young infants. Clin Pharmacol Ther. 2010;87:93–9.
166. Smith PB, Walsh TJ, Hope W, et al. Pharmacokinetics of an elevated dosage of micafungin in premature neonates. Pediatr Infect Dis J. 2009;28:412–5.
167. Pettengell K, Mynhardt J, Kluyts T, Lau W, Facklam D, Buell D. FK463 South African Study Group. Successful treatment of oesophageal candidiasis by micafungin: a novel systemic antifungal agent. Aliment Pharmacol Ther. 2004;20:475–81.
168. de Wet N, Llanos-Cuentas A, Suleiman J, et al. A randomized, double-blind, parallel-group, dose-response study of micafungin compared with fluconazole for the treatment of esophageal candidiasis in HIV-positive patients. Clin Infect Dis. 2004;39: 842–9.
169. de Wet NT, Bester AJ, Viljoen JJ, et al. A randomized, double blind, comparative trial of micafungin (FK463) vs. fluconazole for the treatment of oesophageal candidiasis. Aliment Pharmacol Ther. 2005;21:899–907.
170. Kuse ER, Chetchotisakd P, da Cunha CA, et al. Micafungin versus liposomal amphotericin B for candidaemia and invasive candidosis: a phase III randomised double-blind trial. Lancet. 2007;369: 1519–27.
171. Ostrosky-Zeichner L, Kontoyiannis D, Raffalli J, et al. International, open-label, noncomparative, clinical trial of micafungin alone and in combination for treatment of newly diagnosed and refractory candidemia. Eur J Clin Microbiol Infect Dis. 2005;24:654–61.
172. Denning DW, Marr KA, Lau WM, et al. Micafungin (FK463), alone or in combination with other systemic antifungal agents, for the treatment of acute invasive aspergillosis. J Infect. 2006;53: 337–49.
173. Kontoyiannis DP, Ratanatharathorn V, Young JA, et al. Micafungin alone or in combination with other systemic antifungal therapies in hematopoietic stem cell transplant recipients with invasive aspergillosis. Transpl Infect Dis. 2009;11:89–93.
174. van Burik JA, Ratanatharathorn V, Stepan DE, et al. Micafungin versus fluconazole for prophylaxis against invasive fungal infections during neutropenia in patients undergoing hematopoietic stem cell transplantation. Clin Infect Dis. 2004;39:1407–16.
175. Hiramatsu Y, Maeda Y, Fujii N, et al. Use of micafungin versus fluconazole for antifungal prophylaxis in neutropenic patients receiving hematopoietic stem cell transplantation. Int J Hematol. 2008;88:588–95.
176. Queiroz-Telles F, Berezin E, Leverger G, et al. Micafungin versus liposomal amphotericin B for pediatric patients with invasive candidiasis: substudy of a randomized double-blind trial. Pediatr Infect Dis J. 2008;27:820–6.
177. Sirohi B, Powles RL, Chopra R, et al. A study to determine the safety profile and maximum tolerated dose of micafungin (FK463) in patients undergoing haematopoietic stem cell transplantation. Bone Marrow Transplant. 2006;38:47–51.
178. Cornely O, Maddison P, Ullmann JA. Pooled analysis of safety for micafungin. In: Abstracts of the 47th Interscience Conference on Antimicrobial Agents and Chemotherapy. American Society for Microbiology: abst. M 1175, p. 444 (2007).
179. Mycamine™ Summary of Product Characteristics. European Medicines Agency. 2008. http://www.emea.europa.eu/humandocs/Humans/EPAR/mycamine/mycamine.htm. Acessed 31 Oct 2008.

180. Niwa T, Inoue-Yamamoto S, Shiraga T, Takagi A. Effect of antifungal drugs on cytochrome P450 (CYP) 1A2, CYP2D6, and CYP2E1 activities in human liver microsomes. Biol Pharm Bull. 2005;28:1813–6.
181. Niwa T, Shiraga T, Takagi A. Effect of antifungal drugs on cytochrome P450 (CYP) 2C9, CYP2C19, and CYP3A4 activities in human liver microsomes. Biol Pharm Bull. 2005;28:1805–8.
182. Sakaeda T, Iwaki K, Kakumoto M, et al. Effect of micafungin on cytochrome P450 3A4 and multidrug resistance protein 1 activities, and its comparison with azole antifungal drugs. J Pharm Pharmacol. 2005;57:759–64.
183. Mycamine™ U.S. Prescribers Information. U.S. Food and Drug Administration. 2008. http://www.accessdata.fda.gov/scripts/cder/drugsatfda/index.cfm?fuseaction = Search.Label_ApprovalHistory. Accessed 22 Jan 2008.
184. Hebert MF, Blough DK, Townsend RW, et al. Concomitant tacrolimus and micafungin pharmacokinetics in healthy volunteers. J Clin Pharmacol. 2005;45:1018–24.
185. Keirns J, Sawamoto T, Holum M, Buell D, Wisemandle W, Alak A. Steady-state pharmacokinetics of micafungin and voriconazole after separate and concomitant dosing in healthy adults. Antimicrob Agents Chemother. 2007;51:787–90.

Terbinafine

Peter G. Pappas

Terbinafine is an oral and topical antifungal agent in the allylamine class of antifungal compounds [1]. Discovered in 1983, it is closely related to naftifine. It became available in Europe in 1991, and in 1996 in the United States. Terbinafine is the only oral allylamine available in the United States and is used largely for the treatment of superficial fungal infections, especially those due to dermatophytes. There has been significant interest in developing the drug for the treatment of deep mycoses, either alone or in combination, for disorders such as cryptococcosis, invasive aspergillosis, and other mould infections, but there are only scant clinical data evaluating its efficacy in these settings. Terbinafine is a valuable antifungal drug for the treatment of superficial fungal infections, and has potential as an adjunctive agent in the treatment of selected deep mycoses.

Pharmacodynamics

Mechanism of Action

The mechanism of action of terbinafine is through inhibition of the synthesis of ergosterol, a key sterol component in the plasma membrane of the fungal cell [1, 2]. Terbinafine inhibits squalene epoxidase, the enzyme which catalyzes the conversion of squalene to squalene-2,3 epoxide, a precursor of lanosterol, which in turn is a direct precursor of ergosterol [3, 4]. A deficiency of ergosterol is detrimental to the integrity of the cell membrane resulting in a fungistatic effect similar to that seen with the azole antifungal compounds. In addition to this action, terbinafine also causes excessive intracellular accumulation of squalene, which is believed to exert a further toxic effect on susceptible fungal cells, thereby exerting a fungicidal effect [5]. In this regard, the mechanism of action of terbinafine is distinct from that of the azoles even though both compounds inhibit ergosterol biosynthesis through interruption of the synthesis of its precursors. Terbinafine has a strong affinity for fungal cell enzymes, but unlike the azoles, terbinafine has a very low affinity for the human cytochrome P-450 family of enzymes [6, 7]. This low affinity for the mammalian P-450 enzymes probably accounts for the favorable adverse event profile of terbenafine and the relatively few drug–drug interactions.

Antifungal Spectrum

Terbinafine is a very broad spectrum antifungal agent, exhibiting the best activity against the dermatophytes of all the antifungal agents [8–12]. Terbinafine also demonstrates meaningful in vitro activity against many *Aspergillus* species including *A. fumigatus*, *A. flavus*, *A. niger*, and *A. ustus* [10, 13–15]. Other moulds that appear susceptible based on in vitro testing include many of the dematiaceous fungi such as *Fonsecaea* and *Cladophialophora* species [16] and the agents of eumycetoma [17]. Single case reports of successful therapy with terbinafine in patients with disseminated *Phialophora parasitica* [18], subcutaneous *Exophiala jeanselmei* [19], and *Curvularia lunata* endocarditis [20] suggest clinically relevant antifungal activity against these dematiaceous pathogens. Terbinafine does not consistently demonstrate significant in vitro activity against the hyaline moulds such as *Fusarium* species, *Paecilomyces* spp., *Scedosporium* spp., *Scopulariopsis* spp., or the zygomycetes, but there are reports of successful therapy with terbinafine alone or in combination with other antifungal agents for many of these pathogens [21–25]. The in vitro activity of terbinafine versus selected dermatophytes and moulds is demonstrated in Tables 1–3.

Terbinafine demonstrates good in vitro activity against *C. neoformans* [16, 26], but it has relatively poor activity against other yeasts, including many *Candida* species with

P.G. Pappas (✉)
Division of Infectious Diseases,
University of Alabama at Birmingham, School of Medicine,
Birmingham, AL, USA
e-mail: pappas@uab.edu

C.A. Kauffman et al. (eds.), *Essentials of Clinical Mycology*,
DOI 10.1007/978-1-4419-6640-7_7, © Springer Science+Business Media, LLC 2011

Table 1 Minimum inhibitory concentrations of terbinafine against selected dermatophytes

Organism	MIC range (μg/mL)
Epidermophyton floccosum	0.001–0.05
Microsporum audouinii	0.001–0.04
Microsporum canis	0.0001–0.1
Microsporum gypseum	0.003–0.04
Microsporum persicolor	0.002–0.003
Trichophyton mentagrophytes	0.0001–0.05
Trichophyton mentagrophytes var. *interdigitale*	0.002–0.005
Trichophyton rubrum	0.001–0.15
Trichophyton simii	0.1–0.25
Trichophyton tonsurans	0.003–0.25
Trichophyton violaceum	0.001–0.1
Trichophyton verrucosum	0.001–0.006

MIC, minimum inhibitory concentration

Table 2 Minimum inhibitory concentrations of terbinafine against selected filamentous fungi

Organism	MIC range (μg/mL)
Acremonium spp.	0.25–8
Aspergillus flavus	0.01–1
Aspergillus fumigatus	0.02–5
Aspergillus nidulans	0.02–0.5
Aspergillus niger	0.005–2.5
Aspergillus terreus	0.04–5
Aspergillus ustus	0.1–0.5
Fusarium moniliforme	0.5–10
Fusarium oxysporum	0.25–20
Fusarium solani	1–128
Mucor spp.	64–128
Paecilomyces spp.	1–64
Penicillium spp.	1–5
Pseudallescheria boydii	10–64
Rhizopus spp.	64–100
Scopulariopsis brevicaulis	0.5–8

MIC, minimum inhibitory concentration

the exception of *C. parapsilosis* [27, 28]. Moreover, terbinafine is fungistatic against all of the *Candida* spp. Table 4 summarizes the in vitro activity against selected yeasts.

Terbinafine demonstrates excellent activity against some of the dimorphic fungi, including *Sporothrix schenckii*, against which it exhibits MICs comparable to some of the azole antifungal compounds, including itraconazole [8, 16]. In vitro activity against other dimorphic fungi, such as *Blastomyces dermatitidis*, *Histoplasma capsulatum*, and *Coccidioides* species is good [10, 16]. There are few in vitro or clinical data concerning the use of terbinafine against the other dimorphic fungi, *Penicillium marneffei* and *Paracoccidioides brasiliensis*. The in vitro susceptibility data for these dimorphic pathogens are shown in Table 5. Finally, terbinafine combined with amphotericin B, caspofungin, and selected azoles demonstrates modest additive or synergistic in vitro activity against *Pythium insidiosum* [29–31].

Table 3 Minimum inhibitory concentrations of terbinafine against selected dematiaceous fungi

Organism	MIC range (μg/mL)
Alternaria alternata	0.6–5
Cladophialophora bantianum	0.012–1
Cladosporium carrionii	0.04–1.25
Curvularia lunata	0.2–2
Curvularia fallax	0.25–0.5
Dactylaria constricta	0.01–0.03
Drechslera rostrata	10
Exophilia jeanselmei	0.06–2.5
Fonsecaea compacta	0.04
Fonsecaea pedrosoi	0.04–0.13
Madurella mycetomatis	0.01–1
Madurella grisea	0.01–2.5
Madurella spp.	1–4
Phaeoannellomyces werneckii	0.04–4
Phialophora verrucosa	0.04–0.13
Phialophora parasitica	0.1
Wangiella dermatitidis	0.001–0.08

MIC, minimum inhibitory concentration

Table 4 Minimum inhibitory concentrations of terbinafine against selected yeasts

Organism	MIC range (μg/mL)
Candida albicans	0.03–128
Candida glabrata	10–128
Candida guilliermondii	0.8–128
Candida humicola	1
Candida kefyr	0.5–50
Candida krusei	10–100
Candida parapsilosis	0.03–10
Candida tropicalis	1.2–128
Cryptococcus laurentii	0.08–0.6
Cryptococcus neoformans	0.06–2
Malassezia furfur	0.06–80
Rhodototula rubra	2.5–5
Trichosporon asahii	0.5–128

MIC, minimum inhibitory concentration

Table 5 Minimum inhibitory concentrations of terbinafine against selected dimorphic fungi

Organism	MIC range (μg/mL)
Blastomyces dermatitidis	0.04–1.25
Coccidioides species	0.3–0.6
Histoplasma capsulatum	0.04–0.2
Paracoccidiodes brasiliensis	0.04–0.16
Sporothrix schenckii	0.05–2

MIC, minimum inhibitory concentration

Pharmacokinetics

Oral

Terbinafine for systemic use is only formulated for oral administration. There is no intravenous formulation, in part due to the drug's significant lipophilicity. Terbinafine is well-absorbed following oral dosing with at least 80% bioavailability [32, 33]. The drug demonstrates linear kinetics over a broad range of therapeutic doses with a proportional increase in the area under the curve (AUC) with increasing dose. Peak serum concentrations are achieved within 2 h following oral administration in both adults and children, although at similar doses, peak concentrations are somewhat higher in adults than in children [34]. Peak concentrations in adults following a 125 mg (2 mg/kg) dose range from 0.3 to 0.9 μg/mL, whereas the same dose in children (125 mg or 5 mg/kg) yields peak concentrations ranging between 0.4 and 1.0 μg/mL [34]. Absorption does not appear to be influenced by coadministration of food, antacids, most H-2 receptor antagonists, or proton pump inhibitors. Coadministration with rifampin may, however, significantly increase clearance, and cimetidine can cause a 33% decrease in clearance of terbinafine [7].

The drug is lipophilic and highly bound to plasma proteins (95%), and achieves its highest concentrations in adipose tissue and the keratinous tissues of the skin, nails, hair, and in sebum [35]. Concentrations in these tissues may be tenfold higher than simultaneous levels found in plasma. Because of the unique affinity of terbinafine for keratinous tissue, therapeutic levels can be found in stratum corneum, hair, and nails for up to 12 weeks following discontinuation of therapy. Moreover, measurable concentrations of terbinafine may be found in nail clippings up to 10 months following discontinuation of a limited course (1–4 weeks) of terbinafine [35, 36]. Among the antifungal agents, only itraconazole possesses this unique affinity for keratinous tissue and demonstrates similarly prolonged levels in skin and nails.

Metabolism is primarily hepatic, and at least 15 metabolites have been identified, although none of these demonstrate significant anti-fungal activity [37]. Approximately 80–85% of terbinafine metabolites are excreted in the urine and 15–20% are excreted in the bile. The elimination half-life in normal adults is approximately 26 h [38]. Among patients with significant renal or hepatic dysfunction, drug elimination may be delayed [34]. Accordingly, it has been suggested that the dosing amount be reduced by 50% without altering frequency of administration among patients with either significant renal or hepatic dysfunction.

Topical

Topical terbinafine is widely available as an over-the-counter preparation for milder forms of dermatomycosis and onychomycosis. It is not absorbed systemically in any measurable quantity, but significant levels are achieved in the stratum corneum and the nails although these levels do not approach those achieved with oral terbinafine [39, 40].

Dosing and Administration

Terbinafine is available in 250 mg tablets and in a topical 1% ointment. Because of its extended half-life with oral administration (approximately 26 h), the drug can be dosed once daily. When higher doses (≥1,000 mg per day) are given, it is recommended to split the daily dose to limit gastrointestinal disturbances. Topical therapy is administered twice daily. Duration of therapy for oral terbinafine is dependant on the condition being treated. For most cases of onychomycosis, courses of 3 months may be successful, although courses from 6 to 12 months may be necessary to achieve a lasting response [41]. For sporotrichosis, courses of 3–12 months have been used successfully for patients with uncomplicated cutaneous disease [42, 43]. For other invasive mycoses, few data are available concerning length of oral therapy.

Clinical Uses

Onychomycosis

The term *tinea unguium* refers to nail infections caused by typical dermatophytes whereas *onychomycosis* refers to the broader category of nail, infections that also includes nondermatophytic fungi and yeasts. There is considerable clinical overlap in these two entities and few clinical clues to distinguish from among the wide assortment of causative agents [44]. Several open-label and placebo-controlled studies have been performed to evaluate oral terbinafine for the treatment of onychomycosis [41, 45]. Mycologic response rates for toenail infections treated with terbinafine, 250 mg daily, range between 82% and 92% among patients given 3–6 months of therapy [46, 47]. Clinical cure rates are slightly less than mycologic response rates. For fingernail infections, response rates of 70% at 3 months of therapy and 100% at 6 months have been achieved [48–53]. Surgical or chemical removal of the nail in conjunction with oral terbinafine does not appear to enhance the efficacy of terbinafine alone for onychomycosis [54].

Based on results of comparative trials, terbinafine demonstrates greater efficacy than griseofulvin for both fingernail and toenail onychomycosis [41, 47, 55, 56]. Given the availability of safe and more effective preparations such as terbinafine and itraconazole, griseofulvin has largely fallen into disuse, having been superceded by these two newer oral antifungal agents. Studies comparing itraconazole 200 mg daily and terbinafine 250 mg daily administered for 3 months suggest similar efficacy. These compounds are associated with mycologic cure rates ranging from 67% to 92%, and clinical cure rates from 63% to 80% [41, 45, 57].

Tinea Capitis

Tinea capitis, usually caused by *Trichophyton tonsurans*, is unique among the dermatophytoses in that it does not usually respond to topical antifungal therapy. Terbinafine has potent in vitro activity versus *T. tonsurans* [58]. Accordingly, oral terbinafine has been evaluated for the treatment of children with tinea capitis, effecting clinical cure rates of 80–100% and mycologic cure rates between 90% and 100% [34, 59, 60]. Compared to griseofulvin in randomized, double-blind studies, clinical cure rates are generally higher with terbinafine (90% vs 80%). Mycologic cure rates are similar [41].

Other Superficial Mycoses

For other superficial dermatophyte infections such as tinea corporis, tinea cruris, tinea imbricata, and tinea pedis due to a variety of dermatophytes including *Trichophyton rubrum*, *T. mentagrophytes*, *Microsporum canis*, and *Epidermophyton floccosum*, oral terbinafine is quite effective, but for most patients with these conditions, topical therapy can be used with excellent results. Ordinarily, for patients with superficial mycoses not involving nails and/or scalp, topical therapy with terbinafine is an appropriate alternative to systemic antifungal therapy with terbinafine or itraconazole.

Sporotrichosis

Among the deep mycoses, there has been the most experience with terbinafine for the treatment of sporotrichosis, and there have been limited reports of success with terbinafine at daily doses as low as 125 mg per day for 3–18 months [42, 61–63]. A large randomized double-blind trial compared two doses of terbinafine, 500 and 1,000 mg daily, administered for up to 24 weeks among 63 patients with cutaneous or lymphocutaneous sporotrichosis [43]. Mycological and clinical response rates were 87% with 1,000 mg daily and 52% with 500 mg daily. This success rate is not surprising given the significant concentration of terbinafine in the skin as well as excellent in vitro activity against *S. schenckii*. These response rates with terbinafine are similar to those with itraconazole for the treatment of cutaneous sporotrichosis [64].

Chromoblastomycosis

Chromoblastomycosis is a tropical fungal disease characterized by dense dermal fibrosis associated with organized granulomata. The agents of chromomycosis are typically dematiaceous (pigmented) fungi, and include such organisms as *Fonsecea pedrosoi* and *Cladosporium carrionii*. There has been sporadic use of terbinafine for patients with chromoblastomycosis [65]. In the largest study to date, 42 patients from Madagascar received terbinafine 500 mg daily for up to 1 year, and experienced 12-month mycologic and clinical cure rates of 85% and 74%, respectively [66]. While other experience with terbinafine for this disorder is limited to a small series of case reports [67–69], terbinafine appears to be a promising agent among patients with this very difficult to treat disease.

Fungal Mycetoma

There are at least 16 different fungal organisms that can cause fungal mycetoma. Terbinafine has been used sporadically at doses of 500 or 1,000 mg daily with some encouraging results [70]. For most cases of fungal mycetoma, a combined surgical and antifungal approach is necessary to achieve optimum response. No randomized and controlled studies for this disorder have been performed.

Other Endemic Mycoses

Terbinafine demonstrates excellent in vitro activity versus *H. capsulatum* and *B. dermatitidis*, and a few patients have received terbinafine for treatment of infections due to these organisms with encouraging results [70]. Terbinafine might be considered as potential salvage therapy among patients unable to tolerate any azole drug or amphotericin B. However, given the current availability of very effective azole compounds for these conditions, it is very unlikely that terbinafine will be studied prospectively for treatment of these mycoses.

Combination Therapy for Other Deep Mycoses

One potential use of terbinafine is for combination therapy with other approved antifungal agents for patients with cryptococcosis and invasive mould infections. In vitro data supporting the activity of terbinafine against *C. neoformans* led to the use of terbinafine combined with fluconazole or amphotericin B in selected patients with acute CNS cryptococcosis. No significant drug–drug interactions have been observed and this combined therapeutic approach appears to be well tolerated. Prospective data assessing this approach have been not well documented.

Among patients with invasive mould disease, especially invasive aspergillosis [71], terbinafine has been an attractive potential agent for combination therapy with either amphotericin B or a triazole, such as itraconazole or voriconazole [72]. No prospective randomized studies have been done, but small series and sporadic case reports suggest a favorable response among highly selected patients with a combination of terbinafine with another antifungal agent, usually voriconazole [15, 73]. Up to 2,000 mg per day of terbinafine has been given successfully with stable clinical outcome and has been well tolerated [15, 70].

Adverse Effects

Oral terbinafine appears to be well tolerated in the vast majority of patients, and few drug–drug interactions occur. In the largest study of its kind, adverse effects were assessed in a postmarketing study involving 25,884 patients who had received terbinafine [74]. These data demonstrated that 10.5% of patients experienced a drug-associated adverse event. A more recent survey suggested a lower incidence of significant adverse events (2%) [75]. The most common side effects are gastrointestinal tract symptoms, including nausea, diarrhea, abdominal pain, and dyspepsia, which occurred in about 5% of patients. Skin disorders are the second most common adverse event, affecting fewer than 3% of patients. Most of the cutaneous adverse effects are benign rashes; however, several patients developed erythema multiforme [74], psoriasis [76], and generalized pustular eruptions [77, 78]. Hepatobiliary adverse events have been reported in fewer than 1% of patients and include cholestatic jaundice with mild to moderate hepatocellular dysfunction [79–83]. Terbinafine-induced hepatic failure requiring liver transplantation has been reported [84]. Less commonly reported adverse events include neutropenia [85–87], thrombocytopenia [88], toxic epidermal necrolysis [89], angioedema [74], bullous pemphigoid [90] cutaneous lupus erythematosus [91–94], dermatomyositis [95], and optic atrophy [96].

Despite the frequent concomitant use of other medications, including immunosuppressive agents as well as any other systemic antifungal compounds, terbinafine is an uncommon cause of significant drug–drug interactions [2, 7, 97]. The lack of interaction of terbinafine with the mammalian cytochrome P-450 enzyme system is believed to be responsible for this important characteristic. Unlike the azole antifungal compounds, terbinafine does not appear to significantly alter the metabolism of cyclosporine, tacrolimus, or sirolimus.

Summary

Terbinafine is a broad spectrum oral and topical antifungal agent that possesses a unique mechanism of activity distinct from other available systemic antifungal agents. Most clinical experience with this antifungal has been in the treatment of onychomycosis and other superficial fungal infections, but there is a growing body of experience with terbinafine for the treatment of deeper mycoses, especially cutaneous and lymphocutaneous sporotrichosis. The potential for use of terbinafine as a combination agent with another antifungal drug for the treatment of cryptococcosis and invasive mould disease is intriguing, but remains largely unexplored.

References

1. Petranyi G, Ryder NS, Stutz A. Allylamine derivatives: new class of synthetic antifungal agents inhibiting fungal squalene epoxidase. Science. 1984;224:1239–41.
2. Balfour JA, Faulds D. Terbinafine: a review of its pharmacodynamic and pharmacokinetic properties, and therapeutic potential in superficial mycoses. Drugs. 1992;43:259–84.
3. Ryder NS, Dupont MC. Inhibition of squalene epoxidase by allylamine antimycotic compounds: a comparative study of fungal and mammalian enzymes. Biochem J. 1985;230:765–70.
4. Birnbaum JE. Pharmacology of allylamines. J Am Acad Dermatol. 1990;23:782–5.
5. Ryder NS. Terbinafine: mode of action and properties of the squalene epoxidase inhibition. Br J Dermatol. 1992;126 Suppl 39:2–7.
6. Schuster I. The interaction of representative members from two classes of antimycotics – the azoles and the allylamines – with cytochromes P450 in steroidogenic tissues and liver. Xenobiotica. 1985;15:29–46.
7. Katz HI. Drug interactions of the newer oral antifungal agents. Br J Dermatol. 1999;141 Suppl 56:26–32.
8. Petranyi G, Meingassner JG, Mieth H. Antifungal activity of the allylamine derivative terbinafine in vitro. Antimicrob Agents Chemother. 1987;31:1365–8.
9. Rinaldi MG. In vitro susceptibility of dermatophytes to antifungal drugs. Int J Dermatol. 1993;32:502–3.
10. Ryder NS, Favre B. Antifungal activity and mechanism of action of terbinafine. Rev Contemp Pharmacother. 1997;8:275–87.
11. Arzeni D, Barchiesi F, Compagnuci P, et al. In vitro activity of terbinafine against clinical isolates of dermatophytes. Med Mycol. 1998;36:235–7.
12. Gupta AK, Kohli Y. Clinical and laboratory investigations. In vitro susceptibility testing of ciclopirox, terbinafine, ketoconazole and itraconazole against dermatophytes and nondermatophytes, and in vitro evaluatin of combination antifungal activity. Br J Dermatol. 2003;149:296–305.

13. Schmitt HJ, Bernard EM, Andrade J, Edwards F, Schmitt B, Armstrong D. MIC and fungicidal activity of terbinafine against clinical isolates of *Aspergillus* spp. Antimicrob Agents Chemother. 1987;32:1619–23.
14. Ryder NS, Leitner L. Activity of terbinafine against *Aspergillus* in vitro, in combination with amphotericin B or triazoles. 36th Interscience Conference on Antimicrobial Agents and Chemotherapy. New Orleans: American Society for Microbiology, 1996 Abstract E54.
15. Schiraldi GF, Colombo MD. Potential use of terbinafine in the treatment of aspergillosis. Rev Contemp Pharmacother. 1997;8:349–56.
16. Shadomy S, Espinel-Ingroff A, Gebhart RJ. In vitro studies with SF 86–327, a new orally active allylamine derivative. Sabouraudia. 1985;23:125–32.
17. Venugopal PV, Venugopal TV, Ramakrishna ES, Illavarasin S. Antifungal activity of allylamines against agents of eumycetoma. Indian J Dermatol Venereol Leprol. 1993;59:239–42.
18. Wong PK, Ching WT, Gwon-Chung KJ, Meyer RD. Disseminated *Phialophora parasitica* infection in humans: case report and review. Rev Infect Dis. 1989;11:770–5.
19. Rallis E. Successful treatment of subcutaneous phaeohyphomycosis owing to *Exophiala jeanselmei* with oral terbinafine. Int J Dermatol. 2006;45:1369–70.
20. Bryan CS, Smith CW, Berg DE, Karp RB. *Curvularia lunata* endocarditis treated with terbinafine: case report. Clin Infect Dis. 1993;16:30–2.
21. Chang B, Sun PL, Huang FY, et al. *Paecilomyces lilacinus* peritonitis complicating peritoneal dialysis cured by oral voriconazole and terbinafine combination therapy. J Med Microbiol. 2008;57:1581–4.
22. Sellier P, Monsuez JJ, Lacroix C, et al. Recurrent subcutaneous infection due to *Scopulariopsis brevicaulis* in a liver transplant recipient. Clin Infect Dis. 2000;30:820–3.
23. Bhat SV, Paterson DL, Rinaldi MG, Veldkamp PJ. *Scedosporium prolificans* brain abscess in a patient with chronic granulomatous disease: successful combination therapy with voriconazole and terbinafine. Scand J Infect Dis. 2007;39:87–90.
24. Tong SYC, Peleg AY, Yoong J, Handke R, Szer J, Slavin M. Breakthrough *Scedosporium prolificans* infection while receiving voriconazole prophylaxis in an allogeneic stem cell transplant recipient. Transpl Infect Dis. 2007;9:241–3.
25. Kesson AM, Bellemore MC, O'Mara TJ, Ellis DH, Sorrell TC. *Scedosporium prolificans* osteomyelitis in an immunocompetent child treated with a novel agent, hexadecylphospocholine (miltefosine), in combination with terbinafine and voriconazole: a case report. Clin Infect Dis. 2009;48:1257–61.
26. Hiratani T, Asagi Y, Yamaguchi H. Evaluation of in vitro antimycotic activity of terbinafine, a new allylamine agent. Jpn J Med Mycol. 1991;32:323–32.
27. Ryder NS, Wagner S, Leitner I. In vitro activities of terbinafine against cutaneous isolates of *Candida albicans* and other pathogenic yeasts. Antimicrob Agents Chemother. 1998;42:1057–61.
28. Jessup CJ, Ryder NS, Ghannoum MA. An evaluation of the in vitro activity of terbinafine. Med Mycol. 2000;38:155–9.
29. Cavalheiro AS, Maboni G, de Azevedo MI, et al. In vitro activity of terbinafine combined with caspofungin and azoles against *Pythium insidiosum*. Antimicrob Agents Chemother. 2009;53:2136–8.
30. Cavalheiro AS, Zanette RA, Spader TB, et al. In vitro activity of terbinafine associated to amphotericin B, fluvastatin, rifampicin, metronidazole and ibuprofen against *Pythium insidiosum*. Vet Microbiol. 2009;137:408–11.
31. Brown TA, Grooters AM, Hosgood GL. In vitro susceptibility of *Pythium insidiosum* and a *Lagenidium* sp to itraconazole, posaconazole, voriconazole, terbinafine, caspofungin, and mefenoxam. Am J Vet Res. 2008;69:1463–8.
32. Jensen JC. Clinical pharmacokinetics of terbinafine. Clin Exp Dermatol. 1989;14:110–4.
33. Faergemann J. Pharmacokinetics of terbinafine. Rev Contemp Pharmacother. 1997;8:289–97.
34. Nejjam F, Zagula M, Cabiac MD, Guessous N, Humbert H, Lakhdar H. Pilot study of terbinafine in children suffering from tinea capitis: evaluation of efficacy, safety and pharmacokinetics. Br J Dermatol. 1995;132:98–105.
35. Faergemann J, Zehender H, Denouel J, Hilarious L. Levels of terbinafine in plasma, stratum corneum, dermis-epidermis (without stratum corneum), sebum, hair, and nails during and after 250 mg terbinafine orally once per day for four weeks. Acta Dermatol Venereol. 1993;73:305–9.
36. Faergemann J, Zehender H, Denouel J, Hilarious L. Levels of terbinafine in plasma, stratum corneum, dermis-epidermis without stratum corneum), sebum, hair, and nails during and after 250 mg terbinafine orally once daily for 7 and 14 days. Clin Exp Dermatol. 1994;19:121–6.
37. Humbert H, Cabiac MD, Denouel J, Kirkesseli S. Pharmacokinetics of terbinafine and its five main metabolites in plasma and urine, following a single oral dose in healthy subjects. Biopharm Drug Dispos. 1995;16:685–94.
38. Zehender H, Cabiac MD, Denouel J, Faergemann J, Donatsch P, Kutz K. Elimination kinetics of terbinafine from human plasma and tissue following multiple-dose administration, and comparison with 3 main metabolites. Drug Invest. 1994;8:203–10.
39. Hill S, Thomas R, Smith SG. An investigation of the pharmacokinetics of topical terbinafine 1% cream. Br J Dermatol. 1992;127:396–400.
40. Faergemann J, Zehender H, Boukhabza A, Ganslandt J, Jones TC. Comparison of terbinafine levels in stratum corneum and dermis-epidermis (without stratum corneum) after topical or topical combined with oral therapy in healthy volunteers. J Eur Acad Dermatol Venereol. 1995;5 Suppl 1:S94.
41. Roberts DT. The clinical efficacy of terbinafine in the treatment of fungal infections of nails. Rev Contemp Pharmacother. 1997;8:299–312.
42. Hull PR, Vismer HF. Potential use of terbinafine in the treatment of cutaneous sporotrichosis. Rev Contemp Pharmacother. 1997;8:343–7.
43. Chapman SW, Pappas P, Kauffman C, et al. Comparative evaluation of the efficacy and safety of two doses of terbinafine (500 and 1000 mg day^{-1}) in the treatment of cutaneous or lymphocutaneous sporotrichosis. Mycoses. 2004;47:62–8.
44. Weitzman I, Summerbell RC. The dermatophytes. Clin Microbiol Rev. 1995;8:240–59.
45. Arenas R, Dominguez-Cherit J, Fernandez LM. Open randomized comparison of itraconazole versus terbinafine in onychomycosis. Int J Dermatol. 1995;34:138–43.
46. Hofmann H, Brautigam M, Weidinger G, Zaun H, Lagos II. Treatment of toenail onychomycosis. Arch Dermatol. 1995;131:919–22.
47. Abdel-Rahman SM, Nahata MC. Oral terbinafine: a new antifungal agent. Ann Pharmacother. 1997;31:445–56.
48. Zaias N, Serrano L. The successful treatament of finger *Trichophyton rubrum* onychomycosis with oral terbinafine. Clin Exp Dermatol. 1989;14:120–3.
49. Baudraz-Rosselet F, Rakosi T, Wili PB, Kenzelmann R. Treatment of onychomycosis with terbinafine. Br J Dermatol. 1992;126 Suppl 39:40–6.
50. Goodfield MJ, Andrew L, Evans EG. Short-term treatment of dermatophyte onychomycosis with terbinafine. Br Med J. 1992;304:1151–4.
51. Gupta AK, Cooper EA. Update in antifungal therapy of dermatophytosis. Mycopathology. 2008;166:353–67.
52. Gupta AK, Lynch LE, Kogan N, Cooper EA. The use of an intermittent terbinafine regimen for the treatment of dermatophyte toenail onychomycosis. J Eur Acad Dermatol Venereol. 2009;23:256–62.
53. Criber BJ, Bakshi R. Terbinafine in the treatment of onychomycosis: a review of its efficacy in high-risk populations and in patients with nondermatophyte infections. Br J Dermatol. 2004;150:414–20.

54. Albanese G, DiCintio R, Martini C, Nocoletti A. Short therapy for tinea unguium with terbinafine: four different courses of treatment. Mycoses. 1995;38:211–4.
55. Faergemann J, Anderson C, Hersle K, et al. Double-blind, parallel-group comparison of terbinafine and griseofulvin in the treatment of toenail onychomycosis. J Am Acad Dermatol. 1995;32:750–3.
56. Haneke E, Tausch I, Brautigam M, Weidinger G, Welzel D. Short-duration treatment of fingernail dermatophytosis: a randomized, double-blind study with terbinafine and griseofulvin. J Am Acad Dermatol. 1995;32:72–7.
57. Brautigam M, Nolting S, Schopf RE, Weidinger G. Randomized double-blind comparison of terbinafine and itraconazole for the treatment of toenail tinea infections. Br Med J. 1995;311:919–22.
58. Ghannoum MA, Wraith LA, Cai B, Nyirady J, Isham N. Susceptibility of dermatophyte isolates obtained from a large worldwide terbinafine tinea capitis clinical trial. Br J Dermatol. 2008;159:711–3.
59. Haroon TS, Hussain I, Mahmood A, Nagi AH, Ahman D, Zahid M. An open clinical pilot study of the efficacy and safety of oral terbinafine in dry non-inflammatory tinea capitis. Br J Dermatol. 1992;126 Suppl 39:47–50.
60. Gupta AK, Adamiak A, Cooper EA. The efficacy and safety of terbinafine in children. J Eur Acad Dermatol Venereol. 2003;17:627–40.
61. Hull PR, Vismer HF. Treatment of cutaneous sporotrichosis with terbinafine. Br J Dermatol. 1992;126:51–5.
62. Kudoh K, Kamei E, Terunama A, Nakagawa S, Tagami H. Successful treatment of cutaneous sporotrichosis with terbinafine. J Dermatol Treat. 1996;7:33–5.
63. Coskun B, Saral Y, Akpolat N, Ataseven A, Çiçek D. Sporotrichosis successfully treated with terbinafine and potassium iodide: case report and review of the literature. Mycopathology. 2004;158:53–6.
64. Restrepo A, Robledo J, Gomez I, Tabares AM, Gutierrez R. Itraconazole therapy in lymphangitic and cutaneous sporotrichosis. Arch Dermatol. 1986;122:413–7.
65. Esterre P, Ratsioharana M, Roig P. Potential use of terbinafine in the treatment of chromoblastomycosis. Rev Contemp Pharmacother. 1997;8:357–62.
66. Esterre P, Intani C, Ratsioharana M, Andriantsmahavandy A. A multicenter trial of terbinafine in patients with chromoblastomycosis: effect on clinical and biologic criteria. J Dermatol Treat. 1998;9:529–34.
67. Zhang J, Xi L, Lu C, et al. Successful treatment for chromoblastomycosis caused by *Fonsecaea monophora*: a report of three cases in Guangdong, China. Mycoses. 2008;52:176–81.
68. Queiroz-Telles F, Esterre P, Perez-Blanco M, Vitale RG, Salgado CG, Bonifaz A. Chromoblastomycosis: an overview of clinical manifestations, diagnosis and treatment. Med Mycol. 2009;47:3–15.
69. Zhang JM, Xi LY, Zhang H, et al. Synergistic effects of terbinafine and itraconazole on clinical isolates of *Fonsecaea monophora*. Eur J Dermatol. 2009;19:451–5.
70. Hay RJ. Therapeutic potential of terbinafine in subcutaneous and systemic mycoses. Br J Dermatol. 1999;141 Suppl 56:36–40.
71. Steinbach WJ, Stevens DA, Denning DW. Combination and sequential antifungal therapy for invasive aspergillosis: review of published in vitro and in vivo interactions and 6281 clinical cases from 1966 to 2001. Clin Infect Dis. 2003;37:S188–224.
72. Krishnan-Natesan S, Chandrasekar PH, Manavathu EK, Revankar SG. Successful treatment of primary cutaneous *Aspergillus ustus* infection with surgical debridement and a combination of voriconazole and terbinafine. Diagn Microbiol Infect Dis. 2008;62:443–6.
73. Harari S, Schiraldi GF, de Juli E, Gronda E. Relapsing *Aspergillus bronchitis* in a double lung transplant patient, successfully treated with a new oral antimycotic agent [Letter]. Chest. 1997;111:835–6.
74. Hall M, Monka C, Krupp P, O'Sullivan D. Safety of oral terbinafine: results of a post marketing surveillance study in 25,884 patients. Arch Dermatol. 1997;133:1213–9.
75. Chang CH, Young-Xu Y, Kurth T, Orav JE, Chan AK. The safety of oral antifungal treatments for superficial dermatophytosis and onychomycosis: a meta-analysis. Am J Med. 2007;120:791–8.
76. Gupta AK, Sibbald RG, Knowles SR, Lynde CW, Shear NH. Terbinafine therapy may be associated with the development of psoriasis de novo or its exacerbation: four case reports and a review of drug-induced psoriasis. J Am Acad Dermatol. 1997;36:858–62.
77. Bennett ML, Jorizzo JL, White WL. Generalized pustular eruptions associated with oral terbinafine. Int J Dermatol. 1999;38:596–600.
78. Beltraminelli HS, Lerch M, Arnold A, Bircher AJ, Haeusermann P. Acute generalized exanthematous pustulosis induced by the antifungal terbinafine: case report and review of the literature. Br J Dermatol. 2005;152:780–3.
79. Gupta AK, Del Rosso JQ, Lynde CW, Brown GH, Shear NH. Hepatitis associated with terbinafine therapy: three case reports and a review of the literature. Clin Exp Dermatol. 1998;23:64–7.
80. Conjeevaram G, Vongthavaravat V, Summer R, Koff RS. Terbinafine-induced hepatitis and pancytopenia. Dig Dis Sci. 2001;46:1714–6.
81. Zapata Garrido AJ, Romo AC, Padilla FB. Terbinafine hepatotoxicity. A case report and review of literature. Ann Hepatol. 2003;2:47–51.
82. Ajit C, Suvannasankha A, Zaeri N, Munoz SJ. Terbinafine-associated hepatotoxicity. Am J Med Sci. 2003;325:292–5.
83. Fernandes NF, Geller SA, Fong TL. Terbinafine hepatotoxicity: case report and review of the literature. Am J Gastroenterol. 1998;93:459–60.
84. Perveze Z, Johnson MW, Rubin RA, et al. Terbinafine-induced hepatic failure requiring liver transplantation. Liver Transpl. 2007;13:162–4.
85. Gupta AK, Soori GS, Del Rossa JQ, Bartos PB, Shear NH. Severe neutropenia associated with oral terbinafine therapy. J Am Acad Dermatol. 1998;38:765–7.
86. Shapiro M, Li L, Miller J. Terbinafine-induced neutropenia. Br J Dermatol. 1999;140:1169–99.
87. Kovacs MJ, Alshammari S, Guenther L, Bourcier M. Neutropenia and pancytopenia associated with oral terbinafine. J Am Acad Dermatol. 1994;31:806.
88. Amichai B, Grunwald MH. Adverse drug reactions of the new oral antifungal agents – terbinafine, fluconazole, and itraconazole. Int J Dermatol. 1998;37:410–5.
89. Carstens J, Wendelboe P, Sogaard H, Thestrup-Pederson K. Toxic epidermal necrolysis and erythema multiforme following therapy with terbinafine. Acta Dermatol Venereol. 1994;74:391–2.
90. Aksakal BA, Ozsoy E, Arnavut O, Ali Gürer M. Oral terbinafine-induced bullous pemphigoid. Ann Pharmacother. 2003;37:1625–7.
91. McKay DA, Schofield OM, Benton EC. Terbinafine-induced subacute cutaneous lupus erythematosus. Acta Derm Venereol. 2004;84:472–4.
92. Farhi D, Viguier M, Cosnes A, et al. Terbinafine-induced subacute cutaneous lupus erythematous. Dermatology. 2006;212:59–65.
93. Lorentz K, Booken N, Goerdt S, Goebeler M. Subacute cutaneous lupus erythematosus induced by terbinafine: case report and review of literature. J Dtsch Dermatol Ges. 2008;6:823–7.
94. Hivnor CM, Hudkins ML, Bonner B. Terbinafine-induced subacute cutaneous lupus erythematosus. Cutis. 2008;81:156–7.
95. Magro CM, Schaefer JT, Waldeman J, Knight D, Seilstad K, Hearne D. Terbinafine-induced dermatomyositis: a case report and literature review of drug-induced dermatomyositis. J Cutan Pathol. 2008;35:74–91.
96. Yülek F, Cagil N, Cakmak HB, Akcay EK, Imek A, Kansu T. Bilateral anterior optic neuropathy associated with use of terbinafine. Clin Exp Ophthalmol. 2008;36:488–9.
97. Elewski B, Tavakkol A. Safety and tolerability of oral antifungal agents in the treatment of fungal nail disease: a proven reality. Ther Clin Risk Man. 2005;1:299–306.

Antifungal Pharmacokinetics and Pharmacodynamics

David R. Andes and Alex J. Lepak

The critical role of pharmacokinetics and pharmacodynamics in the selection and dosing of antimicrobial therapeutics, including antifungal agents, has gained increasing recognition [1–4]. The study of pharmacokinetics involves understanding the interaction of a drug with the host, including measurements of absorption, distribution, metabolism, and elimination. The study of antimicrobial pharmacodynamics provides insight into the link between drug pharmacokinetics, in vitro susceptibility, and treatment outcome. Knowledge of the pharmacokinetic/pharmacodynamic index and magnitude associated with efficacy can be helpful for clinicians to predict therapeutic success/failure, guide optimal dosing levels and intervals, aid in susceptibility breakpoint development, guide therapeutic drug monitoring, and limit potential adverse outcomes, including toxicity and the development of resistance [5–8]. Numerous in vitro, animal, and clinical studies have been instrumental in characterizing the pharmacodynamic activity of the clinically available antifungal drug classes, including triazoles, polyenes, flucytosine, and echinocandins [6–18]. The analyses of data with these antifungal drug classes have identified distinct pharmacodynamic characteristics that result in different optimal dosing strategies. Accumulating clinical data have also become available with several antifungals that allow pharmacodynamic data analyses [19–25]. Most often the results of these investigations have corroborated information from experimental models. The following chapter outlines the pharmacodynamic characteristics of antifungals and presents evidence of the clinical relevance of these concepts.

D.R. Andes (✉)
Department of Medicine, and Medical
Microbiology and Immunology, Section of Infectious Diseases,
Madison, WI, USA
e-mail: dra@medicine.wisc.edu

Pharmacokinetic Concepts

Pharmacokinetic studies describe how the body handles a drug, including absorption, distribution, binding to serum and tissue proteins, metabolism, and elimination [1]. Antifungal drug concentrations have been well characterized in numerous body fluids and tissues, including serum, urine, cerebrospinal fluid (CSF), vitreous body, epithelial lining fluid, bronchoalveolar lavage fluid, brain, lung, and kidney. The pharmacokinetic goal of antifungal therapy is to achieve adequate drug concentrations at the site of infection. This begs the rather simplistic question, where is the fungus relative to the antifungal drug? The site of infection for fungal pathogens can range from the bloodstream, where one would expect serum measurements to be of importance, to various tissue sites for which tissue drug concentrations may be of greater interest. Most pathogenic fungi exist primarily in extracellular tissue fluid; thus, even at tissue sites of infection serum measurements serve as a reliable tissue concentration surrogate.

The body sites for which tissue antifungal concentrations have been suggested to be most important include the brain parenchyma and the vitreous body [26]. Outcomes of infection at other tissue sites have correlated well with serum concentrations. For example, Groll and colleagues examined the relationship between efficacy and CSF and brain kinetics for several amphotericin B (AmB) preparations [27]. The CSF concentrations of four polyene compounds were remarkably similar. Brain tissue concentrations of liposomal AmB (LAmB), however, were from six- to tenfold higher than the other polyene preparations. The burden of *Candida* in the brains of rabbits following therapy correlated well with brain tissue penetration of the various drugs.

Another pharmacokinetic factor shown to impact the availability of antimicrobial compounds in tissue is binding to serum proteins such as albumin. In general it is accepted that only unbound (free) drug is pharmacologically active [28, 29]. This is related to the limited ability of protein-bound drug to diffuse across tissue and cellular membranes to reach the drug target. The relevance of protein binding has been

C.A. Kauffman et al. (eds.), *Essentials of Clinical Mycology*,
DOI 10.1007/978-1-4419-6640-7_8, © Springer Science+Business Media, LLC 2011

most clearly demonstrated for drugs from the triazole class, in which there are marked differences in degree of binding among the drugs [1, 11, 12, 15, 30]. The studies demonstrating these findings are discussed later.

Pharmacodynamic Concepts

Pharmacodynamics examines the relationship between pharmacokinetics and outcome. An added dimension of antimicrobial pharmacodynamics is consideration of the drug exposure relative to a measure of in vitro potency or the minimum inhibitory concentration (MIC) (Fig. 1). Three pharmacodynamic indices have been used to describe these relationships, including the peak concentration in relation to the MIC (Cmax/MIC), the area under the concentration curve in relation to the MIC (24 h area under the concentration curve, AUC/MIC), and the time that drug concentrations exceed the MIC expressed as a percentage of the dosing interval (%T>MIC). Knowledge of which of the three pharmacodynamic indices describes antifungal activity provides the basis for determining the frequency with which a drug is most efficaciously administered. For example, if the Cmax/MIC index relationship strongly correlates with activity of drug A, the optimal dosing schedule would provide large infrequent doses. Conversely, if the %T > MIC better describes drug activity, a dosing strategy may include smaller more frequent or even continuous drug administration to prolong the period of time that drug levels exceed the MIC.

Traditionally, three pharmacodynamic questions have been addressed in studies designed to define these concepts. First, what is the pharmacodynamic index associated with treatment efficacy? Second, what is the magnitude of the pharmacodynamic index needed for efficacy, or simply put, how much drug is needed for efficacy? Finally, do the pharmacodynamic results from experimental models predict outcome in patients?

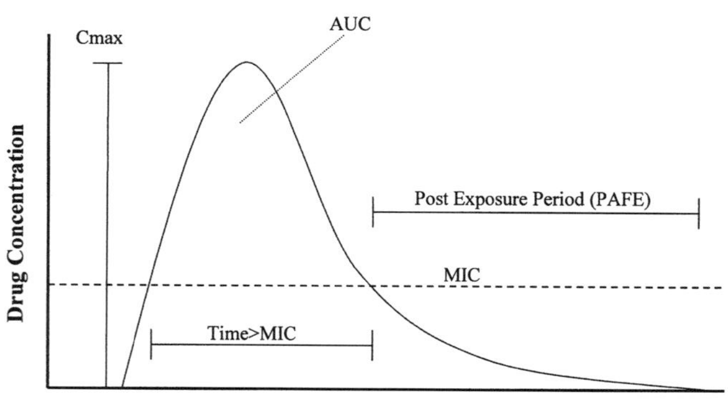

Fig. 1 Pharmacokinetic/pharmacodynamic relationship of antifungal drug concentration over time relative to organism minimum inhibitory concentration (MIC). Pharmacodynamic indices include the maximum or peak drug concentration relative to MIC (Cmax/MIC), the area under the drug concentration curve relative to MIC (AUC/MIC), and time that the concentration of drug exceeds the MIC (Time>MIC). Also represented is the post-exposure period, which represents the time period of drug exposure that is below the MIC in which many antifungals express continued antifungal effect, termed the post-antifungal effect (PAFE)

Concept 1: Impact of Antifungal Concentration on Activity over Time

Two observations have been made in examining the impact of escalating antifungal drug concentrations on fungal viability over time. First is the finding that for some drugs, increasing drug concentrations above the MIC enhances the rate and extent of organism death. When higher concentrations enhance killing, the pharmacodynamic pattern of activity is referred to as concentration-dependent killing. The second observation was noted during periods long after drug exposure (after the antimicrobial is no longer present or present at concentrations below the MIC). For some drugs there is a period of prolonged growth suppression following the initial supra-MIC exposure. This period of growth suppression is termed a post-antifungal effect (PAFE) [31, 32]. Three combinations of these time-kill end point characteristics have been described, and each combination is typically associated with one of the pharmacodynamic indices. The Cmax/MIC is associated with concentration-dependent killing and prolonged PAFEs. The %T>MIC is associated with concentration-independent killing and short PAFEs. The AUC/MIC is associated with prolonged PAFEs and either concentration-dependent or -independent killing.

Concept 2: Impact of Dosing Interval Variation or Fractionation

A second experimental design used to determine which pharmacodynamic index is predictive of efficacy is termed dose fractionation. Traditional dose escalation studies use a single dosing interval. With only a single dosing interval, escalating doses increase the values of all three indices. Dose fractionation studies examine efficacy of various dose levels that are administered by using three or more dosing intervals. In examining treatment results, if the regimens with shorter dosing intervals are more efficacious, the time-dependent index (T>MIC) is the more important index. If the large, infrequently administered dosing regimens are more active, the peak level in relation to the MIC is most predictive. Finally, if the outcome is similar with each of the dosing intervals, the outcome depends on the total dose or the AUC for the dosing regimen.

Concept 3: Pharmacodynamic Target

Knowledge of the pharmacodynamic characteristics of a compound allows one to better design a dosing interval strategy. This knowledge can also be useful to design studies to determine the amount of drug or index magnitude that is associated with treatment efficacy. For example, what pharmacodynamic magnitude of a drug is needed to treat a *Candida* infection? Is this pharmacodynamic magnitude the same as that needed to treat a drug-resistant *Candida* infection? Is the magnitude similar for other fungal species, for different infection sites, in different animal species? The answers to these questions have been explored and most times successfully addressed using a variety of infection models. The results of these studies have demonstrated that the magnitude of a pharmacodynamic index associated with efficacy is similar for drugs within the same class, provided that free drug levels are considered. The pharmacodynamic evaluation of each antifungal drug class and the clinical implications of these studies are detailed in subsequent sections.

Concept 4: Clinical Pharmacodynamics

The final and most important pharmacodynamic question involves determining if the results from the experimental model investigations are helpful for predicting efficacy in patients. The analysis needed for this correlation requires clinical data sets that include drug dose or drug concentration monitoring, organism MIC, and treatment efficacy. These data can be used to determine the pharmacodynamic exposure associated with an acceptable outcome and to determine which treatment end point from preclinical models (e.g., 50% maximal effect or the static dose) correlates with efficacy in patients.

Polyenes

Impact of Antifungal Concentration on Activity over Time

In vitro polyene time-kill studies have been undertaken with numerous yeast and filamentous fungal pathogens [5, 7, 13, 14, 18, 27, 32–37]. The majority of studies have been undertaken with AmB or one of the lipid formulations of this drug. Each of these studies has demonstrated marked concentration-dependent killing and maximal antifungal activity at concentrations exceeding the MIC from two- to tenfold. Several of these in vitro models have also demonstrated prolonged persistent growth suppression following drug exposure and removal (PAFE). The duration of these persistent effects was also linearly related to the concentration of the AmB exposure. For example, the longest periods of in vivo growth suppression were nearly an entire day (>20 h) following a single high dose of AmB in neutropenic mice [14]. For drugs displaying this pattern of activity the Cmax/MIC ratio has most often been the pharmacodynamic index predictive of efficacy.

Impact of Dosing Interval Variation or Fractionation

In vivo dose fractionation studies with AmB in an in vivo *Candida* model demonstrated optimal efficacy when large doses were administered infrequently, and pharmacodynamic analysis of the dose fractionation data illustrate that the Cmax/MIC index best predicts efficacy [14]. With each increase in length of the dosing interval from every 12 h to every 72 h, efficacy was enhanced, and the dose needed to achieve a net static effect was up to tenfold lower when administered with the most widely spaced dosing interval. A similar experimental approach was undertaken in an in vivo *Aspergillus* model [38]. Over a fourfold total dose range, the lung burden of *Aspergillus* was significantly lower when AmB was administered every 72 h compared to every 24 h or every 8 h. The results of these experiments corroborate the importance of the Cmax/MIC pharmacodynamic index and suggest that the pharmacodynamic driver of efficacy is similar among yeast and filamentous fungi.

Pharmacodynamic Target

In vivo study with AmB against multiple *Candida* species in a neutropenic disseminated candidiasis model observed a net static effect (growth inhibition) when the Cmax/MIC ratio approached values of 2–4 [14]. Maximal microbiologic efficacy against these strains in the same model was observed with ratios near 10. Similar investigation of efficacy in a murine pulmonary aspergillosis model demonstrated maximal efficacy with Cmax/MIC exposures in the range of 2–4 [38]. These most recent studies with *Aspergillus* address a critical gap in knowledge and suggest that at least for AmB, both the pharmacodynamic pattern of efficacy and the pharmacodynamic target are similar among fungal species.

It is generally accepted that the lipid formulations of AmB are not as potent in vivo as conventional AmB on a weight (mg/kg) basis. Each of the lipid formulations is complexed to a different lipid and exhibits unique pharmacokinetic characteristics [39]. For example, LamB, which utilizes small unilamellar particles, liposomes, exhibits both high serum and CNS concentrations that are hypothesized to be due to the large serum: CNS gradient relative to the other AmB preparations [27]. Conversely, amphotericin B lipid complex (ABLC) and amphotericin B colloid dispersion (ABCD) achieve higher concentrations in the intracellular space and in organs of the reticuloendothelial system. Several studies have also suggested that ABLC attains higher concentrations in the lung than other formulations [40, 41].

Recent investigations have explored the impact of these pharmacokinetic differences on pharmacodynamic outcomes. For example, a study in an in vivo candidiasis model demonstrated that the difference in potency among the lipid preparations in the lungs, kidneys, and liver were congruent with tissue kinetics in these organs [13]. A novel study in a CNS candidiasis model examined the relationship between kinetics in serum, CSF, and brain parenchyma [27]. The kinetic studies demonstrated no significant difference in CSF concentrations, but higher brain concentrations of LAmB. The brain parenchymal differences in kinetics correlated closely with treatment efficacy in the model for which LAmB appeared to hold an advantage.

Similar investigations in *Aspergillus* pneumonia models have included assessment of lung tissue concentrations [41]. These studies have also suggested a relationship between these lung tissue site concentrations and efficacy. In this case, these pharmacodynamic investigations appear to favor ABLC. Recent studies have also begun to consider compartmental pharmacokinetics in the lung [40]. Specifically, a study in a murine model examined total lung, epithelial lining fluid, and pulmonary macrophage concentrations of each of the AmB preparations. As in previous studies, ABLC produced higher lung concentrations (70-fold higher than serum concentrations); however, a large amount of the compound appeared to reside in the pulmonary alveolar macrophages. The highest epithelial lining fluid concentrations were noted in LAmB-treated animals. Determination of the impact of these pharmacokinetic differences has not yet been reported.

Clinical Relevance

The pharmacokinetics of conventional AmB and the various lipid formulations have been carefully characterized in serum and tissues for several patient populations. Several investigations have attempted to demonstrate a correlation between AmB MIC and outcome [42, 43]. Most of these studies have found it difficult to discern MIC impact. We hypothesize that this is related to the narrow MIC and dose range in these studies, making it difficult to have enough Cmax/MIC or AUC/MIC variation to correlate with outcome. We are aware of only a single investigation that has attempted to correlate individual patient pharmacokinetics, MIC, and outcome with polyenes [44]. The study examined LAmB kinetics and outcome of invasive fungal infections in pediatric patients. In this small study, data from a subset of patients provided detailed kinetics, MIC, and outcome. The results demonstrate a statistically significant relationship between Cmax/MIC ratio and outcome. Maximal efficacy was observed with LAmB serum Cmax/MIC ratios greater than 40. This value is similar to that observed in the animal model studies described earlier when using serum LAmB measurements. This small study demonstrates that pharmacodynamic investigation with a drug from the polyene class can produce meaningful results that are congruent with those from preclinical infection models.

One large clinical study with LAmB tested the impact of dose escalation and observed conflicting results. Cornely et al. compared standard dosing of LAmB (3–5 mg/kg/day) to higher initial doses (10 mg/kg/day) for initial treatment of invasive mold infections [45]. The study was a multicenter, prospective, randomized, double-blinded, trial comparing LAmB administration at 3 mg/kg/day to that of 10 mg/kg/day for the first 14 days of a proven or probable invasive mold infection. After 14 days all patients continued with regular dosing of 3 mg/kg/day. The patient population was overwhelmingly represented by hematologic malignancy (93%), neutropenia (73% at baseline and 90% within 60 days of enrollment), pulmonary site of infection (90%), and aspergillosis as the infecting agent (97%). There was no statistically significant difference in outcomes between the two groups in regard to response rates; however, there were significant differences in renal toxicity, with 31% doubling of creatinine in the high-loading-dose arm versus 14% in the conventional dose arm. In addition, discontinuation of treatment prior to completion of the initial 14 days was higher in the high-dose group (24% vs. 13%). The conclusions from this study are that administration of higher dosages of LAmB for the first 14 days does not improve outcomes and leads to increased risks of toxicity and cost in patients primarily with hematologic malignancy, neutropenia, and pulmonary aspergillosis. From a pharmacodynamic perspective one may speculate (1) that the concentration-effect relationship is either maximal at the 5 mg/kg dose level, (2) that the threefold change in dose level was not enough to discern an efficacy difference, or (3) perhaps more likely, the toxicity of the drug at high concentration outweighed any efficacy benefit.

One additional exploration of AmB dosing regimens has been in the area of toxicodynamics. Investigators have theorized that toxicity, like efficacy, is related to high AmB concentrations. It follows that administration of the total daily dose by continuous infusion would result in lower peak concentrations and thus reduced toxicity. Several small clinical studies have compared toxicity of the continuous infusion dosing strategy with a conventional once-daily regimen [46–49]. For example, Eriksson et al. compared AmB 0.97 mg/kg/day given as a continuous infusion to once-daily administration of the same dosage over 4 h [46]. The continuous regimen resulted in fewer infusion-associated side effects and instances of renal insufficiency. Several case series have reported use of continuous infusion in patients with hematologic malignancies and refractory fever. The majority of these reports note less rise in creatinine than has been reported in historic controls. However, other published experiences have reported conflicting results. Hall et al. observed a similar rate of nephrotoxicity in their use of the continuous-infusion regimen in a cohort of hematology patients with suspected or proven invasive fungal infection [47]. Unfortunately, studies examining the treatment efficacy of this strategy have not been undertaken. Studies from preclinical infection models would predict this strategy would be less effective.

Flucytosine

Impact of Antifungal Concentration on Activity over Time

Several concentration ranging, time-kill investigations have identified a pharmacodynamic pattern of activity distinct from that seen with the polyenes [16–18, 32, 50]. The antifungal activity of flucytosine (5FC) in both in vitro and in vivo *Candida* infection models has been shown to be maximal at concentrations not far above the MIC. Additional exposure to higher concentrations does not impact the extent of organism killing. This pattern of activity is termed time-dependent killing as opposed to the concentration-dependent activity described for amphotericin B. In addition, examination of *Candida* growth following 5FC exposure over a wide concentration range demonstrated organism recovery soon after exposure; thus there were no short or no post-antifungal effects.

Impact of Dosing Interval Variation or Fractionation

5FC in vivo dose fractionation studies in an in vivo candidiasis model similar to those described for AmB demonstrated that efficacy was optimal when drug was administrated in smaller dose levels more frequently [16]. Tenfold less drug was needed for efficacy when administered using the most fractionated dosing strategy by prolonging the time of the antifungal exposure. This time course and dose fractionation result suggests the %T>MIC would be the most predictive index. Consideration of each of the pharmacodynamic indices further demonstrates that the %T>MIC is most closely associated with efficacy.

Pharmacodynamic Target

The index magnitude for which optimal efficacy against *Candida albicans* was noted in a mouse infection model was a time above MIC magnitude of only 40% of the dosing interval (serum concentrations above the MIC for just less than one-half of the dosing interval) [16, 50]. However, as opposed to target studies with other antifungals, the 5FC studies were limited to two strains. However, these studies were corroborated in two independent laboratories. Unfortunately, there has not been a pharmacodynamic study with the most clinically relevant organism and infection site, *Cryptococcus neoformans* and meningitis. Studies using this model may offer critical dosing regimen strategies for this compound with a relatively narrow therapeutic index.

Clinical Relevance

There are no clinical data sets that allow pharmacodynamic analysis with 5FC in regard to treatment efficacy. However, one group of investigators have provided a model of human 5FC pharmacokinetics relative to the %T>MIC target (40–50%) against *Candida* species in a murine model [50]. The group considered the pharmacokinetics of a range of 5FC doses and the MIC distribution for *C. albicans*. Interestingly, doses as low as 25 mg/kg/day (sixfold lower than the currently recommended regimen) would be predicted to achieve the pharmacodynamic target against organisms in the current MIC distribution. Again, the major gap in knowledge for 5FC is characterization in a cryptococcal meningitis model to determine if the pharmacodynamic target is similar.

While pharmacodynamic studies linking 5FC exposure to efficacy have not been adequately explored, examination of toxicodynamic relationships are well established [51–55]. The primary toxicity of 5FC has been associated with high peak concentrations. These studies have shown that bone marrow toxicity is observed when levels in serum exceed 50–60 μg/mL. If one were to consider the human kinetics of the most frequently recommended 5FC dosing of 100 mg/kg/day divided into four doses, each dose of 37.5 mg/kg would remain higher than the MIC for 90% of *C. albicans* isolates tested for more than 10 h. That the pharmacodynamic driver of success and toxicity are different provides an opportunity to design dosing strategies to both optimize treatment efficacy and reduce toxicity. Use of significantly smaller amounts of drug would allow 5FC administration with much less concern about related toxicities. Whether higher concentrations would be optimal for cryptococcal CNS infection remains an important unanswered question.

Triazoles

Impact of Antifungal Concentration on Activity over Time

In vitro and in vivo time-kill studies have been undertaken with all of the clinically available triazole compounds [7, 11, 12, 18, 30, 32, 56–60]. The observations have shown that triazoles exhibit growth inhibition at concentrations near the MIC, much like that observed with 5FC (concentration-independent or time-dependent activity). These investigations have shown that over a wide triazole concentration range (starting below the MIC [sub-MIC] to those more than 200-fold in excess of the MIC), growth of *Candida* organisms are similarly inhibited. In other words, increasing drug concentrations do not enhance antifungal effect.

Furthermore, in vitro studies demonstrated organism regrowth soon after drug removal (i.e., no in vitro post antifungal effect). In vivo studies, however, demonstrated prolonged growth suppression after levels in serum decreased to below the MIC. These prolonged in vivo PAFEs have been theorized to be caused by the profound sub-MIC activity of these drugs (i.e., effect of the triazoles after concentrations fall below the MIC in vivo, similar to those shown in vitro). The pharmacodynamic pattern combination of concentration-independent killing and prolonged PAFEs suggest that the 24 AUC/MIC index is most closely tied to treatment effect.

Impact of Dosing Interval Variation or Fractionation

Dose fractionation studies in several in vivo models with each of the triazole compounds have demonstrated that efficacy is dependent upon the dose, but independent of the dosing frequency. The earliest dose fractionation studies with fluconazole examined the impact of dividing four total dose levels into one, two, or four doses over a 24-h period [60]. The results clearly demonstrated that outcome depended on the total amount of drug or AUC rather than the dosing interval. Subsequent studies with fluconazole, posaconazole, ravuconazole, and voriconazole similarly demonstrated that outcome was independent of fractionation of the total drug exposure supporting the 24-h AUC/MIC as the pharmacodynamic index driving treatment efficacy [11, 12, 15, 30]. These later observations importantly suggest that the pharmacodynamic index associated with efficacy was similar among drugs with a similar mechanism of action, in this case inhibition of ergosterol synthesis.

Pharmacodynamic Target

The usefulness of knowing which index predicts efficacy is being able to then determine the magnitude of the index needed for successful outcome. The most efficient experimental way to define the magnitude of the predictive index is to examine treatment efficacy against organisms with widely varying MICs. These experiments have been difficult for AmB and 5FC, for which the MIC range is fairly narrow for the majority of isolates.

Resistance development has been a clinically relevant issue for the triazoles and *Candida* species. Thus, incorporation of MIC variation into experimental models has been more feasible. For example, the efficacy of posaconazole was examined over a more than 1,000-fold AUC range against 12 *C. albicans* with MICs varying nearly 100-fold [11]. Results from these studies showed that the AUC/MIC exposure associated with treatment efficacy was similar across the group of strains with widely varying MICs. For each of the triazoles examined in these animal model studies, the 24-h AUC/MIC necessary to produce the ED50 corresponds to a value near 25 [11, 12, 15, 30, 61]. This is essentially the same as averaging a drug concentration near the organism MIC for a 24-h period (1 X MIC X 24 h = AUC/MIC of 24) (Table 1).

Similar studies have been undertaken with four triazole compounds that include more than 100 drug/organism combinations for which MICs and dose levels varied more than 1,000-fold each. Two observations from these studies have been particularly relevant. First, for an individual drug, the AUC/MIC target for the triazole was independent of the MIC or the drug resistance mechanism. The second observation was initially less clear. Analysis of treatment outcome among the triazoles with similar strains demonstrated a wide range of dose/MIC and AUC/MIC relationships. However, one major difference among the triazoles is the degree of protein binding with lower values for fluconazole, intermediate values for voriconazole, and high binding with the remaining compounds.

A second look at these relationships, taking into account only free drug concentrations, identified very congruent data plots.

Table 1 Antifungal pharmacodynamic characteristics

Antifungal class	PD characteristic: Concentration dependence	Time dependence	Prolonged PAFE	PD index predictive of efficacy	PD target: Experimental	Clinical
Polyenes	X		X	Cmax/MIC	2–4	
5-FC		X		Time above MIC	≥40%	
Azoles		X	X	AUC/MIC	25	25
Echinocandins	X		X	AUC/MIC	3–5[a]	3–5[a]
					10–20	10–20

[a]PD target magnitude calculated using free drug concentration (i.e.,% drug not protein bound). For the echinocandins, the area under the drug concentration curve(AUC) / minimum inhibitory concentration (MIC) magnitude is different when comparing *C. albicans* to *C. glabrata* or *C. parapsilosis*, with the lower magnitude correlating with the latter two organisms and higher magnitude correlating with *C. albicans*

Calculation of the pharmacodynamic target among triazoles was indeed similar as long as free drug concentrations were considered. The consistency of data with the triazoles demonstrates that when protein binding and hence free drug concentrations are considered, the antifungal pharmacodynamic target is similar among drugs within a mechanistic class, such as triazoles.

The majority of antifungal pharmacodynamic target investigations have been undertaken in *Candida* models. More recently, a model of disseminated aspergillosis has been utilized in these investigations. Mavridou et al. investigated the relationship between posaconazole and voriconazole AUC/MIC and survival in neutropenic mice with disseminated infection with strains of *A. fumigatus* [62, 63]. The group made several important observations. Similar to what has been reported for *Candida* species, the treatment target was similar among four *Aspergillus* strains, which included one wild-type drug-susceptible strain and three strains with reduced azole susceptibility, suggesting that the target is similar among susceptible and resistant strains. Second, the AUC/MIC exposure associated with survival was nearly identical for both of the triazoles when free drug concentrations were considered. Perhaps most interesting, the drug exposure associated with efficacy in these *Aspergillus* models was similar to that described for these drugs in disseminated candidiasis models.

It is clear from multiple epidemiologic investigations that factors other than drug choice or dose impact patient outcome. It has been hypothesized that any of these factors may impact the pharmacodynamic exposure-response relationship. For example, one may intuitively posit that nonneutropenic patients may require less antifungal exposure than neutropenic patients. Several host, pathogen, and infection site factors have begun to be included in pharmacodynamic magnitude studies. For example, a recent study with an investigational triazole (isavuconazole) measured survival rates in mice with and without neutropenia [58]. The dose of isavuconazole needed to produce maximal survival rates was twofold higher in the neutropenic model.

Another host factor of importance for interpretation of preclinical antifungal pharmaocdynamic studies is the impact of the infected animal species. One may expect differences in pharmacokinetics in different animal species to impact the pharmacodynamic target. Consideration of drug exposures in pharmacodynamic terms, relative to the MIC of the organism, however, corrects for interspecies kinetic differences. Simply put, the drug target is in the organism and not in the host and thus host pharmacokinetic differences should not change the antimicrobial exposure the organism needs to see for effect. Studies with fluconazole in mice, rats, and rabbits allow testing of this hypothesis. Results from these treatment studies have shown that the fluconazole AUC/MIC needed to achieve 50% of the maximal microbiologic effect was near 25 and remarkably similar among the mammalian models [15, 60, 64, 65]. This knowledge allows one to hypothesize that results from preclinical animal pharmacodynamic target studies could be used to estimate antifungal dosing efficacy in humans.

Clinical Relevance

The logical next step is to determine if and how the experimental pharmacodynamic studies relate to outcome in patients. Data from antibacterial pharmacodynamics provide a compelling precedence for the predictive value of animal model pharmacodynamics and clinical therapeutic efficacy [1, 4]. The complexities surrounding patients who have fungal disease are well known and undoubtedly contribute to outcomes independent of antifungal pharmacodynamics. The most important confounding host variable is underlying host immune deficiency, which has been shown to be extremely important in influencing patient survival. Despite this limitation, there are several data sets that allow one to consider the relationship between antifungal dose, organism MIC, and clinical outcome [19, 20, 23, 25, 66].

For fluconazole there have been numerous large clinical studies that have provided sufficient data on drug dose, MIC, and outcomes for pharmacodynamic analysis. The earliest and largest (more than 1,000 patients) of these data sets emanated from studies of oropharyngeal candidiasis [20]. Analysis demonstrated that treatment efficacy was maximal with fluconazole exposures relative to the MIC of the infecting *Candida* species near a 24-h AUC/MIC value of 25, congruent with data from the in vivo models. In the largest single analysis, when the fluconazole dose/MIC (AUC/MIC) exceeded 25, clinical success was noted in 91–100% of patients. However, when AUC/MIC was less than 25, clinical failure was noted in 27–35% of patients.

A more contemporary analysis corroborates these findings showing a clinical efficacy of 92% with an AUC/MIC greater than 25, and 9% with values below 25 [23]. These results have been used in the development of in vitro susceptibility breakpoints for fluconazole and other triazoles by the Clinical Laboratory Standards Institute (CLSI). A similar analysis using the European Committee on Antimicrobial Susceptibility Testing (EUCAST) susceptibility method resulted in a twofold higher MIC breakpoint [23]. This difference is due in part to the lower MIC values that are observed using the EUCAST susceptibility media.

A number of data sets from studies of candidemia have allowed similar pharmacodynamic investigation. There is now detailed information on fluconazole pharmacodynamics for more than 600 episodes of candidemia [19, 20, 24, 67, 68]. These data have identified a remarkably similar triazole exposure–clinical response relationship, with both clinical efficacy and patient survival associated with a fluconazole 24-h AUC/MIC ranging from 25 to 50. For example, in study of nearly 90 episodes of candidemia, CART analysis of dose and MIC found that the critical AUC/MIC value associated with patient survival (80% vs. 50%) was the 24-h AUC/MIC value of 25 [19].

A similar clinical analysis is now also available for voriconazole [66]. The dataset includes 1,681 isolates of 16 different *Candida* species from more than 400 subjects during six phase III clinical trials. Analysis demonstrated a strong relationship between MIC and outcome. If one estimates the free drug AUC for the voriconazole regimen used in these trials, the AUC/MIC can then be calculated using the geometric mean MIC for each of the species. Based on this analysis, therapeutic success was observed in 72–85% of cases with 24-h AUC/MIC greater than 25, whereas when AUC/MIC was less than 25, clinical failures were noted in 45% of patients.

Unfortunately, to date there has not been a published dataset for aspergillosis that allows similar analysis. However, there have been several recent voriconazole therapeutic drug monitoring publications that do allow pharmacodynamic estimations for aspergillosis [52, 69–71]. Two studies observed clinical success and patient survival, respectively, with voriconazole serum trough concentrations ranging from 1 to 2 μg/mL for these patients with invasive aspergillosis. If one considers the free drug AUC associated with these trough concentrations and the MIC90 for voriconazole and Aspergillus, the resulting 24-h AUC/MIC value is near 25.

A similar concentration/outcome relationship has also been recently reported for the triazole posaconazole in patients with invasive aspergillosis [72]. In 67 patients with invasive aspergillosis and serum concentration monitoring, the posaconazole average concentration at steady state ranged from 0.13 to 1.25 μg/mL. Maximal clinical response (75%) was observed in the cohort with the highest posaconazole concentration (1.25 μg/mL), while the least successful group (24% success) were found to have the lowest posaconazole serum levels.

Thus, one can use drug monitoring information to examine efficacy from the pharmacodynamic standpoint. It will be critical to include therapeutic drug monitoring in future studies and to include MIC testing when an organism is available.

Echinocandins

Impact of Antifungal Concentration on Activity over Time

Numerous in vitro and in vivo studies with compounds from the echinocandin drug class have been undertaken using *Candida* models [10, 73–81]. Results from these investigations have been consistent. Each of the agents have exhibited pronounced concentration-dependent killing effects and prolonged PAFEs. In vitro time course studies with each of the available echinocandin drugs have demonstrated concentration-dependent killing and prolonged PAFEs similar to those observed with the polyenes. Ernst et al. found that the extent of caspofungin killing of *C. albicans* varied more than 10,000-fold over only a 16-fold rise in concentrations [6]. Over this same range of drug concentrations the investigators observed an increase in the rate of killing and suppression of regrowth that exceeded the 12-h period of study.

Several in vivo studies have confirmed these pharmacodynamic characteristics [10, 74–80]. For example, following single escalating doses of the new echinocandin, aminocandin, marked killing of *C. albicans* was observed when drug levels in serum were more than four times the MIC. The extent of killing increased as concentrations relative to the MIC approached a factor of 10. However, there are a number of reports detailing a concentration-effect ceiling, above which reduced activity is observed. This phenomenon is termed the paradoxical effect [82–85]. Mechanistic evaluation has identified elevated chitin concentrations in strains surviving very high echinocandin concentrations. These findings appear to be strain dependent and occur at concentrations far above those that would occur in patients with current clinical regimens. The clinical relevance of this phenomenon remains unclear.

Impact of Dosing Interval Variation or Fractionation

The earliest dose fractionation studies with the first echinocandin derivative, cilofungin, also demonstrated enhanced efficacy by maximizing serum and tissue concentrations [86]. Subsequent investigations in vivo with newer derivatives against *Candida* species and *A. fumigatus* found that efficacy was maximized by providing large, infrequently administered doses [10, 73, 75, 87]. The total amount of drug necessary to achieve various microbiologic end points over the treatment period was 4.8–7.6-fold smaller when the dosing schedule called for large single doses than when the same amount of total drug was administered in two to six doses. The concentration-dependent killing pattern and results from dose fractionation studies would suggest that either the Cmax/MIC or AUC/MIC would best represent the driving pharmacodynamic index. In vivo studies using serum kinetics suggest that the Cmax/MIC is a better predictor of efficacy. These pharmacodynamic studies with these compounds utilized serum pharmacokinetics.

Recent studies have examined the impact of tissue concentrations at the site of infection. The dose–response relationships were similar in these investigations and support a dosing strategy that involves administration of large doses given infrequently. A recent clinical study with micafungin explored this dosing strategy in an esophageal candidiasis trial [88]. The two micafungin dosing regimens examined included the standard regimen of 150 mg given daily in comparison to a regimen of 300 mg every other day. The total drug exposure or AUC would be similar for the two regimens. Interestingly, clinical and microbiologic efficacy was similar for both regimens, consistent with results from the preclinical models. It will be interesting to see if additional lengthening of the dosing interval can be explored in clinical trials. In animal models studies, the dosing interval has been successfully lengthened to every 7 days while maintaining efficacy [10, 75, 76]. A similar approach has also been undertaken with caspofungin in an in vivo model of aspergillosis [87]. In these dose fractionation studies as well, outcome was optimal with regimens that maximized the drug exposure. Studies in this aspergillosis model further support the contention that antifungal pharmacodynamic relationships for a drug class are similar among fungal organisms.

Pharmacodynamic Target

Recent studies have begun to explore the magnitude of the Cmax/MIC and AUC/MIC indices needed for treatment efficacy. Experiments with anidulafungin against five *C. albicans* isolates demonstrated similar exposure-response relationships when expressed as either the 24-h AUC/MIC or Cmax/MIC indices [10]. The pharmacodynamic target associated with achievement of a static end point corresponded to an anidulafungin-free drug (non-protein bound), 24 h AUC/MIC from 10 to 20. The Cmax/MIC needed to produce this degree of treatment success was a value near 1. Experiments with micafungin and caspofungin with this same group of organisms identified very similar AUC/MIC targets [75]. This compilation of data again supports the premise that the pharmacodynamic target is similar for compounds within a drug class when protein binding is taken into account.

Additional studies were undertaken with groups of organisms from the *C. glabrata* and *C. parapsilosis* species [89]. Susceptibility studies for these two groups demonstrated higher MICs than the *C. albicans* group. One unexpected finding was observed from the in vivo treatment studies. The AUC/MIC pharmacodynamic target for echinocandins against these two *Candida* species was two- to threefold lower than for *C. albicans*.

The approved steady-state regimens for treating invasive candidiasis with these drugs includes 100 mg/day of both anidulafungin and micafungin and 50 mg/day of caspofungin. These regimens produce total and free drug 24-h AUC values in healthy volunteers of 112 mg·h/mL and 1.12 mg·h/mL for anidulafungin, 98 mg·h/mL and 2.94 mg·h/mL for caspofungin, and 126 mg·h/mL and 0.38 mg·h/mL for micafungin. If one considers the pharmacokinetics of the echinocandins and the presented pharmacodynamic targets, the highest MICs for the three *Candida* species that would allow the pharmacodynamic free drug 24-h AUC/MIC (fAUC/MIC) to be met can be estimated. The MIC ceiling based on fAUC/MIC ranging from 5 to 20 would place the susceptibility breakpoint lower than the current CLSI value of 2 μg/mL for each of the drugs. However, the MICs for nearly all of the wild-type strains from surveillance studies would be expected to fall within the "pharmacodynamically susceptible" category based upon the fAUC/MIC targets reported in this study, with the exception of a subset of *C. parapsilosis* isolates.

Pharmacodynamic target investigation against other fungal species has been limited. A single study examined the caspofungin target against a strain of *A. fumigatus* in a murine pulmonary model [87]. Interestingly the caspofungin exposure associated with maximal reduction in organism burden based upon RT-PCR end points was quite similar to that described for efficacy against *C. albicans*.

Clinical Relevance

Most clinical studies with echinocandins have not been extensively examined from the pharmacodynamic standpoint. However, a recent evaluation of three micafungin candidemia trials provided the opportunity to explore the relationship among pharmacokinetics, MIC, and treatment outcome [90]. The dataset included pharmacokinetics from patients with candidemia and outcome in 507 patients. Successful outcome in the entire population was observed with a total drug AUC/MIC greater than 3,000 (success in 98% with AUC/MIC > 3,000 and 84% < 3,000). If one considers the degree of protein binding for micafungin (>99%), the value of 3,000 would be similar to that observed for *C. albicans* in animal model studies. Since the infection model investigations had demonstrated differences among the *Candida* species, subgroup analysis examined the impact of infecting species as well. Interestingly, the AUC/MIC target of patients infected with *C. parapsilosis* was tenfold lower than for the remaining cohort. This difference was even larger than that observed in the animal model experiments. The findings from both the animal model studies and these clinical studies suggest a re-evaluation of current echinocandin susceptibility breakpoints and the consideration of these values at the level of the fungal species.

Combination Therapy

Patient outcomes associated with invasive fungal infections remain less than acceptable. It has been theorized that the combination of two or more antifungal compounds with different mechanisms of action could improve efficacy. The success of the combination of AmB and 5FC for cryptococcal meningitis serves as a critical proof of principle [91]. Numerous in vitro and in vivo infection models have been used to investigate various combinations against *Candida* and *Aspergillus* [57, 92–116]. Combination antifungal therapy continues to be an area of high interest and active investigation. As of 2008 there were >60 in vitro studies, >50 in vivo animal model studies, and >20 case reports or small single-center trials in humans evaluating combination therapy for A*spergillus* infection. The results have been variable, ranging from reduced effects to enhanced effects.

Prior study of antibacterial combinations has demonstrated that consideration of pharmacodynamics can help to decipher these often complex relationships. Even if two drugs together can enhance outcome, it is possible or even likely that this positive interaction is not evident at all drug concentration combinations. Recent in vitro antifungal combination studies using pharmacodynamic analysis have shown this to be the case. Examination of a wide variety of concentration combinations in these studies provides a means to determine not only if drug A and drug B interact in a helpful way, but they allow estimation of the optimal concentrations of each compound. In vivo pharmacodynamic studies should be useful to design clinical trials investigating antifungal drug combination therapy.

An area of intense interest is combination therapy with an echinocandin and a triazole antifungal for *Aspergillus* infections. Numerous in vitro and in vivo studies have examined the impact of this combination. The interpretation of the efficacy data from these investigations have varied from suggesting an enhanced interaction to antagonism. Drug exposure from the standpoint of dose level has been considered in several of these studies. However, extensive pharmacokinetic and pharmacodynamic design and analysis remain, for the most part, unexplored in the area of antifungal combination. The analyses from a few studies suggest the importance of this additional level of investigation. For example, in a study of the combination of caspofungin and voriconazole, the impact of the interaction was dependent upon the dose of the echinocandin; there was enhanced activity with some dosages, but reduced activity with others [117]. Among the unanswered antifungal pharmacodynamic questions, detailed examination of combination therapy is among the most important.

References

1. Craig WA. Pharmacokinetic/pharmacodynamic parameters: rationale for antibacterial dosing of mice and men. Clin Infect Dis. 1998;26:1–10.
2. Andes D. Pharmacokinetics and pharmacodynamics of antifungals. Infect Dis Clin North Am. 2006;20:679–97.
3. Andes D. Clinical utility of antifungal pharmacokinetics and pharmacodynamics. Curr Opin Infect Dis. 2004;17:533–40.
4. Ambrose PG, Bhavnani SM, Rubino CM, et al. Pharmacokinetics-pharmacodynamics of antimicrobial therapy: it's not just for mice anymore. Clin Infect Dis. 2007;44:79–86.
5. Lewis RE, Wiederhold NP, Klepser ME. In vitro pharmacodynamics of amphotericin B, itraconazole, and voriconazole against *Aspergillus*, *Fusarium*, and *Scedosporium* spp. Antimicrob Agents Chemother. 2005;49:945–51.
6. Ernst EJ, Klepser ME, Ernst ME, Messer SA, Pfaller MA. In vitro pharmacodynamic properties of MK-0991 determined by time-kill methods. Diagn Microbiol Infect Dis. 1999;33:75–80.
7. Ernst EJ, Klepser ME, Pfaller MA. Postantifungal effects of echinocandin, azole, and polyene antifungal agents against *Candida albicans* and *Cryptococcus neoformans*. Antimicrob Agents Chemother. 2000;44:1108–11.

8. Ernst EJ, Roling EE, Petzold CR, Keele DJ, Klepser ME. In vitro activity of micafungin (FK-463) against *Candida* spp.: microdilution, time-kill, and postantifungal-effect studies. Antimicrob Agents Chemother. 2002;46:3846–53.
9. Andes D. Use of an animal model of disseminated candidiasis in the evaluation of antifungal therapy. Methods Mol Med. 2005; 118:111–28.
10. Andes D, Diekema DJ, Pfaller MA, et al. In vivo pharmacodynamic characterization of anidulafungin in a neutropenic murine candidiasis model. Antimicrob Agents Chemother. 2008;52:539–50.
11. Andes D, Marchillo K, Conklin R, et al. Pharmacodynamics of a new triazole, posaconazole, in a murine model of disseminated candidiasis. Antimicrob Agents Chemother. 2004;48:137–42.
12. Andes D, Marchillo K, Stamstad T, Conklin R. In vivo pharmacokinetics and pharmacodynamics of a new triazole, voriconazole, in a murine candidiasis model. Antimicrob Agents Chemother. 2003;47:3165–9.
13. Andes D, Safdar N, Marchillo K, Conklin R. Pharmacokinetic-pharmacodynamic comparison of amphotericin B (AMB) and two lipid-associated AMB preparations, liposomal AMB and AMB lipid complex, in murine candidiasis models. Antimicrob Agents Chemother. 2006;50:674–84.
14. Andes D, Stamsted T, Conklin R. Pharmacodynamics of amphotericin B in a neutropenic-mouse disseminated-candidiasis model. Antimicrob Agents Chemother. 2001;45:922–6.
15. Andes D, van Ogtrop M. Characterization and quantitation of the pharmacodynamics of fluconazole in a neutropenic murine disseminated candidiasis infection model. Antimicrob Agents Chemother. 1999;43:2116–20.
16. Andes D, van Ogtrop M. In vivo characterization of the pharmacodynamics of flucytosine in a neutropenic murine disseminated candidiasis model. Antimicrob Agents Chemother. 2000;44: 938–42.
17. Lewis RE, Klepser ME, Pfaller MA. In vitro pharmacodynamic characteristics of flucytosine determined by time-kill methods. Diagn Microbiol Infect Dis. 2000;36:101–5.
18. Ernst EJ, Yodoi K, Roling EE, Klepser ME. Rates and extents of antifungal activities of amphotericin B, flucytosine, fluconazole, and voriconazole against *Candida lusitaniae* determined by microdilution, Etest, and time-kill methods. Antimicrob Agents Chemother. 2002;46:578–81.
19. Baddley JW, Patel M, Bhavnani SM, Moser SA, Andes DR. Association of fluconazole pharmacodynamics with mortality in patients with candidemia. Antimicrob Agents Chemother. 2008;52:3022–8.
20. Rex JH, Pfaller MA, Galgiani JN, et al. Development of interpretive breakpoints for antifungal susceptibility testing: conceptual framework and analysis of in vitro-in vivo correlation data for fluconazole, itraconazole, and candida infections. Subcommittee on Antifungal Susceptibility Testing of the National Committee for Clinical Laboratory Standards. Clin Infect Dis. 1997;24: 235–47.
21. Pfaller MA, Diekema DJ, Ostrosky-Zeichner L, et al. Correlation of MIC with outcome for *Candida* species tested against caspofungin, anidulafungin, and micafungin: analysis and proposal for interpretive MIC breakpoints. J Clin Microbiol. 2008;46:2620–9.
22. Cuesta I, Bielza C, Larranaga P, et al. Data mining validation of fluconazole breakpoints established by the European Committee on Antimicrobial Susceptibility Testing. Antimicrob Agents Chemother. 2009;53:2949–54.
23. Rodriguez-Tudela JL, Almirante B, Rodriguez-Pardo D, et al. Correlation of the MIC and dose/MIC ratio of fluconazole to the therapeutic response of patients with mucosal candidiasis and candidemia. Antimicrob Agents Chemother. 2007; 51:3599–604.
24. Clancy CJ, Yu VL, Morris AJ, Snydman DR, Nguyen MH. Fluconazole MIC and the fluconazole dose/MIC ratio correlate with therapeutic response among patients with candidemia. Antimicrob Agents Chemother. 2005;49:3171–7.
25. Pai MP, Turpin RS, Garey KW. Association of fluconazole area under the concentration-time curve/MIC and dose/MIC ratios with mortality in nonneutropenic patients with candidemia. Antimicrob Agents Chemother. 2007;51:35–9.
26. Kethireddy S, Andes D. CNS pharmacokinetics of antifungal agents. Expert Opin Drug Metab Toxicol. 2007;3:573–81.
27. Groll AH, Giri N, Petraitis V, et al. Comparative efficacy and distribution of lipid formulations of amphotericin B in experimental *Candida albicans* infection of the central nervous system. J Infect Dis. 2000;182:274–82.
28. Kunin CM. Protein binding of antibiotics does affect their antistaphyloccal activity. J Antimicrob Chemother. 1986;17:263.
29. Craig WA, Kunin CM. Significance of serum protein and tissue binding of antimicrobial agents. Annu Rev Med. 1976;27:287–300.
30. Andes D, Marchillo K, Stamstad T, Conklin R. In vivo pharmacodynamics of a new triazole, ravuconazole, in a murine candidiasis model. Antimicrob Agents Chemother. 2003;47:1193–9.
31. Vogelman B, Gudmundsson S, Turnidge J, Leggett J, Craig WA. In vivo postantibiotic effect in a thigh infection in neutropenic mice. J Infect Dis. 1988;157:287–98.
32. Turnidge JD, Gudmundsson S, Vogelman B, Craig WA. The post-antibiotic effect of antifungal agents against common pathogenic yeasts. J Antimicrob Chemother. 1994;34:83–92.
33. Klepser ME, Wolfe EJ, Jones RN, Nightingale CH, Pfaller MA. Antifungal pharmacodynamic characteristics of fluconazole and amphotericin B tested against *Candida albicans*. Antimicrob Agents Chemother. 1997;41:1392–5.
34. Denning DW, Warn P. Dose range evaluation of liposomal nystatin and comparisons with amphotericin B and amphotericin B lipid complex in temporarily neutropenic mice infected with an isolate of *Aspergillus fumigatus* with reduced susceptibility to amphotericin B. Antimicrob Agents Chemother. 1999;43:2592–9.
35. Gavalda J, Martin T, Lopez P, et al. Efficacy of high loading doses of liposomal amphotericin B in the treatment of experimental invasive pulmonary aspergillosis. Clin Microbiol Infect. 2005;11:999–1004.
36. Vitale RG, Meis JF, Mouton JW, Verweij PE. Evaluation of the post-antifungal effect (PAFE) of amphotericin B and nystatin against 30 zygomycetes using two different media. J Antimicrob Chemother. 2003;52:65–70.
37. Warn PA, Morrissey J, Moore CB, Denning DW. In vivo activity of amphotericin B lipid complex in immunocompromised mice against fluconazole-resistant or fluconazole-susceptible *Candida tropicalis*. Antimicrob Agents Chemother. 2000;44:2664–71.
38. Wiederhold NP, Tam VH, Chi J, Prince RA, Kontoyiannis DP, Lewis RE. Pharmacodynamic activity of amphotericin B deoxycholate is associated with peak plasma concentrations in a neutropenic murine model of invasive pulmonary aspergillosis. Antimicrob Agents Chemother. 2006;50:469–73.
39. Adler-Moore JP, Proffitt RT. Amphotericin B lipid preparations: what are the differences? Clin Microbiol Infect. 2008;14 Suppl 4:25–36.
40. Groll AH, Lyman CA, Petraitis V, et al. Compartmentalized intrapulmonary pharmacokinetics of amphotericin B and its lipid formulations. Antimicrob Agents Chemother. 2006;50:3418–23.
41. Lewis RE, Liao G, Hou J, Chamilos G, Prince RA, Kontoyiannis DP. Comparative analysis of amphotericin B lipid complex and liposomal amphotericin B kinetics of lung accumulation and fungal clearance in a murine model of acute invasive pulmonary aspergillosis. Antimicrob Agents Chemother. 2007;51:1253–8.

42. Baddley JW, Marr KA, Andes DR, et al. Patterns of susceptibility of Aspergillus isolates recovered from patients enrolled in the Transplant-Associated Infection Surveillance Network. J Clin Microbiol. 2009;47:3271–5.
43. Park BJ, Arthington-Skaggs BA, Hajjeh RA, et al. Evaluation of amphotericin B interpretive breakpoints for Candida bloodstream isolates by correlation with therapeutic outcome. Antimicrob Agents Chemother. 2006;50:1287–92.
44. Hong Y, Shaw PJ, Nath CE, et al. Population pharmacokinetics of liposomal amphotericin B in pediatric patients with malignant diseases. Antimicrob Agents Chemother. 2006;50:935–42.
45. Cornely OA, Maertens J, Bresnik M, et al. Liposomal amphotericin B as initial therapy for invasive mold infection: a randomized trial comparing a high-loading dose regimen with standard dosing (AmBiLoad trial). Clin Infect Dis. 2007;44:1289–97.
46. Eriksson U, Seifert B, Schaffner A. Comparison of effects of amphotericin B deoxycholate infused over 4 or 24 hours: randomised controlled trial. BMJ. 2001;322:579–82.
47. Hall P, Kennedy G, Morton J, Hill GR, Durrant S. Twenty-four hour continuous infusion of amphotericin B for the treatment of suspected or proven fungal infection in haematology patients. Intern Med J. 2005;35:374.
48. Imhof A, Walter RB, Schaffner A. Continuous infusion of escalated doses of amphotericin B deoxycholate: an open-label observational study. Clin Infect Dis. 2003;36:943–51.
49. Peleg AY, Woods ML. Continuous and 4 h infusion of amphotericin B: a comparative study involving high-risk haematology patients. J Antimicrob Chemother. 2004;54:803–8.
50. Hope WW, Warn PA, Sharp A, et al. Derivation of an in vivo drug exposure breakpoint for flucytosine against *Candida albicans* and Impact of the MIC, growth rate, and resistance genotype on the antifungal effect. Antimicrob Agents Chemother. 2006; 50:3680–8.
51. Kauffman CA, Frame PT. Bone marrow toxicity associated with 5-fluorocytosine therapy. Antimicrob Agents Chemother. 1977;11:244–7.
52. Smith J, Andes D. Therapeutic drug monitoring of antifungals: pharmacokinetic and pharmacodynamic considerations. Ther Drug Monit. 2008;30:167–72.
53. Francis P, Walsh TJ. Evolving role of flucytosine in immunocompromised patients: new insights into safety, pharmacokinetics, and antifungal therapy. Clin Infect Dis. 1992;15:1003–18.
54. Stamm AM, Diasio RB, Dismukes WE, et al. Toxicity of amphotericin B plus flucytosine in 194 patients with cryptococcal meningitis. Am J Med. 1987;83:236–42.
55. Pasqualotto AC, Howard SJ, Moore CB, Denning DW. Flucytosine therapeutic monitoring: 15 years experience from the UK. J Antimicrob Chemother. 2007;59:791–3.
56. Andes D, Forrest A, Lepak A, Nett J, Marchillo K, Lincoln L. Impact of antimicrobial dosing regimen on evolution of drug resistance in vivo: fluconazole and *Candida albicans*. Antimicrob Agents Chemother. 2006;50:2374–83.
57. Ernst EJ, Klepser ME, Pfaller MA. In vitro interaction of fluconazole and amphotericin B administered sequentially against *Candida albicans*: effect of concentration and exposure time. Diagn Microbiol Infect Dis. 1998;32:205–10.
58. Warn PA, Sharp A, Parmar A, Majithiya J, Denning DW, Hope WW. Pharmacokinetics and pharmacodynamics of a novel triazole, isavuconazole: mathematical modeling, importance of tissue concentrations, and impact of immune status on antifungal effect. Antimicrob Agents Chemother. 2009;53:3453–61.
59. Hope WW, Drusano GL, Moore CB, et al. Effect of neutropenia and treatment delay on the response to antifungal agents in experimental disseminated candidiasis. Antimicrob Agents Chemother. 2007;51:285–95.
60. Louie A, Drusano GL, Banerjee P, et al. Pharmacodynamics of fluconazole in a murine model of systemic candidiasis. Antimicrob Agents Chemother. 1998;42:1105–9.
61. Andes D, Lepak A, Nett J, Lincoln L, Marchillo K. In vivo fluconazole pharmacodynamics and resistance development in a previously susceptible *Candida albicans* population examined by microbiologic and transcriptional profiling. Antimicrob Agents Chemother. 2006;50:2384–94.
62. Bruggemann RJ, Mavridou E, Burger DM, Melchers WJG, Verweij P, Mouton JW. Pharmacokinetics/pharmacodynamics of posaconazole in a murine model of disseminated aspergillosis. In: 19th European Congress of Clinical Microbiology and Infectious Diseases (ECCMID), Helsinki, Finland, 16–19 May 2009.
63. Mavridou E, Mouton JW, Mellado E, Melchers WJG, Verweij P. Efficacy of voriconazole against three clinical *Aspergillus fumigatus* isolates with mutations in cyp51A gene. In: 19th European Congress of Clinical Microbiology and Infectious Diseases (ECCMID), Helsinki, Finland, 16–19 May 2009.
64. Rogers TE, Galgiani JN. Activity of fluconazole (UK 49, 858) and ketoconazole against *Candida albicans* in vitro and in vivo. Antimicrob Agents Chemother. 1986;30:418–22.
65. Van t Wout JW, Mattie H, van Furth R. Comparison of the efficacies of amphotericin B, fluconazole, and itraconazole against a systemic *Candida albicans* infection in normal and neutropenic mice. Antimicrob Agents Chemother. 1989;33:147–51.
66. Pfaller MA, Diekema DJ, Rex JH, et al. Correlation of MIC with outcome for Candida species tested against voriconazole: analysis and proposal for interpretive breakpoints. J Clin Microbiol. 2006;44:819–26.
67. Takakura S, Fujihara N, Saito T, Kudo T, Iinuma Y, Ichiyama S. Clinical factors associated with fluconazole resistance and short-term survival in patients with Candida bloodstream infection. Eur J Clin Microbiol Infect Dis. 2004;23:380–8.
68. Lee SC, Fung CP, Huang JS, et al. Clinical correlates of antifungal macrodilution susceptibility test results for non-AIDS patients with severe Candida infections treated with fluconazole. Antimicrob Agents Chemother. 2000;44:2715–8.
69. Andes D, Pascual A, Marchetti O. Antifungal therapeutic drug monitoring: established and emerging indications. Antimicrob Agents Chemother. 2009;53:24–34.
70. Smith J, Safdar N, Knasinski V, et al. Voriconazole therapeutic drug monitoring. Antimicrob Agents Chemother. 2006;50:1570–2.
71. Pascual A, Calandra T, Bolay S, Buclin T, Bille J, Marchetti O. Voriconazole therapeutic drug monitoring in patients with invasive mycoses improves efficacy and safety outcomes. Clin Infect Dis. 2008;46:201–11.
72. Walsh TJ, Raad I, Patterson TF, et al. Treatment of invasive aspergillosis with posaconazole in patients who are refractory to or intolerant of conventional therapy: an externally controlled trial. Clin Infect Dis. 2007;44:2–12.
73. Andes D, Marchillo K, Lowther J, Bryskier A, Stamstad T, Conklin R. In vivo pharmacodynamics of HMR 3270, a glucan synthase inhibitor, in a murine candidiasis model. Antimicrob Agents Chemother. 2003;47:1187–92.
74. Andes D, Safdar N. Efficacy of micafungin for the treatment of candidemia. Eur J Clin Microbiol Infect Dis. 2005;24:662–4.
75. Andes DR, Diekema DJ, Pfaller MA, Marchillo K, Bohrmueller J. In vivo pharmacodynamic target investigation for micafungin against *Candida albicans* and *C. glabrata* in a neutropenic murine candidiasis model. Antimicrob Agents Chemother. 2008;52:3497–503.
76. Gumbo T, Drusano GL, Liu W, et al. Once-weekly micafungin therapy is as effective as daily therapy for disseminated candidiasis in mice with persistent neutropenia. Antimicrob Agents Chemother. 2007;51:968–74.

77. Gumbo T, Drusano GL, Liu W, et al. Anidulafungin pharmacokinetics and microbial response in neutropenic mice with disseminated candidiasis. Antimicrob Agents Chemother. 2006;50:3695–700.
78. Groll AH, Mickiene D, Petraitiene R, et al. Pharmacokinetic and pharmacodynamic modeling of anidulafungin (LY303366): reappraisal of its efficacy in neutropenic animal models of opportunistic mycoses using optimal plasma sampling. Antimicrob Agents Chemother. 2001;45:2845–55.
79. Groll AH, Mickiene D, Petraitis V, et al. Compartmental pharmacokinetics and tissue distribution of the antifungal echinocandin lipopeptide micafungin (FK463) in rabbits. Antimicrob Agents Chemother. 2001;45:3322–7.
80. Hope WW, Mickiene D, Petraitis V, et al. The pharmacokinetics and pharmacodynamics of micafungin in experimental hematogenous Candida meningoencephalitis: implications for echinocandin therapy in neonates. J Infect Dis. 2008;197:163–71.
81. Clancy CJ, Huang H, Cheng S, Derendorf H, Nguyen MH. Characterizing the effects of caspofungin on *Candida albicans*, *Candida parapsilosis*, and *Candida glabrata* isolates by simultaneous time-kill and postantifungal-effect experiments. Antimicrob Agents Chemother. 2006;50:2569–72.
82. Clemons KV, Espiritu M, Parmar R, Stevens DA. Assessment of the paradoxical effect of caspofungin in therapy of candidiasis. Antimicrob Agents Chemother. 2006;50:1293–7.
83. Lewis RE, Albert ND, Kontoyiannis DP. Comparison of the dose-dependent activity and paradoxical effect of caspofungin and micafungin in a neutropenic murine model of invasive pulmonary aspergillosis. J Antimicrob Chemother. 2008;61:1140–4.
84. Stevens DA, Ichinomiya M, Koshi Y, Horiuchi H. Escape of Candida from caspofungin inhibition at concentrations above the MIC (paradoxical effect) accomplished by increased cell wall chitin; evidence for beta-1, 6-glucan synthesis inhibition by caspofungin. Antimicrob Agents Chemother. 2006;50:3160–1.
85. Stevens DA, White TC, Perlin DS, Selitrennikoff CP. Studies of the paradoxical effect of caspofungin at high drug concentrations. Diagn Microbiol Infect Dis. 2005;51:173–8.
86. Walsh TJ, Lee JW, Kelly P, et al. Antifungal effects of the nonlinear pharmacokinetics of cilofungin, a 1, 3-beta-glucan synthetase inhibitor, during continuous and intermittent intravenous infusions in treatment of experimental disseminated candidiasis. Antimicrob Agents Chemother. 1991;35:1321–8.
87. Wiederhold NP, Kontoyiannis DP, Chi J, Prince RA, Tam VH, Lewis RE. Pharmacodynamics of caspofungin in a murine model of invasive pulmonary aspergillosis: evidence of concentration-dependent activity. J Infect Dis. 2004;190:1464–71.
88. Buell D, Kovanda L, Drake T, Fisco C. Alternative day dosing of micafungin in the treatment of esophageal candidiasis. In: 45th Interscience Conference on Antimicrobial Agents and Chemotherapy, Washington, DC, 2005.
89. Andes D, Diekema DJ, Lepak A, Pfaller M, Marchillo K, Bohrmuller J. Identification of the in vivo pharmacodynamic (pd) target for echinocandins against *C. albicans* (CA), *C. glabrata* (CG), and *C. parapsilosis* (CP) in the neutropenic murine disseminated candidiasis model. In: Interscience Conference on Antimicrobial Agents and Chemotherapy, San Francisco, CA, 2009.
90. Andes D, Ambrose PG, Hammel JP, et al. Exposure-response relationships for efficacy of micafungin in patients with invasive candidiasis. In: 49th Interscience Conference on Antimicrobial Agents and Chemotherapy, San Francisco, CA, 2009.
91. Perfect JR, Dismukes WE, Dromer F, et al. Clinical practice guidelines for the management of cryptococcal disease: 2010 update by the Infectious Diseases Society of America. Clin Infect Dis. 2010;50:291–322.
92. Arikan S, Lozano-Chiu M, Paetznick V, Rex JH. In vitro synergy of caspofungin and amphotericin B against *Aspergillus* and *Fusarium* spp. Antimicrob Agents Chemother. 2002;46:245–7.
93. Chaturvedi V, Ramani R, Ghannoum MA, et al. Multilaboratory testing of antifungal combinations against a quality control isolate of *Candida krusei*. Antimicrob Agents Chemother. 2008;52:1500–2.
94. Clemons KV, Espiritu M, Parmar R, Stevens DA. Comparative efficacies of conventional amphotericin b, liposomal amphotericin B (AmBisome), caspofungin, micafungin, and voriconazole alone and in combination against experimental murine central nervous system aspergillosis. Antimicrob Agents Chemother. 2005;49:4867–75.
95. Clemons KV, Stevens DA. Efficacy of micafungin alone or in combination against experimental pulmonary aspergillosis. Med Mycol. 2006;44:69–73.
96. Clemons KV, Stevens DA. Animal models testing monotherapy versus combination antifungal therapy: lessons learned and future directions. Curr Opin Infect Dis. 2006;19:360–4.
97. Demchok JP, Meletiadis J, Roilides E, Walsh TJ. Comparative pharmacodynamic interaction analysis of triple combinations of caspofungin and voriconazole or ravuconazole with subinhibitory concentrations of amphotericin B against *Aspergillus* spp. Mycoses. 2009;53:239–45.
98. Johnson MD, MacDougall C, Ostrosky-Zeichner L, Perfect JR, Rex JH. Combination antifungal therapy. Antimicrob Agents Chemother. 2004;48:693–715.
99. Hope WW, Warn PA, Sharp A, et al. Surface response modeling to examine the combination of amphotericin B deoxycholate and 5-fluorocytosine for treatment of invasive candidiasis. J Infect Dis. 2005;192:673–80.
100. Hope WW, Warn PA, Sharp A, et al. Optimization of the dosage of flucytosine in combination with amphotericin B for disseminated candidiasis: a pharmacodynamic rationale for reduced dosing. Antimicrob Agents Chemother. 2007;51:3760–2.
101. Kirkpatrick WR, Perea S, Coco BJ, Patterson TF. Efficacy of caspofungin alone and in combination with voriconazole in a Guinea pig model of invasive aspergillosis. Antimicrob Agents Chemother. 2002;46:2564–8.
102. Kontoyiannis DP, Hachem R, Lewis RE, et al. Efficacy and toxicity of caspofungin in combination with liposomal amphotericin B as primary or salvage treatment of invasive aspergillosis in patients with hematologic malignancies. Cancer. 2003;98:292–9.
103. Lewis RE, Diekema DJ, Messer SA, Pfaller MA, Klepser ME. Comparison of Etest, chequerboard dilution and time-kill studies for the detection of synergy or antagonism between antifungal agents tested against Candida species. J Antimicrob Chemother. 2002;49:345–51.
104. Lewis RE, Kontoyiannis DP. Micafungin in combination with voriconazole in Aspergillus species: a pharmacodynamic approach for detection of combined antifungal activity in vitro. J Antimicrob Chemother. 2005;56:887–92.
105. Lewis RE, Lund BC, Klepser ME, Ernst EJ, Pfaller MA. Assessment of antifungal activities of fluconazole and amphotericin B administered alone and in combination against *Candida albicans* by using a dynamic in vitro mycotic infection model. Antimicrob Agents Chemother. 1998;42:1382–6.
106. Louie A, Banerjee P, Drusano GL, Shayegani M, Miller MH. Interaction between fluconazole and amphotericin B in mice with systemic infection due to fluconazole-susceptible or -resistant strains of *Candida albicans*. Antimicrob Agents Chemother. 1999;43:2841–7.
107. Louie A, Liu W, Miller DA, et al. Efficacies of high-dose fluconazole plus amphotericin B and high-dose fluconazole plus 5-fluorocytosine versus amphotericin B, fluconazole, and 5-fluorocytosine monotherapies in treatment of experimental endocarditis, endophthalmitis, and pyelonephritis due to *Candida albicans*. Antimicrob Agents Chemother. 1999;43: 2831–40.

108. Marr KA, Boeckh M, Carter RA, Kim HW, Corey L. Combination antifungal therapy for invasive aspergillosis. Clin Infect Dis. 2004;39:797–802.
109. Meletiadis J, Mouton JW, Meis JF, Verweij PE. In vitro drug interaction modeling of combinations of azoles with terbinafine against clinical *Scedosporium prolificans* isolates. Antimicrob Agents Chemother. 2003;47:106–17.
110. Meletiadis J, Mouton JW, Meis JF, Verweij PE. Combination chemotherapy for the treatment of invasive infections by *Scedosporium prolificans*. Clin Microbiol Infect. 2000;6:336–7.
111. Meletiadis J, Mouton JW, Rodriguez-Tudela JL, Meis JF, Verweij PE. In vitro interaction of terbinafine with itraconazole against clinical isolates of *Scedosporium prolificans*. Antimicrob Agents Chemother. 2000;44:470–2.
112. Meletiadis J, Verweij PE, TeDorsthorst DT, Meis JF, Mouton JW. Assessing in vitro combinations of antifungal drugs against yeasts and filamentous fungi: comparison of different drug interaction models. Med Mycol. 2005;43:133–52.
113. Ostrosky-Zeichner L. Combination antifungal therapy: a critical review of the evidence. Clin Microbiol Infect. 2008;14 Suppl 4:65–70.
114. Petraitis V, Petraitiene R, Hope WW, et al. Combination therapy in treatment of experimental pulmonary aspergillosis: in vitro and in vivo correlations of the concentration- and dose- dependent interactions between anidulafungin and voriconazole by Bliss independence drug interaction analysis. Antimicrob Agents Chemother. 2009;53:2382–91.
115. Petraitis V, Petraitiene R, Sarafandi AA, et al. Combination therapy in treatment of experimental pulmonary aspergillosis: synergistic interaction between an antifungal triazole and an echinocandin. J Infect Dis. 2003;187:1834–43.
116. Te Dorsthorst DT, Verweij PE, Meis JF, Punt NC, Mouton JW. In vitro interactions between amphotericin B, itraconazole, and flucytosine against 21 clinical Aspergillus isolates determined by two drug interaction models. Antimicrob Agents Chemother. 2004;48:2007–13.
117. Meletiadis J, Stergiopoulou T, O'Shaughnessy EM, Peter J, Walsh TJ. Concentration-dependent synergy and antagonism within a triple antifungal drug combination against Aspergillus species: analysis by a new response surface model. Antimicrob Agents Chemother. 2007;51:2053–64.

Resistance to Antifungal Drugs

Dominique Sanglard

Fungal infections caused by fungal pathogens are common in immunocompromised hosts. *Candida* spp. comprise the major yeast species recovered from infected individuals; however, other yeast species such as *Cryptococcus neoformans* might also be isolated. Among filamentous fungi causing infections in human, *Aspergillus fumigatus* has a dominant position, and this fungal species is linked to a high mortality [1]. Not only are a restricted number of antifungal agents available to treat these infections, but also resistance to antifungal treatment can occur. Table 1 summarizes the activity of known antifungal agents in several yeast species and *A. fumigatus*.

Antifungal activities are measured using standardized protocols that have been optimized during the past years. The CLSI (Clinical and Laboratory Standards Institute) and EUCAST (European Committee on Antimicrobial Susceptibility Testing) protocols have been published and each details methods for determining the activities of current antifungal agents. Both methods used liquid cultures in cell culture media (RPMI) and antifungal dilutions in the format of 96-well microtiter plates. Other methods have been reported using antifungal gradient strips on agar plates (E-test) or disk diffusion assays. The agreement in the establishment of minimal inhibitory concentration (MIC) values between both methods is over 90% and therefore considered acceptable [2].

Resistance to antifungal treatment can develop on the basis of either clinical or microbiological factors. A persistent infection despite treatment with an antifungal drug at maximal dosage may be described as clinically resistant to the therapeutic agent. The infecting organism may show normal susceptibility to the agent in vitro [3], or clinical resistance to treatment may result from microbial resistance to an agent. Clinical resistance is often the result of complex interactions between an antimicrobial agent and an infecting microbe in a human host. Microbiological resistance can be defined as a shift (a decrease) in antifungal drug susceptibility that can be measured in vitro by appropriate laboratory methods. Resistance to specific antifungal drugs is intrinsic in some yeast pathogens, but can also be acquired either in a transient or permanent manner. The distinction between a susceptible and a resistant fungal isolate can be made when a threshold drug susceptibility value, such as the breakpoint MIC, is reached. In medical practice, breakpoint values could ideally predict the success or the failure of an antifungal treatment. However, experience that has accumulated with different antifungal agents shows that this association cannot always be applied [3]. Table 2 gives breakpoint values established for the main categories of antifungal agents. In this table, an intermediate category is given, the susceptible-dose-dependent MIC (S-DD MIC). Yeasts in this category require higher dosages of the antifungal agent for inhibition. Between CLSI and EUCAST, the breakpoint recommendations vary considerably for two agents, fluconazole and voriconazole [4–6], as summarized in Table 2. These variations are attributed to differences between the two agencies in the patient populations that were analyzed and in a number of parameters related to the activity and pharmacodynamics of antifungal agents.

The breakpoint MIC value of a given fungal pathogen for a specific drug is less relevant for the microbiologist or the molecular biologist because only a modest shift of antifungal drug susceptibility measured by an increase in MIC values can be the consequence of one or several cellular alterations linked to modifications of the genetic material. This chapter will summarize the present situation of antifungal resistance in yeast pathogens and will detail the current understanding of these mechanisms as pertains to clinical situations.

Polyene Resistance

Polyenes belong to a class of natural antifungal compounds discovered in the early 1950s. One of the most successful polyene derivatives, amphotericin B (AmB), is produced by *Streptomyces nodosus* (Fig. 1). AmB can form soluble salts in both basic and acidic environments, is not orally or

D. Sanglard (✉)
Institute of Microbiology, University of Lausanne and University Hospital Center, Lausanne, Switzerland
e-mail: Dominique.sanglard@chuv.ch

C.A. Kauffman et al. (eds.), *Essentials of Clinical Mycology*,
DOI 10.1007/978-1-4419-6640-7_9, © Springer Science+Business Media, LLC 2011

Table 1 Activities of current and emerging antifungal agents against several fungal species

	MIC_{90}[a] (μg/mL)							
Antifungal agent	*C. albicans*	*C. glabrata*	*C. krusei*	*C. parapsilosis*	*C. tropicalis*	*C. neoformans*	*A. fumigatus*	References
Amphotericin B	0.5	1	0.5	0.5	0.5	1	4	[20, 139]
Flucytosine	4	0.5	16–32	1	4	16	>64	[20, 140]
Azoles								
–Fluconazole	1	64	64	2.0	2.0	16	>128	[141, 142]
–Itraconazole	0.25	4.0	2.0	0.5	0.5	1	0.125	[139, 143–146]
–Voriconazole	0.06	2.0	1.0	0.12	0.25	0.25	0.5	
–Posaconazole	0.06	4.0	0.5	0.12	0.25	<0.015	0.031	
–Ravuconazole	0.03	4.0	0.5	0.12	0.25	0.25	1	
Cyclic lipopeptides								
–Caspofungin	0.5	0.5	1	0.5	1	32	0.5 [b]	[147]
–Micafungin	0.0156	0.156	0.125	1	0.0313	>64	0.125 [b]	[148]
–Anidulafungin	0.125	0.5	0.25	4	0.125	>16	0.06 [b]	[149–154]

[a]MIC_{90} is defined as the MIC value to which 90% of a study population belongs

[b]Values are given in MEC (minimal effective concentration)

Table 2 CLSI and EUCAST interpretive breakpoints against *Candida albicans* (in μg/mL)

Antifungal agent	Susceptible	Dose-dependent Susceptible (S-DD) or Intermediate	Resistant
Fluconazole CLSI	≤8	16–32	≥64
Fluconazole EUCAST	≤2	4	>4
Itraconazole	≤0.125	0.25–0.5	≥1
Voriconazole CLSI	≤1	2	≥4
Voriconazole EUCAST	≤0.125	–	>0.125
Flucytosine	≤4	8–16	≥32

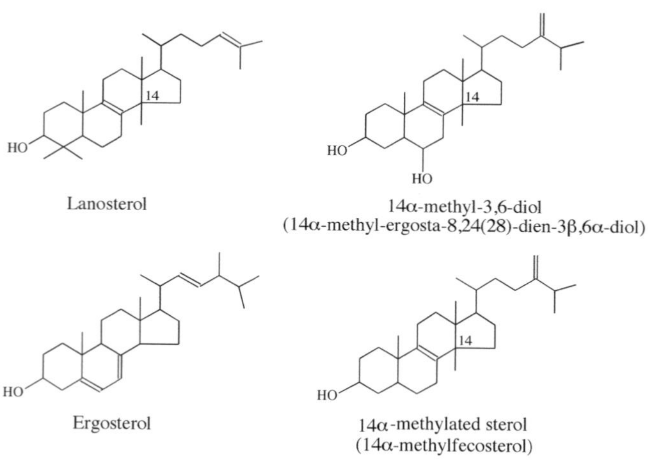

Fig. 1 Major sterol structures

intramuscularly absorbed, and is virtually insoluble in water. The primary mode of action of AmB is to bind ergosterol in the membrane bilayer of susceptible organisms. This interaction is thought to result in the production of aqueous pores consisting of polyene molecules linked to the membrane sterols. This configuration gives rise to a pore-like structure, leakage of vital cytoplasmic components (mono- or divalent cations), and death of the organism. AmB has a strong fungicidal effect on most important yeast pathogens. Time-kill curves have been reported in several studies and showed that AmB induces a 3–4 log decrease in viable counts in a time span of 2–4 h at supra-MIC concentrations.

AmB MICs are dependent on several factors, and among them, the composition of the testing medium is important. Rex et al. [7] recommend the use of a special broth medium (AM3) to determine AmB MICs in *Candida* species. Presently, a standard protocol using AM3 medium has been recommended by the CLSI in the protocol M27-A3. Recently, Peyron et al. [8] evaluated an agar diffusion method using an E-test strip with RPMI or AM3 medium in order to discriminate AmB-resistant from AmB-susceptible *Candida* isolates. AmB MIC_{90} values of various *Candida* species, including *C. albicans*, *C. glabrata*, *C. parapsilosis* and *C. tropicalis*, ranged from 0.25 to 1 μg/mL. AmB fungicidal concentrations are usually 0.5–2 times the MIC in *Candida* species.

Microbiological resistance to AmB can be intrinsic or acquired. Intrinsic resistance to AmB is common for some *C. lusitaniae* [9] and for *Trichosporon* species [10], but acquired resistance during antifungal treatment with AmB is rarely reported for yeast isolates. Some *C. lusitaniae* isolates in vitro are able to undergo rapid switches to AmB resistance when exposed to the drug. Acquired resistance to AmB is often associated with alteration of membrane lipids, especially sterols. Recently, *C. albicans* clinical isolates resistant to AmB were described that lacked ergosterol and accumulated other sterols (3β-ergosta-7,22-dienol and 3β-ergosta-8-enol) typical for a defect in the sterol $\Delta^{5,6}$ desaturase system [11, 12]. Such a defect is known in *S. cerevisiae* harboring a defect of the $\Delta^{5,6}$ desaturase gene *ERG3*. A defect in $\Delta^{8\text{-}7}$ isomerase in a clinical *C. neoformans* isolate from an AIDS patient was linked also with AmB resistance [13]. In *C.*

glabrata, AmB resistance has been reported from clinical samples, and genetic analysis has permitted the identification of mutations in the *ERG6* gene encoding C-24 sterol methyltransferase [14, 15].

Curiously, the disruption of the *ERG3* gene in *C. albicans* is not associated with AmB resistance [16]. This contrasts with the results obtained in clinical strains, which, probably contain other compensatory mutations resulting in AmB resistance. A decrease in the content of cell membrane-associated ergosterol can also cause AmB resistance, because AmB requires the presence of ergosterol to damage fungal cells. Different investigators have supported this possibility by demonstrating that development of inducible resistance, induced by an adaptation mechanism, in a strain of *C. albicans* was accompanied by a decrease in the ergosterol content of the cells and that polyene-resistant *C. albicans* clinical isolates obtained from neutropenic patients had a 74–85% decrease in their ergosterol content [17]. Another mechanism accounting for the resistance of yeast to AmB is thought to be mediated by increased catalase activity, which can contribute to diminish oxidative damage caused by this agent [18].

Flucytosine (5-Fluorocytosine)

Flucytosine (5-FC) belongs to the class of pyrimidine analogues and was developed in the 1950s as a potential antineoplastic agent. Abandoned as anti-cancer drug due to its lack of activity against tumors, it showed, however, good in vitro and in vivo antifungal activity. Because it is highly water-soluble, it can be administered by either oral or intravenous routes [19]. 5-FC is taken up by fungal cells by a cytosine permease and is deaminated by a cytosine deaminase to 5-fluorouracil (5-FU), a potent antimetabolite. 5-FU can be converted to a nucleoside triphosphate and, when incorporated into RNA, causes miscoding. In addition, 5-FU can be converted to a deoxynucleoside, which inhibits thymidilate synthase and thereby DNA synthesis. 5-FC shows little toxicity in mammalian cells, because cytosine deaminase is absent or poorly active in these cells. 5-FU is a potent anticancer agent, but it is impermeable to fungal cells. The conversion of 5-FC to 5-FU by intestinal bacteria is possible, and therefore 5-FC can show toxicity in oral formulations. 5-FC is fungicidal for susceptible fungi. High variability in 5-FC MICs is observed in *Candida* species and *C. neoformans* because of the occurrence of intrinsic resistance. MIC_{90} of 5-FC are in the range of 0.5–4 μg/mL for *Candida* species, including *C. albicans*, *C. parapsilosis*, *C. tropicalis* and *C. glabrata*, and for *C. neoformans* [20].

5-FC is not usually administered as a single agent because of rapid development of resistance. It is therefore used mainly in combination with other agents, particularly AmB. In vitro data regarding the combination of both drugs against *Candida* species and *C. neoformans* are numerous and are contradictory, showing antagonistic, indifferent or synergistic effects [21]. 5-FC is an antifungal agent against which resistance can be intrinsic or acquired. Resistance may occur due to the deficiency or lack of enzymes implicated in the metabolism of 5-FC, or resistance may be due to the deregulation of the pyrimidine biosynthetic pathway, in which products can compete with the fluorinated metabolites of 5-FC. Detailed investigations on the molecular mechanisms of resistance to 5-FC have shown that intrinsic resistance to 5-FC in fungi can be due to a defect in the cytosine permease, as observed in *C. glabrata,* but not in *C. albicans* or *C. neoformans.* Acquired resistance results from a failure to metabolize 5-FC to 5-FUTP (5-fluorouridine triphosphate) and 5-FdUMP (5-fluoro-deoxyuridine monophosphate), or from the loss of feedback control of pyrimidine biosynthesis [22].

Recently, a mutation in the *FUR1* gene encoding uracil phosphoribosyltransferase was reported as a cause of 5-FC resistance. This mutation (cytosine to thymine at position 301) is thought to decrease the conversion of 5-FU, which is produced from deamination of 5-FC, into a toxic metabolite (5-fluorouridine monophosphate) and thus counteracts the action of this compound [23]. Interestingly, this resistance mechanism is enriched in a *C. albicans* subpopulation (clade I), which is one among the five major clades (I, II, III, SA, and E) known in this yeast species. In this population, the *FUR1* mutation can occur in the hetero- or homozygous state and is correlated with increased 5-FC MIC value. In addition to this specific mechanism, a mutation in cytosine deaminase (*FCA1*) has been reported correlating with 5-FC resistance in *C. albicans* [24].

Azoles

Azole antifungal agents discovered in the late 1960s are synthetic compounds belonging to the largest group of antifungal agents. Azole antifungal agents used in medicine are categorized into N-1 substituted imidazoles (ketoconazole, miconazole, clotrimazole) and triazoles (fluconazole, itraconazole, posaconazole, voriconazole, and ravuconazole (Fig. 2). Azoles have a cytochrome P450 as a common cellular target in yeast or moulds (Fig. 3). This cytochrome P450, now referred to as Erg11p, is the product of the *ERG11* gene. The unhindered nitrogen of the imidazole or triazole ring of azole antifungal agents binds to the heme iron of Erg11p as a sixth ligand, thus inhibiting the enzymatic reaction. The affinity of imidazole and triazole derivatives is not only dependent on this interaction, but is also determined by the N-1 substituent, which is actually responsible for the high affinity of azole antifungal agents to their target. Each

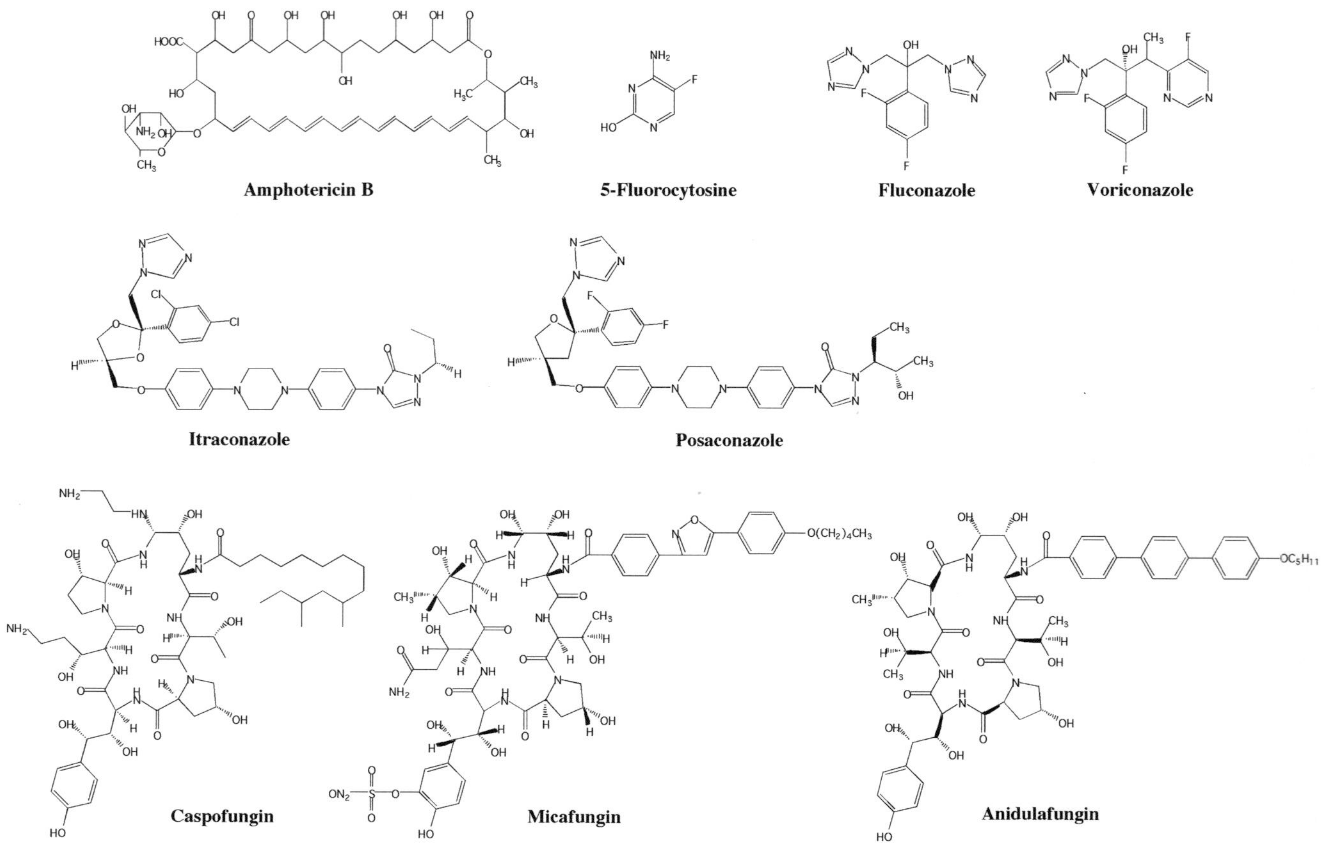

Fig. 2 Chemical structures of major antifungal agents

of these agents has distinct pharmacokinetics and their antifungal efficacies are quite different among yeast and moulds of medical relevance.

Azole antifungals have a broad spectrum of activity. They are active against *Candida* species, *C. neoformans* and dimorphic fungi. Some azole derivatives are more active than others for different fungi. For example, fluconazole is relatively inactive against *C. krusei* or *A. fumigatus* as compared with itraconazole or voriconazole. Posaconazole shows high activity against a large number of filamentous fungi and has a more predictable pharmacodynamic profile than voriconazole; it is also active against fungal pathogens, such as the zygomycetes, which are refractory to other azoles [25]. Azole antifungals are only fungistatic against most yeast species. Against *Candida* infections, fluconazole has demonstrated broad clinical efficacy for mucosal candidiasis, *Candida* urinary tract infections, candidemia, and invasive candidiasis [26].

Reports on resistance to azole antifungal agents were rare until the late 1980s. The first cases of resistance were reported in *C. albicans* after prolonged therapy with miconazole and ketoconazole. Following the use of fluconazole for a wide variety of infections, especially the treatment of mucosal infections in AIDS patients, antifungal resistance to this agent has been more frequent [27]. There are several mechanisms by which yeasts or filamentous fungi can become resistant to azole antifungal agents (Fig. 3).

Resistance by Altered Drug Transport

Failure to accumulate azole antifungals has been identified as a cause of azole resistance in several post-treatment clinical fungal isolates. These isolates include *C. albicans*, *C. glabrata*, *C. krusei*, *C. dubliniensis* and *C. neoformans* [28]. In azole-resistant yeasts, genes encoding ATP Binding Cassette (ABC)-transporters were upregulated as compared to the corresponding azole-susceptible species. So far, only *CDR1* (Candida Drug Resistance 1) and *CDR2* in *C. albicans* [29, 30], *CdCDR1* in *C. dubliniensis* [31, 32], a *CDR1* homologue in *C. tropicalis* [33], *CgCDR1*, *CgCDR2* (also known as *PDH1*) and *CgSNQ2* in *C. glabrata* [34–36] and *AFR1* in *C. neoformans* [37] have been identified as ABC-transporter genes upregulated in azole-resistant isolates.

In *A. fumigatus*, itraconazole is able to induce an ABC-transporter gene, *atrF*; however, the role of this gene in the resistance of clinical isolates to itraconazole is still not established in detail [38]. Heterologous expression of ABC-transporter genes such as *CDR1* and *CDR2*, *CdCDR1*,

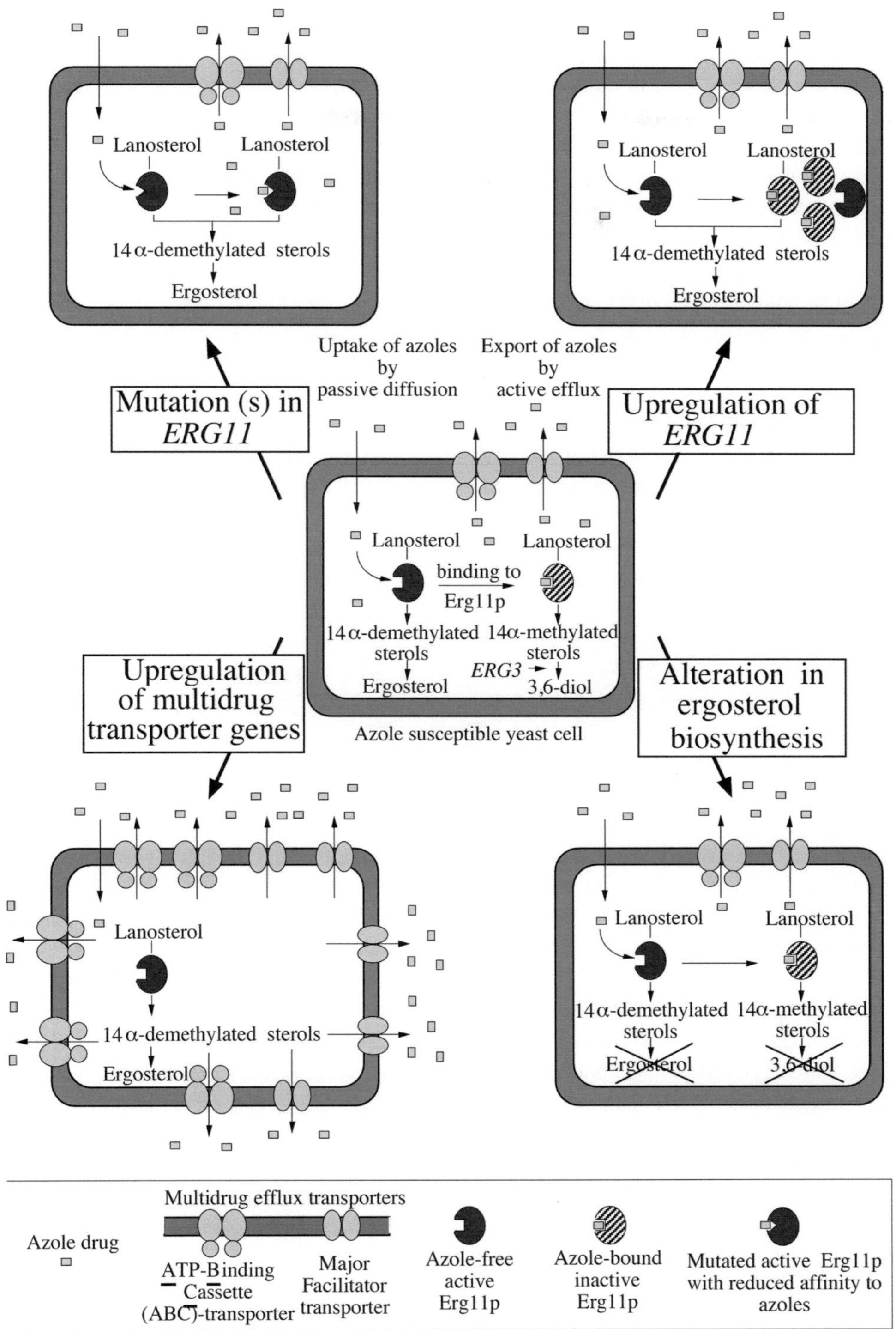

Fig. 3 Schematic view of the four mains resistance mechanisms to azole antifungals in yeast pathogens. Erg11p, the cellular target of azole antifungals, is responsible for the demethylation of lanosterol. 14α-demethlylated sterols serve as further substrates in the formation of ergosterol. When azole drugs bind Erg11p, lanosterol demethylation is blocked and sterol metabolites remains methylated at the position 14α. The toxic metabolite 3,6-diol (14α-methylergosta-8,24(28)-dien-3β,6α-diol) is formed from the action of *ERG3* on 14α-methylfecosterol (see Fig. 2 for sterol structures). Details on specific resistance mechanisms are given in the text

CgCDR1 and *CgCDR2* in *S. cerevisiae* conferred resistance not only to several azole derivatives (fluconazole, itraconazole, ketoconazole) but also to a wide range of compounds, including antifungals and metabolic inhibitors [30, 35, 39].

Several laboratories have also observed that, besides upregulation of ABC-transporter genes, a multidrug transporter gene named *MDR1* (Multidrug Resistance 1), also previously known as *BEN* (Benomyl resistance) and belonging to the family of Major Facilitators, was upregulated in some *C. albicans* azole-resistant clinical isolates. Deletion of *MDR1* in *C. albicans* and also in *C. dubliniensis* isolates with acquired azole resistance by *MDR1* upregulation resulted in a sharp increase of azole susceptibility, thus supporting by this genetic approach, the involvement of this specific gene in azole resistance [40, 41]. Deletion of *MDR1* in an azole-susceptible laboratory strain did not result in a significant increase of azole susceptibility, thus supporting the fact that *MDR1* is almost not expressed in this type of strain and more generally in azole-susceptible clinical isolates [42]. Upregulation of an *MDR1*-like gene has been also observed in a fluconazole-exposed *C. tropicalis* isolate that acquired cross-resistance to fluconazole and itraconazole [33].

In most cases, azole resistance acquired in clinical situations by yeast pathogens by multidrug transporters is maintained over a high number of generations in vitro without drug selection. Azole resistance can however be a reversible phenomenon. Marr and collaborators [43] obtained *C. albicans* isolates that developed azole resistance from bone marrow transplant patients being treated with fluconazole. An increase in the fluconazole MIC was coupled with upregulation of *CDR1*, but was decreased with a parallel decrease in *CDR1* expression in drug-free subculture. Azole-susceptible isolates from this type of patient, when exposed in vitro to fluconazole, developed reversible azole resistance by the same *CDR1* upregulation mechanism. Interestingly, only a portion of individually exposed colonies were rendered less susceptible to fluconazole, thus indicating that hetero-resistance, which was already described in azole-exposed *C. neoformans* isolates, could occur in specific *C. albicans* isolates [44].

Another interesting acquisition of azole resistance by multidrug transporter upregulation in a clinical context has been shown in *C. glabrata*. This yeast could convert to azole resistance by loss of mitochondrial DNA. The phenomenon, also called HFAR, for High Frequency Azole Resistance, because it occurred in vitro at high frequencies, was coupled with upregulation of *CgCDR1* and *CgCDR2* [34]. Interestingly, mitochondrial defects have been reported in several clinical isolates that were exposed to fluconazole during treatment [45, 46].

The molecular basis for the upregulation of multidrug transporters belonging to the ABC and Major Facilitator families has been actively investigated in yeast pathogens. It is believed that the mutation(s) leading to gene upregulation might rather be caused by alterations involving transcription factors. Using the *Renilla* luciferase reporter system fused to *CDR1* and *CDR2* promoters cloned from azole-susceptible isolates, De Micheli et al. [47] showed that their expression was enhanced in an azole-resistant strain, in which these genes are constitutively upregulated. With another reporter system, GFP fused to the *MDR1* promoter from an azole-susceptible strain, Wirsching et al. [48] showed that high fluorescence could be obtained when the chimeric construct was introduced in an azole-resistant strain upregulating *MDR1*.

The systematic dissection of the *CDR1* and *CDR2* promoters allowed the identification of five distinct regulatory elements: the basal expression element (BEE) responsible for basal expression; the drug-responsive element (DRE) required for the response to drugs, such as fluphenazine and estradiol; two steroid responsive elements (SRE) involved in the response to steroid hormones; and the negative regulatory element (NRE) [47, 49, 50]. Internal deletions of the BEE and DRE in the *CDR1* promoter affect basal *CDR1* expression and drug-induced expression, respectively. Conversely, the deletion of the NRE leads to an increase in the basal expression of *CDR1*. In contrast to *CDR1*, the *CDR2* promoter only contains the DRE element [47]. Among these different *cis*-acting elements, only the DRE was shown to be involved not only in the transient up-regulation of both *CDR1* and *CDR2* in response to inducers but also in their constitutive high expression in azole-resistant clinical isolates [47].

The DREs present in the promoter of *CDR* genes contain two CGG triplets which are potentially recognized by Zn_2-Cys_6 transcription factors [51–54]. In order to isolate regulators of *CDR1* and *CDR2*, the *C. albicans* genome was searched for genes encoding proteins with Zn_2-Cys_6 fingers. Interestingly, three of these genes were arranged in tandem near the mating locus (*MTL*), the homozygosity of which is linked to the development of azole resistance in *C. albicans* [55]. Deletion of one of these genes, *TAC1* (transcriptional activator of *CDR* genes), in an azole-susceptible strain led to increased drug susceptibility and to loss of transient *CDR1* and *CDR2* upregulation in presence of inducers. In *C. albicans* clinical isolates resistant to azoles, deletion of *TAC1* abolishes *CDR1* and *CDR2* expression and therefore, drug resistance, demonstrating that *TAC1* is the main mediator of azole resistance due to the upregulation of ABC transporter in *C. albicans* [56]. Tac1p acts by direct binding to the DRE present in the promoter region of both efflux pump genes and induces their expression in response to steroid and several toxic chemicals [47, 56]. Tac1p is not involved in the basal expression of *CDR1* and the transcription factor regulating *CDR1* expression through the BEE element remains to be identified.

Functional dissection studies of the *MDR1* promoter have identified two distinct regulatory regions. The benomyl response element (BRE), also called the *MDR1* drug resistance element (MDRE) is responsible for the constitutive high expression of *MDR1* in fluconazole-resistant isolates [57–59]. This region is also necessary for the inducible expression of *MDR1* in response to benomyl [57, 59]. The second element, the HRE ($\underline{H}_2O_2$ $\underline{r}$esponse $\underline{e}$lement) is involved in the response to oxidative stress agents. In contrast to the BRE, the HRE is not required for constitutive upregulation of *MDR1* in azole-resistant isolates. The HRE region contains two YRE (*YAP1* response element) motifs and the BRE/MDRE contains a perfect match for the Mads-box transcription factor Mcm1p [58, 60, 61]. However there is no direct evidence either for interactions between Yap1p and the HRE and between Mcm1p and the BRE or for the involvement of Yap1p and Mcm1p in the inducible or constitutive expression of *MDR1*.

The molecular basis for the constitutive upregulation of the Major facilitator gene *MDR1* has been recently elucidated. A genome-wide study was undertaken to compare the transcriptional profiles of three different *C. albicans* clinical isolates overexpressing *MDR1* in order to identify genes commonly upregulated with *MDR1*. One of the genes of interest was orf19.7372 since it contained a Zn_2-Cys_6 zinc finger motif of the same type as *TAC1*. Because inactivation of orf19.7372 caused loss of *MDR1* upregulation, the transcription factor was called Mrr1pp (multi-drug resistance regulator) [62]. *MRR1* inactivation in azole-resistant isolates resulted in the loss of *MDR1* expression and increased susceptibility to fluconazole, cerulenin and brefeldin A [62]. Deletion of *MRR1* in a drug-susceptible strain abolished *MDR1* upregulation in presence of inducing chemicals, such as benomyl and H_2O_2, thus demonstrating that Mrr1p mediates both inducible *MDR1* expression and constitutive *MDR1* overexpression in drug-resistant strains [62]. A *MRR1* homolog has been identified in *C. dubliniensis* and was shown responsible for *CdMDR1* expression [63]. Although Mrr1p has not been yet shown to bind directly to the *MDR1* promoter in order to regulate *MDR1* expression, CdMrr1p is able to activate the *MDR1* promoter in the heterologous species *C. albicans*, suggesting that Mrr1p and CdMrr1p recognize the same binding site(s) which should be present in the *MDR1* promoters of both species [63].

The identification of *trans*-acting factors regulating ABC-transporters in pathogenic fungi can also rely on the well-described Pleiotropic Drug Resistance (PDR) network involved in multidrug resistance in *S. cerevisiae*. The two Zn_2-Cys_6 transcription factors *PDR1/PDR3* are master regulators of this network and control multidrug resistance by modifying the expression of several ABC (*PDR5, SNQ2* and *YOR1*)- and MFS (*FLR1, TPO1*)-transporters as well as other genes determining cell membrane composition (*PDR16, RSB1, LPT1*). *In silico* search for *PDR1/PDR3* homologues in the genomes of pathogenic fungi has been performed, and so far only one functional homolog, *CgPDR1*, was described in *C. glabrata* [64]. CgPdr1p has 40% and 35% identity with Pdr1p and Pdr3p, respectively, and could complement a *pdr1Δ S. cerevisiae* mutant strain [65]. Similar to *S. cerevisiae*, the expression of *C. glabrata CgCDR1/2* and *CgSNQ2* genes is regulated by CgPdr1p [64]. Deletion of *CgPDR1* in *C. glabrata* azole-resistant clinical isolates leads to a loss of *CgCDR1*, *CgCDR2* and *CgSNQ2* regulation and to a sharp increase in azole susceptibility, indicating that *CgPDR1* is the main regulator of efflux-mediated azole-resistance in *C. glabrata* [36, 66]. Deletion of *CgPDR1* also abolishes *CgCDR1* and *CgCDR2* up-regulation in presence of fluconazole [66].

It is now well established that *S. cerevisiae* Pdr1p and Pdr3p act through *cis*-acting sites present in the promoters of target genes. The consensus motif is named PDRE (for pleiotropic drug resistance element) and is present in several ABC-transporter gene promoters such as *PDR5*, *SNQ2* and *YOR1* [67]. In *C. glabrata*, a genome-wide study identified genes regulated by *CgPDR1* and, by analysis of the promoters, the sequence 5′-TCC(GA)(CT)GAA-3′ was identified as a strong candidate for *C. glabrata* PDRE. This sequence is found in the promoters of *CgCDR1*, *CgCDR2* and *CgSNQ2* genes, suggesting that CgPdr1p binds directly to PDRE sequences to regulate transcription of target genes [36, 65, 66]. *CgPDR1* contains a PDRE in its promoter suggesting an auto-regulation of its transcription. Consistent with this observation, upregulation of *CgCDR1* and *CgCDR2* is correlated in some azole resistant strains with an increase of *CgPDR1* expression [65, 66]. However, although promoters regions of *CgCDR1*, *CgCDR2*, *CgSNQ2* and *CgPDR1* genes all contain PDRE, they are not simultaneously expressed in clinical azole-resistant isolates [45]. CgPdr1p acts as nuclear receptor by directly binding to diverse drugs and xenobiotics, such as azoles, to activate expression of efflux pumps genes resulting in multidrug resistance [68]. A small portion of the activation domain of CgPdr1p binds directly to the KIX domain of the Mediator co-activator subunit CgGal11p in a xenobiotic-dependent manner in order to activate transcription of target genes [68].

One of the consequences of the involvement of multidrug efflux transporters in resistance to azole antifungals is that these transporters have the ability to mediate cross-resistance to unrelated antifungals or metabolic inhibitors. In order to determine whether or not a given substance is a potential substrate for multidrug efflux transporters, different approaches have been taken. One consists of functional expression of the *C. albicans* multidrug efflux transporters in the baker's yeast *S. cerevisiae* carrying a deletion of the *PDR5* gene [30, 42]. Depending on the acquisition of resistance of *S. cerevisiae* mutants expressing these specific transporters against a given compound, the substance can be considered as a potential substrate for the expressed multidrug transporter. Potential substrates for the multidrug efflux transporters encoded by *CDR1* and *CDR2* include almost all azole antifungals of medical importance, including fluconazole, itraconazole, posaconazole, and voriconazole, and other antifungal agents, such as terbinafine and amorolfine. For the multidrug transporter encoded by *MDR1*, fluconazole was the only relevant substrate among azole antifungals. Several antifungal agents could not be assigned as substrates (AmB, 5-fluorocytosine). Since not only azoles, but other antifungals, such as terbinafine and amorolfine, can be taken simultaneously as substrates by several multidrug efflux transporters, multidrug efflux transporter genes, when overexpressed in clinical yeast isolates, have the potential of mediating cross-resistance to different antifungal agents. Data suggest that the upregulation of *MDR1* is responsible for the specific resistance to fluconazole in *Candida* isolates, and this is consistent with the observation that *MDR1* overexpression in *S. cerevisiae* was only conferring resistance to fluconazole [30].

Resistance to Azole Antifungals Involving Alterations of the Cellular Target

Target alterations are known resistance mechanisms for two classes of antifungal agents, azoles and echinocandins. Resistance mediated by alterations in Erg11/Cyp51, the targets of azoles, has been widely documented involving either mutations or upregulation of their genes. A large number of non-synonymous nucleotide polymorphisms (up to 110, including 100 with unique substitutions) have been described in *ERG11* alleles originating from *C. albicans* azole-resistant isolates. The degree of *ERG11* polymorphism is therefore high and suggests that Erg11p is highly permissive to structural changes resulting from amino acid substitutions. The contribution of each individual mutation to azole resistance is, however, difficult to estimate because *ERG11* mutations often occur in combination (from 2 to 4 combined mutations) in the same allele and because resistance mechanisms are often combined in azole-resistant *C. albicans* isolates [69]. Using different approaches, including heterologous expression in *S. cerevisiae*, enzyme assay in *C. albicans* extracts, and site directed mutagenesis, evidence for their involvement in azole resistance has been provided for at least some of these mutations (F72L, F145L, G464S, Y132F, R467K, S405F) [70–76].

In *A. fumigatus*, itraconazole resistance in clinical isolates is associated with the occurrence of amino acid substitution in Cyp51A, which is the functional ortholog of Erg11p in this fungal species. Interestingly, mutations at position G54 contribute only to itraconazole resistance and not to voriconazole resistance [77, 78]. In contrast, mutations at position M220 confer itraconazole resistance and also high MICs to voriconazole and posaconazole [79]. Similarly, mutations at positions L98 and G138 recently described in Cyp51A conferred cross-resistance to all azoles [79]. The Cyp51A mutation L98H is consistently combined with *cyp51*A upregulation. This mechanism allows cross-resistance to all known azoles [80]. Intriguingly, the L98H substitution and *cyp51*A upregulation mechanisms were also found in isolates of environmental origin, thus raising the question on how azole resistance was acquired in a non-medical environment [81].

In *C. neoformans*, analysis of *ERG11* from a clinical azole-resistant isolate showed a point mutation linked an amino acid substitution G484S that was not observed in the parent azole-susceptible isolate [82]. Recent studies demonstrated that azole resistance in this yeast species can be due to heteroresistance, which is a mechanism by which resistance can be induced or reversed in a portion of a growing population [83].

Upregulation of *ERG11* has been mentioned as a possible cause of azole resistance in a few cases in *C. albicans*, *C. glabrata* clinical isolates and in a single *C. tropicalis* isolate [84]. Upregulation of *ERG11* does not exceed a factor of 3–5 in azole-resistant isolates when compared to *ERG11* expression in related azole-susceptible strains [29, 85–87]. Upregulation of *ERG11* can be achieved in principle by deregulating gene transcription or by gene amplification.

In *S. cerevisiae*, *ERG11* is regulated by two transcriptional activators, Upc2p and Ecm22p, which are members of the Zn_2-Cys_6 transcription factor family [88]. They act through binding to regulatory elements present in the *ERG11* promoter called the Sterol Regulatory Element (SRE). Other SREs are found in genes involved in sterol biosynthesis. A single *C. albicans* gene (*UPC2*) with homology to both *S. cerevisiae* genes, has been identified and characterized [89, 90]. Deletion of *UPC2* in *C. albicans* caused loss of *ERG11* upregulation in response to azole drugs, which occurs otherwise in the parent strain. Promoter deletions and linker scan mutations localized the region important for azole induction to a segment from −224 to −251 upstream of the start codon. This segment contains two 7-bp sequences (5′ TCGTATA 3′) separated by 13-bp [91] forming an imperfect inverted repeat, a typical feature for binding to Zn_2-Cys_6 transcription factors [67]. The Upc2p core binding sequence is conserved between *Candida* and *Saccharomyces*. This core is found in the *ERG11* promoter in a region identified as important for azole induction of *ERG11* expression [90].

As mentioned above, upregulation of *cyp51A* in *A. fumigatus* has been detected in clinical isolates with cross-resistance to several azole antifungal agents. This upregulation is associated with a (L98H) substitution in Cyp51A and with the presence of a 34-bp tandem repeat in the *cyp51A* promoter [80]. This resistance mechanism has been also identified in *A. fumigatus* isolates originating from the environment in the Netherlands. Exposure of environmental isolates to agricultural azole fungicides is suspected as a possible cause of the emergence of such azole-resistant isolates recovered from treated patients [81].

Gain-of-Function Mutations in Regulators of Azole Resistance

The elevated transcription of genes targeted by the transcription factors *TAC1*, *MRR1*, *CgPDR1* and *UPC2* that is observed in azole-resistant clinical isolates is thought to be due to their intrinsic activation. This state of activation, which does not require external stimuli, can be obtained when the transcription factors are modified by mutations, as it is known to occur in several other microorganisms [67, 92]. Consistent with this hypothesis, transcription factor alleles from azole-resistant isolates were shown to confer constitutive high expression of their drug resistance gene targets and thus, azole resistance when expressed in an azole-susceptible background [36, 45, 56, 62, 65, 66, 93–95]. This was first demonstrated in *C. albicans* in which two types of *TAC1* alleles were isolated from clinical isolates: wild-type alleles, which conferred transient *CDR1* and *CDR2* upregulation in response to drugs, and hyperactive alleles, which were isolated from azole-resistant strains and conferred constitutive high *CDR1* and *CDR2* expression and therefore drug resistance to a mutant strain lacking *TAC1* [56, 93]. Sequencing of these alleles revealed that wild-type and hyperactive alleles differed by single point mutations leading to single amino acid substitutions defined as gain-of-function (GOF) mutations.

Several hyperactive alleles from *MRR1*, *CgPDR1* and *UPC2* were identified and harbored GOF mutations. By increasing the number of investigated isolates, the number of GOF for each gene has also considerably increased. Large-scale sequencing of *TAC1* alleles from *C. albicans* clinical isolates has to date identified 39 hyperactive alleles harboring 16 different GOF mutations at 12 distinct positions. Three other GOF mutations introduced by random mutagenesis were also able to confer hyperactivity to a *TAC1* wild type allele [56, 93, 96, 97] (Fig. 4). The majority of these GOF mutations (15) are located in the C-terminal portion of *TAC1* corresponding to a putative transcriptional activation domain, while the remaining mutations are situated in the Middle Homology Region (MHR) and the N-terminal part of the protein, which are regions with no defined function (Fig. 4). How these mutations affect the transcriptional activity of *TAC1* remains unknown. Although other transcription factors have been shown to regulate *CDR1* expression in laboratory studies [50, 98], only mutations in Tac1p have been found to be responsible for *CDR1* and *CDR2* upregulation in clinical *C. albicans* azole-resistant isolates.

Similar to *CDR1/2* upregulation by Tac1p, *MDR1* overexpression is also caused by GOF mutations in its regulator, Mrr1p [62]. So far, 14 distinct GOF have been identified in *MRR1* on 13 distinct positions spanning throughout the open reading frame (Fig. 3) [94]. As for Tac1p, the functional domains of Mrr1p are still unknown. It is therefore difficult to speculate about the molecular mechanism underlying Mrr1p hyperactivity. Nevertheless, GOF mutations were also identified in *CdMRR1*, the *MRR1* homolog of *C. dubliniensis* indicating that GOF mutations affect similarly the activity of Mrr1p in both *C. albicans* and *C. dubliniensis* [63]

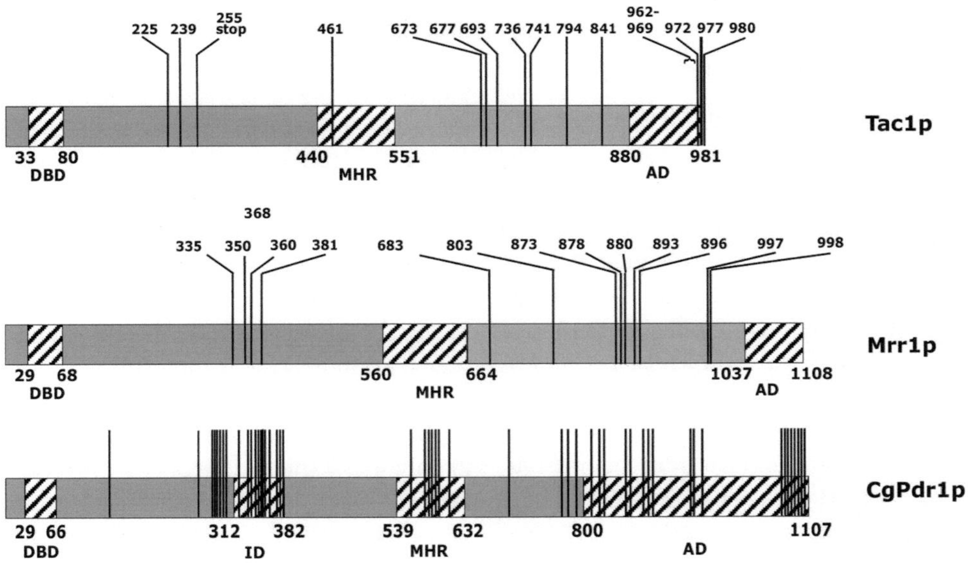

Fig. 4 Positions of gain-of-function mutations in transcriptional activators of azole resistance. Repartition of the GOF mutations (black bars) identified in the transcription factors Tac1p, Mrr1p and CgPdr1p. All GOF mutations are indicated by their position in each activator, with the exception of position 962–969, which indicates a deletion between amino acid position 962–969. Data for *TAC1*, *MRR1* and *CgPDR1* were obtained from published reports [45, 62, 64, 94, 96]. *DBD* DNA binding domain, *ID* inhibitory domain, *MHR* middle homology region, *AD* activation domain

C. glabrata differs from *C. albicans* with respect to the diversity of GOF mutations in *CgPDR1* [45]. Three studies have identified four separate amino acid substitutions in CgPdr1 of azole-resistant strains which are responsible for constitutive high expression of ABC-transporter genes and of *CgPDR1* itself [36, 65, 66]. Large-scale analysis of *CgPDR1* alleles from *C. glabrata* clinical azole-resistant isolates identified 70 alleles, from which only 12 were wild type allele and 58 were hyperactive alleles. These 58 hyperactive alleles contain 58 distinct GOF mutations yielding 57 single amino acids substitutions located at 51 different positions along the protein with some "hot spots" near the N-terminal inhibitory domain, the central MHR domain and the C-terminal activation domain [45].

Up to now, a single *UPC2* GOF has been described in *C. albicans* from an isolate exhibiting high *ERG11* expression levels. Using genome-wide gene expression profiling, it was revealed that *UPC2* and other genes involved in ergosterol biosynthesis to be coordinately upregulated with *ERG11* in a fluconazole-resistant clinical isolate compared with a matched susceptible isolate from the same patient [95]. Sequence analysis revealed that the resistant isolate contained a single-nucleotide substitution in one *UPC2* allele that resulted in a G648D substitution. This substitution aligned functionally to a *UPC2* dominant allele previously obtained from *S. cerevisiae* with a G888D substitution [99]. The hyperactivity conferred by the *C. albicans UPC2* mutant allele may contribute to increase azole resistance by *ERG11* upregulation, but especially when *ERG11* contains already mutations affecting azole binding.

Azole Resistance Mechanisms Involving Alterations in the Ergosterol Biosynthetic Pathway

Analysis of the sterol composition of azole-resistant yeasts has provided several hypotheses on specific alterations of enzymes involved in the complex ergosterol biosynthetic pathway. Accumulation of ergosta-7,22-dienol-3β-ol was observed in two separate azole-resistant *C. albicans* clinical isolates, which is a feature consistent with an absence of sterol $\Delta^{5,6}$ desaturase activity encoded by *ERG3* [11]. The role of *ERG3* in azole resistance originates also from the observation that treatment of a normal yeast cell with azoles inhibits Erg11p and thus results in accumulation of 14α-methylated sterols and 14α-methylergosta-8,24(28)-dien-3β,6α-diol. Formation of this later sterol metabolite is thought to be catalyzed by the *ERG3* gene product (the sterol $\Delta^{5,6}$ desaturase) and thus inactivation of this gene suppresses toxicity and causes azole resistance (Fig. 3). Several azole-resistant isolates originating from *C. albicans* and *C. dubliniensis* have been characterized and contain loss-of function *ERG3* alleles [12, 100, 101]. Other defects of genes participating in ergosterol biosynthesis were recently identified in *C. glabrata*. These involve *ERG6* encoding C-24 sterol methyltransferase, which contains missense or nonsense mutations [14, 15]. Both *ERG6* missense mutations decreased AmB susceptibility but enhanced azole susceptibility. Resistance to AmB can be expected when ergosterol biosynthesis is defective by alteration of genes involved in its biosynthesis. However, *ERG3* defects in clinical isolates or in vitro generated mutants have resulted in only modest MIC shifts as compared to wild type isolates. It is only when *ERG11* is inactivated that high level AmB resistance can be measured [16].

Azole Resistance Mechanism and Their Combination in Clinical Isolates

In some studies investigating resistance mechanisms to azoles in clinical isolates, it was possible to recover sequential isolates from patients treated with these compounds showing a stepwise increase in azole resistance, as measured by susceptibility testing. The stepwise increase in azole resistance indicated that different resistance mechanisms could operate and through sequential addition, explain the increase in azole MIC values. Several examples have been reported documenting the multifactorial basis of azole resistance in clinical isolates. The combination of resistance mechanisms seems to be associated with a high level of azole resistance, resulting for example, in MIC values for fluconazole exceeding 64 μg/mL [86].

Alterations of the target enzymes by several distinct single or multiple mutations and upregulation of multidrug transporters from two different families gives great flexibility for the possibility of a combination of resistance mechanisms. Molecular epidemiology of azole resistance performed mainly with *C. albicans* isolates demonstrated that the diversity of resistance mechanism combinations was high enough that there are only a very few azole resistant isolates with identical patterns of *ERG11* mutations and profiles of multidrug transporter genes expression.

The relative frequency of resistance mechanisms in large populations of azole-resistant isolates has been investigated in only a few studies. Perea et al. [86] showed that 85% of azole-resistant isolates upregulated multidrug transporter genes and that 65% contained *ERG11* mutations linked to azole resistance. Overall, 75% of the azole-resistant isolates manifested a combination of resistance mechanisms. These numbers match our data for isolates from 18 HIV-infected patients, in whom azole-resistant isolates were recovered. Of these isolates, 82% showed upregulation of multidrug transporter genes, 63% contained *ERG11* mutations linked to azole resistance, and 50% showed a combination of resistance mechanisms (D. Sanglard, unpublished). The relative distribution of the type of multidrug transporter genes upregulated in these populations is in favor of the ABC-transporters *CDR1* and *CDR2*; these transporters are upregulated approximately in twice as many azole-resistant isolates than is observed for isolates with *MDR1* upregulation.

Combinations of resistance mechanisms are not always linked with high levels of resistance. In *C. glabrata* azole-resistant isolates, a single resistance mechanism, upregulation of the *CgCDR1* ABC-transporter gene, is responsible for acquisition of high levels of azole resistance. Genetic evidence has also been provided for the occurrence of this single resistance mechanism by deletion of *CgCDR1* in an azole-resistant strain, which results in a decrease of fluconazole MIC values near to those obtained in the parental azole-susceptible isolate [35].

Chromosomal Rearrangements Affecting Multidrug Transporter Expression

In *C. albicans,* high levels of azole resistance usually develop gradually as a result of sequential alterations or combinations of mechanisms due to continuous pressure exerted by the drug. As above explained, the acquisition of GOF mutations in transcriptional activators of drug resistance, including *TAC1*, *MRR1* or *UPC2*, is only a first step in the development of azole resistance. Since these GOF mutations are co-dominant, *C. albicans* needs to carry two hyperactive alleles of each activator in order to develop high levels of azole resistance [56, 93]. These events usually occur from loss of heterozygosity through chromosome loss and reduplication or mitotic recombinations. Moreover, these chromosome alterations can be accompanied by acquisition of extra chromosomal elements to increase gene copy number of transcriptional activators. For example, *TAC1* being located on the left arm of chromosome 5, isochromosome formation with two left arms (i5L) is facilitated. Curiously, *ERG11* is situated near the end of this same chromosome arm and thus i5L formation results in a parallel increase of two major contributor of azole resistance [102, 103]. Retrospective studies have identified in *C. albicans* isolates with high azole resistance a high proportion of isolates harboring the i5L [93, 102].

Chromosome alterations as a mode of gene copy increase of drug resistance genes was also recently documented in *C. glabrata. De novo* mini-chromosome formation was identified in some azole-resistant isolates. In one case, the mini-chromosome included a genome segment containing *CgCDR2*, an ABC-transporter known to contribute to azole resistance [104]. Although the relevance of this specific effect was not demonstrated by genetic approaches, it suggests that *C. glabrata* is also able to adapt to drug resistance by chromosomal rearrangements.

Alternative Mechanisms of Azole Resistance

In addition to the resistance mechanisms described above, alternative pathways for the acquisition of azole resistance can be used by yeast and moulds. One interesting alternative for development of azole resistance uses the ability of fungal pathogens to form biofilms on synthetic or natural surfaces. Biofilms constitute a physical barrier for the efficient penetration of antifungals, which could explain why organisms embedded in these structures become recalcitrant to antifungal action. Measurement of drug susceptibilities in biofilms of *C. albicans* or *C. dubliniensis* yielded high MIC values for azoles and AmB, as compared to planktonic cells. Biofilms still exhibit high susceptibility to caspofungin probably because biofilms contain beta-glucans in their matrix and impairment of glucan synthesis by caspofungin also perturbs biofilm formation [105]. There are at least two situations in which biofilms can form in vivo: when cells grow as multilayers on mucosal surfaces, as seen in oropharyngeal candidiasis, and on synthetic surfaces of catheters. Resistance to antifungal agents by biofilm formation is therefore limited to specific clinical situations.

The molecular basis for antifungal resistance in biofilms is still poorly understood, although several explanations have been provided. Recently published studies suggest that biofilms contain variable proportions of persister cells (phenotypic variants) that are more tolerant to drug action [106]. The term of tolerance is used here to reflect that these cells have the ability to survive to drug action without expressing or using resistance mechanisms, as defined by Lewis [107]. Biofilms also contain heterogeneous cell population at different growth stages, each with different transcriptional activities of genes known to be involved in drug resistance, such as *ERG11*, *CDR1*, *CDR2*, *MDR1*, and thus can contribute transiently to drug resistance [108–110]. Biofilms can also sequester antifungal agents, azoles and AmB, in the polymers of the matrix and thus neutralize their inhibitory effects [111].

Echinocandins

The cell wall is an essential component for the maintenance of turgor of the fungal cell and is absent from mammalian cells. The fundamental components of the cell wall of most fungi comprise chitin, alpha- and beta-linked glucans, mannoproteins, and glycosylphosphatidylinositol (GPI)-anchored proteins. The echinocandins are cyclic lipopeptides that target the biosynthesis of individual cell wall components and are therefore attractive as antifungal drugs. They are non-competitive inhibitors of beta-1,3 glucan synthase, which is part of an enzyme complex that forms the major glucan polymers of most pathogenic fungi. Glucan synthases in *S. cerevisiae* are encoded by 2 separate genes, *FKS1* and *FKS2* [112], whose simultaneous deletion is not viable. *FKS*-like genes have been cloned from other fungal pathogens, including *C. albicans*, *C. neoformans*, and *Paracoccidioides brasiliensis* [113–116].

Synthetic variations on the echinocandin moiety have produced several molecules with improved water solubility, antifungal potency, and efficacy in animal models. The compounds that are currently in clinical use include caspofungin, micafungin, and anidulafungin. Caspofungin is a semisynthetic analogue of pneumocandin Bo and was the first commercialized echinocandin derivative [117]. It is water-soluble and is only available in parenteral form. It has fungicidal activity against a large number of *Candida* spp. and activity against most *Aspergillus* spp. MIC values for these pathogens range between 0.12 and 2 μg/mL. *A. fumigatus* MICs for caspofungin are atypical [118]; requiring other criteria for measuring activity of the echinocandins against *Aspergillus* spp. [119]. The Minimal Effective Concentration (MEC) estimates cell damage assessed by morphological changes seen under the microscope, rather than by a decrease in growth, as classically recorded in standard MIC tests.

Echinocandin resistance was first investigated in the model yeast *S. cerevisiae* with a mutant R560-1C resistant to the semisynthetic pneumocandin derivative, L-733,560. Glucan synthesis catalyzed by a crude membrane fraction prepared from the *S. cerevisiae* was resistant to inhibition by L-733,560. The nearly 50-fold increase in the 50% inhibitory concentration against glucan synthase was paralleled with the increase in whole-cell resistance [120]. Echinocandin resistance has been established in *C. albicans* either by mutagenesis or by spontaneous selection at low frequency of resistant mutants on echinocandin-containing medium. Resistant mutants increased their MIC values to echinocandin derivatives by 50- to 100-fold. The IC_{50} of glucan synthase activity was affected to variable degrees from 4- to over 5,000-fold in these mutants, suggesting that alterations in this enzyme were responsible for resistance. With the cloning of the *FKS1* gene encoding a subunit of beta-1,3 glucan synthase in *C. albicans*, genetic evidence was provided for this possibility since disruption of *FKS1* echinocandin-resistant alleles in *C. albicans* resistant mutant resulted in loss of resistance [113, 115]. These experiments also gave the evidence that echinocandin derivatives were targeting *FKS1* in *C. albicans*. The development of echinocandin resistance was a rare event in *C. albicans*, and it was coupled with reduced virulence in animal models [121].

After several years of clinical use, echinocandin resistance has been reported in several studies. Target alterations have been observed conferring echinocandin resistance essentially by acquisition of mutations in *FKS1* [122]. These mutations are located in two hot-spot regions (HS1, HS2), however HS1, located between residues 641 and 649 of the *C. albicans* Fks1p, is the region with most substitutions [123]. These mutations generally cause cross-resistance to all three echinocandins. *FKS1* modifications in HS1 domains have also been detected in other species including *C. tropicalis* [124], *C. glabrata* [125] and *A. fumigatus* [126]. Intrinsic reduced susceptibility of *C. parapsilosis* is also attributed to natural substitution in the HS1 domain [127]. Several beta-1,3 glucan synthase subunits exist in fungal genomes and therefore mutations in these additional genes can also be targeted by mutations. For example, substitutions in Fks2p from *C. glabrata* are associated with caspofungin resistance [128, 129]. Little is known about the relationship between the altered expression of echinocandin target genes and resistance. It was reported that the activation of the cell integrity pathway by exposure to caspofungin can result in enhanced expression of *FKS* genes [130]. No intrinsic overexpression of *FKS* genes has been yet associated with the acquisition of resistance in *Candida* spp. On the other hand, it was shown that *A. fumigatus* could develop caspofungin resistance by upregulation of *FKS1*. Interestingly, no mutation in this gene could be identified in the resistant isolate [131].

Current Situation with Antifungal Drug Resistance

Antifungal resistance over the last 10–15 years has been seen with fluconazole and itraconazole in oropharyngeal *Candida* infections in patients with AIDS. However, with the introduction of highly active antiretroviral therapy for HIV infection, this disease has markedly decreased [132], and azole-resistant isolates from AIDS patients are now rarely isolated. The extensive use of azole antifungals during the last decade, either for treatment or prophylaxis of fungal diseases, has provided a favorable environment for the emergence of yeast species intrinsically resistant, such as *C. krusei* and *C. glabrata*. Available prospective data from oral and vaginal samples from more than 1,220 women between 1993 and 1995 [133] however, have shown little shift in the spectrum of species. *C. albicans* accounted for 87% of isolates at the start of the study, 84% after 1 year and 83% after 2 years. Recent data published by the same group show that azole MIC_{90} values have not changed over a 2-decade period; however, the percentage of isolates with elevated azole MIC values has increased [134, 135]. The data for HIV-negative patients showed a similar (82–87%) prevalence of *C. albicans*. Therefore, currently, azole usage appears to have little effect in selecting for *Candida* species with intrinsic azole resistance in patients who have mucosal candidiasis.

Large surveillance studies performed in North America and in Europe have looked at the problem of antifungal resistance in disseminated infections. In a review discussing this issue, the main conclusion was that for *C. albicans*, which is the main cause of candidemia, no significant shift in fluconazole or itraconazole MICs has been yet measured [136]. However, a shift towards intrinsically resistant non-*albicans Candida* species has been reported in certain patient populations and in certain institutions. A review of many studies supports a correlation of *C. glabrata* and *C. krusei* prevalence with increasing use of fluconazole [136]. The use of azoles has also resulted in the emergence of uncommon moulds with intrinsic resistance [137], and the acquisition of azole resistance in *A. fumigatus* is a future concern. In the Netherlands, the incidence of *A. fumigatus* species with azole cross-resistance is now as high as 6%. In UK this value was estimated as a high as 8% in 2004 [138]. Some of the azole-resistant isolates were related to others found in the environment in the Netherlands, where triazoles have been used in agriculture for the past 10 years [81].

Physicians faced with the treatment of fungal diseases have seen that fungal pathogens have versatile tools for developing resistance mechanisms. This phenomenon has been amply shown with azole resistance in AIDS patients before the introduction of antiretroviral therapy, and is continuing to be manifested in hospitals in which antifungal agents are commonly prescribed, On the other hand, antifungal agents are now available that have that have improved properties and with new modes of actions that offer attractive alternatives for the treatment of fungal diseases.

References

1. Latge JP. *Aspergillus fumigatus* and aspergillosis. Clin Microbiol Rev. 1999;12:310–50.
2. Arikan S. Current status of antifungal susceptibility testing methods. Med Mycol. 2007;45:569–87.
3. Rex JH, Pfaller MA, Galgiani JN, et al. Development of interpretive breakpoints for antifungal susceptibility testing: Conceptual framework and analysis of in vitro-in vivo correlation data for fluconazole, itraconazole, and *Candida* infections. Subcommittee on Antifungal Susceptibility Testing of the National Committee for Clinical Laboratory Standards. Clin Infect Dis. 1997;24:235–47.
4. Cuesta I, Bielza C, Larranaga P, et al. Data mining validation of fluconazole breakpoints established by the European Committee on Antimicrobial Susceptibility Testing. Antimicrob Agents Chemother. 2009;53:2949–54.
5. EUCAST-AFST (European Committee on Antimicrobial Susceptibility Testing). EUCAST Technical Note on fluconazole. Clin Microbiol Infect. 2008;14:193–5.
6. EUCAST-AFST (European Committee on Antimicrobial Susceptibility Testing). EUCAST Technical Note on voriconazole. Clin Microbiol Infect. 2008;14:985–7.
7. Rex JH, Cooper Jr CR, Merz WG, Galgiani JN, Anaissie EJ. Detection of amphotericin B-resistant *Candida* isolates in a broth-based system. Antimicrob Agents Chemother. 1995;39:906–9.
8. Peyron F, Favel A, Michel-Nguyen A, Gilly M, Regli P, Bolmstrom A. Improved detection of amphotericin B-resistant isolates of *Candida lusitaniae* by Etest. J Clin Microbiol. 2001;39:339–42.
9. Pfaller MA, Messer SA, Hollis RJ. Strain delineation an antifungal susceptibilities of epidemiologically releated and unrelated isolates of *Candida lusitaniae*. Diagnostic Microbiology and Infectious Disease. 1994;20:127–33.
10. Walsh TJ, Melcher GP, Rinaldi MG, et al. *Trichosporon beigelii*, an emerging pathogen resistant to amphotericin B. J Clin Microbiol. 1990;28:1616–22.
11. Nolte FS, Parkinson T, Falconer DJ, et al. Isolation and characterization of fluconazole- and amphotericin B-resistant *Candida albicans* from blood of two patients with leukemia. Antimicrob Agents Chemother. 1997;44:196–9.
12. Chau AS, Gurnani M, Hawkinson R, Laverdiere M, Cacciapuoti A, McNicholas PM. Inactivation of sterol Delta5, 6-desaturase attenuates virulence in Candida albicans. Antimicrob Agents Chemother. 2005;49:3646–51.
13. Kelly SL, Lamb DC, Taylor M, Corran AJ, Baldwin BC, Powderly WG. Resistance to amphotericin B associated with defective sterol delta 8–7 isomerase in a *Cryptococcus neoformans* strain from an AIDS patient. FEMS Microbiol Lett. 1994;122:39–42.
14. Vandeputte P, Tronchin G, Berges T, Hennequin C, Chabasse D, Bouchara JP. Reduced susceptibility to polyenes associated with a missense mutation in the *ERG6* gene in a clinical isolate of *Candida glabrata* with pseudohyphal growth. Antimicrob Agents Chemother. 2007;51:982–90.
15. Vandeputte P, Tronchin G, Larcher G, et al. A nonsense mutation in the *ERG6* gene leads to reduced susceptibility to polyenes in a clinical isolate of *Candida glabrata*. Antimicrob Agents Chemother. 2008;52:3701–9.
16. Sanglard D, Ischer F, Parkinson T, Falconer D, Bille J. Candida albicans mutations in the ergosterol biosynthetic pathway and resistance to several antifungal agents. Antimicrob Agents Chemother. 2003;47:2404–12.
17. Dick JD, Merz WG, Saral R. Incidence of polyene-resistant yeasts recovered from clinical specimens. Antimicrob Agents Chemother. 1980;18:158–63.
18. Sokol-Anderson ML, Brajtburg J, Medoff G. Amphotericin B-induced oxidative damage and killing of *Candida albicans*. J Infect Dis. 1986;154:76–83.
19. Polak A. Mode of action studies. In: Ryley JF, editor. Chemotherapy of fungal Diseases. Berlin: Springer-Verlag; 1990. p. 153–82.
20. Coleman DC, Rinaldi MG, Haynes KA, et al. Importance of *Candida* species other than *Candida albicans* as opportunistic pathogens. Med Mycol. 1998;36:156–65.
21. Groll AH, Piscitelli SC, Walsh TJ. Clinical pharmacology of systemic antifungal agents: a comprehensive review of agents in clinical use, current investigational compounds, and putative targets for antifungal drug development. Adv Pharmacol. 1998;44:343–500.
22. Vanden Bossche H, Marichal P, Odds FC. Molecular mechanisms of drug resistance in fungi. Trends in Microbiology. 1994;2: 393–400.
23. Dodgson AR, Dodgson KJ, Pujol C, Pfaller MA, Soll DR. Clade-specific flucytosine resistance is due to a single nucleotide change in the *FUR1* gene of *Candida albicans*. Antimicrob Agents Chemother. 2004;48:2223–7.
24. Hope WW, Tabernero L, Denning DW, Anderson MJ. Molecular mechanisms of primary resistance to flucytosine in *Candida albicans*. Antimicrob Agents Chemother. 2004;48:4377–86.
25. Smith WJ, Drew RH, Perfect JR. Posaconazole's impact on prophylaxis and treatment of invasive fungal infections: an update. Expert Rev Anti Infect Ther. 2009;7:165–81.

26. Rex JH, Bennett JE, Sugar AM, et al. A randomized trial comparing fluconazole with amphotericin B for the treatment of candidemia in patients without neutropenia. Candidemia Study Group and the National Institute. N Engl J Med. 1994;331:1325–30.
27. White TC, Marr KA, Bowden RA. Clinical, cellular, and molecular factors that contribute to antifungal drug resistance. Clin Microbiol Rev. 1998;11:382–402.
28. Sanglard D, Bille J. Current understanding of the mode of action and of resistance mechanisms to conventional and emerging antifungal agents for treatment of *Candida* infections. In: Calderone R, editor. Candida and Candidiasis. Washington, DC: ASM press; 2002. p. 349–83.
29. Sanglard D, Kuchler K, Ischer F, Pagani JL, Monod M, Bille J. Mechanisms of resistance to azole antifungal agents in *Candida albicans* isolates from AIDS patients involve specific multidrug transporters. Antimicrob Agents Chemother. 1995;39:2378–86.
30. Sanglard D, Ischer F, Monod M, Bille J. Cloning of *Candida albicans* genes conferring resistance to azole antifungal agents: characterization of *CDR2*, a new multidrug ABC-transporter gene. Microbiology. 1997;143:405–16.
31. Moran GP, Sanglard D, Donnelly S, Shanley DB, Sullivan DJ, Coleman DC. Identification and expression of multidrug transporters responsible for fluconazole resistance in *Candida dubliniensis*. Antimicrob Agents Chemother. 1998;42:1819–30.
32. Perea S, Lopez-Ribot JL, Wickes BL, et al. Molecular mechanisms of fluconazole resistance in *Candida dubliniensis* isolates from human immunodeficiency virus-infected patients with oropharyngeal candidiasis. Antimicrob Agents Chemother. 2002;46:1695–703.
33. Barchiesi F, Calabrese D, Sanglard D, et al. Experimental induction of fluconazole resistance in *Candida tropicalis* ATCC 750. Antimicrob Agents Chemother. 2000;44:1578–84.
34. Sanglard D, Ischer F, Bille J. Role of ATP-binding-cassette transporter genes in high-frequency acquisition of resistance to azole antifungals in *Candida glabrata*. Antimicrob Agents Chemother. 2001;45:1174–83.
35. Sanglard D, Ischer F, Calabrese D, Majcherczyk PA, Bille J. The ATP binding cassette transporter gene *CgCDR1* from *Candida glabrata* is involved in the resistance of clinical isolates to azole antifungal agents. Antimicrob Agents Chemother. 1999;43:2753–65.
36. Torelli R, Posteraro B, Ferrari S, et al. The ATP-binding cassette transporter–encoding gene *CgSNQ2* is contributor to the CgPdr1-dependent azole resistance in *Candida glabrata*. Mol Microbiol. 2008;68:186–201.
37. Posteraro B, Sanguinetti M, Sanglard D, et al. Identification and characterization of a *Cryptococcus neoformans* ATP binding cassette (ABC) transporter-encoding gene, *CnAFR1*, involved in the resistance to fluconazole. Mol Microbiol. 2003;47:357–71.
38. Slaven JW, Anderson MJ, Sanglard D, et al. Induced expression of a novel *Aspergillus fumigatus* ABC transporter gene, atrF, in response to itraconazole. Fungal Genet Biol. 2002;36:199–206.
39. Nakamura K, Niimi M, Niimi K, et al. Functional expression of *Candida albicans* drug efflux pump Cdr1p in a *Saccharomyces cerevisiae* strain deficient in membrane transporters. Antimicrob Agents Chemother. 2001;45:3366–74.
40. Wirsching S, Michel S, Morschhauser J. Targeted gene disruption in *Candida albicans* wild-type strains: the role of the *MDR1* gene in fluconazole resistance of clinical *Candida albicans* isolates. Mol Microbiol. 2000;36:856–65.
41. Wirsching S, Moran GP, Sullivan DJ, Coleman DC, Morschhauser J. *MDR1*-mediated drug resistance in *Candida dubliniensis*. Antimicrob Agents Chemother. 2001;45:3416–21.
42. Sanglard D, Ischer F, Monod M, Bille J. Susceptibilities of *Candida albicans* multidrug transporter mutants to various antifungal agents and other metabolic inhibitors. Antimicrob Agents Chemother. 1996;40:2300–5.
43. Marr KA, Lyons CN, Rustad TR, Bowden RA, White TC, Rustad T. Rapid, transient fluconazole resistance in *Candida albicans* is associated with increased mRNA levels of *CDR*. Antimicrob Agents Chemother. 1998;42:2584–9.
44. Marr KA, Lyons CN, Ha K, Rustad TR, White TC. Inducible azole resistance associated with a heterogeneous phenotype in *Candida albicans*. Antimicrob Agents Chemother. 2001;45:52–9.
45. Ferrari S, Ischer F, Calabrese D, et al. Gain of function mutations in *CgPDR1* of *Candida glabrata* not only mediate antifungal resistance but also enhance virulence. PLoS Pathog. 2009;5:e1000268.
46. Brun S, Berges T, Poupard P, et al. Mechanisms of azole resistance in petite mutants of *Candida glabrata*. Antimicrob Agents Chemother. 2004;48:1788–96.
47. De Micheli M, Bille J, Schueller C, Sanglard D. A common drug-responsive element mediates the upregulation of the *Candida albicans* ABC transporters *CDR1* and *CDR2*, two genes involved in antifungal drug resistance. Mol Microbiol. 2002;43:1197–214.
48. Wirsching S, Michel S, Kohler G, Morschhauser J. Activation of the multiple drug resistance gene *MDR1* in fluconazole- resistant, clinical *Candida albicans* strains is caused by mutations in a trans-regulatory factor. J Bacteriol. 2000;182:400–4.
49. Karnani N, Gaur NA, Jha S, et al. SRE1 and SRE2 are two specific steroid-responsive modules of *Candida* drug resistance gene 1 (*CDR1*) promoter. Yeast. 2004;21:219–39.
50. Gaur NA, Puri N, Karnani N, Mukhopadhyay G, Goswami SK, Prasad R. Identification of a negative regulatory element which regulates basal transcription of a multidrug resistance gene *CDR1* of *Candida albicans*. FEMS Yeast Res. 2004;4:389–99.
51. Hikkel I, Lucau-Danila A, Delaveau T, Marc P, Devaux F, Jacq C. A general strategy to uncover transcription factor properties identifies a new regulator of drug resistance in yeast. J Biol Chem. 2003;278:11427–32.
52. Kren A, Mamnun YM, Bauer BE, et al. War1p, a novel transcription factor controlling weak acid stress response in yeast. Mol Cell Biol. 2003;23:1775–85.
53. Mendizabal I, Rios G, Mulet JM, Serrano R, de Larrinoa IF. Yeast putative transcription factors involved in salt tolerance. FEBS Lett. 1998;425:323–8.
54. Schjerling P, Holmberg S. Comparative amino acid sequence analysis of the C6 zinc cluster family of transcriptional regulators. Nucleic Acids Res. 1996;24:4599–607.
55. Rustad TR, Stevens DA, Pfaller MA, White TC. Homozygosity at the *Candida albicans* MTL locus associated with azole resistance. Microbiology. 2002;148:1061–72.
56. Coste AT, Karababa M, Ischer F, Bille J, Sanglard D. *TAC1*, Transcriptional activator of *CDR* genes, is a new transcription factor involved in the regulation of *Candida albicans* ABC transporters *CDR1* and *CDR2*. Eukaryot Cell. 2004;3:1639–52.
57. Raad I, Chatzinikolaou I, Chaiban G, et al. In vitro and ex vivo activities of minocycline and EDTA against microorganisms embedded in biofilm on catheter surfaces. Antimicrob Agents Chemother. 2003;47:3580–5.
58. Riggle PJ, Kumamoto CA. Transcriptional regulation of *MDR1*, encoding a drug efflux determinant, in fluconazole-resistant *Candida albicans* strains through an Mcm1p binding site. Eukaryot Cell. 2006;5:1957–68.
59. Rognon B, Kozovska Z, Coste AT, Pardini G, Sanglard D. Identification of promoter elements responsible for the regulation of *MDR1* from *Candida albicans*, a major facilitator transporter involved in azole resistance. Microbiology. 2006;152:3701–22.
60. Harry JB, Oliver BG, Song JL, et al. Drug-induced regulation of the *MDR1* promoter in *Candida albicans*. Antimicrob Agents Chemother. 2005;49:2785–92.
61. Nguyen DT, Alarco AM, Raymond M. Multiple Yap1p-binding sites mediate induction of the yeast major facilitator *FLR1* gene in

response to drugs, oxidants, and alkylating agents. J Biol Chem. 2001;276:1138–45.

62. Morschhauser J, Barker KS, Liu TT, Bla BWJ, Homayouni R, Rogers PD. The transcription factor Mrr1p controls expression of the *MDR1* efflux pump and mediates multidrug resistance in *Candida albicans*. PLoS Pathog. 2007;3:e164.
63. Schubert S, Rogers PD, Morschhauser J. Gain-of-function mutations in the transcription factor *MRR1* are responsible for overexpression of the *MDR1* efflux pump in fluconazole-resistant *Candida dubliniensis* strains. Antimicrob Agents Chemother. 2008;52:4274–80.
64. Vermitsky JP, Edlind TD. Azole resistance in *Candida glabrata*: coordinate upregulation of multidrug transporters and evidence for a Pdr1-like transcription factor. Antimicrob Agents Chemother. 2004;48:3773–81.
65. Tsai HF, Krol AA, Sarti KE, Bennett JE. *Candida glabrata PDR1*, a transcriptional regulator of a pleiotropic drug resistance network, mediates azole resistance in clinical isolates and petite mutants. Antimicrob Agents Chemother. 2006;50:1384–92.
66. Vermitsky JP, Earhart KD, Smith WL, Homayouni R, Edlind TD, Rogers PD. Pdr1 regulates multidrug resistance in *Candida glabrata*: gene disruption and genome-wide expression studies. Mol Microbiol. 2006;61:704–22.
67. MacPherson S, Larochelle M, Turcotte B. A fungal family of transcriptional regulators: the zinc cluster proteins. Microbiol Mol Biol Rev. 2006;70:583–604.
68. Thakur JK, Arthanari H, Yang F, et al. A nuclear receptor-like pathway regulating multidrug resistance in fungi. Nature. 2008;452:604–9.
69. Marichal P, Koymans L, Willemsens S, et al. Contribution of mutations in the cytochrome P450 14α-demethylase (Erg11p, Cyp51p) to azole resistance in *Candida albicans*. Microbiology. 1999;145:2701–13.
70. Asai K, Tsuchimori N, Okonogi K, Perfect JR, Gotoh O, Yoshida Y. Formation of azole-resistant *Candida albicans* by mutation of sterol 14α−demethylase P450. Antimicrob Agents Chemother. 1999;43:1163–9.
71. Kelly SL, Lamb DC, Kelly DE. Y132H substitution in *Candida albicans* sterol 14alpha-demethylase confers fluconazole resistance by preventing binding to haem. FEMS Microbiol Lett. 1999;180:171–5.
72. Kelly SL, Lamb DC, Loeffler J, Einsele H, Kelly DE. The G464S amino acid substitution in *Candida albicans* sterol 14alpha- demethylase causes fluconazole resistance in the clinic through reduced affinity. Biochem Biophys Res Commun. 1999;262:174–9.
73. Favre B, Didmon M, Ryder NS. Multiple amino acid substitutions in lanosterol 14α-demethylase contribute to azole resistance in *Candida albicans*. Microbiology. 1999;145:2715–25.
74. Sanglard D, Ischer F, Koymans L, Bille J. Amino acid substitutions in the cytochrome P450 lanosterol 14α-demethylase (CYP51A1) from azole-resistant *Candida albicans* clinical isolates contributing to the resistance to azole antifungal agents. Antimicrob Agents Chemother. 1998;42:241–53.
75. Lamb DC, Kelly DE, White TC, Kelly SL. The R467K amino acid substitution in *Candida albicans* sterol 14alpha- demethylase causes drug resistance through reduced affinity. Antimicrob Agents Chemother. 2000;44:63–7.
76. Kudo M, Ohi M, Aoyama Y, Nitahara Y, Chung SK, Yoshida Y. Effects of Y132H and F145L substitutions on the activity, azole resistance and spectral properties of *Candida albicans* sterol 14-demethylase P450 (CYP51): A live example showing the selection of altered P450 through interaction with environmental compounds. J Biochem (Tokyo). 2005;137:625–32.
77. Diaz-Guerra TM, Mellado E, Cuenca-Estrella M, Rodriguez-Tudela JL. A point mutation in the 14alpha-sterol demethylase gene *Cyp51A* contributes to itraconazole resistance in *Aspergillus fumigatus*. Antimicrob Agents Chemother. 2003;47:1120–4.
78. Mann PA, Parmegiani RM, Wei SQ, et al. Mutations in *Aspergillus fumigatus* resulting in reduced susceptibility to posaconazole appear to be restricted to a single amino acid in the cytochrome P450 14alpha-demethylase. Antimicrob Agents Chemother. 2003;47:577–81.
79. Garcia-Effron G, Dilger A, Alcazar-Fuoli L, Park S, Mellado E, Perlin DS. Rapid detection of triazole antifungal resistance in *Aspergillus fumigatus*. J Clin Microbiol. 2008;46:1200–6.
80. Mellado E, Garcia-Effron G, Alcazar-Fuoli L, et al. A new *Aspergillus fumigatus* resistance mechanism conferring in vitro cross-resistance to azole antifungals involves a combination of *cyp51A* alterations. Antimicrob Agents Chemother. 2007;51:1897–904.
81. Snelders E, van der Lee HA, Kuijpers J, et al. Emergence of azole resistance in *Aspergillus fumigatus* and spread of a single resistance mechanism. PLoS Med. 2008;5:e219.
82. Rodero L, Mellado E, Rodriguez AC, et al. G484S amino acid substitution in lanosterol 14-alpha demethylase (*ERG11*) is related to fluconazole resistance in a recurrent *Cryptococcus neoformans* clinical isolate. Antimicrob Agents Chemother. 2003;47:3653–6.
83. Sionov E, Chang YC, Garraffo HM, Kwon-Chung KJ. Heteroresistance to fluconazole in *Cryptococcus neoformans* is intrinsic and associated with virulence. Antimicrob Agents Chemother. 2009;53:2804–15.
84. Vandeputte P, Larcher G, Berges T, Renier G, Chabasse D, Bouchara JP. Mechanisms of azole resistance in a clinical isolate of *Candida tropicalis*. Antimicrob Agents Chemother. 2005;49:4608–15.
85. White TC. Increased mRNA levels of *ERG16*, *CDR*, and *MDR1* correlate with increases in azole resistance in *Candida albicans* isolates from a patient infected with human immunodeficiency virus. Antimicrob Agents Chemother. 1997;41:1482–7.
86. Perea S, Lopez-Ribot JL, Kirkpatrick WR, et al. Prevalence of molecular mechanisms of resistance to azole antifungal agents in *Candida albicans* strains displaying high-level fluconazole resistance isolated from human immunodeficiency virus-infected patients. Antimicrob Agents Chemother. 2001;45:2676–84.
87. Marichal P, Vanden Bossche H, Odds FC, et al. Molecular biological characterization of an azole-resistant *Candida glabrata* isolate. Antimicrob Agents Chemother. 1997;41:2229–37.
88. Vik A, Rine J. Upc2p and Ecm22p, dual regulators of sterol biosynthesis in *Saccharomyces cerevisiae*. Mol Cell Biol. 2001;21: 6395–405.
89. MacPherson S, Akache B, Weber S, De Deken X, Raymond M, Turcotte B. *Candida albicans* zinc cluster protein Upc2p confers resistance to antifungal drugs and is an activator of ergosterol biosynthetic genes. Antimicrob Agents Chemother. 2005;49:1745–52.
90. Silver PM, Oliver BG, White TC. Role of *Candida albicans* transcription factor Upc2p in drug resistance and sterol metabolism. Eukaryot Cell. 2004;3:1391–7.
91. Oliver BG, Song JL, Choiniere JH, White TC. cis-Acting Elements within the Candida albicans ERG11 Promoter Mediate the Azole Response through Transcription Factor Upc2p. Eukaryot Cell. 2007;6:2231–9.
92. Carvajal E, van den Hazel HB, Cybularz-Kolaczkowska A, Balzi E, Goffeau A. Molecular and phenotypic characterization of yeast *PDR1* mutants that show hyperactive transcription of various ABC multidrug transporter genes. Mol Gen Genet. 1997;256:406–15.
93. Coste AT, Turner V, Ischer F, et al. A mutation in Tac1p, a transcription factor regulating *CDR1* and *CDR2*, is coupled with loss of heterozygosity at Chromosome 5 to mediate antifungal resistance in *Candida albicans*. Genetics. 2006;172:2139–56.
94. Dunkel N, Blass J, Rogers PD, Morschhauser J. Mutations in the multidrug resistance regulator *MRR1*, followed by loss of heterozygosity, are the main cause of *MDR1* overexpression in fluconazole-resistant *Candida albicans* strains. Mol Microbiol. 2008;69:827–40.
95. Dunkel N, Liu TT, Barker KS, Homayouni R, Morschhäuser J, Rogers PD. A gain-of-function mutation in the transcription factor Upc2p causes upregulation of ergosterol biosynthesis genes and

increased fluconazole resistance in a clinical *Candida albicans* isolate. Eukaryot Cell. 2008;7:1180–90.

96. Coste A, Crittin J, Bauser C, Rohde B, Sanglard D. Functional analysis of cis- and trans- acting elements of the *Candida albicans* *CDR2* promoter with a novel promoter reporter system. Eukaryot Cell. 2009;8:1250–67.
97. Znaidi S, De Deken X, Weber S, Rigby T, Nantel A, Raymond M. The zinc cluster transcription factor Tac1p regulates PDR16 expression in *Candida albicans*. Mol Microbiol. 2007;66:440–52.
98. Chen CG, Yang YL, Shih HI, Su CL, Lo HJ. CaNdt80 is involved in drug resistance in *Candida albicans* by regulating *CDR1*. Antimicrob Agents Chemother. 2004;48:4505–12.
99. Crowley JH, Leak Jr FW, Shianna KV, Tove S, Parks LW. A mutation in a purported regulatory gene affects control of sterol uptake in *Saccharomyces cerevisiae*. J Bacteriol. 1998;180:4177–83.
100. Pinjon E, Moran GP, Jackson CJ, et al. Molecular mechanisms of itraconazole resistance in *Candida dubliniensis*. Antimicrob Agents Chemother. 2003;47:2424–37.
101. Miyazaki Y, Geber A, Miyazaki H, et al. Cloning, sequencing, expression and allelic sequence diversity of *ERG3* (C-5 sterol desaturase gene) in *Candida albicans*. Gene. 1999;236:43–51.
102. Coste A, Selmecki A, Forche A, et al. Genotypic evolution of azole resistance mechanisms in sequential *Candida albicans* isolates. Eukaryot Cell. 2007;6:1889–904.
103. Selmecki A, Forche A, Berman J. Aneuploidy and isochromosome formation in drug-resistant *Candida albicans*. Science. 2006;313:367–70.
104. Polakova S, Blume C, Zarate JA, et al. Formation of new chromosomes as a virulence mechanism in yeast *Candida glabrata*. Proc Natl Acad Sci U S A. 2009;106:2688–93.
105. Ramage G, Bachmann S, Patterson TF, Wickes BL, Lopez-Ribot JL. Investigation of multidrug efflux pumps in relation to fluconazole resistance in *Candida albicans* biofilms. J Antimicrob Chemother. 2002;49:973–80.
106. LaFleur MD, Kumamoto CA, Lewis K. *Candida albicans* biofilms produce antifungal-tolerant persister cells. Antimicrob Agents Chemother. 2006;50:3839–46.
107. Lewis K. Persister cells, dormancy and infectious disease. Nat Rev Microbiol. 2007;5:48–56.
108. Mukherjee PK, Chandra J, Kuhn DM, Ghannoum MA. Mechanism of fluconazole resistance in *Candida albicans* biofilms: phase-specific role of efflux pumps and membrane sterols. Infect Immun. 2003;71:4333–40.
109. Borecka-Melkusova S, Moran GP, Sullivan DJ, Kucharikova S, Chorvat Jr D, Bujdakova H. The expression of genes involved in the ergosterol biosynthesis pathway in *Candida albicans* and *Candida dubliniensis* biofilms exposed to fluconazole. Mycoses. 2009;52:118–28.
110. Cao YY, Cao YB, Xu Z, et al. cDNA microarray analysis of differential gene expression in *Candida albicans* biofilm exposed to farnesol. Antimicrob Agents Chemother. 2005;49:584–9.
111. Nett J, Lincoln L, Marchillo K, et al. Putative role of beta-1, 3 glucans in *Candida albicans* biofilm resistance. Antimicrob Agents Chemother. 2007;51:510–20.
112. Kurtz MB, Douglas CM. Lipopeptide inhibitors of fungal glucan synthase. J Med Vet Mycol. 1997;35:79–86.
113. Mio T, Adachi-Shimizu M, Tachibana Y, et al. Cloning of the *Candida albicans* homolog of *Saccharomyces cerevisiae* GSC1/FKS1 and its involvement in beta-1, 3-glucan synthesis. J Bacteriol. 1997;179:4096–105.
114. Pereira M, Felipe MS, Brigido MM, Soares CM, Azevedo MO. Molecular cloning and characterization of a glucan synthase gene from the human pathogenic fungus *Paracoccidioides brasiliensis*. Yeast. 2000;16:451–62.
115. Douglas CM, D'Ippolito JA, Shei GJ, et al. Identification of the FKS1 gene of Candida albicans as the essential target of 1, 3-beta-D-glucan synthase inhibitors. Antimicrob Agents Chemother. 1997;41:2471–9.
116. Thompson JR, Douglas CM, Li W, et al. A glucan synthase *FKS1* homolog in *Cryptococcus neoformans* is single copy and encodes an essential function. J Bacteriol. 1999;181:444–53.
117. Onishi J, Meinz M, Thompson J, et al. Discovery of novel antifungal (1, 3)-beta-D-glucan synthase inhibitors. Antimicrob Agents Chemother. 2000;44:368–77.
118. Bowman JC, Hicks PS, Kurtz MB, et al. The antifungal echinocandin caspofungin acetate kills growing cells of *Aspergillus fumigatus* in vitro. Antimicrob Agents Chemother. 2002;46:3001–12.
119. Arikan S, Lozano-Chiu M, Paetznick V, Rex JH. In vitro susceptibility testing methods for caspofungin against *Aspergillus* and *Fusarium* isolates. Antimicrob Agents Chemother. 2001;45:327–30.
120. Douglas CM, Marrinan JA, Li W, Kurtz MB. A *Saccharomyces cerevisiae* mutant with echinocandin-resistant 1, 3-beta- D-glucan synthase. J Bacteriol. 1994;176:5686–96.
121. Frost DJ, Knapp M, Brandt K, Shadron A, Goldman RC. Characterization of a lipopeptide-resistant strain of *Candida albicans*. Can J Microbiol. 1997;43:122–8.
122. Park S, Kelly R, Kahn JN, et al. Specific substitutions in the echinocandin target Fks1p account for reduced susceptibility of rare laboratory and clinical *Candida* sp. isolates. Antimicrob Agents Chemother. 2005;49:3264–73.
123. Perlin DS. Resistance to echinocandin-class antifungal drugs. Drug Resist Updates. 2007;10:121–30.
124. Garcia-Effron G, Kontoyiannis DP, Lewis RE, Perlin DS. Caspofungin-resistant *Candida tropicalis* strains causing breakthrough fungemia in patients at high risk for hematologic malignancies. Antimicrob Agents Chemother. 2008;52:4181–3.
125. Cleary JD, Garcia-Effron G, Chapman SW, Perlin DS. Reduced *Candida glabrata* susceptibility secondary to an *FKS1* mutation developed during candidemia treatment. Antimicrob Agents Chemother. 2008;52:2263–5.
126. Rocha EM, Garcia-Effron G, Park S, Perlin DS. A Ser678Pro substitution in Fks1p confers resistance to echinocandin drugs in *Aspergillus fumigatus*. Antimicrob Agents Chemother. 2007;51:4174–6.
127. Garcia-Effron G, Katiyar SK, Park S, Edlind TD, Perlin DS. A naturally occurring proline-to-alanine amino acid change in Fks1p in *Candida parapsilosis*, *Candida orthopsilosis*, and *Candida metapsilosis* accounts for reduced echinocandin susceptibility. Antimicrob Agents Chemother. 2008;52:2305–12.
128. Thompson GR, Wiederhold NP, Vallor AC, Villareal NC, Lewis JS, Patterson TF. Development of caspofungin resistance following prolonged therapy for invasive candidiasis secondary to *Candida glabrata* infection. Antimicrob Agents Chemother. 2008;52:3783–5.
129. Katiyar S, Pfaller M, Edlind T. *Candida albicans* and *Candida glabrata* clinical isolates exhibiting reduced echinocandin susceptibility. Antimicrob Agents Chemother. 2006;50:2892–4.
130. Reinoso-Martin C, Schuller C, Schuetzer-Muehlbauer M, Kuchler K. The yeast protein kinase C cell integrity pathway mediates tolerance to the antifungal drug caspofungin through activation of Slt2p mitogen-activated protein kinase signaling. Eukaryot Cell. 2003;2:1200–10.
131. Arendrup MC, Perkhofer S, Howard SJ, et al. Establishing in vitro-in vivo correlations for *Aspergillus fumigatus*: The challenge of azoles versus echinocandins. Antimicrob Agents Chemother. 2008;52:3504–11.
132. Martins MD, Lozano-Chiu M, Rex JH. Declining rates of oropharyngeal candidiasis and carriage of *Candida albicans* associated with trends toward reduced rates of carriage of fluconazole-resistant *C. albicans* in human immunodeficiency virus-infected patients. Clin Infect Dis. 1998;27:1291–4.
133. Sobel JD, Ohmit SE, Schuman P, et al. The evolution of *Candida* species and fluconazole susceptibility among oral and vaginal

isolates recovered from human immunodeficiency virus (HIV)-seropositive and at-risk HIV-seronegative women. J Infect Dis. 2000;183:286–93.
134. Shahid Z, Sobel JD. Reduced fluconazole susceptibility of *Candida albicans* isolates in women with recurrent vulvovaginal candidiasis: Effects of long-term fluconazole therapy. Diagn Microbiol Infect Dis. 2009;64:354–6.
135. Bulik CC, Sobel JD, Nailor MD. Susceptibility profile of vaginal isolates of *Candida albicans* prior to and following fluconazole introduction – impact of two decades. Mycoses 2009. Epub ahead of print.
136. Sanglard D, Odds FC. Resistance of *Candida* species to antifungal agents: molecular mechanisms and clinical consequences. Lancet Infect Dis. 2002;2:73–85.
137. Lass-Florl C. The changing face of epidemiology of invasive fungal disease in Europe. Mycoses. 2009;52:197–205.
138. Howard SJ, Cerar D, Anderson MJ, et al. Frequency and evolution of Azole resistance in *Aspergillus fumigatus* associated with treatment failure. Emerg Infect Dis. 2009;15:1068–76.
139. Brandt ME, Pfaller MA, Hajjeh RA, et al. Trends in antifungal drug susceptibility of *Cryptococcus neoformans* isolates in the United States: 1992 to 1994 and 1996 to 1998. Antimicrob Agents Chemother. 2001;45:3065–9.
140. Gehrt A, Peter J, Pizzo PA, Walsh TJ. Effect of increasing inoculum sizes of pathogenic filamentous fungi on MICs of antifungal agents by broth microdilution method. J Clin Microbiol. 1995;33:1302–7.
141. Pfaller MA, Messer SA, Hollis RJ, et al. Trends in species distribution and susceptibility to fluconazole among blood stream isolates of *Candida* species in the United States. Diagn Microbiol Infect Dis. 1999;33:217–22.
142. Pfaller MA, Messer SA, Hollis RJ, et al. In vitro susceptibilities of *Candida* bloodstream isolates to the new triazole antifungal agents BMS-207147, SCH 56592, and voriconazole. Antimicrob Agents Chemother. 1998;42:3242–4.
143. Yildiran ST, Saracli MA, Fothergill AW, Rinaldi MG. In vitro susceptibility of environmental *Cryptococcus neoformans* variety neoformans isolates from Turkey to six antifungal agents, including SCH56592 and voriconazole. Eur J Clin Microbiol Infect Dis. 2000;19:317–9.
144. Yamazumi T, Pfaller MA, Messer SA, Houston A, Hollis RJ, Jones RN. In vitro activities of ravuconazole (BMS-207147) against 541 clinical isolates of *Cryptococcus neoformans*. Antimicrob Agents Chemother. 2000;44:2883–6.
145. Uchida K, Yokota N, Yamaguchi H. In vitro antifungal activity of posaconazole against various pathogenic fungi. Int J Antimicrob Agents. 2001;18:167–72.
146. Mosquera J, Denning DW. Azole cross-resistance in *Aspergillus fumigatus*. Antimicrob Agents Chemother. 2002;46:556–7.
147. Bartizal K, Gill CJ, Abruzzo GK, et al. In vitro preclinical evaluation studies with the echinocandin antifungal MK-0991 (L-743, 872). Antimicrob Agents Chemother. 1997;41:2326–32.
148. Mikamo H, Sato Y, Tamaya T. In vitro antifungal activity of FK463, a new water-soluble echinocandin- like lipopeptide. J Antimicrob Chemother. 2000;46:485–7.
149. Chavez M, Bernal S, Valverde A, Gutierrez MJ, Quindos G, Mazuelos EM. In-vitro activity of voriconazole (UK-109,496), LY303366 and other antifungal agents against oral *Candida* spp. isolates from HIV-infected patients. J Antimicrob Chemother. 1999;44:697–700.
150. Pfaller MA, Messer SA, Coffman S. In vitro susceptibilities of clinical yeast isolates to a new echinocandin derivative, LY303366, and other antifungal agents. Antimicrob Agents Chemother. 1997;41:763–6.
151. Tawara S, Ikeda F, Maki K, et al. In vitro activities of a new lipopeptide antifungal agent, FK463, against a variety of clinically important fungi. Antimicrob Agents Chemother. 2000;44:57–62.
152. Espinel-Ingroff A. Comparison of In vitro activities of the new triazole SCH56592 and the echinocandins MK-0991 (L-743, 872) and LY303366 against opportunistic filamentous and dimorphic fungi and yeasts. J Clin Microbiol. 1998;36:2950–6.
153. Espinel-Ingroff A. In vitro antifungal activities of anidulafungin and micafungin, licensed agents and the investigational triazole posaconazole as determined by NCCLS methods for 12, 052 fungal isolates: review of the literature. Rev Iberoam Micol. 2003;20:121–36.
154. Arikan S, Yurdakul P, Hascelik G. Comparison of two methods and three end points in determination of in vitro activity of micafungin against *Aspergillus* spp. Antimicrob Agents Chemother. 2003;47:2640–3.

Combination Antifungal Therapy

Elizabeth Dodds Ashley and Melissa D. Johnson

Invasive fungal infections continue to cause significant morbidity and mortality among hospitalized patients. In particular, recent studies indicate an increase in the incidence of mould infections among transplant recipients, and *Candida* species have risen to be the third most common pathogen isolated among intensive care unit patients [1, 2]. Advances in modern medical treatment have led to growth in the at-risk population for fungal infections [3]. For example, *Cryptococcus neoformans* has re-emerged as a growing cause of invasive fungal disease due in large part to the development of novel immune therapy for malignancies, rheumatologic disorders, and management of rejection in transplant populations [4]. Unfortunately, these infections are associated with failures and high rates of relapse even when patients receive recommended therapy [5, 6]. Treatment of invasive mycoses continues to be challenging and complicated by the net state of immunosuppression among infected hosts combined with relative lack of efficacy, significant toxicity, drug–drug interactions, and drug resistance associated with available antifungal agents.

Since 2000, the antifungal market has expanded greatly, with FDA approval of three agents belonging to a novel class, the echinocandins, as well as two new agents in the well-established azole class. In addition, clinical development has continued to progress on other new antifungal agents with unique mechanisms of action. These advances have expanded treatment options for patients with invasive mycoses. Given the addition of agents with novel targets of antifungal activity, the permutations available for combination treatment approaches have grown significantly. Unfortunately, while the concept of combination therapy is appealing to clinicians hoping to improve outcomes of patients with systemic mycoses, most of these antifungal combinations have not been evaluated in prospective controlled clinical trials. Numerous in vitro investigations and trials in animal models of fungal infection have been performed. Many of these data are conflicting, however, which further limits our ability to make generalizations or predictions about efficacy of various combinations of antifungal agents in humans with invasive mycoses. It seems clear that combinations will continue to be pursued with vigor in the hopes of improving patient outcomes and identifying optimal therapy for these serious infections.

This chapter summarizes the rationale behind combination antifungal therapy and includes a discussion of the relative benefits and risks of such an approach. Available data from in vitro investigations, animal models of infection and, where possible, human trials are described. We also discuss potential areas for future exploration in this arena.

E. Dodds Ashley (✉)
School of Medicine and Dentistry,
University of Rochester Medical Center, Rochester, NY, USA
e-mail: Elizabeth_doddsashley@urmc.rochester.edu

Rationale for Combination Antifungal Therapy

The rationale for combination antifungal therapy has been discussed extensively in recent literature [7–11]. While combination therapy is commonplace in other disease states such as neoplasms, hypertension, dyslipidemia, and infections, including endocarditis, HIV infection, and mycobacterial disease, its use in fungal infections has been historically confined to cryptococcal meningitis. Since morbidity and mortality of invasive mycoses remain unacceptably high, many clinicians feel justified in pursuing treatments that would hopefully improve patient outcomes.

With that in mind, there are a number of scenarios in which combination antifungal therapy may provide benefit. These include a desire to (1) increase antifungal killing activity of one or more antifungal agents; (2) broaden the spectrum of antifungal activity to cover more pathogens or potentially resistant pathogens; (3) reduce emergence of resistant pathogens; (4) potentially minimize drug-associated toxicities by reducing dosages of antifungal agents in combination; and (5) deliver antifungal agents to multiple body sites, capitalizing on the unique spectrum of activity and/or

C.A. Kauffman et al. (eds.), *Essentials of Clinical Mycology*,
DOI 10.1007/978-1-4419-6640-7_10, © Springer Science+Business Media, LLC 2011

pharmacokinetics of each drug while limiting toxicity [7, 10, 12]. Before being routinely adopted in clinical practice, however, a few potentially detrimental effects of antifungal combinations need to be addressed, including (1) antagonism, (2) increased cost in the absence of proven clinical benefits, and (3) increased potential for drug interactions and/or toxicities [8, 10].

Potential Benefits of Combination Antifungal Therapies

Synergy is defined as increasing activity of one or more agents beyond that expected when using either agent alone. This potential for synergy is perhaps the most compelling argument behind combination antifungal therapy. Classically, combination therapy in the clinical setting has involved simultaneous use of agents that are both considered therapies for the condition being studied, but there are numerous examples of nontraditional agents potentially benefitting antifungal regimens. Each of these will be addressed.

A second paradigm for use of agents in combination includes use of one or more agents to increase antifungal activity of a drug that has insufficient potency when used alone. Each of the antifungal agents released since 2000 has notable gaps in its spectrum of antifungal activity, which makes combinations necessary in order to cover potential causative pathogens or multiple fungi causing infection in some clinical settings. In the case of some fungal infections, often two agents are employed in attempts to avoid the toxicities associated with amphotericin B, as no other available antifungal agent offers the spectrum associated with amphotericin B.

The simultaneous use of flucytosine with other antifungals has been the classic example of a situation in which combination therapy reduces development of resistance to an antifungal agent. Resistance rapidly develops to flucytosine when used alone for systemic fungal infections; numerous investigations have demonstrated that addition of amphotericin B or an azole compound minimizes development of flucytosine resistance [13].

More recent investigations have suggested that HSP90 inhibitors (geldanamycin or radicicol) and/or calcineurin inhibitors (cyclosporine A or tacrolimus) can reduce azole resistance among laboratory strains of *Candida albicans* [14]. This reduction in resistance has been shown for echinocandins, as well, for which inhibition of HSP90 with geldanamycin or calcineurin with cyclosporine A reduced tolerance of *Aspergillus fumigatus* laboratory strains to caspofungin [15]. These agents, given in combination regimens with antifungal drugs, may prevent the development of resistance during prolonged treatment courses, but these theories require more prospective evaluation.

Several antifungal agents have well-established dose-related toxicities. These include nephrotoxicity with amphotericin B as well as visual and hepatic toxicities with voriconazole [16–18]. If synergistic activity could be confirmed between two agents, there is the possibility that lower doses of each agent might be used to reduce the likelihood of these toxicities. For example, in cryptococcal meningitis, lower doses of amphotericin B were successful when combined with flucytosine, and flucytosine dosages were successfully reduced from 150 mg/kg/day to 100 mg/kg/day when flucytosine was combined with amphotericin B [19, 20].

While some in vitro studies have attempted to assess the effect of varying drug concentrations, no published clinical trials have explored varying doses of the antifungal agents in combination to achieve synergy. This seems unlikely to occur based on the necessary sample size and potential risks of undertreatment. It is our opinion that in the clinical setting maximal doses of each agent should be employed and will hopefully result in at least additive, if not synergistic, results.

Another rationale for combination antifungal therapy involves using agents simultaneously to target multiple body sites. This approach has recently been employed in prophylaxis for invasive fungal infections in high-risk bone marrow transplant recipients, with a combination of systemic fluconazole and aerosolized amphotericin B lipid complex [21]. This combination allowed a less-toxic approach to prophylaxis via (1) delivery of amphotericin B directly to the lung (where *Aspergillus* species and other fungi are likely to initiate infection) and (2) delivery of fluconazole systemically to prevent invasive candidiasis and cryptococcosis. Such a strategy has also been proposed as a mechanism to treat both urinary tract fungal infections and systemic fungal infection when susceptibilities do not allow for administration of a single antifungal agent with adequate urinary penetration.

Potential Challenges with Use of Antifungals in Combination

Probably the most obvious concern with using antifungal agents in combination, particularly those with the same biologic target, is attenuation of the antifungal activity of one or both agents. For example, azole antifungals exert their antifungal activity by decreasing the production of ergosterol, the target for amphotericin B [22]. The azoles have, in fact, been implicated in reducing subsequent activity of amphotericin B in in vitro studies of pathogenic fungi, animal models, and human disease [7, 23]. Interestingly, however, this theoretical antagonism has not been consistently observed either in additional in vitro experiments or in human infection [24, 25]. In a prospective, multicenter randomized trial in which amphotericin B or placebo was added to fluconazole for the management of invasive candidiasis there was no difference in the primary outcome of time to failure ($p = 0.08$) [25]. In addition, overall treatment success was higher among those who received the combination of fluconazole and amphotericin B versus fluconazole plus placebo (69% vs 56% respectively, $p = 0.043$) In a study of HIV-associated cryptococcal meningitis, the combination of fluconazole and amphotericin B was associated with similar reduction in colony-forming units (CFU) in cerebrospinal fluid and mortality as amphotericin B alone [24]. While antagonism remains a valid concern for combination therapies, these studies suggest that in vitro findings require validation in vivo.

Increased costs are another concern with use of combination antifungal therapies. Since these medications currently top the drug budgets for many institutions, it is intuitive that if widespread use of combination antifungal therapy is adopted, these expenditures will increase. What is not known at the present time is whether or not these costs will be justified when the other complex variables associated with treatment of invasive fungal infections are considered. Once the clinical role of combination antifungal therapy is more definitively established, pharmacoeconomic studies will be needed.

Polypharmacy arising from the use of agents in combination can result in an increased risk of drug–drug interactions, toxicity, or both. For example, liver enzyme elevations have been associated with both azoles and echinocandins [22]. It is not clear if the risk of liver toxicity is increased when these agents are used concomitantly. Up to now, there are no large clinical trials to demonstrate safe use of this combination.

Many of the nontraditional agents demonstrating potential as part of antifungal combination regimens can prompt drug–drug interactions with coadministered antifungal agents. Renal toxicity has been associated with both polyenes and calcineurin inhibitors. Use of these agents together has been demonstrated to increase risk of renal failure among bone marrow transplant recipients [26]. Severe renal impairment is also a potential contraindication to the use of cyclodextrin-containing intravenous voriconazole or itraconazole, since accumulation of the vehicle may result in renal failure [22].

Drug–drug interactions with azoles via the cytochrome P450 isoenzyme system have been well documented, including cases of rhabdomyolysis when azoles are used with statins [27]. Rifampin has been proposed as a possible agent to potentiate the activity of many antifungal agents. This potent inducer of the hepatic cytochrome P450 enzyme and p-glycoprotein enzyme systems is known to decrease concentrations of many available antifungal agents, including voriconazole, posaconazole, and caspofungin [28, 29]. Calcineurin inhibitors also have important interactions with azoles. Many of these drug–drug interactions will need to be considered if newer alternative agents are employed as part of combination antifungal regimens. At present, the limited human data available for combination antifungal therapy are insufficient to evaluate these potential interactions.

Limitations of Available Studies of Combination Antifungal Therapy

In vitro investigations are by far the most commonly available studies regarding activity of antifungal drugs used in combination. However, there are numerous examples of conflicting data among in vitro investigations of the same antifungal combination for a single pathogen. The reasons for these differences are multifactorial and can in part be explained by variations in drug concentration, susceptibility pattern of the tested pathogen, and differences in experimental conditions. The reasons behind the variability shed light on another major limitation of these studies: namely, the lack of clinical applicability [10]. Often, results of in vitro combinations do not correlate with clinical data based on combinations for treatment of fungal disease. The most frequent example of this is the reported antagonism between amphotericin B and the azoles that arises from the overlapping mechanisms of action for these agents. This antagonism has been noted not only in vitro but also in animal models, but it is not always evident in trials of human disease. Unfortunately, these ex vivo investigations are frequently the only source of information readily available to guide clinicians.

Another significant limitation of these methods is the lack of consideration for the host immune system. The host response, which is essential to successful treatment of fungal disease, is not tested in these in vitro investigations. The addition of human serum to pharmacodynamic models of fungal disease can significantly alter the outcome and change the dynamic profile for the drugs of interest. It is a reasonable extrapolation that the same may be true for studies of combination antifungal therapy.

Animal models are able to overcome many limitations of in vitro studies due to the ability to factor in immune response of the host, although lack of correlation with human studies remains a problem. This is due in part to the difficulty in mimicking human infection in the various animal models of disease. Another confounding variable is the differences in the pharmacokinetic properties of the antifungal drug in animals compared to those properties in humans, making it difficult to determine the appropriate doses needed to simulate human drug exposure. Animal models are also limited in scale in that it is not as easy to run experiments in duplicate as it is with in vitro studies.

Human studies obviously provide the most meaningful data regarding safety and efficacy of combination antifungal therapies. However, these data are very difficult to obtain outside of the setting of individual case experiences. Recruitment to such studies is a major concern, given the large sample size that would be needed to reliably document a significant difference in outcome of combination therapy over traditional monotherapy regimens.

Although there is a rising incidence of invasive fungal infection, the overall number of such infections remains relatively low, thereby limiting the pool of potential subjects. It is also difficult to identify a homogeneous patient population to include in such studies. The risk factors for invasive fungal disease result in an infected population with significant underlying comorbidities, varying states of immunosuppression, and treatment considerations for underlying diseases that often preclude enrollment in a prospective, randomized trial [30].

The high mortality associated with many of these invasive fungal diseases and the uncertainty regarding appropriate treatment have led some to adopt combination therapy as routine practice without supportive clinical trials. In this scenario, questions regarding the ethics of conducting a controlled trial for these infections have been raised. Together, these factors pose significant barriers to completion of prospective evaluations of combination antifungal regimens that to date have not been overcome. Randomized, controlled trials of combination antifungal therapy for the most prevalent invasive fungal infections have been proposed or are currently underway, and we eagerly await the results of such investigations.

Until such data are available, clinicians rely on published human experiences that are primarily limited to case reports or retrospective single-center perspectives. The external validity of each of these small studies is always questioned given the inherent biases associated with the historic control groups and "n of 1" study designs.

Combination Antifungal Therapy for Yeast Infections

Cryptococcal Meningitis

The most common historic use of combination therapy in mycology has been the addition of flucytosine to amphotericin B for treatment of cryptococcal meningitis. This is traditionally associated with in vitro synergy (Table 1) [7, 13, 39]. In some

Table 1 Summary of in vitro and animal data for combination antifungal therapy

Pathogen	Combination	In vitro data	Animal data
Candida spp.	Flucytosine + amphotericin B	Synergy or indifference	Improved survival
	Flucytosine + azoles	Synergy, indifference, or antagonism	Improved clearance, no effect
	Amphotericin B + azoles	Antagonism	No effect, antagonism
	Amphotericin B + rifampin	Synergy	NR
Cryptococcus spp.	Amphotericin B + fluconazole	Indifference	Additive, synergistic
	Amphotericin B + flucytosine	Synergy, additive	Additive, synergistic
	Flucytosine + azole	Additive	Additive, synergistic, indifference
Aspergillus spp.	Amphotericin B + flucytosine	Additive, synergy, indifference	Improved survival or neutral
	Amphotericin B + rifampin	Synergy	NR
	Amphotericin B + echinocandin	Additive, synergy	Improved survival
	Azole + echinocandin	Synergy, additive, Indifference	Reduced mortality, indifference
	Amphotericin B + itraconazole	Antagonism	Antagonism, indifference
Scedosporium spp.	Amphotericin B + micafungin	Synergy to additive	Prolonged survival, decreased fungal burden
	Terbinafine + azole	Synergy	NR
	Amphotericin B + azole	Indifference to additive	NR
	Voriconazole + micafungin	Indifference to synergy	Prolonged survival, decreased fungal burden
	Voriconazole + other azole	Indifference	NR
Zygomycetes	Amphotericin B + rifampin	Additive to synergy	NR
	Amphotericin B + echinocandin	NR	Improved survival
	Amphotericin B + flucytosine	Additive	NR
	Amphotericin B + terbinafine	Additive to synergy	NR
	Voriconazole or itraconazole + terbinafine	Additive to synergy	NR
	Posaconazole + caspofungin	Synergy	NR
	Amphotericin B + posaconazole	Indifference	Prolonged survival
Fusarium spp	Amphotericin B + voriconazole	Antagonism to synergy	NR
	Amphotericin B + caspofungin	Additive to synergy	NR
	Amphotericin B + Anidulafungin	Indifference	NR
	Voriconazole + terbinafine	Synergy	NR
	Itraconazole + terbinafine	Indifference to synergy	NR
	Voriconazole + micafungin	Synergy	NR
	Anidulafungin + azole	Indifference	NR

NR: Not reported in available, published studies

Compiled from references 7, 11, 31-38.

reports, however, an indifferent, or merely additive effect in vitro has been demonstrated with the combination, and in a few cases antagonism has been shown between these two agents [7, 39]. A partial explanation for these conflicting results may be that in the studies which failed to document synergy, low drug concentrations or particularly resistant isolates were utilized [39]. In rabbit and murine models of cryptococcal meningitis caused by flucytosine-susceptible strains of *Cryptococcus neoformans*, improved survival rates and a decrease in organism burden were seen with the combination [7, 40].

Attention has also been given to the role of flucytosine in combination with azole antifungal agents for cryptococcal disease (Table 1). Results in experiments in both animal and ex vivo models trended toward synergistic effects when an azole agent, primarily fluconazole, was given concomitantly with flucytosine [41]. When higher doses of each agent were studied, high success rates were noticed in all treatment groups, making it difficult to interpret any incremental benefit from administering agents in combination.

In a large clinical trial of HIV patients with cryptococcal meningitis, the combination of amphotericin B and flucytosine enabled more rapid clearance of organisms from cerebrospinal fluid as well as reduced rates of relapse when compared to amphotericin B alone [19]. Evidence for this combination is further supported by a randomized trial of HIV-infected patients with cryptococcal meningitis who received one of four treatment regimens: amphotericin B plus flucytosine, amphotericin B alone, amphotericin B plus fluconazole, or a triple combination of amphotericin B, fluconazole, and flucytosine [24]. This study assessed efficacy of these regimens in 64 patients based on rate of reduction in colony-forming units (CFU) of *C. neoformans* at 3, 7, and 14 days after initiating therapy. Interestingly, the combination of amphotericin B and flucytosine was associated with the greatest reduction in CFU compared to the other three regimens. Reduction in CFUs was slightly better with amphotericin B plus fluconazole compared to amphotericin B alone. The triple combination performed similarly to amphotericin B plus fluconazole. Therefore, although antagonism was not demonstrated for amphotericin B plus fluconazole, the other combinations were no better than amphotericin B plus flucytosine as initial management of cryptococcal meningitis [24].

Another randomized trial recently compared initial monotherapy with amphotericin B to combinations of amphotericin B plus low-dose (400 mg daily) or high-dose (800 mg daily) fluconazole for HIV-associated cryptococcal meningitis [42]. After 14 days of treatment, the combination of amphotericin B and high-dose fluconazole was associated with a trend towards more successful outcomes than amphotericin B alone (53.7% vs 41.3%) or amphotericin B plus low-dose fluconazole (53.7% vs 27.1%), but these differences were not statistically significant. The unexpectedly lower rate of early success among those receiving low-dose fluconazole plus amphotericin B could not be explained by other covariates such as baseline CD4 cell count, viral load, or burden of cryptococcal disease. However, these patients had success rates similar to the other treatment groups 42 and 70 days after their initial induction therapy followed by consolidation therapy with daily fluconazole [42]. Another recent study demonstrated an incremental benefit on early fungicidal activity by increasing amphotericin B dosage to 1 mg/kg/day versus 0.7 mg/kg/day, both in combination with flucytosine [43]. This trial was too small to discern differences in toxicity with the higher amphotericin B dose, but the higher dose has been an ongoing concern among clinicians [44]. Amphotericin B plus flucytosine remains the preferred initial (induction) therapy for HIV-associated cryptococcal meningitis in developed nations [45]; amphotericin B plus high-dose fluconazole (800 mg daily) induction therapy may be investigated in future studies as a promising alternative.

Invasive Candidiasis

In vitro experiments and animal models have explored the activity of a variety of antifungal combinations against *Candida* species (Table 1). As with *Cryptococcus*, the combination of amphotericin B and flucytosine has largely appeared synergistic against *Candida* species [7, 31]. Mixed results have been observed with the combination of azoles and flucytosine in vitro, and beneficial impact on survival and tissue burden was observed with such combinations in animal models [7]. Echinocandins have been combined with flucytosine in similar experiments, which have generally reported indifference in vitro [46, 47].

Echinocandins in combination with azoles have often been synergistic or indifferent against *Candida* [47, 48]. Echinocandins have also been combined with amphotericin B in vitro, resulting in synergy or indifference [49, 50]. Caspofungin combined with liposomal amphotericin B in a mouse model of invasive candidal infection resulted in similar rates of survival and tissue burden as monotherapy with either agent, further substantiating indifferent activity [51].

Experience with amphotericin B and azoles against *Candida* has been mostly antagonistic in vitro, with mixed results in animal models based on survival and tissue burden [7, 31]. Sequential exposure has also been problematic for this interaction; pre-exposure to an azole seems to attenuate activity of amphotericin B [7, 52–55]. These findings have led to substantial concern about using combinations of amphotericin B and azole agents in the clinical setting.

Only one large randomized trial has compared FDA-approved combination antifungal therapy to standard therapy in the clinical setting of candidemia/invasive candidiasis [25]. In this study, 219 evaluable patients received fluconazole

(800 mg daily) and for the first 5–6 days also received either placebo or amphotericin B (0.7 mg/kg daily). In the primary analysis of time to failure, the two study groups were similar. Overall treatment success was higher among those who received combination therapy versus monotherapy (69% vs 56%, $p = 0.043$), and more patients receiving fluconazole monotherapy had a higher rate of persistent fungemia (17% persistence with monotherapy vs 6% persistence with combination therapy, $p = 0.02$). On multivariate analysis that controlled for other factors which would impact outcome, such as severity of illness, the combination of fluconazole plus amphotericin B was associated with 38% lower odds of treatment failure.

However, overall mortality at 90 days was similar between treatment groups (approximately 40% in each group). Toxicity associated with amphotericin B was apparent despite the short exposure period in this study, with 23% of patients in the combination therapy group requiring a reduction in dosage versus 3% in the fluconazole/placebo arm. Clearly, no antagonism between amphotericin B and fluconazole was apparent during this study, and there was a trend towards improvement in microbiologic outcomes in patients receiving combination therapy. However, due to the toxicity of this regimen, lack of impact on time to failure, and the emergence of other fungicidal agents such as echinocandins, the combination of amphotericin B and fluconazole is not recommended as first-line therapy for candidemia in the 2009 Infectious Diseases Society of America (IDSA) guidelines [56].

In contrast, combination antifungal therapy is included as part of the IDSA recommendations for management of other forms of invasive candidiasis, which may be particularly difficult to treat and have not been studied in large clinical trials [56]. Specifically, a combination of amphotericin B and flucytosine is recommended for at least the first several weeks of treatment of *Candida* infections of the central nervous system. This recommendation is based on available in vitro data and the pharmacokinetic profile of flucytosine which may optimize concentrations within the CNS.

Similarly, the IDSA guidelines recommend that flucytosine be added to amphotericin B for treating serious cases of *Candida* endophthalmitis. In addition, combination therapy is often considered in initial management of *Candida* endocarditis, and flucytosine can be added to amphotericin B or a lipid formulation for this indication [56]. In a meta-analysis which considered other factors such as surgical intervention, higher mortality was observed among patients who received antifungal monotherapy [57]. A more recent trend has been to add an azole, flucytosine, or even a polyene to echinocandin therapy for *Candida endocarditis*, and some success has been reported with these strategies [58–61]. However, additional data are needed to establish the role of such combinations in the management of this serious *Candida* infection.

Combination Antifungal Therapy for Mould Infections

Aspergillosis

Clinicians are continually striving to improve outcomes for patients with invasive aspergillosis and, toward this end, numerous antifungal combinations have been studied (Table 1). Similar to data for yeast infections, results from in vitro and animal model studies have led to conflicting results [7, 31, 32]. Some of these issues are highlighted in an in vitro study that looked at triple drug combinations for treatment of various species of *Aspergillus* [62]. In vitro testing revealed additive or synergistic effects for most combinations of echinocandins and azoles tested. However, the addition of amphotericin B to these combinations caused wide variations in responses, ranging from enhanced synergy to antagonism. While in vitro experiments such as these can help to shed light on appropriate strategies to improve outcomes associated with invasive aspergillosis, they also highlight the need to base clinical decisions on human data when available.

Perhaps the most attention has focused on combination therapies for aspergillosis that include an echinocandin in combination with another drug class. Unlike concerns for azole and polyene antagonism when given concomitantly, the use of an echinocandin with either an azole or polyene appears to at least have no deleterious effects. In most in vitro models of *Aspergillus* infection, therapy with an echinocandin has shown variable effects ranging from indifferent to synergistic activity [7, 11, 12]. When these combination strategies are further tested in animal models of infection, activity is often improved with lower mortality and less fungal-mediated tissue injury [11, 63].

Interestingly, there have been recent reports that suggest higher echinocandin doses in combination with extended-spectrum triazoles can actually result in antagonistic effects not observed at lower echinocandin doses [63]. While the clinical significance of such findings is unknown, these results serve as another example of the variability of in vitro data.

Limited data are also available for other antifungal combinations, including the use of agents that do not demonstrate appreciable anti-*Aspergillus* activity on their own. Results from studies adding flucytosine or rifampin to amphotericin B or azole therapies typically demonstrate no benefit to additive activity [7, 11]. Terbinafine may have an important role in combination regimens for management of invasive aspergillosis. While terbinafine is reported to have variable effects against *Aspergillus* when combined with amphotericin B [64]; enhanced activity is seen when terbinafine is added to the extended-spectrum triazole agents [64].

Unfortunately, large, prospective clinical trials documenting the efficacy of combination therapy strategies for invasive aspergillosis are lacking. Presently available are smaller clinical experiences that are often retrospective in nature or limited in other methodologic components [7, 11, 65–70]. Many of these have been in the form of case reports. In general, combinations of amphotericin B with the azoles do not appear to significantly improve outcome for studied patients [71–73]. In addition, strategies that include an echinocandin may have some benefit.

Caspofungin has been studied in combination with other antifungal agents in the management of invasive aspergillosis [67, 69]. In a small, single-center, open-label study, patients with pulmonary aspergillosis who were failing therapy with amphotericin B received either voriconazole ($n = 31$) or voriconazole in combination with caspofungin ($n = 16$) [67]. Combination therapy was associated with improved survival relative to a historical cohort of patients who received voriconazole alone. In another study, the combination of caspofungin and voriconazole was used as initial therapy for invasive aspergillosis in a prospective, multicenter cohort of 40 solid-organ transplant recipients compared to a historical cohort of 47 patients who had received a lipid formulation of amphotericin B (LFAB) as primary therapy [69]. Treatment success was 70% among those receiving the combination regimen versus 51% among those who received LFAB ($p = 0.08$). Combination therapy as a salvage approach has also been investigated [68].

Micafungin has been investigated as a single agent or in combination antifungal therapy as primary or salvage regimens in two recent studies [66, 70]. The first study described 225 evaluable adults and children who received micafungin for proven or probable invasive aspergillosis and who had refractory disease or were intolerant of initial antifungal therapy [70]. Micafungin was added to a failing antifungal regimen in 85% of these patients. Complete/partial responses were experienced by 35.6% (8% complete, 27.6% partial) of patients at the end of antifungal therapy, while 53.5% of patients experienced progression of infection. This small study showed no advantage of combination antifungal therapy compared to micafungin alone as either primary therapy (29.4% vs 50%) or salvage therapy (34.5% vs 40.9%).

In a second multicenter retrospective open-label study, 98 adult and pediatric stem cell transplant recipients with invasive aspergillosis (primarily pulmonary disease) received micafungin as a single agent (8%) or in combination with other antifungals (92%) as primary (15%) or salvage (85%) therapy [66]. Amphotericin B or a lipid formulation was most commonly used in conjunction with micafungin. Treatment success was experienced by 26% of patients, who had either complete (5%) or partial (20%) responses. Success rates were 24% among those receiving micafungin in combination with other antifungals, and 38% among the eight patients receiving micafungin alone. Other smaller studies and case series have been performed and suggest that echinocandin combinations may be promising, but conclusive evidence of synergistic effects in combination with other agents for invasive aspergillosis remains to be shown [68, 74, 75].

In the IDSA guidelines for invasive aspergillosis updated in 2008, combination therapy is mentioned, but not endorsed as a first-line treatment option [76]. Combination therapy is provided as an option for patients failing first-line therapies. The guidelines further highlight the critical need for further studies evaluating this therapeutic strategy.

Other Medically Significant Moulds

Medical advances allowing potent immunosuppressive therapy and routine use of antifungal prophylaxis have changed the epidemiology of invasive fungal infections. Several of the more rare fungal pathogens including the Zygomycetes, *Fusarium* species and *Scedosporium* species have emerged as more common pathogens causing disease. These infections are often difficult to treat and combination antifungal therapy is one approach that may offer clinical benefit.

There are in vitro and animal data for combination therapy targeting each of these pathogens (Table 1). For these fungal pathogens, results from in vitro studies are conflicting and, unfortunately, there are limited data available from animal models to further guide therapy. Combinations of amphotericin B and voriconazole together or individually with caspofungin, micafungin, or terbinafine all demonstrated synergistic activity against *Fusarium* species. However combinations including anidulafungin were indifferent in their antifungal effect [11]. Interestingly, the variable susceptibilities observed for different *Fusarium* species may also complicate combination regimens [77]. For *Scedosporium* species, combinations involving micafungin plus amphotericin B, voriconazole, or GM-CSF were consistently associated with improved in vitro activity and more successful end points in the available murine models of infection [33, 78].

Only a limited number of antifungal agents demonstrate appreciable activity against Zygomycetes. Utilizing drugs in combination with minimal to no antifungal activity against these pathogens in vitro may be one way to expand treatment options. For the most part, rifampin, terbinafine, or flucytosine together with amphotericin B result in additive activity [79]. Terbinafine provided synergistic activity when given with extended-spectrum azoles including voriconazole and itraconazole [80]. Posaconazole, in combination with caspofungin, demonstrated synergistic activity against multiple Zygomycetes, but addition of posaconazole to amphotericin B did not improve activity over each agent alone [34, 37]. The few available animal studies for combination therapy of Zygomycetes have confirmed synergy between amphotericin B and all of the echinocandins [35].

The pathophysiology of zygomycosis has led to the exploration of novel combination strategies for this infection. One of these approaches is to utilize iron chelation agents, deferasirox or deferiprone, to augment activity of amphotericin B [81, 82]. This approach is supported by both in vitro and animal models of infection [81, 82].

For treatment of these uncommon fungal pathogens, available human data exist primarily in the form of case reports and case series. Combinations successfully used to treat fusariosis have all incorporated an amphotericin B formulation [83, 84], whereas successful reports of combination treatment for *Scedosporium* species have focused on the use of voriconazole as part of the treatment regimen [85–87].

Much of the available human experience with combination therapy for uncommon mould infections has been obtained in patients with zygomycosis. Many different combinations have been explored for management of individual patients with severe or refractory infections [88, 89]. In one review of 41 cases of rhinocerebral disease, a combination that included an amphotericin B preparation and caspofungin showed improved outcomes, including survival, compared with patients receiving monotherapy regimens [90].

Data regarding safety and preliminary efficacy from prospective trials to evaluate iron chelation in combination with amphotericin B are beginning to emerge [91]. Success was documented in five of eight patients who received this combination; however, the importance of adjunctive surgical management for these patients must be considered [91]. Moreover, not all experiences with iron chelation therapy for zygomycosis have resulted in dramatic success [91, 92].

Future Targets

In the antifungal arena, the concept of combination therapy has been applied to regimens that include one or more agents considered ineffective against the target pathogen. In many cases, the additional drug may not traditionally be used to treat fungal infection. There are numerous examples of agents for different disease states ranging from bacterial infections to cardiovascular disease benefiting patients with fungal disease. Although not a major focus of current treatment strategies for fungal disease, these approaches merit comment.

Statins, quinolones, rifampin, and calcineurin inhibitors are all examples of agents that appear to modulate activity of systemic antifungal agents for mould and yeast infections [93, 94]. Calcineurin inhibitors such as cyclosporine or tacrolimus can render azoles fungicidal [95]. Synergistic activity against *Candida* species has been demonstrated with addition of (1) statins to fluconazole and itraconazole, (2) calcineurin inhibitors cyclosporine and tacrolimus to terbinafine, and (3) quinolones to amphotericin B or fluconazole [96–98]. The quinolone agents can enhance activity of fluconazole even in the setting of fluconazole resistance. Similar results have been seen with the statins and azoles for *C. neoformans* [96]. In vitro evidence of synergy has also been reported for combinations of some nonsteroidal agents (ibuprofen, sodium salicylate, propylparaben, and diclofenac sodium) with fluconazole against some *C. albicans* [99, 100].

Herbal agents may also benefit antifungal therapies. Recent investigations have demonstrated synergy with combinations of berberine and fluconazole or amphotericin B against strains of *C. albicans* in vitro [101, 102]. Berberine has also improved survival when added to amphotericin B in a murine model of disseminated candidiasis [102].

Nontraditional agents may also be beneficial for the treatment of mould infections. Varying results were obtained with quinolones and amphotericin B against *Aspergillus fumigatus* in vitro, but prolonged survival was reported in an animal model with this combination [103]. Combinations of quinolones and fluconazole have also resulted in improved activity against pulmonary mucormycosis in a murine model [93].

The current challenge is that for every positive in vitro or animal in vivo result with combination therapy for fungal disease, there is conflicting evidence, making it very difficult to incorporate these strategies in clinical care. Results may only apply to a very specific group of pathogens. Prospective evaluations of these strategies in treatment of human disease are needed before these approaches can be routinely used in a clinical setting.

References

1. Wisplinghoff H, Bischoff T, Tallent SM, Seifert H, Wenzel RP, Edmond MB. Nosocomial bloodstream infections in US hospitals: analysis of 24, 179 cases from a prospective nationwide surveillance study. Clin Infect Dis. 2004;39:309–17.
2. Nucci M, Marr KA. Emerging fungal diseases. Clin Infect Dis. 2005;41:521–6.
3. Richardson MD. Changing patterns and trends in systemic fungal infections. J Antimicrob Chemother. 2005;56:5–11.
4. Chayakulkeeree M, Perfect JR. Cryptococcosis. Infect Dis Clin North Am. 2006;20:507–44.
5. Spanakis EK, Aperis G, Mylonakis E. New agents for the treatment of fungal infections: clinical efficacy and gaps in coverage. Clin Infect Dis. 2006;43:1060–8.
6. Perfect JR. Management of cryptococcosis: how are we doing? PLoS Med. 2007;4:e47.
7. Johnson MD, MacDougall C, Ostrosky-Zeichner L, Perfect JR, Rex JH. Combination antifungal therapy. Antimicrob Agents Chemother. 2004;48:693–715.
8. Johnson MD, Perfect JR. Combination antifungal therapy: what can and should we expect? Bone Marrow Transplant. 2007; 40:297–306.
9. Ostrosky-Zeichner L. Combination antifungal therapy: a critical review of the evidence. Clin Microbiol Infect. 2008;14 Suppl 4:65–70.

10. Lewis RE, Kontoyiannis DP. Rationale for combination antifungal therapy. Pharmacother. 2001;21:149S–64.
11. Vazquez JA. Clinical practice: combination antifungal therapy for mold infections: much ado about nothing? Clin Infect Dis. 2008;46:1889–901.
12. Baddley JW, Pappas PG. Antifungal combination therapy: clinical potential. Drugs. 2005;65:1461–80.
13. Vermes A, Guchelaar H-J, Dankert J. Flucytosine: a review of its pharmacology, clinical indications, pharmacokinetics, toxicity and drug interactions. J Antimicrob Chemother. 2000;46:171–9.
14. Cowen LE, Lindquist S. Hsp90 potentiates the rapid evolution of new traits: drug resistance in diverse fungi. Science. 2005;309:2185–9.
15. Cowen LE, Singh SD, Köhler JR, et al. Harnessing Hsp90 function as a powerful, broadly effective therapeutic strategy for fungal infectious disease. Proc Natl Acad Sci. 2009;106:2818–23.
16. Imhof A, Schaer DJ, Schwarz U, Schanz U. Neurological adverse events to voriconazole: evidence for therapeutic drug monitoring. Swiss Med Wkly. 2006;136:739–42.
17. Denning DW, Ribaud P, Milpied N, et al. Efficacy and safety of voriconazole in the treatment of acute invasive aspergillosis. Clin Infect Dis. 2002;34:563–71.
18. Harbarth S, Pestotnik SL, Lloyd JF, Burke JP, Samore MH. The epidemiology of nephrotoxicity associated with conventional amphotericin B therapy. Am J Med. 2001;111:528–34.
19. van der Horst CM, Saag MS, Cloud GA, et al. Treatment of cryptococcal meningitis associated with the acquired immunodeficiency syndrome. National Institute of Allergy and Infectious Diseases Mycoses Study Group and AIDS Clinical Trials Group. N Engl J Med. 1997;337:15–21.
20. Bennett JE, Dismukes WE, Duma RJ, et al. A comparison of amphotericin B alone and combined with flucytosine in the treatment of cryptococcal meningitis. N Engl J Med. 1979;301:126–31.
21. Alexander BD, Dodds Ashley ES, Addison RM, Alspaugh JA, Chao NJ, Perfect JR. Non-comparative evaluation of the safety of aerosolized amphotericin B lipid complex in patients undergoing allogeneic hematopoietic stem cell transplantation. Transpl Infect Dis. 2006;8:13–20.
22. Dodds Ashley ES, Lewis R, Lewis JS, Martin C, Andes D. Pharmacology of systemic antifungal agents. Clin Infect Dis. 2006;43:S28–S39.
23. Steinbach WJ, Stevens DA, Denning DW. Combination and sequential antifungal therapy for invasive aspergillosis: review of published in vitro and in vivo interactions and 6281 clinical cases from 1966 to 2001. Clin Infect Dis. 2003;37:188–224.
24. Brouwer AE, Rajanuwong A, Chierakul W, et al. Combination antifungal therapies for HIV-associated cryptococcal meningitis: a randomised trial. Lancet. 2004;363:1764–7.
25. Rex JH, Pappas PG, Karchmer AW, et al. A randomized and blinded multicenter trial of high-dose fluconazole plus placebo versus fluconazole plus amphotericin B as therapy for candidemia and its consequences in nonneutropenic subjects. Clin Infect Dis. 2003;36:1221–8.
26. Kennedy MS, Deeg HJ, Siegel M, Crowley JJ, Storb R, Thomas ED. Acute renal toxicity with combined use of amphotericin B and cyclosporine after marrow transplantation. Transplantation. 1983; 35:211–5.
27. Shaukat A, Benekli M, Vladutiu GD, Slack JL, Wetzler M, Baer MR. Simvastatin-fluconazole causing rhabdomyolysis. Ann Pharmacother. 2003;37:1032–5.
28. Stone JA, Migoya EM, Hickey L, et al. Potential for interactions between caspofungin and nelfinavir or rifampin. Antimicrob Agents Chemother. 2004;48:4306–14.
29. Saad AH, DePestel DD, Carver PL. Factors influencing the magnitude and clinical significance of drug interactions between azole antifungals and select immunosuppressants. Pharmacotherapy. 2006;26:1730–44.
30. Rex JH, Walsh TJ, Nettleman M, et al. Need for alternative trial designs and evaluation strategies for therapeutic studies of invasive mycoses. Clin Infect Dis. 2001;33:95–106.
31. Polak A. The past, present and future of antimycotic combination therapy. Mycoses. 1999;42:355–70.
32. Mukherjee PK, Sheehan DJ, Hitchcock CA, et al. Combination treatment of invasive fungal infections. Clin Microbiol Rev. 2005;18:163–94.
33. Rodriguez MM, Calvo E, Serena C, Marine M, Pastor FJ, Guarro J. Effects of double and triple combinations of antifungal drugs in a murine model of disseminated infection by *Scedosporium prolificans*. Antimicrob Agents Chemother. 2009;53:2153–5.
34. Ibrahim AS, Gebremariam T, Schwartz JA, Edwards Jr JE, Spellberg B. Posaconazole mono-or combination therapy for the treatment of murine zygomycosis. Antimicrob Agents Chemother. 2009; 53:772–5.
35. Ibrahim AS, Gebremariam T, Fu Y, Edwards JE Jr, Spellberg B. Combination echinocandin-polyene treatment of murine mucormycosis. Antimicrob Agents Chemother. 2008;52:1556–8.
36. Spellberg B, Fu Y, Edwards JE, Jr Ibrahim AS. Combination therapy with amphotericin B lipid complex and caspofungin acetate of disseminated zygomycosis in diabetic ketoacidotic mice. Antimicrob Agents Chemother. 2005;49:830–2.
37. Guembe M, Guinea J, Pelaez T, Torres-Narbona M, Bouza E. Synergistic effect of posaconazole and caspofungin against clinical zygomycetes. Antimicrob Agent Chemother. 2007;51:3457–8.
38. Rodriguez MM, Serena C, Marine M, et al. Posaconazole combined with amphotericin B, an effective therapy for a murine disseminated infection caused by *Rhizopus oryzae*. Antimicrob Agents Chemother. 2008;52:3786–8.
39. Hamilton JD, Elliott DM. Combined activity of amphotericin B and 5-fluorocytosine against *Cryptococcus neoformans* in vitro and in vivo in mice. J Infect Dis. 1975;131:129–37.
40. Block ER, Bennett JE. The combined effect of 5-fluorocytosine and amphotericin B in the therapy of murine cryptococcosis. Proc Soc Exp Bio Med. 1973;142:476–80.
41. Allendoerfer R, Marquis AJ, Rinaldi MG, Graybill JR. Combined therapy with fluconazole and flucytosine in murine cryptococcal meningitis. Antimicrob Agents Chemother. 1991;35:726–9.
42. Pappas PG, Chetchotisakd P, Larsen RA, et al. A phase II randomized trial of amphotericin B alone or combined with fluconazole in the treatment of HIV-associated cryptococcal meningitis. Clin Infect Dis. 2009;48:1775–83.
43. Bicanic T, Wood R, Meintjes G, et al. High-dose amphotericin B with flucytosine for the treatment of cryptococcal meningitis in HIV-infected patients: a randomized trial. Clin Infect Dis. 2008; 47:123–30.
44. Powderly WG. Dosing amphotericin B in cryptococcal meningitis. Clin Infect Dis. 2008;47:131–2.
45. Perfect JR, Dismukes WE, Dromer F, et al. Clinical practice guidelines for the management of cryptococcal disease: 2010 update by the infectious Diseases Society of America. Clin Infect Dis 2010;50:291–322.
46. Pai MP, Samples ML, Mercier RC, et al. Activities and ultrastructural effects of antifungal combinations against simulated *Candida* endocardial vegetations. Antimicrob Agents Chemother. 2008; 52:2367–76.
47. Karlowsky JA, Hoban DJ, Zhanel GG, Goldstein BP. In vitro interactions of anidulafungin with azole antifungals, amphotericin B and 5-fluorocytosine against *Candida* species. Int J Antimicrob Agents. 2006;27:174–7.
48. Baltch AL, Bopp LH, Smith RP, Ritz WJ, Michelsen PB. Anticandidal effects of voriconazole and caspofungin, singly and in combination, against *Candida glabrata*, extracellularly and intracellularly in granulocyte-macrophage colony stimulating factor (GM-CSF)-activated human monocytes. J Antimicrob Chemother. 2008;62:1285–90.

49. Barchiesi F, Spreghini E, Tomassetti S, Giannini D, Scalise G. Caspofungin in combination with amphotericin B against *Candida parapsilosis*. Antimicrob Agents Chemother. 2007;51:941–5.
50. Serena C, Marine M, Quindos G, et al. In vitro interactions of micafungin with amphotericin B against clinical isolates of *Candida* spp. Antimicrob Agents Chemother. 2008;52:1529–32.
51. Tunger O, Bayram H, Degerli K, Dinc G, Cetin BC. Comparison of the efficacy of combination and monotherapy with caspofungin and liposomal amphotericin B against invasive candidiasis. Saudi Med J. 2008;29:728–33.
52. Cao B, Tsang PW, Tsang DN, Samaranayake LP, Wang J. A disc plate assay for characterization of the effect of interaction between polyenes and azoles on growth of *Candida albicans* CA12. Microbios. 1996;87:161–7.
53. Lewis RE, Lund BC, Klepser ME, Ernst EJ, Pfaller MA. Assessment of antifungal activities of fluconazole and amphotericin B administered alone and in combination against *Candida albicans* by using a dynamic in vitro mycotic infection model. Antimicrob Agents Chemother. 1998;42:1382–6.
54. Louie A, Liu W, Miller DA, et al. Efficacies of high-dose fluconazole plus amphotericin B and high-dose fluconazole plus 5-fluorocytosine versus amphotericin B, fluconazole, and 5-fluorocytosine monotherapies in treatment of experimental endocarditis, endophthalmitis, and pyelonephritis due to *Candida albicans*. Antimicrob Agents Chemother. 1999;43:2831–40.
55. Sugar AM, Liu X-P. Interactions of itraconazole with amphotericin B in the treatment of murine invasive candidiasis. J Infect Dis. 1998;177:1660–3.
56. Pappas PG, Kauffman CA, Andes D, et al. Clinical practice guidelines for the management of candidiasis: 2009 update by the Infectious Diseases Society of America. Clin Infect Dis. 2009;48:503–35.
57. Steinbach WJ, Perfect JR, Cabell CH, et al. A meta-analysis of medical versus surgical therapy for *Candida* endocarditis. J Infect. 2005;51:230–47.
58. Lye DCB, Hughes A, O'Brien D, Athan E. *Candida glabrata* prosthetic valve endocarditis treated successfully with fluconazole plus caspofungin without surgery: a case report and literature review. Eur J Clin Microbiol Infect Dis. 2005;24:753–5.
59. Lopez-Ciudad V, Castro-Orjales MJ, Leon C, et al Successful treatment of *Candida parapsilosis* mural endocarditis with combined caspofungin and voriconazole. BMC Infect Dis. 2006;6:73.
60. Falcone M, Barzaghi N, Carosi G, et al. *Candida* infective endocarditis: report of 15 cases from a prospective multicenter study. Medicine. 2009;88:160–8.
61. Talarmin JP, Boutoille D, Tattevin P, et al. *Candida* endocarditis: role of new antifungal agents. Mycoses. 2009;52:60–6.
62. Demchok JP, Meletiadis J, Roilides E, Walsh TJ. Comparative pharmacodynamic interaction analysis of triple combinations of caspofungin and voriconazole or ravuconazole with subinhibitory concentrations of amphotericin B against *Aspergillus* spp. Mycoses 2010;53;239–45.
63. Petraitis V, Petraitiene R, Hope WW, et al. Combination therapy in treatment of experimental pulmonary aspergillosis: in vitro and in vivo correlations of the concentration- and dose- dependent interactions between anidulafungin and voriconazole by Bliss independence drug interaction analysis. Antimicrob Agents Chemother. 2009;53:2382–91.
64. Ryder NS, Leitner I. Synergistic interaction of terbinafine with triazoles or amphotericin B against *Aspergillus* species. Med Mycol. 2001;39:91–5.
65. Kontoyiannis DP, Hachem R, Lewis RE, et al. Efficacy and toxicity of caspofungin in combination with liposomal amphotericin B as primary or salvage treatment of invasive aspergillosis in patients with hematologic malignancies. Cancer. 2003;98:292–9.
66. Kontoyiannis DP, Ratanatharathorn V, Young JA, et al. Micafungin alone or in combination with other systemic antifungal therapies in hematopoietic stem cell transplant recipients with invasive aspergillosis. Transpl Infect Dis. 2009;11:89–93.
67. Marr KA, Boeckh M, Carter RA, et al. Combination antifungal therapy for invasive aspergillosis. Clin Infect Dis. 2004; 39:797–802.
68. Maertens J, Glasmacher A, Herbrecht R, et al. Multicenter, noncomparative study of caspofungin in combination with other antifungals as salvage therapy in adults with invasive aspergillosis. Cancer. 2006;107:2888–97.
69. Singh N, Limaye AP, Forrest G, et al. Combination of voriconazole and caspofungin as primary therapy for invasive aspergillosis in solid organ transplant recipients: a prospective, multicenter, observational study. Transplantation. 2006;81:320–6.
70. Denning DW, Marr KA, Lau WM, et al. Micafungin (FK463), alone or in combination with other systemic antifungal agents, for the treatment of acute invasive aspergillosis. J Infect. 2006; 53:337–49.
71. Schaffner A, Böhler A. Amphotericin B refractory aspergillosis after itraconazole: evidence for significant antagonism. Mycoses. 1993;36:421–4.
72. Bajjoka IE, Bailey EM, Vazquez JA, Abouljoud MS. Combination antifungal therapy for invasive aspergillosis infection in liver transplant recipients: report of two patients. Pharmacother. 1999;19:118–23.
73. Kontoyiannis DP, Boktour M, Hanna H, et al. Itraconazole added to a lipid formulation of amphotericin B does not improve outcome of primary treatment of invasive aspergillosis. Cancer. 2005;103:2334–7.
74. Caillot D, Thiébaut A, Herbrecht R, et al. Liposomal amphotericin B in combination with caspofungin for invasive aspergillosis in patients with hematologic malignancies. Cancer. 2007;110:2740–6.
75. Thomas A, Korb V, Guillemain R, et al. Clinical outcomes of lung-transplant recipients treated by voriconazole and caspofungin combination in aspergillosis. J Clin Pharm 2010;35:49–53.
76. Walsh TJ, Anaissie EJ, Denning DW, et al. Treatment of aspergillosis: clinical practice guidelines of the Infectious Diseases Society of America. Clin Infect Dis. 2008;46:327–60.
77. Arikan S, Lozano-Chiu M, Paetznick V, Rex JH. In vitro synergy of caspofungin and amphotericin B against *Aspergillus* and *Fusarium* spp. Antimicrob Agents Chemother. 2002;46:245–7.
78. Ortoneda M, Capilla J, Pujol I, et al. Liposomal amphotericin B and granulocyte colony-stimulating factor therapy in a murine model of invasive infection by *Scedosporium prolificans*. J Antimicrob Chemother. 2002;49:525–9.
79. Dannaoui E, Afeltra J, Meis J, Verweij PE. In vitro susceptibilities of zygomycetes to combinations of antimicrobial agents. Antimicrob Agents Chemother. 2002;46:2708–11.
80. Gómez-López A, Cuenca-Estrella M, Mellado E, Rodríguez-Tudela JL. In vitro evaluation of combination of terbinafine with itraconazole or amphotericin B against Zygomycota. Diagn Microbiol Infect Dis. 2003;45:199–202.
81. Ibrahim AS, Gebermariam T, Fu Y, et al. The iron chelator deferasirox protects mice from mucormycosis through iron starvation. J Clin Invest. 2007;117:2649–57.
82. Spellberg B, Walsh TJ, Kontoyiannis DP, et al. Recent advances in the management of mucormycosis: from bench to bedside. Clin Infect Dis. 2009;48:1743–51.
83. Rothe A, Seibold M, Hoppe TH, et al. Combination therapy of disseminated *Fusarium oxysporum* infection with terbinafine and amphotericin B. Ann Hematol. 2004;83:394–7.
84. Makowsky MJ, Warkentin DI, Savoie ML. Caspofungin and amphotericin B for disseminated *Fusarium verticillioides* in leukemia. Ann Pharmacother. 2005;39:1365–6.
85. Steinbach WJ, Schell WA, Miller JL, Perfect JR. *Scedosporium prolificans* osteomyelitis in an immunocompetent child treated with voriconazole and caspofungin, as well as locally applied polyhexamethylene biguanide. J Clin Microbiol. 2003;41:3981–5.

86. Howden BP, Slavin MA, Schwarer AP, Mijch AM. Successful control of disseminated *Scedosporium prolificans* infection with a combination of voriconazole and terbinafine. Eur J Clin Microbiol Infect Dis. 2003;22:111–3.
87. Gosbell IB, Toumasatos V, Yong J, Kuo RS, Ellis DH, Perrie RC. Cure of orthopaedic infection with *Scedosporium prolificans*, using voriconazole plus terbinafine, without the need for radical surgery. Mycoses. 2003;46:233–6.
88. Rickerts V, Atta J, Herrmann S, et al. Successful treatment of disseminated mucormycosis with a combination of liposomal amphotericin B and posaconazole in a patient with acute myeloid leukaemia. Mycoses. 2006;49:27–30.
89. Gonzalez CE, Couriel DR, Walsh TJ. Disseminated zygomycosis in a neutropenic patient: successful treatment with amphotericin B lipid complex and granulocyte colony-stimulating factor. Clin Infect Dis. 1997;24:192–6.
90. Reed C, Bryant R, Ibrahim AS, et al. Combination polyene caspofungin for treatment of rhino-orbital-cerebral mucormycosis. Clin Infect Dis. 2008;47:364–71.
91. Spellberg B, Andes D, Perez M, et al. Safety and outcomes of open-label deferasirox iron chelation therapy for mucormycosis. Antimicrob Agents Chemother. 2009;53:3122–5.
92. Soummer A, Mathonnet A, Scatton O, et al. Failure of deferasirox, an iron chelator agent, combined with antifungals in a case of severe zygomycosis. Antimicrob Agents Chemother. 2008;52:1585–6.
93. Sugar AM, Liu X-P. Combination antifungal therapy in treatment of murine pulmonary mucormycosis: roles of quinolones and azoles. Antimicrob Agents Chemother. 2000;44:2004–6.
94. Steinbach WJ, Schell WA, Blankenship JR, Onyewu C, Heitman J, Perfect JR. In vitro interactions between antifungals and immunosuppressants against *Aspergillus fumigatus*. Antimicrob Agents Chemother. 2004;48:1664–9.
95. Blankenship JR, Steinbach WJ, Perfect JR, Heitman J. Teaching old drugs new tricks: reincarnating immunosuppressants as antifungal drugs. Curr Opin Investig Drugs. 2003;4:192–9.
96. Chin NX, Weitzman I, Della-Latta P. In vitro activity of fluvastatin, a cholesterol-lowering agent, and synergy with fluconazole and itraconazole against *Candida* species and *Cryptococcus neoformans*. Antimicrob Agents Chemother. 1997;41:850–2.
97. Onyewu C, Blankenship JR, Del Poeta M, Heitman J. Ergosterol biosynthesis inhibitors become fungicidal when combined with calcineurin inhibitors against *Candida albicans*, *Candida glabrata*, and *Candida krusei*. Antimicrob Agents Chemother. 2003;47:956–64.
98. Sugar AM, Liu XP, Chen RJ. Effectiveness of quinolone antibiotics in modulating the effects of antifungal drugs. Antimicrob Agents Chemother. 1997;41:2518–21.
99. Scott EM, Tariq VN, McCrory RM. Demonstration of synergy with fluconazole and either ibuprofen, sodium salicylate, or propylparaben against *Candida albicans* in vitro. Antimicrob Agents Chemother. 1995;39:2610–4.
100. Yücesoy M, ÖKtem IM, Gülay Z. In-vitro synergistic effect of fluconazole with nonsteroidal anti-inflammatory agents against *Candida albicans* strains. J Chemother. 2000;12:385–9.
101. Quan H, Cao YY, Xu Z, et al. Potent in vitro synergism of fluconazole and berberine chloride against clinical isolates of *Candida albicans* resistant to fluconazole. Antimicrob Agents Chemother. 2006;50:1096–9.
102. Han Y, Lee JH. Berberine synergy with amphotericin B against disseminated candidiasis in mice. Biol Pharm Bull. 2005;28:541–4.
103. Nakajima R, Kitamura A, Someya K, Tanaka M, Sato K. In vitro and in vivo antifungal activities of DU-6859a, a fluoroquinolone, in combination with amphotericin B and fluconazole against pathogenic fungi. Antimicrob Agents Chemother. 1995;39:1517–21.

Part III
Mycoses Caused by Yeasts

Candidiasis

Jose A. Vazquez and Jack D. Sobel

Within a few decades, *Candida* species have progressed from infrequent pathogens that were largely considered nuisance contaminants to important and common human pathogens causing a wide spectrum of superficial and deep disease. Superficial infections are frequently community acquired and responsible for considerable morbidity. In contrast, deep seated, invasive, and systemic *Candida* infections are usually nosocomial in origin. The pathogenesis and risk factors for superficial and deep candidiasis, although overlapping, are markedly different; hence, superficial infection uncommonly results in systemic disease. Matching the increased incidence of *Candida* infections has been the availability in the last 2 decades of successive generations of antifungal agents.

Organism

Candida are small (4–6 μm), oval, thin-walled yeast-like fungi that reproduce by budding or fission. On culture media, *Candida* species form smooth, creamy white, glistening colonies. The genus *Candida* is comprised of over 200 species and constitutes an extremely diverse yeast species whose common bond is the absence of a sexual cycle [1]. Only a few species cause disease in humans [2]. Although more than 17 different species of *Candida* have been reported as pathogens, more than 90% of invasive infections are attributed to five species, *Candida albicans*, *Candida glabrata*, *Candida parapsilosis*, *Candida tropicalis*, and *Candida krusei*. Less commonly reported are infections due to *Candida kefyr*, *Candida guilliermondii*, *Candida lusitaniae*, *Candida stellatoidea*, and *Candida dubliniensis*.

J.D. Sobel (✉)
Division of Infectious Diseases, Wayne State University School of Medicine, Detroit Medical Center, Detroit, MI, USA
e-mail: jsobel@med.wayne.edu

Candida albicans remains the major fungal pathogen of humans and the most common cause of mucosal and systemic fungal infection [3], and is the best characterized of the *Candida* species. *Candida glabrata* (synonym: *Torulopsis glabrata)* has become important because of its increasing incidence worldwide and decreased susceptibility to antifungals. Its emergence is largely due to an increased immunocompromised patient population and widespread use of antifungal drugs [4, 5]. In many hospitals, *C. glabrata* is the second most common cause of candidemia following *C. albicans* [3, 6, 7].

Candida parapsilosis in most parts of the world is the third most common cause of candidemia [3], especially in patients with intravenous catheters, prosthetic devices, and intravenous drug use [8, 9]. *Candida parapsilosis* is one of the most common causes of candidemia in neonatal intensive care units [9]. This species produces slime as a virulence factor enabling it to adhere to environmental surfaces and skin of hospital personnel [10]. *Candida tropicalis* is the third or fourth most commonly recovered *Candida* species from blood cultures [3, 11]. Leukemia, prolonged neutropenia, and prolonged intensive care unit (ICU) days are major risk factors for *C. tropicalis* candidemia [11].

Candida krusei is the fifth most common bloodstream isolate. Although less common (1–2%), *C. krusei* is of clinical significance because of its intrinsic resistance to fluconazole and reduced susceptibility to most other antifungal drugs [3]. *Candida krusei* is frequently recovered from patients with hematological malignancies complicated by neutropenia [12–14], tends to be associated with higher mortality rates (49% vs 28% with *C. albicans*), and lower response rates (51% vs 69% with *C. albicans*), and is associated with prior fluconazole use.

Candida kefyr is a rare species that occasionally causes disease in immunocompromised host [3]. *Candida guilliermondii* is another rare species. While infections due to *C. guillermondii* are uncommon, candidemia and invasive disease in the neutropenic host [15], are reported occasionally as is endocarditis in intravenous drug addicts. Of clinical importance is the decreased sensitivity of this species to

C.A. Kauffman et al. (eds.), *Essentials of Clinical Mycology*,
DOI 10.1007/978-1-4419-6640-7_11, © Springer Science+Business Media, LLC 2011

fluconazole and relatively high minimum inhibitory concentrations (MIC) to echinocandins. *Candida lusitaniae* is uncommon (1–2%), but of clinical importance because of intrinsic or secondary resistance acquisition to amphotericin B [16]. This species is typically found in patients with hematological malignancies and those in intensive care units [17].

Candida stellatoidea is a heterogeneous species with at least two confirmed subtypes, I and II [18]. Type I differs from *C. albicans* in several genetic characteristics and is not considered a mutant of *C. albicans*. Type II is a sucrose-negative mutant of *C. albicans* serotype A [18]. Additionally, type II isolates appear to have lower virulence and are slower growers than either type I *C. stellatoidea* or *C. albicans* [19]. *C. stellatoidea* produces germ tubes in vitro, a morphologic characteristic seen only in *C. albicans* and some *C. dubliniensis* strains [2].

Candida dubliniensis is a more recently identified species of *Candida*. Identified initially from the oral cavity of HIV-positive patients [20], *C. dubliniensis* has been recovered from HIV-positive patients throughout the world at rates ranging from 19% to 32% [20] and has also been recovered from 3% to 14% of oral cavities of HIV-negative individuals. This species rarely is associated with candidemia or invasive disease [21, 22]. *C. dubliniensis* is identified by germ tube and chlamydospore production, by an inability to grow at 45 °C, and by using commercially available yeast identification kits [23]. *C. rugosa*, although a rare cause of candidemia, is important because of frequent nystatin and azole-resistance and association with catheters and parenteral nutrition; it is susceptible to amphotericin B and echinocandins [24].

Less common non-*albicans Candida* species are listed in Table 1, and their unique features and diseases are described briefly. Using the strength of molecular identification, cryptic species have been identified within larger species complexes, such as *Candida orthopsilosis*, *Candida metapsilosis*, and *Lodderomyces elongisporus* in the *Candida parapsilosis* complex [25] and *Candida nivariensis* and *Candida bracarensis* in the *Candida glabrata* clade [26, 27]. Similarly, *Candida fermentati* isolates make up a small percentage of the clinical isolates of *C. guillermondii* complex [28].

Pathogenesis

Biologic features that contribute to the ability of *Candida* to cause disease were previously defined phenotypically. Total genome sequencing of *C. albicans* has allowed measurement of the effects of gene knockouts on the virulence of *Candida* in animal models. Genes required for virulence are regulated in response to environmental signals indigenous to the host environment. These signals include temperature, pH, osmotic pressure, and iron and calcium ion concentrations. Adaptation to a changing environment facilitates the ability of *Candida* to survive within the host niche.

Candida albicans undergoes reversible morphological transition between budding, pseudohyphal, and hyphal growth forms [29]. All forms are present in tissue specimens. Yeast cells may be disseminated more effectively, whereas hyphae are thought to promote invasion of epithelial and endothelial tissue and help evade macrophage engulfment [30]. *Candida* double mutants (chp1/chp1, efg1/efg1) that are locked in the yeast form are avirulent in a mouse model [31]. The ability to switch from one form to another appears to have a direct influence on the organism's capacity to cause disease [32]. Drugs that inhibit yeast-hyphal transformation without fungicidal activity have a role in suppressing clinical disease. Multiple genes are recognized as playing a role in morphogenesis, including TUP1 regulated genes [29]. Although the precise nature of the association between fungal morphogenesis and host disease invasion is controversial, it is now accepted that it is the ability to undergo morphogenetic conversion rather than the morphological form itself that is the primary determinant of pathogenicity [33, 34].

The first step in a *Candida* infection is epithelial colonization, which is dependent upon microorganism adherence to epithelial cells and proteins and allows the organism to withstand fluid forces that serve to expel particulates [35]. Adhesive ability of *C. albicans* has been correlated with virulence. A hierarchy exists among *Candida* species, with more frequently isolated pathogenic species exhibiting greater adhesive capacity. Several genes and their products have been identified to play a role in cell adhesion, including the adhesion like sequence (ALS) family of protein encoding cell-surface adhesion glycoproteins (x-agglutinins) and HWP-1, which encodes a protein (Hwp1), an adhesin attaching to buccal epithelial cells [36]. Similarly, candidal adhesion to endothelial cells lining blood vessels is a critical first step in migration of *C. albicans* cells from the circulation into tissues [37].

Invasion of host cells by *Candida* involves penetration and damage of the outer cell envelope. Transmigration is most likely mediated by physical and/or enzymatic processes. Phospholipids and proteins represent the major chemical constituents of the host cell membrane. Phospholipases, by cleaving phospholipids, induce cell lysis and thereby facilitate tissue invasion [38]. Phospholipase activity is concentrated at the hyphal growing tip and extracellular phospholipase is considered necessary for the invasion of tissue. Three genes have been cloned and encode candidal phospholipases. In 1969, Staib first reported that proteolytic activity in *C. albicans* was related to strain pathogenicity [39]. A family of at least nine genes makes up the secreted aspartyl proteinase isoenzymes (SAP) [40]. SAP1 and SAP3 are regulated during

Table 1 Characteristics and disease states associated with the uncommon non-*albicans Candida* species

Candida species	Characteristics/disease states	In vitro susceptibilities AmB	5-FC	Flz	Itz	Clz	Ktz
C. catenulata	A natural contaminant of dairy products, especially camembert cheeses; causes cutaneous, and mucosal infection; candidemia (one case report in a patient with gastric carcinoma who frequently ate cheese)	S	S	DD-S	S		
C. ciferii	Cutaneous, onychomycosis	S	R	R	R	S	S
C. famata	Candidemia, endophthalmitis, peritonitis due to CAPD	S	S	S	S	S	S
C. haemulonii	Candidemia, cutaneous						
C. inconspicua	Candidemia in neutropenics,oropharyngeal, esophageal, and vaginal candidiasis in diabetics and HIV-positive patients	S		R	R		
C. lipolytica	Low virulence, catheter-related candidemia, commonly colonizes the stool, sputum, and mouth, although not associated with mucosal infections	S	S	S	S	S	S
C. norvegensis	Recovered from the GI and respiratory tract, rarely causes candidemia and peritonitis	S	S	DD-S or R	S		S
C. pelliculosa Telomorph: *Hansenula anomola* the sexual state of *Pichia anomola*	The most frequent of the uncommon causes of invasive candidiasis; cases of invasive candidiasis including: candidemia, endocarditis, intraabdominal abscess, pyelonephritis, cerebral ventriculitis	Broad range[a]	S	S	S	S	
C. pulcherrima	Recovered from skin and nails of normal host						
C. rugosa	Associated with nosocomial candidemia and invasive candidiasis in burn patients, neutropenics, and catheter-associated infections	S	S	Broad range[b]	S		S
C. utilis Telomorph: *Hansenula jadinii, Pichia jadinii*	Utilized primarily in industry; a rare cause with only two cases of invasive candidiasis	S		S			
C. viswanathii	Recovered from respiratory tract and rare cause of meningitis						
C. zeylanoides	Low virulence, associated with catheter-related infections and septic arthritis	S		S	S		

S susceptible, *R* resistant, *DD-S* dose dependent susceptible, *MIC* minimum inhibitory concentration, *AmB* amphotericin B, *5-FC* flucytosine, *Flz* fluconazole, *Itz* itraconazole, *Clz* clotrimazole, *Ktz* ketoconazole, *CAPD* continuous ambulatory peritoneal dialysis

[a]Range of MICs of 0.04–1.56 μg/mL

[b]Range of MICs of 2–32 μg/mL

phenotypic transformation. Several studies have confirmed the importance of secreted aspartyl proteinases in the pathogenesis of tissue invasion by *C. albicans*. SAP-gene knockout experiments demonstrate attenuated virulence in both guinea pig and murine models of disseminated candidiasis. The role of *C. albicans* endothelial cell interaction in the pathogenesis of systemic candidiasis was recently reviewed [40].

The ability of *Candida* species to overcome the suppressive effect of antifungal chemotherapy is considered a virulence attribute. Biofilms are defined as structured microbial communities that are attached to a surface and encased in a matrix of exopolymeric material. *Candida* species are frequently found in the normal microbiota of humans, usually in a planktonic form in which they encounter most human surfaces and implanted biomaterials. *Candida* colonization and biofilm formation play an important role in the pathogenesis of superficial and invasive infections because of increased resistance to antifungal therapy and the ability of yeast cells within biofilms to withstand host immune defenses [41]. Devices, such as intravascular catheters, stents, shunts, prostheses, implants, endotracheal tubes, and pacemakers, support *Candida* colonization and biofilm formation [42].

Epidemiology

The last four decades have witnessed a dramatic increase in the incidence of candidemia and invasive candidiasis, originating in tertiary care centers and now observed in virtually all type hospitals [3, 43, 44]. *Candida* species remain the fourth leading cause of nosocomial blood stream infections (BSI) in the United States accounting for 8–10% of all nosocomial BSI's [45]. This translates into approximately 7,000–28,000 episodes annually [7]. It is estimated that approximately two-thirds of all *Candida* BSI are nosocomial [7]; the total annual burden of candidemia in the USA is approximately 10,500–42,000 infections [7, 46]. If one includes all forms of invasive candidiasis, the national burden of invasive candidiasis is approximately 63,000 infections per year [7]. A study estimated the attributable cost in 1997 US dollars of each case of candidemia at $34,000–$44,000, with a national annual total attributable cost for nosocomial candidemia of approximately $800 million in the USA [47].

Studies from 1996 to 2003 show remarkably consistent incidence rates of 22–29 cases per 100,000 US population or 19–24 cases per 10,000 hospital discharges indicating that the incidence has not decreased in the last decade. In contrast using a different data base, Trick et al. studying nosocomial ICU associated candidemia from 1989 to 1989 did demonstrate an absolute decline in frequency of BSI due to *Candida* almost entirely due to an absolute decrease in *C. albicans* BSI [48]. These discrepancies reflect two changes in epidemiology, the absolute and relative reduction in *C. albicans* BSI as well as the shift from ICUs to the general hospital setting. Hajjeh demonstrated that only 36% of *Candida* BSIs occurred in the ICU, and 28% were community onset in nature, an increase of almost 10% over a 5 year period [49].

A recent study based on BSI's from 2006 to 2007 revealed that *Candida* species continued to be the fourth most frequent isolates in healthcare associated infections [50]. In addition to population-based surveillance of candidemia in the USA, similarly designed studies have been performed worldwide, and with the exception of Denmark, the incidence of candidemia in Europe and Canada was significantly lower than the USA. However, in every survey an increase in incidence was documented over the course of the study [7]. Similarly an increase in incidence has been observed in Brazil.

In every surveillance study, risk factors for candidemia appear similar. Higher rates of candidemia occur in infants less than 1 year of age and adults over the age of 65 [49]. In addition, in US studies the incidence was at least fourfold higher among blacks in every age group. Other risk factors that emerged were cancer (71 per 100,000), diabetes (28 per 100,000), as well as the near universality of central venous catheters among patients diagnosed with candidemia [7]. Epidemiologic data indicate that the overall incidence has not decreased and candidemia remains a problem worldwide. Within the hospital setting, not all departments report high rates of candidemia. Patients in ICUs, especially surgical units [51], trauma and burn units, and neonatal ICUs, have the highest rates [52, 53]. Neutropenic patients, previously the highest risk population, are no longer the most vulnerable subpopulation, due to the widespread use of fluconazole prophylaxis during neutropenia.

There has been a recent shift world-wide in the epidemiology of invasive candidiasis, with both a proportional and absolute increase in infections caused by non-*albicans* *Candida* species [7, 50, 54, 55]. The shift was first evident in ICUs. A recent national study in the USA reported the incidence of candidemia caused by non-*albicans Candida* species to be 54.4%, which is higher than the incidence of candidemia caused by *C. albicans*, 45.6% [56]. While not all tertiary care centers report this shift, most highly specialized care centers have noted this trend [57]. On a worldwide basis, *C. albicans* remains the most common species causing invasive disease, but the frequency of isolation is decreasing [7, 48]. The increase has been noted mostly with *C. glabrata*, *C. tropicalis*, and *C. parapsilosis*. In particular, several studies have documented a significant trend towards an increase in *C. glabrata* with increasing patient age and in cancer centers [7, 54, 55, 58, 59]. However, there are worldwide variations in the frequency of isolation of various *Candida* species, and *C. glabrata* remains uncommon in Latin America [7] and in several Western European countries. *C. tropicalis* and

C. parapsilosis are the most common non-*albicans Candida* species in Latin America.

Given the reduced azole sensitivity of *C. glabrata* and several other species, there are profound therapeutic implications. Accordingly, multiple recent studies have been performed in an attempt to recognize risk factors for *C. glabrata* and other non-*albicans Candida* species in order to avoid inappropriate use of antifungal agents. Unfortunately in spite of a plethora of studies, consistent data have not emerged. Several authors have linked institutional or individual fluconazole use in the selection of *C. glabrata*, especially in cancer centers [54, 55, 57, 60]. Increased risk for *C. glabrata* also includes recent major abdominal surgery and older age [61].

Risk factors for *Candida* bloodstream infections include systemic antibiotics, chemotherapy, corticosteroids, presence of intravascular catheters, total parenteral nutrition (TPN), recent abdominal surgery, hospitalization in ICU, malignancy, neutropenia, and prior fungal colonization [52, 53, 62–64]. In a prospective study conducted in six surgical ICUs, multivariate analysis revealed increased risk with prior abdominal surgery, relative risk (RR) of 7.3, acute renal failure (R.R. 4.2), TPN (R.R. 3.6), and use of a triple lumen catheter (R.R. 5.4) as the major risk factors [64]. In contrast to other studies, prior fungal colonization could not be demonstrated as a risk factor, whereas receipt of any systemic antifungal drug was associated with reduced risk [64]. *Candida parapsilosis* is the most frequent cause of *Candida* bloodstream infection in neonates. Neonatal candidemia represents 12% of the cases of candidemia [65].

The source of candidemia remains poorly understood in spite of the aforementioned risk factors. In neutropenic individuals, gut colonization is likely responsible for most cases of candidemia. The gut is also likely to be the source of candidemia following abdominal surgery and in patients without intravascular central catheters. In contrast, in patients with skin colonization and contaminated intravascular catheters, the skin is thought to serve as the source. Other sources include intraabdominal abscesses, peritonitis, and rarely, the urinary tract and contaminated IV solutions. *Candida* species can be recovered from the hospital environment, including food, counter tops, air-conditioning vents, floors, respirators, and from hands of medical personnel [66].

Molecular biology tools have improved our knowledge and understanding of *Candida* epidemiology. Prospective molecular epidemiological studies of *Candida* using longitudinal cultures have shown that individual patients tend to harbor the same genotype of *Candida* over long periods of time [67]. More than 60% of patients with candidemia have positive cultures for the same *Candida* genotype as the genotype isolated from various anatomic sites prior to developing fungemia [67]. DNA typing has also confirmed acquisition of nosocomial *Candida* species from environmental and human sources. *Candida* species have been recovered from 25% to 50% of inanimate surfaces sampled [68], and in several studies, *Candida* was cultured from patients' rooms prior to patient acquisition of the same strain [69]. Surfaces commonly harboring *Candida* spp. were those in contact with hands of personnel or patients. Identical strains of *Candida* have also been recovered from patient food prior to patient acquisition [68, 70]. However, except in outbreak settings, the source of *Candida* species causing infection is usually from the host's endogenous flora.

Clinical Manifestations

Oropharyngeal Candidiasis

Hippocrates is credited with first describing oral thrush in debilitated individuals. Nineteenth-century authorities recognized that thrush invariably arose as a consequence of preexisting illness. The initial discovery of the organism causing thrush was not made until 1839, when Langenbeck described a fungus in buccal aphthae in a case of typhus [71], but it was left to Berg in 1846 to establish a cause–effect relationship between the fungus and oral lesions [72]. The taxonomic confusion continued until 1933 when Berkhout proposed the genus name *Candida*, separating this genus from the universal *Monilia* genus that affects fruit and vegetables [1].

Oropharyngeal candidiasis (OPC) is considered an opportunistic infection caused by a ubiquitous fungal organism that is routinely seen as normal oral flora. The transition from commensal to invasive infection of the oral mucosa is caused by local changes in the microflora or by an inefficient host response system which results in the overgrowth and invasion of *Candida* spp. The prevalence of OPC remains high and continues to increase, because the population of compromised hosts continues to expand [73]. Underlying conditions associated with a greater prevalence of OPC include prematurity, ill-fitting dentures, xerostomia, radiation of the head and neck, uncontrolled diabetes mellitus, hematologic and solid organ malignancies, oral or inhaled corticosteroid use, antimicrobial therapy, and HIV infection [74].

Persistent OPC in infants may be the first manifestation of childhood AIDS or chronic mucocutaneous candidiasis. One group of investigators reported that 28% of cancer patients not receiving antifungal prophylaxis developed OPC [75], and another group observed OPC in 57% of immunocompromised patients [76]. Patients at greatest risk of developing OPC include those receiving corticosteroids and with prolonged neutropenia who are colonized with a *Candida* species [76]. Approximately 80–90% of patients with HIV-infection will develop OPC [77]. In one study, 60% of untreated patients developed an AIDS-related infection or Kaposi's sarcoma within 2 years of the appearance of OPC [78].

Candida albicans remains the most common species responsible for OPC, accounting for 80–90% of cases. The ability of *C. albicans* to adhere to buccal epithelial cells is critical in establishing oral colonization; *C. albicans* adheres better to epithelial cells than non-*albicans Candida* species. Pulsed-field gel electrophoresis of *Candida* strains obtained from HIV-positive patients with OPC compared with isolates recovered from healthy individuals indicate an identical strain distribution frequency, suggesting that HIV-associated candidiasis is not caused by unique or more virulent strains of *Candida*, but from defects in host defenses [79]. Immune defenses against *Candida* depend on appropriate host recognition, followed by activation of antifungal mechanisms in effector cells through pattern-recognition receptors on host cells. This recognition induces intracellular signaling pathways that modulate protective and inflammatory responses, such as expression of costimulatory molecules, release of proinflammatory cytokines and modulation of acquired immunity [80].

Mercante et al. examined the impact of viral load and CD4 cell count on the occurrence of OPC in 160 HIV-positive patients [81], and they identified low HIV viral load (<10,000 copies/mL) as the most important co-variate associated with absence of OPC. Other important variables associated with OPC included age, antiretroviral therapy, and low CD4 cell counts, but only in subjects with HIV viral loads >10,000 copies/mL. In a study comparing current OPC epidemiology from that noted in the pre-HAART era [82], similar epidemiologic findings were noted. Similar to the pre-HAART era, they found a frequency of *Candida* colonization of approximately 50% along with a similar species distribution with *C. albicans* about 85%. As in prior studies, detectable HIV RNA and CD4 count <200 cells/μL were significantly associated with *Candida* colonization of the oral cavity.

Profound differences exist between HIV-positive and negative patients with regard to natural history, diagnosis and management of OPC [83] including an increase in non-*albicans Candida* species recovered from HIV-positive individuals [84]. HIV-positive patients experience recurrent episodes of OPC and esophageal candidiasis as immunodeficiency progresses; these patients may also receive multiple courses of antifungal drugs contributing to antifungal resistance. In these patients, antifungal agents are also less efficacious and take longer to achieve a clinical response. In a prospective study evaluating tissue-associated immune dysfunction in HIV-positive patients with OPC, patients with asymptomatic *Candida* colonization of the oral mucosa and reduced $CD4^+$ cell counts had higher numbers of $CD8^+$ cells throughout the tissue and had normal E-cadherin expression [85]. In contrast, in patients with active OPC, the $CD8^+$ cells tended to accumulate around the epithelial-lamina propria junction with reduced E-cadherin expression. After the resolution of the OPC, the $CD8^+$ cells returned and the E-cadherin expression returned to normal.

Symptoms of oral thrush include a painful mouth, burning tongue and dysphagia. Patients with severe objective intraoral lesions may be asymptomatic. Signs include diffuse erythema with white patches that appear as discrete lesions on the surfaces of the buccal mucosa, palate, oropharynx, tongue, and gums. With some difficulty, the plaques can be wiped off revealing a raw, erythematous and sometimes bleeding base. Constitutional signs of infection are absent. Oropharyngeal candidiasis can impair the quality of life by reduction in fluid or food intake. The most commonly identified form of OPC is termed acute pseudomembranous candidiasis. This form is seen frequently in HIV-positive persons and presents with a whitish-yellow thick curd–like exudate on mucosal surfaces (Fig. 1a). Plaques may be small and discrete or confluent, involving the entire oral mucosa; they consist of necrotic material and desquamated epithelial cells, penetrated by hyphae and yeast cells [86].

Chronic atrophic stomatitis, or denture stomatitis, is the second most common form of OPC. It is frequently asymptomatic, but may be associated with chronic soreness and burning of the mouth. Diffuse erythema and edema of the portion of the palate in contact with dentures is evident (Fig. 1b). The lower denture is rarely involved. Chronic atrophic stomatitis was recorded in 24–60% of denture wearers and is several-fold more frequent in women than in men [87]. *Candida* is detected by culture or microscopy in over 90% of symptomatic subjects. Even in the absence of signs or symptoms, the prevalence of yeast is higher in denture wearers. Maximum concentrations of yeast are found on the denture fitting surface. *Candida* species readily adhere to plastic objects including orthodontic appliances.

Angular cheilitis, or perleche is characterized by soreness, erythema, and fissuring at the corners of the mouth (Fig. 1c). Cheilitis can accompany oral thrush or denture stomatitis, or can appear in the absence of oral disease. Vitamin deficiency and iron-deficiency anemia are also associated with cheilitis, with *Candida* as a secondary colonizer.

Chronic hyperplastic candidiasis or *Candida* leukoplakia is a term used to describe discrete, transparent to whitish raised lesions of variable sizes found on the inner surface of the cheeks and less frequently on the tongue. These lesions are found predominantly in men and are highly associated with smoking. Most leukoplakia lesions are not related to *Candida* infection and may be premalignant. Importantly, there is no known association between *Candida* and either dysplasia or malignancy. Biopsy of *Candida*-related leukoplakia lesions reveals parakeratosis and epithelial hyperplasia with *Candida* invasion. Midline glossitis (median rhomboid glossitis, acute atrophic stomatitis) manifests as symmetrical lesions in the center dorsum of the tongue with erythema and loss of papillae [88].

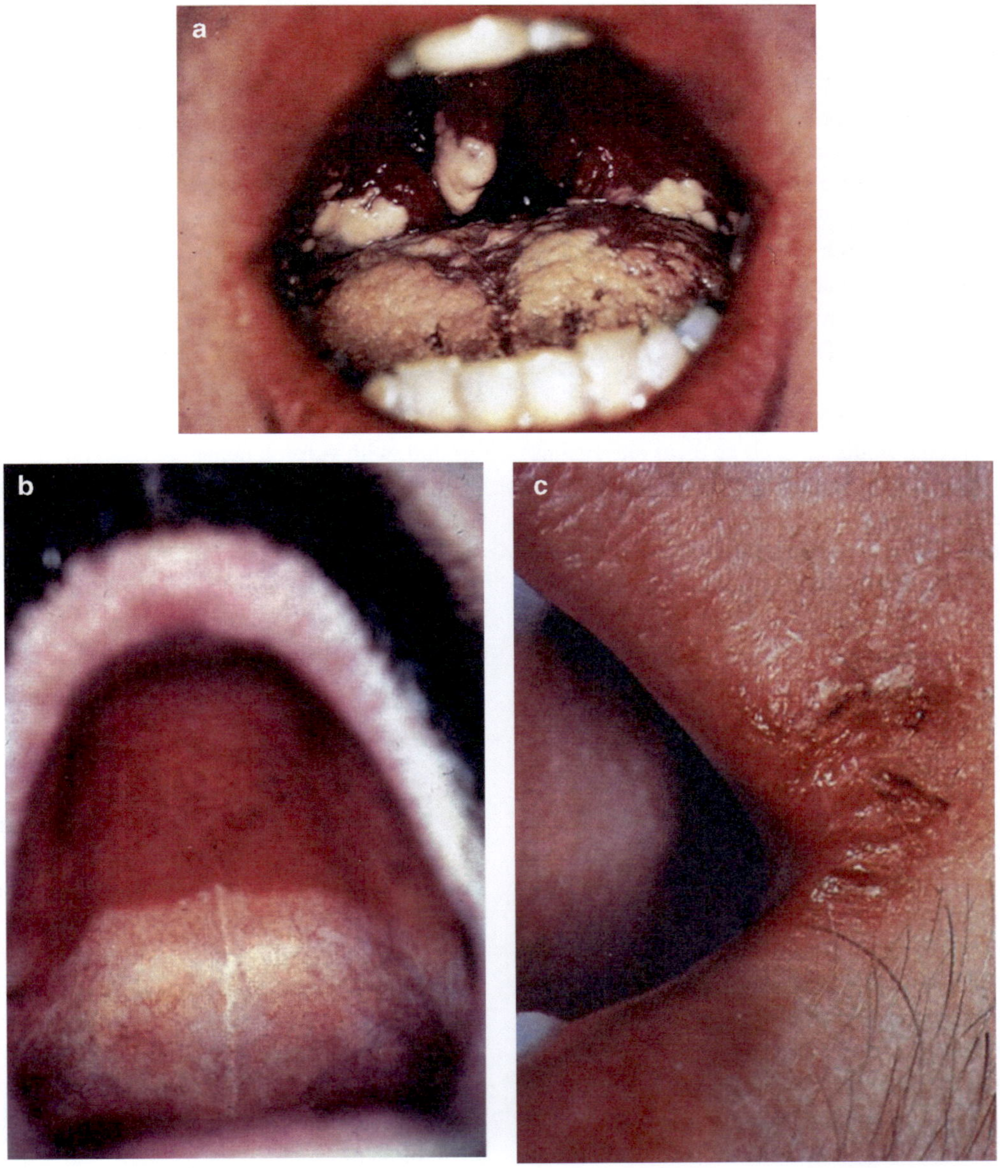

Fig. 1 Oropharyngeal candidiasis demonstrating (**a**) pseudomembranous type, (**b**) atrophic erythematous type associated with denture use, and (**c**) angular cheilitis

Candida species have also been incriminated in an oral "burning mouth" syndrome, characterized by a raw or sore tongue, especially following antibiotic administration. This self-limiting entity, although common, has not been shown to be due to primary or secondary *Candida* infection. Positive smears or cultures for *Candida* can be expected in 20–50% of asymptomatic patients, but these do not prove causality. The etiology of this syndrome is probably multifactorial [79].

Physical signs of OPC are insufficient to allow a reliable diagnosis. Oral lesions resembling candidiasis can occur with severe mucositis accompanying chemotherapy, and can reflect tissue necrosis, viral, or bacterial infections. On the other hand, OPC can complicate herpes simplex virus infections or leukoplakia. Diagnosis requires mycological confirmation, achieved by 10% potassium hydroxide or normal saline microscopic examination. Cultures are not essential for diagnosis and do not distinguish colonization from infection.

Esophageal Candidiasis

The prevalence of *Candida* esophagitis has increased because of AIDS, as well as the increased number of transplant recipients, patients with cancer, and other severely immunocompromised patients. *Candida* are frequently recovered from the esophageal surface and reach the esophagus in oral secretions. Little is known about host and yeast factors operative in the pathogenesis of esophageal candidiasis (EC) and experimental models have not been established. Predisposing factors include exposure to local irradiation, recent cytotoxic chemotherapy, antibiotics, corticosteroids, and neutropenia [79]. The high prevalence of EC in patients with AIDS indicates the critical role of cell mediated immunity. Esophageal candidiasis in an HIV-positive patient may be the first manifestation of AIDS, typically occurring at CD4 counts <100 cells/μL [89].

EC presents with odynophagia, dysphagia, and retrosternal pain. Constitutional findings, such as fever and malaise, occasionally occur. Rarely, epigastric pain is the dominant symptom. Although EC may arise as an extension of OPC, in some series, the esophagus was the only site involved in two-thirds of patients. EC usually occurs in the distal 2/3 of the esophagus. EC in patients with AIDS may be entirely asymptomatic, in spite of extensive esophageal involvement [90]. Esophagitis is classified on the basis of endoscopic appearance: Type I, a few white or beige plagues, up to 2 mm in diameter; Type II, plaques are more numerous, larger than 2 mm in diameter; Type III, confluent, linear and nodular elevated plaques with hyperemia and frank ulceration (Fig. 2) and Type IV, similar to Type III but with increased mucosal friability and occasional narrowing of the lumen [91]. Uncommon complications of esophagitis include perforation, aortic-esophageal fistula, and rarely, extensive necrosis destroying the entire esophageal mucosa. In neutropenic patients, bacteremia and candidemia may arise from EC.

Antifungal therapy is frequently initiated empirically in high-risk patients. A reliable diagnosis of EC can only be made by histological evidence of tissue invasion in biopsy material. The finding of *Candida* within an esophageal lesion by smear or culture or in esophageal brushings does not allow distinction between colonization and infection. Positive esophageal brushings are highly sensitive but nonspecific in the diagnosis of EC. A barium contrast swallow study may reveal shaggy mucosal irregularities and nodular filling defects, but this method of diagnosis has been replaced by endoscopy, which not only provides a rapid and highly sensitive method of diagnosis, but is also the only reliable method of differentiating among the various other causes of esophagitis [89]. The characteristic endoscopic appearance of EC is described as yellow-white plaques on an erythematous background, with varying degrees of ulceration.

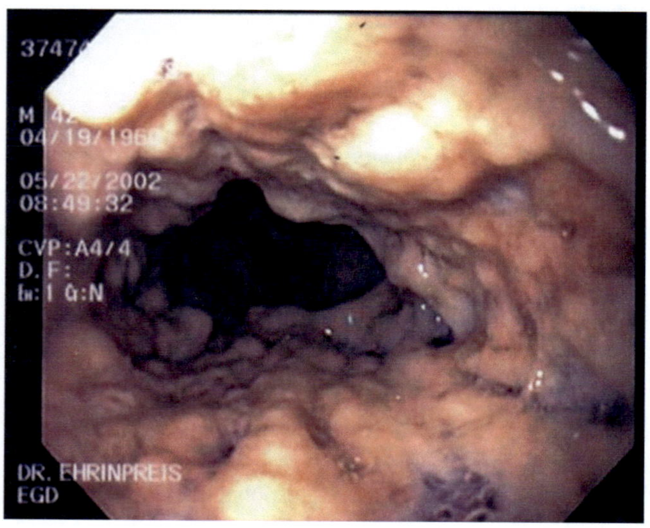

Fig. 2 Type III esophageal candidiasis with confluent plaques

In patients with AIDS and *Candida* esophagitis, gastric involvement is not uncommon and can be manifested by epigastric pain, nausea and vomiting. Most patients are asymptomatic [74, 83]. There is scant information about the need for or efficacy of antifungal therapy.

Cutaneous Candidiasis

Candida can invade any body surface and cause superficial infection of the skin, hair, and nails. Symptomatic mucocutaneous candidiasis will occur if dysfunction or local reduction in host resistance promotes an overgrowth of indigenous flora and there is a breach in the anatomical barriers. Dry intact skin is a potent barrier to fungal invasion, and hydration of the epidermis decreases resistance.

Candida albicans and *C. tropicalis* are the most common causes of superficial infections of the skin and the nails. These organisms favor growth in warm, moist areas such as the skin folds of obese individuals, between the fingers and toes, perineal areas, and genitocrural folds. Infections in these areas occur with much greater frequency in HIV-positive and diabetic patients and are exacerbated by occlusion, moisture, epidermal barrier dysfunction, hormonal manipulation, antibiotic use, and immunosuppression.

Generalized cutaneous candidiasis is a rare form of candidiasis that manifests as a diffuse eruption over the trunk and extremities. Patients have a history of generalized pruritus, with increased severity in the genitocrural folds, anal region, axillae, hands, and feet. Examination reveals a widespread rash that begins as individual vesicles that evolve into large confluent areas [92].

Intertrigo is the most common skin infection due to *Candida*, affecting sites in which skin surfaces are in close proximity providing a warm and moist environment. Infection begins with a vesiculopustular pruritic rash that enlarges and frequently progresses to maceration and erythema. The involved area has a scalloped border with a white rim consisting of necrotic epidermis that surrounds the erythematous macerated base. Satellite lesions are frequently found and may coalesce and extend into larger lesions. Erosio interdigitalis blastomycetica is a form of intertrigo that occurs in the areas between the fingers and toes and manifests as an erythematous painful rash. The affected skin reveals a tender, erythematous area of erosion, that can extend onto the sides of the digits and can be surrounded by maceration [93]. *Candida* folliculitis is predominantly found in the hair follicles and rarely becomes extensive; it should be differentiated from more common bacterial folliculitis.

Candida paronychia and onychomycosis are seen typically in patients with prolonged immersion of extremities in water and in patients with diabetes mellitus. Nail plate infection is generally not due to *Candida* species unless it is associated with congenital candidiasis or chronic mucocutaneous candidiasis [94]. *Candida* paronychia tends to be chronic, presenting as a painful erythematous area around and underneath the nail and nailfold. Physical examination reveals an area of inflammation that is warm, glistening, tense, erythematous, and extends underneath the nail. Chronic manifestations of this infection include loss of seal of the proximal nailfold, nail thickening, ridging, discoloration, and occasional nail loss.

Chronic Mucocutaneous Candidiasis

This syndrome involves multiple superficial sites, primarily the mouth, facial skin, hair and nails, which are simultaneously infected with *Candida* over a prolonged period of time. Chronic mucocutaneous candidiasis (CMC) is not a single disease entity, and is a consequence of multiple defects in host defenses against *Candida*. The final outcome is a chronic, superficial *Candida* infection at sites where *Candida* normally resides as a commensal organism [95]. Chronic mucocutaneous candidiasis is a rare entity; links between increased incidence of CMC and families of Iranian, Jewish or Finnish descent are described [96, 97]. Most CMC infections begin in infancy or the first two decades of life; onset after 30 years of age is rare. Chronic and recurrent infections frequently result in a disfiguring form of CMC called *Candida* granuloma. Most patients with CMC rarely experience visceral or disseminated fungal infections. The most common cause of death is bacterial sepsis.

A wide spectrum of CMC clinical syndromes have been described, based on inheritance as well as clinical factors [95, 98]. Group 1 is chronic oral candidiasis associated with HIV, inhaled steroids and denture-stomatitis. Group 2 comprises CMC associated with endocrinopathy (autosomal recessive) and has also been called "*Candida* endocrinopathy syndrome" or "autoimmune polyendocrinopathy candidiasis syndrome." It is now known to be due to mutations in the autoimmune regulator (AIRE) gene. Group 3 is localized CMC that is characterized by hyperkeratosis and cutaneous horn formation that affects both hands. This group is not associated with endocrine dysfunction. Group 4 is diffuse CMC, and includes patients who have widespread and severe infections and in whom familial factors are unknown or obscure. Group 5 includes CMC associated with thymoma, and usually manifests during the third decade of life. In addition, Group 5 CMC is also associated with myasthenia gravis, hypogammaglobulinemia, red cell aplasia, aplastic anemia, and neutropenia. Group 6 is CMC associated with interstitial keratitis [99]. Group 7 is CMC associated with keratitis, icthyosis, and deafness (KID syndrome).

A variety of *Candida* antigen-specific defects have been described in CMC patients. The commonest abnormality is a negative delayed-type skin test reaction to *Candida* antigen and is evident in 80% of patients tested (controls 16–37%), regardless of the clinical type of CMC. Approximately 70% of patients tested showed defective in vitro lymphocyte blastogenesis in response to *Candida* antigen [100]. A subpopulation of T-suppressor cells that respond to *Candida* mannoproteins by inhibiting T-helper cell function has been described [101]. These investigators reported a serum inhibitory factor in CMC patients that suppressed T-cell function. The majority of patients with CMC have normal or high serum antibodies to *Candida* and no consistent B-cell dysfunction has been reported. T-cell dysfunction is often reversible, with improvement in immunological parameters following clinical remission achieved by antimycotic therapy.

Chronic mucocutaneous candidiasis is frequently associated with endocrinopathies such as hypoparathyroidism (80%), hypoadrenalism (72%), ovarian failure (60%), growth hormone deficiency, gonad insufficiency (15%), diabetes mellitus (12%), and chronic lymphocytic thyroiditis with hypothyroidism (5%) [98]. Autoimmune antibodies may be found to adrenal, thyroid, and gastric tissues, and melanin-producing cells (vitiligo). Other features include thymomas and dental dysplasias, polyglandular autoimmune diseases, and antibodies. The onset of CMC is usually within the first year of life in nonendocrinopathy cases and within the first decade when associated with endocrinopathies. Approximately 90% of all cases of CMC have their onset before the age of 20 years, and about 33% of cases are associated with endocrinopathies.

The earliest lesion to appear is chronic pseudomembranous oral candidiasis. Angular cheilitis and lip fissures can develop and infection can spread to involve the esophagus and larynx. In postmenarchal females, *Candida* vaginitis supervenes, but is not a common feature. These superficial infections tend to be severe, chronic and recurrent in nature. Persistent onychia and paronychia are nearly as common as oral lesions. Lesions of the fingers vary from discoloration and dystrophy of the nails to crusting and hyperkeratotic horns (Fig.3a). Skin lesions, when present, are found mainly on the face, neck, ears, and shoulders, and less often involve the scalp and groin. In severe forms of CMC, there are hyperkeratotic crusts or *Candida* granuloma producing severe disfigurement (Fig. 3b). The latter findings are invariably found in the idiopathic, infant or juvenile-onset cases and rarely in association with endocrinopathy or mature-onset cases. A striking feature of CMC is the lack of invasive candidiasis.

Other associated disorders include autoimmune hepatitis, iron deficiency and malabsorption syndromes, aplastic anemia, hemolytic anemia, pernicious anemia, neutropenia, thrombocytopenia, thymomas, oropharyngeal tumors, and ectodermal abnormalities, such as alopecia and dental dysplasias. Patients with CMC are also prone to superinfections caused by herpes simplex, herpes zoster, bacteremias, disseminated *Mycobacterium avium* infections, dermatophytosis, and occasionally invasive fungal infections.

The evaluation of persons suspected of having any form of CMC should include a complete blood count with differential, lymphocyte phenotyping, T-lymphocyte response to *Candida* and tetanus, skin testing with *Candida*, tetanus, and mumps antigens, lymphokine production by antigen or mitogen-stimulated cells, T and B lymphocyte counts, and serum immunoglobulins. In adults, HIV antibody testing and a chest CT scan to rule out a thymoma should be done [95].

Vulvovaginal Candidiasis

In the USA, *Candida* vaginitis is the second most common vaginal infection. During the childbearing years, 75% of women experience at least one episode of vulvovaginal candidiasis (VVC), and 40–50% of these women experience a second attack [102]. *Candida* is isolated from the genital tract of approximately 10–20% of asymptomatic, healthy women of childbearing age. *Candida* organisms gain access to the vagina from the adjacent perianal area and then adhere to vaginal epithelial cells. *Candida albicans* adheres to vaginal epithelial cells in significantly greater numbers than non-*albicans Candida* species [103].

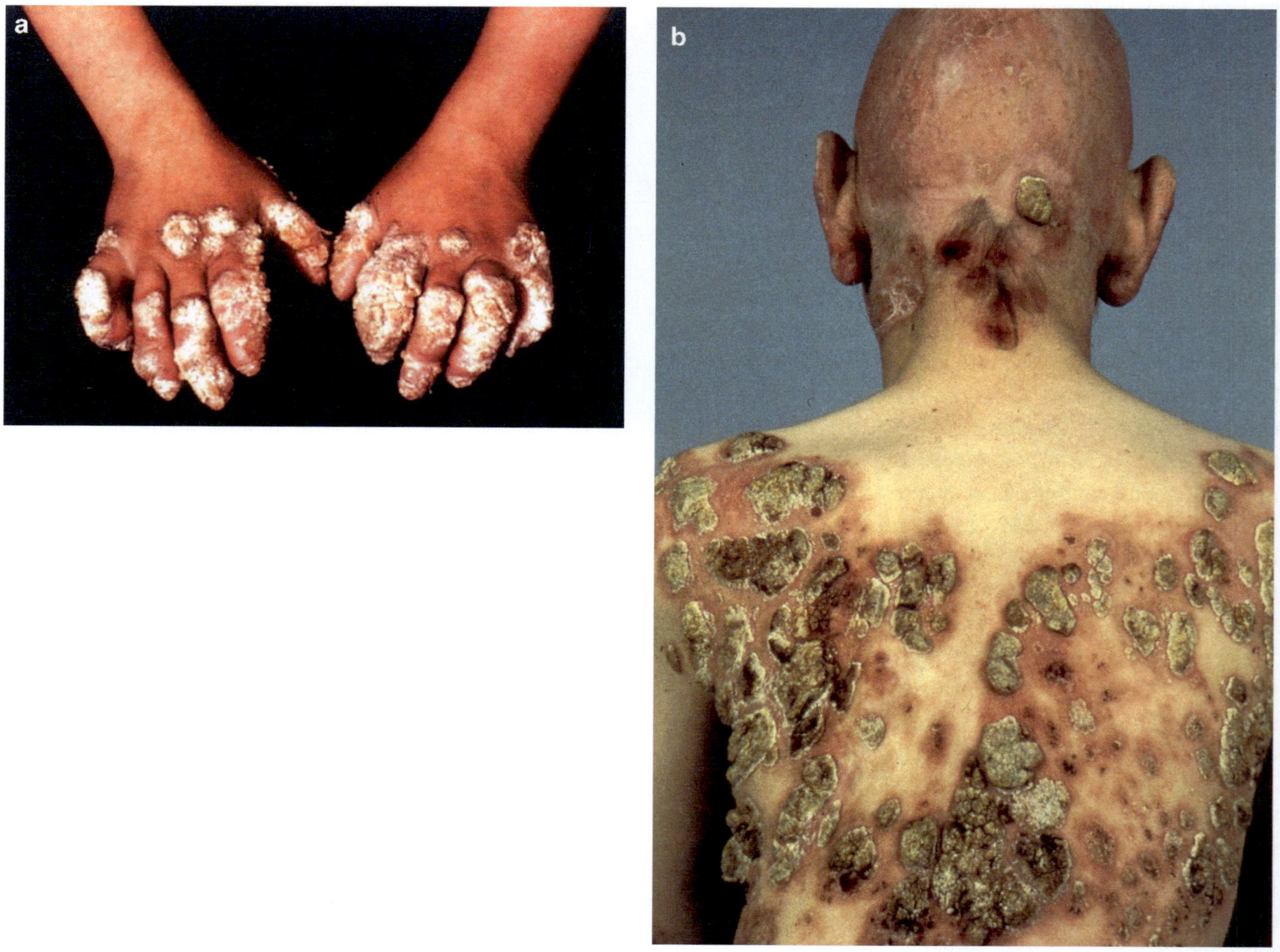

Fig. 3 Chronic mucocutaneous candidiasis showing crusted hyperkeratotic lesions on (**a**) hands and (**b**) trunk and scalp

Several factors, including pregnancy, oral contraceptives with a high estrogen content, and uncontrolled diabetes mellitus, are associated with increased rates of asymptomatic vaginal colonization with *Candida* as well as *Candida* vaginitis (Fig. 4). The hormonal dependence of VVC is illustrated by the fact that *Candida* is seldom isolated from premenarchial girls, and the prevalence of *Candida* vaginitis is lower after the menopause, except in women taking hormone replacement therapy. Other predisposing factors include corticosteroids, antimicrobial therapy, intrauterine devices, and high frequency of coitus.

Germination of *Candida* enhances colonization and tissue invasion. Factors that enhance or facilitate germination, such as estrogen therapy and pregnancy, tend to precipitate symptomatic vaginitis, whereas epithelial cell innate immunity that inhibits germination prevents acute vaginitis in women who are asymptomatic carriers of *Candida*. A precipitating factor that explains the transformation from asymptomatic carriage to symptomatic vaginitis is identified in only a few patients (Fig. 4).

During pregnancy, the incidence of clinical episodes often reaches a maximum in the third trimester, but symptomatic recurrences are common throughout pregnancy. The high levels of reproductive hormones are thought to increase the glycogen content of the vaginal environment and provide a carbon source for *Candida* growth and germination. Estrogens enhance vaginal epithelial cell avidity for *Candida* adherence, and a yeast cytosol receptor or binding system for female reproductive hormones has been documented. In addition, estrogens enhance yeast-mycelial transformation. Low-estrogen oral contraceptives may also cause an increase in *Candida* vaginitis. Hormone replacement therapy may contribute to vaginitis in postmenopausal women. Vaginal colonization with *Candida* is more common in diabetic patients, and poorly controlled diabetes predisposes to symptomatic vaginitis. Glucose tolerance tests have been recommended for women with recurrent vulvovaginal candidiasis (RVVC); however, the yield is low and testing is not justified in otherwise healthy premenopausal women. Diets high in refined sugar may precipitate symptomatic *Candida* vaginitis.

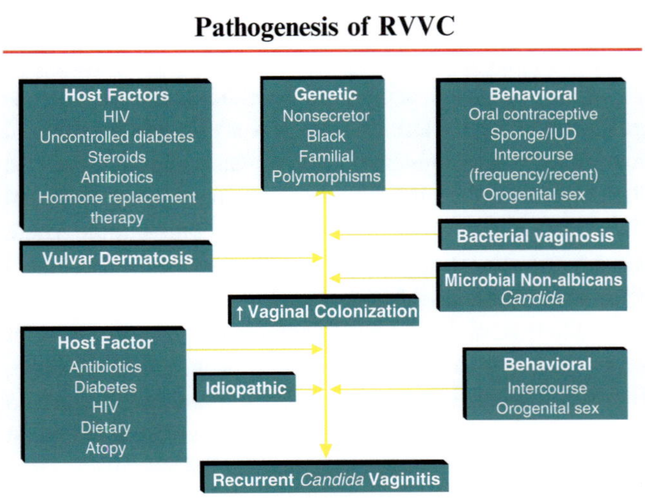

Fig. 4 Pathogenesis of recurrent vulvovaginal candidiasis

Symptomatic VVC is often observed during or after use of systemic or intravaginal antibiotics. Although no antimicrobial agent is free of this complication, the broad-spectrum antibiotics are mainly responsible. They may act by eliminating the normal protective vaginal bacterial flora. *Lactobacillus* spp. provide a colonization-resistance mechanism and prevent germination of *Candida*. However, most women taking antibiotics do not develop *Candida* vaginitis and vaginal depletion of *Lactobacillus* spp. is not associated with increased risk of VVC. Environmental factors that predispose to *Candida* vaginitis may include tight, poorly ventilated clothing and nylon underclothing, which increase perineal moisture and temperature. Chemical contact, local allergy and hypersensitivity reactions may also predispose to symptomatic vaginitis. Iron deficiency is said to predispose to *Candida* infection, but there is no evidence to support this view. In patients who are debilitated or immunosuppressed, oral and vaginal candidiasis correlates well with reduced cell-mediated immunity, as evident in CMC and AIDS. Based on these observations, T-lymphocytes may contribute to normal effective innate vaginal defense mechanisms preventing mucosal invasion by *Candida*.

Several theories have been proposed to explain RVVC [104]. The intestinal reservoir theory is based on recovery of *Candida* on rectal culture in almost 100% of women with vulvovaginal candidiasis. DNA typing of vaginal and rectal cultures obtained simultaneously usually reveals identical strains. However, other studies have shown a lower concordance between rectal and vaginal cultures in patients with RVVC. In a maintenance study of women with RVVC who were receiving ketoconazole, recurrence of *Candida* vaginitis often occurred with no evidence of *Candida* in the rectum. Also, oral nystatin, which reduces intestinal yeast carriage, fails to prevent RVVC. Repeated reintroduction of yeast into the vagina from the gut is therefore no longer considered a likely cause of recurrent *Candida* vaginitis.

The sexual transmission theory is based on the occurrence of penile colonization with *Candida* organisms, which are present in approximately 20% of male partners of women with RVVC, and the observation that infected partners often carry identical *Candida* strains. Oral colonization of partners with an identical strain of *Candida* also occurs, and may be a source of orogenital transmission. However, in most studies involving treatment of partners, there was no reduction in the frequency of episodes of vaginitis.

The vaginal relapse theory to explain RVVC is currently favored. Although antifungal therapy may reduce the number of *Candida* and alleviate signs and symptoms of inflammation, the eradication of *Candida* from the vagina is incomplete because most agents are fungistatic. The small number of organisms that persist in the vagina result in continued carriage of the organism; when host environmental conditions permit, the colonizing organisms increase in number and undergo mycelial transformation, resulting in a new clinical episode. Drug resistance is seldom responsible for RVVC in women infected with *C. albicans*. Current vaginal relapse theories regarding the pathogenesis of RVVC include qualitative and quantitative deficiency in the normal protective vaginal bacterial flora (unproven), and an acquired, often transient, antigen-specific deficiency in local T lymphocyte function that permits unchecked yeast proliferation and germination. Reduced T lymphocyte reactivity to *Candida* antigen may result from the elaboration of prostaglandin E2 by the patient's macrophages which blocks *Candida* antigen-induced lymphocyte proliferation, possibly by inhibiting interleukin-2 production. Abnormal macrophage function could be the result of histamine produced as a consequence of local IgE *Candida* antibodies or a serum factor [105]. Recent evidence of genetic factors that influence epithelial cell susceptibility to colonization (dectin 1 and mannose-binding lectin) are likely critical to pathogenesis of RVVC.

Vulvar pruritus is the most common symptom of VVC. Vaginal discharge is often minimal and sometimes absent. Although described as being typically "cottage cheese-like" in character (Fig. 5), the discharge may vary from watery to homogeneously thick. Vaginal soreness, irritation, vulvar burning, dyspareunia, and external dysuria are other common symptoms. If there is an odor, it is minimal and not offensive. Characteristically, the symptoms are exacerbated during the week before the onset of menses. The onset of menstrual flow brings some relief. Examination reveals erythema and swelling of the labia and vulva, often with discrete pustulopapular peripheral lesions. The cervix is normal and the vaginal mucosa is erythematous with adherent whitish discharge.

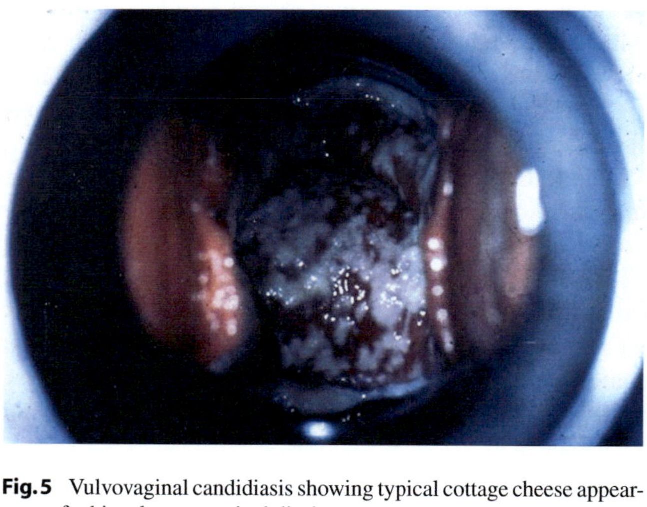

Fig. 5 Vulvovaginal candidiasis showing typical cottage cheese appearance of white clumpy vaginal discharge

In most symptomatic patients with VVC, diagnosis is readily made on the basis of microscopic examination of vaginal secretions. A wet mount with saline has a sensitivity of only 40–60%. A preparation of 10% potassium hydroxide (KOH) is more sensitive (50–70%) in identifying the presence of yeast cells. Patients with *Candida* vaginitis have a normal vaginal pH, 4.0–4.5. A pH > 4.5 suggests the possibility of bacterial vaginosis, trichomoniasis, or mixed infection. Routine cultures are unnecessary, but vaginal culture should be performed in suspicious cases with negative microscopy. Although vaginal culture is the most sensitive method available for detecting *Candida*, a positive culture does not necessarily indicate that *Candida* is responsible for the vaginal symptoms. There is no reliable serological technique for the diagnosis of symptomatic VVC. Commercial tests, including latex agglutination slide tests, are less sensitive than culture and have no advantages over microscopy. Although PCR based diagnosis is now available, its utility is unknown except in excluding the diagnosis of VVC.

Candidemia and Disseminated Candidiasis

Candidemia or systemic candidiasis has been divided into four syndromes, namely, catheter-related candidiasis, acute disseminated candidiasis, chronic disseminated candidiasis (hepatosplenic candidiasis), and deep organ candidiasis [106]. Although hematogenous involvement occurs at some stage in the evolution of each, only the first two syndromes are associated strongly with documented candidemia. Hence use of the term candidemia only as a marker of invasive candidiasis results in the underestimation of the true incidence of invasive candidiasis [106].

Clinical aspects of candidemia are extremely variable. Patients present with fever alone without organ-specific manifestations, or a wide spectrum of symptoms and signs, including fulminant sepsis. Acute candidemia is indistinguishable from bacterial sepsis and septic shock. Clinical manifestations of fungemia are frequently superimposed on those of the underlying illnesses and concomitant bacterial infections, including bacteremia, are not uncommon. There are no specific clinical features of candidemia associated with individual *Candida* species.

At the time of documented candidemia, manifestations of invasive metastatic candidiasis may be present. However, frequently when the latter are evident, blood cultures are no longer positive. Hence, candidemia is a marker, although an insensitive one, of deeply invasive candidiasis [107]. Only 50% of patients with disseminated candidiasis have positive blood cultures [108], and antemortem diagnosis is relatively

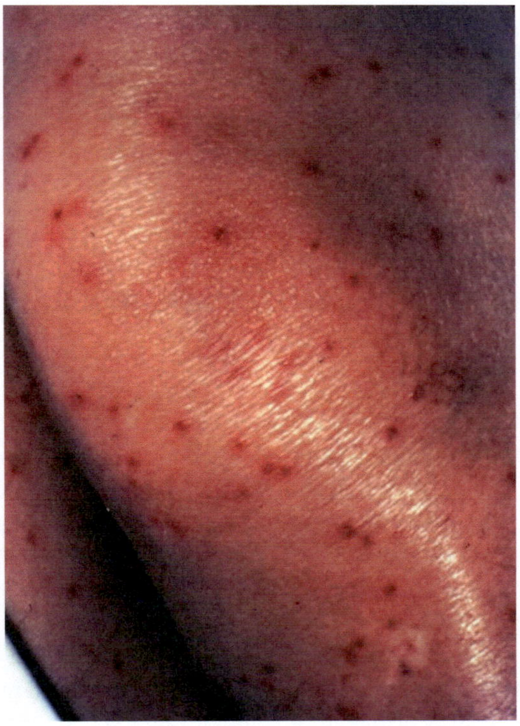

Fig. 6 Papulopustular skin lesions seen in a patient with candidemia

infrequent in the absence of candidemia (15–40%). The likelihood of systemic invasion has been correlated with increasing numbers of positive blood cultures [109] although not all patients with candidemia have the same risk of dissemination. Patients with neutropenia have a significantly higher rate of visceral and cutaneous dissemination [110]. Dissemination to multiple organs often involves skin, kidney, eye, brain, myocardium, liver, spleen, and bone (Fig. 6).

The possibility of asymptomatic disseminated infection drives the treatment principles of candidemia, even when candidemia is transient. Transient candidemia can occur from any source, but frequently it follows intravascular catheter infection with prompt resolution following catheter removal. In most prospective studies of nosocomial candidemia, approximately half the patients will have cleared candidemia within 72 h without receiving systemic fungal therapy. However, they could have seeded into an organ without symptoms appearing until later. Prolonged candidemia, especially when blood cultures remain persistently positive on appropriate antifungal therapy, suggests a persistent focus or source, such as an intravascular catheter, an abscess, or suppurative thrombophlebitis, endocarditis, severe neutropenia, and rarely, antifungal resistance, especially with some non-*albicans Candida* species [7, 111]. At the time of diagnosis of candidemia, physical examination rarely reveals clinical signs of dissemination. However, a thorough examination, including a dilated funduscopic examination, may reveal metastatic infection and is mandatory.

Occasionally, blood cultures obtained via a central catheter may represent contamination, hence the importance of obtaining multiple blood cultures, especially cultures from peripheral vein sites. Nevertheless, febrile patients with a single positive blood culture for *Candida* species should always be considered to have a proven infection. In reviewing 155 episodes of catheter-related candidiasis, investigators observed a similar frequency of autopsy-proven candidiasis whether blood cultures were obtained from a central catheter or a peripheral site [109]. Improving blood culture yield can also be enhanced by increasing blood volume and utilizing newer techniques and media [112]. Given the insensitivity of blood cultures, together with the lack of test for the diagnosis of invasive candidiasis, detection of hematogenous dissemination remains poor.

The crude mortality rates reported in patients with candidemia generally range from 40% to 60% [113–115] with an attributable mortality of 30–40%, exceeding that of most bacteremias [56]. Since 1989, a 50% reduction in national mortality rates for invasive candidiasis has been reported, following a steady increase in mortality in the previous decades reaching 0.62 deaths/100,000 population [116]. A similar decline in rates of death from systemic candidiasis associated with HIV infection occurred (0.04/100,000). The explanation for decreased mortality in both HIV positive and negative patients in spite of increased *Candida* invasive disease may be related to increased awareness, earlier diagnosis, and an enhanced therapeutic armamentarium. If the crude mortality rate of *Candida* BSI is 40%, than 2,800–11,200 deaths each year may be associated with nosocomial candidemia [3]. Infections due to *C. parapsilosis* tend to be associated with reduced lethality (23%), and the highest mortality has been reported for *C. tropicalis* and *C. krusei* [56], especially in neutropenic patients. Candidemia in neutropenic patients is a life-threatening infection that is associated with acute disseminated candidiasis, a sepsis-like syndrome, multiorgan failure, and death.

Candida Eye Infections

Candida organisms gain access to the eye by one of two routes, either direct inoculation during eye surgery or trauma (exogenous), or as the result of hematogenous spread (endogenous) [117, 118]. Any eye structure can be involved, and involvement can be unilateral or bilateral. Endophthalmitis refers to infection of the posterior compartment and can be manifest as chorioretinitis with or without vitritis. Endogenous endophthalmitis occurs in patients with nosocomial candidemia, including neonates, and intravenous drug users [119, 120] *Candida* endophthalmitis should raise the suspicion of concomitant widely disseminated candidiasis.

Estimates of the incidence of eye involvement during candidemia have been as high as 28–37% [121], but recently the incidence appears to be decreasing, perhaps related to the almost uniform treatment of all patients with candidemia. In one prospective study of 50 patients with fungemia, the incidence of ocular candidiasis was 26%, all manifested as chorioretinitis [122]. Several of the patients with an initially negative eye examination developed signs of ocular candidiasis 1–2 weeks later. Not all patients with endophthalmitis have a history of recent candidemia. *Candida albicans* is the commonest species responsible for ocular involvement, but other *Candida* species have been incriminated [123]. In experimental animal models, a tropism of *C. albicans* for chorioretinal blood vessels has been demonstrated.

Symptoms of chorioretinitis are variable and often absent in patients too ill to complain. Symptoms include visual blurring, floaters, scotomata and blindness. Fundoscopic examination usually reveals white, cotton ball-like lesions situated in the chorioretinal layer which may rapidly progress to extend into the posterior vitreous (Fig. 7). Indirect ophthalmoscopy with pupillary dilation is necessary to achieve complete visualization. Ocular lesions require the presence of leukocytes for development; presence of neutropenia inhibits the formation of ocular lesions in experimental rabbit models [124]. All patients with candidemia should have at least one dilated retinal examination early in the course of therapy, preferably performed by an ophthalmologist [106]. This recommendation is particularly important in patients unable to communicate or recognize visual disturbances.

Diagnosis of *Candida* endophthalmitis is usually made on the basis of clinical context and characteristic fundoscopic picture. Aspiration of the anterior chamber is rarely diagnostic whereas vitrectomy, often performed for therapeutic purposes, usually yields positive culture for *Candida* [125]. A diagnostic vitreal aspirate is recommended for patients with endophthalmitis of unknown origin [106]. For candidemic patients with an initially normal fundoscopic examination, some experts recommend a second examination after 2 weeks.

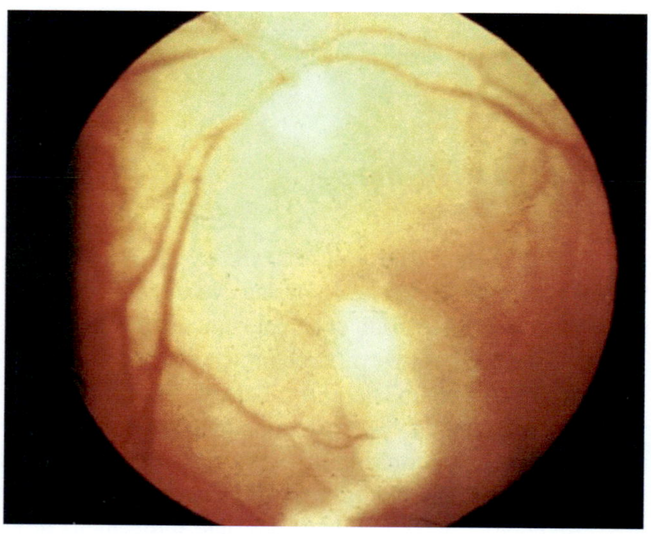

Fig. 7 *Candida* chorioretinitis with vitritis; note white cotton-like lesions extending into the vitreous body

Candida Cardiac and Endovascular Infections

Candida myocarditis is the result of hematogenous dissemination with development of one or more abscesses within the myocardium. Most frequently, abscesses are microabscesses usually diagnosed at autopsy. One group reported 62% of 50 patients with disseminated candidiasis had myocardial involvement at autopsy and other retrospective autopsy studies reported myocardial abscesses in 8–93% [126].

Candida spp. reach the pericardium from adjacent endocarditis or myocarditis but most frequently pericardial involvement is the result of hematogenous seeding or direct inoculation at the time of cardiac surgery [127]. Pericarditis is purulent in nature, resembles bacterial infection, and may be complicated by constrictive disease. Successful therapy requires pericardiectomy in addition to antifungal drugs. Medical therapy alone is associated with an extremely poor prognosis [128].

The advent of prosthetic cardiac valve surgery in the late 1960s together with the worldwide increase in intravenous drug use, especially heroin use, resulted in a dramatic increase in the incidence of *Candida* endocarditis [129]. In a large retrospective review of fungal endocarditis from 1965 to 1995, fungal endocarditis was responsible for fewer than 10% of all cases of infective endocarditis [130]. This review documented the changing epidemiology of fungal endocarditis. Although *C. albicans* was previously responsible for 66% of fungal endocarditis cases, the frequency of fungal endocarditis due to *C. albicans* now accounts for less than half the cases, and infection due to non-*albicans Candida* is as common as that due to *C. albicans* [130]. The increase in non-*albicans Candida* endocarditis reflects the changing epidemiology of nosocomial candidemia, although it would appear that *C. parapsilosis* has a unique tropism for prosthetic endovascular surfaces.

The pathogenesis of *Candida* endocarditis is complex, and several risk factors have been confirmed [130]. *Candida* organisms rarely adhere to and colonize normal valvular endothelium. Predisposing factors include: (1) underlying valvular disease; (2) prosthetic cardiac valves, including homografts, which provide an abnormal surface once coated with platelets and fibronectin for *Candida* adherence; (3) prolonged presence of intravascular catheters, resulting in persistent high inoculum candidemia; (4) heroin addiction, still responsible for sporadic cases and occasional outbreaks of *Candida* endocarditis [129]; (5) other risk factors such as cancer chemotherapy, pre-existing bacterial endocarditis, immunocompromised hosts and temporally related noncardiac surgery, especially abdominal surgery [130]; and (6) low birth weight neonates. *Candida* endocarditis is rare in the setting of granulocytopenia [131]. Possible explanations include the short duration of undiagnosed candidemia together with universal aggressive therapy; however, it is also that the accompanying thrombocytopenia may prevent vegetation formation.

Prosthetic valve endocarditis (PVE) has been the most common form of *Candida* endocarditis. However, Ellis and colleagues in their review concluded that cardiac valve surgery showed the largest decrease in incidence as a risk factor. Most episodes of *Candida* PVE occur within 2 months of valve surgery although endocarditis also occurs much later [132]. Specific risk factors for PVE include complicated surgery, perioperative antibiotics, prolonged postoperative use of catheters, and candidemia even if transient. Damaged endocardium, especially suture line and prosthetic material, serve as foci for *Candida* adherence. Rarely, contamination of homografts and heterografts occurs before insertion. Pacemaker endocarditis due to *Candida* has also been described [133].

Clinical findings and complications of *Candida* endocarditis are similar to those seen with bacterial endocarditis with the exception of increased frequency of large emboli to major vessels in *Candida* endocarditis. Aortic and mitral valve involvement are most common. The classical findings of bacterial endocarditis, including Osler nodes, Janeway lesions, splinter hemorrhages, splenomegaly, hematuria and embolic manifestations have been reported, but some studies have found a reduced incidence of cardiac failure, changing heart murmurs, and splenomegaly [130]. Rarely, polymicrobial *Candida* endocarditis occurs and may follow or accompany bacterial endocarditis. A patient with *Candida* PVE may relapse several years following a putative cure with medical therapy; hence long-term follow-up is necessary [134].

Most patients with *Candida* endocarditis have positive blood cultures. The diagnosis of *Candida* endocarditis is often delayed because blood cultures can be negative. Fungal endocarditis has been noted to be characterized by a long duration of symptoms before hospitalization [130]. Improved diagnosis of *Candida* endocarditis has followed greater awareness of the significance of candidemia, newer blood culture techniques, and more frequent use of echocardiography. Accordingly, increased preoperative diagnosis has been noted in the last decade [130]. Transthoracic and especially transesophogeal echocardiography have made an enormous contribution to facilitating diagnosis and avoiding the usual delay in diagnosis. Visualizing large vegetations in patients with negative blood cultures is strong circumstantial evidence of *Candida* endocarditis. Mycological examination should be performed on all surgically removed emboli.

Mortality of *Candida* endocarditis remains high. Prior to the availability of cardiac surgery, mortality was in excess of 90%. With combined treatment employing surgery and aggressive antifungal therapy, mortality rates <40% can be anticipated.

Noncardiac endovascular *Candida* infections involving large and medium sized arteries and veins have increased with the increased incidence of nosocomial candidemia [135, 136]. Phlebitis is common and often is associated with tunneled subcutaneous catheters. Delay in treatment can result in extensive vascular thrombosis and suppuration and persistent candidemia in spite of treatment with high doses of fungicidal agents. Venous thrombi, even after removal of responsible catheters, impair drug penetration and allow microabscesses to persist within the thrombi with resultant persistent candidemia [137]. For cure, surgical excision of thrombi is often required in addition to prolonged antifungal therapy. Complications include superior vena cava obstruction, tricuspid valve endocarditis, right-sided mural endocarditis, and pulmonary vein thrombosis. Small peripheral vein thrombophlebitis is not uncommon.

Arterial involvement may occur as a result of candidemia seeding prosthetic aortic valves and other large arterial grafts [138]. Uncontrolled diabetes in high-risk patients further facilitates the development of true mycotic aneurysms localized and originating at the graft suture line. In addition to pain, fever, and signs of systemic infection, the mycotic aneurysm may rupture resulting in catastrophic hemorrhage or in large vessel occlusion. *Candida* mycotic aneurysms have been reported in the cerebral circulation, pulmonary arteries following use of Swan-Ganz catheters, iliac vessels of intravenous drug users, and dialysis fistulae.

Chronic Disseminated Candidiasis

Chronic disseminated candidiasis, also termed hepatosplenic candidiasis, develops as a complication of invasive candidiasis during granulocytopenia [139, 140]. Candidemia, the cornerstone of this syndrome, frequently follows *Candida* colonization of the gut, complicated by gastrointestinal mucosa disruption and lamina propria invasion by *Candida*. Many of the patients with chronic disseminated candidiasis have no history of documented candidemia. Following recovery from neutropenia, the *Candida* lesions established during neutropenia do not resolve, but become more prominent, especially in the liver, spleen, and kidneys. At the time of diagnosis, both acute and chronic inflammatory cells are found to surround the outer border of *Candida* pseudohyphae and an expanding zone of tissue necrosis between the inflammatory infiltrate and fungal cells. Occasionally calcification occurs at the center of lesions with nonviable fungal elements. This syndrome is now seen less frequently because of the widespread use of antifungal prophylaxis and early initiation of empirical antifungal therapy for fever in high risk neutropenic patients.

Patients usually have a history of a hematologic malignancy, especially acute leukemia, cytotoxic chemotherapy, and neutropenia for which they were febrile and received antibacterial therapy. After recovery from neutropenia, fever, nausea, vomiting, and right upper quadrant pain occur increase as neutrophils infiltrate foci of *Candida* invasion in liver and spleen. Laboratory findings often include elevation in serum alkaline phosphatase and leukocytosis. Hepatic transaminases are not commonly elevated.

Lesions of chronic disseminated candidiasis can be detected by computed tomography (CT), ultrasonography (US) and magnetic resonance imaging (MRI) (Fig. 8). The characteristic "bulls-eye" lesions are not detectable until neutrophil recovery, and they are not specific for this syndrome. As the lesions resolve during therapy, they may either disappear completely or undergo calcification. Ultrasonography appears to be less sensitive but possibly more specific than CT scanning in demonstrating characteristic target lesions [139, 141]. Diagnosis is confirmed by histopathological examination of hepatic tissue obtained by percutaneous or laparoscopic biopsy. Among *Candida* species, *C. albicans* is most common, and *C. tropicalis* is next most common. This syndrome can be caused by other *Candida* spp. as well as non-*Candida* fungi, such as *Trichosporon* spp., *Fusarium* spp. and *Aspergillus* spp. Metastatic tumors also can simulate the appearance of chronic disseminated candidiasis. Culture of hepatic tissue obtained at biopsy is usually negative, particularly if antifungal therapy has been given.

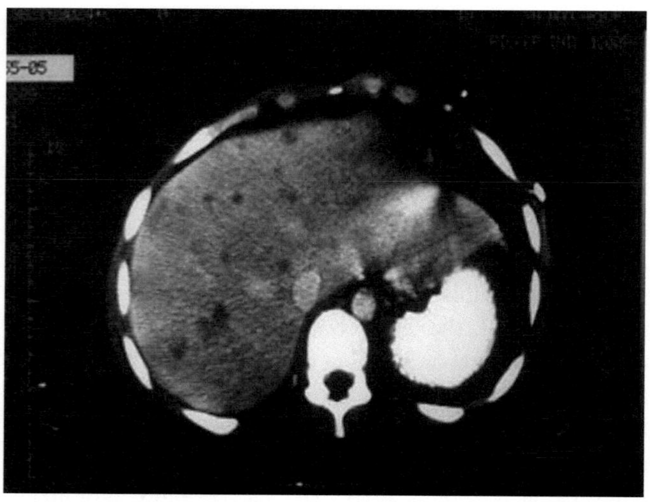

Fig. 8 CT scan of a patient with acute leukemia who had chronic disseminated candidiasis (hepatosplenic candidiasis). Note multiple punched out lesions throughout the liver

Neonatal Candidiasis

Neonatal candidiasis differs from invasive disease in older patients. Neonates present with subtle symptoms. Two distinct *Candida* syndromes are seen in neonates, and especially in preterm, low birth–weight neonates. The most serious of these syndromes is neonatal systemic candidiasis. Developing either via ascending infection of the uterine contents prior to birth or from colonization acquired during passage through the birth canal, hematogenous dissemination of *Candida* presents in the first days or weeks of life with symptoms identical to those of neonatal bacterial sepsis [142, 143]. Involvement of the lung, skin, and particularly the central nervous system (CNS) is common. CNS involvement in the neonate usually manifests as meningoencephalitis and should be assumed to be present in any neonate with candidemia because of the high incidence of this complication. Neurologic defects are common in survivors.

By contrast, neonates with congenital cutaneous candidiasis present within a few hours of birth with a diffuse maculopapular, erythematous rash involving almost any part of the skin [144, 145]. The initial rash can evolve to pustular or vesicular lesions with subsequent desquamation. Culture and microscopic examination of scrapings of the skin reveal *Candida* species, usually *C. albicans*. If the affected neonate is preterm (1,500 g), systemic involvement is frequent and the neonate should be evaluated repeatedly with blood, urine and cerebrospinal fluid (CSF) cultures in order to rule out neonatal systemic candidiasis [142]. In full-term neonates, infection is usually limited to the skin and gastrointestinal tract [146].

Candida Central Nervous System Infections

Candida is the most prevalent cerebral mycosis at postmortem examination and was found in 48% of autopsied subjects with invasive candidiasis [147]. In the same study, less than 25% of the subjects had the diagnosis of CNS involvement made antemortem.Diagnosis is often difficult and frequently delayed in all age groups but especially in preterm low birth weight neonates, resulting in considerable morbidity and mortality. Recently Petraitiene et al. reported the successful use of beta-D-glucan detection in the CSF of rabbits with experimental hematogenous *Candida* meningoencephalitis [148].

Central nervous system candidiasis involves both brain tissue and/or meninges, and, except for occasional association with neurosurgery and head trauma, is invariably the result of hematogenous dissemination [149–151]. In one autopsy study, a correlation between cardiac and cerebral involvement was noted with 80% of patients with myocardial or valve infection also having CNS candidiasis [147]. Cerebral parenchymal infection occurs as a single or multiple micro- or macroabscesses scattered throughout the brain [152]. Rarely, larger abscesses are visualized on CT scan. Other presentations include thrombosis, vasculitis, hemorrhage, fungus balls of both white and gray matter, and mycotic aneurysms. *Candida parapsilosis* has a predilection for cerebral vascular involvement [147]. *Candida* brain abscess presents with a variable picture, including fever, altered mental status (obtundation or coma), and/or focal manifestations depending on size and site of the abscess(es).

Acute *Candida* meningitis presents with meningismus and may be indistinguishable from bacterial infection. *Candida* meningitis has been reported with all species of *Candida*, although a higher representation of *C. tropicalis* has been noted in leukemic children with *Candida* meningitis [153]. In nonneutropenic patients, especially postsurgical patients, meningitis is most commonly caused by *C. albicans*. CSF findings in acute *Candida* meningitis include hypoglycorrhachia, increased protein and variable pleocytosis (mean 600 cells/μL) with lymphocytic dominance. Yeasts are seen on Gram stain in only 40% of patients [147]. Occasional cases that are diagnosed early may present with normal CSF findings. In premature neonates, acute *Candida* meningitis is indistinguishable from bacterial infection or systemic infection, and meningitis is especially severe in this population [154]. Because of the paucity of signs indicating acute meningitis in neonates, and severe morbidity, including hydrocephalus, associated with a delay in diagnosis, lumbar puncture should be obligatory in this high-risk population in the presence of positive blood cultures for *Candida*.

A chronic form of *Candida* meningitis, which may mimic tuberculous or cryptococcal meningitis, has also been reported. Patients present with chronic headache, fever, and nuchal rigidity [150]. Analysis of CSF shows either mononuclear or neutrophilic pleocytosis, elevated protein and hypoglycorrhachia. In one review, only 17% of CSF Gram stains were positive, and only 44% of initial CSF cultures yielded *Candida* species. Overall mortality was 53% [150]. *Candida* species are not uncommon isolates in post-neurosurgical infections, including meningitis and wound or deep surgical-site infections, especially following trauma and in patients with brain tumors [155]. An even more frequent scenario is the patient with fever and positive *Candida* CSF cultures in the presence of an indwelling CSF shunt or device [156]. The clinical significance of a single positive CSF sample drawn through an indwelling device is problematic and a definitive diagnosis may require repeated positive cultures of CSF samples obtained by lumbar puncture. Shunt-associated infections include ventriculitis and meningitis. Anecdotal case reports of *Candida* meningitis following lumbar puncture are extremely rare [157].

Candida Pulmonary Infections

Candida species are frequently found in sputum and aspirates of endotracheal tube secretions, and their role as a possible cause of pulmonary disease is a frequent clinical dilemma. Although invasive lung parenchymal disease due to *Candida* undoubtedly occurs, this is rare. Two forms of *Candida* pneumonia are described [158]. One form is local or diffuse bronchopneumonia as a consequence of bronchogenic spread [159, 160] (Fig. 9). This infrequent event is rarely the consequence of aspiration, even in heavily colonized high-risk patients. The second form is pneumonia resulting from widespread seeding of the lung in a patient with candidemia. The second syndrome is characterized by diffuse, often nodular infiltrates [161]. Other rare clinical manifestations include necrotizing pneumonia, pulmonary mycetoma, and transient infiltrates attributed to allergic bronchopulmonary candidiasis [162].

X-ray and CT scan studies are not useful in diagnosis. Diagnosis of pulmonary candidiasis is extremely difficult and requires biopsy with histopathology demonstrating tissue invasion [163]. Diagnosis cannot be made on the basis of radiologic findings and/or recovery of yeast from sputum or aspirates of endotracheal tube secretions because of the frequency of both upper and lower respiratory tract colonization with *Candida* [164]. Cultures of bronchoalveolar lavage specimens and recovery of *Candida* from lung biopsy specimens are of low sensitivity and specificity and have a

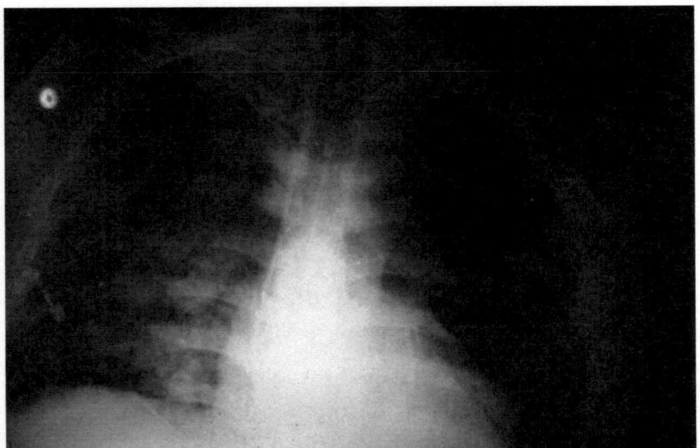

Fig. 9 *Candida* pneumonia, an entity rarely diagnosed ante-mortem

poor positive predictive value. Finally, even when *Candida* infection is confirmed histopathologically, pulmonary invasion is uncommonly of clinical significance and in the few instances of extensive pulmonary involvement, pneumonitis usually occurs in the setting of a terminally ill patient. *Candida* has rarely been reported to cause epiglottitis, laryngitis, and bronchitis [165].

Candida Urinary Tract Infections

Candiduria is a relatively rare finding in otherwise healthy people [166]. The incidence of fungal urinary tract infections, and specifically candiduria, has dramatically increased among hospitalized patients, especially those patients with indwelling drainage devices and those who are immunosuppressed. *Candida* species are the microbial pathogens that are most frequently isolated from the urine samples of patients in surgical ICUs [167].

Diabetes mellitus may predispose patients to candiduria by predisposing them to *Candida* colonization of the vulvovestibular area, enhancing urinary fungal growth in the presence of glycosuria, lowering host resistance to invasion by fungi as a consequence of impaired phagocytic activity, and promoting stasis of urine in a neurogenic bladder. It is likely that antibiotics contribute to colonization by *Candida* species by suppressing endogenous bacterial flora, primarily in the gut and lower genital tract, and possibly in superficial areas adjacent to the urethral meatus. The same risk factors for nosocomial candiduria also predispose to bacteriuria [168, 169]. Candiduria is almost invariably preceded by bacteriuria.

Indwelling urinary catheters serve as a portal of entry for microorganisms into the urinary drainage system. All catheters become colonized if left in place long enough. Other risk factors for candiduria include extremes of age, female sex, use of immunosuppressive agents, intravenous catheters, interruption of urine flow, and radiation therapy [168, 169]. Renal transplantation was previously thought to be a risk factor for ascending infection and candidemia when candiduria was present. However, a nested case-control study of 192 renal transplant recipients who developed candiduria revealed that candidemia occurred in only ten (5%) of patients [170].

The overwhelming majority of fungal infections of the urinary tract involve *Candida* species. In a large multicenter study, *C. albicans* was found in 446 (51.8%) of 861 patients with funguria [169]. The second most common pathogen (found in 134 of patients) was *Candida glabrata*. A second study reported a slightly higher proportion of isolates due to *C. glabrata* [171]. Risk factors for *C. glabrata* infection are similar to those that predispose a patient to *C. albicans* infection [171]. Although *C. albicans* is the most common species encountered, virtually all epidemiologic studies have concluded that non-*albicans Candida* species are also extremely common and more prevalent than in other sites, such as the oropharynx and vagina, possibly as a function of urine composition and pH selecting for non-*albicans* species. In 10% of patients, several species of *Candida* are found simultaneously and candiduria frequently coexists with or follows bacteriuria [171].

Ascending infection is by far the most common route for *Candida* infection of the urinary tract and occurs more often in women due to a shorter urethra and frequent vulvovestibular colonization with *Candida*. Catheterization can cause infection by allowing migration of organisms into the bladder along the external surface of the catheter from the periurethral areas. Ascending infection that originates in the bladder can also lead to infection of the upper urinary tract, especially if vesicoureteral reflux or obstruction of urinary flow occurs, and may result in acute pyelonephritis and, rarely, candidemia. A fungus ball consisting of yeast, hyphal elements, epithelial and inflammatory cells, and, sometimes, renal medullary tissue secondary to papillary necrosis, may complicate infections. The fungus ball tends to be found in dilated areas of the urinary tract, especially in the bladder in the presence of obstruction.

Renal candidiasis most commonly follows hematogenous dissemination of *Candida* to the kidneys. The kidneys are the most commonly involved organ in disseminated candidiasis. *Candida* species have a tropism for the kidneys; one study revealed that 90% of patients with fatal disseminated candidiasis had renal involvement at autopsy. Rarely, isolated hematogenous renal infection after transient candidemia can occur, and often when renal candidiasis is suspected, blood cultures are no longer positive.

The finding of *Candida* organisms in the urine may represent contamination, colonization of the drainage device, or infection. Colonization refers to the asymptomatic adherence of yeast, usually on drainage catheters or other foreign bodies, such as stents and nephrostomy tubes, in the urinary tract and may spuriously result in a high concentration of the organisms on urine culture. Simply finding or culturing the organism does not imply clinical significance, regardless of the concentration of organisms in the urine. In one study, colony counts $\geq 10^4$ cfu/mL of urine were associated with infection in patients without indwelling urinary catheters, but clinically significant renal candidiasis also has been reported with colony counts of only 10^3 cfu/mL of urine [172]. While pyuria supports the diagnosis of infection in the presence of a urinary catheter, pyuria can be explained by mechanical injury of the bladder mucosa by the catheter and is frequently the result of coexistent bacteriuria. Absence of pyuria and low colony counts tend to rule out *Candida* infection, but the low specificity of pyuria and numbers of cfu/mL require that results be interpreted in the clinical context [172].

Rarely, a granular cast containing *Candida* hyphal elements is found, localizing the infection to renal parenchyma. Declining renal function suggests urinary obstruction or renal invasion [166]. For candiduric patients with sepsis, not only is it necessary to obtain blood cultures, but given the frequency that obstruction and stasis coexist, radiographic imaging of the upper tract is essential. Any febrile patient for whom therapy for candiduria is considered necessary should be evaluated to find the anatomic source of candiduria.

Candiduria is most often asymptomatic and usually occurs in hospitalized patients with indwelling catheters and the yeast presence merely represents colonization. These patients usually show none of the signs or symptoms associated with urinary tract infection. Occasionally, patients may present with symptoms of bladder irritation including dysuria, hematuria, frequency, urgency, and suprapubic tenderness. Cystoscopy reveals soft, pearly white, elevated patches with underlying friable mucosa. Hyperemia of the bladder mucosa is common (Fig. 10). Symptomatic *Candida* cystitis is extremely rare in both catheterized and noncatheterized patients, implying that the bladder is relatively resistant to invasion by *Candida* species. Emphysematous cystitis is a rare complication of lower tract infection; prostatic abscess caused by *Candida* species is occasionally seen, especially among patients with diabetes.

Upper urinary tract infection presents with fever, leukocytosis, and costovertebral angle tenderness. On clinical grounds, ascending pyelonephritis and urosepsis with *Candida* species are indistinguishable from bacterial pyelonephritis. Ascending infection almost invariably occurs in the presence of urinary obstruction and stasis, especially in patients with diabetes or nephrolithiasis. *Candida* pyelonephritis is often complicated by local suppurative disease, resulting in pyonephrosis or focal abscess formation and infrequently candidemia. A major complication of upper urinary tract involvement is obstruction caused by fungal balls (bezoars), which can also be visualized by ultrasound. Renal colic may occur with the passage of fungal "stones" which are actually portions of fungal balls.

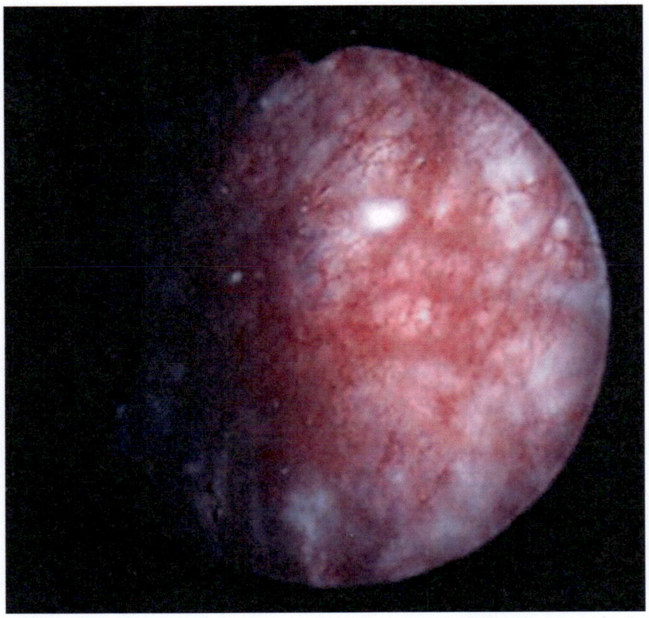

Fig. 10 Appearance of the bladder wall seen through a cystoscope in a patient who had cystitis due to *Candida krusei*

Patients with hematogenous seeding of the kidneys from candidemia may present with high fever, hemodynamic instability, and variable renal insufficiency. Blood cultures are positive for *Candida* in half of these patients. Retinal or skin involvement may suggest dissemination, but candiduria and a decline in renal function may be the only clues to systemic candidiasis in a febrile, high-risk patient. A reliable means for diagnosing invasive candidiasis continues to be elusive.

Candida Abdominal Infections

Candida infection has been increasingly recognized as a cause of abdominal sepsis and is associated with a high mortality rate. Abdominal sepsis may occur as monomicrobial or polymicrobial peritonitis and result in single or multiple abscesses. Translocation of *Candida* across the intact intestinal mucosa has been shown experimentally in animals and human volunteers [173]. Peritoneal contamination with *Candida* species usually follows spontaneous gastrointestinal perforation or surgical opening of the gut [174]. After contamination of the peritoneal cavity, *Candida* organisms do not inevitably result in peritonitis and clinical infection. Peritonitis is more likely to follow proliferation of accompanying bacterial pathogens but can occur with *Candida* alone. Several risk factors have been recognized in the development of peritonitis including recent or concomitant antimicrobial therapy, inoculum size, and surgery for acute pancreatitis [174]. Pancreatic transplantation, especially with enteric drainage, is associated with intraabdominal *Candida* abscess formation [175]. *Candida* species appear to have unique affinity for the inflamed pancreas, resulting in intrapancreatic abscesses or infection of pseudocysts. With *Candida* peritonitis, *Candida* usually remains localized to the peritoneal cavity; dissemination occurs in approximately 25% of patients. Candidemia complicating intraabdominal infection is associated with a high mortality.

The clinical significance of *Candida* isolated from the peritoneal cavity at the time of surgery or in the postoperative period is controversial. Earlier studies concluded that the finding of a positive culture did not require antifungal therapy [176]. In a review of *Candida* isolates from the peritoneal cavity, investigators determined that *Candida* caused intraabdominal infection in 39% (19/49) of patients. In 61%

of patients, *Candida* isolation occurred without signs of peritonitis [174]. Accordingly, in each individual patient, judgment based upon the presence of clinical signs of infection and other risk factors should be taken into consideration in deciding to initiate antifungal therapy [177].

Candida peritonitis complicating chronic ambulatory peritoneal dialysis (CAPD) is more common, but uncommonly results in positive blood cultures and hematogenous dissemination. In a series of patients on CAPD followed for 5 years, fungal peritonitis, most commonly caused by *Candida* species, accounted for 7% of episodes of peritonitis and eight associated deaths [178]. Others have reported that fungal infections account for between 1% and 15% of episodes of peritonitis in patients on CAPD [179]. Few risk factors for CAPD associated fungal peritonitis have emerged except for hospitalization and recent prior episodes of peritonitis and antibacterial therapy. An extraperitoneal site of fungal infection is rarely identified. Clinically, fungal peritonitis cannot be differentiated from bacterial peritonitis except by Gram stain and dialysate culture.

Yeast isolation from the bile is not uncommon, especially following biliary surgery, and has the same significance as asymptomatic bactobilia, that is, colonization without invasion is typical. While a potential source of future infection, the finding of yeast in the bile in itself is not a justification for antifungal therapy [180]. *Candida* is an infrequent cause of cholecystitis and cholangitis usually following extrahepatic biliary tract obstruction [180, 181]. Other risk factors for biliary candidiasis include diabetes, immunosuppression, and abdominal malignancy. A major contributory factor is use of biliary stents placed to relieve obstruction; *Candida* infection usually supervenes when stent drainage is compromised. In this setting, infection is usually polymicrobial and *Candida* is a pathogen that cannot be ignored. An uncommon complication of biliary candidiasis is development of fungus balls in the gall bladder and dilated bile ducts [181]. Candidemia is an infrequent complication of biliary candidiasis. Cholecystitis due to *Candida* has been reported in AIDS patients with cholangiopathy. Morris and colleagues reviewed 31 cases of biliary candidiasis and classified disease as uncomplicated or complicated. Uncomplicated cholecystitis implied that *Candida* organisms were confined to bile and the gall bladder without extrabiliary spread. In contrast, complicated infections implied spread to adjacent structures, including liver and peritoneum. Uncomplicated disease has minimal mortality and cure is achieved by cholecystectomy alone [181].

Candida Musculoskeletal Infections

Candida osteomyelitis has become more common. Most cases result from hematogenous dissemination with seeding of long bones in children and the axial skeleton in adults. Sites of bone infection include the spine, wrist, femur, humerus, and costochondral junctions. Osteomyelitis may present weeks or months following a candidemic episode; hence, at the time of the presentation, blood cultures are usually negative and radiologic findings nonspecific. Diagnosis usually requires percutaneous or open biopsy.

Occasionally, postoperative wound infections may spread to contiguous bone, such as sternum and vertebrae [182]. Regardless of source, manifestations resemble bacterial infection, but run a more insidious course, with a significant delay in diagnosis. Hematogenous vertebral osteomyelitis most commonly affects the lower thoracic or lumbar spine. In one series, 83% of patients had back pain lasting more than 1 month, only 32% presented with fever, and 19% had associated neurologic complications [183]. Species identified were *C. albicans* (57%), *C. tropicalis* (17%), and *C. glabrata* (12%). A prior history of positive blood cultures was present in 51–61% of cases [183].

Candida arthritis also represents a complication of hematogenous candidiasis. It rarely follows local trauma, surgery, or intraarticular injections [184, 185]. Patients with underlying joint disease, such as rheumatoid arthritis and prosthetic joints, are at increased risk. Non-*albicans Candida* species account for a higher than expected frequency of cases of fungal arthritis. *Candida* arthritis can occur in any joint and involves multiple joints in up to 27% of cases. The knee is the most commonly involved joint. Infection resembles bacterial septic arthritis, but frequent delays in diagnosis and suboptimal therapy often lead to chronic infection with secondary bone involvement.

Rarely hematogenous candidiasis may involve single or multiple muscles resulting in *Candida* pyomyositis [186]. Abscesses may be large or small, and this complication is frequently seen in immunosuppressed patients

Diagnosis

Culture and Histopathology

Candida species grow readily when cultures are obtained from body fluids or tissues, and results are usually available in 48–72 h. Isolation of *Candida* species from nonsterile sites such as wounds, skin, urine, sputum, vaginal secretions, and stool is not diagnostic of *Candida* infection. A positive culture only indicates that *Candida* species are present in the tissues examined. On the other hand, positive *Candida* cultures from sterile sites (blood, CSF, pleural fluid, peritoneal fluid) are almost always indicative of infection.

Blood cultures are only positive in 50–60% of autopsy-proven cases of disseminated candidiasis; thus, negative blood cultures do not rule out invasive disease. In one study, the highest sensitivity was achieved using the lysis centrifugation technique [107], but other methods with equal efficacy include the BACTEC high blood volume fungal media and the BacT/Alert system [187, 188]. The sensitivity of blood cultures decreases when patients have received antifungal prophylaxis.

Deep-seated organ *Candida* infection may require tissue biopsy to establish a definitive diagnosis. Tissue samples may contain small numbers of organisms with resultant negative cultures. Tissue sections can be stained with Gomori methenamine silver, methylene blue, or periodic acid-Schiff stains to demonstrate yeasts and hyphae.

Species identification of *Candida* is required for all infections because of the variable susceptibility to antifungal drugs that is species specific. A rapid, but nonspecific identification of *C. albicans* can be made by testing for germ tube production. This test is performed by growing the yeast in calf serum at 37 °C and observing for the formation of hyphae that develop after 60–90 min of incubation [2]. *C. stellatoidea* and *C. dubliniensis* also generate germ tubes, thus eliciting false-positive results. A rapid trehalose test allows for the presumptive identification of *C. glabrata* within a few hours. CHROMagar, a culture media utilized to rapidly identify many common *Candida* species, employs a colorimetric reaction on special agar that allows distinction among *C. albicans*, *C. glabrata*, *C. krusei*, *C. tropicalis*, and several other non-*albicans Candida* species. Commercially available carbohydrate fermentation and assimilation assays allow the identification of the different *Candida* species with more precision.

Non-culture-Based Methods

Serological assays include testing for *Candida* antibodies and antigens. The *Candida* antibody assays are nonstandardized and have no clinical utility. The assay for (1–3)beta-D-glucan in blood appears to have good sensitivity (75–95%) and reportedly a specificity of 88% for fungal infection. This test is not specific for candidiasis, but is also positive for other fungi, such as *Aspergillus*, *Cryptococcus*, *Fusarium*, *Acremonium*, and *Saccharomyces* [189]. In one multicenter study, between 78% and 81% of the 107 patients with proven candidiasis had positive results on the beta-D-glucan assay [190]. In another study, the assay was found to be useful in diagnosing *Candida*-related device biofilm infection [191]. The CSF assay may be useful in *Candida* CNS infections, but requires clinical validation [148].

Polymerase chain reaction (PCR) and DNA probes have the advantage of being able to detect small amounts of *Candida* DNA in either blood or tissues. Despite the fact that PCR assays have been shown to be highly sensitive, they continue to have problems of false-positivity, are technically difficult to perform, and are not yet commercially available.

The *C. albicans* peptide nucleic acid fluorescent in situ hybridization (PNA FISH) assay was first introduced in 2002 for rapid identification of yeast directly from blood cultures [192]. The assay uses PNA probes targeting *C. albicans*-specific rRNA. The test has been shown to have high specificity and sensitivity [192, 193]. A more advanced kit is now available, the *C. albicans*/*C. glabrata* PNA FISH (Advan Dx, Inc, Waburn, MA), which distinguishes between *C. albicans* and *C. glabrata* from blood culture bottles that have signaled positive and demonstrate yeast on Gram staining [194]. A shortened version (1.5 h) has recently been described [195].

In Vitro Susceptibility Testing

Currently available systemic agents with anti-*Candida* activity are amphotericin B, ketoconazole, itraconazole, fluconazole, voriconazole, posaconazole, caspofungin, micafungin, anidulafungin, and flucytosine. The drug of choice depends on the infecting species and the clinical setting. *Candida albicans* is the most susceptible species. The pattern for *C. tropicalis* and *C. parapsilosis* against azoles is quite similar to that for *C. albicans*, with slightly higher MICs for most antifungal drugs. *Candida parapsilosis* tends to have higher MICs and in vitro is less susceptible to all echinocandin agents [3, 196, 197]. *Candida glabrata* tends to have fluconazole MICs that are 16–64-fold higher than those for *C. albicans*. *Candida krusei* isolates have the highest fluconazole and flucytosine MICs of any of the species. In addition, *C. krusei* is also less susceptible to amphotericin B [7].

For three drugs, fluconazole, itraconazole, and flucytosine, interpretive breakpoints when tested by the methods recommended by the Clinical and Laboratory Standards Institute (CLSI) method, CLSI-M27, have been proposed and are summarized in Table 1 [198]. For fluconazole and itraconazole, the designation susceptibility dose dependent (S-DD) implies that susceptibility is dependent on obtaining the maximal possible drug level. For fluconazole, this designation implies use of doses of ≥400 mg/day in adults with normal renal function. Utilizing these breakpoints, *C. albicans*, *C. parapsilosis*, *C. tropicalis*, and *C. lusitaniae* are susceptible to fluconazole, whereas MICs of *C. glabrata* typically are in the S-DD category (Table 2). For itraconazole, *C. glabrata*, *C. krusei*, and *C. lusitaniae* often have MICs in the S-DD category, while the other common *Candida* species are generally susceptible. In general, virtually all azoles, including the latest generation triazoles, voriconazole and posaconazole, are 10–100 times less active against

Table 2 General patterns of susceptibility of *Candida* species (Adapted from [196, 198])

Candida Species	Fluconazole	Itraconazole	Flucytosine	Amphotericin B	Echinocandins
C albicans	S	S	S	S	S
C tropicalis	S	S	S	S	S
C parapsilosis	S	S	S	S	S
C glabrata	S-DD to R	S-DD to R	S	S-I	S
C krusei	R	S-DD to R	I-R	S-I	S
C lusitaniae	S	S	S	S to R	S
	Interpretive breakpoints for isolates of *Candida* (minimum inhibitory concentration, μg/mL)				
Drug	Susceptible (S)	(S-DD or I)	Resistant		
Fluconazole	≤8	S-DD, 16–32	≥64		
Itraconazole	≤0.125	S-DD, 0.25–0.5	≥1		
Flucytosine	≤4	I, 8–16	≥32		
Voriconazole	≤1	S-DD, 2	≥4		
Echinocandins	≤2	–	–		

C. glabrata strains compared to *C. albicans*. Finally, most species, except for *C. krusei*, are susceptible to flucytosine.

Measurement of MICs of amphotericin B utilizing the CLSI-M27 method is unreliable in detecting amphotericin B-resistant isolates [198]. Modifications based on the use of Antibiotic Medium 3 may resolve this problem [198]. Available data indicate that *Candida* isolates with CLSI-M27 amphotericin B MICs of 1 μg/mL are likely resistant to amphotericin B [198].

In contrast to *C. albicans*, the incidence of azole-resistant *Candida* species other than *C. albicans* has increased over the past 10 years [48]. At one end of the spectrum, in a large cancer center there has been a dramatic increase of azole resistant *C. glabrata* (31%) and *C. krusei* (24%), and *C. albicans* was found in only 14% of candidemia episodes. The authors attributed the increase in non-*albicans Candida* species to fluconazole exposure, mainly prophylactic use [57]. Noteworthy, the dramatic increase in non-*albicans Candida* spp. was not seen in patients with solid tumors. *C. krusei* has intrinsic fluconazole resistance, whereas *C. glabrata* resistance is frequently acquired and includes high level resistance (≥64 μg/mL) and intermediate dose-dependent resistance (16–32 μg/mL) Moreover, *C. glabrata* exhibits considerable clinically significant cross resistance between older azole agents (fluconazole and itraconazole) and voriconazole in patients with extensive prior azole drug exposure [148]. Fortunately most tertiary care centers, especially those in Europe, have not documented the same increase in non-*albicans Candida* spp., and both *C. glabrata* and *C. krusei* are predictably sensitive to the echinocandin class of antifungals [199]. Although available for more than 5 years, clinical and in vitro resistance of *Candida* isolates to echinocandins have been remarkably rare. Although *C. parapsilosis* isolates are predictably less susceptible to all three available echinocandins, clinical failure is not common with echinocandin use for this species.

Routine susceptibility testing of all *Candida* isolates is not indicated although all invasive isolates should be identified to the species level. Susceptibility testing is justified in patients with refractory disease, e.g., refractory OPC in AIDS patients or persistent candidemia while on antifungal therapy. Likewise testing of selected isolates from invasive or deep sites might be useful in selecting alternatives to amphotericin B.

Treatment

Oropharyngeal Candidiasis

Oropharyngeal candidiasis may be treated with either topical antifungal agents (nystatin, clotrimazole, miconazole, amphotericin B oral suspension) or systemic oral azole drugs (fluconazole, itraconazole or posaconazole). In patients who are HIV-positive, OPC infections tend to respond more slowly, and about 60% of patients experience a recurrence within 6 months of the initial episode [83]. Guidelines for the prevention and treatment of OPC and EC in HIV-infected adults have been recently published by the United States Publish Health Service and the Infectious Diseases Society of America [106, 200].

Numerous antifungal agents are available for the treatment of OPC. Nystatin solution has been replaced by more active and rapidly acting topical azoles, especially clotrimazole and miconazole [201]. Clotrimazole, 10 mg troches administered five times daily, have been successful in treating mild to moderate OPC [202].

Ketoconazole, 200 mg daily, was the first oral systemic azole used and is highly effective even in debilitated patients including those with malignancy, AIDS, and CMC with cure rates of 80% [203]. However, ketoconazole use has been limited by hepatotoxicity and concerns about the reliability of gastric absorption, especially in patients receiving H2-blockers. A novel addition in the management of OPC has been the approval of miconazole 50 mg muco-adhesive tablets (MBT) [204]. Miconazole MBT is approved in France for the treatment of OPC in the compromised host. In a phase III multicenter study comparing miconazole MBT once daily versus clotrimazole troches five times daily in HIV-positive patients, the MBT was found to be as effective as clotrimazole troches [204]. The MBT is generated from Lauriad technology which is a novel delivery system. This methodology enables the adhesion of the tablet, composed of milk protein concentrate, to the mucous membrane and subsequently allows for the gradual and controlled release of miconazole over a period of 13 h [205].

Itraconazole, fluconazole and posaconazole have markedly improved safety profiles and have become the standard of care, especially for patients with moderate to severe OPC [83, 206].

Posaconazole oral suspension (40 mg/mL) is approved for the treatment of OPC in HIV/AIDS patients [207]. In a randomized, multicenter study comparing posaconazole 100 mg daily to fluconazole 100 mg daily for 14 days in HIV patients with OPC, posaconazole showed clinical success in 92% of patients and demonstrated non-inferiority to fluconazole [207, 208]. These oral drugs are considered equivalent in efficacy. Although most studies on fluconazole efficacy for OPC utilized an initial loading dose of 200 mg followed by 100 mg daily, success has been achieved with 50 mg daily [206]. Fluconazole treatment is characterized by rapid response. Slower response rates have been described with both ketoconazole and miconazole troches in OPC patients with solid tumors [209]. In all published studies, fluconazole 100 mg/day, was at least equal in efficacy and in some studies superior to clotrimazole or ketoconazole [83]. The goal of antifungal therapy in OPC is rapid relief of symptoms, prevention of complications and early relapse following cessation of therapy.

Esophageal Candidiasis

Candida esophagitis requires systemic therapy; topical drugs are of little value. Parenteral therapy is frequently required initially if the patient is unable to take oral medication. Ketoconazole 200 mg bid was shown to be effective in EC [210]. However, ketoconazole has now been replaced by the triazoles, fluconazole, itraconazole and posaconazole because of greater efficacy of the newer triazoles and the adverse side effect profile of ketoconazole. Fluconazole is the standard of care in the management of EC. Oral fluconazole at a dose of 200 mg/day for 14–21 days enjoys a superior safety profile with bioavailability of 92%. In several clinical trials, patients with EC treated with itraconazole oral solution 100–200 mg/day had a clinical response rate of 94%, comparable to the 91% for patients treated with fluconazole tablets 100–200 mg/day [211]. In addition, posaconazole oral suspension 400 mg BID has also been shown to be effective in the management of EC in HIV/AIDS patients [200, 208, 212]. Patients with AIDS are at high risk of developing symptomatic recurrences of EC [213, 214]. Accordingly, many clinicians, following a single episode of EC, begin secondary prophylaxis with either fluconazole, itraconazole or posaconazole. Daily suppressive antifungal therapy with fluconazole 100–200 mg/day is effective in preventing recurrent episodes. However, suppressive therapy should only be used if the recurrences are frequent or are associated with malnutrition due to poor oral intake.

In a randomized, multicenter trial comparing voriconazole to fluconazole for the treatment of EC in 391 immunocompromised patients, voriconazole, 200 mg twice daily, was as effective as fluconazole, 200 mg daily, and well tolerated [215]. Similarly, the echinocandins, anidulafungin, caspofungin, and micafungin, have also proven to be effective in treating EC in HIV-infected patients. Caspofungin 50 mg IV daily was equivalent to amphotericin B 0.5 mg/kg/day in 123 immunocompromised patients with EC. Clinical success was achieved in 74% and 89% of patients receiving caspofungin at 50 mg and 70 mg/day, respectively and in 63% of patients receiving amphotericin B [216]. Anidulafungin 50 mg IV daily showed excellent efficacy when it was compared to fluconazole in the treatment of EC in HIV-infected patients [217]. Micafungin 150 mg IV daily also demonstrated excellent efficacy when compared to fluconazole in a randomized, double-blind study in patients with documented EC [218].

Given the high success rates achieved with fluconazole, itraconazole, posaconazole, voriconazole, and the echinocandins, amphotericin B is now rarely used and generally reserved for endoscopically proven cases of EC that fail azole and echinocandin therapy. Low-dose amphotericin B (0.3–0.5 mg/kg or 10–20 mg daily for 10 days) is often sufficient for moderate disease, but higher doses may be necessary for some patients with AIDS and refractory EC [83, 219].

Refractory Oropharyngeal and Esophageal Candidiasis

Management of fluconazole-resistant OPC and EC is frequently unsatisfactory and any response is short lived, with periodic and rapid recurrences. The clinical impact of antifungal resistance in patients with AIDS has been reviewed [220]. After the onset of fluconazole-resistant thrush, AIDS patients had a median survival of 184 days. Moreover, after the onset of clinical resistance to amphotericin B, the patients had a median survival of only 83 days. Although mucosal candidiasis does not produce death directly, clinical failure acts as a comorbid factor in the rapid demise of these patients and is a marker of severe immunosuppression.

Several studies reveal a good correlation between in vitro susceptibility and response of OPC and EC to antifungal treatment in HIV-infected patients [221, 222]. On the other hand, therapeutic antifungal successes and failures were noted in patients with OPC and *Candida* isolates with both low and high MIC values. Risk factors for the development of fluconazole-resistant mucosal candidiasis in patients with AIDS include greater number of episodes of OPC, lower median CD4 cell count, longer median duration of antifungal therapy, and longer duration of systemic azole exposure [213].

Fluconazole refractory mucocutaneous candidiasis may initially respond to higher doses of fluconazole, 400–800 mg daily, but with a short-term clinical response. Occasionally, fluconazole suspension may be beneficial as a swish and swallow approach [223]. Several studies have demonstrated good response rates with itraconazole oral solution, 200 mg twice daily [224, 225]. Clinical cure or improvement occurred in 55–70% of patients; however, mycological cure rates were only 30% and relapses occurred within a few weeks following treatment cessation. In vitro, ketoconazole and itraconazole cross-resistance is common. Amphotericin B oral suspension is another therapeutic option in patients with azole-refractory mucosal candidiasis [226] but this formulation is no longer available in all countries. In several small studies, clinical improvement rates varied from 50% to 75%, but the relapse rate was high.

Voriconazole and posaconazole have excellent in vitro activity against fluconazole-resistant *C. albicans* isolates [83, 227]. Caspofungin 50 gm daily, micafungin 150 mg daily, and anidulafungin 50 mg daily IV have also demonstrated clinical efficacy [228]. Parenteral amphotericin B, 0.4–0.6 mg/kg daily, is less frequently required. Lipid-based amphotericin B preparations may occasionally prove useful in patients unable to tolerate conventional deoxycholate amphotericin B [229].

Highly active antiretroviral therapy is an essential component of therapy of refractory disease. Treatment with antiretroviral therapy alone without antifungal drugs has been shown to eradicate refractory OPC in patients with advanced HIV infection [230]. Human recombinant granulocyte-macrophage colony-stimulating factor (GM-CSF) has demonstrated encouraging results in patients with refractory OPC and EC [231].

Prevention of Recurrent Oropharyngeal and Esophageal Candidiasis

Chronic suppressive therapy with fluconazole is effective in prevention of OPC in both AIDS [232, 233] and cancer patients [234]. Maintenance fluconazole has been prescribed daily, two or three times weekly, or once weekly. In a large multicenter trial, fluconazole, 200 mg three times weekly, as continuous therapy was compared with fluconazole given only for episodes of acute OPC in patients with advanced HIV infection [235]. The investigators found no differences among the two treatment groups with regard to the development of fluconazole refractory infection. However, continuous fluconazole therapy was associated with fewer cases of OPC and EC and fewer invasive fungal infections. Overall, all of the regimens that have been studied reduced relapse frequency, but have the potential to select for resistant *C. albicans* strains and may be associated with appearance of *C. glabrata*. Given costs of long-term therapy and concern for resistance development, chronic suppressive therapy is only recommended in patients with frequent and disabling recurrences, especially EC, as an alternative to early treatment of each recurrent episode. In spite of numerous reports of refractory mucosal candidiasis due to resistant *C. albicans* during the 1990s, risk of refractory disease in patients receiving maintenance fluconazole and adhering to antiretroviral therapy now appears small [235].

Vulvovaginal Candidiasis

Treatment of VVC predominantly involves use of the imidazole and triazole agents available as topical or oral formulations (Table 3). Azoles achieve higher success rates even over shorter duration of therapy than nystatin vaginal suppositories or creams. Little evidence exists that the choice of formulation of the topical azoles influences cure rates.

Table 3 Azole therapy for vaginal candidiasis

Drug	Formulation	Dosage
Butoconazole	2% cream (5 g)	5 g×3 day
	2% vaginal suppository	1 supp
Clotrimazole	1% cream (5 g)	5 g×7–14 day
	10% cream	1 appl
	100 mg vaginal tablet	1 tab×7 day
	100 mg vaginal tablet	2 tab×3 day
	500 mg vaginal tablet	1 tab once
Miconazole	2% cream (5 g)	5 g×7 day
	100 mg vaginal suppository	1×7 day
	200 mg vaginal suppository	1×3 day
	1,200 mg vaginal suppository	1 supp
Econazole	150 mg vaginal tablet	1 tab×3 day
Fenticonazole	2% cream (5 g)	5 g×7 day
Tioconazole	2% cream (5 g)	5 g×3 day
	6.5% cream (5 g)	5 g once
Terconazole	0.4% cream (5 g)	5 g×7 day
	0.8% cream (5 g)	5 g×3 day
	80 mg vaginal suppository	80 mg×3 day
Fluconazole	150 mg tablet oral	150 mg once
Ketoconazole	200 mg tablet	400 mg×5 day
Itraconazole	100 mg tablet oral	200 mg×3 day

Topical agents previously prescribed for 7–14 days are now available as single dose or short course (3–5 day) regimens. Topical azoles when appropriately prescribed are remarkably free of systemic side effects and toxicity especially in pregnancy [232].

The oral azoles used for systemic therapy are ketoconazole, itraconazole, and fluconazole, but only fluconazole (150 mg given as a single dose) is approved by the FDA for this indication in the United States. Oral azoles have been shown to be at least as effective as topical agents, are more convenient and more popular among users and are free of local side effects [236, 237]. In selecting an antifungal agent, it is useful to define VVC as uncomplicated or complicated disease [238]. The majority of episodes of VVC are uncomplicated (90%). These are sporadic, mild-to-moderate infections caused by *C. albicans* that occur in normal hosts who lack predisposing factors. Uncomplicated infections can be successfully treated with any of the available topical or oral antifungal agents, including short course and single dose regimens.

Complicated infections are defined as those that (1) have a moderate to severe clinical presentation, (2) are recurrent in nature (≥4 episodes per year), (3) are caused by non-*albicans Candida species*, or (4) occur in abnormal hosts, e.g., diabetic patients with poor glucose control. Complicated infections are far less likely to respond to abbreviated courses of therapy [238] and should be treated more intensively for 7–14 days in order to achieve a clinical response. In a study of almost 500 women with complicated VVC, prolonging fluconazole therapy by adding a second dose of 150 mg fluconazole 72 h after the initial dose resulted in significantly higher clinical and mycological cure rates in women with severe VVC [239]. Non-*albicans Candida* species, especially *C. glabrata*, are less susceptible in vitro to azoles, and VVC caused by these species is less likely to respond clinically, especially to short course azole therapy. Encouraging results have been obtained with boric acid 600 mg capsules given vaginally daily for 14 days or topical 17% flucytosine [240].

Vulvovaginal candidiasis in HIV-infected women is incompletely understood. One large study found it to behave in a fashion similar to that in seronegative women [241]. Vaginal carriage of *Candida* is more common in HIV seropositive women, but symptomatic VVC was not more frequent or modestly increased only and did not increase with progressive immunosuppression. Others have, however, noted increased rates of VVC with increasing immunosuppression [242–244]. The differences in results may be due to differences in study design and diagnostic criteria [241, 245]. Longitudinal cohort studies of vaginal candidiasis in HIV-positive women did show a progressive increase in colonization with *C. glabrata* and diminished fluconazole susceptibility [244]. Therapy of VVC in HIV-infected women remains the same as that for seronegative women. Recurrent VVC is usually caused by susceptible strains of *C. albicans*, and resistance is rarely encountered. Although more intensive prolonged induction therapy lasting up to 14 days invariably induces remission, the fungistatic nature of the available agents combined with persistence of the underlying defect makes relapse within 3 months almost inevitable unless a maintenance antifungal regimen is employed. The regimen used most often is fluconazole, 150 mg weekly [246].

Male genital candidiasis presents in two forms, and most commonly as a transient pruritic and erythematous penile cutaneous reaction that may follow unprotected intercourse with exposure to *Candida* antigens present in the partner's vagina and represents a hypersensitivity reaction. Successful treatment entails eradication of yeast in the vagina. True superficial penile *Candida* infection, the second form, occurs infrequently and usually in diabetic and uncircumcised males who develop balanoposthitis that responds promptly to topical or systemic azole therapy.

Cutaneous Candidiasis

Localized cutaneous candidiasis infections may be treated with any number of topical antifungal agents (e.g., clotrimazole, econazole, miconazole, ketoconazole, ciclopirox). *Candida* paronychia requires drainage of the abscess, followed by oral therapy with either fluconazole or itraconazole. However, *Candida* folliculitis, onychomycosis, and extensive cutaneous infections in patients who are immunocompromised require systemic antifungal therapy. For Candida onychomycosis, oral itraconazole appears to be the most efficacious, either 100 mg daily for 3–6 months or as a pulse-dose regimen that requires 200 mg twice daily for 7 days, followed by 3 weeks off therapy. The cycle is repeated every month for 3–6 months [247].

Chronic Mucocutaneous Candidiasis

Oral azoles have revolutionized the prognosis and treatment of CMC. Ketoconazole, fluconazole, and itraconazole induce long treatment-free remissions of CMC and can be used continuously or intermittently in cases requiring chronic maintenance therapy [248, 249]. Over the last decade, a variety of therapeutic approaches aimed at improving cell mediated immunity have been attempted, with inconsistent results and only moderate success as compared to oral azole therapy. Thymus transplantation has been reported to provide improvement in CMC patients suffering from DiGeorge syndrome [250]. White blood cell transfusions produced transient improvement in CMC symptoms only [251]; however, bone marrow transplantation has been successful [252].

Candidemia and Acute Disseminated Candidiasis

The selection of any particular antifungal agent for the treatment of candidemia should take into consideration any recent history of azole exposure, a history of intolerance to antifungals, the *Candida* species involved, available susceptibility data in any particular center, severity of illness, relevant co-morbidities and evidence of involvement of cardiac valves, retina, CNS and/or visceral organs [106]. Early initiation of effective antifungal therapy is critical as evidenced by recent data correlating higher morbidity with delay of appropriate therapy [253, 254].

In the nonneutropenic patient, candidemia is related to the presence of an intravascular catheter in up to 80% of patients [255]. Removal of all intravascular catheters appears to shorten duration of candidemia [114] and has been associated with reduced mortality [256, 257]. Although some patients have even been cured by catheter removal alone [258], many transient episodes of candidemia are associated with hematogenous dissemination leading to end organ involvement, including endophthalmitis and osteomyelitis. Thus, all episodes of candidemia merit antifungal therapy [257, 259]. A dilated fundoscopic examination is important in all candidemic patients [106].

Amphotericin B had been the standard therapy of candidemia [260], but two prospective randomized trials [255, 261] and two retrospective reviews [256, 262], comparing amphotericin B with fluconazole demonstrated that amphotericin B at 0.5–0.6 mg/kg daily and fluconazole at 400 mg daily are highly effective and not significantly different as therapy of candidemia in non-neutropenic patients. In all four studies, the majority of isolates were *C. albicans* and the strength of the data is less for non-*albicans* species, but similar trends hold. Accordingly during the last two decades, fluconazole and amphotericin B have been considered equivalent and both have served as first line therapy for candidemia. Fluconazole should be considered first-line therapy for patients who have mild to moderate illness, who are hemodynamically stable, who have no previous exposure to azoles, and who lack risk factors for *C. glabrata* infection (elderly patients, diabetics, cancer and recent abdominal surgery) [106, 255, 263, 264].

Step-down therapy to fluconazole is reasonable for patients initially responding to amphotericin B or echinocandins provided that the responsible organism is susceptible to fluconazole. For *C. glabrata* fungemia, many experts prefer voriconazole as oral step down treatment. Parenteral voriconazole although shown to be equivalent to amphotericin B in a large multicenter controlled trial is infrequently used for invasive candidiasis, not because of issues of efficacy, but because of frequent drug interactions and adverse effects [265]. There is a little role for itraconazole for candidemia, given similar antifungal activity, ease of administration, superior pharmacokinetics, and better tolerability of fluconazole.

The echinocandins, caspofungin, micafungin, and anidulafungin, have been shown to highly effective for candidemia, achieving ~75% success rates in randomized clinical trials [264, 266, 267]. Because of their efficacy, excellent safety profile, and few drug interactions, echinocandins are now considered by some experts as drugs of first choice for candidemia, especially when fluconazole use is questionable in patients at high risk of infection with *C. glabrata* or *C. krusei*. Somewhat controversial is the selection of either fluconazole or an echinocandin for *C. parapsilosis* candidemia given the higher MICs observed with the entire echinocandin class [268]. Recent guidelines favor the use of fluconazole in this context although clinical data supporting this opinion are absent [106]. Some have found that echinocandins are superior to fluconazole as initial therapy for candidemia [264]. This conclusion remains highly controversial and unlikely to be resolved by future clinical studies comparing the two classes of antifungals.

Voriconazole does not provide predictable activity against fluconazole resistant *C. glabrata* [7], but is useful for patients with fluconazole-resistant *C. krusei*, *C. guilliermondii* or *C. glabrata* with documented voriconazole susceptibility who transition from amphotericin B or echinocandin to oral therapy. Although posaconazole has excellent in vitro activity against most *Candida* species, there are inadequate clinical data to support its use for invasive candidiasis. In addition, the lack of an intravenous preparation prohibits its initial use, although it may be extremely useful for patients when transition to an expanded spectrum oral azole is required to complete therapy.

The required duration of antifungal therapy is undetermined, but therapy is usually continued for approximately 2 weeks after the first negative blood culture in the absence of metastatic complications. With this approach, the rate of subsequent recurrent infection at hematogenously seeded sites is rare [255].

In the neutropenic patient with candidemia, fewer data are available to guide management. Although the gut has been implicated as an occasional source of candidemia in nonneutropenic patients, it appears likely that the gastrointestinal tract is the most common source of candidemia in neutropenic patients [269]. One notable exception is that *C. parapsilosis* fungemia is highly associated with intravascular catheters in cancer patients [8]. Moreover, in neutropenic patients, removal of intravenous catheters, if possible, is still recommended [109]. Recovery of bone marrow function is critical, and no therapeutic approach is consistently successful in the face of persistent leukopenia. Most experience is with amphotericin B at 0.6–1.0 mg/kg daily until recovery of marrow function. The optimal dose of amphotericin

B is not certain, but non-*albicans Candida* species require higher doses (0.8–1.0 mg/kg daily) of amphotericin B, especially *C. krusei* and *C. glabrata*, the two species that also are the least susceptible to fluconazole [270]. Currently, most hematology units use lipid formulations of amphotericin B, 3–5 mg/kg daily, rather than amphotericin B deoxycholate.

Data comparing this approach with fluconazole are limited, but one retrospective matched cohort study found that median daily doses of 400 mg for fluconazole and 0.6 mg/kg for amphotericin B were associated with similar outcomes in a mixed group of neutropenic and nonneutropenic cancer patients [262]. Because of the extensive use of fluconazole as prophylaxis, there is a diminished treatment role for fluconazole among neutropenic patients. In spite of few randomized controlled trials, echinocandins are now considered first line therapy in neutropenic patients in preference to fluconazole [106, 271]. Although data are limited, success rates in neutropenic patients appears similar to those reported in nonneutropenic patients. Because of flucytosine's potential for marrow suppression and the lack of a readily available intravenous formulation, flucytosine is infrequently used.

Patients may develop candidemia while on antifungal therapy, including prophylactic antifungal drugs. Such breakthrough candidemia may be due to infection of an intravascular catheter, in which case the infecting isolate is usually susceptible to the apparently failing drug [272]. In cancer patients, breakthrough candidemia was associated with a higher mortality and occurred more often in the setting of an intensive care unit stay, prolonged neutropenia, and use of corticosteroids [273]. In this setting, immunosuppression should be reduced and factors that might alter antifungal drug delivery or clearance excluded. Intravenous catheters should be changed. Since non-*albicans Candida* species are frequently responsible, the possibility of drug resistance should be considered. If resistance is likely or MIC data document resistance, therapy should be changed to an antifungal drug of a different class.

Central tunneled catheters in febrile neutropenic patients do not require mandatory removal since in this setting alternate vascular access sites are less available and removal is more difficult. Most importantly, such catheters are less likely to be the source of candidemia although they may become infected secondary to bloodstream infection. Occasionally, these valuable access sites may be salvaged using the controversial antibiotic lock method utilizing amphotericin B [274, 275]. However, results are unpredictable. The importance of a positive catheter tip is similarly controversial. In afebrile patients at low risk of candidemia, antifungal treatment does not appear to be indicated. On the other hand, in a high-risk patient with unexplained antibiotic-resistant fever, the finding of a positive catheter tip culture for *Candida* often results in initiation of empirical antifungal therapy.

Chronic Disseminated Candidiasis

In the absence of randomized controlled studies, therapy has usually consisted of prolonged amphotericin B alone; however, this approach has not been uniformly successful [276, 277]. Amphotericin B followed by a protracted course of fluconazole is associated with cure rates of 90% [278, 279]. This regimen is preferred by many experts. Use of fluconazole is sometimes successful when amphotericin B is not. Lipid-based amphotericin B has also been used successfully [280]. Anecdotal case reports indicate successful outcome with caspofungin alone or with azole [281, 282], however failures are also reported. Current recommendations favor a lipid formulation of amphotericin B for 1–2 weeks followed by oral fluconazole, which is continued until there is resolution or calcification of lesions on follow-up CT scans obtained every 2–3 months [106]. Resolution of lesions occurs in the majority of patients within 6 months. Provided that the lesions have stabilized, the patient is clinically improved, and antifungal therapy is continued, stem cell transplantation can be performed and cancer chemotherapeutic agents can be given without relapse occurring [280]. Splenectomy in addition to antifungal therapy is occasionally performed when disease is confined to the spleen.

Adjuvant glucocorticoids may have a role in achieving a prompt resolution of fever, abdominal pain and the inflammatory response in patients refractory to antifungal therapy but prolonged antifungal therapy is still required [283]. Additional studies are still needed before this form of therapy can be recommended.

Neonatal Candidiasis

In infants, failure to promptly remove or replace central venous catheters prolongs candidemia, increases mortality and long term irreversible neurodevelopmental complications [284]. Amphotericin B at 0.5–1.0 mg/kg daily for a total dose of 10–25 mg/kg, with or without flucytosine, is the therapy of choice for neonated candidiasis. The excellent penetration of amphotericin B into the CSF in neonates is presumably part of the reason that amphotericin B alone is often successful [285]. Lipid-formulations of amphotericin B for this condition can be used if urinary tract involvement is excluded. Fluconazole is also attractive in this setting, and has been used successfully at doses of 6–12 mg/kg daily [284, 286–289]. Comparative data between amphotericin B and fluconazole for neonatal candidiasis are lacking, but recommended length of therapy is 3 weeks. Topical and oral therapy with agents such as nystatin or an antifungal azole often are adequate therapy for full-term infants with candidiasis limited to skin and the GI tract [146]. The role of flucytosine in neonates with *Candida* mengitis is questionable and not routinely recommended [284]. Experience with echinocandins is growing, and pharmacokinetic data are now available [284]; nevertheless, until further experience is available, echinocandins use is generally limited to situations in which resistance or toxicity preclude the use of fluconazole or amphotericin B [106].

Candida Urinary Tract Infections

Treatment of candiduria requires differentiating between colonization and superficial and deep tissue infection as well as the anatomical level of infection. Candiduria in catheterized subjects usually represents catheter or superficial bladder colonization only, is extremely common, almost invariably asymptomatic, and of little clinical significance. Asymptomatic candiduria in this context should not be treated since the sequelae of ascending or invasive *Candida* infections are rare [290, 291] and any effects of treatment are short lived [172]. Asymptomatic candiduria should be treated in neutropenic patients and those undergoing elective urinary instrumentation. Treatment was considered in post-renal transplant patients, however, a nested case control study of 192 renal transplant recipients who developed candiduria concluded that treatment with an antifungal agent did not facilitate *Candida* clearance or improve survival [170].

Both prospective [169] and retrospective [292] studies of asymptomatic funguria indicates that neither risk reduction nor antifungal therapy affected morbidity and mortality in hospitalized patients. In a large study of 861 hospitalized patients, only 1.3% of patients developed candidemia [169]. Symptomatic lower urinary tract infections due to *Candida* are rare and should be treated, especially in noncatheterized patients. Therapeutic options include oral fluconazole 200 mg/day for 7–14 days [171], amphotericin B as a 0.3 mg/kg single dose [168], or amphotericin B, 0.3 mg/kg for 5–7 days [293]. Amphotericin B bladder irrigation with a solution of 50 mg amphotericin B in a liter of sterile water through a triple lumen catheter for 7 days is an effective but inconvenient option [294]. Shorter courses may prove to be an alternative [295]. Ketoconazole and itraconazole achieve low urine drug concentrations and yield unreliable results [296], and voriconazole and posaconazole similarly are not excreted into the urine and have not been used for treatment of *Candida* urinary tract infections. Oral flucytosine is rarely indicated because of emergence of resistance during therapy, but has been useful on occasion in eradicating *C. glabrata* infection. The echinocandins are poorly excreted into urine and perhaps have a limited role in treating candiduria associated with invasive urinary candidiasis with fungal parenchymal invasion, for which tissue concentrations of echinocandins may be effective [103].

Ascending pyelonephritis, although uncommon, represents a serious infection that may be complicated by candidemia and disseminated infection [290]. Therapy for this form of *Candida* pyelonephritis consists of relieving any urinary obstruction plus fluconazole or systemic amphotericin B in doses similar to those used for disseminated candidiasis. Finally, candiduria may be the result of renal candidiasis secondary to previous or ongoing candidemia with hematogenous spread. Therapy is identical to that of disseminated candidiasis. A recent retrospective study suggests that organ contamination at the time of renal transplantation can lead to *Candida* infection of the allograft leading to renal arteritis [297].

Ocular Candidiasis

Penetration of amphotericin B into the eye is poor, whereas fluconazole and voriconazole achieve levels in the vitreous body that are approximately 50–75% of serum levels. Amphotericin B, 0.7–1 mg/kg daily, combined with flucytosine, 100 mg/kg daily, is recommended for sight threatening lesions based on early experience [106, 117]. However, systemic therapy alone is not uniformly successful and intravitreal amphotericin B following vitrectomy has been helpful, both as monotherapy or in conjunction with systemic therapy [298–300]. Intravitreal doses of amphotericin B of 5–10 μg are indicated for vision threatening disease [301–303].

Fluconazole diffuses well into all parts of the eye and is an acceptable alternative for less severe disease [304–306]. Fluconazole given as sole therapy for approximately 2 months cured 15 of 16 patients with *Candida* endophthalmitis [307]. Fluconazole was also effective following short courses of amphotericin B. Patients requiring vitrectomy generally have more severe disease, and fluconazole monotherapy was curative when given after vitrectomy. If an ocular implant is present in the infected eye, implant removal appears critical to resolution of the infection [308]. Increasing data are available to show that voriconazole is an effective agent for the treatment of *Candida* endophthalmitis and can be given as an intravitreal injection, as well as systemically for sight threatening disease. The recommended duration of therapy is at least 4–6 weeks, but should be based on repeated examinations that confirm resolution of the lesions.

Candida Cardiac and Endovascular Infections

Medical therapy alone has rarely been curative for cardiac or vascular infections [130, 309–312]. The inability of prolonged courses of high dose amphotericin B to cure either native or prosthetic valve endocarditis [313, 314] has led to the recommendation that patients be treated with a combination of valve replacement and prolonged antifungal therapy [130, 315, 316]. This combined approach remains the latest recommendation of the Infectious Disease Society of America [106]. Post-operative amphotericin B with or without flucytosine is prescribed for at least 6 weeks following surgery [106]. However, due to the high rates of relapse, most clinicians treat for longer than 6 weeks. As an alternative, step down therapy with fluconazole 6–12 mg/kg daily is reasonable with susceptible *Candida* species and with clearance of candidemia. A total course longer than 6 weeks is crucial in patients with perivalvular abscesses and other complications [106].

Most patients are now treated with a lipid formulation of amphotericin B at a dose of 3–5 mg/kg daily to reduce nephrotoxicity. Flucytosine is given at a dose of 100 mg/kg daily in four divided doses with normal renal function. Serum flucytosine levels should be monitored to keep serum drug levels <75 μg/mL.

Case reports of successful medical treatment of *Candida* with echinocandin monotherapy especially caspofungin have appeared [317, 318]. The role of echinocandins has not been fully clarified although there is growing evidence of their use as an alternative to amphotericin B, given their fungicidal activity, rare resistance, and overall safety. Higher doses than normally used for candidemia have been suggested, caspofungin 100–150 mg daily, micafungin 150 mg daily and anidulafungin 100–200 mg daily [106]. Failure with development of resistance to caspofungin, especially with *C. parapsilosis* has been reported [319]. In general, caution is suggested in selecting an echinocandin for *C. parapsilosis*. Fluconazole has been the most frequently employed long-term oral agent, given its superior safety profile [314, 315, 320].

A similar strategy is applicable in children. Medical therapy alone is often pursued in neonates due to their complicated, overlapping medical problems [309, 310, 321]. Effective monotherapy with amphotericin B is more frequently reported in neonates who have disseminated candidiasis with cardiac thrombi and vegetations.

Late recurrence or relapse following medical treatment has been described, even several years after the initial episode [322], emphasizing the need for prolonged follow-up. Chronic suppressive therapy with fluconazole is recommended for patients in whom cardiac surgery is contraindicated [106, 323–325]. Some experts recommend fluconazole suppressive therapy even when successful surgical resection has been performed and followed by 6 weeks of intravenous therapy. This unproven approach is recommended for patients with prosthetic cardiac valves because of high relapse rates and the difficulty involved in repeated cardiac surgeries. In patients with endocarditis caused by fluconazole resistant organisms, such as *C. glabrata* and *C. krusei*, oral voriconazole suppressive therapy is recommended.

There has been a marked reduction in mortality associated with *Candida* endocarditis. In an international multicenter prospective cohort study that included 33 cases of *Candida* endocarditis that were treated between 2000 and 2005, the mortality rate was 30% [326]. These figures are dramatically better than the previous reports of Ellis in 2001 (42–59%) [130]. A recent meta-analysis of 72 of 163 patients who had *Candida* endocarditis between 1980 and 2002, revealed a reduced mortality when patients received combined surgical and medical therapy [327]. Clearly the role of medical therapy alone is improving, and while the prevailing majority opinion advocates a combined approach, a decision should be based on individual case considerations.

Candida infections of transvenous pacemakers require both surgical removal of the infected device and prolonged systemic antifungal therapy for at least 4–6 weeks [133] Purulent *Candida* pericarditis is treated with a combination of surgical drainage (pericardiocentesis or pericardiectomy) together with prolonged antifungal therapy [128, 328]

Persistent candidemia is sometimes due to *Candida* suppurative phlebitis of either central or peripheral veins. In the case of peripheral phlebitis, the involved vein is not always tender, although usually thrombosed. Treatment consists of catheter removal, aspiration, resection, or incision and drainage of the vein, followed by a 14-day course of amphotericin B or fluconazole [135, 137, 329]. When a central vein is involved and surgery is not an option, systemic antifungal therapy may be successful [330, 331]. *Candida* infections of arteriovenous dialysis fistulas are rare, and effective therapy generally requires both antifungal therapy and removal of the fistula.

Candida Abdominal Infections

Removal of the dialysis catheter is usually required for successful therapy of CAPD-related fungal peritonitis [179, 332, 333]. Occasionally, some patients are cured via this maneuver alone [334, 335]. Short courses of parenteral amphotericin B have been used successfully. Intraperitoneal therapy with amphotericin B is associated with abdominal pain and the development of adhesions, and is no longer recommended [336]. Several reports have documented the utility of fluconazole in combination with flucytosine as therapy for dialysis catheter-related peritonitis [333, 337, 338]. Dosages of fluconazole are 100–200 mg daily and dosages of flucytosine are 15 mg/kg after hemodialysis for patients whose catheters have been removed [333, 339].

The potential for *Candida* to cause peritonitis has now been clearly demonstrated [174, 340–342]. While no specific criteria identify the patients in whom *Candida* is significant, factors such as presence of sepsis, multiple operations, pancreatic involvement, and heavy growth of *Candida* from peritoneal cultures strongly suggest that antifungal therapy is indicated [174, 342, 343]. Although amphotericin B has been used in the past, this is rarely indicated now and patients should be treated with fluconazole or an echinocandin [174, 341, 342, 344].

Candida is isolated from the bile in up to 2% of cholecystectomies, but the mere isolation of the organism does not mandate therapy. However, if the patient has biliary obstruction or gangrenous cholecystitis, then isolation of *Candida* merits systemic therapy. Amphotericin B achieves bile concentrations that are two to sevenfold higher than serum concentrations [345]. *Candida* fungus balls can cause biliary obstruction of the collecting system and may require surgical removal. The association between increased mortality and *Candida* superinfections in patients with acute necrotizing pancreatitis [346, 347] provides strong support for the use of an antifungal agent if *Candida* is isolated from pancreatic tissue. After suitable debridement and/or drainage, therapy, usually with fluconazole or an echinocandin, is indicated.

Candida Musculoskeletal Infections

Most investigators recommend amphotericin B as the primary agent for *Candida* osteomyelitis [348–350]. Several groups recommend surgical debridement of infected bone in cases of vertebral osteomyelitis, but not all clinicians agree with that approach [183, 348]. There is no consensus regarding duration of therapy, but treatment is usually continued for at least 2–4 weeks after resolution of clinical signs and symptoms of infection or microbiologic evidence of eradication of infection [106]. One report suggested that amphotericin B might safely be added to bone cement in complicated cases [351]. Several investigators have used a course of amphotericin B, followed by 6–12 months with an azole [348, 350, 352]. There is increasing experience with azole agents and echinocandins for treatment of osteomyelitis [353–356].

Systemic antifungal therapy and joint drainage or joint lavage may be necessary to achieve cure of septic *Candida* arthritis. Open drainage is particularly important in *Candida* infection of the native hip. For infection involving a prosthetic joint, resection arthroplasty is virtually always required [357]. Successful medical treatment with fluconazole for 17 months of a hip prosthesis that was infected with *C. albicans* has been described, but post-therapy follow-up was only 11 months and this type of response appears to be the exception rather than the rule [358]. Most treatment experience for *Candida* arthritis has been with amphotericin B [359]. Substantial synovial fluid levels (20–100% of serum levels) are achieved with amphotericin B. Intraarticular amphotericin B, typically 5–10 mg, has been given at intervals in association with joint aspiration, but may be associated with joint surface irritation [359]. Experience with azole therapy is limited, but a few reports indicate success [357, 360, 361]. Good drug penetration with fluconazole has been documented.

Candida Central Nervous System Infections

No randomized controlled trials have been performed to evaluate the most appropriate therapy. Most experience with the therapy of *Candida* meningitis has been with amphotericin B, often in combination with flucytosine, because of the latter agent's ability to penetrate the blood–brain barrier [362, 363]. Most experts favor lipid-formulations of amphotericin B because of decreased risk of nephrotoxicity [106]. Fluconazole with flucytosine [364], and fluconazole monotherapy have been used [365]. For *Candida* meningitis following neurosurgical procedures, especially in association with CSF devices, such as shunts or drains, device removal plus antifungal therapy is required [366]. For *Candida* meningitis associated with neurosurgery or devices, intravenous amphotericin B is usually effective, but some patients may require the addition of flucytosine or intrathecal amphotericin B [155]. The excellent penetration of fluconazole into the CSF suggests that it might be a useful agent in this setting, although some fluconazole failures have been reported [155, 367].

Treatment of *Candida* brain abscess [151, 368], epidural abscess [369], and intramedullary abscess has been with amphotericin B and flucytosine, occasionally followed by oral azole therapy. Length of therapy has not been defined but experts recommend several weeks of therapy before transition to oral azole therapy. There are no reports of the use of voriconazole or posaconazole for *Candida* CNS infections. Voriconazole achieves excellent levels in CSF [370] but posaconazole CSF levels are low. For the rare case of *C. glabrata* or *C. krusei*, voriconazole seems appropriate therapy after initial treatment with AmB and flucytosine. Echinocandins have been used infrequently for CNS infections and there are reports of both success and failures as well as reports of CNS breakthrough infections after therapy for candidemia [371]. Recently, Hope et al. reported upon micafungin CSF pharmacokinetics in a rat model of neonatal *Candida* meningoencephalitis [372]. Micafungin was not reliably found in the CSF. These agents cannot be currently recommended for CNS candidiasis [106].

Prevention of Invasive Candidiasis in ICU Patients

From 25% to 50% of nosocomial *Candida* infections occur in patients in ICUs 373, particularly those in surgical ICUs [52]. Fluconazole use has increased dramatically in the ICU, both as a prophylactic agent and as empirical therapy in the febrile patient [374–376]. However, multiple studies have failed to show any benefit for prophylaxis, due in part to inclusion of low-risk patients in clinical trials and performance of studies that lacked adequate power [374, 375, 377, 378]. A recently published placebo controlled study utilizing empirical fluconazole for febrile high risk ICU patients failed to show any benefit of empirical antifungal use [379].

Some studies have shown the benefit of fluconazole prophylaxis by either using highly selective entry criteria [177] or enrolling only very high-risk surgical patients [380, 381]. The majority of patients in a surgical ICU are at low risk of invasive *Candida* infection with an approximately 1% overall incidence of candidemia. Patients at highest risk are those who undergo liver transplantation [382, 383], pancreas transplantation [175], and those with persistent or refractory gastrointestinal leakage [177]. While liver and pancreas transplant recipients are easy to identify, as are surgical patients with persistent GI leakage, the group of ICU patients who may benefit from fluconazole prophylaxis remains difficult to select. Recently, investigators have identified critically ill post-surgery patients likely to remain in the ICU for at least 72 h, especially those following abdominal surgery, and in association with acute renal failure, use of intravascular catheters, TPN, and broad-spectrum antibiotics, as a high-risk group [380, 384]. Specific laboratory tests, such as the beta-D-glucan assay, to help identify the patients at highest risk who may benefit from antifungal prophylaxis are currently under study. *Candida* surveillance cultures are currently not widely recommended but are utilized in some medical centers. In summary, fluconazole or echinocandin prophylaxis should only be considered in the ICU setting for high risk patients only in units in which the estimated risk of invasive candidiasis exceeds 10% [60, 61].

In the neonatal ICU setting, it has been shown that prophylactic administration of fluconazole during the first 6 weeks of life is effective in preventing fungal colonization and invasive candidiasis in infants with birth weights <1,000 g [385]. A subsequent randomized multicenter trial performed in nurseries with high rates of invasive candidiasis, confirmed that fluconazole prophylaxis, 3–6 mg/kg twice weekly, in neonates <1,000 g reduced the rates of invasive candidiasis [386]. Similar studies in older infants and children are needed.

References

1. Berkhout CM. DeSchimmelgeschlachter Monilia, Oidium, Vospora, en Torula.; 1923.
2. Odds FC. Ecology of *Candida* and epidemiology of candidosis. In: Odds FC, editor. *Candida* and Candidosis. 2nd ed. London: Bailliere Tindall; 1988.
3. Pfaller MA, Diekema DJ, Jones RN, et al. International surveillance of bloodstream infections due to *Candida* species: frequency of occurrence and in vitro susceptibilities to fluconazole, ravuconazole, and voriconazole of isolates collected from 1997 through 1999 in the SENTRY antimicrobial surveillance program. J Clin Microbiol. 2001;39:3254–9.
4. Fidel Jr PL, Vazquez JA, Sobel JD. *Candida glabrata*: review of epidemiology, pathogenesis, and clinical disease with comparison to *C. albicans*. Clin Microbiol Rev. 1999;12:80–96.
5. Gumbo T, Isada CM, Hall G, Karafa MT, Gordon SM. *Candida glabrata* Fungemia. Clinical features of 139 patients. Medicine (Baltimore). 1999;78:220–7.
6. Pfaller MA, Diekema DJ, Rinaldi MG, et al. Results from the ARTEMIS DISK Global Antifungal Surveillance Study: a 6.5-year analysis of susceptibilities of *Candida* and other yeast species to fluconazole and voriconazole by standardized disk diffusion testing. J Clin Microbiol. 2005;43:5848–59.
7. Pfaller MA, Diekema DJ. Epidemiology of invasive candidiasis: a persistent public health problem. Clin Microbiol Rev. 2007;20:133–63.
8. Girmenia C, Martino P, De Bernardis F, et al. Rising incidence of *Candida parapsilosis* fungemia in patients with hematologic malignancies: clinical aspects, predisposing factors, and differential pathogenicity of the causative strains. Clin Infect Dis. 1996;23:506–14.
9. Levy I, Rubin LG, Vasishtha S, Tucci V, Sood SK. Emergence of *Candida parapsilosis* as the predominant species causing candidemia in children. Clin Infect Dis. 1998;26:1086–8.
10. Sanchez V, Vazquez JA, Barth-Jones D, Dembry L, Sobel JD, Zervos MJ. Nosocomial acquisition of *Candida parapsilosis*: an epidemiologic study. Am J Med. 1993;94:577–82.
11. Kontoyiannis DP, Vaziri I, Hanna HA, et al. Risk factors for *Candida tropicalis* fungemia in patients with cancer. Clin Infect Dis. 2001;33:1676–81.
12. Merz WG, Karp JE, Schron D, Saral R. Increased incidence of fungemia caused by *Candida krusei*. J Clin Microbiol. 1986;24:581–4.
13. Wingard JR, Merz WG, Rinaldi MG, Johnson TR, Karp JE, Saral R. Increase in *Candida krusei* infection among patients with bone marrow transplantation and neutropenia treated prophylactically with fluconazole. N Engl J Med. 1991;325:1274–7.
14. Abbas J, Bodey GP, Hanna HA. *Candida krusei* fungemia. An escalating serious infection in immunocompromised patients. Arch Intern Med. 2000;160:2659–64.
15. Vazquez JA, Lundstrom T, Dembry L, et al. Invasive *Candida guilliermondii* infection: in vitro susceptibility studies and molecular analysis. Bone Marrow Transplant. 1995;16:849–53.
16. Yoon SA, Vazquez JA, Steffan PE, Sobel JD, Akins RA. High-frequency, in vitro reversible switching of *Candida lusitaniae* clinical isolates from amphotericin B susceptibility to resistance. Antimicrob Agents Chemother. 1999;43:836–45.
17. Sanchez V, Vazquez JA, Barth-Jones D, Dembry L, Sobel JD, Zervos MJ. Epidemiology of nosocomial acquisition of *Candida lusitaniae*. J Clin Microbiol. 1992;30:3005–8.
18. Kwon-Chung KJ, Riggsby WS, Uphoff RA, et al. Genetic differences between type I and type II *Candida stellatoidea*. Infect Immun. 1989;57:527–32.
19. Kwon-Chung KJ, Wickes BL, Merz WG. Association of electrophoretic karyotype of *Candida stellatoidea* with virulence for mice. Infect Immun. 1988;56:1814–9.
20. Sullivan D, Coleman D. *Candida dubliniensis*: characteristics and identification. J Clin Microbiol. 1998;36:329–34.
21. Hidalgo JA, Brown W, Vazquez JA. Invasive *Candida dubliniensis* in an HIV-negative patient: a new opportunistic fungal pathogen. Infect Dis Clin Pract. 2000;9:176–9.
22. Sebti A, Kiehn TE, Perlin D, et al. *Candida dubliniensis* at a cancer center. Clin Infect Dis. 2001;32:1034–8.

23. Jabra-Rizk MA, Baqui AA, Kelley JI, Falkler Jr WA, Merz WG, Meiller TF. Identification of *Candida dubliniensis* in a prospective study of patients in the United States. J Clin Microbiol. 1999;37:321–6.
24. Minces LR, Ho KS, Veldkamp PJ, Clancy CJ. *Candida rugosa*: a distinctive emerging cause of candidaemia. A case report and review of the literature. Scand J Infect Dis. 2009;41:1–5.
25. Lockhart SR, Messer SA, Pfaller MA, Diekema DJ. Geographic distribution and antifungal susceptibility of the newly described species *Candida orthopsilosis* and *Candida metapsilosis* in comparison to the closely related species *Candida parapsilosis*. J Clin Microbiol. 2008;46:2659–64.
26. Borman AM, Petch R, Linton CJ, Palmer MD, Bridge PD, Johnson EM. *Candida nivariensis*, an emerging pathogenic fungus with multidrug resistance to antifungal agents. J Clin Microbiol. 2008;46:933–8.
27. Bishop JA, Chase N, Magill SS, Kurtzman CP, Fiandaca MJ, Merz WG. *Candida bracarensis* detected among isolates of *Candida glabrata* by peptide nucleic acid fluorescence in situ hybridization: susceptibility data and documentation of presumed infection. J Clin Microbiol. 2008;46:443–6.
28. Lockhart SR, Messer SA, Pfaller MA, Diekema DJ. Identification and susceptibility profile of *Candida fermentati* from a worldwide collection of *Candida guilliermondii* clinical isolates. J Clin Microbiol. 2009;47:242–4.
29. Brown AJ, Gow NA. Regulatory networks controlling *Candida albicans* morphogenesis. Trends Microbiol. 1999;7:333–8.
30. Grubb SE, Murdoch C, Sudbery PE, Saville SP, Lopez-Ribot JL, Thornhill MH. Adhesion of *Candida albicans* to endothelial cells under physiological conditions of flow. Infect Immun. 2009;77:3872–8.
31. Lo HJ, Kohler JR, DiDomenico B, Loebenberg D, Cacciapuoti A, Fink GR. Nonfilamentous *C. albicans* mutants are avirulent. Cell. 1997;90:939–49.
32. Saville SP, Lazzell AL, Chaturvedi AK, Monteagudo C, Lopez-Ribot JL. Use of a genetically engineered strain to evaluate the pathogenic potential of yeast cell and filamentous forms during *Candida albicans* systemic infection in immunodeficient mice. Infect Immun. 2008;76:97–102.
33. Gow NA, Brown AJ, Odds FC. Fungal morphogenesis and host invasion. Curr Opin Microbiol. 2002;5:366–71.
34. Saville SP, Lazzell AL, Bryant AP, et al. Inhibition of filamentation can be used to treat disseminated candidiasis. Antimicrob Agents Chemother. 2006;50:3312–6.
35. Sundstrom P. Adhesins in *Candida albicans*. Curr Opin Microbiol. 1999;2:353–7.
36. Staab JF, Bradway SD, Fidel PL, Sundstrom P. Adhesive and mammalian transglutaminase substrate properties of *Candida albicans* Hwp1. Science. 1999;283:1535–8.
37. Grubb SE, Murdoch C, Sudbery PE, Saville SP, Lopez-Ribot JL, Thornhill MH. *Candida albicans*-endothelial cell interactions: a key step in the pathogenesis of systemic candidiasis. Infect Immun. 2008;76:4370–7.
38. Leidich SD, Ibrahim AS, Fu Y, et al. Cloning and disruption of caPLB1, a phospholipase B gene involved in the pathogenicity of *Candida albicans*. J Biol Chem. 1998;273:26078–86.
39. Staib F. Proteolysis and pathogenicity of *Candida albicans* strains. Mycopathol Mycol Appl. 1969;37:345–8.
40. Monod M, Togni G, Hube B, Sanglard D. Multiplicity of genes encoding secreted aspartic proteinases in *Candida* species. Mol Microbiol. 1994;13:357–68.
41. Ramage G, Saville SP, Thomas DP, Lopez-Ribot JL. *Candida* biofilms: an update. Eukaryot Cell. 2005;4:633–8.
42. Kojic EM, Darouiche RO. *Candida* infections of medical devices. Clin Microbiol Rev. 2004;17:255–67.
43. Zaoutis TE, Argon J, Chu J, Berlin JA, Walsh TJ, Feudtner C. The epidemiology and attributable outcomes of candidemia in adults and children hospitalized in the United States: a propensity analysis. Clin Infect Dis. 2005;41:1232–9.
44. Sandven P. Epidemiology of candidemia. Rev Iberoam Micol. 2000;17:73–81.
45. Wisplinghoff H, Bischoff T, Tallent SM, Seifert H, Wenzel RP, Edmond MB. Nosocomial bloodstream infections in US hospitals: analysis of 24,179 cases from a prospective nationwide surveillance study. Clin Infect Dis. 2004;39:309–17.
46. Wenzel RP, Gennings C. Bloodstream infections due to *Candida* species in the intensive care unit: identifying especially high-risk patients to determine prevention strategies. Clin Infect Dis. 2005;41 Suppl 6:S389–93.
47. Rentz AM, Halpern MT, Bowden R. The impact of candidemia on length of hospital stay, outcome, and overall cost of illness. Clin Infect Dis. 1998;27:781–8.
48. Trick WE, Fridkin SK, Edwards JR, Hajjeh RA, Gaynes RP. Secular trend of hospital-acquired candidemia among intensive care unit patients in the United States during 1989–1999. Clin Infect Dis. 2002;35:627–30.
49. Hajjeh RA, Sofair AN, Harrison LH, et al. Incidence of bloodstream infections due to *Candida* species and in vitro susceptibilities of isolates collected from 1998 to 2000 in a population-based active surveillance program. J Clin Microbiol. 2004;42:1519–27.
50. Hidron AI, Edwards JR, Patel J, et al. Antimicrobial-resistant pathogens associated with healthcare-associated infections: annual summary of data reported to the National Healthcare Safety Network at the Centers for Disease Control and Prevention, 2006–2007. Infect Control Hosp Epidemiol. 2008;29:996–1011.
51. Vincent JL, Anaissie E, Bruining H, et al. Epidemiology, diagnosis and treatment of systemic *Candida* infection in surgical patients under intensive care. Intensive Care Med. 1998;24:206–16.
52. Beck-Sague C, Jarvis WR. Secular trends in the epidemiology of nosocomial fungal infections in the United States, 1980–1990. National Nosocomial Infections Surveillance System. J Infect Dis. 1993;167:1247–51.
53. Fridkin SK, Jarvis WR. Epidemiology of nosocomial fungal infections. Clin Microbiol Rev. 1996;9:499–511.
54. Abi-Said D, Anaissie E, Uzun O, Raad I, Pinzcowski H, Vartivarian S. The epidemiology of hematogenous candidiasis caused by different *Candida* species. Clin Infect Dis. 1997;24:1122–8.
55. Marr KA, Seidel K, Slavin MA, et al. Prolonged fluconazole prophylaxis is associated with persistent protection against candidiasis-related death in allogeneic marrow transplant recipients: long-term follow-up of a randomized, placebo-controlled trial. Blood. 2000;96:2055–61.
56. Horn DL, Neofytos D, Anaissie EJ, et al. Epidemiology and outcomes of candidemia in 2019 patients: data from the prospective antifungal therapy alliance registry. Clin Infect Dis. 2009;48:1695–703.
57. Hachem R, Hanna H, Kontoyiannis D, Jiang Y, Raad I. The changing epidemiology of invasive candidiasis: *Candida glabrata* and *Candida krusei* as the leading causes of candidemia in hematologic malignancy. Cancer. 2008;112:2493–9.
58. Arendrup MC, Fuursted K, Gahrn-Hansen B, et al. Seminational surveillance of fungemia in Denmark: notably high rates of fungemia and numbers of isolates with reduced azole susceptibility. J Clin Microbiol. 2005;43:4434–40.
59. Pappas PG, Rex JH, Lee J, et al. A prospective observational study of candidemia: epidemiology, therapy, and influences on mortality in hospitalized adult and pediatric patients. Clin Infect Dis. 2003;37:634–43.
60. Playford EG, Marriott D, Nguyen Q, et al. Candidemia in nonneutropenic critically ill patients: risk factors for non-albicans *Candida* spp. Crit Care Med. 2008;36:2034–9.
61. Playford EG, Webster AC, Sorrell TC, Craig JC. Antifungal agents for preventing fungal infections in non-neutropenic critically ill and surgical patients: systematic review and meta-analysis of randomized clinical trials. J Antimicrob Chemother. 2006;57:628–38.

62. Bross J, Talbot GH, Maislin G, Hurwitz S, Strom BL. Risk factors for nosocomial candidemia: a case-control study in adults without leukemia. Am J Med. 1989;87:614–20.
63. Pittet D, Monod M, Suter PM, Frenk E, Auckenthaler R. *Candida* colonization and subsequent infections in critically ill surgical patients. Ann Surg. 1994;220:751–8.
64. Blumberg HM, Jarvis WR, Soucie JM, et al. Risk factors for candidal bloodstream infections in surgical intensive care unit patients: the NEMIS prospective multicenter study. The National Epidemiology of Mycosis Survey. Clin Infect Dis. 2001;33:177–86.
65. Kao AS, Brandt ME, Pruitt WR, et al. The epidemiology of candidemia in two United States cities: results of a population-based active surveillance. Clin Infect Dis. 1999;29:1164–70.
66. Mahayni R, Vazquez JA, Zervos MJ. Nosocomial candidiasis: epidemiology and drug resistance. Infect Agents Dis. 1995;4:248–53.
67. Pfaller MA, Cabezudo I, Hollis R, Huston B, Wenzel RP. The use of biotyping and DNA fingerprinting in typing *Candida albicans* from hospitalized patients. Diagn Microbiol Infect Dis. 1990;13:481–9.
68. Vazquez JA, Sanchez V, Dmuchowski C, Dembry LM, Sobel JD, Zervos MJ. Nosocomial acquisition of *Candida albicans*: an epidemiologic study. J Infect Dis. 1993;168:195–201.
69. Vaudry WL, Tierney AJ, Wenman WM. Investigation of a cluster of systemic *Candida albicans* infections in a neonatal intensive care unit. J Infect Dis. 1988;158:1375–9.
70. Berger C, Frei R, Gratwohl A, Scheidegger C. Bottled lemon juice – a cryptic source of invasive *Candida* infections in the immunocompromised host. J Infect Dis. 1988;158:654–5.
71. Langenbeck B. Auffingung von Pilzer aus der Schleimhaut der Speiserohre einer Typhus-Leiche. Neu Not Geb. Nautur-u-Heilk (Froorief). 1939;12:145–7.
72. Berg FT. GM Torsk hos Barn. Stockholm: LJ Hjerta; 1846.
73. Villar CC, Dongari-Bagtzoglou A. Immune defence mechanisms and immunoenhancement strategies in oropharyngeal candidiasis. Expert Rev Mol Med. 2008;10:e29.
74. Sobel JD, Vazquez JA. Gastrointestinal and hepatic infections. In: Surawicz CM, editor. Fungal Infections of the Gastrointestinal Tract. Philadelphia: WB Saunders; 1995. p. 219–46.
75. Samonis G, Anaissie EJ, Rosenbaum B, Bodey GP. A model of sustained gastrointestinal colonization by *Candida albicans* in healthy adult mice. Infect Immun. 1990;58:1514–7.
76. Yeo E, Alvarado T, Fainstein V, Bodey GP. Prophylaxis of oropharyngeal candidiasis with clotrimazole. J Clin Oncol. 1985;3:1668–71.
77. Feigal DW, Katz MH, Greenspan D, et al. The prevalence of oral lesions in HIV-infected homosexual and bisexual men: three San Francisco epidemiological cohorts. AIDS. 1991;5:519–25.
78. Klein RS, Harris CA, Small CB, Moll B, Lesser M, Friedland GH. Oral candidiasis in high-risk patients as the initial manifestation of the acquired immunodeficiency syndrome. N Engl J Med. 1984;311:354–8.
79. Lamey PJ, Lamb AB. Prospective study of aetiological factors in burning mouth syndrome. Br Med J (Clin Res Ed). 1988;296:1243–6.
80. Whelan WL, Delga JM, Wadsworth E, et al. Isolation and characterization of cell surface mutants of *Candida albicans*. Infect Immun. 1990;58:1552–7.
81. Mercante DE, Leigh JE, Lilly EA, McNulty K, Fidel Jr PL. Assessment of the association between HIV viral load and CD4 cell count on the occurrence of oropharyngeal candidiasis in HIV-infected patients. J Acquir Immune Defic Syndr. 2006;42:578–83.
82. Delgado AC, de Jesus Pedro R, Aoki FH, et al. Clinical and microbiological assessment of patients with a long-term diagnosis of human immunodeficiency virus infection and *Candida* oral colonization. Clin Microbiol Infect. 2009;15:364–71.
83. Vazquez JA. Therapeutic options for the management of oropharyngeal and esophageal candidiasis in HIV/AIDS patients. HIV Clin Trials. 2000;1:47–59.
84. Barchiesi F, Morbiducci V, Ancarani F, Scalise G. Emergence of oropharyngeal candidiasis caused by non-*albicans* species of *Candida* in HIV-infected patients. Eur J Epidemiol. 1993;9:455–6.
85. Fidel PL, Lilly E, Rufener JB, et al. Longitudinal analysis of local immune function in HIV + subjects with oropharyngeal candidiasis. In: Annual Interscience Conference on Antimicrobial Agents and Chemotherapeutics; 2009 9/11-15/2009; San Francisco, 2009. p. Abstract M-365.
86. Letiner T. Oral thrush or acute pseudomembranous candidiasis: a clinical-pathologic study of 44 cases. Oral Surg. 1964;18:27–37.
87. Budtz-Jorgensen E, Stenderup A, Grabowski M. An epidemiologic study of yeasts in elderly denture wearers. Community Dent Oral Epidemiol. 1975;3:115–9.
88. Cernea P, Crepy C, Kuffer R, Mascaro JM, Badillet G, Marie JL. Little known aspects of oral condidiasis. The candidiasis with multiple foci of the oral cavity. Rev Stomatol Chir Maxillofac. 1965;66:103–38.
89. Wheeler RR, Peacock Jr JE, Cruz JM, Richter JE. Esophagitis in the immunocompromised host: role of esophagoscopy in diagnosis. Rev Infect Dis. 1987;9:88–96.
90. Clotet B, Grifol M, Parra O, et al. Asymptomatic esophageal candidiasis in the acquired-immunodeficiency-syndrome-related complex. Ann Intern Med. 1986;105:145.
91. Kodsi BE, Wickremesinghe C, Kozinn PJ, Iswara K, Goldberg PK. *Candida* esophagitis: a prospective study of 27 cases. Gastroenterology. 1976;71:715–9.
92. Alteras I, Feuerman EJ, David M, Shohat B, Livni E. Widely disseminated cutaneous candidosis in adults. Sabouraudia. 1979;17:383–8.
93. Fitzpatrick TB, Johnson RA, Wolff K, Polano MK, Suurmond D. Color atlas and synopsis of clinical dermatology: Common and serious diseases. 3rd ed. New York: McGraw Hill; 1997.
94. Arbegast KD, Lamberty LF, Koh JK, Pergram JM, Braddock SW. Congenital candidiasis limited to the nail plates. Pediatr Dermatol. 1990;7:310–2.
95. Kirkpatrick CH. Chronic mucocutaneous candidiasis. J Am Acad Dermatol. 1994;31:S14–7.
96. Ahonen P, Myllarniemi S, Sipila I, Perheentupa J. Clinical variation of autoimmune polyendocrinopathy-candidiasis-ectodermal dystrophy (APECED) in a series of 68 patients. N Engl J Med. 1990;322:1829–36.
97. Bjorses P, Aaltonen J, Vikman A, et al. Genetic homogeneity of autoimmune polyglandular disease type I. Am J Hum Genet. 1996;59:879–86.
98. Hermans PE, Ritts Jr RE. Chronic mucocutaneous candidiasis. Its association with immunologic and endocrine abnormalities. Minn Med. 1970;53:75–80.
99. Okamoto GA, Hall JG, Ochs H, Jackson C, Rodaway K, Chandler J. New syndrome of chronic mucocutaneous candidiasis. Birth Defects Orig Artic Ser. 1977;13:117–25.
100. Holt PJ, Higgs JM, Munro J, Valdimarsson H. Chronic mucocutaneous candidiasis: a model for the investigation of cell mediated immunity. Br J Clin Pract. 1972;26:331–6.
101. Durandy A, Fischer A, Le Deist F, Drouhet E, Griscelli C. Mannan-specific and mannan-induced T-cell suppressive activity in patients with chronic mucocutaneous candidiasis. J Clin Immunol. 1987;7:400–9.
102. Hurley R, De Louvois J. *Candida* vaginitis. Postgrad Med J. 1979;55:645–7.
103. Sobel JD, Bradshaw SK, Lipka CJ, Kartsonis NA. Caspofungin in the treatment of symptomatic candiduria. Clin Infect Dis. 2007;44:e46–9.

104. Sobel JD. Vulvovaginal candidosis. Lancet. 2007;369:1961–71.
105. Witkin SS. Immunologic factors influencing susceptibility to recurrent candidal vaginitis. Clin Obstet Gynecol. 1991;34:662–8.
106. Pappas PG, Kauffman CA, Andes D, et al. Clinical practice guidelines for the management of candidiasis: 2009 update by the Infectious Diseases Society of America. Clin Infect Dis. 2009;48:503–35.
107. Berenguer J, Buck M, Witebsky F, Stock F, Pizzo PA, Walsh TJ. Lysis-centrifugation blood cultures in the detection of tissue-proven invasive candidiasis. Disseminated versus single-organ infection. Diagn Microbiol Infect Dis. 1993;17:103–9.
108. Hockey LJ, Fujita NK, Gibson TR, Rotrosen D, Montgomerie JZ, Edwards Jr JE. Detection of fungemia obscured by concomitant bacteremia: in vitro and in vivo studies. J Clin Microbiol. 1982;16:1080–5.
109. Lecciones JA, Lee JW, Navarro EE, et al. Vascular catheter-associated fungemia in patients with cancer: analysis of 155 episodes. Clin Infect Dis. 1992;14:875–83.
110. Anaissie EJ, Rex JH, Uzun O, Vartivarian S. Predictors of adverse outcome in cancer patients with candidemia. Am J Med. 1998;104:238–45.
111. Wingard JR. Importance of *Candida* species other than *C. albicans* as pathogens in oncology patients. Clin Infect Dis. 1995;20:115–25.
112. Murray PR. Comparison of the lysis-centrifugation and agitated biphasic blood culture systems for detection of fungemia. J Clin Microbiol. 1991;29:96–8.
113. Wey SB, Mori M, Pfaller MA, Woolson RF, Wenzel RP. Hospital-acquired candidemia. The attributable mortality and excess length of stay. Arch Intern Med. 1988;148:2642–5.
114. Komshian SV, Uwaydah AK, Sobel JD, Crane LR. Fungemia caused by *Candida* species and *Torulopsis glabrata* in the hospitalized patient: frequency, characteristics, and evaluation of factors influencing outcome. Rev Infect Dis. 1989;11:379–90.
115. Fraser VJ, Jones M, Dunkel J, Storfer S, Medoff G, Dunagan WC. Candidemia in a tertiary care hospital: epidemiology, risk factors, and predictors of mortality. Clin Infect Dis. 1992;15:414–21.
116. McNeil MM, Nash SL, Hajjeh RA, et al. Trends in mortality due to invasive mycotic diseases in the United States, 1980–1997. Clin Infect Dis. 2001;33:641–7.
117. Edwards Jr JE, Foos RY, Montgomerie JZ, Guze LB. Ocular manifestations of *Candida* septicemia: review of seventy-six cases of hematogenous *Candida* endophthalmitis. Medicine (Baltimore). 1974;53:47–75.
118. Samiy N, D'Amico DJ. Endogenous fungal endophthalmitis. Int Ophthalmol Clin. 1996;36:147–62.
119. Khan FA, Slain D, Khakoo RA. *Candida* endophthalmitis: focus on current and future antifungal treatment options. Pharmacotherapy. 2007;27:1711–21.
120. Noyola DE, Fernandez M, Moylett EH, Baker CJ. Ophthalmologic, visceral, and cardiac involvement in neonates with candidemia. Clin Infect Dis. 2001;32:1018–23.
121. Brooks RG. Prospective study of *Candida* endophthalmitis in hospitalized patients with candidemia. Arch Intern Med. 1989;149:2226–8.
122. Krishna R, Amuh D, Lowder CY, Gordon SM, Adal KA, Hall G. Should all patients with candidaemia have an ophthalmic examination to rule out ocular candidiasis? Eye. 2000;14(Pt 1):30–4.
123. Joshi N, Hamory BH. Endophthalmitis caused by non-*albicans* species of *Candida*. Rev Infect Dis. 1991;13:281–7.
124. Henderson DK, Hockey LJ, Vukalcic LJ, Edwards Jr JE. Effect of immunosuppression on the development of experimental hematogenous *Candida* endophthalmitis. Infect Immun. 1980;27:628–31.
125. McDonald HR, De Bustros S, Sipperley JO. Vitrectomy for epiretinal membrane with *Candida* chorioretinitis. Ophthalmology. 1990;97:466–9.
126. Franklin WG, Simon AB, Sodeman TM. *Candida* myocarditis without valvulitis. Am J Cardiol. 1976;38:924–8.
127. Rubin RH, Moellering Jr RC. Clinical, microbiologic and therapeutic aspects of purulent pericarditis. Am J Med. 1975;59:68–78.
128. Schrank Jr JH, Dooley DP. Purulent pericarditis caused by *Candida* species: case report and review. Clin Infect Dis. 1995;21:182–7.
129. Rubinstein E, Noriega ER, Simberkoff MS, Holzman R, Rahal Jr JJ. Fungal endocarditis: analysis of 24 cases and review of the literature. Medicine (Baltimore). 1975;54:331–4.
130. Ellis ME, Al-Abdely H, Sandridge A, Greer W, Ventura W. Fungal endocarditis: evidence in the world literature, 1965–1995. Clin Infect Dis. 2001;32:50–62.
131. Chim CS, Ho PL, Yuen ST, Yuen KY. Fungal endocarditis in bone marrow transplantation: case report and review of literature. J Infect. 1998;37:287–91.
132. Nasser RM, Melgar GR, Longworth DL, Gordon SM. Incidence and risk of developing fungal prosthetic valve endocarditis after nosocomial candidemia. Am J Med. 1997;103:25–32.
133. Joly V, Belmatoug N, Leperre A, et al. Pacemaker endocarditis due to *Candida albicans*: case report and review. Clin Infect Dis. 1997;25:1359–62.
134. Galgiani JN, Stevens DA. Fungal endocarditis: need for guidelines in evaluating therapy. Experience with two patients previously reported. J Thorac Cardiovasc Surg. 1977;73:293–6.
135. Friedland IR. Peripheral thrombophlebitis caused by *Candida*. Pediatr Infect Dis J. 1996;15:375–7.
136. Khan EA, Correa AG, Baker CJ. Suppurative thrombophlebitis in children: a ten-year experience. Pediatr Infect Dis J. 1997;16:63–7.
137. Walsh TJ, Bustamente CI, Vlahov D, Standiford HC. Candidal suppurative peripheral thrombophlebitis: recognition, prevention, and management. Infect Control. 1986;7:16–22.
138. Doscher W, Krishnasastry KV, Deckoff SL. Fungal graft infections: case report and review of the literature. J Vasc Surg. 1987;6:398–402.
139. Gorg C, Weide R, Schwerk WB, Koppler H, Havemann K. Ultrasound evaluation of hepatic and splenic microabscesses in the immunocompromised patient: sonographic patterns, differential diagnosis, and follow-up. J Clin Ultrasound. 1994;22:525–9.
140. Anttila VJ, Ruutu P, Bondestam S, et al. Hepatosplenic yeast infection in patients with acute leukemia: a diagnostic problem. Clin Infect Dis. 1994;18:979–81.
141. Semelka RC, Shoenut JP, Greenberg HM, Bow EJ. Detection of acute and treated lesions of hepatosplenic candidiasis: comparison of dynamic contrast-enhanced CT and MR imaging. J Magn Reson Imaging. 1992;2:341–5.
142. Faix RG. Invasive neonatal candidiasis: comparison of albicans and parapsilosis infection. Pediatr Infect Dis J. 1992;11:88–93.
143. Jin Y, Endo A, Shimada M, et al. Congenital systemic candidiasis. Pediatr Infect Dis J. 1995;14:818–20.
144. Almeida Santos L, Beceiro J, Hernandez R, et al. Congenital cutaneous candidiasis: report of four cases and review of the literature. Eur J Pediatr. 1991;150:336–8.
145. Glassman BD, Muglia JJ. Widespread erythroderma and desquamation in a neonate. Congenital cutaneous candidiasis (CCC). Arch Dermatol. 1993;129:899–902.
146. Barone SR, Krilov LR. Neonatal candidal meningitis in a full-term infant with congenital cutaneous candidiasis. Clin Pediatr (Phila). 1995;34:217–9.
147. Lipton SA, Hickey WF, Morris JH, Loscalzo J. Candidal infection in the central nervous system. Am J Med. 1984;76:101–8.
148. Petraitiene R, Petraitis V, Hope WW, et al. Cerebrospinal fluid and plasma (1->3)-beta-D-glucan as surrogate markers for detection and monitoring of therapeutic response in experimental hematogenous *Candida* meningoencephalitis. Antimicrob Agents Chemother. 2008;52:4121–9.
149. Treseler CB, Sugar AM. Fungal meningitis. Infect Dis Clin North Am. 1990;4:789–808.

150. Voice RA, Bradley SF, Sangeorzan JA, Kauffman CA. Chronic candidal meningitis: an uncommon manifestation of candidiasis. Clin Infect Dis. 1994;19:60–6.
151. Burgert SJ, Classen DC, Burke JP, Blatter DD. Candidal brain abscess associated with vascular invasion: a devastating complication of vascular catheter-related candidemia. Clin Infect Dis. 1995;21:202–5.
152. Lai PH, Lin SM, Pan HB, Yang CF. Disseminated miliary cerebral candidiasis. AJNR Am J Neuroradiol. 1997;18:1303–6.
153. McCullers JA, Vargas SL, Flynn PM, Razzouk BI, Shenep JL. Candidal meningitis in children with cancer. Clin Infect Dis. 2000;31:451–7.
154. Fernandez M, Moylett EH, Noyola DE, Baker CJ. Candidal meningitis in neonates: a 10-year review. Clin Infect Dis. 2000;31:458–63.
155. Nguyen MH, Yu VL. Meningitis caused by *Candida* species: an emerging problem in neurosurgical patients. Clin Infect Dis. 1995;21:323–7.
156. Gower DJ, Crone K, Alexander Jr E, Kelly Jr DL. *Candida albicans* shunt infection: report of two cases. Neurosurgery. 1986;19:111–3.
157. Chmel H. *Candida albicans* meningitis following lumbar puncture. Am J Med Sci. 1973;266:465–7.
158. Masur H, Rosen PP, Armstrong D. Pulmonary disease caused by *Candida* species. Am J Med. 1977;63:914–25.
159. Haron E, Vartivarian S, Anaissie E, Dekmezian R, Bodey GP. Primary *Candida* pneumonia. Experience at a large cancer center and review of the literature. Medicine (Baltimore). 1993;72:137–42.
160. Heurlin N, Bergstrom SE, Winiarski J, et al. Fungal pneumonia: the predominant lung infection causing death in children undergoing bone marrow transplantation. Acta Paediatr. 1996;85:168–72.
161. Zeluff BJ. Fungal pneumonia in transplant recipients. Semin Respir Infect. 1990;5:80–9.
162. Lee TM, Greenberger PA, Oh S, Patterson R, Roberts M, Liotta JL. Allergic bronchopulmonary candidiasis: case report and suggested diagnostic criteria. J Allergy Clin Immunol. 1987;80:816–20.
163. von Eiff M, Zuhlsdorf M, Roos N, Hesse M, Schulten R, van de Loo J. Pulmonary fungal infections in patients with hematological malignancies – diagnostic approaches. Ann Hematol. 1995; 70:135–41.
164. el-Ebiary M, Torres A, Fabregas N, et al. Significance of the isolation of *Candida* species from respiratory samples in critically ill, non-neutropenic patients. An immediate postmortem histologic study. Am J Respir Crit Care Med. 1997;156:583–90.
165. Walsh TJ, Gray WC. *Candida* epiglottitis in immunocompromised patients. Chest. 1987;91:482–5.
166. Michigan S. Genitourinary fungal infections. J Urol. 1976;116:390–7.
167. Febre N, Silva V, Medeiros EA, Wey SB, Colombo AL, Fischman O. Microbiological characteristics of yeasts isolated from urinary tracts of intensive care unit patients undergoing urinary catheterization. J Clin Microbiol. 1999;37:1584–6.
168. Fisher JF, Chew WH, Shadomy S, Duma RJ, Mayhall CG, House WC. Urinary tract infections due to *Candida albicans*. Rev Infect Dis. 1982;4:1107–18.
169. Kauffman CA, Vazquez JA, Sobel JD, et al. Prospective multicenter surveillance study of funguria in hospitalized patients. The National Institute for Allergy and Infectious Diseases (NIAID) Mycoses Study Group. Clin Infect Dis. 2000;30:14–8.
170. Safdar N, Slattery WR, Knasinski V, et al. Predictors and outcomes of candiduria in renal transplant recipients. Clin Infect Dis. 2005;40:1413–21.
171. Sobel JD, Kauffman CA, McKinsey D, et al. Candiduria: a randomized, double-blind study of treatment with fluconazole and placebo. The National Institute of Allergy and Infectious Diseases (NIAID) Mycoses Study Group. Clin Infect Dis. 2000;30:19–24.
172. Kozinn PJ, Taschdjian CL, Goldberg PK, Wise GJ, Toni EF, Seelig MS. Advances in the diagnosis of renal candidiasis. J Urol. 1978;119:184–7.
173. Stone HH, Kolb LD, Currie CA, Geheber CE, Cuzzell JZ. *Candida* sepsis: pathogenesis and principles of treatments. Ann Surg. 1974;179:697–711.
174. Calandra T, Bille J, Schneider R, Mosimann F, Francioli P. Clinical significance of *Candida* isolated from peritoneum in surgical patients. Lancet. 1989;2:1437–40.
175. Benedetti E, Gruessner AC, Troppmann C, et al. Intra-abdominal fungal infections after pancreatic transplantation: incidence, treatment, and outcome. J Am Coll Surg. 1996;183:307–16.
176. Peoples JB. *Candida* and perforated peptic ulcers. Surgery. 1986;100:758–64.
177. Eggimann P, Francioli P, Bille J, et al. Fluconazole prophylaxis prevents intra-abdominal candidiasis in high-risk surgical patients. Crit Care Med. 1999;27:1066–72.
178. Rubin J, Kirchner K, Walsh D, Green M, Bower J. Fungal peritonitis during continuous ambulatory peritoneal dialysis: a report of 17 cases. Am J Kidney Dis. 1987;10:361–8.
179. Goldie SJ, Kiernan-Tridle L, Torres C, et al. Fungal peritonitis in a large chronic peritoneal dialysis population: a report of 55 episodes. Am J Kidney Dis. 1996;28:86–91.
180. Ehrenstein BP, Salamon L, Linde HJ, Messmann H, Scholmerich J, Gluck T. Clinical determinants for the recovery of fungal and mezlocillin-resistant pathogens from bile specimens. Clin Infect Dis. 2002;34:902–8.
181. Morris AB, Sands ML, Shiraki M, Brown RB, Ryczak M. Gallbladder and biliary tract candidiasis: nine cases and review. Rev Infect Dis. 1990;12:483–9.
182. Clancy CJ, Nguyen MH, Morris AJ. Candidal mediastinitis: an emerging clinical entity. Clin Infect Dis. 1997;25:608–13.
183. Hendrickx L, Van Wijngaerden E, Samson I, Peetermans WE. Candidal vertebral osteomyelitis: report of 6 patients, and a review. Clin Infect Dis. 2001;32:527–33.
184. Hansen BL, Andersen K. Fungal arthritis. A review. Scand J Rheumatol. 1995;24:248–50.
185. Fukasawa N, Shirakura K. *Candida* arthritis after total knee arthroplasty – a case of successful treatment without prosthesis removal. Acta Orthop Scand. 1997;68:306–7.
186. Belzunegui J, Gonzalez C, Lopez L, Plazaola I, Maiz O, Figueroa M. Osteoarticular and muscle infectious lesions in patients with the human immunodeficiency virus. Clin Rheumatol. 1997;16:450–3.
187. Rowen JL, Tate JM, Nordoff N, Passarell L, McGinnis MR. *Candida* isolates from neonates: frequency of misidentification and reduced fluconazole susceptibility. J Clin Microbiol. 1999;37:3735–7.
188. Wilson ML, Davis TE, Mirrett S, et al. Controlled comparison of the BACTEC high-blood-volume fungal medium, BACTEC Plus 26 aerobic blood culture bottle, and 10-milliliter isolator blood culture system for detection of fungemia and bacteremia. J Clin Microbiol. 1993;31:865–71.
189. Obayashi T, Yoshida M, Mori T, et al. Plasma (1–>3)-beta-D-glucan measurement in diagnosis of invasive deep mycosis and fungal febrile episodes. Lancet. 1995;345:17–20.
190. Ostrosky-Zeichner L, Alexander BD, Kett DH, et al. Multicenter clinical evaluation of the (1–>3) beta-D-glucan assay as an aid to diagnosis of fungal infections in humans. Clin Infect Dis. 2005;41:654–9.
191. Nett J, Lincoln L, Marchillo K, Andes D. Beta-1, 3 glucan as a test for central venous catheter biofilm infection. J Infect Dis. 2007;195:1705–12.
192. Rigby S, Procop GW, Haase G, et al. Fluorescence in situ hybridization with peptide nucleic acid probes for rapid identification of *Candida albicans* directly from blood culture bottles. J Clin Microbiol. 2002;40:2182–6.
193. Wilson DA, Joyce MJ, Hall LS, et al. Multicenter evaluation of a *Candida albicans* peptide nucleic acid fluorescent in situ hybridization probe for characterization of yeast isolates from blood cultures. J Clin Microbiol. 2005;43:2909–12.

194. Shepard JR, Addison RM, Alexander BD, et al. Multicenter evaluation of the *Candida albicans/Candida glabrata* peptide nucleic acid fluorescent in situ hybridization method for simultaneous dual-color identification of *C. albicans* and *C. glabrata* directly from blood culture bottles. J Clin Microbiol. 2008;46:50–5.
195. Gherna M, Merz WG. Identification of *Candida albicans* and *Candida glabrata* within 1.5 hours directly from positive blood culture bottles with a shortened peptide nucleic acid fluorescence in situ hybridization protocol. J Clin Microbiol. 2009;47:247–8.
196. NCCLS. Reference method for broth dilution antifungal susceptibility testing of yeasts. Document M27-A. Wayne: NCCLS, 1997.
197. Kurtz MB, Rex JH. Glucan synthase inhibitors as antifungal agents. Adv Protein Chem. 2001;56:423–75.
198. Rex JH, Pfaller MA, Galgiani JN, et al. Development of interpretive breakpoints for antifungal susceptibility testing: conceptual framework and analysis of in vitro-in vivo correlation data for fluconazole, itraconazole, and candida infections. Subcommittee on Antifungal Susceptibility Testing of the National Committee for Clinical Laboratory Standards. Clin Infect Dis. 1997;24:235–47.
199. Chow JK, Golan Y, Ruthazer R, et al. Factors associated with candidemia caused by non-*albicans Candida* species versus *Candida albicans* in the intensive care unit. Clin Infect Dis. 2008;46:1206–13.
200. Sobel JD, Revankar SG, Vazquez J, Ostrosky-Zeichner L. Mucocutaenous candidiasis in guidelines for prevention and treatment of opportunistic infections in HIV-infected adult and adolescents. MMWR Morb Mortal Wkly Rep. 2008;57:46–9.
201. Kozinn PJ, Taschdjian CL, Dragutsky D. Therapy of oral thrush: a comparative ealuation of gentian violet, mycostatin, and amphotericin B. Monogr Ther. 1957;2:16–24.
202. Shechtman LB, Funaro L, Robin T, Bottone EJ, Cuttner J. Clotrimazole treatment of oral candidiasis in patients with neoplastic disease. Am J Med. 1984;76:91–4.
203. Hughes WT, Bartley DL, Patterson GG, Tufenkeji H. Ketoconazole and candidiasis: a controlled study. J Infect Dis. 1983;147:1060–3.
204. Vazquez JA, Epstein J, Attali P. A multicenter, randomized trial evaluating the efficacy and safety of miconazole mucoadhesive buccal Tablets (MMBT) versus clotrimazole troches (CT) for the treatment of oropharyngeal candidiasis (OPC) in subjects with HIV/AIDS: SMiLES Trial. In: 49th Annual Interscience Conference on Antimicrobial Agents and Chemotherapeutics; Sept 11–15, 2009; San Francisco; 2009.
205. Cardot JM, Chaumont C, Dubray C, Costantini D, Aiache JM. Comparison of the pharmacokinetics of miconazole after administration via a bioadhesive slow release tablet and an oral gel to healthy male and female subjects. Br J Clin Pharmacol. 2004;58:345–51.
206. Hay RJ. Overview of studies of fluconazole in oropharyngeal candidiasis. Rev Infect Dis. 1990;12 Suppl 3:S334–7.
207. Vazquez JA, Skiest DJ, Nieto L, et al. A multicenter randomized trial evaluating posaconazole versus fluconazole for the treatment of oropharyngeal candidiasis in subjects with HIV/AIDS. Clin Infect Dis. 2006;42:1179–86.
208. Skiest DJ, Vazquez JA, Anstead GM, et al. Posaconazole for the treatment of azole-refractory oropharyngeal and esophageal candidiasis in subjects with HIV infection. Clin Infect Dis. 2007;44:607–14.
209. Meunier-Carpentier F, Cruciani M, Klastersky J. Oral prophylaxis with miconazole or ketoconazole of invasive fungal disease in neutropenic cancer patients. Eur J Cancer Clin Oncol. 1983;19:43–8.
210. Fazio RA, Wickremesinghe PC, Arsura EL. Ketoconazole treatment of *Candida* esophagitis – a prospective study of 12 cases. Am J Gastroenterol. 1983;78:261–4.
211. Wilcox CM, Darouiche RO, Laine L, Moskovitz BL, Mallegol I, Wu J. A randomized, double-blind comparison of itraconazole oral solution and fluconazole tablets in the treatment of esophageal candidiasis. J Infect Dis. 1997;176:227–32.
212. Vazquez JA, Skiest DJ, Tissot-Dupont H, Lennox JL, Boparai N, Isaacs R. Safety and efficacy of posaconazole in the long-term treatment of azole-refractory oropharyngeal and esophageal candidiasis in patients with HIV infection. HIV Clin Trials. 2007;8:86–97.
213. Maenza JR, Keruly JC, Moore RD, Chaisson RE, Merz WG, Gallant JE. Risk factors for fluconazole-resistant candidiasis in human immunodeficiency virus-infected patients. J Infect Dis. 1996;173:219–25.
214. Maenza JR, Merz WG, Romagnoli MJ, Keruly JC, Moore RD, Gallant JE. Infection due to fluconazole-resistant *Candida* in patients with AIDS: prevalence and microbiology. Clin Infect Dis. 1997;24:28–34.
215. Ally R, Schurmann D, Kreisel W, et al. A randomized, double-blind, double-dummy, multicenter trial of voriconazole and fluconazole in the treatment of esophageal candidiasis in immunocompromised patients. Clin Infect Dis. 2001;33:1447–54.
216. Villanueva A, Arathoon EG, Gotuzzo E, Berman RS, DiNubile MJ, Sable CA. A randomized double-blind study of caspofungin versus amphotericin for the treatment of candidal esophagitis. Clin Infect Dis. 2001;33:1529–35.
217. Krause DS, Simjee AE, van Rensburg C, et al. A randomized, double-blind trial of anidulafungin versus fluconazole for the treatment of esophageal candidiasis. Clin Infect Dis. 2004;39:770–5.
218. de Wet NT, Bester AJ, Viljoen JJ, et al. A randomized, double blind, comparative trial of micafungin (FK463) vs. fluconazole for the treatment of oesophageal candidiasis. Aliment Pharmacol Ther. 2005;21:899–907.
219. Medoff G, Dismukes WE, Meade 3rd RH, Moses JM. A new therapeutic approach to *Candida* infections. A preliminary report. Arch Intern Med. 1972;130:241–5.
220. Koletar SL, Weed HG, Raimundo MB. Thrush unresponsive to treatment with fluconazole in HIV-infected patients. In: First National Conference on Human Retroviruses; 1994; Washington, DC; 1994.
221. Cameron ML, Schell WA, Bruch S, Bartlett JA, Waskin HA, Perfect JR. Correlation of in vitro fluconazole resistance of *Candida* isolates in relation to therapy and symptoms of individuals seropositive for human immunodeficiency virus type 1. Antimicrob Agents Chemother. 1993;37:2449–53.
222. Quereda C, Polanco AM, Giner C, et al. Correlation between in vitro resistance to fluconazole and clinical outcome of oropharyngeal candidiasis in HIV-infected patients. Eur J Clin Microbiol Infect Dis. 1996;15:30–7.
223. Martins MD, Rex JH. Fluconazole suspension for oropharyngeal candidiasis unresponsive to tablets. Ann Intern Med. 1997;126:332–3.
224. Eichel M, Just-Nubling G, Helm EB, Stille W. Itraconazole suspension in the treatment of HIV-infected patients with fluconazole-resistant oropharyngeal candidiasis and esophagitis. Mycoses. 1996;39 Suppl 1:102–6.
225. Cartledge JD, Midgley J, Gazzard BG. Itraconazole cyclodextrin solution: the role of in vitro susceptibility testing in predicting successful treatment of HIV-related fluconazole-resistant and fluconazole-susceptible oral candidosis. AIDS. 1997;11:163–8.
226. Nguyen MT, Weiss PJ, LaBarre RC, Miller LK, Oldfield EC, Wallace MR. Orally administered amphotericin B in the treatment of oral candidiasis in HIV-infected patients caused by azole-resistant *Candida albicans*. AIDS. 1996;10:1745–7.
227. Ruhnke M, Schmidt-Westhausen A, Trautmann M. In vitro activities of voriconazole (UK-109, 496) against fluconazole-susceptible and -resistant *Candida albicans* isolates from oral cavities of patients with human immunodeficiency virus infection. Antimicrob Agents Chemother. 1997;41:575–7.
228. Vazquez JA, Schranz JA, Clark K, Goldstein BP, Reboli A, Fichtenbaum C. A phase 2, open-label study of the safety and efficacy

of intravenous anidulafungin as a treatment for azole-refractory mucosal candidiasis. J Acquir Immune Defic Syndr. 2008;48:304–9.
229. Brajtburg J, Powderly WG, Kobayashi GS, Medoff G. Amphotericin B: delivery systems. Antimicrob Agents Chemother. 1990;34:381–4.
230. Zingman BS. Resolution of refractory AIDS-related mucosal candidiasis after initiation of didanosine plus saquinavir. N Engl J Med. 1996;334:1674–5.
231. Swindells S. Pilot study of adjunctive GM-CSF (yeast derived) for fluconazole-resistant oral candidiasis in HIV-infection. Infect Dis Clin Pract. 1997;6:278–9.
232. Powderly WG, Finkelstein D, Feinberg J, et al. A randomized trial comparing fluconazole with clotrimazole troches for the prevention of fungal infections in patients with advanced human immunodeficiency virus infection. NIAID AIDS Clinical Trials Group. N Engl J Med. 1995;332:700–5.
233. Schuman P, Capps L, Peng G, et al. Weekly fluconazole for the prevention of mucosal candidiasis in women with HIV infection. A randomized, double-blind, placebo-controlled trial. Terry Beirn Community Programs for Clinical Research on AIDS. Ann Intern Med. 1997;126:689–96.
234. Philpott-Howard JN, Wade JJ, Mufti GJ, Brammer KW, Ehninger G. Randomized comparison of oral fluconazole versus oral polyenes for the prevention of fungal infection in patients at risk of neutropenia. Multicentre Study Group. J Antimicrob Chemother. 1993;31:973–84.
235. Goldman M, Cloud GA, Wade KD, et al. A randomized study of the use of fluconazole in continuous versus episodic therapy in patients with advanced HIV infection and a history of oropharyngeal candidiasis: AIDS Clinical Trials Group Study 323/Mycoses Study Group Study 40. Clin Infect Dis. 2005;41:1473–80.
236. Sobel JD, Brooker D, Stein GE, et al. Single oral dose fluconazole compared with conventional clotrimazole topical therapy of *Candida* vaginitis. Fluconazole Vaginitis Study Group. Am J Obstet Gynecol. 1995;172:1263–8.
237. Nurbhai M, Grimshaw J, Watson M, Bond C, Mollison J, Ludbrook A. Oral versus intra-vaginal imidazole and triazole anti-fungal treatment of uncomplicated vulvovaginal candidiasis (thrush). Cochrane Database Syst Rev 2007:CD002845.
238. Sobel JD, Faro S, Force RW, et al. Vulvovaginal candidiasis: epidemiologic, diagnostic, and therapeutic considerations. Am J Obstet Gynecol. 1998;178:203–11.
239. Sobel JD, Kapernick PS, Zervos M, et al. Treatment of complicated *Candida* vaginitis: comparison of single and sequential doses of fluconazole. Am J Obstet Gynecol. 2001;185:363–9.
240. Sobel JD, Chaim W, Nagappan V, Leaman D. Treatment of vaginitis caused by *Candida glabrata*: use of topical boric acid and flucytosine. Am J Obstet Gynecol. 2003;189:1297–300.
241. Schuman P, Sobel JD, Ohmit SE, et al. Mucosal candidal colonization and candidiasis in women with or at risk for human immunodeficiency virus infection. HIV Epidemiology Research Study (HERS) Group. Clin Infect Dis. 1998;27:1161–7.
242. Rhoads JL, Wright DC, Redfield RR, Burke DS. Chronic vaginal candidiasis in women with human immunodeficiency virus infection. JAMA. 1987;257:3105–7.
243. Duerr A, Sierra MF, Feldman J, Clarke LM, Ehrlich I, DeHovitz J. Immune compromise and prevalence of *Candida* vulvovaginitis in human immunodeficiency virus-infected women. Obstet Gynecol. 1997;90:252–6.
244. Sobel JD, Ohmit SE, Schuman P, et al. The evolution of *Candida* species and fluconazole susceptibility among oral and vaginal isolates recovered from human immunodeficiency virus (HIV)-seropositive and at-risk HIV-seronegative women. J Infect Dis. 2001;183:286–93.
245. White MH. Is vulvovaginal candidiasis an AIDS-related illness? Clin Infect Dis. 1996;22 Suppl 2:S124–7.
246. Sobel JD, Wiesenfeld HC, Martens M, et al. Maintenance fluconazole therapy for recurrent vulvovaginal candidiasis. N Engl J Med. 2004;351:876–83.
247. Rex JH, Walsh TJ, Sobel JD, et al. Practice guidelines for the treatment of candidiasis. Infectious Diseases Society of America. Clin Infect Dis. 2000;30:662–78.
248. Hay RJ, Clayton YM. Fluconazole in the management of patients with chronic mucocutaneous candidosis. Br J Dermatol. 1988;119:683–4.
249. Burke WA. Use of itraconazole in a patient with chronic mucocutaneous candidiasis. J Am Acad Dermatol. 1989;21:1309–10.
250. Aiuti F, Businco L, Gatti RA. Reconstitution of T-cell disorders following thymus transplantation. Birth Defects Orig Artic Ser. 1975;11:370–6.
251. Kirkpatrick CH, Rich RR, Graw Jr RG, Smith TK, Mickenberg I, Rogentine GN. Treatment of chronic mucocutaneous moniliasis by immunologic reconstitution. Clin Exp Immunol. 1971;9:733–48.
252. Hoh MC, Lin HP, Chan LL, Lam SK. Successful allogeneic bone marrow transplantation in severe chronic mucocutaneous candidiasis syndrome. Bone Marrow Transplant. 1996;18:797–800.
253. Morrell M, Fraser VJ, Kollef MH. Delaying the empiric treatment of candida bloodstream infection until positive blood culture results are obtained: a potential risk factor for hospital mortality. Antimicrob Agents Chemother. 2005;49:3640–5.
254. Garey KW, Rege M, Pai MP, et al. Time to initiation of fluconazole therapy impacts mortality in patients with candidemia: a multi-institutional study. Clin Infect Dis. 2006;43:25–31.
255. Rex JH, Bennett JE, Sugar AM, et al. A randomized trial comparing fluconazole with amphotericin B for the treatment of candidemia in patients without neutropenia. Candidemia Study Group and the National Institute. N Engl J Med. 1994;331:1325–30.
256. Nguyen MH, Peacock Jr JE, Tanner DC, et al. Therapeutic approaches in patients with candidemia. Evaluation in a multicenter, prospective, observational study. Arch Intern Med. 1995;155:2429–35.
257. Luzzati R, Amalfitano G, Lazzarini L, et al. Nosocomial candidemia in non-neutropenic patients at an Italian tertiary care hospital. Eur J Clin Microbiol Infect Dis. 2000;19:602–7.
258. Klein JJ, Watanakunakorn C. Hospital-acquired fungemia. Its natural course and clinical significance. Am J Med. 1979; 67:51–8.
259. Edwards Jr JE, Bodey GP, Bowden RA, et al. International conference for the development of a consensus on the management and prevention of severe candidal infections. Clin Infect Dis. 1997;25:43–59.
260. Meunier F. Management of candidemia. N Engl J Med. 1994;331:1371–2.
261. Phillips P, Shafran S, Garber G, et al. Multicenter randomized trial of fluconazole versus amphotericin B for treatment of candidemia in non-neutropenic patients. Canadian Candidemia Study Group. Eur J Clin Microbiol Infect Dis. 1997;16:337–45.
262. Anaissie EJ, Vartivarian SE, Abi-Said D, et al. Fluconazole versus amphotericin B in the treatment of hematogenous candidiasis: a matched cohort study. Am J Med. 1996;101:170–6.
263. Rex JH, Pappas PG, Karchmer AW, et al. A randomized and blinded multicenter trial of high-dose fluconazole plus placebo versus fluconazole plus amphotericin B as therapy for candidemia and its consequences in nonneutropenic subjects. Clin Infect Dis. 2003;36:1221–8.
264. Reboli AC, Rotstein C, Pappas PG, et al. Anidulafungin versus fluconazole for invasive candidiasis. N Engl J Med. 2007; 356:2472–82.
265. Kullberg BJ, Sobel JD, Ruhnke M, et al. Voriconazole versus a regimen of amphotericin B followed by fluconazole for candidaemia in non-neutropenic patients: a randomised non-inferiority trial. Lancet. 2005;366:1435–42.

266. Kuse ER, Chetchotisakd P, da Cunha CA, et al. Micafungin versus liposomal amphotericin B for candidaemia and invasive candidosis: a phase III randomised double-blind trial. Lancet. 2007; 369:1519–27.
267. Mora-Duarte J, Betts R, Rotstein C, et al. Comparison of caspofungin and amphotericin B for invasive candidiasis. N Engl J Med. 2002;347:2020–9.
268. Bennett JE. Echinocandins for candidemia in adults without neutropenia. N Engl J Med. 2006;355:1154–9.
269. Nucci M, Colombo AL. Risk factors for breakthrough candidemia. Eur J Clin Microbiol Infect Dis. 2002;21:209–11.
270. Goldman M, Pottage Jr JC, Weaver DC. *Candida krusei* fungemia. Report of 4 cases and review of the literature. Medicine (Baltimore). 1993;72:143–50.
271. Betts R, Glasmacher A, Maertens J, et al. Efficacy of caspofungin against invasive *Candida* or invasive *Aspergillus* infections in neutropenic patients. Cancer. 2006;106:466–73.
272. Blumberg EA, Reboli AC. Failure of systemic empirical treatment with amphotericin B to prevent candidemia in neutropenic patients with cancer. Clin Infect Dis. 1996;22:462–6.
273. Uzun O, Ascioglu S, Anaissie EJ, Rex JH. Risk factors and predictors of outcome in patients with cancer and breakthrough candidemia. Clin Infect Dis. 2001;32:1713–7.
274. Arnow PM, Kushner R. *Malassezia furfur* catheter infection cured with antibiotic lock therapy. Am J Med. 1991;90:128–30.
275. Viale P, Petrosillo N, Signorini L, Puoti M, Carosi G. Should lock therapy always be avoided for central venous catheter-associated fungal bloodstream infections? Clin Infect Dis. 2001;33:1947–8.
276. Haron E, Feld R, Tuffnell P, Patterson B, Hasselback R, Matlow A. Hepatic candidiasis: an increasing problem in immunocompromised patients. Am J Med. 1987;83:17–26.
277. Kontoyiannis DP, Luna MA, Samuels BI, Bodey GP. Hepatosplenic candidiasis. A manifestation of chronic disseminated candidiasis. Infect Dis Clin North Am. 2000;14:721–39.
278. Anaissie E, Bodey GP, Kantarjian H, et al. Fluconazole therapy for chronic disseminated candidiasis in patients with leukemia and prior amphotericin B therapy. Am J Med. 1991;91:142–50.
279. Kauffman CA, Bradley SF, Ross SC, Weber DR. Hepatosplenic candidiasis: successful treatment with fluconazole. Am J Med. 1991;91:137–41.
280. Walsh TJ, Whitcomb PO, Revankar SG, Pizzo PA. Successful treatment of hepatosplenic candidiasis through repeated cycles of chemotherapy and neutropenia. Cancer. 1995;76:2357–62.
281. Sora F, Chiusolo P, Piccirillo N, et al. Successful treatment with caspofungin of hepatosplenic candidiasis resistant to liposomal amphotericin B. Clin Infect Dis. 2002;35:1135–6.
282. Hubel K, Chemnitz J, Brochhagen HG, Cornely OA. Successful treatment of chronic disseminated candidiasis with caspofungin and itraconazole in a patient with progressive acute leukemia and prolonged neutropenia. Int J Hematol. 2004;79:289–92.
283. Legrand F, Lecuit M, Dupont B, et al. Adjuvant corticosteroid therapy for chronic disseminated candidiasis. Clin Infect Dis. 2008;46:696–702.
284. Benjamin Jr DK, Stoll BJ, Fanaroff AA, et al. Neonatal candidiasis among extremely low birth weight infants: risk factors, mortality rates, and neurodevelopmental outcomes at 18 to 22 months. Pediatrics. 2006;117:84–92.
285. Baley JE, Meyers C, Kliegman RM, Jacobs MR, Blumer JL. Pharmacokinetics, outcome of treatment, and toxic effects of amphotericin B and 5-fluorocytosine in neonates. J Pediatr. 1990;116:791–7.
286. Viscoli C, Castagnola E, Fioredda F, Ciravegna B, Barigione G, Terragna A. Fluconazole in the treatment of candidiasis in immunocompromised children. Antimicrob Agents Chemother. 1991;35:365–7.
287. Driessen M, Ellis JB, Cooper PA, et al. Fluconazole vs. amphotericin B for the treatment of neonatal fungal septicemia: a prospective randomized trial. Pediatr Infect Dis J. 1996;15:1107–12.
288. Wainer S, Cooper PA, Gouws H, Akierman A. Prospective study of fluconazole therapy in systemic neonatal fungal infection. Pediatr Infect Dis J. 1997;16:763–7.
289. Huang YC, Lin TY, Lien RI, et al. Candidaemia in special care nurseries: comparison of albicans and parapsilosis infection. J Infect. 2000;40:171–5.
290. Ang BS, Telenti A, King B, Steckelberg JM, Wilson WR. Candidemia from a urinary tract source: microbiological aspects and clinical significance. Clin Infect Dis. 1993;17:662–6.
291. Coullioud D, Van der Auwera P, Viot M, Lasset C. Prospective multicentric study of the etiology of 1051 bacteremic episodes in 782 cancer patients. CEMIC (French-Belgian Study Club of Infectious Diseases in Cancer). Support Care Cancer. 1993;1:34–46.
292. Simpson C, Blitz S, Shafran SD. The effect of current management on morbidity and mortality in hospitalised adults with funguria. J Infect. 2004;49:248–52.
293. Fan-Havard P, O'Donovan C, Smith SM, Oh J, Bamberger M, Eng RH. Oral fluconazole versus amphotericin B bladder irrigation for treatment of candidal funguria. Clin Infect Dis. 1995;21:960–5.
294. Sanford JP. The enigma of candiduria: evolution of bladder irrigation with amphotericin B for management–from Anecdote to Dogma and a lesson from Machiavelli. Clin Infect Dis. 1993;16:145–7.
295. Leu HS, Huang CT. Clearance of funguria with short-course antifungal regimens: a prospective, randomized, controlled study. Clin Infect Dis. 1995;20:1152–7.
296. Wong-Beringer A, Jacobs RA, Guglielmo BJ. Treatment of funguria. JAMA. 1992;267:2780–5.
297. Albano L, Bretagne S, Mamzer-Bruneel MF, et al. Evidence that graft-site candidiasis after kidney transplantation is acquired during organ recovery: a multicenter study in France. Clin Infect Dis. 2009;48:194–202.
298. Shah CP, McKey J, Spirn MJ, Maguire J. Ocular candidiasis: a review. Br J Ophthalmol. 2008;92:466–8.
299. Martinez-Vazquez C, Fernandez-Ulloa J, Bordon J, et al. *Candida albicans* endophthalmitis in brown heroin addicts: response to early vitrectomy preceded and followed by antifungal therapy. Clin Infect Dis. 1998;27:1130–3.
300. Results of the Endophthalmitis Vitrectomy Study. A randomized trial of immediate vitrectomy and of intravenous antibiotics for the treatment of postoperative bacterial endophthalmitis Endophthalmitis Vitrectomy Study Group. Arch Ophthalmol 1995;113:1479–96.
301. Stern GA, Fetkenhour CL, O'Grady RB. Intravitreal amphotericin B treatment of *Candida* endophthamitis. Arch Ophthalmol. 1977;95:89–93.
302. Perraut Jr LE, Perraut LE, Bleiman B, Lyons J. Successful treatment of *Candida albicans* endophthalmitis with intravitreal amphotericin B. Arch Ophthalmol. 1981;99:1565–7.
303. Brod RD, Flynn Jr HW, Clarkson JG, Pflugfelder SC, Culbertson WW, Miller D. Endogenous *Candida* endophthalmitis. Management without intravenous amphotericin B. Ophthalmology. 1990;97:666–72. disc: 72–4.
304. Savani DV, Perfect JR, Cobo LM, Durack DT. Penetration of new azole compounds into the eye and efficacy in experimental *Candida* endophthalmitis. Antimicrob Agents Chemother. 1987;31:6–10.
305. O'Day DM, Foulds G, Williams TE, Robinson RD, Allen RH, Head WS. Ocular uptake of fluconazole following oral administration. Arch Ophthalmol. 1990;108:1006–8.
306. Urbak SF, Degn T. Fluconazole in the treatment of *Candida albicans* endophthalmitis. Acta Ophthalmol (Copenh). 1992;70:528–9.

307. Akler ME, Vellend H, McNeely DM, Walmsley SL, Gold WL. Use of fluconazole in the treatment of candidal endophthalmitis. Clin Infect Dis. 1995;20:657–64.
308. Kauffman CA, Bradley SF, Vine AK. *Candida* endophthalmitis associated with intraocular lens implantation: efficacy of fluconazole therapy. Mycoses. 1993;36:13–7.
309. Zenker PN, Rosenberg EM, Van Dyke RB, Rabalais GP, Daum RS. Successful medical treatment of presumed *Candida* endocarditis in critically ill infants. J Pediatr. 1991;119:472–7.
310. Faix RG. Nonsurgical treatment of *Candida* endocarditis. J Pediatr. 1992;120:665–6.
311. Melamed R, Leibovitz E, Abramson O, Levitas A, Zucker N, Gorodisher R. Successful non-surgical treatment of *Candida tropicalis* endocarditis with liposomal amphotericin-B (AmBisome). Scand J Infect Dis. 2000;32:86–9.
312. Aaron L, Therby A, Viard JP, Lahoulou R, Dupont B. Successful medical treatment of *Candida albicans* in mechanical prosthetic valve endocarditis. Scand J Infect Dis. 2003;35:351–2.
313. Utley JR, Mills J, Roe BB. The role of valve replacement in the treatment of fungal endocarditis. J Thorac Cardiovasc Surg. 1975;69:255–8.
314. Nguyen MH, Nguyen ML, Yu VL, McMahon D, Keys TF, Amidi M. *Candida* prosthetic valve endocarditis: prospective study of six cases and review of the literature. Clin Infect Dis. 1996;22:262–7.
315. Muehrcke DD. Fungal prosthetic valve endocarditis. Semin Thorac Cardiovasc Surg. 1995;7:20–4.
316. Muehrcke DD, Lytle BW, Cosgrove 3rd DM. Surgical and long-term antifungal therapy for fungal prosthetic valve endocarditis. Ann Thorac Surg. 1995;60:538–43.
317. Jimenez-Exposito MJ, Torres G, Baraldes A, et al. Native valve endocarditis due to *Candida glabrata* treated without valvular replacement: a potential role for caspofungin in the induction and maintenance treatment. Clin Infect Dis. 2004;39:e70–3.
318. Rajendram R, Alp NJ, Mitchell AR, Bowler IC, Forfar JC. *Candida* prosthetic valve endocarditis cured by caspofungin therapy without valve replacement. Clin Infect Dis. 2005;40:e72–4.
319. Moudgal V, Little T, Boikov D, Vazquez JA. Multiechinocandin- and multiazole-resistant *Candida parapsilosis* isolates serially obtained during therapy for prosthetic valve endocarditis. Antimicrob Agents Chemother. 2005;49:767–9.
320. Cancelas JA, Lopez J, Cabezudo E, et al. Native valve endocarditis due to *Candida parapsilosis*: a late complication after bone marrow transplantation-related fungemia. Bone Marrow Transplant. 1994;13:333–4.
321. Mayayo E, Moralejo J, Camps J, Guarro J. Fungal endocarditis in premature infants: case report and review. Clin Infect Dis. 1996;22:366–8.
322. Johnston PG, Lee J, Domanski M, et al. Late recurrent *Candida* endocarditis. Chest. 1991;99:1531–3.
323. Roupie E, Darmon JY, Brochard L, Saada M, Rekik N, Brun-Buisson C. Fluconazole therapy of candidal native valve endocarditis. Eur J Clin Microbiol Infect Dis. 1991;10:458–9.
324. Hernandez JA, Gonzalez-Moreno M, Llibre JM, Aloy A, Casan CM. Candidal mitral endocarditis and long-term treatment with fluconazole in a patient with human immunodeficiency virus infection. Clin Infect Dis. 1992;15:1062–3.
325. Castiglia M, Smego Jr RA, Sames EL. *Candida* endocarditis and amphotericin B intolerance: Potential role for fluconazole. Infect Dis Clin Pract. 1994;3:248–53.
326. Baddley JW, Benjamin Jr DK, Patel M, et al. *Candida* infective endocarditis. Eur J Clin Microbiol Infect Dis. 2008;27:519–29.
327. Steinbach WJ. Antifungal agents in children. Pediatr Clin North Am. 2005;52:895–915.
328. Rabinovici R, Szewczyk D, Ovadia P, Greenspan JR, Sivalingam JJ. *Candida* pericarditis: clinical profile and treatment. Ann Thorac Surg. 1997;63:1200–4.
329. Torres-Rojas JR, Stratton CW, Sanders CV, et al. Candidal suppurative peripheral thrombophlebitis. Ann Intern Med. 1982;96:431–5.
330. Jarrett F, Maki DG, Chan CK. Management of septic thrombosis of the inferior vena cava caused by *Candida*. Arch Surg. 1978;113:637–9.
331. Strinden WD, Helgerson RB, Maki DG. *Candida* septic thrombosis of the great central veins associated with central catheters. Clinical features and management. Ann Surg. 1985;202:653–8.
332. Montenegro J, Aguirre R, Gonzalez O, Martinez I, Saracho R. Fluconazole treatment of candida peritonitis with delayed removal of the peritoneal dialysis catheter. Clin Nephrol. 1995;44:60–3.
333. Michel C, Courdavault L, al Khayat R, Viron B, Roux P, Mignon F. Fungal peritonitis in patients on peritoneal dialysis. Am J Nephrol. 1994;14:113–20.
334. Bayer AS, Blumenkrantz MJ, Montgomerie JZ, Galpin JE, Coburn JW, Guze LB. *Candida* peritonitis. Report of 22 cases and review of the English literature. Am J Med. 1976;61:832–40.
335. Sugar AM. Antifungal therapy in CAPD peritonitis-do we have a choice? Semin Dial. 1991;4:145–6.
336. Arfania D, Everett ED, Nolph KD, Rubin J. Uncommon causes of peritonitis in patients undergoing peritoneal dialysis. Arch Intern Med. 1981;141:61–4.
337. Levine J, Bernard DB, Idelson BA, Farnham H, Saunders C, Sugar AM. Fungal peritonitis complicating continuous ambulatory peritoneal dialysis: successful treatment with fluconazole, a new orally active antifungal agent. Am J Med. 1989;86:825–7.
338. Corbella X, Sirvent JM, Carratala J. Fluconazole treatment without catheter removal in *Candida albicans* peritonitis complicating peritoneal dialysis. Am J Med. 1991;90:277.
339. Eisenberg ES. Intraperitoneal flucytosine in the management of fungal peritonitis in patients on continuous ambulatory peritoneal dialysis. Am J Kidney Dis. 1988;11:465–7.
340. Solomkin JS, Simmons RL. *Candida* infection in surgical patients. World J Surg. 1980;4:381–94.
341. Solomkin JS, Flohr AB, Quie PG, Simmons RL. The role of *Candida* in intraperitoneal infections. Surgery. 1980;88:524–30.
342. Alden SM, Frank E, Flancbaum L. Abdominal candidiasis in surgical patients. Am Surg. 1989;55:45–9.
343. Rantala A, Lehtonen OP, Kuttila K, Havia T, Niinikoski J. Diagnostic factors for postoperative candidosis in abdominal surgery. Ann Chir Gynaecol. 1991;80:323–8.
344. Aguado JM, Hidalgo M, Ridriguez-Tudela JL. Successful treatment of candida peritonitis with fluconazole. J Antimicrob Chemother. 1994;34:847.
345. Adamson PC, Rinaldi MG, Pizzo PA, Walsh TJ. Amphotericin B in the treatment of *Candida* cholecystitis. Pediatr Infect Dis J. 1989;8:408–11.
346. Hoerauf A, Hammer S, Muller-Myhsok B, Rupprecht H. Intra-abdominal *Candida* infection during acute necrotizing pancreatitis has a high prevalence and is associated with increased mortality. Crit Care Med. 1998;26:2010–5.
347. Grewe M, Tsiotos GG, Luque de-Leon E. Sarr MG. Fungal infection in acute necrotizing pancreatitis. J Am Coll Surg. 1999;188:408–14.
348. Gathe Jr JC, Harris RL, Garland B, Bradshaw MW, Williams Jr TW. *Candida* osteomyelitis. Report of five cases and review of the literature. Am J Med. 1987;82:927–37.
349. Ferra C, Doebbeling BN, Hollis RJ, Pfaller MA, Lee CK, Gingrich RD. *Candida tropicalis* vertebral osteomyelitis: a late sequela of fungemia. Clin Infect Dis. 1994;19:697–703.
350. Almekinders LC, Greene WB. Vertebral *Candida* infections. A case report and review of the literature. Clin Orthop Relat Res 1991:174–8.
351. Marra F, Robbins GM, Masri BA, et al. Amphotericin B-loaded bone cement to treat osteomyelitis caused by *Candida albicans*. Can J Surg. 2001;44:383–6.

352. Sugar AM, Saunders C, Diamond RD. Successful treatment of *Candida* osteomyelitis with fluconazole. A noncomparative study of two patients. Diagn Microbiol Infect Dis. 1990;13:517–20.
353. Bannatyne RM, Clarke HM. Ketoconazole in the treatment of osteomyelitis due to *Candida albicans*. Can J Surg. 1989;32:201–2.
354. Hennequin C, Bouree P, Hiesse C, Dupont B, Charpentier B. Spondylodiskitis due to *Candida albicans*: report of two patients who were successfully treated with fluconazole and review of the literature. Clin Infect Dis. 1996;23:176–8.
355. Dan M, Priel I. Failure of fluconazole therapy for sternal osteomyelitis due to *Candida albicans*. Clin Infect Dis. 1994;18:126–7.
356. Arranz-Caso JA, Lopez-Pizarro VM, Gomez-Herruz P, Garcia-Altozano J, Martinez-Martinez J. *Candida albicans* osteomyelitis of the zygomatic bone. A distinctive case with a possible peculiar mechanism of infection and therapeutic failure with fluconazole. Diagn Microbiol Infect Dis. 1996;24:161–4.
357. Tunkel AR, Thomas CY, Wispelwey B. *Candida* prosthetic arthritis: report of a case treated with fluconazole and review of the literature. Am J Med. 1993;94:100–3.
358. Merrer J, Dupont B, Nieszkowska A, De Jonghe B, Outin H. *Candida albicans* prosthetic arthritis treated with fluconazole alone. J Infect. 2001;42:208–9.
359. Bayer AS, Guze LB. Fungal arthritis. I. *Candida* arthritis: diagnostic and prognostic implications and therapeutic considerations. Semin Arthritis Rheum. 1978;8:142–50.
360. Katzenstein D. Isolated *Candida* arthritis: report of a case and definition of a distinct clinical syndrome. Arthritis Rheum. 1985;28:1421–4.
361. Weers-Pothoff G, Havermans JF, Kamphuis J, Sinnige HA, Meis JF. *Candida tropicalis* arthritis in a patient with acute myeloid leukemia successfully treated with fluconazole: case report and review of the literature. Infection. 1997;25:109–11.
362. Smego Jr RA, Perfect JR, Durack DT. Combined therapy with amphotericin B and 5-fluorocytosine for *Candida* meningitis. Rev Infect Dis. 1984;6:791–801.
363. Buchs S, Pfister P. *Candida* meningitis. Course, prognosis and mortality before and after introduction of the new antimycotics. Mykosen. 1983;26:73–81.
364. Marr B, Gross S, Cunningham C, Weiner L. Candidal sepsis and meningitis in a very-low-birth-weight infant successfully treated with fluconazole and flucytosine. Clin Infect Dis. 1994;19:795–6.
365. Gurses N, Kalayci AG. Fluconazole monotherapy for candidal meningitis in a premature infant. Clin Infect Dis. 1996;23:645–6.
366. Chiou CC, Wong TT, Lin HH, et al. Fungal infection of ventriculoperitoneal shunts in children. Clin Infect Dis. 1994;19:1049–53.
367. Cruciani M, Di Perri G, Molesini M, Vento S, Concia E, Bassetti D. Use of fluconazole in the treatment of *Candida albicans* hydrocephalus shunt infection. Eur J Clin Microbiol Infect Dis. 1992;11:957.
368. Black JT. Cerebral candidiasis: case report of brain abscess secondary to *Candida albicans*, and review of literature. J Neurol Neurosurg Psychiatry. 1970;33:864–70.
369. Bonomo RA, Strauss M, Blinkhorn R, Salata RA. *Torulopsis* (*Candida*) *glabrata*: a new pathogen found in spinal epidural abscess. Clin Infect Dis. 1996;22:588–9.
370. Lutsar I, Roffey S, Troke P. Voriconazole concentrations in the cerebrospinal fluid and brain tissue of guinea pigs and immunocompromised patients. Clin Infect Dis. 2003;37:728–32.
371. Liu KH, Wu CJ, Chou CH, et al. Refractory candidal meningitis in an immunocompromised patient cured by caspofungin. J Clin Microbiol. 2004;42:5950–3.
372. Hope WW, Mickiene D, Petraitis V, et al. The pharmacokinetics and pharmacodynamics of micafungin in experimental hematogenous *Candida* meningoencephalitis: implications for echinocandin therapy in neonates. J Infect Dis. 2008;197:163–71.
373. Rangel-Frausto MS, Wiblin T, Blumberg HM, et al. National epidemiology of mycoses survey (NEMIS): variations in rates of bloodstream infections due to *Candida* species in seven surgical intensive care units and six neonatal intensive care units. Clin Infect Dis. 1999;29:253–8.
374. Garbino T, Lew D, Romand JA. Fluconazole prevents severe *Candida* spp. infections in high risk critically ill patients. In: Paper presented at the American Society Microbiology. Washington, DC; 1997.
375. Rocco TR, Simms HH. Inadequate proof of adverse outcome due to the use of fluconazole in critically ill patients. Arch Surg. 2000;135:1114.
376. Gleason TG, May AK, Caparelli D, Farr BM, Sawyer RG. Emerging evidence of selection of fluconazole-tolerant fungi in surgical intensive care units. Arch Surg. 1997;132:1197–201. discussion 202.
377. Savino JA, Agarwal N, Wry P, Policastro A, Cerabona T, Austria L. Routine prophylactic antifungal agents (clotrimazole, ketoconazole, and nystatin) in nontransplant/nonburned critically ill surgical and trauma patients. J Trauma. 1994;36:20–5. discussion 5–6.
378. Ables AZ, Blumer NA, Valainis GT, Godenick MT, Kajdasz DK, Yuko Y. Fluconazole prophylaxis of severe candida infection in trauma and postsurgical patients: A prospective, double-blind, randomized, placebo-controlled trial. Infect Dis Clin Pract. 2000;9:169–75.
379. Schuster MG, Edwards Jr JE, Sobel JD, et al. Empirical fluconazole versus placebo for intensive care unit patients: a randomized trial. Ann Intern Med. 2008;149:83–90.
380. Pelz RK, Hendrix CW, Swoboda SM, et al. Double-blind placebo-controlled trial of fluconazole to prevent candidal infections in critically ill surgical patients. Ann Surg. 2001;233:542–8.
381. Piarroux R, Grenouillet F, Balvay P, et al. Assessment of preemptive treatment to prevent severe candidiasis in critically ill surgical patients. Crit Care Med. 2004;32:2443–9.
382. Kung N, Fisher N, Gunson B, Hastings M, Mutimer D. Fluconazole prophylaxis for high-risk liver transplant recipients. Lancet. 1995;345:1234–5.
383. Tollemar J, Hockerstedt K, Ericzon BG, Jalanko H, Ringden O. Liposomal amphotericin B prevents invasive fungal infections in liver transplant recipients. A randomized, placebo-controlled study. Transplantation. 1995;59:45–50.
384. Ostrosky-Zeichner L, Sable C, Sobel J, et al. Multicenter retrospective development and validation of a clinical prediction rule for nosocomial invasive candidiasis in the intensive care setting. Eur J Clin Microbiol Infect Dis. 2007;26:271–6.
385. Kaufman D, Boyle R, Hazen KC, Patrie JT, Robinson M, Donowitz LG. Fluconazole prophylaxis against fungal colonization and infection in preterm infants. N Engl J Med. 2001;345:1660–6.
386. Manzoni P, Stolfi I, Pugni L, et al. A multicenter, randomized trial of prophylactic fluconazole in preterm neonates. N Engl J Med. 2007;356:2483–95.

Cryptococcosis

John W. Baddley and William E. Dismukes

Cryptococcosis is a systemic mycosis caused by the encapsulated yeast *Cryptococcus neoformans*, an organism found in soil and often associated with pigeon droppings. Infection involves most frequently the lungs or central nervous system and, less frequently, the blood, skin, skeletal system, and prostate. Because the incidence of cryptococcosis is greatly increased in immunocompromised patients, especially among patients with AIDS or organ transplant recipients, cryptococcosis is considered an opportunistic fungal infection. Treatment of cryptococcosis is based on anatomic site of disease, severity of disease, and the underlying immune status of the patient. Cryptococcal meningitis is treated with induction therapy of amphotericin B with or without flucytosine, followed by a prolonged course of fluconazole. For pulmonary disease alone, fluconazole is effective therapy in most patients. Chronic maintenance therapy with fluconazole may be required in HIV-infected patients or transplant patients who remain immunosuppressed.

Organism

More than 40 species of the genus *Cryptococcus* have been described, but few are recognized as causing infection in humans [1]. The predominant pathogen is *C. neoformans*, but two other species, *C. albidus*, and *C. laurentii*, have been reported to rarely cause disease in humans [2–4]. *Cryptococcus neoformans* is a round or oval encapsulated yeast, measuring approximately 4–6 μm in diameter in clinical specimens, and having a capsule ranging in size from 1 to >30 μm. In specimens isolated from nature, organisms tend to be smaller and poorly encapsulated [5].

Cryptococcus neoformans is grouped into serotypes A, B, C, D, and AD hybrids based on antigenic determinates on the polysaccharide capsule, with serotype A most common. *Cryptococcus neoformans* var. *neoformans* has included serotypes A, D, and AD, and *C. neoformans* var. *gattii* included serotypes B and C. It has been proposed to further simplify the classification of *Cryptococcus* into pathogenic varieties: *C. neoformans* var. *grubii* and *C. neoformans* var. *neoformans*. *C. neoformans* var. *gattii* has been reclassified as *C. gattii*, a species distinct from *C. neoformans* [6]. The *C. neoformans* varieties differ somewhat in epidemiology, ecology, and certain biochemical properties. In contrast to *C. neoformans*, *C. gattii* uncommonly infects AIDS patients, is found primarily in tropical areas, and is able to assimilate malate. The epidemiology of *C. gattii* is evolving with its emergence in Vancouver, Canada and the Pacific Northwest United States since 1999 [7–9]. For a more detailed description of differences among pathogenic cryptococci , see these two comprehensive references [10, 11].

The sexual, or perfect, state of *C. neoformans*, *Filobasidiella neoformans*, a basidiomycete, can be demonstrated by mating the fungus under certain defined conditions [12]. In this perfect state, mycelia are produced which bear basidiospores 1–3 μm in size. The perfect state has not yet been demonstrated in patients or in nature, so the importance of inhalation of basidiospores in disease acquisition is unknown.

C. neoformans produces white to cream-colored, smooth, mucoid colonies when grown on solid culture media such as blood agar or Sabouraud's dextrose agar. The amount of mucoidness of the colonies is related to the thickness of the capsule. Growth of *Cryptococcus* usually occurs in 36–72 h and is typically slower than that of *Candida* or *Saccharomyces* species under the same conditions. *C. neoformans* grows at 37°C, whereas nonpathogenic species of *Cryptococcus* do not. A distinguishing feature of *C. neoformans* is the ability to produce melanin. On selective media supplemented with niger seed (birdseed agar), smooth brown colonies are formed after several days of incubation. Color reactions on solid media are also useful to distinguish between *C. neoformans* var. *neoformans* or *grubii* and *C. gattii*. For example, colonies of *C. gattii* on canavanine-glycine-bromthymol blue (CGB) agar turn the agar blue, while colonies of *C. neoformans* do not elicit a color change [13].

J.W. Baddley (✉)
Division of Infectious Diseases, Birmingham VA Medical Center, University of Alabama at Birmingham School of Medicine, Birmingham, AL, USA
e-mail: jbaddley@uab.edu

C.A. Kauffman et al. (eds.), *Essentials of Clinical Mycology*,
DOI 10.1007/978-1-4419-6640-7_12, © Springer Science+Business Media, LLC 2011

Epidemiology

C. neoformans is ubiquitous in the environment. The organism was isolated initially in nature from peach juice in 1894 by Francisco Sanefelice, and was first isolated from soil by Emmons in 1951 [14]. *C. neoformans* was isolated from pigeon excrement in 1955, and has since been isolated from multiple geographic sites worldwide, many of which are contaminated by pigeon or other bird excrement. Pigeon droppings are commonly colonized with *C. neoformans*, and may contain greater than 10^6 organisms per gram of fecal material. Pigeons do not appear to develop cryptococcal disease, perhaps due to the pigeon's high body temperature [15]. Although *C. neoformans* is isolated most frequently from pigeon excreta and soil, it has been isolated less commonly from other sources, including fruits and vegetables, decaying wood, dairy products, and excrement from a wide variety of avian species [16].

In contrast to the numerous geographic sites of isolation of *C. neoformans*, the isolation of *C. gattii* has been more restricted [14]. *C. gattii* has been isolated from leaves, wood, bark, and air associated with *Eucalyptus camaldulensis* (red river gum) and few other types of trees, but has not been isolated from bird droppings [16–18]. The distribution of *E. camaldulensis*, in tropical and subtropical regions such as Southern California, Australia, Southeast Asia, Central Africa, and Brazil, corresponds to areas where cases of cryptococcosis due to *C. gattii* are recognized as endemic [14, 19]; however, infections caused by *C. gattii* occur in areas without eucalyptus trees, suggesting an additional unidentified environmental source [20].

Because *C. neoformans* is isolated primarily from pigeon droppings and soil, the assumption has been made that infection arises via aerosolized particles from pigeon excrement. This hypothesis has been difficult to confirm, as most patients who develop cryptococcosis do not recall a history of recent exposure to pigeons or their excreta. Exposure to *C. neoformans*, on the basis of serum antibody levels or skin testing, is common among pigeon handlers; however, the incidence of active cryptococcal infections among this population does not appear to be increased [21, 22]. No particular occupational predisposition to cryptococcosis is currently recognized, although data from population-based surveillance suggest that outdoor occupations may be associated with an increased risk of cryptococcosis [23]. Association with pigeons, pigeon excrement, soil, or dust does not appear to increase the likelihood of proven cryptococcosis [23].

In the majority of cases, infection with *C. neoformans* is thought to be caused by inhalation of the organism, either in yeast form or perhaps as basidiospores, from an environmental source such as bird droppings or soil. Evidence for this mechanism of acquisition is supported by isolation of cryptococci measuring less than 4 μm, ideal for alveolar deposition, from aerosols associated with soil and pigeon excreta [5, 24]. Unlike other mycoses transmitted by aerosolized particles, outbreaks of cryptococcosis from a particular environmental source rarely, if ever, occur [14, 25]. Although lung infection can follow acute inhalation of *Cryptococcus* organisms, in most cases disease occurs as a reactivation of dormant infection.

C. neoformans has been isolated frequently from pulmonary and skin cultures of healthy, asymptomatic individuals, but this fungal organism is not regarded as normal microbial flora in animals or humans [26, 27]. Rarely, skin infection can occur after local inoculation, but in most cases, skin disease results from blood-borne dissemination after an initial lung focus of infection. Person-to-person transmission via inhalation of aerosols has not yet been documented, but in several cases, other sources of presumed human-to-human transmission have been described [28–31]. In one report, a recipient of a corneal transplant from a donor with cryptococcosis developed cryptococcal endophthalmitis more than 2 months after transplantation [28]. In a second case, a healthcare worker developed cryptococcal skin lesions at the site of an inoculation of blood from a patient with cryptococcemia [29]. A more recent case was described in which the recipient of a lung transplant developed cryptococcal left lower lobe pneumonia 2 days after transplantation [30]. Endotracheal cultures from postoperative day 2 were positive for *C. neoformans*, although donor lung cultures were positive only for *Rhodotorula* species; however, development of pulmonary cryptococcosis this early in the post-transplant period suggests transmission by the donor organ. Evidence supporting zoonotic transmission of *Cryptococcus* has been reported [32–34]. In one description, a clinical isolate from a renal transplant recipient with cryptococcal meningitis was indistinguishable on the basis of molecular genotyping from an isolate present in the feces of the patient's pet cockatoo [32].

Cryptococcosis occurs in many patients without a recognized immunologic defect, but the large majority of patients have a predisposing factor or underlying disease [5]. Evidence is convincing that patients with defects in T cell–mediated immunity are at increased risk of developing cryptococcal infection. Predisposing conditions include AIDS, systemic corticosteroids, organ transplantation, lymphoreticular malignancies, diabetes mellitus, pregnancy, and sarcoidosis independent of steroid use (Table 1) [10, 35–39]. With the advent of newer immunosuppressive therapies, especially TNF-α inhibitors and monoclonal antibodies such as alemtuzumab, cryptococcosis is emerging in other patient populations [40–43]. Prior to the AIDS epidemic, up to 50% of patients with cryptococcosis had no recognized T cell immune defect or dysfunction [44, 45]. In a recent observational study of 306 HIV-negative patients with cryptococcosis, 21% had no significant immune dysfunction or other

Table 1 Underlying diseases associated with cryptococcosis

HIV
Corticosteroids
Organ transplantation
Malignancy
CD4 T-cell lymphopenia
Connective tissue disease
Renal failure
Cirrhosis
Chronic lung disease
Immunosuppressive agents (monoclonal antibodies, TNF-α inhibitors)
Diabetes mellitus
Pregnancy
Sarcoidosis
Sytemic lupus erythematosus
Rheumatoid arthritis

predisposing condition to cryptococcosis [35]. In contrast, among patients with a predisposing condition, chronic organ disease and glucocorticosteroid use were most common [35]. Idiopathic CD4 lymphocytopenia has also been associated with cryptococcosis in patients with no other predisposing conditions for cryptococcosis [46, 47].

Before the era of highly active antiretroviral therapy (HAART), the prevalence of cryptococcosis among patients with AIDS was estimated to be between 5% and 10% [48, 49] Data from four United States geographic areas, prior to use of HAART, showed the annual incidence of cryptococcosis among patients with AIDS to range from 17 to 66 cases per 1,000 persons [23]. In contrast, among non-HIV-infected persons, the annual incidence ranged from 0.2 to 0.9 per 100,000 persons. In Europe, the prevalence of cryptococcosis among AIDS patients is lower than that in the United States [50, 51].

Although the widespread use of HAART has lowered the incidence of cryptococcosis cases in medically developed countries, the incidence and mortality rate of cryptococcosis are still extremely high in areas in which there is limited access to HAART and/or healthcare [50–55]. In Africa and other developing areas, the prevalence of cryptococcosis in patients with AIDS approaches 30% and is often an AIDS-defining illness [56]. A recent study estimated that the global burden of HIV-associated cryptococcosis approximates 1 million cases annually worldwide, resulting in more than 600,000 deaths per year by 3 months after infection [57].

Pathogenesis

Once *C. neoformans* is inhaled, transient colonization of the airways occurs before subsequent spread and establishment of respiratory infection. Given the widespread presence of *Cryptococcus* in the environment, exposure is likely common. However, the incidence of infection is very low, suggesting that most people mount an appropriate host response when exposed to the organism. *Cryptococcus*, after it enters the body of a susceptible host, can produce latent infection or acute disease. Development of disease appears to depend on inoculum of inhaled organisms, virulence of the organism, and interaction with the host's cellular immune response. As noted earlier, host defense, especially cell-mediated immunity, is fundamental to protection from cryptococcal infections and is important in containing infection and producing granulomatous inflammation [58].

After inhalation of the organism, the first line of defense is the alveolar macrophage, followed by recruitment of other inflammatory cells via chemokines and cytokines such as IL-12, IL-18, and monocyte chemotactic protein-1 [39]. In addition, complement-mediated phagocytosis appears to have an important role in initial defense [59]. In vitro, alveolar macrophages are able to bind and phagocytize *C. neoformans* in the presence of human serum containing opsonins such as C3 [60]. Macrophages from patients with HIV infection tend to be impaired or defective in both oxidative-dependent and oxidative-independent killing of *C. neoformans* [61].

If initial defense mechanisms in alveoli are ineffective, cryptococci reach the bloodstream and disseminate to other organs, such as the central nervous system (CNS) or prostate. In such sites, additional defense mechanisms are needed to thwart progressive infection. In vitro and in animal models, other cells, including neutrophils, natural-killer cells, macrophage-like microglial cells, and T cell lymphocytes can kill or inhibit growth of cryptococci [62]. Cytokines, especially interleukin-2 and interferon-γ, released by phagocytic cells and lymphocytes, also appear to play an important role in enhancing the killing of *C. neoformans* [10].

The role of humoral immunity in protection against cryptococcal infections is controversial, but increasing data indicate that this facet of the immune response may play an important role. Antibodies to capsular constituents facilitate clearance of cryptococcal antigen, enhancing antibody-dependent cell-mediated killing and increasing antifungal activity of leukocytes and natural killer cells [63, 64]. In addition, an anti-beta-glucan monoclonal antibody has been shown to inhibit growth and capsule formation of *C. neoformans* [65].

Among several factors of virulence and pathogenicity for *C. neoformans* and *C. gattii*, the best characterized include the polysaccharide capsule, thermotolerance (ability to grow at 37°C), melanin pigment production, mannitol production, and soluble extracellular constituents. Several in-depth reviews are recommended for more detailed information about factors of virulence, genetics, and pathogenicity [10, 66–68]. For a particular *C. neoformans* isolate, virulence is attributed to these different factors plus the interaction of the host's immune responses. Three of these factors will be discussed below.

The polysaccharide capsule of *C. neoformans* is composed of a backbone of α-1,3-D-mannopyranose units with single residues of β-D-xylopyranosyl and β-D-glucuronopyranosyl, and referred to as glucuronoxylomannan (GXM). The capsule appears to be the key virulence factor for *C. neoformans*; acapsular mutants are typically avirulent, whereas encapsulated isolates have varying degrees of virulence [69]. The capsule may sometimes protect the organism from host defenses. Phenotypic switching in *Cryptococcus* can occur in vivo during chronic infection, allowing for changes in the polysaccharide capsule and cell wall that affect the yeast's ability to resist phagocytosis [70]. Encapsulated *C. neoformans* cells are not phagocytized or killed by neutrophils, monocytes, or macrophages to the same degree as acapsular mutants [71]. In addition, highly encapsulated strains are less able to stimulate T-cell proliferation, and do not enhance the production of cytokines as well as poorly encapsulated or acapsular strains [72, 73].

Melanin production also appears to be an important virulence factor of *C. neoformans*, based on in vitro and animal in vivo systems. For example, the role of melanin was first demonstrated when naturally occurring *C. neoformans* mutants lacking melanin were found to be less virulent in mice than melanin-producing strains [74]. Melanin is deposited in the inner cell wall of *C. neoformans*, and may resist oxidation or reactive nitrogen intermediates produced by phagocytes [75].

Another virulence mechanism of *Cryptococcus* is its ability to survive within either alkaline or acidic environment of the phagolysosome of phagocytic cells, or bloodstream, thereby allowing it to survive and disseminate. Recent studies suggest glycosphingolipid glucosylceramide is essential for fungal growth in extracellular environments [76, 77].

Clinical Manifestations

Pulmonary Infection

Pulmonary cryptococcal involvement can manifest in a variety of ways, ranging from asymptomatic airway colonization or infection to fulminant respiratory failure with acute respiratory distress syndrome (ARDS) [78, 79]. Most patients are asymptomatic, or will have only mild-to-moderate symptoms such as dyspnea, cough, malaise, pleuritic chest pain, night sweats or, rarely, hemoptysis [80–82]. Constitutional symptoms, such as fever, night sweats, and weight loss are less common in HIV-negative patients unless extrapulmonary disease is also present [80].

In the immunologically normal host, a diagnosis of respiratory colonization with *Cryptococcus* can be made on the basis of a positive respiratory tract culture without evidence of pulmonary symptoms or abnormalities on chest radiography. Limited data suggest that patients with colonization often have underlying pulmonary pathology, such as chronic obstructive pulmonary disease [27]. The diagnosis of colonization, particularly in the immunocompromised patient, must be interpreted with caution. Because of the propensity of *Cryptococcus* for dissemination to the central nervous system (CNS), a thorough evaluation for extrapulmonary sites of cryptococcal involvement in the immunocompromised host is recommended [83].

The radiographic features of pulmonary cryptococcosis are varied and influenced by the degree of immunosuppression of the patient. Findings may reveal lobar, patchy infiltrates (Fig. 1); single or multiple nodular lesions (Fig. 2); interstitial infiltrates; mediastinal or hilar adenopathy

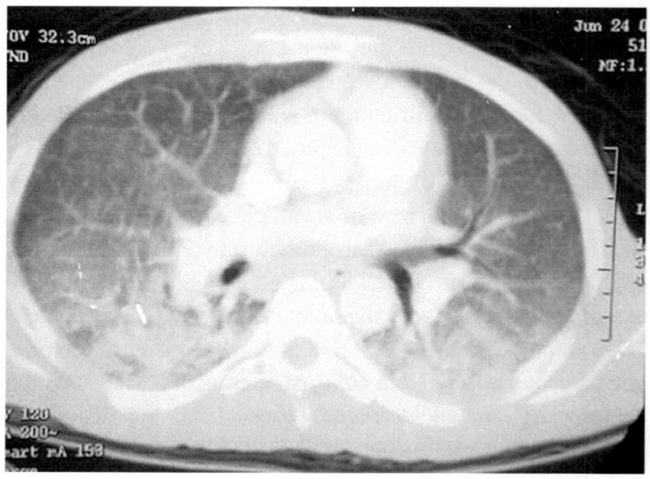

Fig. 1 CT showing severe bilateral cryptococcal lobar pneumonia and prominent adenopathy in an AIDS patient

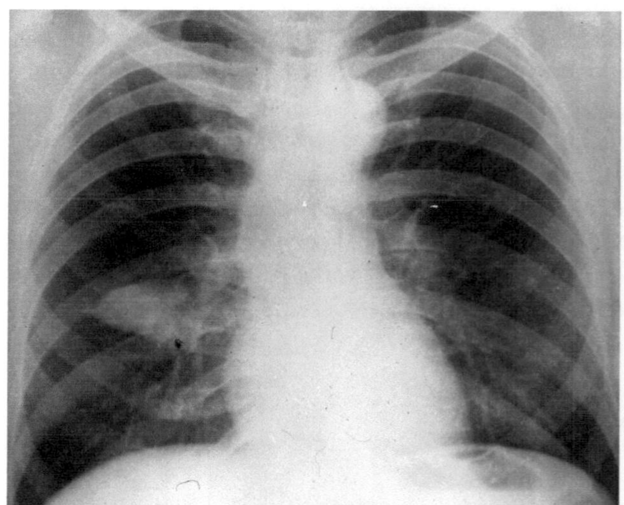

Fig. 2 Well-circumscribed small mass/nodule in patient with underlying systemic lupus erythematosus treated with corticosteroids

(Fig. 3); circumscribed mass lesions (0.5–7 cm) (Fig. 4); or less commonly, pleural effusions or cavitary lesions (Fig. 5) [80, 84]. Radiographically, *C. gattii* infection manifests as focal pulmonary disease and may be mistaken for malignancy [85, 86]. In HIV-negative patients, solitary or multiple pulmonary nodules may be seen in 60–80% of patients [80, 83, 87]. Focal or multifocal airspace consolidation is the next most common radiographic pattern among HIV-negative patients and is present in 10–30% of cases [80, 83, 88]. In contrast, in patients with AIDS, the most common radiographic abnormalities are diffuse, interstitial infiltrates, and lobar, often mass-like, infiltrates [89, 90]. Pulmonary nodules are less common, but are more likely to cavitate than nodules in patients without immune compromise.

Comparison of pulmonary cryptococcal infection in AIDS patients versus HIV-negative patients reveals other important distinctions. In AIDS patients, pulmonary disease plus other sites of involvement are more common. These patients may have a more rapid clinical course, often associated with increased mortality [90, 91]. The majority of AIDS patients with cryptococcal pneumonia have constitutional symptoms, in part explained by increased frequency of concomitant extrapulmonary sites of cryptococcal infection, for example, dissemination to the CNS [90]. The finding of pulmonary

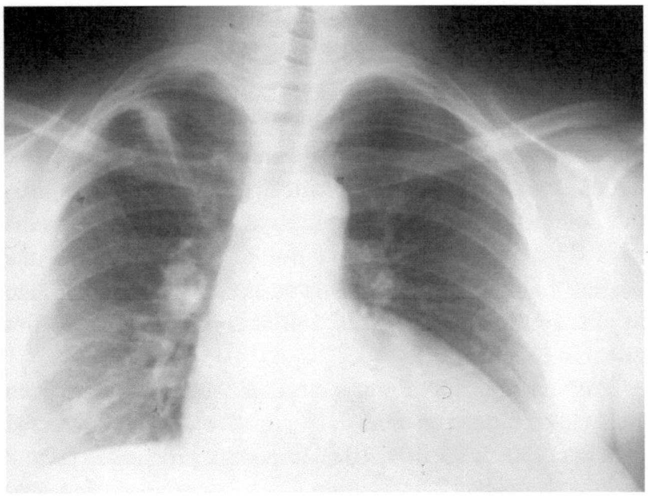

Fig. 3 Cryptococcal lung disease manifest as prominent bilateral hilar adenopathy plus nodule in right upper lobe and patchy pneumonitis in right lower lobe in immunocompetent host

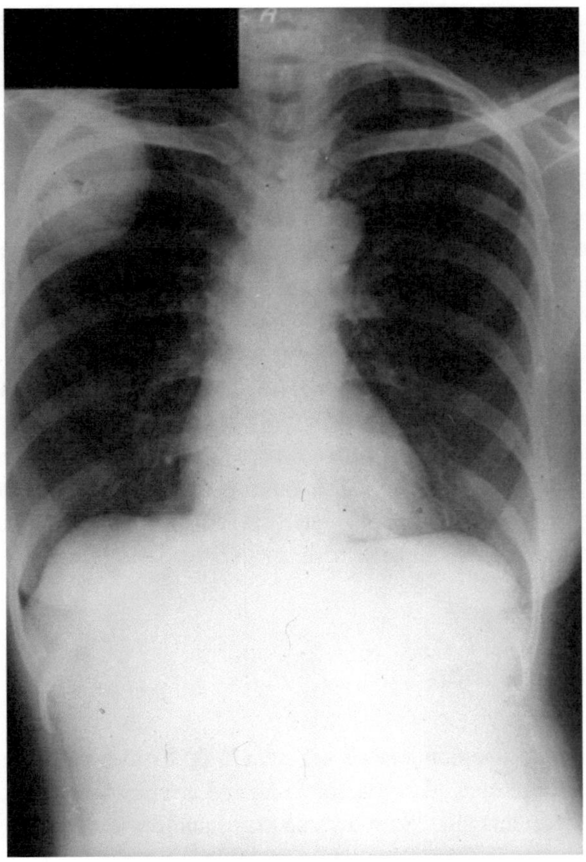

Fig. 4 Large, well-circumscribed cryptococcal mass lesion in right upper lobe of immunocompetent host. Mass was excised surgically

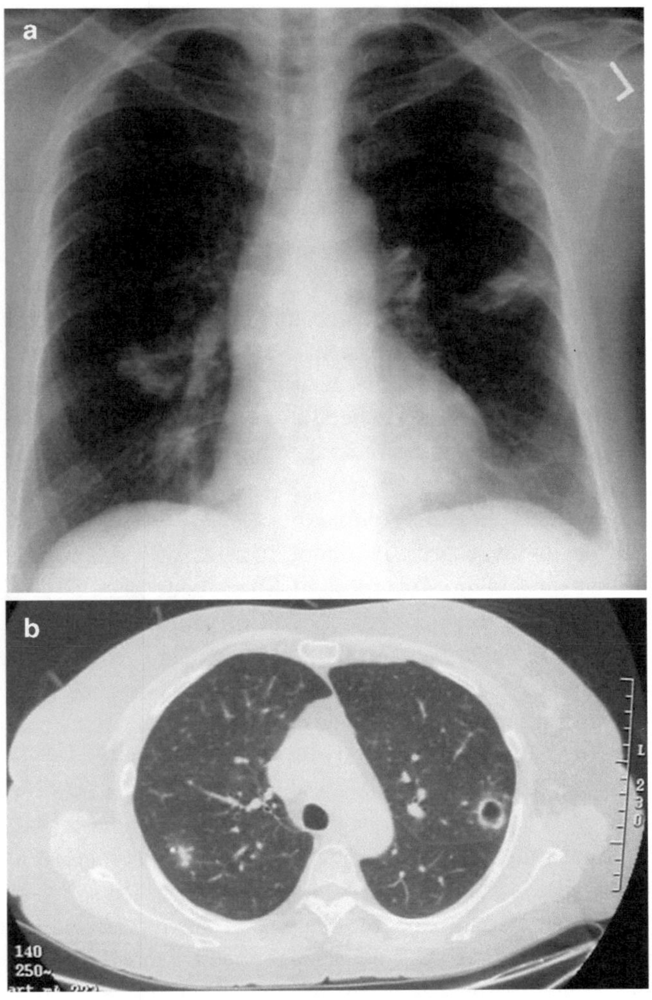

Fig. 5 (**a**) Cryptococcal lung disease manifest as several irregular nodules. (**b**) Note cavitation of left lung nodule shown on CT scan

cryptococcosis in an AIDS patient warrants thorough evaluation for CNS disease, even in the asymptomatic patient.

Central Nervous System Infection

The most common clinical manifestation of cryptococcosis is CNS infection, manifested typically as meningitis, which can be subacute or chronic. The clinical presentation and course of cryptococcal meningitis vary greatly and are often related to the immune status or underlying condition of the patient. In general, the signs and symptoms of cryptococcal meningitis among AIDS patients and HIV-negative patients are similar; however, in AIDS patients, onset tends to be more acute, and the course more rapidly progressive, perhaps explained by poor inflammatory response and the high burden of organisms in these patients. A wide range of symptoms and signs can be seen with CNS cryptococcosis, but complaints are often mild or nonspecific and include headache, nausea and vomiting, and malaise. In some instances, patients are even asymptomatic. Altered mental status, somnolence, and obtundation may signify advanced disease and a poor prognosis [92]. Fever is typically low-grade, and is more likely to be present in HIV-infected patients [92, 93]. Unlike in bacterial meningitis, meningismus is uncommon. Cranial nerve dysfunction may occur in up to 30% of patients, and may result from increased intracranial pressure, cryptococcal invasion of cranial nerves, or brain parenchymal lesions (cryptococcomas). The most common symptoms and signs of cranial nerve involvement include decreased visual acuity, blindness, diplopia, hearing loss, and facial weakness. Seizures, often a reflection of increased intracranial pressure or focal mass lesions, tend to occur later in the course of disease.

Increased intracranial pressure associated with cryptococcal meningitis, especially among patients with AIDS, is a prominent finding. An opening CSF pressure of >250 mm H_2O is found in approximately half of patients with AIDS [94–96]. In AIDS patients, high yeast burden is felt to be a contributing factor to increased intracranial pressures [96]. Cryptococci may cause outflow obstruction by blocking passage of CSF across arachnoid villi. In addition, soluble cryptococcal capsular polysaccharide may accumulate in arachnoid villi, leading to alterations in CSF drainage [94]. Consequently, routine assessment of suspected cryptococcal meningitis should always include manometry. Imaging of the brain is also important to evaluate for hydrocephalus and potential mass lesions; MRI is more effective than CT imaging in identifying lesions [97, 98]. In a recent study evaluating neuroimaging findings in transplant patients with cryptococcosis, outcomes tended to be worse in patients with parenchymal lesions when compared with meningitis or hydrocephalus [99].

Among HIV-negative patients with *C. gattii* infection, intracranial infection is associated with more complications, especially cerebral cryptococcomas, than in patients with *C. neoformans* infection [86, 100]. In AIDS patients, other causes of brain lesions, such as *Toxoplasma gondii* and lymphoma, should be considered. Among AIDS patients with cryptococcal meningitis and increased intracranial pressure, hydrocephalus is an uncommon finding on brain imaging [101]. By contrast, in HIV-negative patients with subacute or chronic cryptococcal meningitis, the course is more likely complicated by hydrocephalus caused by obstruction of flow due to inflammation of the basilar meninges [102]. However, normal ventricular size in the setting of increased intracranial pressure is not uncommon [103].

Prognostic factors for cryptococcal meningitis have been well characterized in both HIV-negative and HIV-infected patients [45, 92, 93, 104, 105]. Important prognostic factors include the patient's underlying disease or predisposing condition, the burden of organisms, titers of CSF cryptococcal antigen, mental status at baseline, and the ability to mount an inflammatory response in CSF [92]. For example, in AIDS patients, fewer white blood cells on initial lumbar puncture may signify poor prognosis [92]. Cryptococcal antigen detection in the CSF may be of prognostic value in certain patient populations. In HIV-negative patients with meningitis, a CSF cryptococcal antigen of ≥ 1:8 at the conclusion of ≥1 month of therapy correlated with likelihood of relapse [45]. Likewise, in AIDS patients, higher titers of CSF cryptococcal antigen (> 1:1024) at baseline are predictive of poorer outcomes [92]. In AIDS patients with meningitis, serial measurement of cryptococcal antigen titers obtained during acute therapy or prolonged suppression has little role in management [106, 107].

Among treated patients with cryptococcal meningitis, mortality rates vary from 5% to 25%, and most deaths occur within the first few weeks of illness [92–94, 108]. Data suggest that mortality in AIDS patients due to cryptococcosis appears to be decreasing, but still remains a common outcome in resource-limited settings [57, 109].

Skin Infection

Cryptococcal skin lesions are seen in up to 15% of patients with disseminated cryptococcosis, and are most common in HIV patients [10]. Skin disease may manifest as a variety of cutaneous lesions, including pustules, papules, purpura, ulcers, cellulitis, superficial granulomas or plaques, abscesses, and sinus tracts [10, 39]. Cases of necrotizing cellulitis have also been described [110]. In AIDS patients, umbilicated papules resembling molluscum contagiosum are present frequently (Fig. 6) [111]. Cellulitis, characterized by prominent erythema and induration, is often present in patients receiving systemic corticosteroids or other immunosuppressive therapy (Fig. 7) [112]. Cryptococcal skin lesions have resulted rarely from local inoculation, predominately due to laboratory accidents, but the majority of skin lesions result from disseminated infection [113]. Primary cutaneous cryptococcosis appears to be a distinct entity [114].

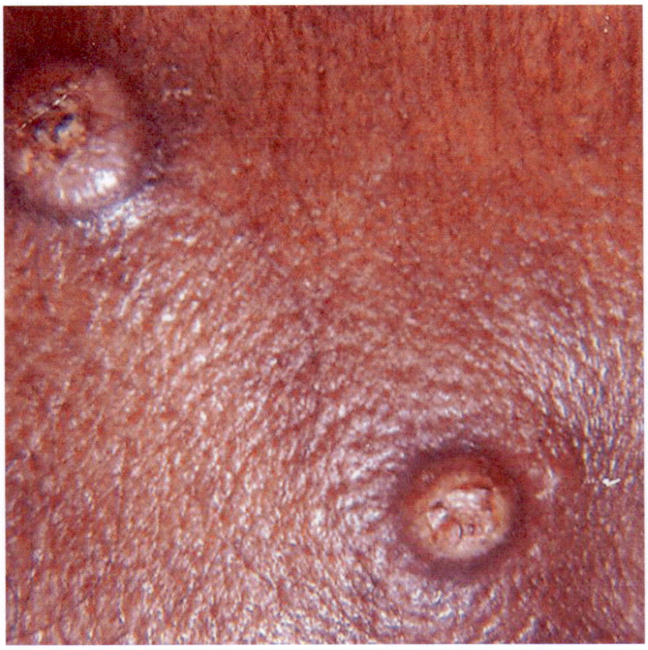

Fig. 6 Molluscum contagiosum–like umbilicated papules due to cryptococcosis in the skin of an AIDS patient

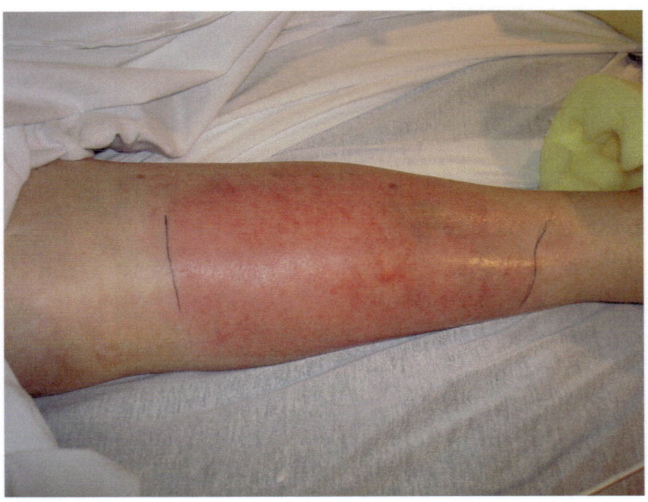

Fig. 7 Cryptococcal cellulitis in a corticosteroid-treated lung transplant patient

Osteoarticular Infection

Cryptococcal lesions of the skeletal system are present in fewer than 10% of patients with disseminated cryptococcosis [115, 116]. Lesions often manifest with soft tissue swelling and tenderness, but lack of symptoms is not uncommon. A single skeletal site is involved most often, with vertebral infection occurring most frequently [115]. On radiography, well-circumscribed, osteolytic lesions, which may resemble malignancy, are seen. Cryptococcal septic arthritis is rare, and most often involves the knee joint [117].

Other Sites of Infection

Cryptococcal infection can involve many other sites and organ systems. Because of the frequency of positive blood cultures and disseminated disease, particularly in AIDS patients, infection may involve virtually any organ. Not infrequently, cryptococcemia in the absence of a proven organ site is discovered [118]. Additional nonmeningeal, extrapulmonary sites of involvement include the prostate, kidneys, muscle, liver, thyroid, sinuses, peritoneum, adrenals, esophagus, heart and aorta, and eyes [39, 119–121]. The prostate gland may also serve as a "sanctuary" for *Cryptococcus* pre- and posttreatment [122, 123]. In one series of HIV-infected patients treated successfully for cryptococcal meningitis, cultures of urine were positive in 9 (22%) of 41 patients at the end of therapy [123].

Immune Reconstitution Inflammatory Syndrome

Immune reconstitution inflammatory syndrome (IRIS) has become an important phenomenon in patients with AIDS and cryptococcal meningitis and recently among transplant recipients [124–127]. IRIS may occur following introduction of HAART in the setting of AIDS with the restoration of CD4 cells or decreasing immunosuppressive therapy in transplant recipients with the reversal of a predominantly Th2 to a Th1 proinflammatory response [128, 129]. Usually, IRIS occurs in one of two scenarios: (1) after starting HAART in patients with cryptococcosis or (2) as a paradoxical effect in patients on HAART during cryptococcal treatment.

The incidence of IRIS is estimated to be between 4 and 16 cases per 100 person-years among AIDS patients [126] and has a prevalence of 4.8% among solid organ transplant recipients [127]. In a recent prospective study evaluating IRIS among 65 HIV patients with cryptococcal meningitis who started HAART after initiation of antifungal treatment, IRIS developed in 11(17%) patients at a median of 29 days from starting HAART [124]. Patients with IRIS had greater immune responses with HAART (on the basis of T cell recovery) than non-IRIS patients, and IRIS did not appear to be associated with increased mortality rates [124]. Among organ transplant recipients, IRIS has occurred more frequently in patients receiving potent immunosuppressive therapy such as tacrolimus, mycophenolate mofetil, and prednisone when compared with other less immunosuppressive regimens [127].

IRIS may occur within a few days to many months after HAART administration [125]. IRIS typically manifests as meningitis, cryptococcomas, lymphadenitis, or hydrocephalus. Often, symptoms can be confused as signs of treatment failure or disease caused by other opportunistic infections. A positive culture of blood, CSF, or tissue for *C. neoformans*, obtained during evaluation for IRIS, excludes this diagnosis and indicates active cryptococcal infection.

As of yet, there is no reliable way to establish the diagnosis of IRIS; however, risk factors for development of IRIS among AIDS patients include previously unrecognized HIV infection, CD4 cell count <7 cells/μL, fungemia, higher CSF opening pressure, glucose and white blood cell counts, and HAART initiation with 2 months of cryptococcosis diagnosis [125, 126]. Levels of CSF proinflammatory cytokines do not appear to distinguish IRIS patients from those with cryptococcal meningitis alone [124].

Diagnosis

The diagnosis of cryptococcosis can be made by using several methods. A definitive diagnosis is made by culture and identification of the organism from a sterile site. Clinical specimens can be examined with an India ink preparation, a rapid test which is performed by mixing an equal amount of CSF or other fluid and nigrosin or Pelikan India ink on a slide. After adding a coverslip and upon viewing, the polysaccharide capsule of *Cryptococcus* will exclude the ink particles and appear as a halo around the organism (Fig. 8). In patients with cryptococcal meningitis, a positive India ink preparation showing budding yeasts surrounded by a capsule is a useful presumptive test for diagnosis. In AIDS patients with cryptococcal meningitis, India ink preparation of CSF will be positive in 60–80% of cases [92, 93], whereas in HIV-negative patients the positivity rate is lower [35, 130]. Presumptive diagnosis of cryptococcosis can also be made by wet preparations of clinical samples or with the use of Gram stain. However, with these methods, the appearance of cryptococci may be highly variable; therefore, culture should be used for confirmation. Although not specific for the cryptococcal cell wall, Calcofluor white staining may be useful, particularly if few yeast cells are present.

The presumptive diagnosis of cryptococcosis is frequently made on examination of tissue sections. On routine hematoxylin and eosin staining, *C. neoformans* is difficult to identify. However, Gomori-methenamine silver or periodic acid-Schiff staining does allow identification; the organism can be recognized by its oval shape, and narrow-based budding. With the use of mucicarmine staining (Fig. 9), the organism will stain rose to burgundy in color and help differentiate *C. neoformans* from other yeasts, especially *Blastomyces dermatiditis* and *Histoplasma capsulatum*.

The diagnosis of cryptococcal meningitis is easier to establish than the diagnosis of pulmonary cryptococcosis. If cryptococcal meningitis is suspected, a lumbar puncture should be performed. Abnormalities in CSF commonly include elevated opening pressure, hypoglycorrhachia, elevated protein, and a lymphocytic pleocytosis. In AIDS patients with cryptococcal meningitis, the CSF formula

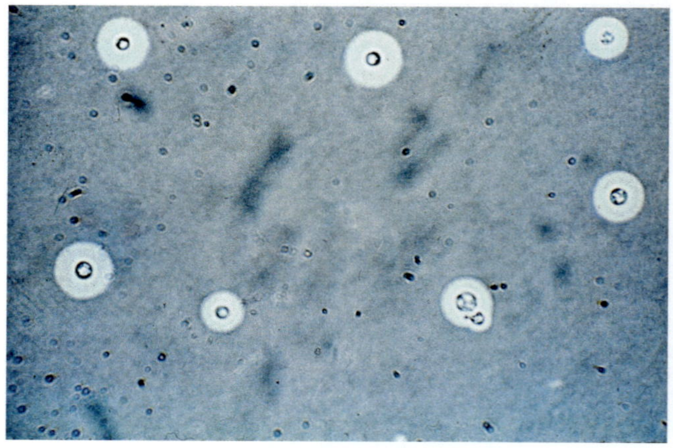

Fig. 8 India ink preparation showing *Cryptococcus neoformans* in cerebrospinal fluid. Note budding yeast form and distinct outline of cell walls and surrounding capsules

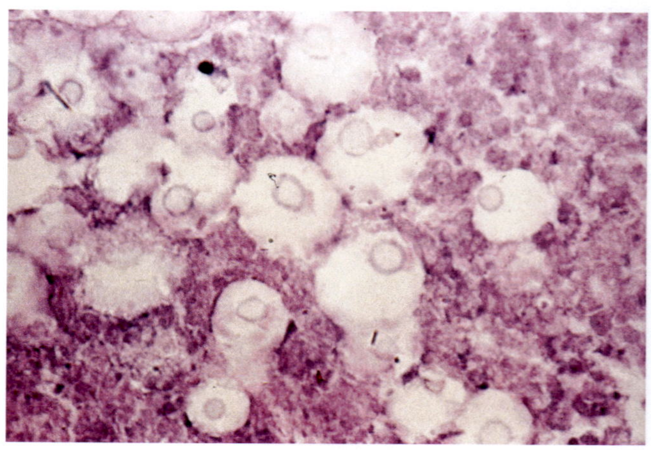

Fig. 9 Mucicarmine stain of brain parenchyma showing numerous densely packed encapsulated cryptococci. Note variable size of capsules

may be normal or show only minimal abnormalities [92]. However, elevated opening pressure is common and may be seen in 50–70% of AIDS patients [94, 96]. In AIDS patients, lack of white blood cells in the CSF is not unusual and may reflect decreased or absent inflammatory response; furthermore, few white blood cells in CSF is a poor prognostic sign [92].

The detection of cryptococcal polysaccharide antigen in CSF or serum is useful in patients with suspected cryptococcosis. After infection is established, cryptococcal polysaccharide becomes solubilized in fluids and can be detected by latex agglutination and quantified. Any positive cryptococcal antigen titer in CSF should be correlated with clinical findings. A titer of ≥ 1:4 strongly suggests cryptococcal infection, particularly in the immunocompromised patient. In cryptococcal meningitis, antigen testing is highly sensitive and specific, and may be particularly useful if CSF cultures are negative. Cryptococcal antigen is found in CSF in >90% and in serum in >70% of patients with cryptococcal meningitis. In AIDS patients with cryptococcal meningitis, sensitivity of the CSF antigen test is even greater (approaching 95–99%) and titers are often higher, up to10^6 [92, 93]. The utility of antigen testing is limited in patients with pulmonary cryptococosis. Among HIV-negative patients with pulmonary cryptococcosis, serum cryptococcal antigen will be positive in 25–56% of cases [35, 131].

With cryptococcal antigen testing, it is important to use proper controls to eliminate errors in testing. The presence of rheumatoid factor may cause a false-positive result when serum is tested, as will the presence of polysaccharide from *Trichosporon asahii* (*beigelii*) or use of inactivated pronase for testing [132]. In addition, false-negative cryptococcal antigen results, although rare, may be due to low numbers of organisms invading the CSF, infection by poorly or non-encapsulated strains, high titers of antigen (prozone phenomenon), low titers of antigen, or immune complexes [10].

Either routine bacteriologic or fungal media will facilitate culture of *C. neoformans*. Colonies are usually detected after 2–7 days of growth. In patients with AIDS and cryptococcal meningitis, blood and CSF cultures will be positive in 55% and 95%, respectively [92, 93]. In a recent study of HIV-negative patients with cryptococcal meningitis, CSF cultures were positive in 89% of patients tested [35]. For blood cultures, the lysis-centrifugation (isolator) technique appears to be the most sensitive method to identify *C. neoformans* [133]. Use of canavanine-glycine-bromthymol blue (CGB) agar will help to distinguish *C. gattii* from other *Cryptococcus* species, as colonies of *C. gattii* will turn the agar blue, while other species do not elicit a color change [13].

The methods of in vitro antifungal susceptibility testing for *C. neoformans* against a variety of antifungal agents have been standardized, although interpretive breakpoints for the antifungal agents against *C. neoformans* have yet to be defined [134]. Most *C. neoformans* isolates appear susceptible to available antifungal agents, including amphotericin B, flucytosine, fluconazole, itraconazole, voriconazole, and posaconazole [135–137]. However, the echinocandin class of antifungals has poor activity against *C. neoformans* [138]. Several reports indicate the potential for microbiologic resistance to fluconazole and clinical failure among patients with cryptococcosis [124, 139–141]. Susceptibility testing should be reserved for patients who have failed primary therapy, for those who relapse after apparently successful primary therapy, and for those who develop cryptococcosis with a history of recent exposure to an azole agent.

Treatment

The treatment of cryptococcosis is decided on the basis of sites of involvement and the underlying immunologic status of the patient. The treatment recommendations and references herein are closely aligned with recent consensus guidelines from the Infectious Diseases Society of America [142]. Please refer to these guidelines for more information. For patients with pulmonary disease, the aims of therapy are to eradicate disease and to prevent dissemination to the CNS. For patients with CNS disease, the aims of therapy are to eradicate or control the infection, adequately manage elevated intracranial pressure, and prevent long-term neurologic sequelae. Prior to 1950, before the availability of amphotericin B, surgical intervention for pulmonary disease was the only therapeutic option available, and cryptococcosis was associated with high mortality rates.

With the availability of amphotericin B in the 1950s and its use as a single agent for cryptococcosis, outcomes were significantly improved, but adverse reactions to amphotericin B were frequently encountered. Flucytosine was found to be an effective drug in vitro for cryptococcosis, and became available for clinical use in 1972 [143]. It was used with moderate success for cryptococcal meningitis and pneumonia; however, single-drug therapy with flucytosine led to rapid emergence of resistance, and flucytosine use as a single agent has, for the most part, been abandoned [143]. Combination therapy with amphotericin B and flucytosine, first employed in a large clinical trial in 1979, resulted in treatment success in 60–85% of patients [45, 130]. In addition, the availability of the triazoles in the early 1990s led to simplification of the primary regimen for cryptococcal meningitis, utilizing, for example, shorter courses of combination amphotericin B and flucytosine followed by prolonged oral therapy with azoles, primarily fluconazole, and good efficacy [92, 93]. Recently, studies of another combination therapy, amphotericin B and fluconazole, have shown encouraging results [144, 145].

Treatment of the HIV-Negative Patient

Pulmonary Infection

The presentation of pulmonary cryptococcosis in the HIV-negative patient can vary widely, ranging from colonization, to asymptomatic disease, to fulminant pneumonia or ARDS [81]. Treatment data from clinical trials among HIV-negative patients with pulmonary infection are limited, and questions remain about which populations require therapy and the optimal dosage and duration of therapy (Table 2) [35, 146, 149]. The only prospective data concerning the treatment of pulmonary cryptococcosis are available from trials involving CNS infections among HIV-negative patients, where resolution of pulmonary disease was not a trial end point [45, 130]. Although few studies, particularly in the era of effective azole therapy, have addressed risk factors for CNS dissemination among patients with pulmonary cryptococcal infection, most authorities recommend lumbar puncture in immunocompromised patients and those with systemic symptoms [81, 83, 142]. A recent study of 166 HIV-negative patients with pulmonary disease identified high-dose corticosteroids, weight loss, headache, and altered mental status as baseline predictors of meningitis [83].

In patients with normal immunologic function and colonization (defined as positive respiratory tract cultures with negative chest radiograph and absence of symptoms), observation is recommended. Immunocompetent patients with an abnormal chest radiograph and asymptomatic disease or mild disease often have done well without therapy, as was common prior to the availability of oral azole antifungals [81, 147, 156]. However, with the availability of oral azole therapy, most immunocompetent patients with pulmonary disease are treated [82].

In contrast, all patients with immune compromise and colonization should receive therapy. If a decision to treat is made, oral fluconazole at a dosage of 400 mg/day for 6–12 months is recommended [146, 148, 149]. In HIV-negative patients with immunocompromising conditions and asymptomatic or mild-to-moderate disease, treatment should be initiated both to prevent CNS dissemination as well as to eradicate symptoms [81, 131]. Fluconazole at a dosage of 400 mg daily is a suitable regimen and is associated with improvement in >80% of cases [35, 146, 149]. Therapy should continue beyond resolution of symptoms and chest radiographic abnormalities. Most experts recommend therapy for 6–12 months' duration [142, 146, 149].

The optimal length of therapy has not yet been determined from clinical trials, but factors to be considered include resolution of symptoms and radiographic findings, persistent immunosuppression, underlying disease, and duration of elevated serum cryptococcal antigen titer. Itraconazole, 200–400 mg daily; voriconazole, 200 mg twice daily; or posaconazole, 400 mg twice daily can be used as alternatives if fluconazole is unavailable or contraindicated [151, 152]. However, there

Table 2 Treatment of cryptococcal Infection in the HIV-negative patient

Pulmonary disease

- A. Colonization[a]
  - 1. Observation in the immunocompetent patient
  - 2. Fluconazole 400 mg daily for 6–12 months
- B. Asymptomatic or minimally symptomatic disease
  - 1. Fluconazole 200–400 mg/day for 6–12 months [35, 146–148]
  - Alternative: Close observation without therapy is a consideration
- C. Mild-to-moderate disease
  - 1. Fluconazole 200–400 mg/day for 6–12 months [35, 146–149]
  - Alternative: (1) Itraconazole 200–400 mg/day for 6–12 months [150]
    - (2) Voriconazole 200 mg twice daily or posaconazole 400 mg twice daily for 6–12 months [151, 152]
- D. Severe or progressive disease, or azole drug not an option
  - Amphotericin B 0.5–1.0 mg/kg/day for a total dose of 1–2 g. This may be followed by oral fluconazole in selected patients [35, 81, 146]
  - Alternative: (1) Regimens similar to those used for CNS disease, as described below
    - (2) Surgical resection in selected cases refractory to therapy

CNS disease

- Amphotericin B 0.5–1.0 mg/kg/day plus flucytosine 100 mg/kg/day for 2–4 weeks followed by fluconazole 400 mg/day, for 8–10 weeks [93]
- Amphotericin B, 0.5–1.0 mg/kg/day plus flucytosine 100 mg/kg/day for 6–10 weeks [45, 130]
- *Note*: Lipid formulations of amphotericin B (liposomal AmB 3–6 mg/kg/day or ABLC 5 mg/kg/day) may be substituted in patients with intolerance to amphotericin B deoxycholate) [153–155]
- Adjunctive therapy: see text

Maintenance therapy

- Fluconazole 200 mg/day for at least 6 months should be considered for patients with persistent immunosuppression, i.e., transplant recipients [129]

[a]Colonization is defined as a positive respiratory tract culture without signs or symptoms of pulmonary disease or radiographic abnormalities

are few data examining these drugs for the treatment of pulmonary cryptococcosis, much of which evaluates use after treatment failure or drug intolerance.

For HIV-negative patients with severe pulmonary disease or progressive disease, or for whom azole therapy is not an option, most experts would recommend an amphotericin B formulation, with or without flucytosine, as initial therapy for 2–6 weeks, followed by fluconazole [142]. For organ transplant recipients, given the risk of nephrotoxicity associated with concurrent AmB and calcineurin inhibitors, lipid formulations of AmB as induction therapy are preferable for severe non-CNS disease [129].

The role of surgery in patients with pulmonary cryptococcosis is limited [35, 131, 147]. Surgical intervention for pulmonary cryptococcosis may be required for removal of large mass lesions or areas of persistent focal radiographic abnormalities that are refractory to antifungal therapy.

CNS Infection

Early studies among HIV-negative patients with CNS cryptococcosis were important in defining the efficacy of combination therapy with amphotericin B and flucytosine and duration of therapy among immunocompromised patients [45, 130]. In the first prospective study of cryptococcal meningitis in 50 HIV-negative patients, combination therapy with low-dose amphotericin B (0.3 mg/kg/day) plus high-dose flucytosine (150 mg/kg/day) given for 6 weeks was compared to amphotericin B therapy alone (0.4 mg/kg/day) given for 10 weeks [130]. Combination therapy resulted in higher rates of cure and improvement, fewer relapses, and more rapid sterilization of CSF ($P < .001$). Adverse reactions to flucytosine occurred in 11 (32%) of 34 patients, necessitating discontinuation of flucytosine in 6. While the authors concluded that combination therapy was superior to amphotericin B alone, concerns were expressed about the low dosage of amphotericin B and high dosage of flucytosine used in the two arms of the study.

The next prospective study attempted to better address duration of therapy among HIV-negative patients with cryptococcal meningitis by comparing combination therapy with amphotericin B (0.3 mg/kg/day) and flucytosine (150 mg/kg/day) for 4 versus 6 weeks [45]. Note that the treatment regimens employed here were similar to those used in the initial trial [130]. In the second study, 91 patients were randomized to receive either 4 (45 patients) or 6 (46 patients) weeks of therapy. Among randomized patients treated for 4 weeks, cure or improvement was noted in 75%, compared with 85% cure or improvement among patients treated for 6 weeks. Patients who received 4 weeks of therapy had a higher relapse rate (27%) when compared with patients who received 6 weeks of therapy (16%). Toxicities of the regimens in both groups were similar and were most often azotemia, leukopenia, and diarrhea. Among 23 nonrandomized transplant recipients who were protocol-adherent, 16 (70%) of 23 were cured or improved, but 7 (30%) relapsed. From this study, significant baseline predictors of a favorable response included headache, normal mental status, and a CSF white cell count above 20/mm^3. The authors concluded that important considerations in determining duration of therapy should include the patient's underlying disease and immune status and severity of meningitis.

Few other studies are available which address treatment of cryptococcal CNS disease in HIV-negative patients, and none have been randomized or controlled [35, 146]. Dromer and colleagues reviewed retrospectively 83 cases of meningeal and extrameningeal cryptococcosis in HIV-negative French patients, with emphasis on the comparison of efficacy of amphotericin B and fluconazole [146]. Patients with more severe infections, such as meningitis, or those with higher CSF cryptococcal antigen titers, were more likely to receive amphotericin B. However, a subgroup of 25 patients received fluconazole alone for cryptococcal meningitis; 68% were cured with this regimen. A more recent retrospective study by Pappas and colleagues reported findings in 306 patients from 15 US medical centers [35]. As in the Dromer study, patients with CNS disease were more likely to receive amphotericin B, alone or in combination. The most common regimen employed was induction therapy with amphotericin B and flucytosine, followed by consolidation therapy with fluconazole as described for HIV-infected patients. Of 107 patients who received induction therapy with amphotericin B and flucytosine, 90 (84%) were cured or improved. In this study, only 8 of 154 patients with meningitis were treated with fluconazole alone; 7 were cured or improved.

Many of the treatment recommendations for HIV-negative patients with CNS cryptococcal disease have been extrapolated from results of more recent studies in HIV-infected patients [92, 93, 153, 154]. Specific issues addressed by these studies include use of higher doses of amphotericin B (0.5–1.0 mg/kg/day) [92, 93, 155]; substitution of lipid amphotericin B formulations in patients with renal insufficiency [153–155]; and treatment with an "induction" regimen of amphotericin B plus flucytosine for 2 weeks followed by a "consolidation" regimen with fluconazole for an additional 8–12 weeks [93]. For details on these studies, see the section on treatment of CNS disease in HIV-infected patients. For organ transplant recipients, given the risk of nephrotoxicity associated toxicity with concurrent AmB and calcineurin inhibitors, lipid formulations of AmB as induction therapy are preferable for CNS and severe non-CNS disease [129]. The authors favor the "induction/consolidation" approach for the treatment of cryptococcal meningitis in HIV-negative patients, especially for organ transplant recipients [93, 142].

For CNS infections caused by *C. gattii*, treatment recommendations are similar for those patients with CNS infection secondary to *C. neoformans*. However, because of the frequency of cerebral cryptococcomas in patients with *C. gattii*, management is best guided by imaging studies.

Other Sites of Infection

HIV-negative patients present infrequently with cryptococcal disease at other sites in the absence of pulmonary or CNS infection. Other infections may include skin lesions, abscesses, cryptococcemia, or positive urine cultures. Among solid organ transplant patients, it has been observed that those who received tacrolimus were less likely to have central nervous system involvement and more likely to have skin, soft-tissue, or osteoarticular involvement when compared to patients receiving non tacrolimus-based immunosuppression [157]. In HIV-negative patients, few studies address treatment for these entities [35]. For the majority of patients, treatment is recommended; however, no preferred regimen has been identified. In a retrospective review of 40 HIV-negative patients with cryptococcal disease at non-CNS and nonpulmonary sites, 36 (90%) received antifungal therapy, and 25 (63%) were successfully treated [35]. Multiple regimens were used: 20 evaluable patients received amphotericin B alone or in combination with flucytosine or fluconazole, and 12 (60%) of these 20 were cured or improved; 12 other patients received fluconazole alone and all were cured or improved.

Maintenance Therapy

Although no prospective studies have addressed the use of maintenance or suppressive therapy for HIV-negative patients who have been successfully treated for cryptococcal disease, many experts recommend 6–12 months of additional maintenance therapy with oral fluconazole, 200 mg/day, for selected patients who remain persistently immunocompromised after initial treatment. Among solid organ transplant recipients, the relapse rate of cryptococcosis after 6 months of maintenance therapy is minimal [129]. A recent observation noted that cryptococcal CNS parenchymal lesions may persist radiographically for months or years after completion of therapy, and do not necessarily signify relapse or recurrence of disease [158].

Treatment of the HIV-infected Patient

Pulmonary Infection

The diagnosis of cryptococcal pneumonia in HIV-infected patients is difficult, as the clinical signs and symptoms and radiographic findings can often be nonpecific and mimic disease by other pathogens. Because HIV-related cryptococcal pneumonia is associated frequently with dissemination, a systematic evaluation with blood and CSF cultures and CSF and serum cryptococcal antigen testing is recommended in HIV-infected patients with a positive respiratory tract culture for *Cryptococcus* [142]. Because there have been no controlled trials that evaluate the treatment of pulmonary cryptococcal infection in HIV-infected patients, the treatment of choice and duration of therapy have yet to be elucidated (Table 3).

HIV-infected patients who are asymptomatic, or have mild-to-moderate symptoms with positive respiratory tract cultures, may be good candidates for therapy with oral fluconazole, 200–400 mg daily. Itraconazole, 200–400 mg daily, may be used as a second-line oral therapy [150]. For patients with severe or progressive pulmonary disease, or for patients who cannot tolerate azole therapy, treatment should be similar to recommendations for CNS disease, as described below, and in Table 3.

Length of therapy for cryptococcal pneumonia should be 6–12 months. For HIV-infected patients on HAART with CD4 count >100 cells/μL and decreasing or stable cryptococcal antigen titers (≤ 1:512), discontinuation of maintenance therapy can be considered [166]. For a detailed discussion of this topic, see the section on maintenance therapy under treatment of the HIV-infected patient with CNS infection.

CNS Infection

Many important trials focusing on the treatment of cryptococcal meningitis have been conducted in the HIV-infected population during the last two decades. These studies have demonstrated the efficacy of higher doses of amphotericin B used as primary induction therapy, the safety and efficacy of oral azole antifungal drugs in the treatment of CNS disease, and the importance of adequate management of elevated intracranial pressure associated with cryptococcal meningitis. The principle of rapid fungicidal activity should be the focus of the induction strategy, and a sterile CSF culture at 2 weeks, associated with a favorable outcome, as in previous studies, should be a goal [93, 169].

Based on success rates of 75–85% in earlier studies of combination therapy with amphotericin B and flucytosine among HIV-negative patients with cryptococcal meningitis [45, 130], AIDS patients with CNS disease were treated initially with combination therapy for prolonged periods. However, early reports during the late 1980s suggested that use of flucytosine in HIV-infected patients was frequently associated with cytopenias, and offered no survival benefit or improvement in relapse rate when compared to single therapy with amphotericin B [170]. Because of concerns for flucytosine toxicity, decreased success rates, and the evolving

Table 3 Treatment of cryptococcal infection in the HIV-infected patient

Pulmonary disease
A. Asymptomatic or mild-to-moderate disease
Fluconazole 400 mg/day for 6–12 months depending on immune reconstitution[a] [88, 91, 148]
Alternatives: Itraconazole 400 mg/day 6–12 months depending on immune reconstitution[a] [150]
Fluconazole 400 mg/day plus flucytosine 100 mg/kg/day for 10 weeks [159]
B. Severe, progressive disease
Regimens similar to those for CNS disease (see below)
CNS disease
Amphotericin B 0.7–1.0 mg/kg/day plus flucytosine 100 mg/kg/day for 2 weeks followed by fluconazole 400 mg/day for 8–12 weeks [92, 93]
Alternative: Itraconazole 400 mg/day may be substituted for fluconazole
Amphotericin B 0.7–1.0 mg/kg/day for 4–6 weeks [92]
Amphotericin B 0.7 mg/kg/day plus fluconazole 800 mg/day for ≥8 weeks [145]
Note: Lipid formulations of amphotericin B (liposomal AmB 3–6 mg/kg/day or ABLC 5 mg/kg/day) may be substituted in patients with intolerance to amphotericin B deoxycholate) [153–155]
Fluconazole 400 mg/day plus flucytosine 100 mg/kg/day for 10 weeks [159, 160]
Fluconazole 800–1200 mg/day for 10–12 weeks [161, 162]
Itraconazole 200 mg/day for 10–12 weeks [150, 163]
Maintenance therapy[a]
Fluconazole 200 mg/day [106, 164, 165]
Alternatives: Amphotericin B 1 mg/kg/week [106]
Itraconazole 200–400 mg/day [165]

[a]Lifelong maintenance therapy may be discontinued in selected patients who achieve immune reconstitution with highly active antiretroviral therapy [166–168]

availability of the potent oral azoles fluconazole and itraconazole, subsequent studies evaluated novel regimens for primary therapy of CNS cryptococcal disease [92, 163, 171].

In a small study in the late 1980s of 21 patients with AIDS and cryptococcal meningitis, Larsen and colleagues compared combination therapy with amphotericin B (0.7–1.0 mg/kg/day) plus flucytosine (150 mg/kg/day) to fluconazole (400 mg/day) alone [171]. Clinical and mycologic failure was more common in patients who received fluconazole, particularly in patients with severe disease. In fact, the study was discontinued prematurely because of the higher mortality rate in fluconazole-treated patients. An important finding in this study was the successful treatment in all six patients who received higher doses of amphotericin B as part of the combination regimen. In a second small study of 28 patients with presumed cryptococcal meningitis by De Gans and colleagues, reported in 1992, itraconazole, 200 mg twice daily, was compared to combination therapy with amphotericin B (0.3 mg/kg/day) plus flucytosine (150 mg/kg/day), both administered for 6 weeks [163]. Among patients who received itraconazole, 5 (42%) of 12 achieved a complete response, compared with all 10 patients who received amphotericin B plus flucytosine.

In contrast to these two small trials, two large sequential trials were conducted jointly by the National Institute of Allergy and Infectious Diseases (NIAID) Mycoses Study Group (MSG) and the NIAID AIDS Clinical Trials Group (ACTG) in the 1990s. The initial trial compared amphotericin B (0.3 mg/kg/day) with fluconazole (200 mg/day) in the treatment of AIDS-associated cryptococcal meningitis [92]. Flucytosine as combination therapy with amphotericin B was optional, and was utilized in only nine patients. Treatment was successful in 34% of 131 fluconazole recipients, compared with 40% of 63 amphotericin B recipients. The mortality rate was similar in both groups: 18% in patients who received fluconazole versus 14% in patients who received amphotericin B ($P = .48$). However, the mortality rate during the first 2 weeks was higher among patients receiving fluconazole, and conversion of CSF cultures to negative was less rapid in fluconazole-treated patients. While this study showed no significant difference between the two arms, the results emphasized the need for a more effective primary regimen for the treatment of cryptococcal meningitis.

The second joint study was conducted to evaluate higher doses of amphotericin B, lower doses of flucytosine, and the safety and efficacy of oral azoles in the treatment of AIDS-associated CNS cryptococcosis [93]. Patients were randomized to receive 2 weeks of induction therapy with combination amphotericin B (0.7 mg/kg/day) plus flucytosine (100 mg/kg/day) (202 patients) or amphotericin B alone (0.7 mg/kg/day) (179 patients). At the end of 2 weeks of therapy, if entry criteria were met, patients were again randomized to receive 8 weeks of consolidation treatment with oral fluconazole, 400 mg/day, or oral itraconazole, 400 mg/day. At the end of 2 weeks, CSF cultures for *C. neoformans* were negative in 60% of patients who received combination amphotericin B and flucytosine, compared with 51% of amphotericin B alone treated patients ($P = 0.06$). However, clinical outcomes at 2 weeks did not differ significantly between the two groups. At the end of the 10-week induction and consolidation treatment period, clinical responses were also similar between the two groups, with 68% of fluconazole-treated patients responding, compared with 70% response among itraconazole-treated patients. Negative CSF cultures were observed in 72% of patients who received fluconazole, compared with 60% of patients who received itraconazole. The addition of flucytosine in the first 2 weeks and treatment with fluconazole over the next 8 weeks were independently associated with CSF sterilization. The use of higher-dose amphotericin B plus lower-dose flucytosine was associated with more effective CSF sterilization and decreased mortality at 2 weeks when compared with previous studies of combination therapy. Fluconazole and itraconazole were both effective as consolidation therapy, although fluconazole appeared to lead to more rapid CSF sterilization. This trial established the concept of "induction" and "consolidation" therapy as an attractive and effective treatment regimen for CNS cryptococcosis.

Additional evidence supporting the efficacy of amphotericin B plus flucytosine as induction therapy treatment was obtained from a randomized trial that evaluated four different antifungal regimens. Sixty-four AIDS patients with first episode cryptococcal meningitis were randomized to receive primary therapy with amphotericin B (0.7 mg/kg daily), amphotericin B (0.7 mg/kg plus flucytosine 100 mg/kg daily), amphotericin B (0.7 mg/kg plus fluconazole 400 mg daily), or a triple-drug regimen consisting of amphotericin B, flucytosine, and fluconazole at the above doses [172]. The primary end point of this study was the rate of reduction in CSF cryptococcal colony-forming units from serial quantitative CSF cultures obtained on days 3, 7, and 14 of treatment. Amphotericin B plus flucytosine achieved clearance of cryptococci from CSF significantly faster than amphotericin B alone, amphotericin B plus fluconazole, and triple-drug therapy. Logistic regression analysis demonstrated that cerebral dysfunction and high counts of *C. neoformans* per milliliter of CSF at baseline were independently associated with early mortality.

A recent cohort study with 208 HIV-positive and -negative patients with cryptococcal meningitis also showed the success of amphotericin B plus flucytosine therapy for 14 days over any other induction regimen among patients with severe cryptococcosis [173]. The risk of failure was 26% in the combination group, compared with 56% with other treatments ($P < 0.001$). Less than 14 days of flucytosine was also independently associated with treatment failure at 3 months in 168 cases of cryptococcosis [173]. A third trial evaluated amphotericin B (0.7 mg/kg/day vs 1.0 mg/kg/day) combined with flucytosine; the regimen utilizing higher-dose amphotericin B was more fungicidal with manageable toxicity, but there was no difference in 2- and 10-week mortality [108].

For HIV-infected patients with cryptococcal meningitis and renal insufficiency, lipid formulations of amphotericin B may be substituted. Clinical experience suggests that combination therapy with lipid formulations of amphotericin B is effective; however, only a few trials have evaluated these formulations [153–155, 174]. The optimal dosages of lipid formulations of amphotericin B have not yet been determined. Response rates of 66–86% were seen in patients receiving amphotericin B lipid complex [153, 174], and in 80% of patients receiving liposomal amphotericin B at a dose of 4 mg/kg/day [155]. An additional study with liposomal amphotericin B showed clinical response in 18 (78%) of 23 patients [154].

Although less well studied, other therapeutic options for CNS cryptococcal disease in HIV-infected patients have been employed, but are considered second-line options to the induction/consolidation options above. In a very recent study of 143 randomized patients, the combination use of amphotericin B (0.7 mg/kg/day) plus fluconazole (800 mg/day) demonstrated satisfactory outcomes compared to amphotericin B alone and may be a reasonable approach to therapy in settings where flucytosine is not available or contraindicated [145]. In this phase II study, the 14-day end point of success in the amphotericin B alone, amphotericin B plus fluconazole 400 mg/day (6 mg/kg), and amphotericin B plus fluconazole 800 mg/day (12 mg/kg) was 41%, 27%, and 54%, respectively. If this combination is used, the higher fluconazole dose is recommended. Combination therapy with fluconazole and flucytosine appears more effective than fluconazole alone, but is also more toxic [159, 160]. Primary therapy with either fluconazole or itraconazole alone administered for 10–12 weeks has also been evaluated in several trials, with variable responses [92, 150, 161–163]. If fluconazole is used alone, then higher daily doses should be administered. Notably, low success rates at 800 mg/day have been substantially improved with 1,200–2,000 mg/day [175]. When using higher daily doses of fluconazole, divided doses are recommended to minimize gastrointestinal toxicity.

Maintenance Therapy

After initial successful treatment of cryptococcal meningitis in AIDS patients, high relapse rates have been demonstrated in patients who did not receive lifelong suppressive or chronic maintenance therapy [164]. A placebo-controlled trial evaluated the effectiveness of fluconazole as maintenance therapy for AIDS patients who received successful therapy for cryptococccal meningitis with amphotericin B with or without flucytosine [164]. Relapse occurred in 15% of patients in the placebo group, compared with 0% in fluconazole-treated patients, thereby establishing the need for maintenance therapy in this population.

Subsequently, a randomized comparative trial conducted by the NIAID-MSG and NIAID-ACTG demonstrated the superior efficacy of oral fluconazole (200 mg daily) to intravenous amphotericin B (1 mg/kg weekly) for maintenance therapy [106]. Relapses of symptomatic cryptococcal disease were seen in 18% and 2% of patients receiving amphotericin B and fluconazole, respectively ($P < .001$). In addition, patients receiving amphotericin B had more frequent adverse events and associated bacterial infections.

The NIAID-MSG and NIAID-ACTG conducted another trial comparing oral fluconazole (200 mg daily) with oral itraconazole (200 mg daily) for 12 months as maintenance therapy for CNS cryptococcal disease [165]. Fluconazole proved to be superior; the trial was terminated prematurely after interim analysis revealed that 23% of itraconazole-treated patients relapsed, compared with only 4% of fluconazole-treated patients ($P = .006$). Furthermore, the trial showed that risk of relapse was increased if the patient had not received flucytosine during the initial 2 weeks of primary therapy for cryptococcal meningitis ($P = .04$). These studies established fluconazole as the drug of choice for maintenance of cryptococcal disease in HIV-infected patients.

Until recently, maintenance or lifelong suppressive therapy has been recommended for all AIDS patients after successful completion of therapy for acute cryptococcosis [166]. Studies suggest that risk of recurrence of cryptococcosis in AIDS patients is low, provided patients have successfully completed primary therapy for cryptococcosis, are free of symptoms of cryptococcosis, and have achieved immune reconstitution with HAART therapy [167, 168, 176]. For example, a prospective, multicenter trial conducted among 42 AIDS patients in Thailand randomized patients to continue or discontinue maintenance fluconazole therapy when the CD4 cell count had increased to >100 cells/μL and an undetectable HIV RNA level had been sustained for 3 months [168]. At a median of 48 weeks of observation, there were no episodes of relapse of cryptococcal meningitis in either group.

A second retrospective multicenter study was conducted among 100 patients with AIDS living in six different countries [167]. Inclusion criteria were a proven diagnosis of cryptococcal meningoencephalitis, a CD4 cell count of >100 cells/μL while receiving HAART, and the subsequent discontinuation of maintenance antifungal therapy. No relapse or death occurred during a median period of 26.1 months when patients were receiving both HAART and maintenance therapy for cryptococcal meningitis. After discontinuation of maintenance therapy, four relapses occurred (incidence 1.53 cases per 100 person-years) during a median period of observation of 28.4 months. This illustrates that careful follow-up of patients who discontinue maintenance therapy is necessary.

Collectively, these results indicate that maintenance therapy for cryptococcal meningitis may be safely discontinued in most patients (1) responding to HAART with a CD4 cell count >100/μL and an undetectable or low HIV RNA level sustained for ≥3 months and (2) receiving at least 1 year of antifungal drug exposure with close patient follow-ups and serial cryptococcal serum antigen tests. Reinstitution of fluconazole maintenance therapy should be considered if CD4 count drops below 100/μL and/or serum cryptococcal antigen titer rise. Some authorities recommend a lumbar puncture to confirm CSF sterility prior to discontinuation of maintenance therapy.

The decision of when to initiate HAART in the treatment of coinfection with *Cryptococcus* and HIV to avoid IRIS remains uncertain. Recent studies suggest earlier initiation of HAART within 2 weeks may be possible without triggering an unacceptable increase in the frequency or severity of IRIS [177]. In some clinical settings, long delays in HAART can place patients at risk for dying of other complications of HIV infection. It is also important to anticipate complications of drug interactions with HAART and antifungal drugs.

Adjunctive Therapy

As mentioned previously, elevated intracranial pressure is a common finding in cryptococcal meningoencephalitis, especially among patients with AIDS. Furthermore, a very high opening pressure at baseline may be associated with more frequent headaches and meningismus, pathologic reflexes, early death, and overall increased mortality rates [94]. The treatment of persistent elevated intracranial pressure is aimed at reducing CSF volume, either by repeated lumbar puncture or lumbar or ventricular drainage. If intracranial pressures cannot be adequately reduced with frequent lumbar punctures, lumbar drain placement or ventriculostomy may be necessary for CSF removal [102]. Intraventricular shunting, via ventriculoperitoneal shunt, is often reserved for patients with hydrocephalus or persistently elevated pressures. In HIV-negative patients with persistently increased intracranial pressure and no evidence of hydrocephalus on imaging studies, placement of a ventriculoperitoneal shunt may also be life-saving [103]. Moreover, shunting is not typically associated with dissemination of cryptococcal infection into the peritoneum or bloodstream [102]. Medical therapy including the use of acetazolamide, mannitol, or corticosteroids is not useful in the management of increased intracranial pressure in cryptococcal meningoencephalitis [178].

Prevention and Control

Prevention of cryptococcal disease is difficult because *C. neoformans* is ubiquitous in the environment and only causes sporadic disease. Because of the morbidity and mortality associated with CNS cryptococcal disease, and the increased incidence of cryptococcosis in patients with advanced HIV infection, primary prophylaxis has been studied in AIDS patients in several prospective trials [179, 180]. Although fluconazole and itraconazole have been shown to reduce the frequency of primary cryptococcal disease among those who have CD4 counts <50 cells/μL, a survival benefit has not been established. In addition, concern exists for the development of azole-resistant fungi if widespread antifungal prophylaxis is employed. For these reasons and the concern for drug interactions, medication compliance, and costs, primary prophylaxis for crytococcosis is not routinely recommended [179, 180]. However, in areas in which availability of HAART is limited, HIV drug resistance is high, and incidence of cryptococcal disease is very high, prophylaxis or pre-emptive strategies with use of serum cryptococcal antigen might be considered [181].

Asymptomatic cryptococcal antigenemia is a well-documented clinical condition in advanced HIV disease, and its prevalence has ranged between 4% and 12% per year in certain populations [182–186]. Antigenemia preceded symptoms of meningitis by a median of 22 days in one study in Uganda and, when not detected, made appearance of disease unlikely over the subsequent year [187]. Cryptococcal antigenemia has been shown to be associated with increased mortality rates among those initiating HAART, and persons with antigenemia are at theoretical risk for the "unmasking" form of cryptococcal IRIS [128]. The precise management of asymptomatic antigenemia remains uncertain, but an aggressive diagnostic and pre-emptive therapeutic stance may be warranted in areas with increased incidence.

References

1. de Hoog G. Atlas of Clinical Fungi. 2nd ed. Washington, DC: American Society for Microbiology Press; 2001.
2. Johnson LB, Bradley SF, Kauffman CA. Fungaemia due to *Cryptococcus laurentii* and a review of non-neoformans cryptococcaemia. Mycoses. 1998;41:277–80.
3. Khawcharoenporn T, Apisarnthanarak A, Mundy LM. Non-neoformans cryptococcal infections: a systematic review. Infection. 2007;35:51–8.
4. Kordossis T, Avlami A, Velegraki A, et al. First report of *Cryptococcus laurentii* meningitis and a fatal case of *Cryptococcus albidus* cryptococcaemia in AIDS patients. Med Mycol. 1998;36:335–9.
5. Neilson JB, Fromtling RA, Bulmer GS. *Cryptococcus neoformans*: size range of infectious particles from aerosolized soil. Infect Immun. 1977;17:634–8.
6. Franzot SP, Salkin IF, Casadevall A. *Cryptococcus neoformans* var. *grubii:* separate varietal status for *Cryptococcus neoformans* serotype A isolates. J Clin Microbiol. 1999;37:838–40.
7. Kidd SE, Hagen F, Tscharke RL, et al. A rare genotype of *Cryptococcus gattii* caused the cryptococcosis outbreak on Vancouver Island (British Columbia, Canada). Proc Natl Acad Sci USA. 2004;101:17258–63.
8. Chambers C, MacDougall L, Li M, Galanis E. Tourism and specific risk areas for *Cryptococcus gattii*, Vancouver Island, Canada. Emerg Infect Dis. 2008;14:1781–3.
9. Byrnes 3rd EJ, Bildfell RJ, Frank SA, Mitchell TG, Marr KA, Heitman J. Molecular evidence that the range of the Vancouver Island outbreak of *Cryptococcus gattii* infection has expanded into the Pacific Northwest in the United States. J Infect Dis. 2009; 199:1081–6.
10. Mitchell TG, Perfect JR. Cryptococcosis in the era of AIDS–100 years after the discovery of *Cryptococcus neoformans*. Clin Microbiol Rev. 1995;8:515–48.
11. Kwon-Chung KJ, Bennett JE. Epidemiologic differences between the two varieties of *Cryptococcus neoformans*. Am J Epidemiol. 1984;120:123–30.
12. Kwon-Chung KJ. A new species of Filobasidiella, the sexual state of *Cryptococcus neoformans* B and C serotypes. Mycologia. 1976; 68:943–6.
13. Min KH, Kwon-Chung KJ. The biochemical basis for the distinction between the two *Cryptococcus neoformans* varieties with CGB medium. Zbl Bakt Mik Hyg. 1986;261:471–80.
14. Levitz SM. The ecology of *Cryptococcus neoformans* and the epidemiology of cryptococcosis. Rev Infect Dis. 1991;13:1163–9.
15. Emmons CW. Saprophytic sources of *Cryptococcus neoformans* associated with the pigeon (*Columba livia*). Am J Hyg. 1955;62: 227–32.
16. Girish Kumar KCP, Prabu D, Mitani H, Mikami Y, Menon T. Environmental isolation of *Cryptococcus neoformans* and *Cryptococcus gattii* from living trees in Guindy National Park, Chennai, South India. Mycoses. 2010;53:262–4.
17. Refojo N, Perrotta D, Brudny M, Abrantes R, Hevia AI, Davel G. Isolation of *Cryptococcus neoformans* and *Cryptococcus gattii* from trunk hollows of living trees in Buenos Aires City, Argentina. Med Mycol. 2009;47:177–84.
18. Granados DP, Castaneda E. Isolation and characterization of *Cryptococcus neoformans* varieties recovered from natural sources in Bogota, Colombia, and study of ecological conditions in the area. Microb Ecol. 2005;49:282–90.
19. Ellis DH, Pfeiffer TJ. Natural habitat of *Cryptococcus neoformans* var. *gattii*. J Clin Microbiol. 1990;28:1642–4.
20. Chen SC, Currie BJ, Campbell HM, et al. *Cryptococcus neoformans* var. *gattii* infection in northern Australia: existence of an environmental source other than known host eucalypts. Trans R Soc Trop Med Hyg. 1997;91:547–50.
21. Fink JN, Barboriak JJ, Kaufman L. Cryptococcal antibodies in pigeon breeders' disease. J Allergy. 1968;41:297–301.
22. Newberry Jr WM, Walter JE, Chandler Jr JW, Tosh FE. Epidemiologic study of *Cryptococcus neoformans*. Ann Intern Med. 1967;67:724–32.
23. Hajjeh RA, Conn LA, Stephens DS, Cryptococcal Active Surveillance Group, et al. Cryptococcosis: population-based multistate active surveillance and risk factors in human immunodeficiency virus-infected persons. J Infect Dis. 1999;179:449–54.
24. Powell KE, Dahl BA, Weeks RJ, Tosh FE. Airborne *Cryptococcus neoformans*: particles from pigeon excreta compatible with alveolar deposition. J Infect Dis. 1972;125:412–5.
25. Swinne D, Deppner M, Laroche R, Floch JJ, Kadende P. Isolation of *Cryptococcus neoformans* from houses of AIDS-associated cryptococcosis patients in Bujumbura (Burundi). AIDS (London). 1989;3:389–90.
26. Duperval R, Hermans PE, Brewer NS, Roberts GD. Cryptococcosis, with emphasis on the significance of isolation of *Cryptococcus neoformans* from the respiratory tract. Chest. 1977;72:13–9.
27. Tynes B, Mason KN, Jennings AE, Bennett JE. Variant forms of pulmonary cryptococcosis. Ann Intern Med. 1968;69:1117–25.
28. Beyt Jr BE, Waltman SR. Cryptococcal endophthalmitis after corneal transplantation. N Engl J Med. 1978;298:825–6.

29. Glaser JB, Garden A. Inoculation of cryptococcosis without transmission of the acquired immunodeficiency syndrome. N Engl J Med. 1985;313:266.
30. Kanj SS, Welty-Wolf K, Madden J, et al. Fungal infections in lung and heart-lung transplant recipients. Report of 9 cases and review of the literature. Medicine. 1996;75:142–56.
31. de Castro LE, Sarraf OA, Lally JM, Sandoval HP, Solomon KD, Vroman DT. *Cryptococcus albidus* keratitis after corneal transplantation. Cornea. 2005;24:882–3.
32. Nosanchuk JD, Shoham S, Fries BC, Shapiro DS, Levitz SM, Casadevall A. Evidence of zoonotic transmission of *Cryptococcus neoformans* from a pet cockatoo to an immunocompromised patient. Ann Intern Med. 2000;132:205–8.
33. Lagrou K, Van Eldere J, Keuleers S, et al. Zoonotic transmission of *Cryptococcus neoformans* from a magpie to an immunocompetent patient. J Intern Med. 2005;257:385–8.
34. Shrestha RK, Stoller JK, Honari G, Procop GW, Gordon SM. Pneumonia due to *Cryptococcus neoformans* in a patient receiving infliximab: possible zoonotic transmission from a pet cockatiel. Respir Care. 2004;49:606–8.
35. Pappas PG, Perfect JR, Cloud GA, et al. Cryptococcosis in human immunodeficiency virus-negative patients in the era of effective azole therapy. Clin Infect Dis. 2001;33:690–9.
36. Vilchez RA, Irish W, Lacomis J, Costello P, Fung J, Kusne S. The clinical epidemiology of pulmonary cryptococcosis in non-AIDS patients at a tertiary care medical center. Medicine. 2001;80:308–12.
37. Sun HY, Wagener MM, Singh N. Cryptococcosis in solid-organ, hematopoietic stem cell, and tissue transplant recipients: evidence-based evolving trends. Clin Infect Dis. 2009;48:1566–76.
38. Kontoyiannis DP, Peitsch WK, Reddy BT, et al. Cryptococcosis in patients with cancer. Clin Infect Dis. 2001;32:e145–50.
39. Chayakulkeeree M, Perfect JR. Cryptococcosis. Infect Dis Clin N Am. 2006;20:507–44.
40. Hage CA, Wood KL, Winer-Muram HT, Wilson SJ, Sarosi G, Knox KS. Pulmonary cryptococcosis after initiation of anti-tumor necrosis factor-alpha therapy. Chest. 2003;124:2395–7.
41. Silveira FP, Husain S, Kwak EJ, et al. Cryptococcosis in liver and kidney transplant recipients receiving anti-thymocyte globulin or alemtuzumab. Transpl Infect Dis. 2007;9:22–7.
42. Peleg AY, Husain S, Kwak EJ, et al. Opportunistic infections in 547 organ transplant recipients receiving alemtuzumab, a humanized monoclonal CD-52 antibody. Clin Infect Dis. 2007;44:204–12.
43. Munoz P, Giannella M, Valerio M, et al. Cryptococcal meningitis in a patient treated with infliximab. Diagn Microbiol Infect Dis. 2007;57:443–6.
44. Lewis JL, Rabinovich S. The wide spectrum of cryptococcal infections. Am J Med. 1972;53:315–22.
45. Dismukes WE, Cloud G, Gallis HA, et al. Treatment of cryptococcal meningitis with combination amphotericin B and flucytosine for four as compared with six weeks. N Engl J Med. 1987;317:334–41.
46. Zonios DI, Falloon J, Huang CY, Chaitt D, Bennett JE. Cryptococcosis and idiopathic CD4 lymphocytopenia. Medicine (Baltimore). 2007;86:78–92.
47. Duncan RA, von Reyn CF, Alliegro GM, Toossi Z, Sugar AM, Levitz SM. Idiopathic CD4+ T-lymphocytopenia – four patients with opportunistic infections and no evidence of HIV infection. N Engl J Med. 1993;328:393–8.
48. Currie BP, Casadevall A. Estimation of the prevalence of cryptococcal infection among patients infected with the human immunodeficiency virus in New York City. Clin Infect Dis. 1994;19:1029–33.
49. Dismukes WE. Antifungal therapy: from amphotericin B to present. Trans Am Clin Climatol Assoc. 1993;104:166–77. discussion 77–9.
50. Dromer F, Mathoulin S, Dupont B, Laporte A, French Cryptococcosis Study Group. Epidemiology of cryptococcosis in France: a 9-year survey (1985–1993). Clin Infect Dis. 1996;23:82–90.
51. Dromer F, Mathoulin-Pelissier S, Fontanet A, Ronin O, Dupont B, Lortholary O. Epidemiology of HIV-associated cryptococcosis in France (1985–2001): comparison of the pre- and post-HAART eras. AIDS (London). 2004;18:555–62.
52. Mirza SA, Phelan M, Rimland D, et al. The changing epidemiology of cryptococcosis: an update from population-based active surveillance in 2 large metropolitan areas, 1992–2000. Clin Infect Dis. 2003;36:789–94.
53. Chen SC. Cryptococcosis in Australasia and the treatment of cryptococcal and other fungal infections with liposomal amphotericin B. J Antimicrob Chemother. 2002;49 Suppl 1:57–61.
54. Hakim JG, Gangaidzo IT, Heyderman RS, et al. Impact of HIV infection on meningitis in Harare, Zimbabwe: a prospective study of 406 predominantly adult patients. AIDS (London). 2000;14:1401–7.
55. Jarvis JN, Boulle A, Loyse A, et al. High ongoing burden of cryptococcal disease in Africa despite antiretroviral roll out. AIDS (London). 2009;23:1182–3.
56. Heyderman RS, Gangaidzo IT, Hakim JG, et al. Cryptococcal meningitis in human immunodeficiency virus-infected patients in Harare, Zimbabwe. Clin Infect Dis. 1998;26:284–9.
57. Park BJ, Wannemuehler KA, Marston BJ, Govender N, Pappas PG, Chiller TM. Estimation of the current global burden of cryptococcal meningitis among persons living with HIV/AIDS. AIDS (London). 2009;23:525–30.
58. Goldman D, Lee SC, Casadevall A. Pathogenesis of pulmonary *Cryptococcus neoformans* infection in the rat. Infect Immun. 1994;62:4755–61.
59. Kwon-Chung KJ, Kozel TR, Edman JC, et al. Recent advances in biology and immunology of *Cryptococcus neoformans*. J Med Vet Mycol. 1992;30 Suppl 1:133–42.
60. Bolanos B, Mitchell TG. Phagocytosis of *Cryptococcus neoformans* by rat alveolar macrophages. J Med Vet Mycol. 1989;27: 203–17.
61. Harrison TS, Levitz SM. Mechanisms of impaired anticryptococcal activity of monocytes from donors infected with human immunodeficiency virus. J Infect Dis. 1997;176:537–40.
62. Levitz SM, Mathews HL, Murphy JW. Direct antimicrobial activity of T cells. Immunol Today. 1995;16:387–91.
63. Casadevall A. Antibody immunity and invasive fungal infections. Infect Immun. 1995;63:4211–8.
64. Lendvai N, Casadevall A, Liang Z, Goldman DL, Mukherjee J, Zuckier L. Effect of immune mechanisms on the pharmacokinetics and organ distribution of cryptococcal polysaccharide. J Infect Dis. 1998;177:1647–59.
65. Rachini A, Pietrella D, Lupo P, et al. An anti-beta-glucan monoclonal antibody inhibits growth and capsule formation of *Cryptococcus neoformans* in vitro and exerts therapeutic, anticryptococcal activity in vivo. Infect Immun. 2007;75:5085–94.
66. Buchanan KL, Murphy JW. What makes *Cryptococcus neoformans* a pathogen? Emerg Infect Dis. 1998;4:71–83.
67. Ma H, May RC. Virulence in *Cryptococcus* species. Adv Appl Microbiol. 2009;67:131–90.
68. Heitman J, Kozel T, Kwon-Chung J, Perfect J, Casadevall A, editors. *Cryptococcus*: From human pathogen to model yeast. Washington, DC: American Society for Microbiology Press; 2010.
69. Chang YC, Kwon-Chung KJ. Complementation of a capsule-deficient mutation of *Cryptococcus neoformans* restores its virulence. Mol Cell Biol. 1994;14:4912–9.
70. Guerrero A, Jain N, Goldman DL, Fries BC. Phenotypic switching in *Cryptococcus neoformans*. Microbiology. 2006;152:3–9.
71. Bulmer GS, Sans MD. *Cryptococcus neoformans*. 3. Inhibition of phagocytosis. J Bacteriol. 1968;95:5–8.
72. Levitz SM, Tabuni A, Kornfeld H, Reardon CC, Golenbock DT. Production of tumor necrosis factor alpha in human leukocytes stimulated by *Cryptococcus neoformans*. Infect Immun. 1994;62: 1975–81.

73. Collins HL, Bancroft GJ. Encapsulation of *Cryptococcus neoformans* impairs antigen-specific T-cell responses. Infect Immun. 1991;59:3883–8.
74. Kwon-Chung KJ, Polacheck I, Popkin TJ. Melanin-lacking mutants of *Cryptococcus neoformans* and their virulence for mice. J Bacteriol. 1982;150:1414–21.
75. Wang Y, Aisen P, Casadevall A. *Cryptococcus neoformans* melanin and virulence: mechanism of action. Infect Immun. 1995;63: 3131–6.
76. Rittershaus PC, Kechichian TB, Allegood JC, et al. Glucosylceramide synthase is an essential regulator of pathogenicity of *Cryptococcus neoformans*. J Clin Invest. 2006;116:1651–9.
77. Garcia J, Shea J, Alvarez-Vasquez F, et al. Mathematical modeling of pathogenicity of *Cryptococcus neoformans*. Mol Syst Biol. 2008;4:183.
78. Visnegarwala F, Graviss EA, Lacke CE, et al. Acute respiratory failure associated with cryptococcosis in patients with AIDS: analysis of predictive factors. Clin Infect Dis. 1998;27:1231–7.
79. Murray RJ, Becker P, Furth P, Criner GJ. Recovery from cryptococcemia and the adult respiratory distress syndrome in the acquired immunodeficiency syndrome. Chest. 1988;93:1304–6.
80. Chang WC, Tzao C, Hsu HH, et al. Pulmonary cryptococcosis: comparison of clinical and radiographic characteristics in immunocompetent and immunocompromised patients. Chest. 2006;129: 333–40.
81. Kerkering TM, Duma RJ, Shadomy S. The evolution of pulmonary cryptococcosis: clinical implications from a study of 41 patients with and without compromising host factors. Ann Intern Med. 1981;94:611–6.
82. Pappas PG. Therapy of cryptococcal meningitis in non-HIV-infected patients. Curr Infect Dis Rep. 2001;3:365–70.
83. Baddley JW, Perfect JR, Oster RA, et al. Pulmonary cryptococcosis in patients without HIV infection: factors associated with disseminated disease. Eur J Clin Microbiol Infect Dis. 2008;27: 937–43.
84. Roebuck DJ, Fisher DA, Currie BJ. Cryptococcosis in HIV negative patients: findings on chest radiography. Thorax. 1998;53:554–7.
85. Oliveira Fde M, Severo CB, Guazzelli LS, Severo LC. *Cryptococcus gattii* fungemia: report of a case with lung and brain lesions mimicking radiological features of malignancy. Rev Inst Med Trop São Paulo. 2007;49:263–5.
86. Speed B, Dunt D. Clinical and host differences between infections with the two varieties of *Cryptococcus neoformans*. Clin Infect Dis. 1995;21:28–34.
87. Khoury MB, Godwin JD, Ravin CE, Gallis HA, Halvorsen RA, Putman CE. Thoracic cryptococcosis: immunologic competence and radiologic appearance. Am J Roentgenol. 1984;142:893–6.
88. Shirley RM, Baddley JW. Cryptococcal lung disease. Curr Opin Pulm Med. 2009;15:254–60.
89. Woodring JH, Ciporkin G, Lee C, Worm B, Woolley S. Pulmonary cryptococcosis. Semin Roentgenol. 1996;31:67–75.
90. Cameron ML, Bartlett JA, Gallis HA, Waskin HA. Manifestations of pulmonary cryptococcosis in patients with acquired immunodeficiency syndrome. Rev Infect Dis. 1991;13:64–7.
91. Meyohas MC, Roux P, Bollens D, et al. Pulmonary cryptococcosis: localized and disseminated infections in 27 patients with AIDS. Clin Infect Dis. 1995;21:628–33.
92. Saag MS, Powderly WG, Cloud GA, The NIAID Mycoses Study Group and the AIDS Clinical Trials Group, et al. Comparison of amphotericin B with fluconazole in the treatment of acute AIDS-associated cryptococcal meningitis. N Engl J Med. 1992;326:83–9.
93. van der Horst CM, Saag MS, Cloud GA, National Institute of Allergy and Infectious Diseases Mycoses Study Group and AIDS Clinical Trials Group, et al. Treatment of cryptococcal meningitis associated with the acquired immunodeficiency syndrome. N Engl J Med. 1997;337:15–21.
94. Graybill JR, Sobel J, Saag M, The NIAID Mycoses Study Group and AIDS Cooperative Treatment Groups, et al. Diagnosis and management of increased intracranial pressure in patients with AIDS and cryptococcal meningitis. Clin Infect Dis. 2000;30: 47–54.
95. Pappas PG. Managing cryptococcal meningitis is about handling the pressure. Clin Infect Dis. 2005;40:480–2.
96. Bicanic T, Brouwer AE, Meintjes G, et al. Relationship of cerebrospinal fluid pressure, fungal burden and outcome in patients with cryptococcal meningitis undergoing serial lumbar punctures. AIDS (London). 2009;23:701–6.
97. Fujita NK, Reynard M, Sapico FL, Guze LB, Edwards Jr JE. Cryptococcal intracerebral mass lesions: the role of computed tomography and nonsurgical management. Ann Intern Med. 1981; 94:382–8.
98. Charlier C, Dromer F, Leveque C, et al. Cryptococcal neuroradiological lesions correlate with severity during cryptococcal meningoencephalitis in HIV-positive patients in the HAART era. PloS. 2008;3:e1950.
99. Singh N, Lortholary O, Dromer F, et al. Central nervous system cryptococcosis in solid organ transplant recipients: clinical relevance of abnormal neuroimaging findings. Transplantation. 2008;86:647–51.
100. Mitchell DH, Sorrell TC, Allworth AM, et al. Cryptococcal disease of the CNS in immunocompetent hosts: influence of cryptococcal variety on clinical manifestations and outcome. Clin Infect Dis. 1995;20:611–6.
101. Popovich MJ, Arthur RH, Helmer E. CT of intracranial cryptococcosis. Am J Roentgenol. 1990;154:603–6.
102. Park MK, Hospenthal DR, Bennett JE. Treatment of hydrocephalus secondary to cryptococcal meningitis by use of shunting. Clin Infect Dis. 1999;28:629–33.
103. Liliang PC, Liang CL, Chang WN, Lu K, Lu CH. Use of ventriculoperitoneal shunts to treat uncontrollable intracranial hypertension in patients who have cryptococcal meningitis without hydrocephalus. Clin Infect Dis. 2002;34:E64–8.
104. Diamond RD, Bennett JE. Prognostic factors in cryptococcal meningitis. A study in 111 cases. Ann Intern Med. 1974;80:176–81.
105. Lu CH, Chang WN, Chang HW, Chuang YC. The prognostic factors of cryptococcal meningitis in HIV-negative patients. J Hosp Infect. 1999;42:313–20.
106. Powderly WG, Saag MS, Cloud GA, The NIAID AIDS Clinical Trials Group and Mycoses Study Group, et al. A controlled trial of fluconazole or amphotericin B to prevent relapse of cryptococcal meningitis in patients with the acquired immunodeficiency syndrome. N Engl J Med. 1992;326:793–8.
107. Powderly WG, Cloud GA, Dismukes WE, Saag MS. Measurement of cryptococcal antigen in serum and cerebrospinal fluid: value in the management of AIDS-associated cryptococcal meningitis. Clin Infect Dis. 1994;18:789–92.
108. Bicanic T, Wood R, Meintjes G, et al. High-dose amphotericin B with flucytosine for the treatment of cryptococcal meningitis in HIV-infected patients: a randomized trial. Clin Infect Dis. 2008;47: 123–30.
109. McNeil MM, Nash SL, Hajjeh RA, et al. Trends in mortality due to invasive mycotic diseases in the United States, 1980–1997. Clin Infect Dis. 2001;33:641–7.
110. Baer S, Baddley JW, Gnann JW, Pappas PG. Cryptococcal disease presenting as necrotizing cellulitis in transplant recipients. Transpl Infect Dis 2009.
111. Pema K, Diaz J, Guerra LG, Nabhan D, Verghese A. Disseminated cutaneous cryptococcosis. Comparison of clinical manifestations in the pre-AIDS and AIDS eras. Arch Intern Med. 1994;154: 1032–4.
112. Anderson DJ, Schmidt C, Goodman J, Pomeroy C. Cryptococcal disease presenting as cellulitis. Clin Infect Dis. 1992;14:666–72.

113. Casadevall A, Mukherjee J, Yuan R, Perfect J. Management of injuries caused by *Cryptococcus neoformans*-contaminated needles. Clin Infect Dis. 1994;19:951–3.
114. Neuville S, Dromer F, Morin O, Dupont B, Ronin O, Lortholary O. Primary cutaneous cryptococcosis: a distinct clinical entity. Clin Infect Dis. 2003;36:337–47.
115. Behrman RE, Masci JR, Nicholas P. Cryptococcal skeletal infections: case report and review. Rev Infect Dis. 1990;12:181–90.
116. Nottebart HC, McGehee RF, Utz JP. *Cryptococcus neoformans* osteomyelitis: case report of two patients. Sabouraudia. 1974;12: 127–32.
117. Stead KJ, Klugman KP, Painter ML, Koornhof HJ. Septic arthritis due to *Cryptococcus neoformans*. J Infect. 1988;17:139–45.
118. Perfect JR. Cryptococcosis. Infect Dis Clin N Am. 1989;3:77–102.
119. Braman RT. Cryptococcosis (torulosis) of prostate. Urology. 1981;17:284–5.
120. Crump JR, Elner SG, Elner VM, Kauffman CA. Cryptococcal endophthalmitis: case report and review. Clin Infect Dis. 1992;14: 1069–73.
121. Leavitt AD, Kauffman CA. Cryptococcal aortitis. Am J Med. 1988;85:108–10.
122. Staib F, Seibold M, L'Age M, et al. *Cryptococcus neoformans* in the seminal fluid of an AIDS patient. A contribution to the clinical course of cryptococcosis. Mycoses. 1989;32:171–80.
123. Larsen RA, Bozzette S, McCutchan JA, Chiu J, Leal MA, Richman DD, et al. Persistent *Cryptococcus neoformans* infection of the prostate after successful treatment of meningitis. Ann Intern Med. 1989;111:125–8.
124. Bicanic T, Meintjes G, Rebe K, et al. Immune reconstitution inflammatory syndrome in HIV-associated cryptococcal meningitis: a prospective study. J Acquir Immune Defic Syndr. 2009;51: 130–4.
125. Lortholary O, Fontanet A, Memain N, Martin A, Sitbon K, Dromer F. Incidence and risk factors of immune reconstitution inflammatory syndrome complicating HIV-associated cryptococcosis in France. AIDS (London). 2005;19:1043–9.
126. Shelburne 3rd SA, Darcourt J, White Jr AC, et al. The role of immune reconstitution inflammatory syndrome in AIDS-related *Cryptococcus neoformans* disease in the era of highly active antiretroviral therapy. Clin Infect Dis. 2005;40:1049–52.
127. Singh N, Lortholary O, Alexander BD, et al. An immune reconstitution syndrome-like illness associated with *Cryptococcus neoformans* infection in organ transplant recipients. Clin Infect Dis. 2005;40:1756–61.
128. Shelburne SA, Visnegarwala F, Darcourt J, et al. Incidence and risk factors for immune reconstitution inflammatory syndrome during highly active antiretroviral therapy. AIDS. 2005;19:399–406.
129. Singh N, Dromer F, Perfect JR, Lortholary O. Cryptococcosis in solid organ transplant recipients: current state of the science. Clin Infect Dis. 2008;47:1321–7.
130. Bennett JE, Dismukes WE, Duma RJ, et al. A comparison of amphotericin B alone and combined with flucytosine in the treatment of cryptococcal meningitis. N Engl J Med. 1979;301:126–31.
131. Aberg JA, Mundy LM, Powderly WG. Pulmonary cryptococcosis in patients without HIV infection. Chest. 1999;115:734–40.
132. Campbell CK, Payne AL, Teall AJ, Brownell A, Mackenzie DW. Cryptococcal latex antigen test positive in patient with *Trichosporon beigelii* infection. Lancet. 1985;2(8445):43–4.
133. Tarrand JJ, Guillot C, Wenglar M, Jackson J, Lajeunesse JD, Rolston KV. Clinical comparison of the resin-containing BACTEC 26 Plus and the Isolator 10 blood culturing systems. J Clin Microbiol. 1991;29:2245–9.
134. Reference method for broth dilution antifungal susceptibility testing of yeasts: approved standard, 3rd edn., M23-A3. Wayne: Clinical Laboratory Standards Institute, 2008.
135. Brandt ME, Pfaller MA, Hajjeh RA, et al. Trends in antifungal drug susceptibility of *Cryptococcus neoformans* isolates in the United States: 1992 to 1994 and 1996 to 1998. Antimicrob Agents Chemother. 2001;45:3065–9.
136. Pfaller MA, Diekema DJ, Gibbs DL, et al. Results from the ARTEMIS DISK Global Antifungal Surveillance Study, 1997 to 2007: 10.5-year analysis of susceptibilities of noncandidal yeast species to fluconazole and voriconazole determined by CLSI standardized disk diffusion testing. J Clin Microbiol. 2009;47:117–23.
137. Torres-Rodriguez JM, Alvarado-Ramirez E, Murciano F, Sellart M. MICs and minimum fungicidal concentrations of posaconazole, voriconazole and fluconazole for *Cryptococcus neoformans* and *Cryptococcus gattii*. J Antimicrob Chemother. 2008;62:205–6.
138. Bartizal K, Gill CJ, Abruzzo GK, et al. In vitro preclinical evaluation studies with the echinocandin antifungal MK-0991 (L-743, 872). Antimicrob Agents Chemother. 1997;41:2326–32.
139. Aller AI, Martin-Mazuelos E, Lozano F, et al. Correlation of fluconazole MICs with clinical outcome in cryptococcal infection. Antimicrob Agents Chemother. 2000;44:1544–8.
140. Armengou A, Porcar C, Mascaro J, Garcia-Bragado F. Possible development of resistance to fluconazole during suppressive therapy for AIDS-associated cryptococcal meningitis. Clin Infect Dis. 1996;23:1337–8.
141. Witt MD, Lewis RJ, Larsen RA, et al. Identification of patients with acute AIDS-associated cryptococcal meningitis who can be effectively treated with fluconazole: the role of antifungal susceptibility testing. Clin Infect Dis. 1996;22:322–8.
142. Perfect JR, Dismukes WE, Dromer F, et al. Clinical practice guidelines for the management of cryptococcal disease: 2010 update by the Infectious Disease Society of America. Clin Infect Dis. 2010;50:291–322.
143. Hospenthal DR, Bennett JE. Flucytosine monotherapy for cryptococcosis. Clin Infect Dis. 1998;27:260–4.
144. Harrison TS. Amphotericin B plus fluconazole for HIV-associated cryptococcal meningitis. Clin Infect Dis. 2009;48:1784–6.
145. Pappas PG, Chetchotisakd P, Larsen RA, et al. A phase II randomized trial of amphotericin B alone or combined with fluconazole in the treatment of HIV-associated cryptococcal meningitis. Clin Infect Dis. 2009;48:1775–83.
146. Dromer F, Mathoulin S, Dupont B, Brugiere O, Letenneur L, French Cryptococcosis Study Group. Comparison of the efficacy of amphotericin B and fluconazole in the treatment of cryptococcosis in human immunodeficiency virus-negative patients: retrospective analysis of 83 cases. Clin Infect Dis. 1996;22 Suppl 2:S154–60.
147. Nadrous HF, Antonios VS, Terrell CL, Ryu JH. Pulmonary cryptococcosis in nonimmunocompromised patients. Chest. 2003;124: 2143–7.
148. Jarvis JN, Harrison TS. Pulmonary cryptococcosis. Semin Respir Crit Care Med. 2008;29:141–50.
149. Yamaguchi H, Ikemoto H, Watanabe K, Ito A, Hara K, Kohno S. Fluconazole monotherapy for cryptococcosis in non-AIDS patients. Eur J Clin Microbiol Infect Dis. 1996;15:787–92.
150. Denning DW, Tucker RM, Hanson LH, Hamilton JR, Stevens DA. Itraconazole therapy for cryptococcal meningitis and cryptococcosis. Arch Intern Med. 1989;149:2301–8.
151. Raad II, Graybill JR, Bustamante AB, et al. Safety of long-term oral posaconazole use in the treatment of refractory invasive fungal infections. Clin Infect Dis. 2006;42:1726–34.
152. Perfect JR, Marr KA, Walsh TJ, et al. Voriconazole treatment for less-common, emerging, or refractory fungal infections. Clin Infect Dis. 2003;36:1122–31.
153. Sharkey PK, Graybill JR, Johnson ES, et al. Amphotericin B lipid complex compared with amphotericin B in the treatment of cryptococcal meningitis in patients with AIDS. Clin Infect Dis. 1996;22:315–21.

154. Coker RJ, Viviani M, Gazzard BG, et al. Treatment of cryptococcosis with liposomal amphotericin B (AmBisome) in 23 patients with AIDS. AIDS (London, England). 1993;7:829–35.
155. Leenders AC, Reiss P, Portegies P, et al. Liposomal amphotericin B (AmBisome) compared with amphotericin B both followed by oral fluconazole in the treatment of AIDS-associated cryptococcal meningitis. AIDS (London). 1997;11:1463–71.
156. Hammerman KJ, Powell KE, Christianson CS, et al. Pulmonary cryptococcosis: clinical forms and treatment. A Center for Disease Control Cooperative Mycoses study. Am Rev Respir Dis. 1973;108:1116–23.
157. Husain S, Wagener MM, Singh N. *Cryptococcus neoformans* infection in organ transplant recipients: variables influencing clinical characteristics and outcome. Emerg Infect Dis. 2001;7:375–81.
158. Hospenthal DR, Bennett JE. Persistence of cryptococcomas on neuroimaging. Clin Infect Dis. 2000;31:1303–6.
159. Larsen RA, Bozzette SA, Jones BE, et al. Fluconazole combined with flucytosine for treatment of cryptococcal meningitis in patients with AIDS. Clin Infect Dis. 1994;19:741–5.
160. Mayanja-Kizza H, Oishi K, Mitarai S, et al. Combination therapy with fluconazole and flucytosine for cryptococcal meningitis in Ugandan patients with AIDS. Clin Infect Dis. 1998;26:1362–6.
161. Menichetti F, Fiorio M, Tosti A, et al. High-dose fluconazole therapy for cryptococcal meningitis in patients with AIDS. Clin Infect Dis. 1996;22:838–40.
162. Haubrich RH, Haghighat D, Bozzette SA, Tilles J, McCutchan JA, The California Collaborative Treatment Group. High-dose fluconazole for treatment of cryptococcal disease in patients with human immunodeficiency virus infection. J Infect Dis. 1994;170:238–42.
163. de Gans J, Portegies P, Tiessens G, et al. Itraconazole compared with amphotericin B plus flucytosine in AIDS patients with cryptococcal meningitis. AIDS (London). 1992;6:185–90.
164. Bozzette SA, Larsen RA, Chiu J, California Collaborative Treatment Group, et al. A placebo-controlled trial of maintenance therapy with fluconazole after treatment of cryptococcal meningitis in the acquired immunodeficiency syndrome. N Engl J Med. 1991;324:580–4.
165. Saag MS, Cloud GA, Graybill JR, National Institute of Allergy and Infectious Diseases Mycoses Study Group, et al. A comparison of itraconazole versus fluconazole as maintenance therapy for AIDS-associated cryptococcal meningitis. Clin Infect Dis. 1999;28:291–6.
166. Kaplan JE, Benson C, Holmes KH, Brooks JT, Pau A, Masur H. Guidelines for prevention and treatment of opportunistic infections in HIV-infected adults and adolescents: recommendations from CDC, the National Institutes of Health, and the HIV Medicine Association of the Infectious Diseases Society of America. MMWR. 2009;58:1–207.
167. Mussini C, Pezzotti P, Miro JM, et al. Discontinuation of maintenance therapy for cryptococcal meningitis in patients with AIDS treated with highly active antiretroviral therapy: an international observational study. Clin Infect Dis. 2004;38:565–71.
168. Vibhagool A, Sungkanuparph S, Mootsikapun P, et al. Discontinuation of secondary prophylaxis for cryptococcal meningitis in human immunodeficiency virus-infected patients treated with highly active antiretroviral therapy: a prospective, multicenter, randomized study. Clin Infect Dis. 2003;36:1329–31.
169. Bicanic T, Meintjes G, Wood R, et al. Fungal burden, early fungicidal activity, and outcome in cryptococcal meningitis in antiretroviral-naive or antiretroviral-experienced patients treated with amphotericin B or fluconazole. Clin Infect Dis. 2007;45:76–80.
170. Chuck SL, Sande MA. Infections with *Cryptococcus neoformans* in the acquired immunodeficiency syndrome. N Engl J Med. 1989;321:794–9.
171. Larsen RA, Leal MA, Chan LS. Fluconazole compared with amphotericin B plus flucytosine for cryptococcal meningitis in AIDS. A randomized trial. Ann Intern Med. 1990;113:183–7.
172. Brouwer AE, Rajanuwong A, Chierakul W, et al. Combination antifungal therapies for HIV-associated cryptococcal meningitis: a randomised trial. Lancet. 2004;363:1764–7.
173. Dromer F, Bernede-Bauduin C, Guillemot D, Lortholary O. Major role for amphotericin B-flucytosine combination in severe cryptococcosis. PloS. 2008;3:2870.
174. Baddour LM, Perfect JR, Ostrosky-Zeichner L. Successful use of amphotericin B lipid complex in the treatment of cryptococcosis. Clin Infect Dis. 2005;40 Suppl 6:S409–13.
175. Longley N, Muzoora C, Taseera K, et al. Dose response effect of high-dose fluconazole for HIV-associated cryptococcal meningitis in southwestern Uganda. Clin Infect Dis. 2008;47:1556–61.
176. Aberg JA, Price RW, Heeren DM, Bredt B. A pilot study of the discontinuation of antifungal therapy for disseminated cryptococcal disease in patients with acquired immunodeficiency syndrome, following immunologic response to antiretroviral therapy. J Infect Dis. 2002;185:1179–82.
177. Zolopa A, Andersen J, Komarow L, et al. Immediate vs. deferred ART in the setting of a randomized strategy trial ACTG A5164. 15th Conference on Retroviruses and Opportunistic Infections. February, 2008. Boston. Abstract 142.
178. Newton PN, le Thai H, Tip NQ, et al. A randomized, double-blind, placebo-controlled trial of acetazolamide for the treatment of elevated intracranial pressure in cryptococcal meningitis. Clin Infect Dis. 2002;35:769–72.
179. McKinsey DS, Wheat LJ, Cloud GA, National Institute of Allergy and Infectious Diseases Mycoses Study Group, et al. Itraconazole prophylaxis for fungal infections in patients with advanced human immunodeficiency virus infection: randomized, placebo-controlled, double-blind study. Clin Infect Dis. 1999;28:1049–56.
180. Powderly WG, Finkelstein D, Feinberg J, NIAID AIDS Clinical Trials Group, et al. A randomized trial comparing fluconazole with clotrimazole troches for the prevention of fungal infections in patients with advanced human immunodeficiency virus infection. N Engl J Med. 1995;332:700–5.
181. Jarvis JN, Lawn SD, Vogt M, Bangani N, Wood R, Harrison TS. Screening for cryptococcal antigenemia in patients accessing an antiretroviral treatment program in South Africa. Clin Infect Dis. 2009;48:856–62.
182. Tassie JM, Pepper L, Fogg C, et al. Systematic screening of cryptococcal antigenemia in HIV-positive adults in Uganda. J Acquir Immune Defic Syndr. 2003;33:411–2.
183. Nelson MR, Bower M, Smith D, Reed C, Shanson D, Gazzard B. The value of serum cryptococcal antigen in the diagnosis of cryptococcal infection in patients infected with the human immunodeficiency virus. J Infect. 1990;21:175–81.
184. Desmet P, Kayembe KD, De Vroey C. The value of cryptococcal serum antigen screening among HIV-positive/AIDS patients in Kinshasa, Zaire. AIDS (London). 1989;3:77–8.
185. Liechty CA, Solberg P, Were W, et al. Asymptomatic serum cryptococcal antigenemia and early mortality during antiretroviral therapy in rural Uganda. Trop Med Int Health. 2007;12:929–35.
186. Micol R, Lortholary O, Sar B, et al. Prevalence, determinants of positivity, and clinical utility of cryptococcal antigenemia in Cambodian HIV-infected patients. J Acquir Immune Defic Syndr. 2007;45:555–9.
187. French N, Gray K, Watera C, et al. Cryptococcal infection in a cohort of HIV-1-infected Ugandan adults. AIDS (London). 2002; 16:1031–8.

Rhodotorula, Saccharomyces, Malassezia, Trichosporon, Blastoschizomyces, and Sporobolomyces

Jose A. Vazquez

Yeasts are found ubiquitously in nature in association with plants, mammals, and insects. Humans are continually exposed to multiple genera of yeasts via various routes. Depending on the interaction between host mucosal defense mechanisms and fungal virulence factors, yeast colonization may be transient or persistent and either systemic or local disease can ensue.

Yeast organisms are usually of low virulence and frequently require a significant alteration or reduction in host defenses prior to tissue invasion. Recently, because of the increased population of immunocompromised patients and the use of azole prophylaxis, the frequency of infections due to non-*Candida* yeast infections has increased in frequency [1, 2].

Rhodotorulosis

Rhodotorulosis results from infection with the genus *Rhodotorula* [3]. Although the yeast is recovered worldwide from a variety of sources, infection is generally only seen in the immunocompromised host [3–5].

Mycology

The fungi from the genus *Rhodotorula* are imperfect basidiomycetous yeasts belonging to the family Cryptococcaceae [3, 4]. There are eight species in the genus *Rhodotorula* [5–7]. *Rhodotorula rubra (R. mucilaginosa)* is the species most frequently associated with human infection [5, 8]. The other less commonly isolated species include *R. glutinis*, *R. pilimanae*, *R. pallida*, *R. aurantiaca*, *R. minuta* (syn, *R. marina*) [5]. The majority of *Rhodotorula* species produce red-to-orange colonies due to the presence of carotenoid pigments [3, 4] (Fig. 1). The yeast is mucoid, encapsulated, rarely forms mycelia, and readily grows on almost all types of culture media. *Rhodotorula* is very similar to *Cryptococcus* in rate of growth, cell size and shape, presence of capsule, and the ability to split urea. Differences include the inability of *Rhodotorula* to assimilate inositol and to ferment sugars [3, 4]. *Rhodotorula* can be differentiated from other red-pigmented yeast, such as *Sporobolomyces*, by the lack of ballistospore formation.

In vitro susceptibility studies (Table 1) reveal that currently approved antifungals have a wide degree of activity against *Rhodotorula* [9–15]. *Rhodotorula* spp. are susceptible to amphotericin B, and minimum inhibitory concentrations (MIC) range from 0.25 to 1.0 μg/mL [9–11]. *Rhodotorula* are less susceptible to azoles; MICs to fluconazole range from 0.5 to 64 μg/mL; itraconazole, 0.25–16 μg/mL; ketoconazole, 0.4–0.8 μg/mL; posaconazole 0.5–4.0 μg/mL; voriconazole 0.25–4.0 μg/mL; and isavuconazole 0.03–0.125 μg/mL [9–15]. In addition, *Rhodotorula* species are susceptible to flucytosine, MIC range 0.06–0.5 μg/mL [11]. In contrast, *Rhodotorula* spp. appear to be intrinsically resistant to the echinocandins; MICs to caspofungin range from 16 to >16 μg/mL and to micafungin from 16 to 64 μg/mL [9, 10].

Epidemiology

Rhodotorula species are commonly recovered from seawater, plants, air, food (cheese and milk products, fruit juices) [3, 4, 16], and occasionally from humans. They are frequently recovered as an airborne laboratory contaminant [3, 4, 16]. Additionally, *Rhodotorula* are commonly recovered from shower curtains, bathtub–wall junctions, and toothbrushes. In humans, *Rhodotorula* spp. have been recovered from the skin [17], nails [18, 19], respiratory tract, urinary tract [17, 18], gastrointestinal tract [20], and bloodstream [19, 21, 22].

R. rubra and *R. glutinis* account for approximately 0.5% of yeasts isolated from the oral cavity and more than 12% of yeast isolates from stool and rectal swabs [23]. It is important

J.A. Vazquez (✉)
Division of Infectious Diseases Henry Ford Hospital,
Wayne State University School of Medicine, Detroit, MI, USA
e-mail: jvazque1@hfhs.org

C.A. Kauffman et al. (eds.), *Essentials of Clinical Mycology*,
DOI 10.1007/978-1-4419-6640-7_13, © Springer Science+Business Media, LLC 2011

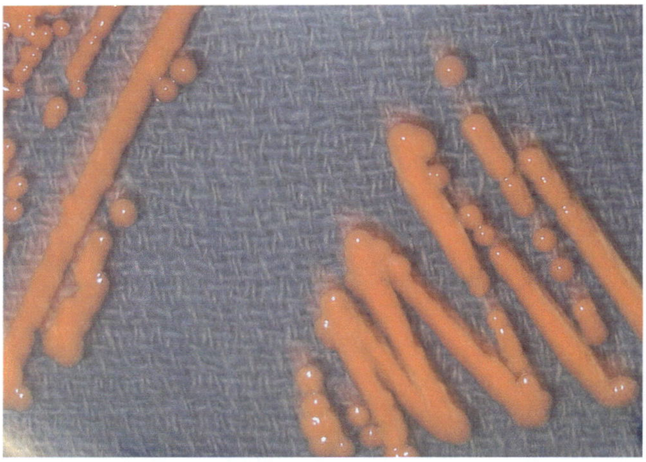

Fig. 1 Glistening smooth moist colonies of *Rhodotorula rubra*. The color can range from deep coral to pink to salmon. The colony borders are usually smooth, but also can be mucoid

Table 1 In vitro antifungal susceptibilities of *Rhodotorula* spp. [9–15]

Yeast	Antifungal Agent	MIC Range μg/mL
Rhodutorula spp.	Amphotericin B	0.25–1.0
	Itraconazole	0.25–16
	Fluconazole	0.5–64
	Voriconazole	0.25–4.0
	Posaconazole	0.5– 4.0
	Ravuconazole	0.25–2.0
	Isavuconazole	0.03–0.125
	Caspofungin	8–>16
	Micafungin	16–64
	Flucytosine	0.06–0.5

to note that the recovery of *Rhodotorula* species from human sources, especially mucosal sites, has frequently been of questionable clinical significance, although isolation from numerous sterile body sites has now been described [24].

Catheter-related infection is the most common form of infection associated with *Rhodotorula* [5, 25]. The most common underlying risk factors include hematologic and solid organ malignancies, chronic renal failure, continuous ambulatory peritoneal dialysis, cirrhosis, use of total parenteral nutrition, cirrhosis, neutropenia, corticosteroids, HIV infection, and solid organ and stem cell transplantation [5, 9, 25].

Clinical Manifestations

Clinical signs and symptoms of *Rhodotorula* infection are nonspecific, and vary from subtle and mild to severe, including septic shock. *Rhodotorula* have been incriminated in a wide spectrum of infections, including fungemia [5, 9, 19, 22, 26–29], endocarditis [30], peritonitis [31], meningitis and ventriculitis [5, 24], prosthetic joint infection [32], endophthalmitis [5] and disseminated disease [5, 33].

Rhodotorula fungemia is the most common form of infection. In most cases, it is associated with intravascular catheters in patients receiving either chemotherapy or long-term antimicrobials [5, 8, 9, 19, 22, 25, 26, 34, 35]. Fever is the most frequent manifestation associated with fungemia.

Endocarditis. A fatal case of aortic valve endocarditis in a patient with underlying rheumatic heart disease has been described [26]. In addition, a second case of endocarditis in a 7-year-old boy, who was treated successfully with 5-flucytosine, has also been reported [30].

Central Nervous System Infections. Several cases of meningitis and ventriculitis have been described [5]. *R. rubra* was reported in a fatal case of meningitis in a patient with acute leukemia [36]. The patient presented with epistaxis, frontal headaches, right tympanic membrane perforation, followed by fever and chills. The organism was recovered from the cerebrospinal fluid (CSF) on culture, and seen on an India ink stain. The patient was treated with amphotericin B, but did not respond. In a second case of meningitis, *R. rubra* was recovered from the CSF of an HIV-positive patient [24]. The diagnosis was made with a positive CSF culture for *R. rubra*. The patient responded clinically to 15 days of flucytosine, but relapsed 8 months later. *R. rubra* also has been implicated in a case of postoperative ventriculitis in a woman with benign meningioma. The patient was treated successfully with flucytosine and amphotericin B [37].

Peritonitis. Several cases of *R. rubra* peritonitis have been described in patients undergoing continuous ambulatory peritoneal dialysis [5, 31]. Environmental cultures revealed a possible common source outbreak. In all patients, the symptoms were subtle and intermittent at first, and consisted of abdominal pain, anorexia, nausea, and occasional diarrhea. *Rhodotorula* is easily recovered from peritoneal fluid, thereby providing early identification and appropriate antifungal therapy.

Diagnosis

In the majority of proven infections, *Rhodotorula* is recovered from a sterile site of infection. In these cases, the decision to attribute a causal role to *Rhodotorula* is relatively simple, and the patient should be treated appropriately for an invasive fungal infection. A more difficult situation is when the organism is recovered from body sites that may normally harbor *Rhodotorula* species, especially in the absence of signs or symptoms of infection. In this setting, it is necessary to establish true infection instead of colonization.

Rhodotorula species grow readily in blood cultures and any media suitable for yeast, such as Sabouraud dextrose agar. There are no serologic diagnostic tests available.

Treatment

It is difficult to assess the role of antifungal therapy in patients with infection due to the genus *Rhodotorula*. Optimal management of patients with indwelling catheters infected with *Rhodotorula* has not been well defined. There are several reports that document clearance of fungemia and resolution of infection by removing the intravascular catheter in the absence of antifungal therapy [5, 8, 9, 19, 35]. On the other hand, several reports suggest antifungal treatment alone may suffice [5, 14, 19]. Although there are no clinical trials evaluating the best antifungal to use in infections due to *Rhodotorula* spp., in vitro assays have demonstrated that amphotericin B has the best activity [8, 10, 11]. It is important to note that *Rhodotorula* are intrinsically resistant to echinocandins and are relatively resistant to most azoles except for isavuconazole [10–13]. Given that infections due to *Rhodotorula* can be severe and life threatening, it is probably best to manage these infections aggressively by discontinuing the indwelling venous catheter, if possible, and treating with amphotericin B.

Saccharomyces

Saccharomyces is an ascomycetous yeast that is widespread in nature and is occasionally part of the normal flora of the human gastrointestinal and genitourinary tracts [17, 38]. The species includes *S. cerevisiae, S. fragilis,* and *S. carlsbergensis. S. cerevisiae,* also known as brewer's yeast or baker's yeast, has been reported to cause infection in humans. *S. cerevisiae* is better known for its commercial uses, i.e., beer and wine production, health food supplementation, and recently by its use in DNA recombinant technology, than as a human pathogen [3]. *S. cerevisiae* has been found to be a cause of mucosal and disseminated infection in humans, primarily in immunocompromised hosts [38–43].

Mycology

Cells are oval to spherical, measure 3–9 μm by 5–20 μm, and exist as multilateral budding cells as either haploids or diploids [3, 4]. Cells may form short chains and elongate as rudimentary pseudohyphae or form no pseudohyphae. Ascospores, one to four in number, are in either tetrahedral or linear arrangements and are gram-negative (vegetative cells are gram-positive). Colonies are smooth, moist, and either white or cream-colored.

Saccharomyces are almost invariably nonpathogenic. Kiehn and coworkers reviewed more than 3,300 yeast cultures from cancer patients and found only 19 isolates of *S. cerevisiae* [19]. In a more recent review from the University of Minnesota bone marrow transplant program, only two *S. cerevisiae* infections were found out of 138 documented fungal infections over a 15-year period [44].

In the majority of situations the organism is nonpathogenic due to innate low virulence. In early experimental studies, subcutaneous inoculation with *S. cerevisiae* was neither lethal nor invasive for normal and cortisone-treated mice [45]. More recent studies have demonstrated that some clinical isolates of *S. cerevisiae* in CD-1 mice can proliferate and resist clearance in vivo, supporting the role of *S. cerevisiae* as a cause of clinical infection [46].

Epidemiology

Recovery of *Saccharomyces* from human mucosal surfaces rarely is of clinical significance. On the other hand, isolation from sterile body sites has now been described [44, 47]. *Saccharomyces* has been recovered from the bloodstream, lungs, peritoneal cavity, esophagus, urinary tract, and vagina [38, 43, 44, 47].

Recent DNA typing studies evaluating the relatedness between clinical strains and commercial strains of *S. cerevisiae* have demonstrated that commercial products may be a contributing factor in human colonization and infection [48]. Four women suffering from recurrent *S. cerevisiae* vaginitis had exposure to bread dough that contained *S. cerevisiae* genotypes that were identical to those found in the vagina. Furthermore, the husband of one of the women, who worked at a pizza shop, was also colonized subungually by the same strain of *S. cerevisiae* recovered from his wife's vagina [42]. Recently, Cassone et al. reported an outbreak of *S. cerevisiae* subtype *S. boulardii* fungemia among three intensive care unit patients that were in proximity to patients receiving the lyophilized preparation of *S. cerevisiae* [49]. The authors speculated that the yeast colonized the ICU and eventually colonized the skin of those patients, leading to catheter-associated fungemia.

The risk factors associated with *Saccharomyces* infections are similar to the risk factors associated with candidemia and systemic candidiasis, including central venous catheters, neutropenia, antimicrobials, and gastrointestinal tract surgery [39, 41, 50, 51]. There have also been several reports of *S. cerevisiae* fungemia in HIV-positive individuals [52]. Possible portals of entry for invasive disease include the oropharynx, gastrointestinal tract, and skin [51].

Clinical Manifestations

Clinical signs and symptoms of infection are nonspecific and vary from subtle and mild to severe. *Saccharomyces* species have been incriminated in bloodstream infections [3, 39, 43, 50, 51], endocarditis [53, 54], peritonitis [43, 55, 56], disseminated disease [43, 47, 51], pneumonia [39], urinary tract infection [47, 51] and vaginitis [38, 42]. Fungemia, the most common form of infection, is seen in the immunocompromised host and is associated with intravascular catheters, chemotherapy, and antimicrobials [41, 51]. Manifestations are similar to those of systemic candidiasis and candidemia. Fever is the most frequent symptom associated with fungemia, and in the majority of cases, the patients have survived with treatment.

Resp*iratory Tract Infections*. Four suspected cases of pneumonia due to *S. cerevisiae* have been reported. In three out of the four, the patients had underlying hematologic malignancies, and the diagnosis was made on biopsy of lung tissue [39, 43, 51]. There have also been two cases of empyema. In one patient, the empyema resulted from a complication during sclerotherapy for esophageal varices [57].

Peritonitis. There have been two surgical cases in which *S. cerevisiae* was recovered from the peritoneal fluid of symptomatic patients [39, 51]. In both patients, the organism was recovered after surgery for a malignant neoplasm. Both were cured with surgical drainage and antifungal therapy. There has been one reported case of cholecystitis in a patient with diabetes mellitus [58]. *S. cerevisiae* was recovered from the gallbladder and from the stone inside the gallbladder. The patient did well postcholecystectomy and required no antifungal therapy.

Endocarditis. Three documented cases of endocarditis have been reported [43, 51, 53]. All were associated with prosthetic valves, and two were in intravenous heroin users. All three patients were apparently cured with antifungal therapy; in only one patient was the valve replaced.

Genitourinary Tract Infections. There have been three reported cases of urinary tract infections due to *S. cerevisiae* [47, 51]. One patient had bilateral ureteral obstruction and developed fungus balls due to *S. cerevisiae*. Two renal abscesses associated with fungemia have also been documented [51].

Vaginitis due to *S. cerevisiae* has been reported in 17 women, including 9 women with symptomatic vaginitis indistinguishable from that caused by *C. albicans* [38, 42]. All patients had a history of chronic vaginitis unresponsive to standard antifungal drugs, and all but two had systemic or local predisposing factors. Additionally, 8 other women were reported with refractory vaginitis due to *S. cerevisiae* [42].

Diagnosis

The decision to attribute a causal role to *S. cerevisiae* is simple when the organism is isolated from a normally sterile body site, and the patient should be treated for an invasive fungal infection. Diagnostic difficulty occurs when the organism is recovered from body sites that may be colonized by *Saccharomyces,* especially in the absence of symptoms of infection. In this setting, it is necessary to establish true infection instead of colonization with this organism.

S. cerevisiae readily grows in blood cultures and on Sabouraud dextrose media. No serologic diagnostic tests are available to assist in the diagnosis.

Treatment

As with many nonpathogenic yeast infections, it is difficult to assess the role of antifungal therapy in patients with infection due to the genus *Saccharomyces*. Optimal management of patients with prosthetic valve infections and infected indwelling catheters has not been established. There are several reports that document clearance of fungemia and resolution of infection by removing the intravascular catheter without providing antifungal therapy [39, 43, 51]. Most experts advocate the removal of the indwelling catheter and the use of antifungal agents [51]. Although in vitro susceptibility tests have not been standardized, *Saccharomyces* are susceptible to most antifungal drugs, including amphotericin B, 5-flucytosine, ketoconazole, fluconazole, itraconazole, voriconazole, posaconazole, and isavuconazole (Table 2) [12, 13, 38]. However, most *Saccharomyces* isolates have higher MICs to most antifungal drugs than does *Candida albicans*.

Malassezia Infections

Malassezia furfur (*Pityrosporum orbiculare*, *P. ovale*) and other *Malassezia* are common yeasts frequently found on normal human skin [3, 4]. *Malassezia* are well known to cause superficial skin infections such as tinea (pityriasis) versicolor, dermatophytosis, and folliculitis; occasionally in

Table 2 In vitro antifungal susceptibilities of *Saccharomyces cerevisiae* [12, 13, 38]

Yeast	Antifungal Agent	MIC Range µg/mL
Saccharomyces cerevisiae	Amphotericin B	0.5–2.0
	Itraconazole	0.25–1.0
	Fluconazole	0.5–16
	Voriconazole	0.06–0.25
	Posaconazole	0.12–1.0
	Isavuconazole	0.03–1.0
	Caspofungin	0.25–1.0
	Anidulafungin	0.03–0.25
	Flucytosine	0.06–0.12

the immunocompromised host they cause fungemia and disseminated infection [3, 4].

Mycology

The genus *Malassezia* consists of several species, including *M. furfur* and *M. pachydermatis*. *M. furfur* is a dimorphic lipophilic yeast that cannot synthesize medium- or long-chain fatty acids and has strict in vitro requirements for exogenous fatty acids of the C_{12} and C_{14} series [59]. *M. furfur* and other *Malassezia* exist primarily in the yeast form, but may form filamentous structures on the skin when the organism is associated with superficial infections [60].

Because of its nutritional requirements, *M. furfur* is not frequently isolated from clinical specimens in the microbiology laboratory unless its presence is suspected and special preparations are made. *M. pachydermatis* is generally associated with infections in dogs, where it produces otitis externa [59]. Recently, this species of *Malassezia* has been found on the skin of dog owners whose animals had an active infection. This species has occasionally been implicated in human infections [61, 62].

Both organisms, when grown under favorable conditions, produce clusters of oval to round, thick-walled yeast cells, with unipolar buds that form repeatedly from the same pole of the parent cell, giving rise to the characteristic "collarette" at the bud site. The cells measure approximately 6 μm in their largest dimension [3, 4, 60, 63].

Optimal growth for *M. furfur* occurs between 35°C and 37°C. Media such as Sabouraud dextrose agar, chocolate agar, trypticase soy agar with 5% sheep blood all require the addition of supplements such as olive oil in order to permit growth of this organism [64]. *M. pachydermatis* does not require exogenous lipids for growth and can be recovered on standard fungal media. In addition, *M. pachydermatis* does not have known filamentous forms [60]. Colonies are dry and white to creamy in color [3, 4].

Although in vitro susceptibility assays have not been standardized (Table 3), the majority of *M. furfur* strains appear to be susceptible to most antifungals, including amphotericin B (MIC range 0.12–16 μg/mL), ketoconazole (MIC range 0.03–1 μg/mL), fluconazole (MIC range 0.5–32 μg/mL), itraconazole (MIC range 0.03–0.06 μg/mL), voriconazole (MIC range 0.03–16), posaconazole (MIC range 0.03–32 μg/mL) [12, 65–68]. Most isolates are intrinsically resistant to flucytosine (MIC ≥ 64 μg/mL) [65–68].

Table 3 In vitro antifungal susceptibilities of *Malassezia* spp. [12, 65–68]

Yeast	Antifungal Agent	MIC Range μg/mL
Malassezia spp.	Amphotericin B	0.12–6.0
	Itraconazole	0.03–0.06
	Fluconazole	0.5–32
	Voriconazole	0.03–16
	Posaconazole	0.03–32
	Isavuconazole	0.03–1.0
	Flucytosine	≥64

Epidemiology

Malassezia frequently colonizes the skin of normal hosts over the scalp, shoulders, chest, and back [64]. The distribution of colonization correlates with oily areas of the skin due to the organism's requirement for exogenous fatty acids, which it obtains from sebum. The highest incidence of colonization has been found in young teenagers, with rates greater than 90% [63]. The low incidence of colonization in preadolescent children has been postulated to be due to immature sebum production.

Isolation of *M. furfur* from newborns is reported to be less than 10% in nonintensive care settings. However, isolation of *M. furfur* has been reported to be greater than 80% in neonatal intensive care units [60, 64, 69]. The reason for this increased colonization rate may be because sick infants are handled frequently by adult personnel who are colonized [67].

Risk factors that correlate with increased colonization rates in neonates include prematurity, duration of hospitalization in the intensive care unit, use of occlusive dressings, and prolonged use of antimicrobials [60, 70]. Although the epidemiology of disseminated infection has not been well studied, there are several risk factors frequently associated with deep-seated infection due to *M. furfur*. These include prematurity, central venous catheters [60, 71–73], total parenteral nutrition, parenteral lipid preparations [71–73], and immunocompromised state [60].

Molecular epidemiologic studies using PCR-mediated DNA fingerprinting have concluded that within the neonatal intensive care unit there is longitudinal persistence of both *M. furfur* and *M. pachydermatis* strains [74].

Clinical Manifestations

Malassezia produces superficial skin infections, such as tinea (pityriasis) versicolor and a distinctive folliculitis and, on occasion, deep-seated or hematogenous infection [67]. The first reported case of systemic infection was described in 1981 in a premature neonate who developed vasculitis while on lipid therapy [61]. Since then, numerous reports have described disseminated infection due to *M. furfur* [60, 67].

The manifestations of disseminated or deep-seated infection vary from subclinical and mild symptoms, such as fever, to sepsis with multiorgan dysfunction [60, 63, 67]. Although the majority of these infections are seen in premature infants, they may occur occasionally in the immunocompromised adult. Commonly reported signs and symptoms of systemic infection other than fever include bradycardia and respiratory distress (50%), apnea (37%), hepatosplenomegaly (25%), and lethargy (12%) [69]. Laboratory findings include leukocytosis and thrombocytopenia, and chest radiographs usually reveal bilateral pulmonary infiltrates [69]. Although not commonly recognized, pneumonia due to *M. furfur* has been reported on several occasions in patients who have received a stem cell transplant [75]. In all four cases reported, the organisms were recovered from the bronchoalveolar lavage (BAL) specimen. In addition, all patients had central venous catheters and all had been receiving TPN. Deep-seated organ dissemination is rare.

Diagnosis

The diagnosis of disseminated infection sometimes can be made by Gram stain of the buffy coat of blood. The budding yeast cells also can be observed using stains, such as Giemsa, periodic acid–Schiff (PAS), or Calcofluor [3, 4]. Blood cultures will usually be negative, unless the infection is suspected and the laboratory adds sterile olive oil to the media. Recovery of the organism may be enhanced by using lysis centrifugation blood culture tubes to support the growth of the yeast [76]. In addition, palmitic acid (3%) supplementation may improve the recovery of *Malassezia* [76].

Treatment

Management of *M. furfur* fungemia and disseminated infection is controversial. Most authorities recommend prompt removal of the central venous catheter and discontinuation of intravenous lipids [60, 63, 67]. In most cases without deep-seated infection, removal of the central venous catheter and discontinuation of lipids is all that is needed to clear the infection. This treatment approach accomplishes two objectives: eradication of the nidus of infection and removal of the nutritional requirements of the organism. If fungemia persists or there is evidence of deep-seated infection, antifungal therapy should be initiated. Fortunately, *Malassezia* species are susceptible to azoles and polyenes (Table 3) [60, 63, 65, 67]. Although randomized clinical trials have not been undertaken, in most situations either fluconazole (400 mg/day) or amphotericin B (0.7 mg/kg/day) intravenously should be sufficient to eradicate the infection.

Trichosporonosis

Infections due to the genus *Trichosporon* may be classified as superficial or deep [77, 78]. Superficial infection of the hair shafts, generally due to *Trichosporon asahii* (*T. beigelii*), is commonly known as white piedra because of the soft white nodules characteristic of this infection. Deep-seated or disseminated *Trichosporon* infections have been recognized in the compromised host with increasing frequency over the past decade and are life-threatening.

The organism now known as *T. asahii* was first described in 1865 by Beigel, who identified it as the causative agent of hair shaft infection [79]. The first reported case of disseminated infection appears to be a 39-year-old woman who had adenocarcinoma of the lung and who developed a brain abscess [78].

Mycology

The genus *Trichosporon*, initially described by Behrend, currently contains two main species: *T. asahii* (formerly, *T. beigelii, T. cutaneum*) [79] and *Blastoschizomyces capitatus*, previously called *T. capitatum* or *Geotrichum capitatum* [3, 4, 77, 80, 81]. Gueho and colleagues have also suggested that the species known as *T. asahii* may include several different *Trichosporon* species with epidemiologic and pathogenic differences [80]. In 1991, investigators using isoenzyme delineation and Polymerase chain reaction (PCR) DNA fingerprinting techniques suggested that the strains that generally produce superficial infections are distinctly different from those strains that produce invasive disease [82].

Trichosporon species are characterized by true hyphae, pseudohyphae, arthroconidia, and blastoconidia and are commonly found in soil, animals, and on human skin [3, 4, 77]. *T. asahii* grows readily on Sabouraud dextrose agar as rapidly growing, smooth, shiny gray to cream-colored yeast-like colonies with cerebriform radiating furrows that become dry and membranous with age [3, 4] (Fig. 2).

T. asahii is readily identified using commercially available carbohydrate assimilation assays. Over 30 species of Trichosporon have been identified. Although *T. asahii* is the most commonly recovered species, other species associated with invasive infection include, *T. inkin,* which has been recovered in association with peritonitis, osteomyelitis, endocarditis, and urinary tract, cutaneous, and subcutaneous infections [83], and *T. mycotoxinivorans,* which has been associated with pneumonia in patients with cystic fibrosis [84].

In 1963, investigators described the presence of common antigens between *T. asahii* and *Cryptococcus neoformans* [85]. Immunodiagnosis of trichosporonosis using the

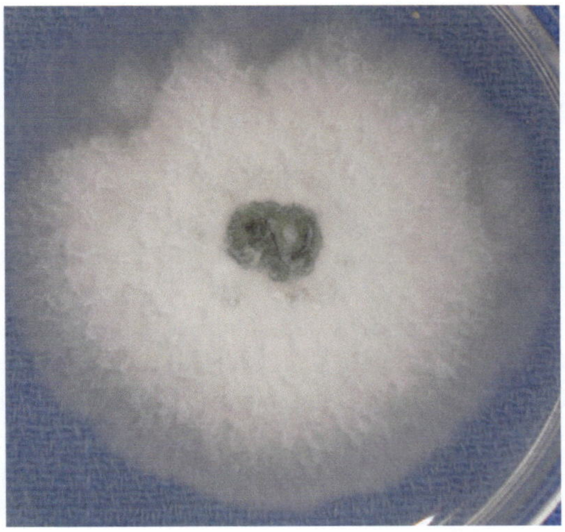

Fig. 2 Growth of *Trichosporon asahii* on Sabouraud's dextrose agar. Although initially cream colored, with age the colony becomes wrinkled and its center becomes heaped up and darkens to a greenish gray color

anticryptococcal latex-agglutination test of the serum has also been reported [86, 87].

Epidemiology

While *T. asahii* is generally found in the soil, it may also be recovered from air, rivers and lakes, sewage, and bird droppings [77, 88]. It rarely colonizes the inanimate environment, but may occasionally colonize the mucosal surfaces of the oropharynx, the lower gastrointestinal tract, and the skin in approximately 4% of humans [23, 89].

There have been more than 100 documented cases of disseminated infection due to *T. asahii* [3, 4, 77, 89–92]. In most cases the major risk factors included underlying neoplastic disease (acute leukemia, chronic leukemia, multiple myeloma, solid tumors) and neutropenia [92–97]. In patients who do not have cancer and are not neutropenic, the major risk factors include corticosteroids, prosthetic valve surgery, solid organ transplantation (kidney, heart, liver), chronic active hepatitis, antimicrobials, cystic fibrosis, and intravenous drug use [90, 98–100]. In the majority of cases, the proposed portal of entry appears to be the respiratory tract, gastrointestinal tract, central venous catheters, or percutaneous vascular devices [84, 88, 90, 99, 100].

Clinical Manifestations

Trichosporonosis can be classified into superficial infections such as white piedra (hair shaft), onychomycosis and otomycosis, and invasive infection. Invasive infection can be further divided into localized deep tissue infection and disseminated (hematogenous) infection.

Deep tissue infection results from the invasion of *Trichosporon* into nonmucosal tissues. The infection may involve a single organ infection or multiple organs. The most frequently affected organ is the lungs, representing approximately 33% of localized deep tissue infections [99–101]. Other sites of deep organ infection include the peritoneum [99–102], heart valves (natural and prosthetic) [83, 92], eyes [103], brain, liver, and spleen [104], stomach [105], kidneys [96], uterine tissue, gallbladder [97, 106], and central nervous system (chronic fungal meningitis) [88, 107].

The clinical spectrum of disseminated infection resembles systemic candidiasis and includes fungemia associated with organ infection [99, 100, 108]. Disseminated infections may be either acute or chronic. Acute disseminated trichosporonosis frequently has a sudden onset and progresses rapidly, primarily in patients who are persistently neutropenic with fungemia characterized by persistent fever despite broad-spectrum antibacterial agents. Patients frequently develop cutaneous lesions (33%), pulmonary infiltrates (30–60%), and hypotension, with renal and ocular involvement [99, 100, 108].

The metastatic cutaneous lesions begin as an erythematous rash with raised papules on the trunk and the extremities. As the infection progresses, the rash evolves into macronodular lesions, followed by central necrosis of the nodules and, rarely, the formation of hemorrhagic bullae [109]. Pulmonary infiltrates frequently accompany the disseminated infection and may manifest as a lobar consolidation, bronchopneumonia, or a reticulonodular pattern [88, 108].

Renal involvement in disseminated infection is quite common and occurs in approximately 75% of the cases. Renal disease may manifest as proteinuria, hematuria, red blood cell casts, acute renal failure, and glomerulonephritis [88, 89]. Urine cultures are frequently positive for *Trichosporon* and should suggest disseminated disease in a neutropenic patient.

Chorioretinitis is frequently seen in disseminated disease and may cause decreased or complete loss of vision due to retinal vein occlusion and retinal detachment [110]. In experimental studies, *Trichosporon* has been found to have tropism for the choroid and retina [110, 111]. However, unlike candidal endophthalmitis, *Trichosporon* usually infects uveal tissues, including the iris, but spares the vitreous [88, 110].

During disseminated infection, virtually any tissue in the body may be infected with *Trichosporon*. The organs that have been documented to be involved include the liver, spleen, gastrointestinal tract, lymph nodes, myocardium, bone marrow, pleura, brain, adrenal gland, thyroid gland, and skeletal muscle [90, 111–115].

In chronic disseminated trichosporonosis, symptoms may be present for several weeks to months and include persistent fever despite broad-spectrum antimicrobial therapy [111].

This infection is similar to the entity known as chronic disseminated (hepatosplenic) candidiasis and tends to be a chronic infection of the liver, spleen, and other tissues after recovery from neutropenia [116, 117]. Laboratory studies frequently reveal an elevated alkaline phosphatase. Imaging the abdomen with either a CT scan or MR reveals hepatic or splenic lesions compatible with abscesses. If lesions are demonstrated, a biopsy is needed to confirm the diagnosis.

Diagnosis

The diagnosis is made with a biopsy sent for histopathology and for culture of the skin or involved organs. On histopathologic examination, the unique feature of *Trichosporon* infection is the array of fungal forms, including yeasts, arthroconidia, hyphae, and pseudohyphae that are seen in tissues (Fig. 3). Blood cultures may also be useful in diagnosing disseminated infection and, on occasion, in deep-tissue infection. *Trichosporon* will grow readily in blood culture and on fungal-specific media such as Sabouraud dextrose agar [3, 88]. The presence of *Trichosporon* in the urine of a high-risk patient should increase the suspicion of disseminated infection.

There are no standardized serologic assays for *Trichosporon*, but the serum latex agglutination test for *C. neoformans* may be positive in patients with trichosporonosis [85]. The initial clinical observations suggesting the usefulness of this test was reported by McManus and coworkers, who demonstrated a positive serum latex agglutination test for *C. neoformans* in several patients with disseminated *Trichosporon* infection [87].

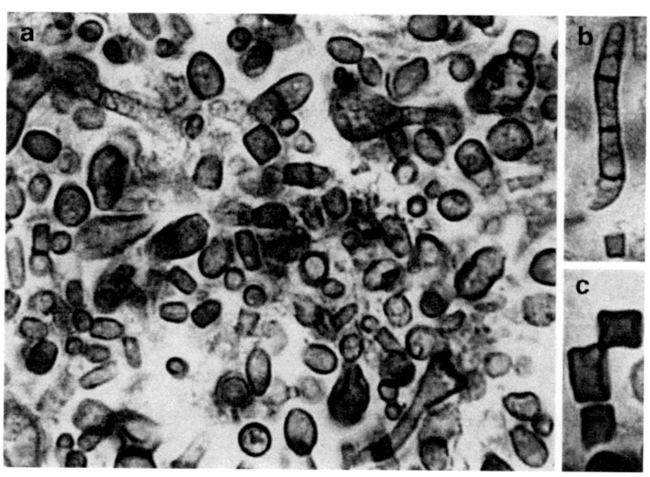

Fig. 3 Fungal forms noted in the lung obtained at autopsy of a patient who died of disseminated *Trichosporon asahii* infection. (**a**) view showing hyphae, pseudohyphae, arthroconidia, and blastospores (yeasts); (**b**) higher magnification showing hyphae (2,800×); (**c**) higher magnification showing arthroconidia (2,800×)

Treatment

Trichosporonosis has a mortality rate of 60–70%. The underlying disease, persistent neutropenia, and concurrent infections contribute to overall mortality. The initial step in the management of disseminated *Trichosporon* infection should be to decrease or reverse immunosuppression. Optimal therapy has not been established. Until recently, most patients received amphotericin B, occasionally in combination with flucytosine [111]. Several investigators, however, have reported amphotericin B tolerant and resistant isolates of *T. asahii* [88, 108].

Although there are no clinical trials, there are several antifungal options currently available. In vitro susceptibility studies and animal models suggest that azoles and not polyenes or echinocandins are more effective in the eradication of *Trichosporon* species in neutropenic and nonneutropenic models [10–13, 92, 118–122]. In vitro susceptibility studies of *T. asahii* (Table 4) reveal fluconazole MIC_{50} of 8.0 μg/mL (MIC range 4–64 μg/mL) and itraconazole MIC_{50} of 0.25 μg/mL (range 0.12–16 μg/mL) [13, 119]. In the same study, amphotericin B MIC_{50} for *T. asahii* was 4.0 μg/mL (range 1.0–8.0 μg/mL) [12, 13, 119]. Although there are no established breakpoints to define susceptibility, the majority of the *Trichosporon* spp. evaluated thus far demonstrate relatively high MICs to the polyenes and echinocandins with relatively low MICs to the newer azoles [10–13, 122].

It is important to note that the newer triazoles – voriconazole, posaconazole, isavuconazole, and ravuconazole – have demonstrated broader and more potent in vitro activity against most *Trichosporon* species than the older azoles [10–13, 119]. All four triazoles have demonstrated excellent in vitro activity against most isolates of *Trichosporon* (Table 4). Voriconazole MIC_{50} 0.25 μg/mL (range 0.03–0.25 μg/mL), posaconazole MIC_{50} 1 μg/mL (range 0.25–1 μg/mL), isavuconazole MIC_{50} 0.125 μg/mL (range 0.03–0.25 μg/mL), and ravuconazole MIC_{50} 4 μg/mL (range 0.25–16 μg/mL) [10–13, 119, 122].

In a murine model of disseminated trichosporonosis, it was found that combination therapy with micafungin and

Table 4 In vitro antifungal susceptibilities of *Trichosporon asahii* [10–13, 119, 122]

Yeast	Antifungal Agent	MIC Range μg/mL
Trichosporon asahii	Amphotericin B	1.0–8.0
	Itraconazole	0.12–16
	Fluconazole	4.0–64
	Voriconazole	0.03–0.25
	Posaconazole	0.25–1.0
	Ravuconazole	0.06–0.12
	Isavuconazole	0.03–1.0
	Caspofungin	≥64
	Flucytosine	16–≥64

amphotericin B demonstrated a synergistic effect leading to prolonged survival time and decreased renal fungal burden when compared with either agent alone. In addition, the combination of micafungin and fluconazole also reduced the renal fungal burden when compared with monotherapy [123]. Combination therapy with fluconazole and amphotericin B has been used successfully in a bone marrow transplant recipient who developed breakthrough trichosporonosis while receiving prophylaxis against invasive fungal infection with caspofungin [124].

Although there are limited clinical data, one possible therapeutic approach would be to use voriconazole 200–300 mg twice daily in a patient with disseminated trichosporonosis. It may be clinically useful to determine in vitro susceptibilities as a helpful adjunct in the management of this serious infection, especially in light of recent case reports describing multidrug resistant *T. asahii* infections [121–125].

Blastoschizomyces capitatus

Infections due to *Blastoschizomyces capitatus*, although not as common as *T. asahii*, have been recognized in the immunocompromised host over the past 20–25 years [126, 127]. Most cases appear to be very similar to either disseminated candidiasis or disseminated *T. asahii* infection [3, 4].

Mycology

B. capitatus, formerly *Trichosporon capitatum* (syn. *G. capitatum)* is difficult to differentiate from *G. candidum* and *T. asahii* [3, 4, 79–81]. *B. capitatus* produces smooth to wrinkled, raised hyaline colonies with short and finely funiculose aerial mycelium. Hyphae are septate and branching and often form annelloconidia instead of arthroconidia [127].

In vitro susceptibility studies (Table 5) indicate that *B. capitatus* is susceptible to amphotericin B (MIC_{90} 0.62 μg/mL, range 0.125–64 μg/mL); less susceptible to azoles such as fluconazole (MIC_{90} 32 μg/mL), ketoconazole (MIC_{90} 3.12 μg/mL, range 0.04–32 μg/mL); and susceptible to itraconazole (MIC_{90} 0.25 μg/mL). Most isolates are resistant to flucytosine (MIC range 0.04–≥64 mg/mL) [14, 128]. The newer triazoles – voriconazole and posaconazole – demonstrate good in vitro activity [11, 12, 15, 129].

Table 5 In vitro antifungal susceptibilities of *Blastoschizomyces capitatus* and *Sporobolomyces* spp. [11, 12, 14, 15, 128, 129]

Yeast	Antifungal Agent	MIC Range μg/mL
Blastoschizomyces capitatus	Amphotericin B	0.06–64
	Itraconazole	0.25–0.50
	Fluconazole	4.0–32
	Voriconazole	0.06–0.25
	Posaconazole	0.12–0.25
	Flucytosine	0.04–≥64
Sporobolomyces	Amphotericin B	0.12–1.0
	Fluconazole	1.0–64
	Itraconazole	1.0–2.0
	Voriconazole	0.25–4.0

Epidemiology

B. capitatus is found in wood and poultry but has also been recovered from sputum and normal intact skin [3, 4]. Geographically, *B. capitatus* differs from *T. asahii*, with *B. capitatus* infections found more commonly in Europe and *T. asahii* infections found in North America [77, 127]. In most cases, the major risk factors include neutropenia and underlying hematologic malignancies [127]. The portal of entry is unknown, but is suspected to be the respiratory tract, gastrointestinal tract, and possibly infected central venous catheters [3, 4, 77, 127].

Clinical Manifestations

B. capitatus infection may involve a single organ or multiple organs and may be associated with fungemia. The most frequently affected organs are the lungs, liver, skin, and central nervous system. In addition, other involved organs include the spleen, epididymis, kidney, gastrointestinal tract, vertebral body and disc, and prosthetic heart valves [14].

The clinical spectrum of disseminated infection is similar to that of systemic candidiasis and includes fungemia with or without organ infection [14, 127]. Generally, the manifestations begin with fever unresponsive to antibacterial therapy in a neutropenic patient. In addition, in the largest series from Italy, many patients presented with pulmonary disease characterized by cavitary lung lesions and focal hepatosplenic lesions [126]. Skin lesions similar to those found in systemic candidiasis were also seen. Less commonly described infections include endocarditis, especially involving prosthetic valves, urinary tract infection, vertebral osteomyelitis with discitis of the lumbar spine, cerebritis, and brain abscess [111, 127–131].

Diagnosis

Diagnosis is made by positive blood cultures or by biopsy with histopathology and culture of the skin or affected organs. In a series from Italy, blood cultures were positive in 20 of 22 cases [127]. *B. capitatus* will grow easily in blood culture bottles and on fungal-specific media such as Sabouraud dextrose agar [3, 4]. Although skin lesions are common, fungal stains and cultures of these lesions are usually negative [3, 4, 127].

Treatment

Disseminated infections with *B. capitatus* have mortality rates between 60% and 70% [127]. Underlying disease, persistent neutropenia, and concurrent infections are significant contributing factors to overall mortality. Optimal therapy has not been established. Until recently, most patients received amphotericin B [111]. The initial step in the management of disseminated infection should be to decrease or reverse the immunocompromised state. Since most isolates are susceptible to amphotericin B, the recommended therapy is amphotericin B at a dose of 1.0–1.5 mg/kg/day [14]. Based on their excellent in vitro activity, voriconazole and posaconazole are suitable alternatives for therapy [15, 128, 129].

Sporobolomyces

Sporobolomyces are yeast-like organisms that belong to the family Sporobolomycetaceae. These yeasts, which are found throughout the world in soil, bark, and decaying organic material, rarely have been associated with infections in humans. There are seven known species of *Sporobolomyces*, but only three have been reported to cause human disease, *S. salmonicolor, S. holsaticus*, and *S. roseus*. To date, there have been six cases of documented *Sporobolomyces* infections: a nasal polyp, one case of dermatitis, one case of infected skin blisters, one case of Madura foot, and two cases of disseminated infection (lymph node and bone marrow) in patients with AIDS [132–134]. Despite the fact that *Sporobolomyces* are saprophytic, these case reports indicate the potential ability of these organisms to produce invasive infection in humans, especially, in an immunocompromised host.

Sporobolomyces produces pink–orange colonies due to the production of carotenoid pigments, and should be differentiated from *R. rubra*, which also produces a similar color [3, 4]. The genus *Sporobolomyces* is differentiated from other yeast by their reproductive ballistoconidia [135]. In vitro susceptibility studies (Table 5) show that *S. salmonicolor* is susceptible to amphotericin B, fluconazole, and ketoconazole. All patients reported thus far have responded to therapy with either amphotericin B or ketoconazole [14].

References

1. Safdar A, Singhal S, Mehta J. Clinical significance of non-*Candida* fungal blood isolation in patients undergoing high-risk allogeneic hematopoietic stem cell transplantation (1993–2001). Cancer. 2004;100:2456–61.
2. Kontoyiannis DP. Echinocandin-based initial therapy in fungemic patients with cancer: A focus on recent guidelines of the Infectious Diseases Society of America. Clin Infect Dis. 2009;49:638–40.
3. Kwon-Chung KJ, Bennett JE. Infections due to *Trichosporon* and other miscellaneous yeast-like fungi. In: Kwon-Chung KJ, Bennett JE, editors. Medical Mycology. 1st ed. Philadelphia: Lea & Febiger; 768. p. 782–1992.
4. Rippon JW. Medical Mycology. The pathogenic fungi and Pathogenic actinomycetes. 3rd ed. Philadelphia: W. B. Saunders; 1988. p. 148–52.
5. Tuon FF, Costa SF. Rhodotorula infection. A systematic review of 128 cases from the literature. Rev Iberoam Micol. 2008;25:135–40.
6. Fell JW, Tallman AS, Ahearn DG. *Rhodotorula* Harrison. In: Kreiger-van Rij NJW, editor. The Yeasts: A Taxonomic Study. 3rd ed. Amsterdam: Elsevier Science Publishers; 1984. p. 893–905.
7. Fell JW, Boekhout T, Fonseca A, Scorzetti G, Statzelli-Tallman A. Biodiversity and systematics of basidiomycetous yeast as determined by large-subunit rDNA D1/D2 domain sequence analysis. Int J Syst Evol Microbiol. 2000;50:1351–71.
8. Dubuc de Almeida GM, Figueiredo Costa S, Melhem M, et al. *Rhodotorula* spp, isolated from blood cultures:clinical and microbiological aspects. Med Mycol. 2008;46:547–56.
9. Zaas AK, Boyce M, Schell W, et al. Risk of fungemia due to *Rhodotorula* and antifungal susceptibility testing of *Rhodotorula* isolates. J Clin Microbiol. 2003;41:5233–5.
10. Serena C, Pastor FJ, Ortoneda M, Capilla J, Nolard N, Guarro J. In vitro antifungal susceptibilities of uncommon basidiomycetous yeasts. Antimicrobiol Agent Chemother. 2004;48:2724–6.
11. Diekema DJ, Petroelje B, Messer SA, Hollis RJ, Pfaller MA. Activities of available and investigational agents against *Rhodotorula* species. J Clin Microbiol. 2005;43:476–8.
12. Pfaller MA, Diekema DJ, Gibbs DL, et al. Results from the ARTEMIS DISK global antifungal surveillance study, 1997 to 2007: 10.5-year analysis of suceptibilities of noncandidal yeast species to fluconazole and voriconazole determined by CLSI standardized disk diffusion testing. J Clin Microbiol. 2009;47:117–23.
13. Thompson GR, Wiederhold NP, Sutton DA, Fothergill A, Patterson TE. In vitro activity of isavuconazole against *Trichosporon*, *Rhodotorula*, *Geotrichum*, *Saccharomyces* and *Pichia* species. J Antimicrob Chemother. 2009;64:79–83.
14. Hazen KC. New and emerging yeast pathogens. Clin Microbiol Rev. 1995;8:462–78.
15. Espinel-Ingroff A. In vitro activity of the new triazole voriconazole (UK-109, 496) against opportunistic filamentous and dimorphic fungi and common and emerging yeast pathogens. J Clin Microbiol. 1998;36:198–202.
16. Volz PA, Jerger DE, Wurzburger AJ, Hiser JL. A preliminary study of yeasts isolated from marine habitats at Abaco Island, the Bahamas. Mycopathol Mycol Appl. 1974;54:313–6.
17. Mackenzie DWH. Yeasts from human sources. Sabouraudia. 1961;1:8–14.
18. Ahearn DG, Jannach JR, Roth FJ. Speciation and densities of yeasts in human urine specimens. Sabouraudia. 1966;5:110–9.
19. Kiehn TE, Gorey E, Brown AE, Edwards FF, Armstrong D. Sepsis due to *Rhodotorula* related to use of indwelling central venous catheters. Clin Infect Dis. 1992;14:841–6.
20. Saez H. Etude ecologique sur les *Rhodotorula* des homotherms. Rev Med Vet. 1979;130:903–8.

21. Kares L, Biava MF. Levures isolees dans les hemocultures de 1962 a Mar 1979 in laboratoire de mycologie du CHU de Nancy. Bull Soc Fr Mycol Med. 1979;8:153–5.
22. Anaissie E, Bodey GP, Kantarjiani H, et al. New spectrum of fungal infections in patients with cancer. Rev Infect Dis. 1989;11:369–78.
23. Rose HD, Kurup VP. Colonization of hospitalized patients with yeast-like organisms. Sabouraudia. 1977;15:251–6.
24. Gyaurgieva OH, Bogomolova TS, Gorshkova GI. Meningitis caused by *Rhodotorula rubra* in an HIV-infected patient. J Med Vet Mycol. 1996;34:357–9.
25. Tuon FF, Duboc de Almeida GM, Costa SF. Central venous catheter-associated fungemia due to *Rhodotorula* spp. – a systematic review. Med Mycol. 2007;45:441–7.
26. Louria DB, Greenberg SM, Molander DW. Fungemia caused by certain nonpathogenic strains of the family Cryptococcaceae. N Engl J Med. 1960;263:1281–4.
27. Shelbourne PF, Carey RJ. *Rhodotorula* fungemia complicating staphylococcal endocarditis. JAMA. 1962;180:38–42.
28. Leeber DA, Scher I. *Rhodotorula* fungemia presenting as "endotoxic" shock. Arch Intern Med. 1969;123:78–81.
29. Young RC, Bennett JE, Geelhoed GW, Levine AS. Fungemia with compromised host resistance: a study of 70 cases. Ann Intern Med. 1974;80:605–12.
30. Naveh YA, Friedman A, Merzbach D, Hashman N. Endocarditis caused by *Rhodotorula* successfully treated with 5-flucytosine. Br Heart J. 1975;37:101–4.
31. Eisenberg ES, Alpert BE, Weiss RA, Mittman N, Soeiro R. *Rhodotorula rubra* peritonitis in patients undergoing continuous ambulatory peritoneal dialysis. Am J Med. 1983;75:349–52.
32. Savini V, Sozio F, Catavitello C, et al. Femoral prosthesis infection by *Rhodotorula mucilaginosa*. J Clin Microbiol. 2008;46:3544–5.
33. Rusthoven JJ, Feld R, Tuffnell PG. Systemic infection by *Rhodotorula* spp. in the immunocompromised host. J Infect. 1984;8:241–6.
34. Louria DB, Blevins A, Armstrong D, Burdick R, Lieberman P. Fungemia caused by non-pathogenic yeasts. Arch Intern Med. 1967;119:247–52.
35. Braun DK, Kauffman CA. *Rhodotorula* fungaemia: A life-threatening complication of indwelling central venous catheters. Mycoses. 1992;35:305–8.
36. Pore RS, Chen J. Meningitis caused by *Rhodotorula*. Sabouraudia. 1976;14:331–5.
37. Donald FE, Sharp JF. *Rhodotorula rubra* ventriculitis. J Infect. 1988;16:187–91.
38. Sobel JD, Vazquez J, Lynch M, Meriwether C, Zervos MJ. Vaginitis due to *Saccharomyces cerevisiae*: Epidemiology, clinical aspects, and therapy. Clin Infect Dis. 1993;16:93–9.
39. Cimolai N, Gill MJ, Church D. *Saccharomyces cerevisiae* fungemia: Case report and review of the literature. Diagn Microbiol Infect Dis. 1987;8:113–7.
40. Tawfik OW, Papasian C, Dixon AY, Potter LM. *Saccharomyces cerevisiae* pneumonia in a patient with acquired immune deficiency syndrome. J Clin Microbiol. 1989;27:1689–91.
41. Nielsen H, Stenderup J, Bruun B. Fungemia with Saccharomycetaceae. Report of four cases and review of the literature. Scand J Infect Dis. 1990;22:581–4.
42. Nyirjesy P, Vazquez JA, Ufberg DD, Sobel JD, Boikov DA, Buckley HR. *Saccharomyces cerevisiae* vaginitis: transmission from yeast used in baking. Obstet Gynecol. 1995;86:326–9.
43. Enache-Angoulvant A, Hennequin C. Invasive Saccharomyces infection: a comprehensive review. Clin Infect Dis. 2005;41: 1559–68.
44. Morrison VA, Haake RJ, Weisdorf DJ. The spectrum of non-*Candida* fungal infections following bone marrow transplantation. Medicine (Baltimore). 1993;72:78–89.
45. Holzschu DL, Chandler FW, Ajello L, Ahearn DG. Evaluation of industrial yeast for pathogenicity. Sabouradia. 1979;17:71–8.
46. Clemons KV, McCusker JH, Davis RW, Stevens DA. Comparative pathogenesis of clinical and non-clinical isolates of *Saccharomyces cerevisiae*. J Infect Dis. 1994;169:859–67.
47. Eng RH, Drehmel R, Smith SM, Goldstein EJC. *Saccharomyces cerevisiae* infections in man. Sabouraudia. 1984;22:403–7.
48. McCullough MJ, Clemens KV, Farina C, McCusker JH, Stevens DA. Epidemiological investigation of vaginal *Saccharomyces cerevisiae* isolates by a genotypic method. J Clin Microbiol. 1998;36:557–62.
49. Cassone M, Serra P, Mondello F, et al. Outbreak of *Saccharomyces cerevisiae* subtype *boulardii* fungemia in patients neighboring those treated with a probiotic preparation of the organism. J Clin Microbiol. 2003;41:5340–43.
50. Eschete ML, West BC. *Saccharomyces cerevisiae* septicemia. Arch Intern Med. 1980;140:1539–44.
51. Aucott JN, Fayen J, Grossnicklas H, Morrissey A, Lederman MM, Salata RA. Invasive infection with *Saccharomyces cervisiae*: report of three cases and review. Rev Infect Dis. 1990;12:406–11.
52. Sethi N, Mandell W. *Saccharomyces* fungemia in a patient with AIDS. NY State J Med. 1988;88:278–79.
53. Stein PD, Folkens AT, Hruska KA. *Saccharomyces* fungemia. Chest. 1970;58:173–5.
54. Rubinstein E, Noriega ER, Simberkoff MS, Holzman R, Rahal JJ. Fungal endocarditis: analysis of 24 cases and review of the literature. Medicine (Baltimore). 1997;54:331–44.
55. Canafax DM, Mann HJ, Dougherty SH. Postoperative peritonitis due to *Saccharomyces cerevisiae* treated with ketoconazole. Drug Intell Clin Pharm. 1982;16:698–99.
56. Dougherty SH, Simmons RL. Postoperative peritonitis caused by *Saccharomyces cerevisiae*. Arch Surg. 1982;117:248–49.
57. Chertow GM, Marcantonio ER, Wells RG. *Saccharomyces cerevisiae* empyema in a patient with esophago-pleural fistula complicating variceal sclerotherapy. Chest. 1991;99:1518–19.
58. Katras T, Hollier PP, Stanton PE. Calculous cholecystitis associated with *Saccharomyces cerevisiae*. Infect Med. 1992;9:38–9.
59. Nazzaro-Porro MN, Passi S, Caprilli F, Morpurgo G. Growth requirements and lipid metabolism of *Pityrosporum orbiculare*. J Invest Dermatol. 1976;66:178–82.
60. Marcon MJ, Powell DA. Human infections due to *Malassezia* spp. Clin Microbiol Rev. 1992;5:101–19.
61. Redline RW, Dahms BB. *Malassezia* pulmonary vasculitis in an infant on long-term intralipid therapy. N Engl J Med. 1981;305: 1395–8.
62. Gueho E, Simmons RB, Pruitt WR, Meyer SA, Ahearn DG. Association of *Malassezia pachydermatis* with systemic infections of humans. J Clin Microbiol. 1987;25:1789–90.
63. Marcon MJ, Powell DA. Epidemiology, diagnosis and management of *M. furfur* systemic infection. Diagn Microbiol Infect Dis. 1987;10:161–75.
64. Ingham E, Cunningham AC. *Malassezia furfur*. J Med Vet Mycol. 1993;31:265–88.
65. Velegraki A, Alexopoulos EC, Kritikou S, Gaitanis G. Use of fatty acid RPMI 1640 media for testing susceptibilities of eight *Malassezia* species to the new triazole posaconazole and to six established antifungal agents by modified NCCLS M27-A2 microdilution method and E test. J Clin Microbiol. 2004;42:3589–93.
66. Faergemann J. In vitro and in vivo activities of ketoconazole and itraconazole against *Pityrosporum orbiculare*. Antimicrob Agents Chemother. 1984;26:773–4.
67. Klotz SA. *Malassezia furfur*. Infect Dis Clin N Am. 1989;3:53–63.
68. Gupta AK, Kohli Y, Li A, Faergemann J, Summerbell RC. In vitro susceptibility of the seven *Malassezia* species to ketoconazole, voriconazole, itraconazole and terbinafine. Br J Dermatol. 2000;142:758–65.

69. Powell DA, Hayes J, Durrell DE, Miller M, Marcon MJ. *Malassezia furfur* skin colonization of infants hospitalized in intensive care units. J Pediatr. 1987;111:217–20.
70. Roberts W. *Pityrosporum orbiculare*: incidence and distribution on clinically normal skin. Br J Dermatol. 1969;81:264–9.
71. Garcia CR, Johnston BL, Corvi G, Walker LJ, George L. Intravenous catheter-associated *Malassezia furfur* fungemia. Am J Med. 1987;83:790–2.
72. Weiss SJ, Schoch PE, Cunha BA. *Malassezia furfur* fungemia associated with central venous catheter lipid emulsion infusion. Heart Lung. 1991;20:87–90.
73. Barber GR, Brown AE, Kiehn TE, Edwards FF, Armstrong D. Catheter-related *Malassezia furfur* fungemia in immunocompromised patients. Am J Med. 1993;95:365–70.
74. van Belkum A, Boekhout T, Bosboom R. Monitoring spread of *Malassezia* infections in a neonatal intensive care unit by PCR-medicated genetic typing. J Clin Microbiol. 1994;32:2528–32.
75. Blaes AH, Cavert WP, Morrison VA. *Malassezia*: is it a pulmonary pathogen in the stem cell transplant population. Transpl Infect Dis. 2009;11:313–7.
76. Nelson SC, Yau YCW, Richardson SE, Matlow AG. Improved detection of *Malassezia* species in lipid-supplemented peds plus blood culture bottles. J Clin Microbiol. 1995;33:1005–7.
77. Chagas-Neto TC, Chaves GM, Colombo AL. Update on the genus *Trichosporon*. Mycopathologia. 2008;166:121–32.
78. Watson KC, Kallichurum S. Brain abscess due to *Trichosporon cutaneum*. J Med Microbiol. 1970;3:191–3.
79. Behrend G. Ubertrichomycosis nodosa. Berlin Lin Wochenschr. 1890;27:464.
80. Gueho E, de Hoog GS, Smith MT, Meyer SA. DNA relatedness, taxonomy, and medical significance of *Geotrichum capitatum*. J Clin Microbiol. 1997;25:1191–4.
81. Salkin IF, Gordon MA, Samsonoff WA, Rieder CL. *Blastoschizomyces capitatus*, a new combination. Mycotaxon. 1985;22:375–80.
82. Kemeker BJ, Lehman PF, Lee JW, Walsh TJ. Distinction of deep vs. superficial clinical and non-clinical environmental isolates of *Trichosporon beigelii* by isoenzymes and restriction fragment length polymorphisms of rDNA generated by the polymerase chain reaction. J Clin Microbiol. 1991;29:1677–83.
83. Ramos JM, Cuenca-Estrella M, Gutierrez F, Elia M, Rodriguez-Tudela JL. Clinical case of endocarditis due to *Trichosporon inkin* and antifungal susceptibility profile of the organism. J Clin Microbiol. 2004;42:2341–44.
84. Hickey PW, Sutton DA, Fothergill AW, et al. *Trichosporon mycotoxinivorans*, a novel respiratory pathogen in patients with cystic fibrosis. J Clin Microbiol. 2009;47:3091–97.
85. Seeliger HPR, Schroter R. A serologic study on the antigenic relationship of the form genus *Trichosporon*. Sabouraudia. 1963;2:248–50.
86. Campbell CK, Payne AL, Teall AJ, Brownell A, Mackenzie DW. Cryptococcal latex antigen test positive in a patient with *Trichosporon beigelii*. Lancet. 1985;2:43–4.
87. McManus EJ, Bozdech MJ, Jones JM. Role of the latex agglutination test for cryptococcal antigen in diagnosing disseminated infection with *Trichosporon beigelii*. J Infect Dis. 1985;151: 1167–9.
88. Walsh TJ, Melcher GP, Lee JW, Pizzo PA. Infections due to *Trichosporon* species: new concepts in mycology, pathogenesis, diagnosis and treatment. Curr Top Med Mycol. 1993;5:79–113.
89. Haupt HM, Merz WG, Beschorner WE, Vaughan WP, Saral R. Colonization and infection with *Trichosporon* species in the immunosuppressed host. J Infect Dis. 1983;147:199–203.
90. Ebright JR, Fairfax MR, Vazquez JA. *Trichosporon asahii*, a non-*Candida* yeast that caused fatal septic shock in a patient without cancer or neutropenia. Clin Infect Dis. 2001;33:28–30.
91. Krcmery V, Mateicka F, Kunova A, et al. Hematogenous trichosporonosis in cancer patients: report of 12 cases including 5 during prophylaxis with itraconazole. Support Care Cancer. 1999;7:39–43.
92. Keay S, Denning D, Stevens DA. Endocarditis due to *Trichosporon beigelii*: In-vitro susceptibility of isolates and review. Rev Infect Dis. 1991;13:383–6.
93. Fisher DJ, Christy C, Spafford P, Maniscalo WM, Hardy DJ, Graman PS. Neonatal *Trichosporon beigelii* infection. Report of a cluster of cases in a neonatal intensive care unit. Pediatr Infect Dis J. 1993;12:149–55.
94. Mirza SH. Disseminated *Trichosporon beigelii* infection causing skin lesions in a renal transplant patient. J Infect. 1993;27:67–70.
95. Hajjeh RA, Blumberg HM. Bloodstream infection due to *Trichosporon beigelii* in a burn patient: Case report and review of therapy. Clin Infect Dis. 1995;20:913–6.
96. Lussier N, Laverdiere M, Delorme J, Weiss K, Dandavino R. *Trichosporon beigelii* funguria in renal transplant recipients. Clin Infect Dis. 2000;31:1299–301.
97. Chan RM, Lee P, Wroblewski J. Deep-seated trichosporonosis in an immunocompetent patient: A case report of uterine trichosporonosis. Clin Infect Dis. 2000;31:621–5.
98. Netsvyetayeva I, Swoboda-Kopec E, Paczek L, et al. *Trichosporon asahii* as a prospective pathogen in solid organ transplant recipients. Mycoses. 2009;52:263–5.
99. Ruan SY, Chien JY, Hsueh PR. Invasive trichosporonosis caused by *Trichosporon asahii* and other unusual Trichosporon species at a medical center in Taiwan. Clin Infect Dis. 2009;49:e11–7.
100. Da Silva Rodrigues G, de Faria RR Ubatuba, Silva Guazzelli L, de Mattos Oliveira F, Severo LC. Infeccion nosocomial por *Trichosporon asahii*:revision clinica de 22 casos. Rev Iberoam Micol. 2006;23:85–9.
101. Marin J, Chiner E, Franco J, Borras R. *Trichosporon beigelii* pneumonia in a neutropenic patient. Eur J Clin Microbiol Infect Dis. 1989;8:631–3.
102. Cheng IKP, Fang G, Chan T, Chan PC, Chan MK. Fungal peritonitis complicating peritoneal dialysis: Report of 27 cases and review of the literature. Quart J Med. 1989;71:407–16.
103. Sheikh HA, Mahgoub S, Badi K. Postoperative endophthalmitis due to *Trichosporon cutaneum*. Br J Ophthalmol. 1986;58:591–4.
104. Bhansali S, Karanes K, Palutke W, Crane L, Kiel R, Ratanatharathorn V. Successful treatment of disseminated *Trichosporon beigelii* (cutaneum) infection with associated splenic involvement. Cancer. 1986;58:1630–2.
105. Szili M, Domjan L. Primary gastric mycosis caused by *Trichosporon cutaneum*. Mykosen. 1982;25:189–93.
106. Patel SA, Borges MC, Batt MD, Rosenblate HJ. *Trichosporon* cholangitis associated with hyperbilirubinemia, and findings suggesting primary sclerosing cholangitis on endoscopic retrograde cholangiopancreatography. Gastroenterology. 1990;85:84–7.
107. Surmont I, Vergauwen B, Marcelis L, Verbist L, Verhoef G, Boogaerts M. First report of chronic meningitis caused by *Trichosporon beigelii*. Eur J Clin Microbiol Infect Dis. 1990;9:226–9.
108. Walsh TJ, Melcher GP, Rinaldi MG, et al. *Trichosporon beigelii*, an emerging pathogen resistant to amphotericin B. J Clin Microbiol. 1990;28:1616–22.
109. Yung CW, Hanauer SB, Fretzin D, Rippon JW, Shapiro C, Gonzalez M. Disseminated *Trichosporon beigelii* (*cutaneum*). Cancer. 1981;48:2107–11.
110. Walsh TJ, Orth DH, Shapiro CM, Levine RA. Metastatic fungal chorioretinitis developing during *Trichosporon* sepsis. Ophthalmology. 1982;89:152–6.
111. Walsh TJ. Trichosporonosis. Infect Dis Clin North Am. 1989;3: 43–52.
112. Walsh TJ, Newman KR, Moody M, Wharton R, Wade JC. Trichosporonosis in patients with neoplastic disease. Medicine (Baltimore). 1986;65:268–79.

113. Ito T, Ishikawa Y, Fujii R, et al. Disseminated *Trichosporon capitatum* infection in a patient with acute leukemia. Cancer. 1988; 61:585–8.
114. Mochizuki T, Sugiura H, Watanabe S, Takada M, Hodohara K, Kushima R. A case of disseminated trichosporonosis: A case report and immunohistochemical identification of fungal elements. J Med Vet Mycol. 1988;26:343–9.
115. Liu KL, Herbrecht R, Bergerat JP, Koenig H, Waller J, Oberling F. Disseminated *Trichosporon capitatum* infection in a patient with acute leukemia undergoing bone marrow transplantation. Bone Marrow Transplant. 1990;6:219–21.
116. Thaler M, Pastakia B, Shawker TH, O'Leary TO, Pizzo PA. Hepatic candidiasis in cancer patients: The evolving picture of the syndrome. Ann Intern Med. 1988;108:88–100.
117. Meyer MH, Letscher-Bru V, Waller J, Lutz P, Marcellin L, Herbrecht R. Chronic disseminated *Trichosporon asahii* infection in a leukemic child. Clin Infect Dis. 2002;35:e22–e5.
118. Walsh TJ, Lee JW, Melcher GP, et al. Experimental *Trichosporon* infection in persistently granulocytopenic rabbits: Implications for pathogenesis, diagnosis, and treatment of an emerging opportunistic mycosis. J Infect Dis. 1992;166:121–33.
119. Paphitou NI, Ostrosky-Zeichner L, Paetznick VL, Rodriguez JR, Chen E, Rex JH. In vitro antifungal susceptibilities of *Trichosporon* species. Antimicrob Agents Chemother. 2002;46:1144–6.
120. Anaissie E, Gokaslan A, Hachem R, et al. Azole therapy for trichosporonosis: clinical evaluation of eight patients, experimental therapy for murine infection, and review. Clin Infect Dis. 1992;15:781–87.
121. Matsue K, Uryu H, Koseki M, Asada N, Takeuchi M. Breakthrough trichosporonosis in patients with hematologic malignancies receiving micafungin. Clin Infect Dis. 2006;42:753–7.
122. Mazuelos EM, Rodriguez-Tudela JL. Actividad in vitro de anidulafungina. Comparacion con actividad de otras equinocandinas. Enferm Infecc Microbiol Clín. 2008;26:7–13.
123. Serena C, Pastor FJ, Gilgado F, Mayayo E, Guarro J. Efficacy of micafungin in combination with other drugs in a murine model of disseminated trichosporonosis. Antimicrob Agent Chemother. 2005;49:497–502.
124. Goodman D, Pamer E, Jakubowski A, Morris C, Sepkowitz. Breakthrough trichosporonosis in a bone marrow transplant recipient receiving caspofungin acetate. Clin Infect Dis. 2002;35: e35–e6.
125. Wolf DG, Falk R, Hacham M, et al. Multidrug-resistant *Trichosporon asahii* infection of nongranulocytopenic patients in three intensive care units. J Clin Microbiol. 2001;39:4420–5.
126. Gemeinhardt H. Lungenpathogenitat von *Trichosporon capitatum* beim menschen. Zentrablatt fur Bakteriolgie (Series A). 1965;196: 121–33.
127. Martino P, Venditti M, Micozzi A, et al. *Blastoschizomyces capitatus*: an emerging cause of invasive fungal disease in leukemia patients. Rev Infect Dis. 1990;12:570–82.
128. D'Antonio D, Piccolomini R, Fioritoni G, et al. Osteomyelitis and intervertebral discitis caused by *Blastoschizomyces capitatus* in a patient with acute leukemia. J Clin Microbiol. 1994;32:224–7.
129. Espinel-Ingroff A. Comparison of in vitro activities of the new triazole SCH56592 and the echinocandins MK-0991 (L-743, 872) and LY303366 against opportunistic filamentous and dimorphic fungi and yeast. J Clin Microbiol. 1998;36:2950–6.
130. Polacheck I, Salkin IF, Kitzes-Cohen, Raz R. Endocarditis caused by *Blastoschizomyces capitatus* and taxonomic review of the genus. J Clin Microbiol. 1992;30:2318–22.
131. D'Antonio D, Mazzoni A, Iacone A, et al. Emergence of fluconazole-resistant strains of *Blastoschizomyces capitatus* causing nosocomial infections in cancer patients. J Clin Microbiol. 1996;34:753–5.
132. Bergman AG, Kauffman CA. Dermatitis due to *Sporobolomyces* infection. Arch Dermatol. 1984;120:1059–60.
133. Plazas J, Portilla J, Boix V, Perez-Mateo M. *Sporobolomyces salmonicolor* lymphadenitis in an AIDS patient: pathogen or passenger? AIDS. 1994;8:387–98.
134. Morris JT, Beckius M, McAllister CK. *Sporobolomyces* infection in an AIDS patient. J Infect Dis. 1991;164:623–4.
135. Fell JW, Tallman AS. Genus 13. *Sporobolomyces* Kluyver et van Niel. In: Kreiger-van Rij NJW, editor. The Yeasts: a Taxonomic Study. 3rd ed. Amsterdam: Elsevier Science Publishers; 1984. p. 911–20.

Part IV
Mycoses Caused by Moulds

Aspergillosis

Thomas F. Patterson

The opportunistic mold *Aspergillus* is the etiologic agent responsible for a variety of infections and conditions referred to as aspergillosis. These manifestations include a spectrum of diseases from allergic responses to the organism (allergic bronchopulmonary aspergillosis), to colonization with *Aspergillus* spp. (aspergilloma or fungus ball and other superficial conditions, such as external ear colonization) and invasive infection (invasive pulmonary aspergillosis and other clinical syndromes of tissue invasion).

The importance of *Aspergillus* as a clinically important pathogen has increased dramatically. Invasive aspergillosis is a significant cause of morbidity and mortality in high-risk patients [1–3]. The increased number of cases of invasive aspergillosis is due to the fact that a greater number of patients are at risk for this disease, including patients undergoing hematopoietic stem cell or solid organ transplantation and the use of corticosteroids and other immunosuppressive therapies. Management of invasive aspergillosis remains difficult due to the limited sensitivity of diagnostic tests and is further compounded by the fact that antifungal agents must be begun promptly if therapy is likely to be successful [3]. Cultures may not always be positive in patients with invasive aspergillosis, but it is important to recognize that a positive culture result in a high-risk patient may suggest the presence of infection. Recent developments in non-culture-based methods allow early diagnosis of infection, which can be used to initiate early antifungal therapy. Radiology may also be useful in establishing a presumptive diagnosis of infection [4]. Even when antifungal therapy is begun promptly, outcomes of therapy remain poor, particularly in patients with disseminated disease and in those with persistent immunosuppression [1, 3, 5]. Significant advances in the therapy of aspergillosis have been reported, and guidelines using currently available drugs have been published [3].

T.F. Patterson (✉)
Division of Infectious Diseases, The University of Texas Health Science Center at San Antonio,
San Antonio, TX, USA
e-mail: patterson@uthscsa.edu

Historic Review

Micheli in Florence first recognized *Aspergillus* in 1729 [6]. In his historic monograph *Nova Geneva Plantarum*, Micheli, a priest, noted the resemblance between the spore-bearing head of the organism he described as *Aspergillus* and an aspergillum used to sprinkle holy water (with the name derived from the Latin *aspergo*, to sprinkle) [6, 7]. Later, Rayer and Montagne identified *Aspergillus candidus* from a bird air sac in 1842, but the first detailed microscopic descriptions of *Aspergillus* were provided in 1856 by Virchow, who also published the first detailed descriptions of human infection [8, 9]. Virchow examined tissues described in earlier reports of animal disease by Bennett in 1844 and Sluyter in 1847 and concluded the organisms were closely related to those that he observed in human infection [10]. Fresenius introduced the term *aspergillosis* in 1863 in his work describing avian infection [11].

Initial descriptions of clinical cases (some of which were likely colonization) were detailed in workers that had been occupationally exposed to the organism, and the association was made with infection and certain occupations, such as pigeon feeders, wig combers, farmers, feed-mill workers, and others exposed to dust or grains [5]. Others noted the potential for *Aspergillus* to colonize or invade cavities that formed following other diseases such as tuberculosis. Deve described fungus balls due to *Aspergillus* (aspergilloma) in 1938 [12]. The potential for allergic reactions to the organisms in the form of allergic bronchopulmonary aspergillosis was described by Hinson and colleagues in 1952 [13]. It was not until the mid-1950s, with the introduction of immunosuppressive agents such as corticosteroids and cytotoxic chemotherapy, that the first occurrences of invasive aspergillosis in immunocompromised hosts were recognized [14]. In recent decades the use of immunosuppressive therapies in increasing numbers of patients has resulted in a dramatic global increase in the numbers of invasive infections due to *Aspergillus* [15].

C.A. Kauffman et al. (eds.), *Essentials of Clinical Mycology*,
DOI 10.1007/978-1-4419-6640-7_14, © Springer Science+Business Media, LLC 2011

Mycology

After the initial early descriptions of the organism, *Aspergillus flavus* was formally named in 1809 [16]. Thom and Church first classified the genus in 1926 with 69 *Aspergillus* species in 11 groups [17–19]. The term "group" has now been replaced with "section," although this nomenclature is not common in clinical mycology laboratories [20]. With the use of molecular techniques to identify fungi, the number of species of aspergilli has increased to over 250 species in seven subgenera and multiple sections [21, 22]. However, phenotypic methods and DNA internal transcribed spacer sequencing only identify isolates within a section, so the recommendation for clinical laboratories is to report species as members of a "species complex." [22].

Most species of *Aspergillus* reproduce asexually, but a teleomorph, or sexual form, has been identified for pathogenic species, including *Aspergillus fumigatus* with its recently described teleomorph *Neosartorya fumigata*, *Aspergillus nidulans* (teleomorph *Emericella nidulans*), and *Aspergillus vitis* (teleomorph *Eurotium amstelodami*) [23, 24]. The generic name *Aspergillus* is generally applied to all species regardless of their teleomorphs, rather than separating the organisms into a limited number of new and unfamiliar species based on discovery of a sexual state along with the majority of isolates without a teleomorph identified [25]. The taxonomy of *Aspergillus* has been extensively revised with reclassification and identification of species based on molecular studies such as sequencing of ribosomal genes, beta-tubulin, or calmodulin [26]. These studies have allowed more natural subgroupings and more accurate identification of species but will undoubtedly continue to cause revisions in *Aspergillus* nomenclature.

The genus *Aspergillus* is classified as an anamorphic member (asexual form) of the family Trichocomaceae of the form class Hyphomycetes in the phylum Deuteromycota. The teleomorphs of *Aspergillus* species are classified in seven genera in the order Eurotiales in the phylum Ascomycota [21]. Identification of the genus *Aspergillus* and of common pathogenic species is not usually difficult, but species-level identification can be more challenging, particularly for atypical or poorly sporulating isolates. Misidentification of these "cryptic" members of *Aspergillus* sections is common [27].

The most common species causing invasive infection are members of the *A. fumigatus*, *A. flavus*, *A. niger*, and *A. terreus* species complexes. Recent studies have shown continued emergence of less common species, including less pathogenic species as etiologic agents of invasive infection (Table 1). With more prolonged and profound immunosuppression, the list of rare species causing invasive infection continues to increase and includes: *A. alabamensis*, *A. alliaceus* (teleomorph *Petromyces alliaceus*), *A. avenaceus*, *A. caesiellus*, *A. candidus*, *A.carneus*, *A. chevalieri*, *A.clavatus*, *A. calidoustus*, *A. flavipes*, *A. fumigataffinis*, *A. glaucus*, *A. granulosus*, *A. lentulus*, *A. novofumigatus*, *A. nidulans*, *A. ochraceus*, *A. oryzae*, *A. puniceus*, *A. pseudodeflectus*, *A. restrictus*, *A. sydowii*, *A. quadrilineatus*, *A. tamarii*, *A. tubingensis*, *A. versicolor*, *A. vitus*, *A.wentii*, *Neosartorya pseudofischeri*, and many others, although the authenticity of some has been questioned [20, 21, 28–31].

Table 1 Identification of *Aspergillus* species in 261 cases of invasive infection [1]

Species	Number (%)
Aspergillus fumigatus	173 (66)
A. flavus	36 (14)
A. niger	17 (7)
A. terreus	11 (4)
A. versicolor	2
A. nidulans	1
A. oryzae	1
A. glaucus	1
Not specified or not identified	19 (7)

Pathogenic *Aspergillus* species grow easily and rapidly at a broad range of culture temperatures and on a wide variety of media, although blood cultures are rarely positive. Growth of pathogenic species at 37 °C is a feature that usually differentiates the pathogenic from nonpathogenic isolates. *A. fumigatus* is able to grow at temperatures up to 50 °C, which, in addition to morphology, can be used to identify that species [29]. Most *Aspergillus* species will initially appear as small, fluffy white colonies within 48 h of culture. Presumptive identification at the genus level is usually performed based on morphologic characteristics without difficulty, although species-level identification of unusual species may be significantly more difficult, particularly if sporulation is slow.

Microscopic features and colony morphology for *A. fumigatus*, *A. flavus*, *A. terreus*, and *A. niger* are shown in Figs. 1 and 2, respectively. Species identification of *Aspergillus* is important, as differences in pathogenicity as well as susceptibility occur. Key features of the four species most frequently associated with clinical manifestations of disease are outlined below.

Aspergillus fumigatus (see Figs. 1a and 2a), the most common pathogen in the section *Fumigati* is the most frequent species to cause invasive aspergillosis historically, comprising up to 90% of the isolates. *A. fumigatus* has been less prevalent in some recent reports [1, 32, 33]. The organism is found widespread in nature – in soil, on decaying vegetation, in the air, and in water supplies [34]. Thermotolerance permits a wide range of suitable host conditions. Colonies are a gray-green color with a woolly to cottony texture [29]. Hyphae are septate and hyaline with columnar conidial heads. Conidiophores are smooth-walled, uncolored, and uniseriate with closely compacted phialides only on the upper portion of

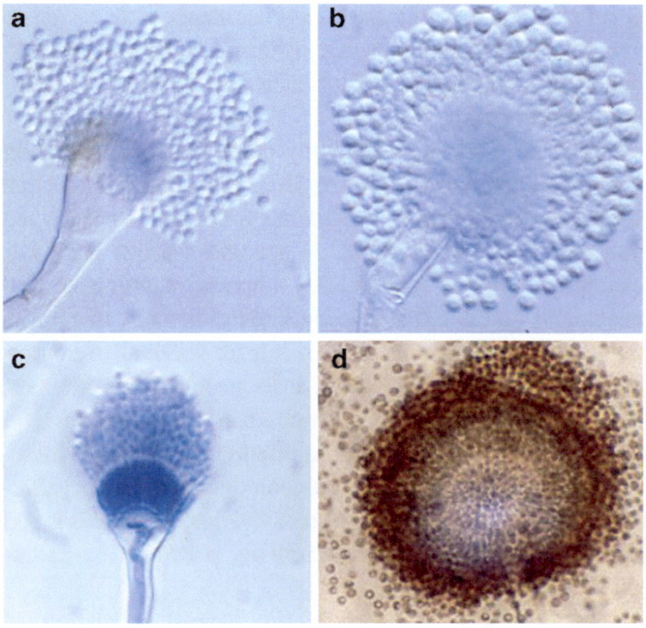

Fig. 1 Microscopic characteristics of *Aspergillus* species fruiting structures. (**a**) *Aspergillus fumigatus* (**b**) *A. flavus* (**c**) *A. terreus* (**d**) *A. niger* (all magnifications ×420) (Photomicrographs kindly provided by Dr. Deanna Sutton)

the vesicle. Conidia are smooth to finely roughened and are 2–3 μm in diameter. Hyphae, which are strongly angioinvasive, may not always branch at a 45° angle. Fruiting heads rarely occur in clinical specimens in sites exposed to air [29].

Other "cryptic" members in the section *Fumigati* that are pathogenic in humans have been described, including *A. lentulus*, *A. fumigataffinis*, *A. novofumigatus*, and others. These species sporulate poorly and, in contrast to *A. fumigatus*, fail to grow at 50 °C but do grow at 10 °C [27, 30]. Identification of these species can be clinically relevant, as some species, such as *A. lentulus*, exhibit decreased antifungal susceptibility [35]. When these species are only identified phenotypically, they should be referred to as members of the *A. fumigatus* species complex.

Aspergillus flavus (see Figs. 1b and 2b) is found in soil and decaying vegetation. Colonies are olive to lime green and grow at a rapid rate. This species is typically biseriate with rough conidiophores and smooth conidia 3–6 μm that serve to distinguish the species. Some isolates are uniseriate. The organism is a common cause of sinusitis as well as invasive infection in immunosuppressed hosts. *Aspergillus flavus* is also responsible for a mycotoxicosis, as the species produces

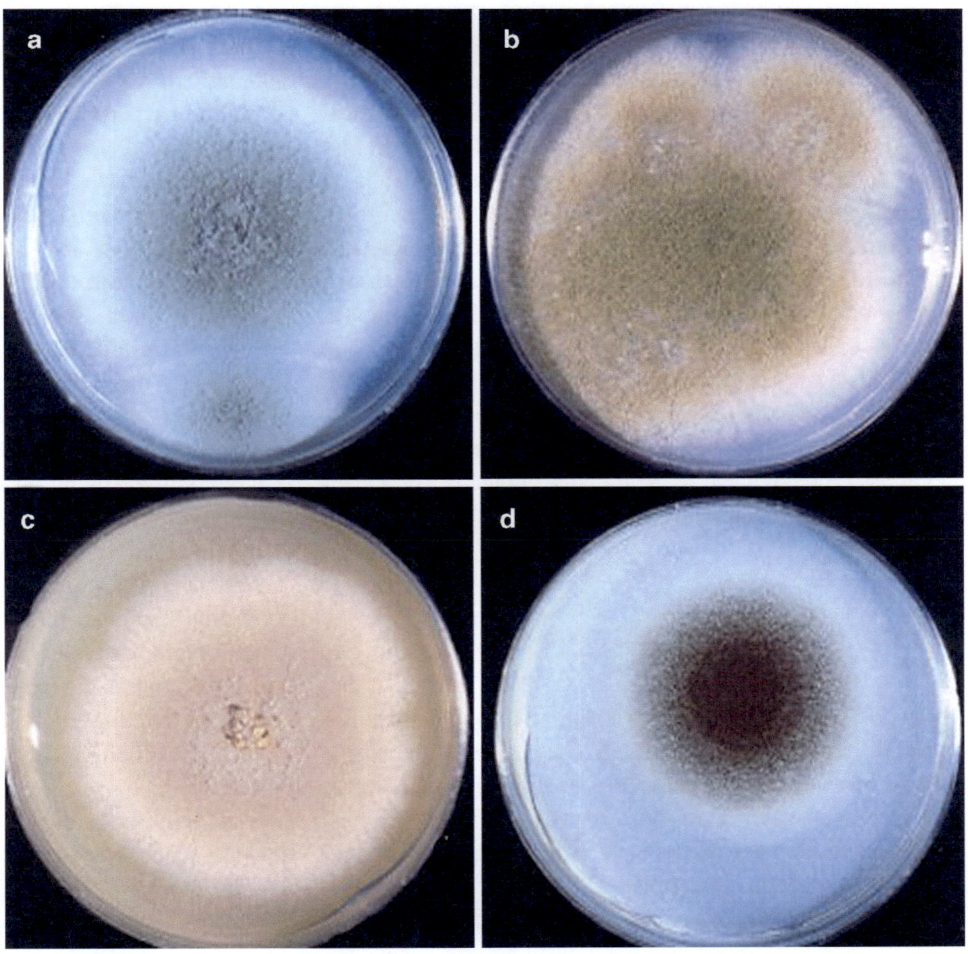

Fig. 2 Colony morphology of *Aspergillus* species. (**a**) *Aspergillus fumigatus* (**b**) *A. flavus* (**c**) *A. terreus* (**d**) *A. niger* (Colony photographs kindly provided by Dr. Deanna Sutton)

a potent aflatoxin [19]. If characterized by morphology alone, *A. flavus* and other species in the section *Flavi* should be referred to as members of the *Aspergillus flavus* species complex.

Aspergillus terreus (see Figs. 1c and 2c) is common in tropical and subtropical habitats and has been increasingly reported as a cause of invasive infection in immunocompromised hosts [36]. Colonies are buff to beige to cinnamon [29]. Conidial heads are biseriate and columnar. Conidiophores are smooth-walled and hyaline. Globose, sessile accessory conidia are frequently produced on submerged hyphae. Conidia are small (2–2.5 μm). The colony color and fruiting structures are characteristic for this species, notable for its decreased susceptibility to amphotericin B [37]. Molecular characterization has shown that *A. terreus* is also a species complex.

Aspergillus niger (see Figs. 1d and 2d) is widespread in soil and on plants and is common in foods such as pepper. Colonies are initially white but quickly become black with the production of the fruiting structures. It grows rapidly with a pale yellow reverse side. Like other *Aspergillus* species, hyphae are hyaline and septate. Conidial heads are biseriate and cover the entire vesicle. Conidia are brown to black and are very rough (4–5 μm) [29]. The species, which is commonly associated with colonization and otic infections, produces oxalate crystals in clinical specimens [38]. This species complex also contains several related species.

Other less common species of *Aspergillus* also cause invasive infection [1, 33]. Some species cause infections in certain epidemiologic settings, such as *A. nidulans*, which is an important cause of invasive infection in patients with chronic granulomatous disease and may be resistant to amphotericin B [39]. Another species of clinical relevance is *A. calidoustus*, a species in the section *Usti*, which grows at 37 °C and was formerly called *A. ustus*, a species which fails to grow at 37 °C. This species is often resistant to multiple antifungal drugs and has been associated with invasive infection in severely immunosuppressed patients [32]. These less pathogenic species must be recognized as potentially clinically significant pathogens in susceptible hosts [20].

Pathogenesis and Host Defenses

Aspergillus infection is typically acquired through inhalation of conidia into the lungs, although other routes of exposure, such as oral or aerosol exposure to contaminated water, may also occur [40]. Cutaneous exposure through surgical wounds, contaminated intravenous catheters, and arm boards can lead to cutaneous infections [41].

Invasive aspergillosis is uncommon in immunocompetent patients, although infection in apparently normal hosts does occur [1]. Hence, despite the ubiquitous nature of the organism and frequent exposures to *Aspergillus* conidia, normal host defenses do not readily permit invasive pulmonary aspergillosis to occur.

Aspergillus species commonly produce toxins, including aflatoxins, ochratoxin A, fumagillin, and gliotoxin, that can contribute to clinical manifestations following exposure and may contribute to virulence in specific settings [19]. For example, gliotoxin significantly impacts macrophage and neutrophil function, but in experimental models, disruption of gliotoxin production did not impact survival in neutropenic animals [42]. However, in nonneutropenic animals, deletion of gliotoxin genes resulted in prolonged survival [43] and, as such, may be more important in invasive infection that develops in nonneutropenic patients. Other pathogenic factors include production of a variety of proteases and phospholipases, which are commonly produced by pathogenic strains [44, 45].

The first line of host defense against inhalation of *Aspergillus* conidia is ciliary clearance of the organism from the airways, limiting access to deep lung structures for larger, less pathogenic conidia. In the pulmonary tissues, the alveolar macrophage is a potent defense, capable of ingesting and killing inhaled *Aspergillus* conidia [46]. The hydrophobic rodlet layer on the conidial cell surface immunologically protects *Aspergillus* against activation of the host innate immune cell response [47]. After germination, the major line of defense against both swollen conidia and hyphae is the polymorphonuclear leukocyte. Recent studies in experimental models have shown the importance of early neutrophil influx in preventing conidial germination and limiting hyphal invasion [48]. Hyphae are too large to be effectively ingested, and hyphal damage occurs extracellularly [49].

Swollen conidia and hyphae are both able to fix complement, which is important in phagocytic killing of the organism. Notably, *A. fumigatus* produces a complement inhibitor, which may play a role in its pathogenicity [50]. Host defenses against *Aspergillus* may be enhanced by opsonization of conidia with complement or other molecules such as mannose-binding protein or surfactant proteins [51]. A deficiency in mannose-blinding lectin has been associated with increased risk for invasive pulmonary aspergillosis [52]. Antibody responses due to prior exposures to *Aspergillus* are common, but antibodies are not protective against invasive infection nor are they useful for diagnosis of infection, due to the fact few immunosuppressed patients are able to mount an antibody response even in the setting of invasive disease [53].

The NADPH oxidase in phagocytes is essential in host defenses against *Aspergillus* species, as demonstrated by the increased susceptibility of patients with chronic granulomatous disease, an inherited disorder of NADPH oxidase, to *Aspergillus* infections [54]. Corticosteroids play a major role in increasing susceptibility to *Aspergillus* by decreasing oxidative killing of the organisms and also by increasing hyphal growth rate [55]. Corticosteroids impair alveolar macrophage function and reduce neutrophil killing of hyphae, which may be reversed to some degree with the use of interferon-γ or with administration of granulocyte or granulocyte-macrophage growth factors [56].

T helper (Th) cytokines have important roles in innate and adaptive defense against *Aspergillus*. In a murine model of invasive aspergillosis, a Th1 response induced by administration of soluble interleukin-4 was associated with a favorable response [57]. Pathogen recognition receptors, including toll-like receptors (TLRs) and dectin-1, also mediate innate defenses against *Aspergillus* [58]. Recognition of *Aspergillus* by TLR2 and dectin-1 results in activation of intracellular pathways leading to proinflammatory cytokine production [59, 60]. These events provide initial host defenses against *Aspergillus* and bridge innate and acquired immunity [61]. Recently, polymorphisms in host genes, including TLR4 haplotypes and plasminogen gene alleles, have been associated with increased susceptibility to invasive aspergillosis in patients undergoing hematopoietic stem cell transplantation [62, 63]. Improved understanding of host defenses could lead to identification and targeted management of patients with increased susceptibility to invasive disease.

In contrast to the deficient host defense responses in invasive infection, in noninvasive allergic forms of aspergillosis such as allergic bronchopulmonary aspergillosis (ABPA) or allergic sinusitis, the pathogenesis often relates to exuberant inflammatory host responses to the organism [64]. The immune responses in ABPA that occur in both asthmatic patients and in those with cystic fibrosis is a Th2 response [65]. ABPA begins with an allergic inflammatory response that follows after inhalation of *Aspergillus* conidia into the bronchi, where they germinate and form hyphae [66]. Colonizing hyphae then release allergens that are processed by HLA-DR2 or HLA-DR5 antigen-presenting cells. The resultant Th2 inflammatory response in bronchial tissue leads to excessive mucin production, recruitment of eosinophils, intermittent bronchial obstruction, and eventually bronchiectasis in some patients [65].

Similarly, the pathogenesis of aspergilloma or fungus ball due to *Aspergillus* is not well defined but also seems to be associated with host responses to chronic colonization. In aspergilloma, the organism does not usually invade the tissues, but it colonizes a pulmonary cavity. Although tissue invasion resulting in a chronic necrotizing form of aspergillosis can occur, the pathogenic features leading from colonization to invasive disease are not clearly understood [67]. Chronic forms of pulmonary aspergillosis have been linked to subtle immune defects, including polymorphisms in mannose-binding protein or surfactant [68].

Epidemiology

Aspergillus species are ubiquitous saprophytic molds that are found worldwide in a variety of habitats. They are found in soil, water, and food and are particularly common in decaying vegetation. Exposure to the organisms occurs worldwide and throughout the year, although higher ambient concentrations of *Aspergillus* conidia in autumn and winter have been suggested [69]. The inoculum for establishing infection is not known. Presumably persons with normal pulmonary defense mechanisms can withstand even extensive exposure without any manifestation of disease, while severely immunocompromised hosts are likely to develop disease with lower inocula.

Patients at highest risk for invasive aspergillosis include those with prolonged neutropenia; recipients of hematopoietic stem cell transplants or solid organ transplants, especially lung transplants; patients with advanced AIDS; and those with chronic granulomatous disease [1, 58]. Other patients at risk include those on chronic corticosteroids or tumor necrosis factor antagonists [70], those with chronic lung disease, and, more recently described, patients with nontraditional risk factors in the intensive care unit [71].

Prolonged neutropenia is a major risk factor for invasive aspergillosis [72]. Without recovery from neutropenia, response to even aggressive antifungal therapy is unlikely [1]. Nevertheless, with changing patterns of immunosuppressive therapy, patients are less likely to remain neutropenic for extended periods of time, and the use of growth factors has further limited the duration of neutropenia. An index that considers the duration and depth of neutropenia has been developed to predict risk of invasive mycoses in patients with recurrent or persistent episodes of neutropenia [73].

In recent surveys, other immunosuppressive conditions have emerged as important risk factors for invasive aspergillosis, and the time period for risk of invasive aspergillosis in a variety of hosts is now greatly extended. In patients receiving hematopoietic stem cell transplants, the period at risk extends for more than 100 days after immunosuppression [74–76]. The extended period of risk reflects long-term complications of high-dose corticosteroid therapy and other immunosuppressive agents for chronic graft-versus-host disease, especially following non-myeloablative transplant procedures.

Patients undergoing allogeneic hematopoietic stem cell transplantation and those with hematologic malignancies, such as acute myelogenous leukemia, are at highest risk for developing invasive infection [1]. Even among high-risk patients there is substantial heterogeneity of risk. For example, in patients with acute myelogenous leukemia, the incidence of invasive aspergillosis ranges from as low as 2% to as high as 25% or more, with a mean incidence of approximately 4–7% [77–80]. Among patients who have received a solid organ transplant, those undergoing lung transplantation are at particular risk for *Aspergillus* infection. The clinical presentation ranges from an ulcerative tracheobronchitis to disseminated infection [81, 82]. The increased risk in these patients is due to the transplanted organ being exposed to the environment, altered ciliary clearance, and the fact that many of these patients are colonized prior to transplantation [82]. Invasive aspergillosis in liver transplant recipients typically involves pulmonary infection, occurs late in the post-transplantation period, and is associated with a lower mortality rate, as compared to those who develop aspergillosis earlier after liver transplantation.

Outbreaks of invasive aspergillosis have occurred in patients exposed to *Aspergillus* in association with construction and other environmental risks [83]. Air filtration and infection control measures, such as construction barriers that reduce risks by limiting exposure to aerosols, have been shown to reduce the incidence of infection. Air filtration with high-efficiency particulate air (HEPA) filters has been recommended as the standard of care in bone marrow transplant units during the period of most severe neutropenia in order to reduce the rates of nosocomial infection [69, 84]. However, in the most severely immunosuppressed patients, aspergillosis may still occur, either as a result of endogenous reactivation of infection or due to other exposures, perhaps even related to aerosols of contaminated water [40, 84, 85]. Stem cell and solid organ transplant patients who are at greatest risk for invasive aspergillosis frequently receive substantial portions of their care outside the hospital setting; however, control of air quality in those settings is not possible.

Clinical Syndromes

The clinical presentation of diseases produced by *Aspergillus* species is diverse and generally reflect the underlying immune status of the host and the host's response to the organism [86]. The syndromes of aspergillosis range from asymptomatic colonization, superficial or saprophytic infection, allergic responses to the organism, and acute or subacute invasive disease [3].

Saprophytic and Superficial Aspergillosis

Pulmonary Aspergilloma

A pulmonary fungus ball due to *Aspergillus* (aspergilloma) is characterized by chronic, extensive colonization of *Aspergillus* species in a pulmonary cavity or ectatic bronchus. Fungus balls may also develop in other sites, such as the maxillary or ethmoid sinus, or even in the upper jaw following endodontic treatment [87]. Typically *Aspergillus* fungus balls in the lung develop in cavities as a result of pre-existing infections or diseases, such as tuberculosis, histoplasmosis, sarcoidosis, bullous emphysema, fibrotic lung disease or, rarely, *Pneumocystis jiroveci* pneumonia. The diagnosis of a pulmonary fungus ball, which can also be due to other molds, is usually made radiographically with the appearance of a solid round mass inside a cavity. The detection of *Aspergillus* antibodies are further evidence that the radiographic findings are consistent with a diagnosis of fungus ball due to *Aspergillus;* biopsy is not usually undertaken [3, 88].

Although the presence of a fungus ball due to *Aspergillus* may be relatively asymptomatic, in some patients tissue invasion may occur, leading to invasive pulmonary aspergillosis or a subacute chronic necrotizing form of the disease [3, 67]. Hemoptysis is a common clinical symptom and can lead to a fatal complication. Hemoptysis has been reported as the cause of death in up to 26% of patients with aspergilloma [88]. Management of aspergilloma is determined by the frequency and severity of hemoptysis, and by evaluation for risk factors that are associated with a poor prognosis. Complications are more likely in patients with severe underlying lung disease, immunosuppression, or extensive disease suggested by high titers of *Aspergillus* antibody. In these settings, specific therapies may be needed earlier in the course of management in order to avoid potential life-threatening hemoptysis [88].

Chronic Forms of Pulmonary Aspergillosis

The spectrum of aspergillosis of the lower respiratory tract includes diseases previously referred to as "semi-invasive pulmonary aspergillosis" and chronic necrotizing pulmonary aspergillosis [86]. The chronic and progressive nature of infection with *Aspergillus* species in some patients has led some authors to describe pulmonary aspergillosis along a continuum [67]. Chronic necrotizing pulmonary aspergillosis is the descriptive term applied to cavitary lung disease, chronic respiratory symptoms, and the presence of serum-precipitating antibodies to *Aspergillus*. Direct invasion of *Aspergillus* into the lung parenchyma without angioinvasion occurs, and this form of infection is described as a subacute or non-angioinvasive form of disease [67]. The term chronic cavitary pulmonary aspergillosis, sometimes referred to as "complex aspergilloma" in the surgical literature, has been applied to the formation and expansion of multiple pulmonary cavities [89]. Some of these patients have been described as having subtle defects in host defenses including polymorphisms in mannose-binding lectin [68]. It is currently unclear if these distinctions of chronic pulmonary aspergillosis will provide assistance in guiding management.

Other Superficial or Colonizing Conditions

Aspergillus is associated with fungal balls of the sinuses without tissue invasion [87]. The maxillary sinus is the site most commonly involved. Clinical presentation is similar to that for any chronic sinusitis with chronic nasal discharge, sinus congestion, and pain. The diagnosis of a fungal ball is suggested on CT scan of the sinuses; positive cultures for *Aspergillus*, usually *A. fumigatus* or *A. flavus*, are obtained by aspiration of material from the sinuses. Management is usually directed at surgical removal of the lesion and confirmation that the fungal ball has not caused bony erosion.

Otomycosis is a condition of superficial colonization by *Aspergillus*, most typically *A. niger* [90]. The usual clinical presentation is that of an external otitis media with ear pain and drainage. Examination of the ear canal may reveal the black conidiophores of *A. niger*. Treatment involves cleaning debris from the ear canal and the topical administration of a variety of agents, including cleansing solutions and topical antifungal agents. Voriconazole has also been beneficial in anecdotal case reports [91].

Other superficial or colonizing conditions due to *Aspergillus* include onychomycosis, which can be a chronic condition not responsive to antifungal agents directed at yeasts. Culture confirmation of *Aspergillus* as the etiologic agent may be useful in this setting.

Aspergillus species may also colonize the airways without causing disease in patients with a variety of lung conditions. A survey of clinical laboratories showed that a large number of isolates of *Aspergillus* are not associated with infection [33]. Many of those isolates come from sputum samples of patients without apparent invasive disease, although the role of *Aspergillus* in causing symptoms of occasional hemoptysis and bronchitis in those patients is unclear.

Allergic Manifestations of Disease

Allergic Bronchopulmonary Aspergillosis

ABPA is a chronic allergic response to colonization with *Aspergillus*. Classic criteria for establishing a diagnosis include (1) episodic bronchial obstruction (asthma); (2) peripheral eosinophilia; (3) immediate skin test reactivity to *Aspergillus* antigen; (4) precipitating *Aspergillus* antibodies; (5) elevated serum immunoglobulin E (IgE); (6) history of or presence of pulmonary infiltrates; and (7) central bronchiectasis [64, 92]. The detection of the first six criteria establishes a likely diagnosis, while the presence of all seven confirms the condition. Other secondary features that may be present include sputum cultures yielding *Aspergillus*, brown mucus plugs in expectorated sputum, elevated specific IgE antibodies against *Aspergillus*, late skin test reactivity to *Aspergillus*, and reactions following intrabronchial challenge with *Aspergillus* [64, 93].

In ABPA, typically the initiating event is for an asthmatic patient to develop an allergic reaction to inhaled *Aspergillus*. Following that reaction, mucus plugs develop in the bronchi and can be detected by the presence of hyphae in sputa. The impacted mucus causes atelectasis, which in turn causes transient pulmonary infiltrates; repeated bronchial reactions ultimately lead to bronchiectasis in the proximal bronchi. Characteristic "ring signs" (circular or oblong densities) or "tram lines" (parallel shadows) are seen on chest radiographs. These findings result from chronic peribronchial inflammation around dilated bronchi [64].

ABPA is reported to occur in up to 14% of patients with steroid-dependent asthma [64] and is also particularly common in patients colonized with *Aspergillus*, including patients with cystic fibrosis who have a 7% prevalence of ABPA [65]. In cystic fibrosis patients undergoing lung transplantation, the presence of *Aspergillus* colonization is an important risk factor for developing invasive pulmonary aspergillosis.

This form of aspergillosis typically progresses through a series of stages which are helpful in delineating appropriate management of the condition: (1) acute; (2) remission; (3) exacerbation; (4) steroid-dependent asthma; and (5) fibrosis [64, 93]. The initial acute stage is usually responsive to corticosteroid therapy, which may lead to a period of asymptomatic remission. Most patients will experience exacerbations and may eventually become steroid dependent. Late-stage manifestations include pulmonary fibrosis that may be associated with substantially reduced pulmonary function and are associated with a poor long-term prognosis. Management of ABPA is directed at reducing acute asthmatic symptoms and avoiding end-stage fibrotic complications. Corticosteroid therapy is commonly used for treating exacerbations, although few randomized trials have been conducted to evaluate its use. Increasing serum IgE levels, worsening or new infiltrates, or worsening findings on spirometry suggest that steroids may be helpful [3]. The role of antifungal agents is limited, although itraconazole appears to be beneficial in reducing symptoms and allowing a reduction in the use of corticosteroids. A randomized double-blind, placebo-controlled trial showed that itraconazole, 200 mg daily, for 16 weeks significantly reduced daily corticosteroid use, reduced levels of serum IgE, and improved exercise tolerance and pulmonary function [94].

Other Allergic Manifestations

Allergic responses can also contribute to symptoms of sinusitis [95]. Allergic sinusitis is similar in its presentation to sinusitis complicated with fungal balls due to *Aspergillus*.

Frequently, in patients with allergic sinusitis, polyposis or eosinophil-rich mucin-containing Charcot-Leyden crystals are seen [95]. Management is largely directed at confirming lack of invasive infection and in aerating the sinus. The use of steroids or antifungal agents has not been conclusively demonstrated to be of benefit [3].

Invasive Syndromes Caused by Aspergillus

Infection with *Aspergillus* is usually acquired through inhalation of airborne conidia that invade the lung tissue in the absence of an effective monocytic or neutrophilic immune response [96]. The major clinical presentation is invasive pulmonary aspergillosis, which arises from spread of the organism from a primary pulmonary inoculum or from the paranasal sinuses. Hyphal invasion into blood vessels is common, occurring in approximately a third of patients. Nonpulmonary sites become infected by contiguous spread or via hematogenous spread to the central nervous system, occurring in 10–40% of severely immunosuppressed patients, such as those undergoing allogeneic hematopoietic stem cell transplantation, or to other organs, including the liver, spleen, kidney, skin, bone, and heart [1, 5].

Response to antifungal therapy depends on several factors, including the immune status of the host and extent of the infection at time of diagnosis. Favorable responses, defined as those with complete resolution of signs and symptoms and those with partial responses, have been historically seen in fewer than 40% of treated patients (Table 2) [1]. Even more striking are the extremely poor responses seen in the most highly immunosuppressed patients. For example, in a survey of 595 patients with invasive aspergillosis, favorable responses were seen in only 13% of patients undergoing allogeneic bone marrow transplantation [1]. Similarly poor responses have been reported in severely immunosuppressed patients in other series [97–101]. Extent of infection also correlates with likelihood of a favorable outcome: in patients with disseminated infection, favorable responses decrease to fewer than 20% and are frequently fewer than 10% in patients with central nervous system disease who remain immunosuppressed [1].

Table 2 Favorable responses in invasive aspergillosis: role of immunosuppression and extent of disease [1]

Underlying disease (*n*)	Complete/ partial responses (%)
Overall (595)	37
Severe immunosuppression (363)	28
Allogeneic BMT (151)	13
Hematologic malignancy (212)	39
Less severe immunosuppression (232)	51

Site of infection (*n*)	Complete/ partial responses (%)
Pulmonary (330)	40
Disseminated (without CNS) (114)	18
Central nervous system (34)	9

BMT bone marrow transplant, *CNS* central nervous system

As might be predicted, the mortality rate of patients with invasive aspergillosis correlates with the immune status of the host and extent of disease. Lin and colleagues reviewed 1941 patients from 50 series of invasive aspergillosis and found an overall mortality rate of 60%, which rose to more than 80% in patients with severe immunosuppression and almost 90% in those with central nervous system involvement [2]. More effective therapies and improved diagnostic strategies have been associated with more successful outcomes and improved survival [102, 103] although outcomes in patients with disseminated infection or persistent immunosuppression remain poor [101, 104].

Invasive Pulmonary Aspergillosis

Invasive pulmonary aspergillosis is the most common manifestation of invasive aspergillosis. The temporal pattern of infection is closely linked to changes in circulating neutrophils, including both the degree and the duration of severe neutropenia. A significant number of patients are colonized at the time of admission or develop sinus or airway colonization with *Aspergillus* shortly after hospitalization, suggesting prior community-acquired colonization or infection [84, 85]. The disease rarely manifests before 10–12 days of profound neutropenia.

The most frequent symptoms include progressive dry cough, fever despite therapy with broad-spectrum antibiotics (although fever may not be present in patients receiving corticosteroids), dyspnea, and pleuritic chest pain. Notably, extensive infection can develop before symptoms are prominent, which emphasizes the importance of clinical suspicion to establish the diagnosis early. Other manifestations include hemoptysis and pneumothorax. Invasive pulmonary aspergillosis may resemble a pulmonary embolism with sudden onset of chest pain and difficulty breathing. The physical examination is often not helpful.

Laboratory studies usually reflect neutropenia and thrombocytopenia secondary to chemotherapy. Occasional nonspecific findings include elevation in bilirubin and lactate dehydrogenase, coagulation abnormalities, elevation in C-reactive protein and fibrinogen. Patients with more widespread pulmonary involvement may develop respiratory failure characterized by hypoxemia with compensatory hyperventilation, hypocapnea, and respiratory alkalosis. The prognosis of patients with focal nodular pulmonary lesions is more favorable; limited disease may respond to antifungal therapy and also be amenable to adjunctive surgical intervention [3, 4, 105, 106].

Initially, plain chest radiographs often show few abnormalities [107]. With progression of the infection, diffuse

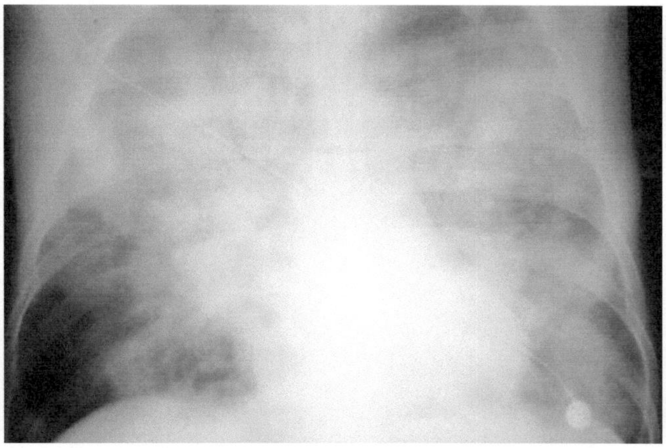

Fig. 3 Chest radiograph showing diffuse pulmonary infiltrates of invasive pulmonary aspergillosis

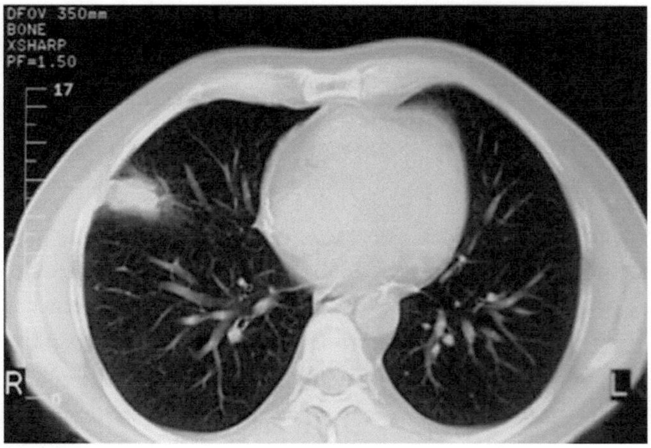

Fig. 4 Computed tomography of chest showing "halo" sign of low attenuation surrounding a nodular lung lesion in early invasive pulmonary aspergillosis

nodular pulmonary infiltrates typically occur and are readily seen on chest radiographs (Fig. 3). Other pulmonary lesions include pleural-based, wedge-shaped densities and cavities. Pleural effusions have been considered rare [5], but recent studies suggest that pleural effusions are more common than has been recognized, although their relationship with infection has not been established [99, 108].

Chest CT scans are more sensitive for detecting early infection and in establishing the extent of infection. The presence of a "halo" of low attenuation surrounding a nodular lesion is an early finding and has been used as a marker for initiating early antifungal therapy (Fig. 4) [99, 107, 108]. Later in the course of infection, nodular lesions can cavitate, usually in temporal association with recovery of neutrophils, producing an "air-crescent" sign (Fig. 5). Despite the utility of these radiographic findings, it should be recognized that their validity has been established in high-risk, neutropenic, and hematopoietic stem cell transplant patients. In other groups, including solid organ transplant patients, other opportunistic etiologic agents can

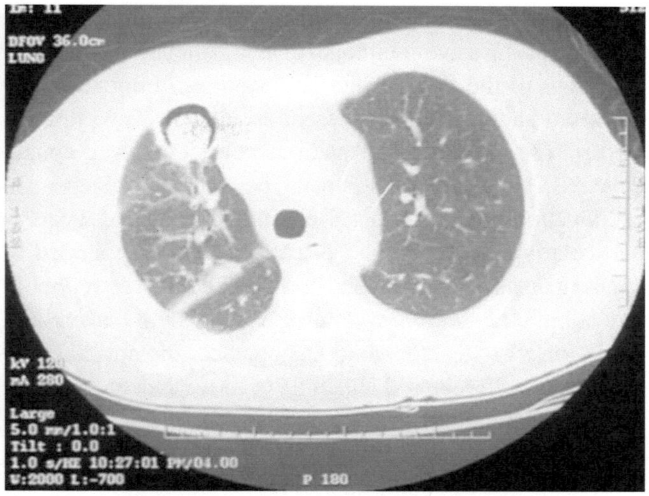

Fig. 5 Computed tomography of chest showing classic "air crescent" sign of invasive aspergillosis

clearly cause similar findings; consequently, CT findings should be interpreted with caution.

Tracheobronchitis

Aspergillus infection of the airways is more common in patients in patients undergoing lung transplantation and in those with advanced AIDS [81, 109]. The syndromes in these patients range from colonization, which is particularly common in lung transplant recipients, to extensive pseudomembranous or ulcerative tracheobronchitis that occurs at the suture line of the transplant [110, 111]. Symptoms of tracheobronchitis may be mild and can be confused with other causes, including rejection in lung transplantation. Typically these patients have cough, fever, and dyspnea along with chest pain and hemoptysis. In more severe disease, unilateral wheezes or stridor may develop due to local obstruction [5].

Plain radiographs are not sensitive for the diagnosis of tracheobronchitis, and clinical suspicion combined with change in pulmonary functional capacity are early clues for the diagnosis. Bronchoscopy with biopsy to document tissue invasion is needed to establish the diagnosis of invasive *Aspergillus* tracheobronchitis. Therapy with systemic antifungal agents is usually given for a prolonged period of time. Aerosols of amphotericin B deoxycholate are difficult to administer and are poorly tolerated, but aerosols of lipid formulations amphotericin B have been successfully used for localized disease [112].

Sinusitis

Involvement of the nasal passages or sinuses is also a relatively classic manifestation of invasive aspergillosis that may appear as isolated syndromes or, more commonly, in the context of invasive pulmonary aspergillosis. *Aspergillus* infections of the sinuses and nasal cavities in immunocompromised patients usually present as acute invasive rhinosinusitis. The clinical manifestations consist of fever, cough, epistaxis, sinus discharge, facial pain, and headache. On examination, identification of anesthetic areas and ulcers is particularly important. The disease can quickly spread to adjacent areas, such as palate, orbit, and brain. The mortality rate is high, ranging from 20% in patients with leukemia in remission who are undergoing maintenance therapy, to 100% in patients with relapsed leukemia or those undergoing stem cell transplantation [3]. Plain radiographs are not sensitive for the diagnosis and do not distinguish fungal etiologies from other causes of sinusitis. Sinus CT scans are useful for establishing extent of infection and determining local invasion of bone and soft tissues. Diagnosis is established presumptively from culture of sinus or nasal material but requires tissue to document invasive disease.

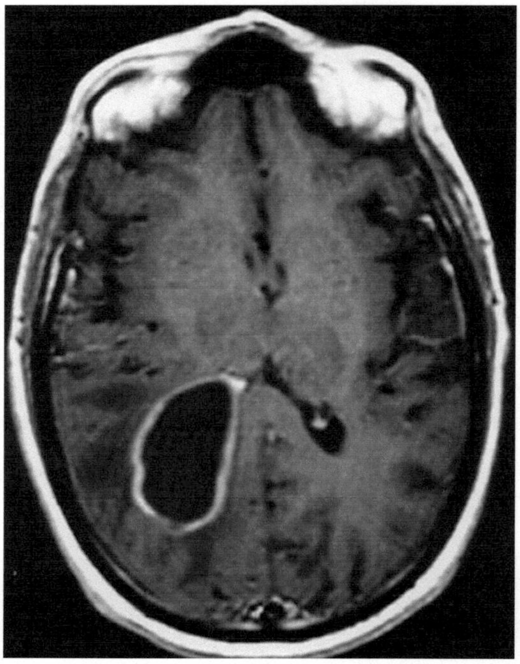

Fig. 6 Brain abscess of invasive aspergillosis with ring enhancement and extensive edema

Disseminated Infection

Widely disseminated invasive aspergillosis is a frequent end-stage complication of refractory pulmonary aspergillosis. In patients with severe immunosuppression, including patients with profound neutropenia, extensive graft-versus-host disease, and progressive underlying malignancy, infection can disseminate rapidly and involve virtually every organ system, as seen in autopsy series. In patients with extensive disease, favorable responses to therapy are uncommon, and mortality rates approach 90% [2, 101, 104].

Cerebral Aspergillosis

Cerebral aspergillosis is one of the most dreaded complications of disseminated aspergillosis; historically, the mortality rates were greater than 90%, although recent studies have suggested better responses with aggressive antifungal therapy and surgical intervention [2, 113]. Cerebral aspergillosis occurs in as many as 10–20% of all cases of invasive aspergillosis, and is usually associated with disseminated disease [1, 5, 113]. In severely immunosuppressed patients, such as those undergoing hematopoietic stem cell transplantation, *Aspergillus* is a major cause of brain abscess; in one series, 58% of lesions that were biopsied revealed aspergillosis [114]. Isolated cerebral aspergillosis can occur in immunocompetent patients, in whom it is associated with a slightly better prognosis provided the diagnosis is made early and surgical drainage or extirpation is performed. *Aspergillus* meningitis is rare.

The clinical presentation of cerebral aspergillosis is characterized by focal neurologic signs, alteration in mental status, and headaches. Fever may occur but is usually related to other concomitant infections. On CT scan of the brain, *Aspergillus* lesions appear similar to other infectious causes of brain abscess and manifest ring enhancement of the abscess along with surrounding edema (Fig. 6). Magnetic resonance imaging may reveal additional lesions. Although the diagnosis of cerebral aspergillosis is confirmed by biopsy, the etiology can be inferred in patients who have widely disseminated infection. However, in highly immunosuppressed patients, including those with organ or stem cell transplants or advanced AIDS, the differential diagnosis is very broad and includes bacterial brain abscesses, toxoplasmosis, other fungi, tuberculosis, and lymphoma. Consequently, a presumptive diagnosis should be entertained with caution. The outcome of cerebral aspergillosis has been almost universally fatal. Recent studies have reported overall responses of 35% after therapy with voriconazole and surgical intervention, although responses in patients with persistent immunosuppression are still extremely poor [113].

Cutaneous Disease

Skin involvement by *Aspergillus* can either represent disseminated hematogenous spread or local infection associated with an intravenous catheter insertion site or the skin areas covered by adhesive dressings [3]. While most cutaneous lesions occur in patients with neutropenia or in other immunocompromised patients, including neonates, *Aspergillus* can also invade burns or surgical wounds [3]. Clinically, the lesion shows an area of rapidly increasing erythema with a necrotic, often ulcerated, center and can resemble ecthyma gangrenosum. Pathologically, there is invasion of blood vessels and cutaneous ulceration. In patients with cutaneous disease as a manifestation of widespread disseminated aspergillosis, a skin biopsy is a relatively easy method to obtain tissue to establish the diagnosis.

Osteomyelitis

Aspergillus osteomyelitis is an uncommon manifestation of invasive aspergillosis. Bony involvement can occur in the setting of local extension from a pulmonary, sinus, or brain lesion, resulting in extensive infection that is often refractory to therapy. *Aspergillus* osteomyelitis can also be seen as a complication of disseminated infection or as a primary infection in certain risk groups, such as patients with chronic granulomatous disease or intravenous drug users [3]. With primary infection, the spine, usually the lumbar area, is often affected [115]. The lesions can be seen on plain radiographs as well as on CT scan or MR imaging, which are useful to stage the infection and guide needle biopsy of the lesion. Favorable responses, as high as 55%, have been reported in one review of the use of voriconazole for *Aspergillus* osteomyelitis. Long-term therapy and surgical intervention are frequently needed in those not responding to medical management [116].

Other Invasive Infections

Invasive aspergillosis in a variety of other sites has been reported in case reports or small series [5]. Endocarditis due to *Aspergillus* can occur on either native or prosthetic heart valves. The diagnosis of endocarditis due to *Aspergillus* is particularly difficult, as blood cultures usually remain negative despite extensive disease. The prognosis for *Aspergillus* endocarditis is poor even with surgical intervention, although successful therapy with voriconazole alone has been reported [117]. Pericarditis can also occur, usually secondary to local extension from the lungs or in the setting of disseminated disease, and can be complicated by cardiac tamponade [5].

Other unusual sites of *Aspergillus* infection include the eye (keratitis, endophthalmitis), gastrointestinal tract, and kidneys, although invasive infection has been observed in virtually all body sites [5, 118]. *Aspergillus* keratitis is frequently associated with trauma or corneal surgery [119]. The diagnosis of fungal keratitis is established with smears showing hyphae that are indistinguishable from other molds, such as *Fusarium*. Cultures are required to confirm the diagnosis. Therapy is usually with amphotericin B or natamycin drops, but data supporting their use are limited [3]. In anecdotal cases, voriconazole has been successfully administered systemically as well as topically [3, 120].

Diagnosis

The diagnosis of invasive aspergillosis is established presumptively on clinical grounds and confirmed by growth of the organism in culture and histopathology. Non-culture-based tests offer the potential for a more rapid diagnosis. However, non-culture-based tests remain relatively insensitive, and invasive procedures are often reluctantly performed, so that many patients have a presumptive diagnosis based on clinical suspicion alone. The clinical syndrome of acute dyspnea, pleuritic chest pain, and hemoptysis that results from angioinvasion of pulmonary vessels by the fungus is an important but usually late clue to the diagnosis.

A number of approaches can be utilized to obtain tissue samples for invasive aspergillosis. For pulmonary lesions and other sites, such as soft tissue or bone, a fine-needle biopsy can be attempted and guided by CT to increase the diagnostic yield and avoid a more invasive procedure. Bronchoscopy with bronchoalveolar lavage (BAL) and transbronchial biopsy is useful in establishing a specific diagnosis and in evaluating for other pathogens in these high-risk patients. Brain lesions that are not accessible can be presumptively identified by establishing the presence of invasive pulmonary or disseminated aspergillosis [3].

Histopathology

The diagnosis of invasive aspergillosis is proven with hyphal invasion of tissue specimens together with a positive culture for *Aspergillus* species [121]. Hyphal elements and morphology are usually easily demonstrated in infected tissues using stains such as Gomori methenamine silver or periodic acid–Schiff (see Fig. 7). *Aspergillus* hyphae are typically hyaline, septate, 3–6 μm wide with parallel cross-walls, and dichotomously branched at acute angles [29]. These features usually allow distinction from Zygomycetes, which are much broader, exhibit right-angle branching, and are rarely or sparsely septate. Agents of phaeohyphomycosis can be distinguished due to their black or darkly pigmented hyphae due to melanin that stains with the Fontana-Masson stain [122]. However, it is important to note that a number of pathogenic moulds, including *Scedosporium*, *Fusarium*, *Geotrichum*, *Scopulariopsis*, and others will have virtually identical appearances to *Aspergillus* species on histopathology. Although specific immunohistochemical stains using fluorescent antibodies to *Aspergillus* can distinguish the organism, as can polymerase

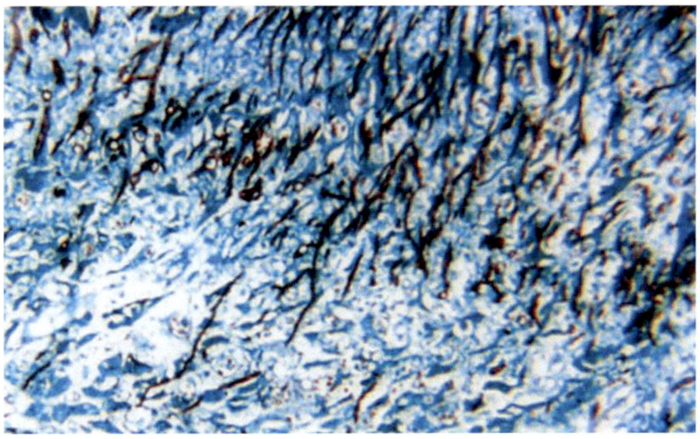

Fig. 7 Lung tissue section showing thin, acutely branching hyphae on Grocott-Gomori methenamine silver (*GMS*) stain invading pulmonary tissues (original magnification ×420)

chain reaction (PCR)–based approaches, these methods are not widely available for routine clinical use [123].

Culture and Susceptibility

Cultures for *Aspergillus* in respiratory samples can be used to diagnose invasive infection in high-risk patients [124]. In patients with high rates of infection, such as patients with neutropenia or those undergoing stem cell transplantation, the presence of *Aspergillus* in a respiratory sample, particularly if obtained from BAL fluid, is highly suggestive of the diagnosis of invasive aspergillosis [121]. In contrast, blood cultures are rarely positive for *Aspergillus*. These features have led the joint European Organization for Research and Treatment of Cancer/Mycoses Study Group (EORTC/MSG) panel to propose that positive BAL cultures in conjunction with clinical illness and pulmonary infiltrates in neutropenic or allogeneic hematopoietic stem cell transplant patients constitute adequate criteria for a diagnosis of probable invasive pulmonary aspergillosis [121].

Genus-specific identification and susceptibility testing are becoming more important as antifungal therapies are increasingly directed at specific pathogens. For example, voriconazole is active against most *Aspergillus* species but is not active against Zygomycetes [125]. Similarly, the echinocandins are not active in vitro against Zygomycetes and have limited direct activity against moulds other than *Aspergillus*. Culture of the organism will also allow susceptibility testing to be performed.

Susceptibility testing for moulds, including *Aspergillus*, has been validated, although there are limited data correlating susceptibility results with clinical activity [3]. Antifungal resistance to azoles has been reported for a limited number of isolates, which correlates with lack of clinical response in experimental infection in animal models and in some patients [126, 127]. Multi-triazole resistance, including the spread of a single resistance mechanism, has been reported in *Aspergillus* strains [126–128]. In isolates obtained since 1999, prevalence of resistance ranged from 1.7% to 6% [128]. Not all resistant isolates are cross-resistant to other azoles in vitro so testing various antifungals may be useful [126, 127]. Some species, such as *A. terreus*, are resistant to amphotericin B and susceptible to azoles, so testing of that species could also be of potential clinical utility [37]. Nevertheless, the need for routine susceptibility testing of *Aspergillus* is limited at the present time [3].

Radiographic Studies

Radiographic findings can also be useful to suggest a diagnosis of *Aspergillus* infection. Plain chest radiographs are too insensitive to make the diagnosis, as extensive pulmonary disease may be present with few findings on chest films. In neutropenic and hematopoietic stem cell transplant patients with invasive aspergillosis and other angioinvasive moulds, chest CT scans often demonstrate lesions that are not visible on plain radiographs. A "halo" of low attenuation surrounding a nodular lung lesion in a high-risk patient has been associated with an early diagnosis of infection (Fig. 4) [4]. A nodular lesion may subsequently undergo cavitation to form an "air crescent" sign that is associated with aspergillosis; this radiographic sign occurs later in the course of illness, usually after recovery of neutrophils (Fig. 5) [4]. The presence of a CT "halo" sign as a trigger to begin presumptive therapy in high-risk patients resulted in favorable responses, particularly when combined with detection of circulating levels of serum galactomannan [129]. It should also be recognized that pulmonary lesions can increase in volume over the first 7 days of therapy even with an eventual clinical response so that radiographic progression does not necessarily mean progression of the infection [4].

Non-Culture-Based Methods

Non-culture-based methods have been used to establish a rapid diagnosis of invasive aspergillosis. Detection of antibody to *Aspergillus* was evaluated for diagnosis of invasive disease, but a large proportion of patients have antibodies caused by prior asymptomatic exposure to ubiquitous *Aspergillus* conidia and immunosuppressed patients do not develop a prompt antibody response to infection [53]. Thus, non-culture-based diagnostics have been targeted to *Aspergillus* antigens or metabolites and, more recently, to molecular targets associated with invasive infection.

Detection of galactomannan (GM) in serum and more recently in other body fluids, especially BAL, has played an important role in the non-culture-based diagnosis of invasive aspergillosis [130]. The current EIA assay (Platelia *Aspergillus*, Sanofi Diagnostics Pasteur, Marnes-la-Coquette, France; BioRad, Redmond, WA) utilizes a monoclonal antibody to GM and has been extensively validated in experimental models and in clinical studies [130]. Sensitivity for detecting invasive aspergillosis has been reported as high as 89% with a specificity of 92% in high-risk hematopoietic stem cell transplant patients [131]. Other studies have found lower sensitivity ranging as low as 40–50%, particularly in the setting of mould-active antifungal prophylaxis or therapy and when serial samples were not used for testing [132, 133]. An index of positivity in serum of 0.5 is now recommended, particularly in high-risk patients [130, 133, 134]. False-positive results have been seen in some patients, including neonates and pediatric patients, and are thought to be due to dietary intake or the presence of cross-reacting antigens from bacteria such as *Bifidobacterium.* False-positive findings have also occurred in patients receiving antibiotics, particularly piperacillin-tazobactam, and in some other fungal infections, such as histoplasmosis [130, 135–137]. Although the method has been used to test other body fluids, such as cerebrospinal fluid and BAL fluid, these samples have been less extensively studied compared to serum [138, 139]. In one study, detection of GM in BAL fluid increased the sensitivity, compared to serum, from 47% to 85% [140], and BAL was the only sample that was positive in other studies [141, 142]. However, false-positive results have been reported in patients with *Aspergillus* colonization and with the use of fluids used for BAL that contain GM, such as plasmalyte [143, 144]. Studies are ongoing to establish the clinical utility and cut-off threshold for positivity in nonserum samples.

Another non-culture-based method approved for clinical use is detection of serum (1$\rightarrow$3) beta-D-glucan using an amebocyte limulus lysate test [145–148]. This assay detects cell wall beta-glucans and, as such, is not specific for *Aspergillus* but is also positive in infections due to other fungi, including *Candida* and moulds other than *Aspergillus*. Although there are limited clinical studies to support the use of this assay in invasive aspergillosis, its use is included in the EORTC/MSG definitions for establishing a diagnosis of invasive fungal infection [121].

The use of PCR to establish a molecular basis for diagnosis has also been evaluated in invasive aspergillosis [149, 150], but a number of features still limit its utility. There are no externally validated methods, and a variety of targets and techniques have been utilized [151]. A recent meta-analysis of published results of PCR studies showed a sensitivity of 75% and a specificity of 87% when two positive samples were used to establish a positive result. For a single sample, this rose to a sensitivity of 88% at the cost of reduced specificity of 75% [152]. Levels of circulating PCR product in serum or blood are low, but promising results have been seen, particularly when combined with other diagnostic methods [153, 154].

Treatment

Historically, therapy with amphotericin B deoxycholate was the recommended therapy for invasive aspergillosis, but outcomes using this agent were extremely poor, particularly in severely immunosuppressed patients and those with extensive infection. Overall response rates of <40% and mortality rates >60% were common [1, 2]. Fortunately, an extensive effort has resulted in development of new drugs to meet this unmet medical need [155]. Antifungal agents with activity against *Aspergillus* have been developed, and these drugs have substantially improved the armamentarium for use in invasive aspergillosis. These include voriconazole, posaconazole, liposomal amphotericin B, amphotericin B lipid complex, caspofungin, micafungin, and anidulafungin, (Table 3).

Triazole Antifungals

Voriconazole, a potent, broad-spectrum, triazole antifungal, has become the recommended primary therapy for most patients with invasive aspergillosis [3]. In vitro, voriconazole demonstrates fungicidal activity against clinically relevant *Aspergillus* species, including *A. terreus* [167]. Voriconazole, which is available in both oral and parenteral forms, is approved for the primary therapy of invasive aspergillosis based on a randomized trial comparing voriconazole to amphotericin B deoxycholate followed by other licensed antifungal therapy [99]. In this trial, successful outcomes occurred in 52% of voriconazole-treated patients as compared to only 31% in patients receiving amphotericin B. Importantly, benefit was demonstrated in patients at high risk for mortality, such as stem cell transplant recipients and those with extrapulmonary disease, including central nervous system involvement [99, 168]. A survival advantage with voriconazole versus standard therapy was shown [99]. The benefit of voriconazole has also been demonstrated in adult and pediatric patients receiving salvage therapy for invasive aspergillosis [169, 170]. In addition, voriconazole has shown efficacy in difficult to treat aspergillosis, including successful therapy in 35% of patients with central nervous system infection and in 52% of patients with bone infection [113, 116].

Although voriconazole is generally well tolerated and exhibits favorable pharmacokinetics, there are a number of

Table 3 Antifungal agents for invasive aspergillosis

Class/agent	Route of administration	Dose	Comment
Azoles			
Voriconazole	IV/oral	6 mg/kg q12h × 2 loading dose IV; 4 mg/kg q12hr (IV); 200 mg q12h (PO); 7 mg/kg twice daily for children <11 year	Recommended primary therapy of invasive aspergillosis in most patients; improved survival as compared with amphotericin B [3, 99]
Posaconazole	Oral	200 mg 4× daily; 200 mg 3× daily for prophylaxis	Efficacy in salvage therapy and prophylaxis; well-tolerated; variable bioavailability [77, 80, 156, 157]
Itraconazole	Oral	200 mg bid	Improved bioavailability with oral solution; toxicity limits utility in immunosuppressed patients [1, 158]
Isavuconazole	IV/Oral	Investigational	Phase III comparative trials in progress; activity in experimental infection [159]
Polyenes			
Amphotericin B deoxycholate	IV	1.0–1.5 mg/kg/day	Previous "gold standard" therapy; significant toxicity; limited efficacy in high-risk patients [160, 161]
Liposomal amphotericin	IV	3–5 mg/kg/day	Recommended as alternative primary therapy in some patients; well tolerated; minimal infusion reactions or nephrotoxicity; 3 mg/kg/day as effective as 10 mg/kg/day as primary therapy of invasive pulmonary aspergillosis [106]
Amphotericin B lipid complex	IV	5 mg/kg/day	Indicated for invasive mycoses intolerant or refractory to standard therapy [162]
Echinocandins			
Caspofungin	IV	70 mg load, then 50–70 mg/day	Approved for use in patients with invasive aspergillosis refractory to or intolerant of standard therapy; well tolerated in clinical trials; not recommended for primary therapy; anecdotal role in combination therapy [97, 101, 163]
Micafungin	IV	100 mg/day	Efficacy in salvage therapy [164]
Anidulafungin	IV	200 mg load, then 100 mg/day	Efficacy in vitro and in experimental infection; [165, 166] combination clinical study with voriconazole in progress

considerations, including substantial drug-drug interactions, especially with drugs metabolized through cytochrome P450 3A4 isoenzymes. These include the immunsuppressive agents' cyclosporine, tacrolimus, and sirolimus. The latter agent is contraindicated because voriconazole leads to a substantial increase in sirolimus serum concentrations. The most common adverse event associated with voriconazole is a transient and reversible visual disturbance, which has been reported in approximately one-third of patients receiving the drug [99, 171]. This effect, which is dose related, is described as an altered or increased light perception that is temporary and is not associated with sequelae. Other adverse events have been less common, including liver abnormalities in 15% of patients, skin rash in 6%, nausea and vomiting in 2% and anorexia in 1%.

A major advantage of voriconazole is the ability to administer the drug both orally and parenterally. In some patients receiving oral drugs, weight-based dosing may be beneficial [3]. Therapeutic drug monitoring for voriconazole has been recommended in patients with toxicity as well as those with progressive infection, as drug levels higher than 6 μg/mL are more likely to be associated with toxicity, and levels <2 μg/mL are more likely to be associated with inadequate therapeutic responses [172]. Voriconazole is primarily metabolized through cytochrome 2C19 so that some patient groups, particularly non-Indian Asian patients, have significant reductions in voriconazole metabolism and increases in serum concentrations [171]. Voriconazole is linear in its metabolism in pediatric patients; a dose of 7 mg/kg twice daily produces levels in pediatric patients similar to those in adults receiving the standard dosage [3, 173].

Posaconazole, currently available in only an oral formulation, has been shown to have activity against *Aspergillus* in vitro as well as in vivo studies [3, 156]. Posaconazole is approved for use in prophylaxis against *Aspergillus* and has activity in salvage therapy as well. Posaconazole exhibits saturable absorption so that oral loading doses are not possible. This may impact its use for primary therapy, as steady-state levels make not be achieved for up to a week [171]. In a salvage study of invasive aspergillosis in patients refractory to or intolerant of conventional antifungal therapy, favorable responses were seen in 42% of patients receiving posaconazole as compared to only 26% of patients receiving conventional therapy [156]. An important observation in this study was the improved outcomes associated with higher serum levels of posaconazole. In a separate study, posaconazole levels <0.7 μg/mL were reported for 70% of samples, and 16% of samples had undetectable levels. Accordingly, measurement of serum levels in critically ill patients is advised [157].

Posaconazole has been generally well tolerated; however, in one large trial in patients with acute leukemia or myelodysplasia, there was more toxicity shown in those receiving posaconazole prophylaxis than in those receiving fluconazole or itraconazole prophylaxis [77]. Posaconazole undergoes glucuronidation by the liver and has the capacity for drug-drug interactions through inhibition of CYP450 3A4 isoenzymes, although liver toxicity appears less common than with other azoles [171].

Itraconazole is approved for salvage therapy of aspergillosis, but its utility is limited by its toxicity and unfavorable pharmacokinetic profile. Itraconazole is currently available in an oral capsule formulation, which is poorly bioavailable, and an oral suspension, which offers better absorption but has limited gastrointestinal tolerability [171]. An intravenous itraconazole preparation is no longer available. In less immunosuppressed patients who are able to take oral therapy, itraconazole has been shown to be effective and is usually used for those who have saprophytic or allergic diseases associated with *Aspergillus* and as step-down therapy for patients who were initially treated with an intravenous antifungal agent [1].

Isavuconazole is an investigational triazole in clinical development which is a broad-spectrum agent with activity in vitro and in vivo against *Aspergillus* species and is available orally as well as intravenously [159]. Isavuconazole is currently undergoing evaluation in comparative trials for invasive aspergillosis.

Polyenes

Overall response rates for amphotericin B deoxycholate, which was the recommended therapy for invasive aspergillosis for more than 40 years, were favorable in only about 25% of patients. Among severely immunosuppressed patients, such as those undergoing hematopoietic stem cell transplantation, response rates were favorable in only 10–15% [1, 99]. A number of studies have demonstrated the limited efficacy and significant dose-limiting toxicities, including higher mortality rates and overall higher costs of care, associated with amphotericin B deoxycholate when given in high doses for mould infections, such as those due to *Aspergillus* [160, 161].

Recommendations regarding the role of lipid formulations of amphotericin B in invasive aspergillosis are limited because few randomized trials have been conducted with these agents [3]. One early trial with amphotericin B colloidal dispersion showed similar efficacy compared with amphotericin B deoxycholate and less renal toxicity, but the colloidal dispersion formulation was associated with more toxicity than other lipid formulations, did not improve outcomes, and is rarely clinically used [98]. Other studies have established the improved efficacy and reduced toxicity of the lipid-based agents in salvage settings, and all lipid formulations are approved for this indication [3].

A meta-analysis of studies using lipid formulations of amphotericin B showed reduced nephrotoxicity and favorable results as salvage therapy for invasive aspergillosis [174]. A recent clinical trial of primary therapy for invasive pulmonary aspergillosis compared the utility of two doses of liposomal amphotericin B (3 mg/kg daily vs 10 mg/kg daily) for 2 weeks followed by standard therapy [106]. In this study, similar efficacy was observed in both groups (46% and 50% in the low and high initial dose therapy, respectively), with more kidney and liver toxicity in the high-dose group. Thus, these results suggest that liposomal amphotericin B can be recommended as primary therapy in patients for whom voriconazole is contraindicated because of underlying hepatic toxicity or because of concerns with drug interactions [3].

Echinocandins

The echinocandins all have activity against *Aspergillus* [165, 175, 176]. These agents, which are administered intravenously, target glucan synthase, the enzyme that is needed for synthesis of beta-1,3-glucan in fungal cell walls [177]. FDA-approved agents in this class are caspofungin, micafungin, and anidulafungin. Caspofungin is approved for treatment of patients refractory to or intolerant of standard therapies for invasive aspergillosis [3]. In an open-label trial for such patients, caspofungin was demonstrated to produce satisfactory clinical responses in 41% (22/54) of patients studied [97]. Micafungin has also been evaluated in a salvage setting with similar clinical results [164].

The echinocandins are not fungicidal against *Aspergillus* species, but do significantly alter growth of the hyphae [177]. In a recent study evaluating caspofungin as primary therapy for invasive aspergillosis, overall responses were disappointingly low (33%), suggesting that echinocandins should not be used as first-line therapy for invasive aspergillosis [101]. An important point is that all of the echinocandins have been extremely well tolerated with few clinically significant adverse events.

Combination Therapy

The clinical availability of several antifungal drugs and drug classes with activity against *Aspergillus* has increased interest in combination antifungal therapy for this potentially lethal disease. Early studies in this area were performed in experimental animal models and in vitro and showed antagonism between amphotericin B and ketoconazole, an early imidazole with limited *Aspergillus* activity [178]. This antagonism occurred with pretreatment of *Aspergillus* with the imidazole, reducing cell wall ergosterol and eliminating the site of action of amphotericin B. However, studies with newer azoles have not consistently shown this antagonistic effect [179].

Other combinations have been evaluated, including amphotericin B and rifampin, amphotericin B and flucytosine, and others, such as terbinafine [180]. Problems with rifampin combined with azoles include increased metabolism of the azole drugs, which obviates their use and makes this combination unattractive. Similarly, flucytosine has limited activity against *Aspergillus* and can cause pancytopenia that worsens immunosuppression. Recent animal model studies and retrospective anecdotal clinical reports have demonstrated the potential efficacy of reducing the burden of infection by using echinocandins in combination with triazoles or polyene therapy [163, 166, 175, 181]. Although clinical studies using combination antifungal therapy are in progress, at present the routine use of combination therapy for primary therapy of invasive aspergillosis is not recommended [3].

Adjunctive Therapies

The role of adjunctive therapies for management of invasive aspergillosis has not been well studied. Surgical removal of isolated pulmonary nodules prior to additional immunosuppressive therapies has been shown to improve outcome of infection [105, 107]. In other cases, medical therapy with voriconazole alone may be successful without the need for surgery [3]. Other therapies, such as granulocyte transfusions, granulocyte and granulocyte-macrophage colony-stimulating factors, and interferon-gamma have been shown in anecdotal reports to improve outcomes in individual patients. Currently, these approaches are not recommended for routine use because improved responses and survival rates have not been conclusively demonstrated [3].

Approach to Management

Guidelines for treating invasive aspergillosis have been recently published by the Infectious Diseases Society of America [3]. There are still a limited number of randomized clinical trials to guide recommendations for therapy. Gaps in knowledge exist in a number of difficult situations, such as selection of therapy for patients in whom primary therapy is not successful and when to consider using combination therapy. Nevertheless, the guidelines suggest that in high-risk patients a prompt diagnosis and aggressive antifungal therapy may improve the outcome of this disease [3]. Unfortunately, even aggressive antifungal therapy is unlikely to be successful unless the underlying state of immunosuppression of the patient improves. Diagnostic measures such as cultures from respiratory samples, CT scans, and non-culture-based methods can all be used to facilitate earlier and more precise diagnosis.

Voriconazole is the recommended primary therapy in most patients. Lipid formulations of amphotericin B are recommended as alternative primary therapy in patients for whom voriconazole is contraindicated. A number of options exist for salvage therapy, including triazole antifungals, such as posaconazole or voriconazole, lipid formulations of amphotericin B, and the echinocandins. Combination therapy is not recommended for routine use as primary therapy but may be considered in patients with progressive infection, pending completion of ongoing clinical trials. Optimal duration of therapy is unknown, but improvement in underlying immunosuppression is critical to a successful outcome.

Prevention and Prophylaxis

Prevention of invasive aspergillosis in high-risk patients remains a difficult challenge. Outbreaks of *Aspergillus* infections have been linked to hospital construction, contaminated ventilations systems, operating rooms, and contaminated water [40, 69, 85]. It is important to recognize that high-risk immunosuppressed patients now spend much of their treatment course in the outpatient setting; consequently, community-acquired infection is also common [85]. Prevention of nosocomial aspergillosis in the highest-risk populations is difficult even when state-of-the-art air control systems, such as point-of-use HEPA filters, frequent air exchanges, and positive-pressure ventilation, are used [69, 83] High-risk patients also can have exposures in the hospital setting outside of the protective environment of their hospital room [84].

Antifungal prophylaxis using agents with activity against *Aspergillus* has been limited due to lack of available agents and the toxicity of amphotericin B. Agents evaluated for prophylaxis include low-dose amphotericin B, low-dose lipid formulations of amphotericin B, and nasal and aerosolized forms of amphotericin B. None of these have been conclusively demonstrated to have efficacy in large, randomized clinical trials. Itraconazole has been suggested to have benefit in preventing mold infections, but poor tolerance by high-risk patients has limited its use [158, 182]. Itraconazole was shown to reduce the incidence of invasive aspergillosis in a long-term single-arm study in patients with chronic granulomatous disease [183]. Similarly, aerosolized liposomal amphotericin B reduced breakthrough infection in a single-center study [184].

Two randomized trials have established the safety and efficacy of posaconazole in high-risk patients. Posaconazole, when compared with fluconazole, in patients with severe graft-versus-host disease, reduced the number of breakthrough *Aspergillus* infections [80]. In another study, in patients with acute myelogenous leukemia or myelodysplasia, posaconazole was compared to fluconazole or itraconazole [77]. In that study, posaconazole reduced breakthrough mycoses, including aspergillosis, and improved survival rates. There were more serious adverse events in patients receiving posaconazole, but prophylaxis was generally well tolerated. Thus, posaconazole prophylaxis is recommended for patients at highest risk for invasive aspergillosis [3].

References

1. Patterson TF, Kirkpatrick WR, White M, I3 Aspergillus Study Group, et al. Invasive aspergillosis. Disease spectrum, treatment practices, and outcomes. Medicine (Baltimore). 2000;79:250–60.
2. Lin SJ, Schranz J, Teutsch SM. Aspergillosis case – fatality rate: systematic review of the literature. Clin Infect Dis. 2001;32:358–66.
3. Walsh TJ, Anaissie EJ, Denning DW, et al. Treatment of aspergillosis: clinical practice guidelines of the Infectious Diseases Society of America. Clin Infect Dis. 2008;46:327–60.
4. Caillot D, Couaillier JF, Bernard A, et al. Increasing volume and changing characteristics of invasive pulmonary aspergillosis on sequential thoracic computed tomography scans in patients with neutropenia. J Clin Oncol. 2001;19:253–9.
5. Denning DW. Invasive aspergillosis. Clin Infect Dis. 1998; 26:781–803.
6. Micheli P. Nova plantarum genra juxta Tournefortii methodum disposita. Florence: Bernardo Paperini; 1729.
7. Mackenzie DW. Aspergillus in man. In: Vanden Bossche H, Mackenzie DWR, Cauwenbergh G, editors. Proceedings of the Second International Symposium on Topics in Mycology; 1987. Antwerp, Belgium: University of Antwerp; 1987. p. 1–8.
8. Kwon-Chung KJ. *Aspergillus*: Diagnosis and description of the genus. In: Vanden Bossche H, Mackenzie DWR, Cauwenbergh G, editors. Proceedings of the Second International Symposium on Topics in Mycology; 1987. Antwerp: University of Antwerp; 1987. p. 11–21.
9. Virchow V. Breitage zur lehre von den beim menschen vorkommenden pfanzlichen parasiten. Virchows Archiv 1856:557.
10. Kwon-Chung KJ, Bennett JE. Medical Mycology. Philadelphia: Lea & Febiger; 1992.
11. Fresenius G. Beitrage zur Mykologie. Frankfurt: HL Bronner; 1863.
12. Deve F. Une nouvelle forme anatomoradiologique de mycose pulmonaire primitive: le megamycetome intrabronchetasique. Arch Med Chir Appl Respir. 1938;13:337–61.
13. Hinson K, Moon A, Plummer N. Broncho-pulmonary aspergillosis. A review and a report of eight new cases. Thorax. 1952;7:317–33.
14. Rankin N. Disseminated aspergillosis and moniliasis associated with agranulocytosis and antibiotic therapy. Br Med J. 1953;183:918–9.
15. Groll AH, Shah PM, Mentzel C, Schneider M, Just-Nuebling G, Huebner K. Trends in the postmortem epidemiology of invasive fungal infections at a university hospital. J Infect. 1996;33:23–32.
16. Link H. Observations in ordines plantarum naturales. Gesellschaft Naturforschender Freunde zu Berlin, Magazin. 1809;3:1.
17. Thom C, Church M. The Aspergilli. Baltimore: Williams & Wilkins; 1926.
18. Raper B, Fennel J. The Genus *Aspergillus*. Baltimore: Williams & Wilkins; 1965.
19. Patterson TF. Chapter 258. *Aspergillus* species. In: Mandell GL, Bennett JE, Dolin R, editors. Mandell, Douglas, and Bennett's Principles and Practice of Infectious Diseases. 7th ed. Philadelphia, PA: Churchill Livingstone Elsevier; 2009. p. 3241–55.
20. Sutton DA. Rare and emerging agents of hyalohyphomycosis. Curr Fungal Infect Reports. 2008;2:134–42.
21. Summerbell R. Ascomycetes. *Aspergillus*, *Fusarium*, *Sporothrix*, *Piedraia*, and Their Relatives. In: Howard DH, editor. Pathogenic Fungi in Humans and Animals. 2nd ed. New York: Marcel Dekker; 2003. p. 237–498.
22. Balajee SA, Houbraken J, Verweij PE, et al. *Aspergillus* species identification in the clinical setting. Stud Mycol. 2007;59:39–46.
23. Klich M, Pitt J. A laboratory guide to common *Aspergillus* species and their teleomorphs. North Ryde, New South Wales, Australia: Commonwealth Scientific and Industrial Research Organization; 1988.
24. O'Gorman CM, Fuller HT, Dyer PS. Discovery of a sexual cycle in the opportunistic fungal pathogen Aspergillus fumigatus. Nature. 2009;457:471–4.
25. Pitt JI, Samson RA. *Nomenclatural* considerations in naming species of *Aspergillus* and its teleomorphs. Stud Mycol. 2007;59:67–70.
26. Geiser DM, Klich MA, Frisvad JC, Peterson SW, Varga J, Samson RA. The current status of species recognition and identification in *Aspergillus*. Stud Mycol. 2007;59:1–10.
27. Balajee SA, Nickle D, Varga J, Marr KA. Molecular studies reveal frequent misidentification of *Aspergillus fumigatus* by morphotyping. Eukaryot Cell. 2006;5:1705–12.
28. Pitt J. The current role of *Aspergillus* and *Penicillium* in human and animal health. J Med Vet Mycol. 1994;1:17–21.
29. Sutton DA, Fothergill AW, Rinaldi MG, editors. Guide to Clinically Significant Fungi. 1st ed. Baltimore: Williams & Wilkins; 1998.
30. Balajee SA, Gribskov JL, Hanley E, Nickle D, Marr KA. *Aspergillus lentulus* sp. nov., a New Sibling Species of A. fumigatus. Eukaryot Cell. 2005;4:625–32.
31. Balajee SA, Baddley JW, Peterson SW, et al. *Aspergillus alabamensis*, a new clinically relevant species in the section Terrei. Eukaryot Cell. 2009;8:713–22.
32. Sutton DA, Fothergill AW, Rinaldi MG. *Aspergillus in vitro* antifungal susceptibility data: New millennium trends (abstract 16). In: Abstracts of Advances Against Aspergillosis, September 9–11, 2004, San Francisco, CA; 2004.
33. Perfect JR, Cox GM, Lee JY, et al. The impact of culture isolation of *Aspergillus* species: a hospital-based survey of aspergillosis. Clin Infect Dis. 2001;33:1824–33.
34. Anaissie EJ, Stratton SL, Dignani MC, et al. Pathogenic *Aspergillus* species recovered from a hospital water system: A 3-year prospective study. Clin Infect Dis. 2002;34:780–9.
35. Balajee SA, Imhof A, Gribskov JL, Marr KA. Determination of antifungal drug susceptibilities of *Aspergillus* species by a fluorescence-based microplate assay. J Antimicrob Chemother. 2005;55:102–5.
36. Steinbach WJ, Benjamin Jr DK, Kontoyiannis DP, et al. Infections due to *Aspergillus terreus*: a multicenter retrospective analysis of 83 cases. Clin Infect Dis. 2004;39:192–8.
37. Steinbach WJ, Perfect JR, Schell WA, Walsh TJ, Benjamin Jr DK. In vitro analyses, animal models, and 60 clinical cases of invasive *Aspergillus terreus* infection. Antimicrob Agents Chemother. 2004;48:3217–25.
38. Geyer SJ, Surampudi RK. Photo quiz - Birefringent crystals in a pulmonary specimen. Clin Infect Dis. 2002;34(481):551–2.
39. Kontoyiannis DP, Lewis RE, May GS, Osherov N, Rinaldi MG. *Aspergillus nidulans* is frequently resistant to amphotericin B. Mycoses. 2002;45:406–7.
40. Anaissie EJ, Costa SF. Nosocomial aspergillosis is waterborne. Clin Infect Dis. 2001;33:1546–8.

41. Walsh TJ. Primary cutaneous aspergillosis – An emerging infection among immunocompromised patients. Clin Infect Dis. 1998; 27:453–7.
42. Cramer Jr RA, Gamcsik MP, Brooking RM, et al. Disruption of a nonribosomal peptide synthetase in *Aspergillus fumigatus* eliminates gliotoxin production. Eukaryot Cell. 2006;5:972–80.
43. Spikes S, Xu R, Nguyen CK, et al. Gliotoxin production in *Aspergillus fumigatus* contributes to host-specific differences in virulence. J Infect Dis. 2008;197:479–86.
44. Latge JP. *Aspergillus fumigatus* and aspergillosis. Clin Microbiol Rev. 1999;12:310–50.
45. Alp S, Arikan S. Investigation of extracellular elastase, acid proteinase and phospholipase activities as putative virulence factors in clinical isolates of *Aspergillus* species. J Basic Microbiol. 2008;48:331–7.
46. Schaffner A, Douglas H, Braude A. Selective protection against *conidia* by mononuclear and against mycelia by polymorphonuclear phagocytes in resistance to *Aspergillus*. Observations on these two lines of defense in vivo and in vitro with human and mouse phagocytes. J Clin Invest. 1982;69:617–31.
47. Aimanianda V, Bayry J, Bozza S, et al. Surface hydrophobin prevents immune recognition of airborne fungal spores. Nature. 2009;460:1117–21.
48. Mircescu MM, Lipuma L, van Rooijen N, Pamer EG, Hohl TM. Essential role for neutrophils but not alveolar macrophages at early time points following *Aspergillus fumigatus* infection. J Infect Dis. 2009;200:647–56.
49. Levitz SM, Selsted ME, Ganz T, Lehrer RI, Diamond RD. In vitro killing of spores and hyphae of *Aspergillus fumigatus* and *Rhizopus oryzae* by rabbit neutrophil cationic peptides and bronchoalveolar macrophages. J Infect Dis. 1986;154:483–9.
50. Washburn RG, Gallin JI, Bennett JE. Oxidative killing of *Aspergillus fumigatus* proceeds by parallel myeloperoxidase-dependent and -independent pathways. Infect Immun. 1987;55:2088–92.
51. Crosdale DJ, Poulton KV, Ollier WE, Thomson W, Denning DW. Mannose-binding lectin gene polymorphisms as a susceptibility factor for chronic necrotizing pulmonary aspergillosis. J Infect Dis. 2001;184:653–6.
52. Lambourne J, Agranoff D, Herbrecht R, et al. Association of mannose-binding lectin deficiency with acute invasive aspergillosis in immunocompromised patients. Clin Infect Dis. 2009;49:1486–91.
53. Young RC, Bennett JE. Invasive aspergillosis. Absence of detectable antibody response. Am Rev Resp Dis 1971;104:710–6.
54. Segal BH, Romani LR. Invasive aspergillosis in chronic granulomatous disease. Med Mycol. 2009;47 Suppl 1:S282–90.
55. Ng T, Robson G, Denning DW. Hydrocortisone-enchanced growth of *Aspergillus spp* implications for pathogenesis. Microbiology. 1994;140:2475–80.
56. Roilides E, Uhlig K, Venzon D, Pizzo PA, Walsh TJ. Prevention of corticosteroid-induced suppression of human polymorphonuclear leukocyte-induced damage of *Aspergillus fumigatus* hyphae by granulocyte colony-stimulating factor and gamma interferon. Infect Immun. 1993;61:4870–7.
57. Cenci E, Perito S, Enssle KH, et al. Th1 and Th2 cytokines in mice with invasive aspergillosis. Infect Immun. 1997;65:564–70.
58. Segal BH. Aspergillosis. N Engl J Med. 2009;360:1870–84.
59. Meier A, Kirschning CJ, Nikolaus T, Wagner H, Heesemann J, Ebel F. Toll-like receptor (TLR) 2 and TLR4 are essential for Aspergillus-induced activation of murine macrophages. Cell Microbiol. 2003;5:561–70.
60. Marr KA, Balajee SA, Hawn TR, et al. Differential role of MyD88 in macrophage-mediated responses to opportunistic fungal pathogens. Infect Immun. 2003;71:5280–6.
61. Mambula SS, Sau K, Henneke P, Golenbock DT, Levitz SM. Toll-like receptor (TLR) signaling in response to *Aspergillus fumigatus*. J Biol Chem. 2002;277:39320–6.
62. Bochud PY, Chien JW, Marr KA, et al. Toll-like receptor 4 polymorphisms and aspergillosis in stem-cell transplantation. N Engl J Med. 2008;359:1766–77.
63. Zaas AK, Liao G, Chien JW, et al. Plasminogen alleles influence susceptibility to invasive aspergillosis. PLoS Genet. 2008;4:e1000101.
64. Agarwal R. Allergic bronchopulmonary aspergillosis. Chest. 2009;135:805–26.
65. Stevens DA, Moss RB, Kurup VP, et al. Allergic bronchopulmonary aspergillosis in cystic fibrosis–state of the art: cystic Fibrosis Foundation Consensus Conference. Clin Infect Dis. 2003;37 Suppl 3:S225–64.
66. Greenberger PA. Allergic bronchopulmonary aspergillosis. J Allergy Clin Immunol. 2002;110:685–92.
67. Hope WW, Walsh TJ, Denning DW. The invasive and saprophytic syndromes due to Aspergillus spp. Med Mycol. 2005;43 Suppl 1:S207–38.
68. Vaid M, Kaur S, Sambatakou H, Madan T, Denning DW, Sarma PU. Distinct alleles of mannose-binding lectin (MBL) and surfactant proteins A (SP-A) in patients with chronic cavitary pulmonary aspergillosis and allergic bronchopulmonary aspergillosis. Clin Chem Lab Med. 2007;45:183–6.
69. Partridge-Hinckley K, Liddell GM, Almyroudis NG, Segal BH. Infection control measures to prevent invasive mould diseases in hematopoietic stem cell transplant recipients. Mycopathologia. 2009;168(6):329–37.
70. Warris A, Bjorneklett A, Gaustad P. Invasive pulmonary aspergillosis associated with infliximab therapy. N Engl J Med. 2001; 344:1099–100.
71. Meersseman W, Van Wijngaerden E. Invasive aspergillosis in the ICU: an emerging disease. Intensive Care Med. 2007;33:1679–81.
72. Gerson SL, Talbot GH, Hurwitz S, Strom BL, Lusk EJ, Cassileth PA. Prolonged granulocytopenia: the major risk factor for invasive pulmonary aspergillosis in patients with acute leukemia. Ann Intern Med. 1984;100:345–51.
73. Portugal RD, Garnica M, Nucci M. Index to predict invasive mold infection in high-risk neutropenic patients based on the area over the neutrophil curve. J Clin Oncol. 2009;27:3849–54.
74. Baddley JW, Stroud TP, Salzman D, Pappas PG. Invasive mold infections in allogeneic bone marrow transplant recipients. Clin Infect Dis. 2001;32:1319–24.
75. Wald A, Leisenring W, van Burik J-A, Bowden RA. Epidemiology of *Aspergillus* infections in a large cohort of patients undergoing bone marrow transplantation. J Infect Dis. 1997;175:1459–66.
76. Marr KA, Carter RA, Crippa F, Wald A, Corey L. Epidemiology and outcome of mould infections in hematopoietic stem cell transplant recipients. Clin Infect Dis. 2002;34:909–17.
77. Cornely OA, Maertens J, Winston DJ, et al. Posaconazole vs. fluconazole or itraconazole prophylaxis in patients with neutropenia. N Engl J Med. 2007;356:348–59.
78. De Pauw BE, Donnelly JP. Prophylaxis and aspergillosis – has the principle been proven? N Engl J Med. 2007;356:409–11.
79. Pagano L, Caira M, Candoni A, et al. The epidemiology of fungal infections in patients with hematologic malignancies: the SEIFEM-2004 study. Haematologica. 2006;91:1068–75.
80. Ullmann AJ, Lipton JH, Vesole DH, et al. Posaconazole or fluconazole for prophylaxis in severe graft-versus-host disease. N Engl J Med. 2007;356:335–47.
81. Paterson DL, Singh N. Invasive aspergillosis in transplant recipients. Medicine (Baltimore). 1999;78:123–38.
82. Gavalda J, Len O, San Juan R, et al. Risk factors for invasive aspergillosis in solid-organ transplant recipients: a case-control study. Clin Infect Dis. 2005;41:52–9.
83. Haiduven D. Nosocomial aspergillosis and building construction. Med Mycol 2009;47:S210–6.
84. Patterson JE, Peters J, Calhoon JH, et al. Investigation and control of aspergillosis and other filamentous fungal infections in solid organ transplant recipients. Transpl Infect Dis. 2000;2:22–8.

85. Patterson JE, Zidouh A, Miniter P, Andriole VT, Patterson TF. Hospital epidemiologic surveillance for invasive aspergillosis: patient demographics and the utility of antigen detection. Infect Control Hosp Epidemiol. 1997;18:104–8.
86. Thompson GR 3rd, Patterson TF. *Pulmonary aspergillosis*. Semin Respir Crit Care Med. 2008;29:103–10.
87. Ferguson BJ. Fungus balls of the paranasal sinuses. Otolaryngol Clin North Am. 2000;33:389–98.
88. Kauffman CA. Quandary about treatment of aspergillomas persists. Lancet. 1996;347:1640.
89. Denning DW, Riniotis K, Dobrashian R, Sambatakou H. Chronic cavitary and fibrosing pulmonary and pleural aspergillosis: case series, proposed nomenclature change, and review. Clin Infect Dis. 2003;37 Suppl 3:S265–80.
90. Kaur R, Mittal N, Kakkar M, Aggarwal AK, Mathur MD. Otomycosis: a clinicomycologic study. Ear Nose Throat J. 2000;79:606–9.
91. Parize P, Chandesris MO, Lanternier F, et al. Antifungal therapy of *Aspergillus invasive otitis externa*: efficacy of voriconazole and review. Antimicrob Agents Chemother. 2009;53:1048–53.
92. Rosenberg M, Patterson R, Mintzer R, Cooper B, Roberts MC, Harris K. Clinical and immunologic criteria for the diagnosis of allergic bronchopulmonary aspergillosis. Ann Intern Med. 1977;86:405–14.
93. Patterson R, Greenberger PA, Radin RC, Roberts M. Allergic bronchopulmonary aspergillosis: staging as an aid to management. Ann Intern Med. 1982;96:286–91.
94. Stevens DA, Schwartz HJ, Lee JY, et al. A randomized trial of itraconazole in allergic bronchopulmonary aspergillosis. N Engl J Med. 2000;342:756–62.
95. DeShazo RD, Chapin K, Swain RE. Fungal sinusitis. N Engl J Med. 1997;337:254–9.
96. Latge JP. The pathobiology of *Aspergillus fumigatus*. Trends Microbiol. 2001;9:382–9.
97. Maertens J, Raad I, Petrikkos G, et al. Efficacy and safety of caspofungin for treatment of invasive aspergillosis in patients refractory to or intolerant of conventional antifungal therapy. Clin Infect Dis. 2004;39:1563–71.
98. Bowden R, Chandrasekar P, White MH, et al. A double-blind, randomized, controlled trial of amphotericin B colloidal dispersion versus amphotericin B for treatment of invasive aspergillosis in immunocompromised patients. Clin Infect Dis. 2002;35:359–66.
99. Herbrecht R, Denning DW, Patterson TF, et al. Voriconazole versus amphotericin B for primary therapy of invasive aspergillosis. N Engl J Med. 2002;347:408–15.
100. Kontoyiannis DP, Ratanatharathorn V, Young JA, et al. Micafungin alone or in combination with other systemic antifungal therapies in hematopoietic stem cell transplant recipients with invasive aspergillosis. Transpl Infect Dis. 2009;11:89–93.
101. Viscoli C, Herbrecht R, Akan H, et al. An EORTC Phase II study of caspofungin as first-line therapy of invasive aspergillosis in haematological patients. J Antimicrob Chemother. 2009;64:1274–81.
102. Pagano L, Caira M, Candoni A, et al. Invasive aspergillosis in patients with acute myeloid leukemia: a SEIFEM-2008 registry study. Haematologica. 2009;95(4):644–50.
103. Neofytos D, Horn D, Anaissie E, et al. Epidemiology and outcome of invasive fungal infection in adult hematopoietic stem cell transplant recipients: analysis of multicenter prospective antifungal therapy (PATH) alliance registry. Clin Infect Dis. 2009;48:265–73.
104. Parody R, Martino R, Sanchez F, Subira M, Hidalgo A, Sierra J. Predicting survival in adults with invasive aspergillosis during therapy for hematological malignancies or after hematopoietic stem cell transplantation: single-center analysis and validation of the Seattle, French, and Strasbourg prognostic indexes. Am J Hematol. 2009;84:571–8.
105. Yeghen T, Kibbler CC, Prentice HG, et al. Management of invasive pulmonary aspergillosis in hematology patients: a review of 87 consecutive cases at a single institution. Clin Infect Dis. 2000;31:859–68.
106. Cornely OA, Maertens J, Bresnik M, et al. Liposomal amphotericin B as initial therapy for invasive mold infection: a randomized trial comparing a high-loading dose regimen with standard dosing (AmBiLoad trial). Clin Infect Dis. 2007;44:1289–97.
107. Caillot D, Casasnovas O, Bernard A, et al. Improved management of invasive pulmonary aspergillosis in neutropenic patients using early thoracic computed tomographic scan and surgery. J Clin Oncol. 1997;15:139–47.
108. Greene RE, Schlamm HT, Oestmann JW, et al. Imaging findings in acute invasive pulmonary aspergillosis: clinical significance of the halo sign. Clin Infect Dis. 2007;44:373–9.
109. Denning DW, Follansbee SE, Scolaro M, Norris S, Edelstein H, Stevens DA. Pulmonary aspergillosis in the acquired immunodeficiency syndrome. N Engl J Med. 1991;324:654–62.
110. Hadjiliadis D, Howell DN, Davis RD, et al. Anastomotic infections in lung transplant recipients. Ann Transplant. 2000;5:13–9.
111. Singh N, Paterson DL. *Aspergillus* infections in transplant recipients. Clin Microbiol Rev. 2005;18:44–69.
112. Palmer SM, Drew RH, Whitehouse JD, et al. Safety of aerosolized amphotericin B lipid complex in lung transplant recipients. Transplantation. 2001;72:545–8.
113. Schwartz S, Ruhnke M, Ribaud P, et al. Improved outcome in central nervous system aspergillosis, using voriconazole treatment. Blood. 2005;106:2641–5.
114. Hagensee ME, Bauwens JE, Kjos B, Bowden RA. Brain abscess following marrow transplantation: experience at the Fred Hutchinson Cancer Research Center, 1984–1992. Clin Infect Dis. 1994;19:402–8.
115. Vinas PC, King PK, Diaz FG. Spinal *aspergillus* osteomyelitis. Clin Infect Dis. 1999;28:1223–9.
116. Mouas H, Lutsar I, Dupont B, et al. Voriconazole for invasive bone aspergillosis: a worldwide experience of 20 cases. Clin Infect Dis. 2005;40:1141–7.
117. Reis LJ, Barton TD, Pochettino A, et al. Successful treatment of *Aspergillus* prosthetic valve endocarditis with oral voriconazole. Clin Infect Dis. 2005;41:752–3.
118. Halpern M, Szabo S, Hochberg E, et al. Renal aspergilloma: an unusual cause of infection in a patient with the acquired immunodeficiency syndrome. Am J Med. 1992;92:437–40.
119. Rahimi F, Hashemian MN, Rajabi MT. *Aspergillus fumigatus keratitis* after laser in situ keratomileusis: a case report and review of post-LASIK fungal keratitis. Eye (Lond). 2007;21:843–5.
120. Bunya VY, Hammersmith KM, Rapuano CJ, Ayres BD, Cohen EJ. Topical and oral voriconazole in the treatment of fungal keratitis. Am J Ophthalmol. 2007;143:151–3.
121. De Pauw B, Walsh TJ, Donnelly JP, et al. Revised definitions of invasive fungal disease from the European Organization for Research and Treatment of Cancer/Invasive Fungal Infections Cooperative Group and the National Institute of Allergy and Infectious Diseases Mycoses Study Group (EORTC/MSG) Consensus Group. Clin Infect Dis. 2008;46:1813–21.
122. Dixon DM, Polak-Wyss A. The medically important dematiaceous fungi and their identification. Mycoses. 1991;34:1–18.
123. Kaufman L, Standard PG, Jalbert M, Cole GT. Immunohistologic identification of *Aspergillus* spp. and other hyaline fungi by using polyclonal fluorescent antibodies. J Clin Microbiol. 1997;35:2206–9.
124. Horvath JA, Dummer S. The use of respiratory-tract cultures in the diagnosis of invasive pulmonary aspergillosis. Am J Med. 1996;100:171–8.
125. Pfaller MA, Messer SA, Hollis RJ, Jones RN. Antifungal activities of posaconazole, ravuconazole, and voriconazole compared to those of itraconazole and amphotericin B against 239 clinical isolates of *Aspergillus* spp. and other filamentous fungi: report from SENTRY antimicrobial surveillance program, 2000. Antimicrob Agents Chemother. 2002;46:1032–7.

126. Verweij PE, Mellado E, Melchers WJ. Multiple-triazole-resistant aspergillosis. N Engl J Med. 2007;356:1481–3.
127. Mosquera J, Denning DW. Azole cross-resistance in *Aspergillus fumigatus*. Antimicrob Agents Chemother. 2002;46:556–7.
128. Snelders E, van der Lee HA, Kuijpers J, et al. Emergence of azole resistance in *Aspergillus fumigatus* and spread of a single resistance mechanism. PLoS Med. 2008;5:e219.
129. Maertens J, Theunissen K, Verhoef G, et al. Galactomannan and computed tomography-based preemptive antifungal therapy in neutropenic patients at high risk for invasive fungal infection: a prospective feasibility study. Clin Infect Dis. 2005;41:1242–50.
130. Mennink-Kersten MA, Donnelly JP, Verweij PE. Detection of circulating galactomannan for the diagnosis and management of invasive aspergillosis. Lancet Infect Dis. 2004;4:349–57.
131. Maertens J, Verhaegen J, Lagrou K, Van Eldere J, Boogaerts M. Screening for circulating galactomannan as a noninvasive diagnostic tool for invasive aspergillosis in prolonged neutropenic patients and stem cell transplantation recipients: a prospective validation. Blood. 2001;97:1604–10.
132. Herbrecht R, Letscher-Bru V, Oprea C, et al. *Aspergillus* galactomannan detection in the diagnosis of invasive aspergillosis in cancer patients. J Clin Oncol. 2002;20:1898–906.
133. Marr KA, Balajee SA, McLaughlin L, Tabouret M, Bentsen C, Walsh TJ. Detection of galactomannan antigenemia by enzyme immunoassay for the diagnosis of invasive aspergillosis: variables that affect performance. J Infect Dis. 2004;190:641–9.
134. Maertens J, Theunissen K, Verbeken E, et al. Prospective clinical evaluation of lower cut-offs for galactomannan detection in adult neutropenic cancer patients and haematological stem cell transplant recipients. Br J Haematol. 2004;126:852–60.
135. Mennink-Kersten MA, Klont RR, Warris A, Op den Camp HJ, Verweij PE. *Bifidobacterium* lipoteichoic acid and false ELISA reactivity in *Aspergillus* antigen detection. Lancet. 2004;363:325–7.
136. Viscoli C, Machetti M, Cappellano P, et al. False-positive galactomannan platelia *Aspergillus* test results for patients receiving piperacillin-tazobactam. Clin Infect Dis. 2004;38:913–6.
137. Wheat LJ, Hackett E, Durkin M, et al. Histoplasmosis-associated cross-reactivity in the BioRad Platelia *Aspergillus* enzyme immunoassay. Clin Vaccine Immunol. 2007;14:638–40.
138. Viscoli C, Machetti M, Gazzola P, et al. *Aspergillus* galactomannan antigen in the cerebrospinal fluid of bone marrow transplant recipients with probable cerebral aspergillosis. J Clin Microbiol. 2002;40:1496–9.
139. Klont RR, Mennink-Kersten MA, Verweij PE. Utility of *Aspergillus* antigen detection in specimens other than serum specimens. Clin Infect Dis. 2004;39:1467–74.
140. Becker MJ, Lugtenburg EJ, Cornelissen JJ, Van Der Schee C, Hoogsteden HC, De Marie S. Galactomannan detection in computerized tomography-based broncho-alveolar lavage fluid and serum in haematological patients at risk for invasive pulmonary aspergillosis. Br J Haematol. 2003;121:448–57.
141. Musher B, Fredricks D, Leisenring W, Balajee SA, Smith C, Marr KA. *Aspergillus* galactomannan enzyme immunoassay and quantitative PCR for diagnosis of invasive aspergillosis with bronchoalveolar lavage fluid. J Clin Microbiol. 2004;42:5517–22.
142. Bergeron A, Belle A, Sulahian A, et al. Contribution of galactomannan antigen detection in bronchoalveolar lavage to the diagnosis of invasive pulmonary aspergillosis in patients with hematologic malignancies. Chest 2009. 2010;137:410–5.
143. Husain S, Clancy CJ, Nguyen MH, et al. Performance characteristics of the platelia *Aspergillus* enzyme immunoassay for detection of *Aspergillus* galactomannan antigen in bronchoalveolar lavage fluid. Clin Vaccine Immunol. 2008;15:1760–3.
144. Hage CA, Reynolds JM, Durkin M, Wheat LJ, Knox KS. Plasmalyte as a cause of false-positive results for *Aspergillus* galactomannan in bronchoalveolar lavage fluid. J Clin Microbiol. 2007;45:676–7.
145. Ostrosky-Zeichner L, Alexander BD, Kett DH, et al. Multicenter clinical evaluation of the (1−>3) beta-D-glucan assay as an aid to diagnosis of fungal infections in humans. Clin Infect Dis. 2005;41:654–9.
146. Parker Jr JC, McCloskey JJ, Knauer KA. Pathobiologic features of human candidiasis: a common deep mycosis of the brain, heart and kidney in the altered host. J Clin Pathol. 1976;5:991–1000.
147. Senn L, Robinson JO, Schmidt S, et al. 1, 3-Beta-D-glucan antigenemia for early diagnosis of invasive fungal infections in neutropenic patients with acute leukemia. Clin Infect Dis. 2008;46:878–85.
148. Obayashi T, Negishi K, Suzuki T, Funata N. Reappraisal of the serum (1−>3)-beta-D-glucan assay for the diagnosis of invasive fungal infections–a study based on autopsy cases from 6 years. Clin Infect Dis. 2008;46:1864–70.
149. White PL, Linton CJ, Perry MD, Johnson EM, Barnes RA. The evolution and evaluation of a whole blood polymerase chain reaction assay for the detection of invasive aspergillosis in hematology patients in a routine clinical setting. Clin Infect Dis. 2006;42:479–86.
150. Loeffler J, Hebart H, Brauchle U, Schumacher U, Einsele H. Comparison between plasma and whole blood specimens for detection of *Aspergillus* DNA by PCR. J Clin Microbiol. 2000;38:3830–3.
151. Donnelly JP. Polymerase chain reaction for diagnosing invasive aspergillosis: getting closer but still a ways to go. Clin Infect Dis. 2006;42:487–9.
152. Mengoli C, Cruciani M, Barnes RA, Loeffler J, Donnelly JP. Use of PCR for diagnosis of invasive aspergillosis: systematic review and meta-analysis. Lancet Infect Dis. 2009;9:89–96.
153. Cuenca-Estrella M, Meije Y, Diaz-Pedroche C, et al. Value of serial quantification of fungal DNA by a real-time PCR-based technique for early diagnosis of invasive Aspergillosis in patients with febrile neutropenia. J Clin Microbiol. 2009;47:379–84.
154. Costa C, Costa JM, Desterke C, Botterel F, Cordonnier C, Bretagne S. Real-time PCR coupled with automated DNA extraction and detection of galactomannan antigen in serum by enzyme-linked immunosorbent assay for diagnosis of invasive aspergillosis. J Clin Microbiol. 2002;40:2224–7.
155. Patterson TF. New agents for treatment of invasive aspergillosis. Clin Infect Dis. 2002;35:367–9.
156. Walsh TJ, Raad I, Patterson TF, et al. Treatment of invasive aspergillosis with posaconazole in patients who are refractory to or intolerant of conventional therapy: an externally controlled trial. Clin Infect Dis. 2007;44:2–12.
157. Thompson GR 3rd, Rinaldi MG, Pennick G, Dorsey SA, Patterson TF, Lewis 2nd JS. Posaconazole therapeutic drug monitoring: a reference laboratory experience. Antimicrob Agents Chemother. 2009;53:2223–4.
158. Marr KA, Crippa F, Leisenring W, et al. Itraconazole versus fluconazole for prevention of fungal infections in patients receiving allogeneic stem cell transplants. Blood. 2004;103:1527–33.
159. Warn PA, Sharp A, Denning DW. In vitro activity of a new triazole BAL4815, the active component of BAL8557 (the water-soluble prodrug), against Aspergillus spp. J Antimicrob Chemother. 2006;57:135–8.
160. Bates DW, Su L, Yu DT, et al. Mortality and costs of acute renal failure associated with amphotericin B therapy. Clin Infect Dis. 2001;32:686–93.
161. Wingard JR, Kubilis P, Lee L, et al. Clinical significance of nephrotoxicity in patients treated with amphotericin B for suspected or proven aspergillosis. Clin Infect Dis. 1999;29:1402–7.
162. Walsh TJ, Hiemenz JW, Seibel NL, et al. Amphotericin B lipid complex for invasive fungal infections: analysis of safety and efficacy in 556 cases. Clin Infect Dis. 1998;26:1383–96.
163. Marr KA, Boeckh M, Carter RA, Kim HW, Corey L. Combination antifungal therapy for invasive aspergillosis. Clin Infect Dis. 2004;39:797–802.

164. Denning DW, Marr KA, Lau WM, et al. Micafungin (FK463), alone or in combination with other systemic antifungal agents, for the treatment of acute invasive aspergillosis. J Infect. 2006;53:337–49.
165. Pfaller MA, Boyken L, Hollis RJ, et al. In vitro susceptibility of clinical isolates of *Aspergillus* spp. to anidulafungin, caspofungin, and micafungin: a head-to-head comparison using the CLSI M38-A2 broth microdilution method. J Clin Microbiol. 2009; 47:3323–5.
166. Spreghini E, Orlando F, Santinelli A, et al. Anidulafungin in combination with amphotericin B against *Aspergillus fumigatus*. Antimicrob Agents Chemother. 2009;53:4035–9.
167. Espinel-Ingroff A, Johnson E, Hockey H, Troke P. Activities of voriconazole, itraconazole and amphotericin B in vitro against 590 moulds from 323 patients in the voriconazole Phase III clinical studies. J Antimicrob Chemother. 2008;61:616–20.
168. Denning DW, Ribaud P, Milpied N, et al. Efficacy and safety of voriconazole in the treatment of acute invasive aspergillosis. Clin Infect Dis. 2002;34:563–71.
169. Perfect JR, Marr KA, Walsh TJ, et al. Voriconazole treatment for less-common, emerging, or refractory fungal infections. Clin Infect Dis. 2003;36:1122–31.
170. Walsh TJ, Lutsar I, Driscoll T, et al. Voriconazole in the treatment of aspergillosis, scedosporiosis and other invasive fungal infections in children. Pediatr Infect Dis J. 2002;21:240–8.
171. Dodds Ashley ES, Lewis R, Lewis JS, Martin C, Andes D. Pharmacology of systemic antifungal agents. Clin Infect Dis. 2006;43:S29–39.
172. Smith J, Safdar N, Knasinski V, et al. Voriconazole therapeutic drug monitoring. Antimicrob Agents Chemother. 2006;50:1570–2.
173. Walsh TJ, Karlsson MO, Driscoll T, et al. Pharmacokinetics and safety of intravenous voriconazole in children after single- or multiple-dose administration. Antimicrob Agents Chemother. 2004;48:2166–72.
174. Barrett JP, Vardulaki KA, Conlon C, et al. A systematic review of the antifungal effectiveness and tolerability of amphotericin B formulations. Clin Ther. 2003;25:1295–320.
175. Kirkpatrick WR, Perea S, Coco BJ, Patterson TF. Efficacy of caspofungin alone and in combination with voriconazole in a Guinea pig model of invasive aspergillosis. Antimicrob Agents Chemother. 2002;46:2564–8.
176. Petraitis V, Petraitiene R, Groll AH, et al. Comparative antifungal activities and plasma pharmacokinetics of micafungin (FK463) against disseminated candidiasis and invasive pulmonary aspergillosis in persistently neutropenic rabbits. Antimicrob Agents Chemother. 2002;46:1857–69.
177. Bowman JC, Hicks PS, Kurtz MB, et al. The antifungal echinocandin caspofungin acetate kills growing cells of *Aspergillus fumigatus* in vitro. Antimicrob Agents Chemother. 2002;46:3001–12.
178. Schaffner A, Frick PG. The effect of ketoconazole on amphotericin B in a model of disseminated aspergillosis. J Infect Dis. 1985;151:902–10.
179. Meletiadis J, Stergiopoulou T, O'Shaughnessy EM, Peter J, Walsh TJ. Concentration-dependent synergy and antagonism within a triple antifungal drug combination against *Aspergillus* species: analysis by a new response surface model. Antimicrob Agents Chemother. 2007;51:2053–64.
180. Steinbach WJ, Stevens DA, Denning DW. Combination and sequential antifungal therapy for invasive aspergillosis: review of published in vitro and in vivo interactions and 6281 clinical cases from 1966 to 2001. Clin Infect Dis. 2003;37 Suppl 3:S188–224.
181. Petraitis V, Petraitiene R, Sarafandi AA, et al. Combination therapy in treatment of experimental pulmonary aspergillosis: synergistic interaction between an antifungal triazole and an echinocandin. J Infect Dis. 2003;187:1834–43.
182. Winston DJ, Maziarz RT, Chandrasekar PH, et al. Intravenous and oral itraconazole versus intravenous and oral fluconazole for long-term antifungal prophylaxis in allogeneic hematopoietic stem-cell transplant recipients. A multicenter, randomized trial. Ann Intern Med. 2003;138:705–13.
183. Gallin JI, Alling DW, Malech HL, et al. Itraconazole to prevent fungal infections in chronic granulomatous disease. N Engl J Med. 2003;348:2416–22.
184. Rijnders BJ, Cornelissen JJ, Slobbe L, et al. Aerosolized liposomal amphotericin B for the prevention of invasive pulmonary aspergillosis during prolonged neutropenia: a randomized, placebo-controlled trial. Clin Infect Dis. 2008;46:1401–8.

Mucormycosis and Entomophthoramycosis (Zygomycosis)

Ashraf S. Ibrahim, John E. Edwards, Jr, Scott G. Filler, and Brad Spellberg

Previously the term zygomycosis was used to refer to infections caused by fungi belonging to the phylum Zygomycota, class Zygomycetes, orders Mucorales and Entomophthorales. However, a more recent classification based on molecular phylogenetic studies of rRNA, tef1, and rpb1, has abolished the class Zygomycetes and instead distributes fungi previously in the phylum Zygomycota into the phylum Glomeromycota and four subphyla, including Mucoromycotina, Kickxellomycotina, Zoopagomycotina, and Entomophthoromycotina (Table 1) [1]. Therefore, the term zygomycosis, which has been used by clinicians and mycologists for decades, is no longer relevant to fungal taxonomy. Both terms, mucormycosis and zygomycosis, are used throughout this book, reflecting the recent changes in nomenclature and the slower evolution of clinical parlance.

Fungi of the subphylum Mucormycotina, order Mucorales, are distributed into six families, all of which can cause cutaneous and deep infections in immunocompromised patients (Fig. 1) [2]. In contrast, the subphylum Entomophthoromycotina, order Entomophthorales, contains two families of organisms that cause subcutaneous and mucocutaneous infections primarily in immunocompetent children (Fig. 1) [3]. Because infections caused by organisms of the order Mucorales differ both clinically and pathologically from infections caused by organisms of the order Entomophthorales, we use the term mucormycosis to refer to infections caused by organisms belonging to the order Mucorales and entomophthoramycosis for infections caused by organisms of the order Entomophthorales. This chapter will be devoted to the more common problem of mucormycosis, and a small section at the end of the chapter deals with entomophthoramycosis.

Mycology

Fungi of the order Mucorales are classified into six different families based on morphologic analysis of the fungi, including the presence and location of rhizoids, the presence of apophyses, and the morphology of the columellae [3]. Other taxonomically relevant features include carbohydrate assimilation and the maximal growth temperature. Because the diseases caused by the different families of Mucorales are clinically indistinguishable from each other, laboratory confirmation of the identity of the causative agent is the only way to differentiate among these fungi. The identification of organisms isolated from patients with mucormycosis to the species level is necessary to clarify the epidemiology of this infection and may be helpful in predicting susceptibility to different antifungal drugs.

Fungi in the family Mucoraceae are isolated more frequently from patients with mucormycosis than any other family. *Rhizopus oryzae* (*Rhizopus arrhizus*) is the most common cause of infection, representing approximately 70% of all cases, followed by *Rhizopus microsporus* var. *rhizopodiformis* [2, 4]. Other, less frequently isolated species of the Mucoraceae family that cause a similar spectrum of infections include *Absidia corymbifera, Apophysomyces elegans, Mucor* species, and *Rhizomucor pusillus* [2, 5]. Other organisms, such as *Cunninghamella bertholletiae* in the Cunninghamellaceae family have been increasingly isolated from patients with pulmonary, disseminated, and cutaneous mucormycosis [6–9]. Additionally, *Saksenaea vasiformis* in the Saksenaceae family has been reported as a cause of cutaneous [10], subcutaneous [11, 12], rhinocerebral [13], and disseminated infections [14, 15]. Rare cases of mucormycosis

A.S. Ibrahim (✉)
Division of Infectious Diseases, Harbor-UCLA Research and Education Institute, Torrance, CA, USA
e-mail: Ibrahim@labiomed.org

C.A. Kauffman et al. (eds.), *Essentials of Clinical Mycology*,
DOI 10.1007/978-1-4419-6640-7_15, © Springer Science+Business Media, LLC 2011

Table 1 New taxonomy of fungi previously belonging to the phylum *Zygomycota* (Adapted from [1])

Rank	Taxon
Phylum	Glomeromycota
Subphylum	Mucoromycotina
Order	Mucorales, Endogonales, Mortierellales
Subphylum	Entomophthoromycotina
Order	Entomophthorales
Subphylum	Zoopagomycotina
Order	Zoopagales
Subphylum	Kickxellomycotina
Order	Kickxellales, Dimargaritales, Harpellales, Asellariales

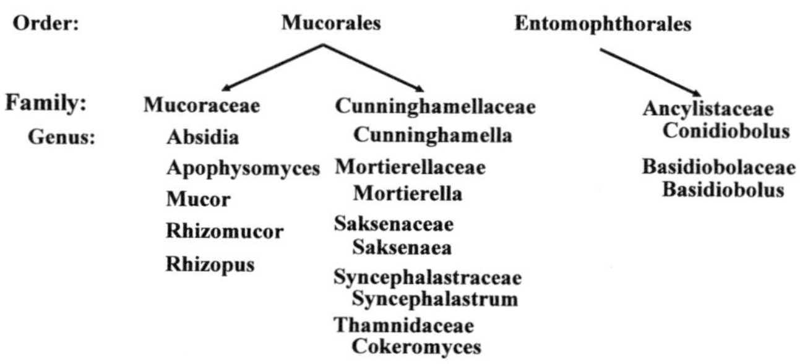

Fig. 1 Families of the order Mucorales (Adapted from [2])

have been reported due to *Cokeromyces recurvatus* in the Thamnidiaceae family [16], *Mortierella* species in the Mortierellaceae family [2] and *Syncephalastrum* species in the Syncephalastraceae family [17].

Epidemiology

Agents of mucormycosis are ubiquitous and thermotolerant organisms that usually grow in decaying matter, including bread, vegetables, fruits, and seeds. They can also be recovered from soil, compost piles, and animal excreta. Most of the Mucorales can grow and sporulate abundantly on any carbohydrate-containing source. Abundant growth with sporulation is usually seen in culture media within 2–5 days. The spores are easily airborne, and Mucorales are readily recovered as contaminants in laboratory cultures. Indeed, the ability of *R. microsporus* var. *rhizopodiformis* to grow on nonsterile wooden sticks used for culturing stool samples from immunocompromised patients has led to misdiagnosis of patients with gastrointestinal mucormycosis [18].

Members of the Mucorales cause both localized and disseminated infections in immunocompromised patients. Only rare case reports of invasive mucormycosis in apparently normal hosts have been described [19, 20], although local cutaneous infections may occur in patients who have had traumatic implantation of soil or plant material [21]. Allergic pulmonary disease does occur in immunocompetent hosts and reflects an acute hypersensitivity immune response illness rather than invasive disease [22, 23].

Mucormycosis is relatively uncommon in neutropenic patients compared to other fungal infections. However, there has been an alarming rise in the incidence of mucormycosis at major transplant centers. For example, at the Fred Hutchinson Cancer Research Center, Marr et al. described a greater than two-fold increase in the number of cases from 1985–1989 to 1995–1999 [24]. Kontoyiannis et al. described a similar increase in the incidence of mucormycosis at MD Anderson Cancer Center over a similar time span [25]. In fact, in high-risk patients the prevalence of mucormycosis has been described to be as high as 3% [26, 27], and up to 8% in autopsied patients with leukemia [28]. Because the number of iatrogenically immunocompromised patients continues to rise, it is likely that the incidence of mucormycosis will also increase [2, 4].

The major risk factors for mucormycosis include uncontrolled diabetes mellitus and other forms of metabolic acidosis, treatment with corticosteroids, especially in patients who have received an organ or bone marrow transplant, have experienced trauma or burns, have malignant hematologic disorders, or have received deferoxamine therapy to chelate iron in iron overload states. The underlying causes influence the clinical manifestations of the disease. For example, diabetics in ketoacidosis usually develop rhinocerebral mucormycosis, although other forms of the disease, such as pulmonary or disseminated infections may occur, whereas patients with malignant hematologic disease, lymphoma, or severe neutropenia usually develop pulmonary mucormycosis [4]. Both rhinocerebral and pulmonary mucormycosis are acquired through inhalation [2, 29]. Other routes of infection include direct implantation into skin, causing local cutaneous infection, and ingestion of contaminated food, which leads to gastrointestinal mucormycosis in highly immunocompromised patients and premature neonates.

Pathogenesis

Host Defenses

The pathogenesis of mucormycosis has been investigated in both in vitro and in animal models. Animal models have included mice or rabbits with mild diabetic ketoacidosis induced by streptozotocin or alloxan, cortisone-treated mice, neutropenic mice, and deferoxamine-treated animals. Inhalation of Mucorales spores by immunocompetent animals does not result in the development of mucormycosis [30]. In contrast, when the animals are immunosuppressed by corticosteroids or by induction of diabetes, the animals die from progressive pulmonary and hematogenously disseminated infection [30, 31].

The ability of inhaled spores to germinate and form hyphae in the host is critical for establishing infection. Bronchoalveolar macrophages harvested from lungs of immunocompetent mice are able to ingest and inhibit germination of *R. oryzae* spores, preventing progression of the disease [30]. However, these bronchoalveolar macrophages have limited capacity to kill the organism; viable organisms can still be recovered from the phagolysosomes. In contrast, bronchoalveolar macrophages of immunosuppressed mice are unable to prevent germination of the spores in vitro or after intranasal infection [30].

Severely neutropenic patients are at increased risk for developing mucormycosis. In contrast, patients with the acquired immunodeficiency syndrome (AIDS) do not seem to be at increased risk for developing mucormycosis [3]. These findings suggest that neutrophils, but not necessarily T lymphocytes, are critical for inhibiting fungal spore proliferation. Recruitment of neutrophils to sites of infection occurs in response to fungal constituents and activation of the alternative complement pathway [32, 33]. Both mononuclear and polymorphonuclear phagocytes of normal hosts kill Mucorales by generating oxidative metabolites and the cationic peptides, defensins [30, 34, 35]. In the presence of hyperglycemia and low pH, as found in patients with diabetic ketoacidosis, phagocytes are dysfunctional and have impaired chemotaxis and defective intracellular killing by both oxidative and nonoxidative mechanisms [36]. The exact mechanisms by which ketoacidosis, diabetes, and corticosteroids impair the function of these phagocytes remain unknown. Furthermore, phagocyte dysfunction alone cannot explain the high incidence of mucormycosis in patients with diabetic ketoacidosis because the incidence of mucormycosis in these patients is increased much more than infections caused by other pathogens [3–5]. Therefore, Mucorales must possess unique virulence traits that enable the organism to survive in this subset of patients.

The Role of Iron in Pathogenesis

It has recently been discovered that a specific factor that uniquely predisposes patients in diabetic ketoacidosis to mucormycosis is the level of available unbound iron in serum [37, 38]. Iron is required by virtually all microbial pathogens for growth and virulence [39]. In mammalian hosts, very little serum iron is available to microorganisms because it is highly bound to host carrier proteins, such as transferrin [37]. Sequestration of serum iron is a major host defense mechanism against microbes in general and Mucorales in particular, because *Rhizopus* grows poorly in normal serum unless exogenous iron is added [37, 38]. Furthermore, the bacterial siderophore, deferoxamine, predisposes patients to *Rhizopus* infection by acting as a xenosiderophore, which supplies previously unavailable iron to the fungus [38]. The mechanism by which *Rhizopus* obtains iron from the iron-deferoxamine complex involves binding of this complex to the mold, followed by active reduction of the iron by the fungus, resulting in release of iron from deferoxamine and subsequent transport of the reduced iron intracellularly [40]. This transport is likely mediated by iron permeases. Administration of deferoxamine worsens survival of guinea pigs infected with *Rhizopus* but not *Candida albicans* [38, 40, 41]. Additionally, in vitro studies of radiolabeled iron uptake from deferoxamine in serum show that *Rhizopus* is able to incorporate eightfold and 40-fold more iron than is *Aspergillus fumigatus* and *C. albicans,* respectively [38].

As mentioned previously, patients with diabetic ketoacidosis are at high risk of developing rhinocerebral mucormycosis [3–5]. These patients have elevated levels of available iron in their serum, and such serum supports growth of *R. oryzae* at acidic pH (7.3–6.88) but not at alkaline pH (7.7–8.38) [37]. Sera that did not support *R. oryzae* growth at acidic pH had less available iron than sera that supported fungal growth. Furthermore, adding exogenous iron to sera allowed *R. oryzae* to grow profusely at acidic conditions but not at pH$\geq$7.4. Finally, simulated acidotic conditions decreased the iron-binding capacity of sera collected from normal volunteers, suggesting that acidosis temporarily disrupts the capacity of transferrin to bind iron, probably by proton-mediated displacement of ferric iron from transferrin [42].

Recent animal data showed that mice with diabetic ketoacidosis were protected from *Rhizopus* infection by administering iron chelators, such as deferiprone and deferasirox [43, 44], that are not utilized by *Mucorales* as xenosiderophores. These studies lend support to the hypothesis that increased susceptibility of patients with diabetic ketoacidosis to mucormycosis is likely due in part to an elevation in available serum iron.

Fungi can obtain iron from the host by using low-molecular-weight iron chelators (siderophores) or high-affinity iron permeases [39, 45]. Because the siderophores of *Rhizopus* species are very inefficient at obtaining iron from serum [38, 40], it is believed that these siderophores contribute very little to the ability of this organism to grow in patients who are receiving deferoxamine or who have diabetic ketoacidosis. The high-affinity iron permeases are able to transport serum iron intracellularly, and are therefore likely to be critical for the survival of the organism in susceptible hosts. Indeed recent data show that the high-affinity iron permease (*rFTR1*) is expressed by *R. oryzae* during murine infection. Inhibition of *rFTR1* gene expression by RNA-i or reduction of *rFTR1* copy number by gene disruption reduces the virulence of the fungus in animal models of mucormycosis [46].

A third mechanism by which fungi can obtain iron from the host is through utilization of hemin [47, 48]. The *Rhizopus* genome project revealed two homologues (RO3G_07326 and RO3G_13316) of the heme oxygenase (CaHMX1) [49]. These two *R. oryzae* homologues may enable *R. oryzae* to obtain iron from host hemoglobin, and might explain the angioinvasive nature of *R. oryzae*.

Mucorales–Endothelial Cell Interactions

A hallmark of mucormycosis is the virtually uniform presence of extensive angioinvasion with resultant vessel thrombosis and tissue necrosis [4, 50]. This angioinvasion likely contributes to the capacity of the organism to hematogenously disseminate to other target organs. Therefore, damage of and penetration through endothelial cells or the extracellular matrix proteins lining blood vessels is likely a critical step in *R. oryzae*'s pathogenetic strategy. An earlier study showed that *R. oryzae* can adhere to the extracellular matrix laminin and type IV collagen [51]. More recently, it has been shown that *R. oryzae* spores and hyphae are able to damage human umbilical vein endothelial cells in vitro [52]. It has also been shown that injury requires adherence of the fungus to endothelial cells followed by invasion into the cells. Adherence to endothelial cells is believed to be mediated by a specific receptor since it was found to be saturable [52]. Glucose-regulated protein (GRP78) acts as a receptor which mediates penetration through and damage of endothelial cells by Mucorales. GRP78 (also known as BiP/HSPA5) is a member of the HSP70 protein family, and some of it is located on the cell surface [53]. It is a key regulator of the unfolded protein response (UPR) [54].

Interestingly, elevated concentrations of glucose and iron consistent with those noted during diabetic ketoacidosis enhanced surface GRP78 expression and resulting penetration through and damage of endothelial cells by Mucorales in a receptor-dependent manner. Mice with diabetic ketoacidosis have enhanced susceptibility to mucormycosis and have increased expression of GRP78 in the sinus, lungs, and brains when compared with normal mice. Anti-GRP78 immune serum protects mice in DKA from mucormycosis [55]. These observations provide novel insight into the etiology of the unique susceptibility of diabetic ketoacidosis patients to mucormycosis and could provide a foundation for novel therapeutic interventions.

Mycotoxins

Rhizopus species are also known for their ability to produce mycotoxins, such as the macrocyclic polyketide metabolite, rhizoxin, as well as the cyclic peptides, rhizonins A and B [56]. A recent study demonstrated that the mycotoxin rhizoxin is not biosynthesized by *Rhizopus* itself, but rather by an intracellular, symbiotic bacterium of the genus *Burkholderia* [57]. This bacterium is sensitive to antibiotics belonging to the fluoroquinolone family. For example, rhizoxin production is completely abrogated when *Rhizopus* is grown in media containing 40 μg/mL of ciprofloxacin [57]. Rhizoxin has long been known to be crucial to the plant pathogenic strategy of *Rhizopus,* but it does not appear to have a substantive role in causing mammalian disease. Organisms that have been rendered bacteria-free by ciprofloxacin treatment or those that cannot produce rhizoxin because of the absence of *Burkholderia* are still pathogenic in mouse and fruit fly models of infection [58].

Other putative virulence factors include the ability of *Rhizopus* to secrete lytic enzymes, including aspartic proteinases [59]. Additionally, *Rhizopus* species have an active ketone reductase system which may be an additional virulence factor that functions by enhancing growth in the acidic and glucose-rich environment seen in ketoacidotic states [60]. To date, none of these potential virulence factors have been definitively proven to be essential for the development of mucormycosis.

Clinical Manifestations

Based on clinical presentation and the involvement of a particular anatomic site, mucormycosis can be divided into at least five categories: (1) rhinocerebral, (2) pulmonary, (3) cutaneous, (4) gastrointestinal, and (5) disseminated.

Rhinocerebral

Rhinocerebral mucormycosis is the most common form of the disease, representing between one third to one half of all cases [61]. About 70% of cases of rhinocerebral (occasionally referred to as craniofacial) mucormycosis are found in diabetic patients with ketoacidosis [4, 62]. Rhinocerebral mucormycosis is increasingly being encountered in patients receiving high doses of corticosteroids, such as those with rheumatologic disorders, and those who have received an organ transplant [61, 63–65].

The initial presentation is often consistent with sinusitis, including facial pain, unilateral headache, proptosis, and soft tissue swelling. Fever is frequently, but not invariably, present. The infection may rapidly extend into the neighboring tissues. Infected tissues are initially erythematous, then violaceous, and ultimately black as tissue infarction develops (Fig. 2).

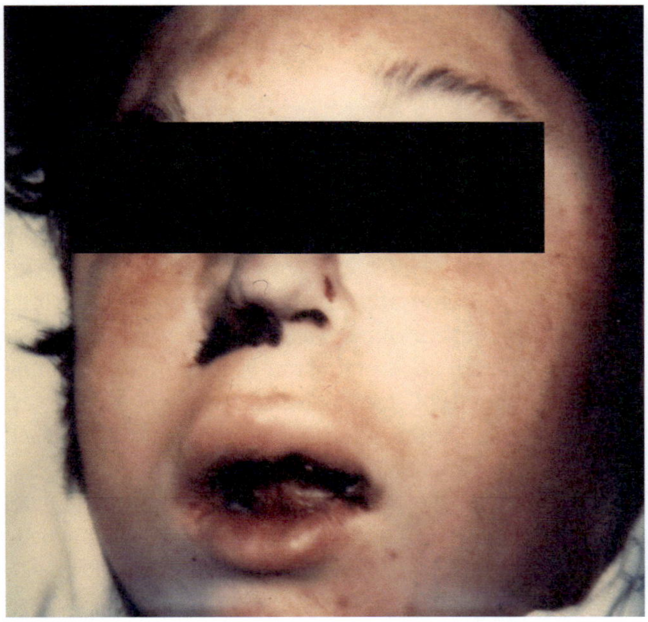

Fig. 2 Rhinocerebral mucormycosis in a pregnant woman who had diabetic ketoacidosis. Note bilateral swelling and infarction of skin of nose and infranasal tissue. There was also gangrenous ulceration of the palate

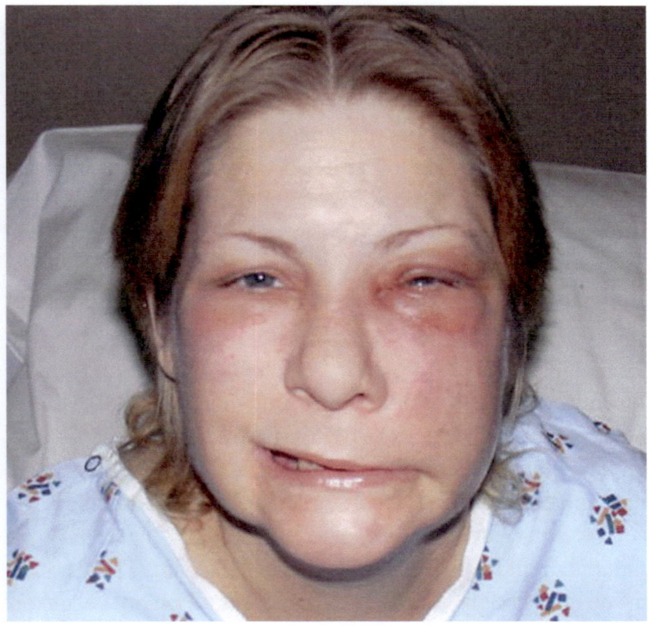

Fig. 3 Rhinocerebral mucormycosis in a patient who had diabetic ketoacidosis. Note swelling, erythema, proptosis, ptosis, and peripheral left facial nerve palsy

Infection can sometimes extend from the sinuses into the mouth and produce painful, necrotic ulcerations of the hard palate. If untreated, infection usually spreads from the ethmoid sinus to the orbit, resulting in loss of extraocular muscle function, proptosis, and chemosis. Involvement of the optic nerve is manifested by blurred vision and eventually blindness. The trigeminal nerve may be affected, resulting in ptosis and pupillary dilation. Cranial nerve findings represent extensive infection and portend a grave prognosis (Fig. 3).

Infection can spread posteriorly from the orbit or sinuses to the central nervous system. Clinicians should consider the possibility of mucormycosis of the central nervous system in patients with diabetic ketoacidosis with mental status changes that persist after metabolic abnormalities have been corrected. The angioinvasive nature of the fungus may result in cavernous sinus and internal carotid artery thrombosis [66], and occasionally may lead to hematogenous dissemination of the infection [61, 67].

Prior to the availability of antifungal agents, rhinocerebral mucormycosis was almost universally fatal [67]. Although the mortality rate associated with rhinocerebral disease remains high, cure is likely when diagnosed early and treated aggressively with surgery and antifungal agents [68, 69]. Disease limited to the sinuses or orbit has a mortality rate of <40% with aggressive therapy, whereas disease extending into the central nervous system results in mortality rates >60%. The nature of the underlying disease and the reversibility of immune dysfunction are the most important determinants of survival. One study showed that among patients with rhinocerebral disease, survival was 75%, 60%, and 20% for patients with no underlying immunosuppression, diabetes, and immunosuppression, respectively [70].

Pulmonary

Pulmonary mucormycosis occurs most commonly in patients with profound and prolonged neutropenia, such as that noted in patients with leukemia or recipients of a hematopoietic stem cell transplant. Such patients have usually received broad-spectrum antibiotics for unremitting fever [24, 71]. Patients with diabetic ketoacidosis can also develop pulmonary mucormycosis, although infections in these patients may be less fulminant and follow a more subacute course than is typically seen in patients with neutropenia [72, 73]. Pulmonary mucormycosis may develop as a result of inhalation or by hematogenous or lymphatic spread. Symptoms include fever, dyspnea, and cough. Angioinvasion results in tissue necrosis associated with hemoptysis, which may be fatal if a large blood vessel is involved [74, 75]. If infection is not treated, hematogenous dissemination to the contralateral lung and other organs occurs frequently. Patients with untreated pulmonary mucormycosis usually succumb to complications of disseminated disease [73]. When it occurs in isolation, pulmonary mucormycosis associated mortality is approximately 50–70%; it is almost universally fatal if a manifestation of disseminated disease [73, 76].

Cutaneous

Cutaneous mucormycosis can occur following traumatic implantation of soil or plant material, such as occurs after motor vehicle accidents. In diabetic or immunocompromised patients, cutaneous lesions may arise at an insulin injection or catheter insertion site [77]. A large epidemic of cutaneous mucormycosis was reported in patients who had contaminated surgical dressings applied to their skin [78, 79]. Cutaneous mucormycosis may also occur in burn patients [80].

Although this form of disease usually arises from primary inoculation of the infection site, it sometimes is due to disseminated disease. These two routes of infection have distinct clinical presentations. Primary infection produces an acute inflammatory response with purulence, abscess formation, tissue swelling, and necrosis. The lesions may appear red and indurated, and often progress to black eschars. The necrotic tissue may slough and produce large ulcers. Primary cutaneous disease, which may be polymicrobial, is usually rapidly progressive even in the face of appropriate debridement and medical treatment. Occasionally, aerial mycelia may be visible on the surface of the cutaneous lesion. This form of cutaneous disease can be very invasive locally, and penetrate from the cutaneous and subcutaneous tissues into the adjacent fat, muscle, fascia, and bone. Cutaneous and subcutaneous disease may lead to necrotizing fasciitis, which has a mortality rate approaching 80% [81–83]. Secondary vascular invasion may also lead to hematogenously disseminated infection of the deep organs. When cutaneous mucormycosis results from hematogenously disseminated infection, the lesion typically begins as an erythematous, indurated, and painful cellulitis, progressing to an ulcerative lesion covered by a black eschar (Fig. 4).

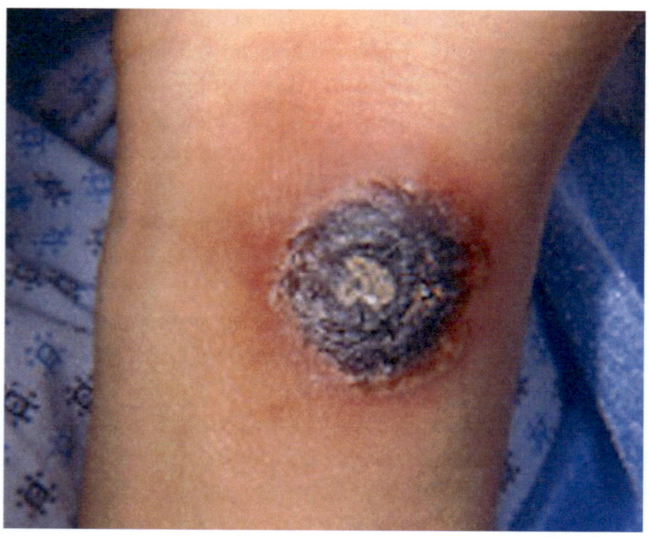

Fig. 4 Cutaneous mucormycosis in a patient who had acute leukemia. Note the black eschar with surrounding erythema. The lesion was quite painful (Courtesy of Dr. Dimitrios Kontoyiannis)

Gastrointestinal

Mucormycosis of the gastrointestinal tract is rare, but it is increasingly encountered in nosocomial settings. It is thought to arise from ingestion of the fungi. In the past, this was seen almost exclusively among patients who were extremely malnourished, especially infants and children [84, 85]. More recently, nosocomial infections have been described in neutropenic or other critically ill patients, sometimes resulting from primary contamination of a medication or from the contaminated wooden applicator sticks used to mix medication slurries. Symptoms of gastrointestinal mucormycosis are varied and depend on the affected site. Abdominal pain and symptoms of intestinal obstruction such as distention, nausea, and vomiting are the most common symptoms. Fever and hematochezia may also occur. The diagnosis is usually made by biopsy of the involved area during surgery or endoscopy.

Disseminated

Hematogenously disseminated mucormycosis may originate from any primary site of infection. Pulmonary mucormycosis in severely neutropenic patients has the highest incidence of dissemination. Less commonly, dissemination can arise from the gastrointestinal tract, the sinuses, or cutaneous lesions, particularly in burn patients. The most common site of dissemination is the brain, but metastatic lesions may be found in any organ, especially the spleen, heart, and skin. Cerebral infection following dissemination is distinct from rhinocerebral mucormycosis, and results in abscess formation and infarction. Patients may present with an insidious onset of neurologic symptoms, or with more sudden development of focal neurologic deficit, altered mental status, and coma. The mortality rate associated with dissemination to the brain approaches 100% [86]. With or without central nervous system involvement, disseminated mucormycosis has a mortality rate >90% [76]. Agents of Mucorales may cause infection in virtually any body site. Central nervous system involvement in the absence of sinus infection, endocarditis, and pyelonephritis occur occasionally, usually in the context of intravenous drug use [87–90]. Other reports have described mucormycosis in osteoarticular structures, mediastinum, trachea, superior vena cava, and as a cause of external otitis [91–97].

Diagnosis

A high index of suspicion is required to make the diagnosis of mucormycosis. Autopsy series demonstrate that up to half of cases are diagnosed postmortem [98, 99]. Because the

Mucorales are environmental isolates, establishing a definitive diagnosis requires a positive culture from a sterile site obtained by a needle aspirate or a tissue biopsy or histopathologic evidence of invasive disease [4]. A probable diagnosis of mucormycosis can be established by culture from a nonsterile site, such as sputum or bronchoalveolar lavage, in a patient with appropriate risk factors and clinical and radiographic evidence of disease.

Despite the fact that the Mucorales grow quite quickly on laboratory culture media, cultures may be negative in up to half of patients with mucormycosis. The primary reason for negative cultures from affected tissues is that the organism is killed during tissue grinding, which is routinely used to process tissue specimens for culture in clinical microbiology laboratories. When mucormycosis is a diagnostic consideration, the clinical microbiology laboratory should be notified so that tissue for culture may be placed in whole sections or cubes in the center of a culture plate, rather than subjected to routine homogenization prior to inoculation on artificial media.

There are no reliable serologic or skin tests for mucormycosis; the diagnosis is usually made by examination of biopsy or cytologic material. The characteristic histologic appearance is the presence of wide, ribbon-like, aseptate hyphae that branch at right angles (Fig. 5). The organisms are often surrounded by extensive necrotic debris. Other fungi including *Aspergillus, Fusarium, or Scedosporium* species may appear similar to Mucorales on biopsy, but these molds are usually thinner, septate, and branch at acute angles. The genus and species of the infecting organism are determined by morphologic identification and sporulation patterns of the fungi isolated in culture.

Routine imaging with CT may be an insensitive means of determining the extent of disease among patients with rhino-orbital-cerebral disease, sometimes demonstrating only sinus involvement [100]. MRI is more sensitive than CT scans for

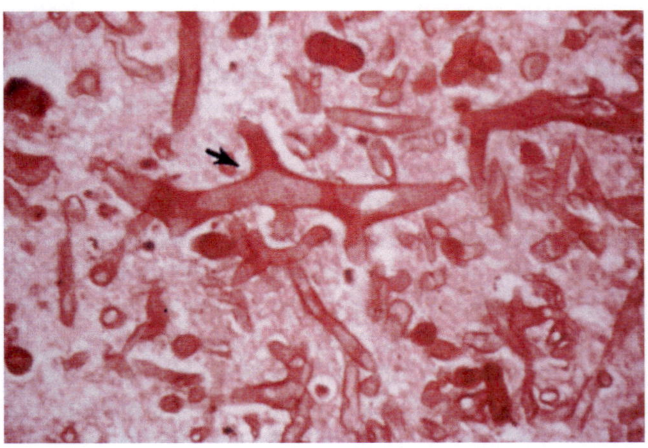

Fig. 5 Periodic acid–Schiff stain of excised tissue from the sinus of a patient with rhinocerebral mucormycosis. Note the wide, ribbon-like hyphae that branch at right angles and that do not show septae

detecting orbital and CNS involvement [100]. Only rarely is a retro-orbital mass seen on CT scans among patients with orbital mucormycosis and proptosis.

CT scans are useful for early detection of pulmonary mucormycosis, particularly in patients with cancer. By logistic regression, pulmonary mucormycosis in patients with cancer could be distinguished from aspergillosis on the basis of the presence of sinusitis, multiple (≥10) nodules by CT scan, and pleural effusion [101]. Also, a recent retrospective study reported that seven of eight immunocompromised patients treated at a cancer center who had a "reverse halo" sign (focal area of ground-glass attenuation surrounded by a ring of consolidation) on chest CT scan had mucormycosis rather than infections with other molds [102]. The reverse halo sign was seen early in the disease course of these patients. Further refinement of radiographic techniques for distinguishing mucormycosis from other infectious and noninfectious diseases is an important area of future research.

The diagnosis of disseminated disease is made difficult because patients are usually ill with multiple comorbid conditions and virtually always have negative blood cultures. In the appropriate patient, evidence of infarction in multiple organs should suggest a diagnosis of mucormycosis. Other disseminated mycoses, especially aspergillosis, may present with an identical clinical picture. Patients with suspected disseminated mucormycosis should undergo a careful search for unexplained cutaneous lesions for biopsy.

Treatment

Four factors are critical for eradicating mucormycosis: rapidity of diagnosis; reversal of the underlying predisposing factors, if possible; appropriate surgical debridement of infected tissue; and appropriate antifungal therapy. Early diagnosis is important because small, focal lesions can often be surgically excised before they progress to involve critical structures or disseminate. Moreover, early initiation of polyene therapy within 5 days of diagnosis has been associated with improvement in survival [103]. Hence, establishing an early diagnosis of mucormycosis and early appropriate therapeutic intervention is critical to optimize long-term outcomes. Correcting or controlling predisposing problems is also essential for improving the treatment outcome. In diabetic ketoacidotic patients, hyperglycemia and acidemia should be corrected. Discontinuation of deferoxamine or immunosuppressive therapy, particularly corticosteroids, should be strongly considered when the diagnosis of mucormycosis is made.

Surgical debridement of the infected and necrotic tissue should be performed on an urgent basis. In rhinocerebral mucormycosis, early surgical excision of the infected sinuses and appropriate debridement of the retro-orbital space can often prevent extension into the eye and obviate the need for enucleation. It is important to emphasize that during orbital surgery among patients with presumed mucormycosis, it is necessary to biopsy the extraocular muscles, since they may appear normal despite extensive fungal involvement. Repeated surgical exploration of the sinuses and orbit may be necessary to ensure that all necrotic tissue has been debrided and the infection has not progressed. Among patients with pulmonary mucormycosis, surgical treatment plus antifungal therapy greatly improves outcome compared to the use of antifungal therapy alone [73]. Moreover, surgery was found to be an independent variable predicting a favorable outcome in patients with mucormycosis [104].

Polyenes

Amphotericin B deoxycholate (AmB-d) is the only antifungal agent approved for the treatment of mucormycosis [3–5]. Because many Mucorales isolates are either relatively or highly resistant to AmB-d, high doses of this drug are required. AmB-d should be administered at 1.0–1.5 mg/kg/day initially. However, this dose is frequently associated with significant nephrotoxicity. Thus, lipid formulations of AmB have become preferred agents for this infection because they are significantly less nephrotoxic and can be safely administered at higher doses for a longer period of time when compared to AmB-d [100, 105]. Several recent studies demonstrate the efficacy of these agents. In one study, amphotericin B lipid complex (ABLC) resulted in a 71% success rate as salvage therapy for mucormycosis [106]. Primary treatment with liposomal amphotericin B (LAmB) was associated with a 67% (16/24) survival rate, compared to 39% (24/62) survival with AmB-d ($p=0.02$) in cancer patients with mucormycosis. [76] Additionally, animal studies have demonstrated that high-dose LAmB (15 mg/kg/day) is more efficacious than AmB (1 mg/kg/day) in treating diabetic ketoacidotic mice infected with *R. oryzae* [107].

Recent animal data suggest that LAmB may be preferred to ABLC for treating central nervous system mucormycosis. In a comparative pharmacokinetic study in rabbits, LAmB achieved brain tissue levels of >5-fold greater than ABLC [108]. While LAmB and ABLC are similarly effective in neutropenic mice, LAmB is superior to ABLC in mice with diabetic ketoacidosis, primarily due to superior clearance of the fungus from the brain [109]. A recent retrospective series in patients with rhino-orbital-cerebral mucormycosis receiving ABLC as primary therapy found that these patients had inferior outcomes when compared to patients receiving either AmB-d or LAmB, confirming these observations in animals [100].

Azoles

Itraconazole is the first marketed azole drug that showed promising in vitro activity against *Absidia,* but not against *Rhizopus* spp., the most common pathogens isolated from clinical cases [110]. Therefore, itraconazole plays almost no role in treating mucormycosis. Fluconazole and the second-generation broad-spectrum triazole, voriconazole, are not active against Mucorales in vitro [110]. Indeed the prophylactic and therapeutic use of voriconazole in transplant patients has been associated with breakthrough disseminated mucormycosis [27, 111–115]. In fact, a recent study demonstrated that in vitro pretreatment of *Mucorales* with voriconazole, increased the virulence of these organisms in murine and fly models of mucormycosis [31].

Posaconazole was approved recently by the Food and Drug Administration (FDA) for prophylaxis in patients with prolonged neutropenia and for stem cell transplant patients with severe GVHD and also for treatment of esophageal candidiasis. Posaconazole has enhanced in vitro activity against *Mucorales*, with reported MIC_{90} of 0.25–8 μg/mL, with *Rhizopus* spp. having the highest MIC (MIC_{90} 8 μg/mL) [110, 116–118]. In febrile neutropenic patients and in those with invasive fungal infections, oral posaconazole, 400 mg twice daily, results in serum levels consistently <1 μg/mL, with considerable patient-to-patient variability [119–122]. Therefore, pharmacokinetic/pharmacodynamic data raise concerns about the reliability of achieving adequate in vivo levels of oral posaconazole to treat mucormycosis, especially infection caused by *Rhizopus* species.

Animal data assessing the role of posaconazole in treating experimental mucormycosis raise concerns about the efficacy of this drug. For example, in neutropenic mice infected with *Mucor* species, posaconazole was significantly less effective than AmB-d [123]. Similarly, Dannaoui and colleagues [124] found that posaconazole was less effective than AmB-d in treating mice infected with *Rhizopus microsporus* or *Absidia,* and it had no activity in mice infected with *R. oryzae,* which causes >70% of clinical cases of mucormycosis [4, 100, 104]. In two more recent studies, posaconazole monotherapy was also no better than AmB-d placebo for treatment of *R. oryzae* infection in neutropenic or DKA mice [125, 126].

Based on the available animal data and the absence of clinical data, posaconazole monotherapy cannot currently be recommended as primary treatment of mucormycosis. In contrast, available clinical data from open-label salvage studies suggest that posaconazole is a reasonable option for patients with mucormycosis who are refractory to or intolerant of polyenes [127, 128]. It is also commonly used as "step-down" therapy for stable patients who have initially responded to a polyene, but there are no prospective studies exploring this approach to therapy.

Antifungal Combination Therapy

All approved echinocandins, including caspofungin, micafungin, and anidulafungin, have minimal activity against agents of mucormycosis when tested in vitro [129, 130]. However, it is known that *R. oryzae* has the 1,3 β-glucan synthase target enzyme for echinocandins [49], and this enzyme can be inhibited by these agents [131]. In the murine model of disseminated mucormycosis, caspofungin has limited activity against *R. oryzae* [131]. Furthermore, in diabetic ketoacidotic mice infected with *R. oryzae*, combination caspofungin plus ABLC therapy markedly improves survival rates compared to caspofungin alone or placebo [132]. Combination therapy with LAmB plus either micafungin or anidulafungin improves survival rates in neutropenic and diabetic ketoacidotic mice with disseminated mucormycosis [133]. The mechanism by which echinocandins improve the outcome of mucormycosis infection when combined with lipid formulations of AmB is unknown, but it could be related to the enhanced exposure of β glucan on the fungal surface, which in part results in enhanced immune stimulation [134, 136]. Alternatively, echinocandins might affect certain virulence factors of *Mucorales* that are as yet unidentified.

In a recent small retrospective study, combination therapy with lipid formulations of AmB plus caspofungin was associated with significantly improved outcomes for rhino-orbital-cerebral mucormycosis in diabetic patients compared to polyene monotherapy [100]. By multivariate analysis, only combination therapy was significantly associated with superior outcomes (OR = 10.9 for success vs. monotherapy, $p = 0.02$).

Because the data are very limited, further clinical studies are necessary to determine the usefulness of echinocandin combination therapy in patients with mucormycosis. If used in a combination regimen, dose escalation of echinocandins is not advisable due to possible paradoxical loss of efficacy, as has been noted in murine mucormycosis at doses ≥ 3 mg/kg/day [131, 133].

Iron Chelation Therapy

The iron chelators deferiprone and deferasirox have been shown to have activity in murine mucormycosis [43, 44]. Deferasirox, which is currently approved to treat iron overload in transfusion-dependent anemias [135], is fungicidal for clinical isolates of Mucorales in vitro, with an MIC_{90} of 6.25 μg/mL [136]. The drug exhibits time-dependent killing, with killing occurring at 12–24 h of drug exposure. Based on trough serum levels >15 μg/mL in patients treated with deferasirox at 20 mg/kg/day [137, 138], it should be feasible to maintain deferasirox serum levels in excess of the MICs of Mucorales. In diabetic ketoacidotic mice with disseminated mucormycosis, deferasirox is as effective as LAmB therapy, and combination deferasirox-LAmB therapy synergistically improves survival rates [136]. In particular, combination therapy results in a 100-fold decrease in brain fungal burden compared to monotherapy.

Based on these animal data, deferasirox was used successfully as salvage therapy in a patient with advanced rhinocerebral mucormycosis who had progressive brainstem disease despite LAmB therapy [139]. A study describing adjunctive therapy with deferasirox given to eight patients with mucormycosis suggested that the drug is safe and possibly efficacious, based on the observation that seven of eight patients survived the infection [140]. One study reported the failure of salvage deferasirox in a patient who had undergone partial colectomy to resect mucormycosis [141]. This failure might be attributed to the poor bioavailability of the oral iron chelator in the context of abdominal surgery.

Currently, a double-blind, randomized, placebo-controlled, phase II study of adjunctive deferasirox therapy (20 mg/kg/day for 14 days) with LAmB for mucormycosis is ongoing. Additional clinical data will be necessary to gain a more comprehensive safety and efficacy profile for this drug in combination with antifungals.

Posaconazole Combination Therapy

Two recent preclinical studies evaluated the efficacy of posaconazole combination therapy for murine mucormycosis. In the first study, Rodriguez et al. found that combining posaconazole with AmB-d enhanced the survival rate of neutropenic mice infected with *R. oryzae* only when compared to a subtherapeutic dose (0.3 mg/kg/day) of AmB-d monotherapy [126]. In contrast, combination therapy was not superior to a standard dose of AmB-d monotherapy (0.8 mg/kg/day). In the second study, combination posaconazole plus LAmB did not improve survival rates compared to LAmB monotherapy in either neutropenic or diabetic ketoacidotic mice with mucormycosis [125]. To date, no clinical studies have evaluated the combination of posaconazole and polyene for primary therapy for mucormycosis.

Hyperbaric Oxygen Treatment

Some case reports have suggested that hyperbaric oxygen may be a beneficial adjunct to the standard surgical and medical antifungal therapy of mucormycosis, particularly for patients with rhinocerebral disease. In a small retrospective study of patients with rhinocerebral mucormycosis, two of six patients who received hyperbaric oxygen died, whereas four of seven patients who received only standard debridement and amphotericin B died. It is hypothesized that hyperbaric oxygen might be useful for treating mucormycosis in conjunction with standard therapy because higher oxygen pressure improves the ability of neutrophils to kill the organism [142]. Additionally, high oxygen pressure inhibits the germination of fungal spores and growth of mycelia in vitro [143].

Cytokine Treatment

Proinflammatory cytokines, such as interferon-gamma and granulocyte-monocyte colony-stimulating factor (GM-CSF), enhance the ability of granulocytes to damage the agents of mucormycosis [144]. Case reports have described survival of patients with mucormycosis treated with adjunctive recombinant G-CSF and GM-CSF or with recombinant interferon-gamma in conjunction with lipid formulations of AmB [145–149]. G-CSF-mobilized granulocyte transfusions have been increasingly used for refractory mycoses, including mucormycosis [150, 151]. The reported experience with granulocyte transfusions is limited to anecdotal reports, but such transfusions may be lifesaving in persistently neutropenic hosts with mucormycosis.

Entomophthoramycosis

Mycology

The order Entomophthorales includes two histopathologically similar, but clinically and mycologically distinct, genera: *Basidiobolus* and *Conidiobolus* [2, 3, 5]. Both basidiobolomycosis and conidiobolomycosis present mainly as subcutaneous infections in immunocompetent hosts. However, both of these infections occasionally disseminate in both immunocompetent and immuncompromised hosts [2]. Basidiobolomycosis is caused by *Basidiobolus ranarum*. Previous descriptions of this organism have used the synonyms *B. haptosporus, B. meristosporus,* or *B. heterosporus* [2]; however, *B. ranarum* is currently considered the preferred name. Infection with this organism tends to involve the trunk and limbs. In contrast, conidiobolomycosis (also known as rhinophycomycosis, rhinoentomophthoromycosis, or nasofacial zygomycosis) is caused by *Conidiobolus coronatus* or *Conidiobolus incongruous,* and primarily involves the nose and soft tissues of the face [152, 153].

Epidemiology

Basidiobolomycosis is predominantly a disease of childhood and adolescence and is only occasionally seen in adults [5]. In contrast, conidiobolomycosis almost always afflicts adults [154, 155]. Both diseases occur primarily in the tropical and subtropical regions of Africa and Southeast Asia [2]. Rare cases have been seen in other parts of the world. Although entomophthoramycosis occurs mainly in healthy individuals, some cases have occurred in immunocompromised hosts [156–158].

The agents of entomophthoramycosis are normally found in soil throughout the world. *Basidiobolus ranarum* is found in decaying vegetation, soil, and the gastrointestinal tracts of reptiles, fish, amphibians and bats [159]. Similarly, *C. coronatus* is found in soil, decaying vegetation, insects, and in the gastrointestinal contents of lizards and toads [2, 160, 161]. Although the agents of entomophthoramycosis are ubiquitous, clinically apparent infection is rare. Only 150 cases were estimated to occur worldwide in 1991 [162], raising the possibility that rather than a chance event, the individuals who develop this infection have a subtle defect in host immunity to this group of organisms.

The mode of transmission for *B. ranarum* is assumed to be through minor skin trauma and insect bites [163]. Fungal spores are found in bristles of mites and are probably carried by other insects. Infected insects are ingested by reptiles and amphibians, which subsequently pass the spores in their excreta [164]. *Basidiobolus ranarum* may be present on "toilet leaves" that are used for skin cleaning after a bowel movement. Thus, direct inoculation of the perineum may occur from these contaminated leaves. Consistent with this theory is the finding that the infection most commonly occurs in the buttocks, thigh, and perineum [163]. *Basidiobolus ranarum* occasionally causes rhinocerebral infections in hyperglycemic patients, suggesting that it may also be acquired by inhalation [156].

Conidiobolomycosis occurs eight times more frequently in males and is most common in individuals who work outdoors in the tropical and subtropical rain forests of Africa and Southeast Asia. The mode of transmission of conidiobolomycosis has not been clearly established. The predilection of the organism to infect the head and face suggests that the route of inoculation is via inhalation of spores or through minor trauma to the nose or face [154]. It is also possible that this infection is transmitted by insect bites [152].

Conidiobolomycosis is also a zoonotic infection, occurring in horses and mules [152].

Clinical Manifestations

Basidiobolomycosis typically presents as a chronic infection of the subcutaneous tissue of the arms, legs, trunk, or buttocks [165] and is characterized by the presence of firm painless nodular subcutaneous lesions that spread locally. The infection is slowly progressive if not treated, but may also heal spontaneously [166]. Although dissemination is uncommon [167], deeper invasion of the muscles beneath the subcutaneous infected areas [168] as well as widespread dissemination [169] have been reported. Rarely, *B. ranarum* infects the gastrointestinal tract, typically the stomach, duodenum, and colon [170–172]. Symptoms of gastrointestinal basidiobolomycosis include fever, abdominal pain, diarrhea, constipation, weight loss, and, less commonly, chills and rigors. Angioinvasive disease similar to that noted in mucormycosis has been described [169, 173] Polypoidal mass in the paranasal sinuses with extradural extension has been reported as a rare complication [174].

Infections with *Conidiobolus* present most commonly as chronic sinusitis. The infection initially manifests with swelling of the inferior nasal turbinates. Untreated, infection extends to the adjacent facial and subcutaneous tissues and the paranasal sinuses. Swelling of the nose, mouth, and perinasal tissue ensues, resulting in nasal congestion and drainage, sinus pain, and epistaxis [175]. Severe generalized facial swelling may develop [3]. The presence of subcutaneous nodules in the eyebrows, upper lip, and cheeks may be quite disfiguring, especially if there is regional lymph node involvement and subsequent lymphedema [176]. Rarely, infection can involve the pharynx and larynx, resulting in dysphagia and airway obstruction. Unlike mucormycosis, conidiobolomycosis usually does not spread to the central nervous system [167]. Disseminated infections are rare, but have been reported in both immunocompetent and immunocompromised patients [154].

Diagnosis

In endemic areas of entomophthoramycosis, basidiobolomycosis and conidiobolomycosis can most easily be distinguished from one another by the anatomic location of the infection and the age of the patient. The diagnosis is best made by biopsy of the infected subcutaneous or submucosal tissue. Both diseases have similar histopathology. The hyphae, which are broad, thin-walled, and occasionally septate, are best visualized with hematoxylin and eosin staining because of the presence of Splendore-Hoeppli eosinophilic material [167]. Other stains such as periodic acid–Schiff and Gomori methenamine silver are less effective in staining the Entomophthorales [3, 170]. Hyphae are surrounded by eosinophils, lymphocytes, and plasma cells. The presence of eosinophils is an important histopathologic finding for entomophthoramycosis. Angioinvasion with subsequent tissue necrosis and infarction are rarely seen [3]. The agents of entomophthoramycosis cannot be identified at the species level by histopathology; thus specimens must be cultured if species identification is to be performed.

Treatment

No single drug has been proven to be effective in treating all cases of entomophthoramycosis. Saturated solution of potassium iodide (SSKI), trimethoprim-sulfamethoxazole, AmB-d azoles, and a combination of these agents have been used with varying success. Because of the rarity of the infections, none of these treatment regimens have been directly compared. Furthermore, some cases of entomophthoramycosis may resolve without treatment. SSKI has traditionally been used in the treatment of entomophthoramycosis, with mixed clinical results [160, 177, 178] The mechanism of action of SSKI is not known. Therapy with SSKI should be administered for at least 3 months at 1.5–2.0 g daily. Trimethoprim-sulfamethoxazole has fewer side effects than SSKI; however, it must be administered at high doses for a longer period of time [179, 180]. Fluconazole [181] and itraconazole [182] have been used successfully to treat entomophthoramycosis, but there has been more experience with ketoconazole [152, 162, 179]. Anecdotally, months of continuous treatment with ketoconazole or multiple courses of shorter-course therapy are required for resolution of the infection [152, 179]. Amphotericin B is usually not the first choice of treatment, but is often used as salvage therapy. Some isolates of *B. ranarum* and *Conidiobolus* species are susceptible to AmB in vitro, while other isolates are resistant [183]. There are anecdotal reports of successful therapy with SSKI combined with trimethoprim-sulfamethoxazole [154], ketoconazole [152, 184], or fluconazole [152] in patients in whom single-drug therapy had failed. Terbinafine combined with either AmB-d or itraconazole has also been successful [185, 186] Experience with lipid formulations of AmB is limited.

In addition to antifungal therapy, surgical removal of accessible nodules and reconstruction of grossly deformed tissues should be performed when possible. Unfortunately, relapses of infection may occur following surgery [5].

References

1. Hibbett DS, Binder M, Bischoff JF, et al. A higher-level phylogenetic classification of the Fungi. Mycol Res. 2007;111:509–47.
2. Ribes JA, Vanover-Sams CL, Baker DJ. Zygomycetes in human disease. Clin Microbiol Rev. 2000;13:236–301.
3. Sugar AM. Agents of Mucormycosis and Related Species. In: Mandell GL, Bennett JE, Dolin R, editors. Principles and practice of infectious diseases. 6th ed. Philadelphia: Elsevier; 2005. 2979.
4. Spellberg B, Edwards Jr J, Ibrahim A. Novel perspectives on mucormycosis: pathophysiology, presentation, and management. Clin Microbiol Rev. 2005;18:556–69.
5. Kwon-Chung KJ, Bennett JE. Mucormycosis. In: Medical mycology. Philadelphia: Lea & Febiger; 1992. p. 524–59.
6. Cohen-Abbo A, Bozeman PM, Patrick CC. *Cunninghamella* infections: review and report of two cases of *Cunninghamella* pneumonia in immunocompromised children. Clin Infect Dis. 1993;17:173–7.
7. Kontoyianis DP, Vartivarian S, Anaissie EJ, Samonis G, Bodey GP, Rinaldi M. Infections due to *Cunninghamella bertholletiae* in patients with cancer: report of three cases and review. Clin Infect Dis. 1994;18:925–8.
8. Kwon-Chung KJ, Young RC, Orlando M. Pulmonary mucormycosis caused by *Cunninghamella elegans* in a patient with chronic myelogenous leukemia. Am J Clin Pathol. 1975;64:544–8.
9. Motohashi K, Ito S, Hagihara M, Maruta A, Ishigatsubo Y, Kanamori H. Cutaneous zygomycosis caused by *Cunninghamella bertholletiae* in a patient with chronic myelogenous leukemia in blast crisis. Am J Hematol. 2009;84:447–8.
10. Bearer EA, Nelson PR, Chowers MY, Davis CE. Cutaneous zygomycosis caused by *Saksenaea vasiformis* in a diabetic patient. J Clin Microbiol. 1994;32:1823–4.
11. Lye GR, Wood G, Nimmo G. Subcutaneous zygomycosis due to *Saksenaea vasiformis*: rapid isolate identification using a modified sporulation technique. Pathology. 1996;28:364–5.
12. Pritchard RC, Muir DB, Archer KH, Beith JM. Subcutaneous zygomycosis due to *Saksenaea vasiformis* in an infant. Med J Australia. 1986;145:630–1.
13. Gonis G, Starr M. Fatal rhinoorbital mucormycosis caused by *Saksenaea vasiformis* in an immunocompromised child. Pediatr Infect Dis J. 1997;16:714–6.
14. Hay RJ, Campbell CK, Marshall WM, Rees BI, Pincott J. Disseminated zygomycosis (mucormycosis) caused by *Saksenaea vasiformis*. J Infect. 1983;7:162–5.
15. Torell J, Cooper BH, Helgeson NG. Disseminated *Saksenaea vasiformis* infection. Am J Clin Pathol. 1981;76:116–21.
16. Kemna ME, Neri RC, Ali R, Salkin IF. *Cokeromyces recurvatus*, a mucoraceous zygomycete rarely isolated in clinical laboratories. J Clin Microbiol. 1994;32:843–5.
17. Kamalam A, Thambiah AS. Cutaneous infection by *Syncephalastrum*. Sabouraudia. 1980;18:19–20.
18. Verweij PE, Voss A, Donnelly JP, de Pauw BE, Meis JF. Wooden sticks as the source of a pseudoepidemic of infection with *Rhizopus microsporus* var. *rhizopodiformis* among immunocompromised patients. J Clin Microbiol. 1997;35:2422–3.
19. Al-Asiri RH, Van Dijken PJ, Mahmood MA, Al-Shahed MS, Rossi ML, Osoba AO. Isolated hepatic mucormycosis in an immunocompetent child. Am J Gastroenterol. 1996;91:606–7.
20. Del Valle Zapico A, Rubio Suárez A, Mellado Encinas P, Morales Angulo C, Cabrera Pozuelo E. Mucormycosis of the sphenoid sinus in an otherwise healthy patient. Case report and literature review. J Laryngol Otol. 1996;110:471–3.
21. Petrikkos G, Skiada A, Sambatakou H, et al. Mucormycosis: ten-year experience at a tertiary-care center in Greece. Eur J Clin Microbiol Infect Dis. 2003;22:753–6.
22. O'Connell MA, Pluss JL, Schkade P, Henry AR, Goodman DL. *Rhizopus*-induced hypersensitivity pneumonitis in a tractor driver. J Allergy Clin Immunol. 1995;95:779–80.
23. Wimander K, Belin L. Recognition of allergic alveolitis in the trimming department of a Swedish sawmill. Eur J Respir Dis Suppl. 1980;107:163–7.
24. Marr KA, Carter RA, Crippa F, Wald A, Corey L. Epidemiology and outcome of mould infections in hematopoietic stem cell transplant recipients. Clin Infect Dis. 2002;34:909–17.
25. Kontoyiannis DP, Wessel VC, Bodey GP, Rolston KV. Zygomycosis in the 1990s in a tertiary-care cancer center. Clin Infect Dis. 2000;30:851–6.
26. Maertens J, Demuynck H, Verbeken EK, et al. Mucormycosis in allogeneic bone marrow transplant recipients: report of five cases and review of the role of iron overload in the pathogenesis. Bone Marrow Transplant. 1999;24:307–12.
27. Marty FM, Cosimi LA, Baden LR. Breakthrough zygomycosis after voriconazole treatment in recipients of hematopoietic stem-cell transplants. N Engl J Med. 2004;350:950–2.
28. Greenberg RN, Scott LJ, Vaughn HH, Ribes JA. Zygomycosis (mucormycosis): emerging clinical importance and new treatments. Curr Opin Infect Dis. 2004;17:517–25.
29. Lueg EA, Ballagh RH, Forte V. Analysis of the recent cluster of invasive fungal sinusitis at the Toronto Hospital for Sick Children. J Otolaryngol. 1996;25:366–70.
30. Waldorf AR, Ruderman N, Diamond RD. Specific susceptibility to mucormycosis in murine diabetes and bronchoalveolar macrophage defense against *Rhizopus*. J Clin Invest. 1984;74:150–60.
31. Lamaris GA, Ben-Ami R, Lewis RE, Chamilos G, Samonis G, Kontoyiannis DP. Increased virulence of Zygomycetes organisms following exposure to voriconazole: a study involving fly and murine models of zygomycosis. J Infect Dis. 2009;199:1399–406.
32. Diamond RD, Krzesicki R, Epstein B, Jao W. Damage to hyphal forms of fungi by human leukocytes in vitro. A possible host defense mechanism in aspergillosis and mucormycosis. Am J Pathol. 1978;91:313–28.
33. Marx RS, Forsyth KR, Hentz SK. Mucorales species activation of a serum leukotactic factor. Infect Immun. 1982;38:1217–22.
34. Waldorf AR. Pulmonary defense mechanisms against opportunistic fungal pathogens. Immunol Ser. 1989;47:243–71.
35. Diamond RD, Haudenschild CC, Erickson NF. Monocyte-mediated damage to *Rhizopus oryzae* hyphae in vitro. Infect Immun. 1982;38:292–7.
36. Chinn RY, Diamond RD. Generation of chemotactic factors by *Rhizopus oryzae* in the presence and absence of serum: relationship to hyphal damage mediated by human neutrophils and effects of hyperglycemia and ketoacidosis. Infect Immun. 1982;38:1123–9.
37. Artis WM, Fountain JA, Delcher HK, Jones HE. A mechanism of susceptibility to mucormycosis in diabetic ketoacidosis: transferrin and iron availability. Diabetes. 1982;31:1109–14.
38. Boelaert JR, de Locht M, Van Cutsem J, et al. Mucormycosis during deferoxamine therapy is a siderophore-mediated infection. In vitro and in vivo animal studies. J Clin Invest. 1993;91:1979–86.
39. Howard DH. Acquisition, transport, and storage of iron by pathogenic fungi. Clin Microbiol Rev. 1999;12:394–404.
40. de Locht M, Boelaert JR, Schneider YJ. Iron uptake from ferrioxamine and from ferrirhizoferrin by germinating spores of *Rhizopus microsporus*. Biochem Pharmacol. 1994;47:1843–50.
41. Boelaert JR, Van Cutsem J, de Locht M, Schneider YJ, Crichton RR. Deferoxamine augments growth and pathogenicity of *Rhizopus*, while hydroxypyridinone chelators have no effect. Kidney Int. 1994;45:667–71.
42. Ibrahim AS, Spellberg B, Edwards Jr J. Iron acquisition: a novel perspective on mucormycosis pathogenesis and treatment. Curr Opin Infect Dis. 2008;21:620–5.

43. Ibrahim AS, Edwards JE, Jr, Fu Y, Spellberg B. Deferiprone iron chelation as a novel therapy for experimental mucormycosis. J Antimicrob Chemother. 2006;58:1070–3.
44. Ibrahim AS, Gebermariam T, Fu Y, et al. The iron chelator deferasirox protects mice from mucormycosis through iron starvation. J Clin Invest. 2007;117:2649–57.
45. Stearman R, Yuan DS, Yamaguchi-Iwai Y, Klausner RD, Dancis A. A permease-oxidase complex involved in high-affinity iron uptake in yeast. Science. 1996;271:1552–7.
46. Ibrahim AS, Gebermariam T, Lin L, Luo G, Husseiny MI, Skory CD, Fu Y, French SW, Edwards JE, Jr, Spellberg B. The high affinity iron permeasc is a key virulence factor required for *Rhizopus oryzae* pathogenesis. Mol Microbiol. 2010;77:587–604.
47. Santos R, Buisson N, Knight S, Dancis A, Camadro JM, Lesuisse E. Haemin uptake and use as an iron source by *Candida albicans*: role of CaHMX1-encoded haem oxygenase. Microbiology. 2003;149:579–88.
48. Worsham PL, Goldman WE. Quantitative plating of *Histoplasma capsulatum* without addition of conditioned medium or siderophores. J Med Vet Mycol. 1988;26:137–43.
49. Ma LJ, Ibrahim AS, Skory C, et al. Genomic analysis of the basal lineage fungus *Rhizopus oryzae* reveals a whole-genome duplication. PLoS Genet. 2009;5:e1000549.
50. Ibrahim AS, Edwards JE, Jr, Filler SG. Zygomycosis. In: Dismukes WE, Pappas PG, Sobel JD, editors. Clinical mycology. New York: Oxford University Press; 2003. p. 241–51.
51. Bouchara JP, Oumeziane NA, Lissitzky JC, Larcher G, Tronchin G, Chabasse D. Attachment of spores of the human pathogenic fungus *Rhizopus oryzae* to extracellular matrix components. Eur J Cell Biol. 1996;70:76–83.
52. Ibrahim AS, Spellberg B, Avanessian V, Fu Y, Edwards JE, Jr. *Rhizopus oryzae* adheres to, is phagocytosed by, and damages endothelial cells in vitro. Infect Immun. 2005;73:778–83.
53. Wang M, Wey S, Zhang Y, Ye R, Lee AS. Role of the unfolded protein response regulator GRP78/BiP in development, cancer and neurological disorders. Antioxidants Redox Signal. 2009;11:2307–16.
54. Ni M, Lee AS. ER chaperones in mammalian development and human diseases. FEBS Lett. 2007;581:3641–51.
55. Liu M, Spellberg B, Phan QT, Fu Y, Lec AS, Edwards JE Jr. Filler SG, Ibrahim AS. The endothelial cell receptor GRP78 is required for macormycosis pathogenesis in diabetic mice. J Clin Invest; 2010;120:1914–1924.
56. Jennessen J, Nielsen KF, Houbraken J, et al. Secondary metabolite and mycotoxin production by the *Rhizopus microsporus* group. J Agric Food Chem. 2005;53:1833–40.
57. Partida-Martinez LP, Hertweck C. Pathogenic fungus harbours endosymbiotic bacteria for toxin production. Nature. 2005;437:884–8.
58. Ibrahim AS, Gebremariam T, Liu M, et al. Bacterial endosymbiosis is widely present among zygomycetes but does not contribute to the pathogenesis of mucormycosis. J Infect Dis. 2008;198:1083–90.
59. Farley PC, Sullivan PA. The *Rhizopus oryzae* secreted aspartic proteinase gene family: an analysis of gene expression. Microbiology. 1998;144(Pt 8):2355–66.
60. Anand VK, Alemar G, Griswold Jr JA. Intracranial complications of mucormycosis: an experimental model and clinical review. Laryngoscope. 1992;102:656–62.
61. Pillsbury HC, Fischer ND. Rhinocerebral mucormycosis. Arch Otolaryngol. 1977;103:600–4.
62. McNulty JS. Rhinocerebral mucormycosis: predisposing factors. Laryngoscope. 1982;92:1140–3.
63. Peterson KL, Wang M, Canalis RF, Abemayor E. Rhinocerebral mucormycosis: evolution of the disease and treatment options. Laryngoscope. 1997;107:855–62.
64. Yanagisawa E, Friedman S, Kundargi RS, Smith HW. Rhinocerebral phycomycosis. Laryngoscope. 1977;87:1319–35.
65. Abedi E, Sismanis A, Choi K, Pastore P. Twenty-five years' experience treating cerebro-rhino-orbital mucormycosis. Laryngoscope. 1984;94:1060–2.
66. Lowe Jr JT, Hudson WR. Rhincerebral phycomycosis and internal carotid artery thrombosis. Arch Otolaryngol. 1975;101:100–3.
67. LeCompte PM, Miessner WA. Mucormycosis of the central nervous system associated with hemochromatosis. Am J Pathol. 1947;23:673–6.
68. Bullock JD, Jampol LM, Fezza AJ. Two cases of orbital phycomycosis with recovery. Am J Ophthalmol. 1974;78:811–5.
69. Parfrey NA. Improved diagnosis and prognosis of mucormycosis. A clinicopathologic study of 33 cases. Medicine. 1986;65:113–23.
70. Blitzer A, Lawson W, Meyers BR, Biller HF. Patient survival factors in paranasal sinus mucormycosis. Laryngoscope. 1980;90:635–48.
71. Morrison VA, McGlave PB. Mucormycosis in the BMT population. Bone Marrow Transplant. 1993;11:383–8.
72. Rothstein RD, Simon GL. Subacute pulmonary mucormycosis. J Med Vet Mycol. 1986;24:391–4.
73. Tedder M, Spratt JA, Anstadt MP, Hegde SS, Tedder SD, Lowe JE. Pulmonary mucormycosis: results of medical and surgical therapy. Ann Thorac Surg. 1994;57:1044–50.
74. Harada M, Manabe T, Yamashita K, Okamoto N. Pulmonary mucormycosis with fatal massive hemoptysis. Acta Pathol Jpn. 1992;42:49–55.
75. Watts WJ. Bronchopleural fistula followed by massive fatal hemoptysis in a patient with pulmonary mucormycosis. A case report. Arch Intern Med. 1983;143:1029–30.
76. Gleissner B, Schilling A, Anagnostopolous I, Siehl I, Thiel E. Improved outcome of zygomycosis in patients with hematological diseases? Leuk Lymphoma. 2004;45:1351–60.
77. Kerr OA, Bong C, Wallis C, Tidman MJ. Primary cutaneous mucormycosis masquerading as pyoderma gangrenosum. Br J Dermatol. 2004;150:1212–3.
78. Gartenberg G, Bottone EJ, Keusch GT, Weitzman I. Hospital-acquired mucormycosis (*Rhizopus rhizopodiformis*) of skin and subcutaneous tissue: epidemiology, mycology and treatment. N Engl J Med. 1978;299:1115–8.
79. Mead JH, Lupton GP, Dillavou CL, Odom RB. Cutaneous *Rhizopus* infection. Occurrence as a postoperative complication associated with an elasticized adhesive dressing. J Am Med Assoc. 1979;242:272–4.
80. Ledgard JP, van Hal S, Greenwood JE. Primary cutaneous zygomycosis in a burns patient: a review. J Burn Care Res. 2008;29:286–90.
81. Boyd AS, Wiser B, Sams HH, King LE. Gangrenous cutaneous mucormycosis in a child with a solid organ transplant: a case report and review of the literature. Pediatr Dermatol. 2003;20:411–5.
82. Kordy FN, Al-Mohsen IZ, Hashem F, Almodovar E, Al Hajjar S, Walsh TJ. Successful treatment of a child with posttraumatic necrotizing fasciitis caused by *Apophysomyces elegans*: case report and review of literature. Pediatr Infect Dis J. 2004;23:877–9.
83. Prasad RM, Bose SM, Vaiphei K, Verma GR. Post operative abdominal wall mucormycosis mimicking as bacterial necrotising fasciitis. J Postgrad Med. 2003;49:187–8.
84. Amin SB, Ryan RM, Metlay LA, Watson WJ. *Absidia corymbifera* infections in neonates. Clin Infect Dis. 1998;26:990–2.
85. Sharma MC, Gill SS, Kashyap S, et al. Gastrointestinal mucormycosis–an uncommon isolated mucormycosis. Indian J Gastroenterol. 1998;17:131–3.
86. Straatsma BR, Zimmerman LE, Gass JDM. Phycomycosis: a clinicopathologic study of fifty-one cases. Lab Invest. 1962;11:963–85.
87. Woods KF, Hanna BJ. Brain stem mucormycosis in a narcotic addict with eventual recovery. Am J Med. 1986;80:126–8.
88. Virmani R, Connor DH, McAllister HA. Cardiac mucormycosis. A report of five patients and review of 14 previously reported cases. Am J Clin Pathol. 1982;78:42–7.

89. Tuder RM. Myocardial infarct in disseminated mucormycosis: case report with special emphasis on the pathogenic mechanisms. Mycopathologia. 1985;89:81–8.
90. Vesa J, Bielsa O, Arango O, Lladó C, Gelabert A. Massive renal infarction due to mucormycosis in an AIDS patient. Infection. 1992;20:234–6.
91. Maliwan N, Reyes CV, Rippon JW. Osteomyelitis secondary to cutaneous mucormycosis. Report of a case and a review of the literature. Am J Dermatopathol. 1984;6:479–81.
92. Pierce PF, Wood MB, Roberts GD, Fitzgerald Jr RH, Robertson C, Edson RS. *Saksenaea vasiformis* osteomyelitis. J Clin Microbiol. 1987;25:933–5.
93. Leong ASY. Granulomatous mediastinitis due to *Rhizopus* species. Am J Clin Pathol. 1978;70:103–7.
94. Connor BA, Anderson RJ, Smith JW. Mucor mediastinitis. Chest. 1979;75:524–6.
95. Andrews DR, Allan A, Larbalestier RI. Tracheal mucormycosis. Ann Thorac Surg. 1997;63:230–2.
96. Helenglass G, Elliott JA, Lucie NP. An unusual presentation of opportunistic mucormycosis. Br Med J (Clin Res ed). 1981;282: 108–9.
97. Ogunlana EO. Fungal air spora at Ibadan, Nigeria. Appl Microbiol. 1975;29:458–63.
98. Mori T, Egashira M, Kawamata N, et al. Zygomycosis: two case reports and review of reported cases in the literature in Japan. Nippon Ishinkin Gakkai Zasshi. 2003;44:163–79.
99. Tietz HJ, Brehmer D, Jänisch W, Martin H. Incidence of endomycoses in the autopsy material of the Berlin Charité Hospital. Mycoses. 1998;41 Suppl 2:81–5.
100. Reed C, Bryant R, Ibrahim AS, et al. Combination polyene-caspofungin treatment of rhino-orbital-cerebral mucormycosis. Clin Infect Dis. 2008;47:364–71.
101. Chamilos G, Marom EM, Lewis RE, Lionakis MS, Kontoyiannis DP. Predictors of pulmonary zygomycosis versus invasive pulmonary aspergillosis in patients with cancer. Clin Infect Dis. 2005;41:60–6.
102. Wahba H, Truong MT, Lei X, Kontoyiannis DP, Marom EM. Reversed halo sign in invasive pulmonary fungal infections. Clin Infect Dis. 2008;46:1733–7.
103. Chamilos G, Lewis RE, Kontoyiannis DP. Delaying amphotericin B-based frontline therapy significantly increases mortality among patients with hematologic malignancy who have zygomycosis. Clin Infect Dis. 2008;47:503–9.
104. Roden MM, Zaoutis TE, Buchanan WL, et al. Epidemiology and outcome of zygomycosis: a review of 929 reported cases. Clin Infect Dis. 2005;41:634–53.
105. Walsh TJ, Finberg RW, Arndt C, et al. Liposomal amphotericin B for empirical therapy in patients with persistent fever and neutropenia. National Institute of Allergy and Infectious Diseases Mycoses Study Group. N Engl J Med. 1999;340:764–71.
106. Walsh TJ, Hiemenz JW, Seibel NL, et al. Amphotericin B lipid complex for invasive fungal infections: analysis of safety and efficacy in 556 cases. Clin Infect Dis. 1998;26:1383–96.
107. Ibrahim AS, Avanessian V, Spellberg B, Edwards Jr JE. Liposomal amphotericin B, and not amphotericin B deoxycholate, improves survival of diabetic mice infected with *Rhizopus oryzae*. Antimicrob Agents Chemother. 2003;47:3343–4.
108. Groll AH, Giri N, Petraitis V, et al. Comparative efficacy and distribution of lipid formulations of amphotericin B in experimental *Candida albicans* infection of the central nervous system. J Infect Dis. 2000;182:274–82.
109. Ibrahim AS, Gebremariam T, Husseiny MI, et al. Comparison of lipid amphotericin B preparations in treating murine zygomycosis. Antimicrob Agents Chemother. 2008;52:1573–6.
110. Sun QN, Fothergill AW, McCarthy DI, Rinaldi MG, Graybill JR. In vitro activities of posaconazole, itraconazole, voriconazole, amphotericin B, and fluconazole against 37 clinical isolates of zygomycetes. Antimicrob Agents Chemother. 2002;46:1581–2.
111. Blin N, Morineau N, Gaillard F, et al. Disseminated mucormycosis associated with invasive pulmonary aspergillosis in a patient treated for post-transplant high-grade non-Hodgkin's lymphoma. Leuk Lymphoma. 2004;45:2161–3.
112. Imhof A, Balajee SA, Fredricks DN, Englund JA, Marr KA. Breakthrough fungal infections in stem cell transplant recipients receiving voriconazole. Clin Infect Dis. 2004;39:743–6.
113. Kobayashi K, Kami M, Murashige N, Kishi Y, Fujisaki G, Mitamura T. Breakthrough zygomycosis during voriconazole treatment for invasive aspergillosis. Haematologica 2004;89:ECR42.
114. Kontoyiannis DP, Lionakis MS, Lewis RE, et al. Zygomycosis in a tertiary-care cancer center in the era of Aspergillus-active antifungal therapy: a case-control observational study of 27 recent cases. J Infect Dis. 2005;191:1350–60.
115. Oren I. Breakthrough zygomycosis during empirical voriconazole therapy in febrile patients with neutropenia. Clin Infect Dis. 2005;40:770–1.
116. Pfaller MA, Messer SA, Hollis RJ, Jones RN. Antifungal activities of posaconazole, ravuconazole, and voriconazole compared to those of itraconazole and amphotericin B against 239 clinical isolates of *Aspergillus* spp. and other filamentous fungi: report from SENTRY Antimicrobial Surveillance Program, 2000. Antimicrob Agents Chemother. 2002;46:1032–7.
117. Lass-Florl C, Mayr A, Perkhofer S, et al. Activities of antifungal agents against yeasts and filamentous fungi: assessment according to the methodology of the European Committee on Antimicrobial Susceptibility Testing. Antimicrob Agents Chemother. 2008;52: 3637–41.
118. Arikan S, Sancak B, Alp S, Hascelik G, McNicholas P. Comparative in vitro activities of posaconazole, voriconazole, itraconazole, and amphotericin B against *Aspergillus* and *Rhizopus*, and synergy testing for *Rhizopus*. Med Mycol. 2008;12:1–7.
119. Ullmann AJ, Cornely OA, Burchardt A, et al. Pharmacokinetics, safety, and efficacy of posaconazole in patients with persistent febrile neutropenia or refractory invasive fungal infection. Antimicrob Agents Chemother. 2006;50:658–66.
120. Krishna G, Martinho M, Chandrasekar P, Ullmann AJ, Patino H. Pharmacokinetics of oral posaconazole in allogeneic hematopoietic stem cell transplant recipients with graft-versus-host disease. Pharmacotherapy. 2007;27:1627–36.
121. Krishna G, Parsons A, Kantesaria B, Mant T. Evaluation of the pharmacokinetics of posaconazole and rifabutin following co-administration to healthy men. Curr Med Res Opin. 2007;23:545–52.
122. Krishna G, Sansone-Parsons A, Martinho M, Kantesaria B, Pedicone L. Posaconazole plasma concentrations in juvenile patients with invasive fungal infection. Antimicrob Agents Chemother. 2007;51:812–8.
123. Sun QN, Najvar LK, Bocanegra R, Loebenberg D, Graybill JR. In vivo activity of posaconazole against *Mucor* spp. in an immunosuppressed-mouse model. Antimicrob Agents Chemother. 2002;46: 2310–2.
124. Dannaoui E, Meis JF, Loebenberg D, Verweij PE. Activity of posaconazole in treatment of experimental disseminated zygomycosis. Antimicrob Agents Chemother. 2003;47:3647–50.
125. Ibrahim AS, Gebremariam T, Schwartz JA, Edwards Jr JE, Spellberg B. Posaconazole mono- or combination therapy for treatment of murine zygomycosis. Antimicrob Agents Chemother. 2009;53:772–5.
126. Rodriguez MM, Serena C, Marine M, Pastor FJ, Guarro J. Posaconazole combined with amphotericin B, an effective therapy for a murine-disseminated infection caused by *Rhizopus oryzae*. Antimicrob Agents Chemother. 2008;52:3786–8.
127. van Burik JA, Hare RS, Solomon HF, Corrado ML, Kontoyiannis DP. Posaconazole is effective as salvage therapy in zygomycosis:

a retrospective summary of 91 cases. Clin Infect Dis. 2006; 42:e61–5.
128. Greenberg RN, Mullane K, van Burik JA, et al. Posaconazole as salvage therapy for zygomycosis. Antimicrob Agents Chemother. 2006;50:126–33.
129. Diekema DJ, Messer SA, Hollis RJ, Jones RN, Pfaller MA. Activities of caspofungin, itraconazole, posaconazole, ravuconazole, voriconazole, and amphotericin B against 448 recent clinical isolates of filamentous fungi. J Clin Microbiol. 2003;41:3623–6.
130. Espinel-Ingroff A. In vitro antifungal activities of anidulafungin and micafungin, licensed agents and the investigational triazole posaconazole as determined by NCCLS methods for 12, 052 fungal isolates: review of the literature. Rev Iberoam Micol. 2003;20:121–36.
131. Ibrahim AS, Bowman JC, Avanessian V, et al. Caspofungin inhibits *Rhizopus oryzae* 1, 3-beta-D-glucan synthase, lowers burden in brain measured by quantitative PCR, and improves survival at a low but not a high dose during murine disseminated zygomycosis. Antimicrob Agents Chemother. 2005;49:721–7.
132. Spellberg B, Fu Y, Edwards Jr JE, Ibrahim AS. Combination therapy with amphotericin B lipid complex and caspofungin acetate of disseminated zygomycosis in diabetic ketoacidotic mice. Antimicrob Agents Chemother. 2005;49:830–2.
133. Ibrahim AS, Gebremariam T, Fu Y, Edwards Jr JE, Spellberg B. Combination echinocandin-polyene treatment of murine mucormycosis. Antimicrob Agents Chemother. 2008;52:1556–8.
134. Lamaris GA, Lewis RE, Chamilos G, et al. Caspofungin-Mediated beta-Glucan Unmasking and Enhancement of Human Polymorphonuclear Neutrophil Activity against Aspergillus and Non-Aspergillus Hyphae. J Infect Dis. 2008;198:186–92.
135. Cappellini MD. Iron-chelating therapy with the new oral agent ICL670 (Exjade). Best Pract Res Clin Haematol. 2005;18:289–98.
136. Ibrahim AS, Gebermariam T, Fu Y, et al. The iron chelator deferasirox protects mice from mucormycosis through iron starvation. J Clin Invest. 2007;117:2649–57.
137. Piga A, Galanello R, Forni GL, et al. Randomized phase II trial of deferasirox (Exjade, ICL670), a once-daily, orally-administered iron chelator, in comparison to deferoxamine in thalassemia patients with transfusional iron overload. Haematologica. 2006;91:873–80.
138. Miyazawa K, Ohyashiki K, Urabe A, et al. A safety, pharmacokinetic and pharmacodynamic investigation of deferasirox (Exjade, ICL670) in patients with transfusion-dependent anemias and iron-overload: a Phase I study in Japan. Int J Hematol. 2008;88:73–81.
139. Reed C, Ibrahim A, Edwards Jr JE, Walot I, Spellberg B. Deferasirox, an iron-chelating agent, as salvage therapy for rhinocerebral mucormycosis. Antimicrob Agents Chemother. 2006;50: 3968–9.
140. Spellberg B, Andes D, Perez M, et al. Safety and outcomes of open-label deferasirox iron chelation therapy for mucormycosis. Antimicrob Agents Chemother. 2009;53:3122–5.
141. Soummer A, Mathonnet A, Scatton O, et al. Failure of deferasirox, an iron chelator agent, combined with antifungals in a case of severe zygomycosis. Antimicrob Agents Chemother. 2008;52:1585–6.
142. Couch L, Theilen F, Mader JT. Rhinocerebral mucormycosis with cerebral extension successfully treated with adjunctive hyperbaric oxygen therapy. Arch Otolaryngol Head Neck Surg. 1988;114: 791–4.
143. Robb SM. Reactions of fungi to exposure to 10 atmospheres pressure of oxygen. J Gen Microbiol. 1966;45:17–29.
144. Gil-Lamaignere C, Simitsopoulou M, Roilides E, Maloukou A, Winn RM, Walsh TJ. Interferon- gamma and Granulocyte-Macrophage Colony-Stimulating Factor Augment the Activity of Polymorphonuclear Leukocytes against Medically Important Zygomycetes. J Infect Dis. 2005;191:1180–7.
145. Abzug MJ, Walsh TJ. Interferon-gamma and colony-stimulating factors as adjuvant therapy for refractory fungal infections in children. Pediatr Infect Dis J. 2004;23:769–73.
146. Gonzalez CE, Couriel DR, Walsh TJ. Disseminated zygomycosis in a neutropenic patient: successful treatment with amphotericin B lipid complex and granulocyte colony-stimulating factor. Clin Infect Dis. 1997;24:192–6.
147. Kullberg BJ, Anaissie EJ. Cytokines as therapy for opportunistic fungal infections. Res Immunol. 1998;149:478–88. discussion 515.
148. Ma B, Seymour JF, Januszewicz H, Slavin MA. Cure of pulmonary *Rhizomucor pusillus* infection in a patient with hairy-cell leukemia: role of liposomal amphotericin B and GM-CSF. Leuk Lymphoma. 2001;42:1393–9.
149. Mastroianni A. Paranasal sinus mucormycosis in an immunocompetent host: efficacy and safety of combination therapy with Liposomal Amphotericin B and adjuvant rHuGM-CSF. Infez Med. 2004;12:278–83.
150. Grigull L, Beilken A, Schmid H, et al. Secondary prophylaxis of invasive fungal infections with combination antifungal therapy and G-CSF-mobilized granulocyte transfusions in three children with hematological malignancies. Support Care Cancer. 2006;14:783–6.
151. Slavin MA, Kannan K, Buchanan MR, Sasadeusz J, Roberts AW. Successful allogeneic stem cell transplant after invasive pulmonary zygomycosis. Leuk Lymphoma. 2002;43:437–9.
152. Thakar A, Baruah P, Kumar S, Sharma MC. Rhinophycomycosis. J Laryngol Otol. 2001;115:493–6.
153. Yang X, Li Y, Zhou X, et al. Rhinofacial conidiobolomycosis caused by *Conidiobolus coronatus* in a Chinese rice farmer. Mycoses. 2010;53(4):369–73.
154. Gugnani HC. Entomophthoromycosis due to *Conidiobolus*. Eur J Epidemiol. 1992;8:391–6.
155. Martinson FD. Chronic phycomycosis of the upper respiratory tract. Rhinophycomycosis entomophthorae. Am J Trop Med Hyg. 1971;20:449–55.
156. Dworzack DL, Pollock AS, Hodges GR, Barnes WG, Ajello L, Padhye A. Zygomycosis of the maxillary sinus and palate caused by *Basidiobolus haptosporus*. Arch Intern Med. 1978;138:1274–6.
157. Walsh TJ, Renshaw G, Andrews J, et al. Invasive zygomycosis due to *Conidiobolus incongruus*. Clin Infect Dis. 1994;19:423–30.
158. Tan DC, Hsu LY, Koh LP, Goh YT, Koh M. Severe conidiobolomycosis complicating induction chemotherapy in a patient with acute lymphoblastic leukaemia. Br J Haematol. 2005;129:447.
159. Okafor JI, Testrake D, Mushinsky HR, Yangco BG. A *Basidiobolus* sp. and its association with reptiles and amphibians in southern Florida. Sabouraudia. 1984;22:47–51.
160. Rippon JW. Medical mycology. 2nd ed. Philadelphia: The W.B. Saunders Company; 1982. p. 303–14.
161. Dreschler C. Two new species of *Conidiobolus* found in the plant detritus. Am J Bot. 1960;47:368–77.
162. Costa AR, Porto E, Pegas JR, et al. Rhinofacial zygomycosis caused by *Conidiobolus coronatus*. A case report. Mycopathologia. 1991;115:1–8.
163. Cameroon HM. Entomophthoromycosis. In: Mahgoub ES, editor. Tropical mycoses. Beerse: Janssen Research Council; 1990. p. 186–98.
164. Dreschler C. Supplementary development stages of *Basidiobolus ranarum* and *Basidiobolus haptosporus*. Mycologia. 1956;48: 655–77.
165. Goodman NL, Rinaldi MG. Agents of zygomycosis. In: Balows A, Hausler WJ, Herrmann KL, Isenberg HD, Shadomy HJ, editors. Manual of clinical microbiology. 5th ed. Washington: ASM Press; 1991. p. 674–92.
166. Bittencourt AL, Arruda SM, de Andrade JA, Carvalho EM. Basidiobolomycosis: a case report. Pediatr Dermatol. 1991;8: 325–8.
167. Chandler FW, Watts JC. Pathologic diagnosis of fungal infections. Chicago: ASCP Press; 1987. p. 85–95.
168. Kamalam A, Thambiah AS. Muscle invasion by *Basidiobolus haptosporus*. Sabouraudia. 1984;22:273–7.

169. van den Berk GE, Noorduyn LA, van Ketel RJ, van Leeuwen J, Bemelman WA, Prins JM. A fatal pseudo-tumour: disseminated basidiobolomycosis. BMC Infect Dis. 2006;6:140.
170. Pasha TM, Leighton JA, Smilack JD, Heppell J, Colby TV, Kaufman L. Basidiobolomycosis: an unusual fungal infection mimicking inflammatory bowel disease. Gastroenterology. 1997; 112:250–4.
171. Al Jarie A, Al-Mohsen I, Al Jumaah S, et al. Pediatric gastrointestinal basidiobolomycosis. Pediatr Infect Dis J. 2003;22: 1007–14.
172. Hussein MR, Musalam AO, Assiry MH, Eid RA, El Motawa AM, Gamel AM. Histological and ultrastructural features of gastrointestinal basidiobolomycosis. Mycol Res. 2007;111:926–30.
173. Bigliazzi C, Poletti V, Dell'Amore D, Saragoni L, Colby TV. Disseminated basidiobolomycosis in an immunocompetent woman. J Clin Microbiol. 2004;42:1367–9.
174. Singh R, Xess I, Ramavat AS, Arora R. Basidiobolomycosis: a rare case report. Indian J Med Microbiol. 2008;26:265–7.
175. Onuigbo WI, Gugnani HC, Okafor BC, Misch KA. Nasal entomophthorosis in an Igbo from Nigeria. J Laryngol Otol. 1975; 89:657–61.
176. Ravisse P, Destombes P, Le Gonidec G. 10 new clinical cases of mycoses caused by Entomophorales in Cameroon. Bull Soc Pathol Exot Filiales. 1976;69:33–40.
177. Bittencourt AL, Serra G, Sadigursky M, Araujo MG, Campos MC, Sampaio LC. Subcutaneous zygomycosis caused by *Basidiobolus haptosporus*: presentation of a case mimicking Burkitt's lymphoma. Am J Trop Med Hyg. 1982;31:370–3.
178. Okafor BC, Gugnani HC, Jacob A. Nasal entomophthorosis with laryngeal involvement. Mykosen. 1983;26:471–7.
179. Drouhet E, Dupont B. Laboratory and clinical assessment of ketoconazole in deep-seated mycoses. Am J Med. 1983;74:30–47.
180. Restrepo A. Treatment of tropical mycoses. J Am Acad Dermatol. 1994;31:S91–102.
181. Barro-Traore F, Ouedraogo D, Konsem T, et al. Conidiobolomycosis, a rare fungal tumor: a case report in Ouagadougou, Burkina Faso. Bull Soc Pathol Exot. 2008;101:14–6.
182. Mathew R, Kumaravel S, Kuruvilla S, et al. Successful treatment of extensive basidiobolomycosis with oral itraconazole in a child. Int J Dermatol. 2005;44:572–5.
183. Yangco BG, Okafor JI, TeStrake D. In vitro susceptibilities of human and wild-type isolates of *Basidiobolus* and *Conidiobolus* species. Antimicrob Agents Chemother. 1984;25:413–6.
184. Mukhopadhyay D, Ghosh LM, Thammayya A, Sanyal M. Entomophthoromycosis caused by *Conidiobolus coronatus*: clinicomycological study of a case. Auris Nasus Larynx. 1995;22:139–42.
185. Foss NT, Rocha MR, Lima VT, Velludo MA, Roselino AM. Entomophthoramycosis: therapeutic success by using amphotericin B and terbinafine. Dermatology. 1996;193:258–60.
186. Fischer N, Ruef C, Ebnother C, Bachli EB. Rhinofacial *Conidiobolus coronatus* infection presenting with nasal enlargement. Infection. 2008;36:594–6.

Hyalohyphomycoses (Hyaline Moulds)

Harrys A. Torres and Dimitrios P. Kontoyiannis

The hyalohyphomycoses, or hyaline moulds, are human infections caused by soil-dwelling and plant saprophytic moulds [1]. Hyalohyphomycosis encompasses a loose artificial classification system since it does not refer to a specific taxonomic classification [2]. Agents of hyalohyphomycosis include non-melanin-producing, nondematiaceous moulds, which typically appear on histopathologic sections as colorless, hyaline, or light-colored septate hyphae [3]. These hyphae are either branched or unbranched, and occasionally they are toruloid [1, 3, 4]. Important human pathogens included in this group are *Aspergillus*, *Penicillium*, *Fusarium*, *Scopulariopsis*, *Pseudallescheria*, *Scedosporium*, *Acremonium*, *Paecilomyces*, and *Trichoderma* species (Table 1) [1, 3, 5–8].

The hyaline moulds are identified at the genus and species levels largely on the basis of morphology of their reproductive structures, including phialides (fertile cells) and conidia (spores) [4]. Molecular methods, such as polymerase chain reaction (PCR)-based techniques, show promise as diagnostic aids in the early detection of hyalohyphomycetes. The general characteristics of the heterogeneous group of fungi causing hyalohyphomycosis are listed in Table 2.

Hyaline moulds uncommonly cause human disease. In immunocompetent hosts, they predominantly cause localized infections, but in severely compromised hosts, they have now emerged as a cause of severe and frequently fatal deep-seated infections. Most severe cases of hyalohyphomycosis occur in patients with hematologic malignancies or in hematopoietic stem cell transplant (HSCT) or solid organ transplant recipients. Most of these organisms exhibit broad-spectrum resistance to existing antifungal drugs, and recovery from immunosuppression is critical for clinical response. This chapter focuses only on hyaline moulds that have been recognized as emerging pathogens. The most common pathogen in this group, *Aspergillus,* is discussed in a separate chapter.

D.P. Kontoyiannis (✉)
Department of Internal Medicine,
The University of Texas, MD Anderson Cancer Center,
Houston, TX, USA
e-mail: dkontoyi@mdanderson.org

Fusarium Species

Epidemiology

Fusarium derives its name from its fusiform conidia [9]. Long known as plant pathogens, these ubiquitous moulds are common in decomposing organic matter and soil [10, 11]. *Fusarium* species cause fusariosis, a life-threatening opportunistic mycotic infection that is being increasingly recognized worldwide [11–13]. The epidemiologic distribution of fusariosis is not homogeneous; from 50% to 85% of all cases have been reported from the USA [14, 15]. It is not clear whether this reflects a unique ecologic niche for these fungi or is at least partially due to the increased recognition of this infection in the USA. Outside the USA, most cases of fusariosis have been reported in the Mediterranean region (Spain, France, Italy, and Israel) or in subtropical countries such as Brazil. [14, 16–19] Within the USA, the distribution of fusariosis is not homogeneous in that most cases have been reported from only a few centers [14]. In fact, *Fusarium* species have emerged in some tertiary cancer centers as the second most common filamentous fungal pathogen after *Aspergillus* [11].

In a small study from a Brazilian cancer center, *Fusarium* species were identified as the most common mould causing fungemia in HSCT recipients [20]. Not surprisingly, the cumulative incidence of fusariosis among HSCT recipients varies according to the type of transplantation. The incidence among recipients of allogeneic HLA–mismatched related donor transplants is 4 times the incidence among recipients of allogeneic HLA–compatible related donor transplants and 10 times the incidence among recipients of autologous transplants [21]. *Fusarium* infection tends to vary seasonally. The infection is most prevalent in autumn in France and most prevalent in summer in Texas, Israel, and Italy [17]. This may reflect sporulation efficiency of *Fusarium* species during these seasons [17].

The portals of entry for *Fusarium* infection include the respiratory tract, digestive tract, and the skin, periungual regions, or burns, and vascular catheters [15]. The predominant mode of infection is inhalation into the lungs or upper

C.A. Kauffman et al. (eds.), *Essentials of Clinical Mycology*,
DOI 10.1007/978-1-4419-6640-7_16, © Springer Science+Business Media, LLC 2011

Table 1 Agents of hyalohyphomycosis

Acremonium spp.[a]	*Microsphaeropsis* spp.
Aphanoascus spp.	*Myriodontium* spp.
Aspergillus spp.	*Nannizziopsis* spp.
Arthrographis spp.	*Neocosmospora* spp.
Beauveria spp.	*Paecilomyces* spp.[a]
Cephalotheca spp.	*Penicillium* spp.
Cerinosterus spp.	*Onychocola* spp.
Chrysonilia spp.	*Ovadendron* spp.
Chrysosporium spp.	*Pseudallescheria* spp.[a]
Colletotrichum spp.	*Scedosporium* spp.[a]
Coprinus spp.	*Schizophyllum* spp.
Cylindrocarpon spp.	*Scopulariopsis* spp.[a]
Fusarium spp.[a]	*Scytalidium* spp.
Geotrichum spp.[a]	*Tritirachium* spp.
Gibberella spp.	*Trichoderma* spp.[a]
Gymnascella spp.	*Tubercularia* spp.
Lecythophora spp.	*Verticillium* spp.
Metarhizium spp.	*Volutella* spp.
Microsphaeropsis spp.	

[a]Emerging pathogens discussed in this chapter

Table 2 General characteristics of agents of hyalohyphomycosis

Ubiquitous, soil saprophytes
Acquisition: lung, skin, foreign bodies
Normally community-acquired but sporadically acquired nosocomially
Rare cause of infection
Predominantly cause localized infections in immunocompetent hosts following traumatic inoculation
Uncommon causes of allergic sinusitis or asthma
Uncommon but emerging cause of severe and frequently fatal focal respiratory or disseminated opportunistic infections in severely compromised hosts
Most cases occur in patients with hematologic malignancies, hematopoietic stem cell transplant recipients, or solid organ recipients
Resemble *Aspergillus* species in tissue (potential for misidentification)
Several hyalohyphomycetes (e.g., *Fusarium* species, *Scedosporium* species, *Acremonium* species, *Scopulariopsis* species, and *Trichoderma* species) can grow in blood cultures
Most organisms exhibit broad-spectrum resistance to existing antifungal drugs
Aggressive surgical intervention may improve survival rates
Recovery of immune function essential to survival

airways [22]. Therefore, not surprisingly, most cases of fusariosis are considered community acquired. However, *Fusarium* species can also cause nosocomial infections, such as postoperative endophthalmitis or peritonitis associated with dialysis catheters [15, 22]. The water distribution system has been implicated as a reservoir of *Fusarium* species [23, 24]. Some cases of fusariosis in hospital patients coincided with construction work [25], but others have reported that the most likely source of *Fusarium* infection is the external environment rather than a nosocomial source [26].

The genus *Fusarium* currently includes over 100 species, at least 12 of which are human pathogens [27, 28]. Among these, the most common human pathogens are *F. solani* (responsible for 50% of reported *Fusarium* infections in humans), *F. oxysporum* (14%), *F. verticillioides* (also known as *F. moniliforme*) (10–11%), and *F. proliferatum* (5%); much less common pathogens are *F. dimerum*, *F. chlamydosporum*, *F. nygamai*, *F. napiforme*, *F. semitectum*, *F. equiseti*, *F. thapsinum*, *F. sacchari*, *F. decemcellulare*, *F. incarnatum*, *F. falciforme*, and *F. polyphialidicum* [18, 27, 29–31]. This uneven distribution of *Fusarium* species might be related to the relatively higher virulence of some species, such as *F. solani*, as evidenced by findings in a murine model of fusariosis [32].

The species distribution may vary geographically. For example, in a recent study of isolates sequentially collected from 1985 to 2007 from 75 patients with *Fusarium* infections diagnosed in two hospitals in northern Italy, 41% of the isolates were *F. verticillioides*, 25% were *F. solani*, 13% were *F. proliferatum*, and 12% were *F. oxysporum* [28]. In this study, the distribution of the *Fusarium* species also differed according to patients' clinical presentations, with *F. verticillioides* accounting for 57% of the isolates from immunocompromised patients [28].

Pathogenesis

Fusarium species have the remarkable ability of being effective broad-spectrum pathogens against prokaryotic bacteria, such as *Pseudomonas*, and plants and mammals. The pathogenesis of infection by *Fusarium* species is related to the mould's ability to produce mycotoxins or to cause direct invasive disease [33]. Of note, similar to zygomycetes and *Aspergillus* species, *Fusarium* species are highly angiotropic and angioinvasive, causing hemorrhagic infarction and tissue necrosis, especially in pancytopenic hosts [10, 11].

The mycotoxins produced by *Fusarium* species include trichothecenes, such as T-2 toxin, deoxynivalenol, fumonisins, zearalenones, fusaric acid, and apicidin [34, 35]. The molecular events that control the production of such toxins are unknown. The ability of *Fusarium* species to produce these toxins has been associated with crop destruction [11] and with human or animal mycotoxicoses, such as alimentary toxic aleukia [33, 36]. Fumonisins commonly contaminate maize and maize products worldwide and have recently been linked to consumption of maize-based tortillas [37]. The ingestion of grains contaminated with these mycotoxins may cause allergic symptoms or lead to cancer, such as esophageal cancer after long-term consumption [33, 34, 38]. In addition, exposure to fumonisins may play a role in human birth defects [35]. Several mycotoxins induce leukopenia and bone marrow destruction and suppress platelet aggregation [33]. Whether their production also contributes to prolonged chemotherapy-induced myelosuppression remains unclear [10, 15]. There are no data on whether mycotoxins are overexpressed in strains causing invasive human fusariosis [33, 34].

Granulocytes and macrophages play essential roles in the immune defense against fusariosis. Granulocytes inhibit growth of hyphae, while macrophages inhibit both germination of conidia and growth of hyphae [11, 33]. Neutropenia seems to be the critical factor in the development of invasive fusariosis [11, 34]. In a recent series from a comprehensive cancer center, 82% of patients with fusariosis were neutropenic, and 75% of patients with fusariosis had an absolute neutrophil count < 100/uL [39]. However, other host factors besides quantitative granulocyte counts or qualitative neutrophil defects could influence the development of fusariosis in immunocompromised patients [14, 40–43]. For example, patients with refractory aplastic anemia have a low incidence of *Fusarium* infection, and fusariosis is uncommon in patients with chronic granulomatous disease. Proven disseminated fusariosis has been reported in patients with solid tumors in the absence of neutropenia.

Corticosteroids add to the immune-impaired state, predisposing to invasive fusariosis [11, 34]. Human interleukin-15 seems to play an important role in the immunomodulation of host response to *Fusarium* infection [44]. A recent study analyzing factors affecting the virulence of fusariosis in *Drosophila melanogaster* experimental models found that *F. moniliforme* infection was associated with a more acute infection and higher mortality rates when injected into *Toll*-deficient flies than when injected into wild-type flies [45]. This finding is consistent with findings that the virulence of *Fusarium* species seems to be higher than that of other hyalohyphomycetes, such as *Aspergillus* species, *Scedosporium apiospermum,* and *S. prolificans* [45, 46]. Finally, *Fusarium* species can adhere to Silastic catheters; infections of central venous catheters, continuous ambulatory peritoneal dialysis catheters, and contact lenses have been reported [33].

Clinical Manifestations

Fusarium species can cause localized or disseminated infections [15, 22]. Host factors play a crucial role in determining the severity and type of infection. Studies of *Fusarium* infection in immunocompetent patients include mostly localized infections of the eyes, gastrointestinal tract, skin and nails, peritoneum, and lungs [17]. Interestingly, in a retrospective study from Israel, 68 of 89 (76%) patients were immunocompetent [17]. These patients tended to be older than immunocompromised patients and had a high prevalence of underlying diseases, such as ischemic heart disease, diabetes mellitus, peripheral vascular disease, and chronic renal failure [17]. Clinical manifestations of fusariosis according to different underlying conditions are described in Table 3.

Fusarium species (especially *F. solani*) are the most frequent cause of fungal keratitis [33]. Endophthalmitis by contiguous extension to the anterior chamber is a feared complication of severe *Fusarium* keratitis [47]. In the USA, Singapore, and Hong Kong, an outbreak of *Fusarium* keratitis occurred from 2004 to 2006 among wearers of contact lenses. A case control study of 164 of these cases noted a strong association with use of one particular brand of contact lens solution [48]. Most (94%) of the confirmed case patients wore soft contact lenses [48]. It was determined that extrinsic contamination of the lens solution and the lens cases occurred with multiple different strains of *Fusarium,* and that this particular solution was not fungistatic [48]. This outbreak caused substantial morbidity, and many patients had visual loss, requiring corneal transplantation [48].

Fusarium species can cause localized infections of the nails and skin [3, 22]. *Fusarium* is increasingly recognized as a cause of paronychia in profoundly neutropenic patients [11], and *Fusarium* onychomycosis can lead to disseminated fusariosis in immunocompromised patients. [15, 33, 49] *Fusarium* infections commonly involve the extremities, especially the skin of the lower limbs, which is involved in more than 50% of patients [17]. *Fusarium* species are also a well-known cause of eumycetoma [50], and they cause colonization and infection of burn wounds [51], granulomas,

Table 3 Clinical manifestations of fusariosis according to underlying condition

Underlying condition	Clinical manifestations
Acute leukemia or other hematologic malignancy	FUO, sinopulmonary infection, catheter-associated fungemia, disseminated infection, osteoarticular infections
Hematopoietic stem cell transplant	Disseminated infection, pneumonia, sinusitis, meningoencephalitis
Solid organ transplant	Cutaneous infection, lung abscess, liver abscess, peritonitis, disseminated infection
Solid tumors	Onychomycosis, localized soft-tissue infection, disseminated infection (rare)
Severe burns	Burn-wound colonization or wound infection, necrotizing local infection, disseminated infection
Miscellaneous conditions[a]	Onychomycosis, invasive intranasal infection, endophthalmitis, disseminated infection
Immunocompetent host[b]	Osteomyelitis, keratitis, endophthalmitis, chronic invasive rhinosinusitis

FUO fever of unknown origin

[a]Diabetes mellitus, chronic renal failure, myasthenia

[b]Following trauma or surgery

ulcers, and panniculitis. [33] A case of intractable cutaneous fusariosis with erythematous facial plaques and deep dermal infiltrates in the absence of immunosuppression has been described [52].

In profoundly immunocompromised patients, *Fusarium* species cause four patterns of infection: refractory fever of unknown origin, sinopulmonary infection, disseminated infection, and a variety of focal single-organ infections. The usual initial presentation of invasive fusariosis is a persistent fever in a profoundly neutropenic patient [36].

Pulmonary involvement can manifest either nodular or cavitary lesions or both [12]. In a recent study of 20 patients with hematologic malignancies and pulmonary fusariosis, nodules or masses were the most common findings on chest computed tomography (CT) scan, seen in 82% of patients, and mimicked findings with pulmonary aspergillosis. Halo sign, a common finding in pulmonary aspergillosis, was not seen in pulmonary fusariosis. CT scans are more sensitive than chest radiography in the early detection of pulmonary fusariosis in patients with hematologic malignancies [53]. *Fusarium* pneumonia has also been reported after lung transplantation [19]. However, the pathogenic role of *Fusarium* isolate in the respiratory tract of other immunocompromised patients, such as those with HIV infection, is less clear.

Sinopulmonary fusariosis is clinically indistinguishable from the more common invasive aspergillosis. Pneumonia or other focal invasive infection due to *Fusarium* species can disseminate in the setting of continuous, profound immunosuppression. Almost any organ can be involved, including the skin, lung, kidney, spleen, liver, brain, bone marrow, heart, pancreas, eye, nose, palate, sinuses, or gastrointestinal tract [3, 15, 33, 54–57]. Since *Fusarium* species are often resistant to antifungal agents, breakthrough fusariosis occurring during empiric or prophylactic therapy with amphotericin B, fluconazole, itraconazole, ketoconazole, or caspofungin in neutropenic patients is not uncommon [11, 12, 15, 58–61].

Disseminated fusariosis represents the end of the spectrum of the infection caused by *Fusarium* species. Disseminated *Fusarium* infection was first reported almost 30 years ago [62]. Since then, the incidence of disseminated invasive fusariosis has increased significantly [10, 13, 33, 34]. Neutropenic patients with hematologic malignancies (especially acute leukemia), allogeneic HSCT recipients, and patients with extensive burns are at increased risk of disseminated fusariosis [3, 15, 58]. Patients with hematologic malignancies account for 90% of the reported cases of disseminated fusariosis [34]. Infection typically occurs during a prolonged period of neutropenia [12, 15, 54]. Among allogeneic HSCT recipients, a trimodal distribution of fusariosis incidence is observed: there is a first peak before engraftment, a second peak at a median of 2 months after transplantation, and a third peak 1 year after transplantation [21]. The second peak occurs approximately 1 month earlier than the corresponding peak for aspergillosis (median time to diagnosis after transplantation, 64 days for fusariosis vs. 100 days for aspergillosis) [21]. Almost half of all cases of disseminated fusariosis are caused by *F. solani*; the next most common causes are *F. oxysporum* and *F. moniliforme* [12, 15, 33].

The clinical setting and manifestations of severe fusariosis in immunosuppressed patients mimic those in patients with aspergillosis [53]. However, some distinct differences can be seen. For example, blood cultures are positive in 50–70% of patients with disseminated fusariosis but in fewer than 6% of patients with invasive aspergillosis [15]. Whereas skin lesions are the hallmark of disseminated fusariosis, occurring in 60–90% of cases, skin lesions occur in <10% of patients with disseminated aspergillosis [15, 33, 63]. Patients with neutropenia have a higher rate of disseminated skin lesions than do patients without neutropenia [64]. Types of lesions seen in patients with disseminated fusariosis include subcutaneous nodules, palpable and nonpalpable purpura, red or gray macules, red or gray papules, macules or papules with progressive central necrosis with central, flaccid pustules, vesicles, and hemorrhagic bullae [15, 33, 63] (Fig. 1). These skin lesions can involve any site but most often involve the extremities [63, 64]. These lesions, especially the

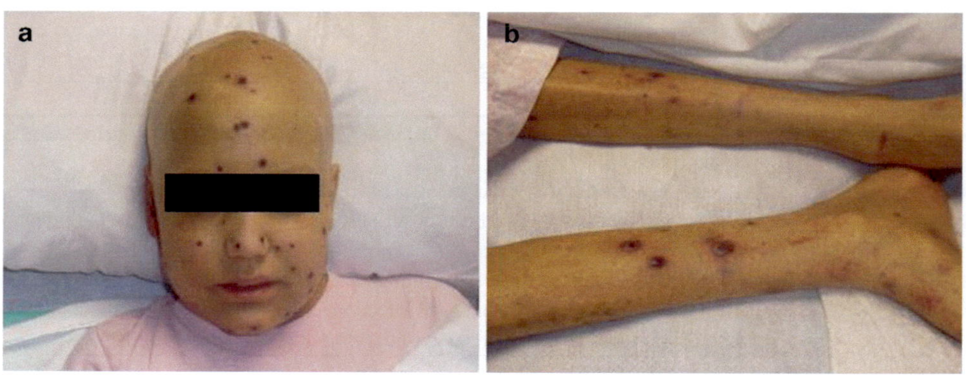

Fig. 1 Characteristic skin lesions of disseminated fusariosis in a hematopoietic stem cell transplant recipient showing (**a**) tender subcutaneous nodules and (**b**) macules and papules simultaneously showing various stages of evolution and progressive central necrosis

subcutaneous nodules, are often tender, and most patients have lesions at various stages of evolution [12, 63]. The number of disseminated skin lesions can range from 4 to more than 30 [63]. Skin lesions are an important potential source of diagnostic tissue [64].

Fusarium infections in immunosuppressed solid organ transplant recipients (kidney, lung, liver, and heart-liver) receiving a prolonged course of corticosteroids tend to remain localized; these patients have a better outcome than do allogeneic HSCT recipients who have graft-versus-host disease and are receiving corticosteroids [65–67].

Other presentations of invasive fusariosis in immunocompromised hosts include osteomyelitis, septic arthritis, myositis, foot abscesses, sinusitis, endocarditis, myocarditis, external otitis, peritonitis, brain abscesses, breast abscess, cystitis, meningoencephalitis, and chronic hepatic infection [10, 11, 15, 33, 56, 68].

Laboratory Diagnosis

The histopathologic picture of fusariosis similar to that caused by other invasive moulds, most importantly *Aspergillus* species [3]. Biopsy of lesions reveals extensive necrosis surrounding the fungal elements, which are characterized as dichotomously branching, acutely angular septate hyphae. This picture is not reliably distinguishable from those of other hyaline moulds, including *Aspergillus* species [11, 15, 66]. Immunohistologic staining of tissues has been used successfully for diagnosing selected cases [3].

Culture is an important tool in the diagnosis of *Fusarium* infection. *Fusarium* colonies begin as a white patch, which quickly develops a pink, purple, or yellow center with a lighter periphery. *Fusarium* species may produce three types of spores: macroconidia, microconidia, and chlamydospores [33]. The morphology of the macroconidia (canoe-shaped) is key for characterizing the genus *Fusarium* (Fig. 2a) [15, 33, 59]. If macroconidia are not present in a culture, identifying *Fusarium* species is difficult, and confusion with other genera, such as *Acremonium*, *Cylindrocarpon*, or *Verticillium*, may occur [11, 15, 59]. In addition to the morphology of the macroconidia, the morphology of the conidiophores bearing the microconidia and the presence of chlamydospores are important features [33] (Fig. 2b).

Key features for differentiating the various *Fusarium* species include color of the colony, length and shape of the macroconidia, and number, shape, and arrangement of microconidia. However, differentiating species is difficult, because of their propensity for rapid morphologic change [10, 33, 57]. Traditional identification based on morphologic methods is cumbersome, laborious, and time-consuming, and must be reserved for trained mycologists [27]. *Fusarium* isolates involved in human infections do not always have morphologic characteristics that allow their identification [27]. As a consequence, in 33–50% of cases of fusariosis, *Fusarium* isolates are misdiagnosed or not detected [28].

A reference laboratory is the best resource for identifying *Fusarium* species. To enhance diagnostic potential, molecular methods such as PCR-based techniques can be used to complement conventional isolation techniques, such as blood cultures. PCR techniques with the use of universal primers, genus-specific probes, or probes based on single-stranded conformational polymorphism may distinguish *Fusarium* from other moulds and identify specific *Fusarium* species in many different types of samples, including blood, bronchoalveolar lavage fluid, skin or nail specimens, ocular samples, urine, and pericardial fluid [18, 27–29, 69–71]. While less sensitive than morphologic methods, in situ hybridization directed against rRNA sequences provides a rapid and accurate method of distinguishing *Fusarium* from organisms such as *Aspergillus* and *Pseudallescheria* that have similar or identical morphologic features on light microscopy. [72] Rapid molecular methods are being developed, and they will probably replace the morphologic methods in the future [27].

Definitive diagnosis of fusariosis relies on the recovery of *Fusarium* species from infected tissues or blood cultures [3, 36] (Fig. 2c). *Fusarium* species are more readily isolated from blood cultures than are *Aspergillus* species [15, 22]. While *Fusarium* species are a well-recognized cause of true fungemia, *Aspergillus* species recovered from blood cultures typically reflect pseudofungemia [73]. One explanation for the frequent presence of *Fusarium* species in the blood is that they can produce many dispersive conidia, which can grow in cultures taken from blood. This phenomenon is a characteristic of yeasts but not of most common pathogenic moulds [15]. *Fusarium* species can also be recovered from urine in the setting of disseminated fusariosis [55].

Susceptibility In vitro

Interpreting minimum inhibitory concentrations (MICs) for moulds has long been problematic [74], and applying in vitro susceptibility to hyalohyphomycetes is no exception. There are no established breakpoints of susceptibility or resistance of moulds to various classes of antifungals. Therefore, moulds, including agents of hyalohyphomycosis, should not be routinely tested for susceptibility [74].

Fusarium species are among the most drug-resistant fungi [66], and among *Fusarium* species, *F. solani* is considered the most resistant [15, 75, 76]. A standardized broth-microdilution MIC method for testing the susceptibility of filamentous fungi, including *Fusarium* species, to antifungals is

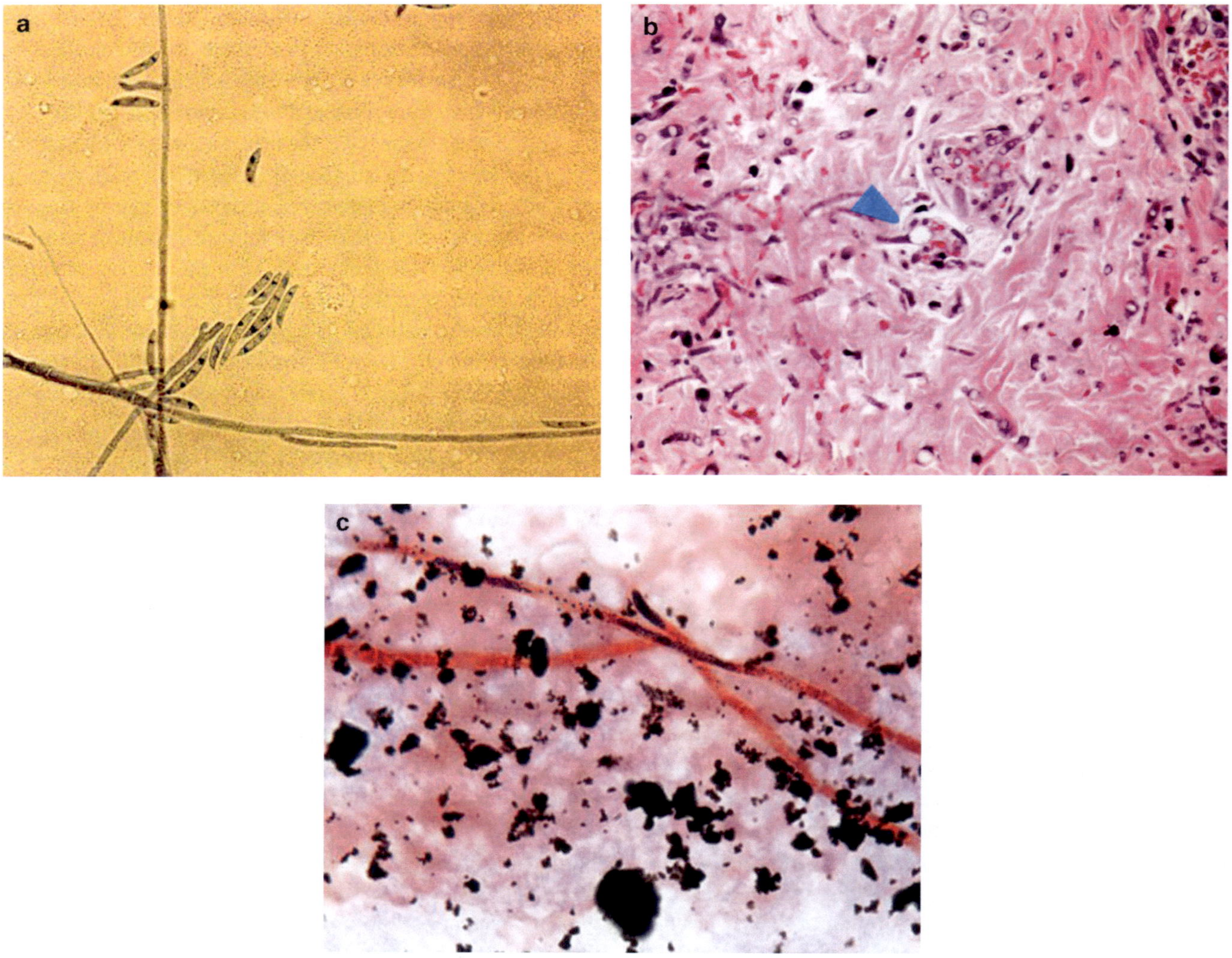

Fig. 2 Microscopic features of *Fusarium* species showing (**a**) characteristic canoe-shaped morphology of macroconidia (Lactophenol cotton blue stain, 400X; (**b**) presence of chlamydospores in subcutaneous tissue (H&E stain, 400X) and (**c**) Gram stain from blood culture bottle showing hyphae (100X) (Courtesy of Dr. A. Wanger, University of Texas, Health Science Center at Houston)

available [77]. However, in vitro susceptibility or resistance to antifungal agents may not predict the clinical outcome of *Fusarium* infection [15, 33].

Fusarium isolates are resistant to the antifungal agents miconazole, ketoconazole, flucytosine, fluconazole, itraconazole, and nikkomycin Z [3, 54, 55, 75, 78–81]. Voriconazole, ravuconazole, and posaconazole show variable activity in vitro and in animal models [79, 82–84]. However, these triazoles have no significant in vitro fungicidal effects on *F. solani* [27, 79, 82].

Other reports have shown that voriconazole, ravuconazole, and posaconazole exhibit species-dependent fungistatic activity against *Fusarium* species, especially the non-*solani Fusarium* species; voriconazole appears to be the most potent of the three drugs [85–87]. However, against *Fusarium* species as a group, voriconazole is not more active than amphotericin B [85]. In a recent study with 13 isolates of *F. solani*, 10 isolates had voriconazole MICs $\geq$4 μg/mL (MIC range 1.0–16.0 μg/mL) [88], and in a series evaluating the in vitro susceptibilities to antifungals of 75 *Fusarium* isolates from Italian patients, the majority of *F. solani* isolates exhibited high azole MICs. In contrast, all *F. verticillioides* isolates were inhibited by posaconazole, 90% were inhibited by voriconazole, and 84% were inhibited by itraconazole. Amphotericin B was active at $\leq$2 μg/mL against 70 of the 75 isolates tested [28]. Other studies show consistent activity of amphotericin B against *Fusarium* species in vitro [27], and in a rabbit model amphotericin B lipid complex and, to a lesser degree, deoxycholate amphotericin B additively augmented the fungicidal activity of pulmonary alveolar macrophages against conidia of *F. solani* [89].

Terbinafine shows some in vitro activity against some isolates of non-*solani Fusarium* species [34, 78]. A study of the in vitro activity of 11 antifungal drugs against 24 isolates of *F. verticillioides* showed that terbinafine was the most active drug [18]. However, terbinafine exhibits a species-dependent fungistatic activity in vitro, and in other studies, showed no activity against most of the *Fusarium* isolates [27]. The in vitro activity of isavuconazole, a promising novel broad-spectrum triazole in late-stage clinical development, was recently compared with that of voriconazole in 20 *Fusarium* isolates. Both drugs showed limited activity [90].

Amphotericin B and natamycin are the most active agents against *Fusarium* species in vitro and in vivo [3, 10, 15, 82]. Liposomal amphotericin B at high doses (10–20 mg/kg/day) significantly reduces tissue burden in the liver and spleen of immunocompetent mice infected with *F. verticillioides* [91].

Fusarium species are resistant to the glucan synthesis inhibitors caspofungin, anidulafungin, micafungin, and the new investigational echinocandin aminocandin [15, 18, 81, 92–95]. One possible explanation is that *Fusarium* species may possess less 1,3-β-D-glucan than 1,6-β-glucan or other non-1,3-β-D-glucans [93]. A recent study found that exposure to a subinhibitory concentration of caspofungin (0.0625 μg/mL) resulted in an increase in β-glucan exposure that was associated with a significant increase in human polymorphonuclear neutrophil-mediated hyphal damage of *F. solani* and *F. oxysporum* [96].

Pentamidine had significant in vitro activity against five *F. solani* isolates and five non-*F. solani* isolates, with non-*F. solani* isolates being more susceptible than *F. solani* isolates [97]. Pentamidine was fungicidal against all non-*F. solani* isolates, whereas it had fungistatic effects against four of the five *F. solani* isolates [97].

In view of the innate resistance of *Fusarium* species to antifungals alone, combinations of antifungals have been studied. The activities of eight antifungal combinations were tested against 38 isolates of *Fusarium* species collected from patients with keratomycosis. Synergism was obtained with amphotericin B plus terbinafine and with amphotericin B plus itraconazole. Antagonism was shown with natamycin plus some azoles and with natamycin plus terbinafine. For terbinafine-based combinations, indifference was the most common interaction [98].

In one study, no interactions were observed for the combination of amphotericin B and voriconazole for most *Fusarium* isolates obtained from deep-seated infections [31]. Terbinafine combined with different azoles showed synergistic activity against 3 isolates of *F. verticillioides* [99], and a combination of terbinafine and voriconazole was synergistic against 15 isolates of *F. solani*. The MIC for terbinafine alone was 256 μg/mL, and for voriconazole alone was from 2 to 16 μg/mL, whereas with the combination, the MICs were 1 μg/mL and 0.25–1 μg/mL, respectively [31]. Finally, a study that evaluated the in vitro interaction of six antifungal drugs in pair combinations against 11 strains of *Fusarium* species showed that the most remarkable combinations were amphotericin B plus itraconazole against *F. solani*, amphotericin B plus ravuconazole against *F. verticillioides*, and amphotericin B plus voriconazole and amphotericin B plus terbinafine against *F. oxysporum* [99].

Despite the lack of activity of caspofungin alone, the in vitro combination of caspofungin and amphotericin B appears to be either synergistic or additive against some *Fusarium* isolates [100] (Kontoyiannis, unpublished data). Additionally, in vitro synergy has been shown between amphotericin B and rifampin [101], and additive interaction has been demonstrated between amphotericin B and azithromycin [102]. However, these combinations have not been shown to be useful in treating human infection.

Treatment

Fusarium infections in immunocompetent hosts are frequently localized infections that might not require systemic therapy [17]. However, in some cases, surgery plus systemic antifungal therapy may be needed to achieve a favorable outcome [71, 103]. In view of the relative rarity of human infections caused by *Fusarium* species, information about human infections has been derived from case reports or uncontrolled case series. Furthermore, analysis of these reports has been confounded by lack of reporting of other factors critical for response, such as the recovery of neutrophil count. Therefore, the optimal management of fusariosis is not well defined [15, 59].

The treatment of disseminated fusariosis in heavily immunosuppressed patients, in particular, has been disappointing; reported mortality and morbidity rates exceed 75% [12, 15]. In one study of HSCT recipients, the median duration of survival after diagnosis of fusariosis was 13 days, and only 13% of patients remained alive 90 days after diagnosis [21]. Among patients with hematologic malignancies and HSCT recipients, the failure rate was 81% in the 32 patients with disseminated or pulmonary fusariosis versus 40% in the 10 patients with localized soft tissue or sinus fusariosis [60]. Relapse after subsequent episodes of neutropenia has also been reported [12]. Some principles of therapy are listed in Table 4.

The most important factors predicting the outcome of *Fusarium* infection are the extent of the infection and the

Table 4 Principles of therapy in fusariosis

Early aggressive treatment with high doses of lipid amphotericin B
Low threshold for switching to voriconazole or posaconazole
Antifungal combination therapy (e.g., lipid amphotericin B + voriconazole) might be considered
Rapid tapering of corticosteroids, if possible
Consideration for G-CSF-primed granulocyte transfusions
Long duration of antifungal therapy, which should be individualized
Removal of catheter for catheter-associated fungemia
Debridement of devitalized tissue with localized disease (onychomycosis, sinusitis, abscess)

recovery of immunosuppression of the host [3, 12, 33]. In a multiple logistic regression analysis of 89 patients with fusariosis, chronic renal failure, hematologic malignancy, burns, and disseminated infections were independently associated with poor outcome [17]. In a more recent series of 44 patients with fusariosis, fungemia was the only independent risk factor for 12-week mortality [39]. Neutrophil recovery and infection limited to skin and soft tissue are significantly associated with improved survival rates in patients with fusariosis. [39] Persistent neutropenia was present in all 19 patients with hematologic malignancies and invasive fusariosis in whom antifungal therapy failed [104]. In a multicenter study in patients with hematologic malignancies, persistent neutropenia and therapy with corticosteroids were the only predictors of poor response in 84 patients [105], and in another multicenter study of HSCT recipients, persistent neutropenia was the only significant predictor of poor outcome [21].

One of the most important clinical aspects of severe *Fusarium* infection is the relative lack of responsiveness of this fungus to either amphotericin B deoxycholate or a lipid formulation of amphotericin B in the setting of profound immunosuppression [10, 15]. Higher doses of amphotericin B deoxycholate (1.0–1.5 mg/kg) or lipid formulations of amphotericin B (at least 5 mg/kg/day) have been administered to transiently stabilize fusariosis [11]. Walsh and coworkers reported that in 11 patients with fusariosis, including some with disseminated disease, there was an 82% response rate (complete or partial) to amphotericin B lipid complex (5 mg/kg/day). However, confounding factors, including neutrophil recovery, immunosuppressive tapering, and adjunctive surgical therapy, were not specifically addressed [106]. Successful treatment of disseminated fusariosis has been reported using higher doses of liposomal amphotericin B (9 mg/kg/day) [107], and with amphotericin B lipid complex at daily doses from 1.8 to 10.0 mg/kg/day. In the latter study, 12 patients (46%) were considered to have been cured or to have improved, and 3 had disease that was considered to be stable. Better outcomes were highly dependent on correction of neutropenia [108].

Voriconazole and posaconazole have shown preclinical activity against *Fusarium* species and provide some hope for management of this severe infection [88, 109]. However, on the basis of recent data showing that the voriconazole susceptibility ranges for *F. solani* are wide, elevated dose levels of voriconazole or even combination therapy should be considered to treat fusariosis [88]. Salvage treatment data suggest that voriconazole therapy may be successful in some patients, including those with unresolved chemotherapy-induced neutropenia [110]. Small series have noted successful outcomes when fusariosis was treated with voriconazole alone or in combination with other antifungals [111, 112]. Individual case reports have documented successful therapy with voriconazole, failure with voriconazole, and breakthrough fusariosis during voriconazole prophylaxis in patients with prolonged immunosuppression [113–117].

The experience at our institution indicates that the response rate to posaconazole in patients with fusariosis refractory to or intolerant of standard therapy approaches 50% [114]. In a multicenter, open-label retrospective trial of 21 patients with proven or probable invasive fusariosis treated with posaconazole as salvage therapy, the overall rate of successful outcome was 48%. The success rate was 67% in leukemia patients who recovered from myelosuppression, but only 20% in leukemia patients with persistent neutropenia and in 17% HSCT recipients [115]. Another report described successful use of posaconazole as salvage therapy for fusariosis in two solid organ transplant recipients [116].

In a recent series of 44 patients with fusariosis, most patients (84%) received combination antifungal therapy (typically a lipid formulation of amphotericin B and a triazole) for a mean duration of 28 days [39]. Despite that, 54% failed treatment at 12 weeks [39], Case reports describing the efficacy of combination antifungal therapy with amphotericin B formulations with voriconazole are increasingly reported [117, 118]. There have been a few reports of good response of fusariosis to caspofungin, either alone or combined with amphotericin B, although resolution of fusariosis in these patients coincided with neutrophil recovery [119, 120]. Several patients have responded to the combination of liposomal amphotericin B and terbinafine, although recovery of neutrophils had also occurred [121, 122].

A history of invasive fusariosis should not be an absolute contraindication to subsequent HSCT, provided that there is an objective response of the infection to antifungal therapy. The most important factors associated with a favorable outcome in HSCT recipients with invasive fusariosis are the resolution of myelosuppression and the absence of severe graft-versus-host disease [12].

The mainstay of treatment for keratitis or corneal ulcers caused by *Fusarium* species remains topical natamycin [123, 124]. However, failures are not uncommon [125]. Successful salvage therapy with amphotericin B lipid complex or with topical and systemic posaconazole have been described [47, 125]. Vitrectomy with intravitreal and intravenous administration of amphotericin B and oral flucytosine has been used to treat *Fusarium* endophthalmitis with variable results [126–128], and experience is increasing with the use of voriconazole for this disease [129]. Most patients who have *Fusarium* keratitis should have keratoplasty with removal of the contaminated lens, in addition to topical treatment with natamycin or other antifungal agents [33].

Some patients with mycetoma due to *Fusarium* species respond to itraconazole [130]. Interestingly, the application of high-concentration nystatin powder (6,000,000 units/g) has been reported to halt the progression of invasive *Fusarium* infection in severely burned pediatric patients [131].

Adjunctive Therapy

A few small uncontrolled series have shown that patients with peritonitis following placement of continuous ambulatory peritoneal dialysis catheters or with central venous catheter–related fungemia have a good outcome when the catheter is removed [10, 33]. Early recognition of *Fusarium* infection, followed by early aggressive therapy and catheter or indwelling venous port removal can prevent dissemination of infection [15]. A child with *F. solani* endocarditis, possibly catheter-associated, remained stable following removal of the catheter and neutrophil recovery. This patient received no surgical intervention, but a combination of liposomal amphotericin B plus voriconazole was administered for 11 months despite the in vitro resistance of the organism to all available antifungal agents [132].

In immunocompetent patients, *Fusarium* onychomycosis should be treated with removal of the infected keratin and topical or systemic antimycotic therapy [33, 133]. Nail avulsion followed by application of ciclopirox ointment and bifonazole ointment or 8% ciclopirox nail lacquer has been reported to be effective [133]. In patients with hematologic malignancies, *Fusarium* onychomycosis should be treated aggressively with nail removal and systemic antifungal therapy.

Surgical resection of necrotic tissue, when possible, is an important component of therapy against fusariosis [33, 71, 134]. Other potentially beneficial adjuvant therapeutic strategies include shortening the duration of neutropenia with recombinant granulocyte colony-stimulating factor (G-CSF) and granulocyte-macrophage colony-stimulating factor (GM-CSF) and performing granulocyte transfusion from G-CSF- and GM-CSF-stimulated donors [11, 12, 15]. The use of G-CSF and GM-CSF has been associated with earlier recovery of neutropenia and improved survival rates in patients with invasive fungal infection, including fusariosis [15, 135]. In profoundly neutropenic patients with fusariosis, granulocyte transfusion results in a favorable response rate of 33–50% [15, 136]. However, confounding factors, such as remission from an underlying malignancy, recovery of neutrophil counts, and differences in extent of disease (localized instead of disseminated fusariosis) might cause the effects of this procedure to be overestimated. The independent contribution of granulocyte transfusions is uncertain at the moment [59].

Other potential adjuvant therapies include interferon-γ and interleukin-15, which enhance hyphal damage by neutrophils against *F. solani* and *F. oxysporum*, suggesting a positive effect of these cytokines on the immune response against fusariosis [44, 137, 138]. A patient with disseminated fusariosis was treated successfully using combination antifungal therapy (voriconazole plus micafungin) plus immune augmentation with donor granulocyte transfusions, recombinant interferon γ-1b, and GM-CSF [139].

Scedosporium apiospermum/Pseudallescheria boydii

The genus *Scedosporium* includes *S. apiospermum/Pseudallescheria boydii* and *S. prolificans*. The taxonomy of this genus is rather complex [140]. At this time, *P. boydii* is considered a species complex with considerable variability. *S. apiospermum* is the anamorph (asexual state) of *P. boydii*, and *S. prolificans* is a totally different species within the genus [140]. To further complicate this taxonomy, molecular studies have indicated that *P. boydii* and *S. apiospermum* are distinct species [141] and have also shown the presence of the newly described species, *S. aurantiacum* [142]. When molecular identification was used, *S. aurantiacum* comprised 45% of the Australian "*S. apiospermum*" isolates, and there was documented genetic variability within *S. aurantiacum* [142]. However, preliminary observations indicate that the epidemiology and clinical relevance of *S. aurantiacum* may be similar to that of *S. apiospermum* [142]. In this section, we therefore discuss the *S. apiospermum/P. boydii* species complex together.

Epidemiology and Pathogenesis

S. apiospermum can be isolated from a wide variety of natural substrates, including water, sewage, soil, swamps, waterlogged pastures, coastal tidelands, and poultry and cattle manure [3, 143]. *S. apiospermum* is distributed worldwide [144, 145]. *S. apiospermum* causes both localized and disseminated infections. The portal of entry is the lung, the paranasal sinuses, or the skin following traumatic inoculation [140, 143, 146]. In animal models, T-lymphocyte-dependent immune processes play no major role in resistance to *S. apiospermum* [147]. In a recent in vitro study, exposure to a subinhibitory concentration of caspofungin resulted in a marked increase in β-glucan exposure that was associated with a significant increase in human polymorphonuclear neutrophil-mediated hyphal damage of *S. apiospermum* [96]. Polymorphonuclear neutrophil–induced damage was further augmented by the addition of anti–β-glucan antibody [96].

Clinical Manifestations

Scedosporiosis comprises a wide spectrum of clinical diseases. *S. apiospermum/P. boydii* is the leading cause of eumycetoma in North America and Western countries [50, 143, 146]. Other presentations of scedosporiosis include corneal ulcers, keratitis, chorioretinitis, endophthalmitis, otitis, sinusitis, pneumonia, endocarditis, meningitis, cerebritis, arthritis, osteomyelitis, and skin, lung, and thyroid abscesses in both immunosuppressed and normal hosts [144, 148–150]. Because it is found in water, *S. apiospermum* can cause pneumonia, brain abscesses, osteomyelitis, and disseminated disease in victims of near-drowning [143, 145, 151] and tsunami survivors [152]. *S. apiospermum/P. boydii* isolated from the upper or lower respiratory tract could represent transient local colonization, bronchopulmonary saprobic involvement, fungus ball formation, or invasive infection [140]. Conditions that alter the innate host defense mechanisms, such as neutropenia, corticosteroid therapy, and chronic granulomatous disease, can lead to invasive fungal infection in a patient whose respiratory tract is colonized [140].

Scedosporium infections may mimic more common infections in immunologically intact hosts; for example, a lymphocutaneous presentation can mimic sporotrichosis [144], and chronic lymphadenitis resembles tuberculous lymphadenitis [153]. Bone and joint infections following puncture wounds of the extremities suffered while gardening have also been associated with scedosporiosis [154]. Likewise, *S. apiospermum* arthritis is most often associated with puncture wounds, lacerations, bicycle injuries, and podiatric surgery [144]. *S. apiospermum* is a rare cause of fungal infection in intravenous drug abusers [155]. In recent years, an association of *S. apiospermum* with cystic fibrosis has been reported, with some patients having asymptomatic colonization, but others developing a picture indistinguishable from that of allergic bronchopulmonary aspergillosis [145].

In profoundly immunosuppressed patients, rapidly progressive severe sinopulmonary, sino-orbital, or disseminated *S. apiospermum* infection has been reported [36, 144, 146]. Maxillary sinuses are the most common site of *S. apiospermum* sinusitis [144, 148]. In immunocompromised hosts, especially in neutropenic patients, hematogenous dissemination as a complication of *S. apiospermum* pneumonia can involve almost any organ [143]. Manifestations include thyroid, brain, or renal abscesses; meningitis; osteomyelitis; endophthalmitis; tenosynovitis; and skin and subcutaneous disease [143, 144, 156, 157]. Among organ transplant recipients, the median time from transplantation to onset of *S. apiospermum* infection was 4 months (range, 0.5–158 months) [158].

Laboratory Diagnosis

Because *S. apiospermum*, like other agents of hyalohyphomycoses, is histologically similar to *Aspergillus* species, scedosporiosis cannot be distinguished from invasive aspergillosis on the basis of histopathology alone [3]. Diagnosis is confirmed if cultures of biopsy specimens demonstrate masses of septate hyphae with terminal oval brown conidia [146]. True fungemia has been reported in the setting of scedosporiosis, especially in patients with disseminated infection [159].

Besides culture methods, serologic procedures, specific counterimmunoelectrophoresis or immunodiffusion antibody assays have been reported to be reliable for both diagnosing and prognostically evaluating the various forms of scedosporiosis [144, 160]. However, these techniques are not specific enough to diagnose *S. apiospermum* infection because of cross-reactions with *Aspergillus* and other pathogens and false-negative results [160, 161].

PCR-based assays appear to be useful in the rapid diagnosis of infections caused by *S. apiospermum*, even before fungal cultures become positive [162]. In situ hybridization directed against rRNA sequences, while less sensitive than morphology, is highly accurate and may help to distinguish *S. apiospermum* from organisms such as *Fusarium* species or *Aspergillus* species in histologic sections [72].

Susceptibility In vitro

Ketoconazole, fluconazole, itraconazole, amphotericin B, and voriconazole, have variable activity against *S. apiospermum.* [85, 160] Amphotericin B and nystatin do not have fungicidal activity against *S. apiospermum.* [82, 163] Itraconazole has been reported to have activity in vitro (MIC 0.25–0.7 μg/mL) [153, 160], as have miconazole [144] and posaconazole [79]. Among the azoles, the most potent in vitro activity is observed with voriconazole (median MIC_{50} of 0.25 μg/mL) [140]. In a recent study of *S. apiospermum* clinical isolates, 11 of 28 (36%) *S. apiospermum* isolates had itraconazole MICs of ≥ 1.0 μg/mL, and 26 of 28 (93%) *S. apiospermum* isolates had amphotericin B MICs of ≥ 2.0 μg/mL, and 90% of isolates were inhibited by 1 μg/mL voriconazole [164]. In other in vitro studies, the voriconazole MICs for *S. apiospermum* ranged from 0.06 to 4.0 μg/mL [88, 111], with voriconazole MICs ≥ 4 μg/mL observed in only 1 of 57 isolates [88]. In an in vitro and in vivo activity report of itraconazole, fluconazole, and posaconazole against 30 clinical isolates of *S. apiospermum*, posaconazole was the most active drug [165]. Echinocandins also showed antifungal activity against *S. apiospermum*, with caspofungin being the most active (median MIC 0.5 μg/mL) and anidulafungin being the second most active (median MIC 1 μg/mL) [140]. Micafungin showed low minimum effective concentration values (≤ 2μg/mL) for 32 of 36 (88.9%) isolates of *S. apiospermum* [95], but the in vivo antifungal efficacy of echinocandins has not been demonstrated [36].

In in vitro studies of combination therapy, combinations of amphotericin B and azole agents exhibited a positive effect against 15–25% of *S. apiospermum* isolates, and synergy between azole agents and echinocandins was detected for a few isolates [166]. A combination of voriconazole with micafungin was synergistic against 33% of *S. apiospermum* isolates [167]; in another report, amphotericin B and micafungin were synergistic for 31.6% of *S. apiospermum* isolates [168]. In an immunosuppressed mouse model, posaconazole was more effective than itraconazole and as effective as fluconazole in preventing death and significantly reducing the fungal load of *P. boydii* from tissues; however, neither drug was able to eradicate the fungus from the tissues [165].

Treatment

Mortality rates have been reported to be as high as 80% for patients with *S. apiospermum* infection [145, 169], and the mortality rate after near-drowning is high (70%), even in immunocompetent hosts [170]. Disseminated infection caused by *S. apiospermum* is associated with a poor prognosis. In a recent series from Italy on acute leukemia patients with disseminated *S. apiospermum* infection, four of five patients died of infection despite administration of amphotericin B or voriconazole [169]. In patients with hematologic malignancies or HSCT recipients, mortality due to *S. apiospermum* infection was associated with dissemination, fungemia, intensive care unit admission, APACHE II score >11, prolonged and persistent neutropenia, and breakthrough *Scedosporium* infection [171]. In a review of transplant recipients with *S. apiospermum* infection, survival rates were greater among those receiving voriconazole, but this difference was not statistically significant [158].

The virulence and antifungal drug resistance of *S. apiospermum* as well as the occurrence of infection during neutropenia contribute to the poor outcome [13, 159]. Because amphotericin B lacks in vitro activity against most *Scedosporium* isolates and results in poor in vivo therapeutic responses, it has been hypothesized that prior use of amphotericin B, by eliminating other more susceptible fungi, predisposes patients to *Scedosporium* infections [160]. *S. apiospermum* is best treated with voriconazole or posaconazole. There is lack of in vitro/in vivo correlation in these complex cases, and most data on therapy is obtained from case reports or small case series. In a small number of patients from a cancer center, 5 of 6 survivors received posaconazole or voriconazole, and only 1 of 12 patients who died received a triazole [171].

In the largest published study to date on scedosporiosis, successful responses to voriconazole therapy were seen in 45 (64%) of 70 *S. apiospermum*–infected patients [164]. In this study, all nine successfully treated central nervous system infections were due to *S. apiospermum*, and one patient was coinfected with *S. prolificans* [164]. Successful treatment of *S. apiospermum* endophthalmitis with systemic plus intravitreal voriconazole combined with vitrectomy has been described [172]. A patient with multiple brain abscesses caused by *S. apiospermum* that progressed despite neurosurgical drainage and treatment with itraconazole, amphotericin B, and ketoconazole was successfully treated with posaconazole [173].

Reversing the underlying cause of immunosuppression with G-CSF or GM-CSF and performing aggressive surgical intervention are essential to survival for patients with invasive scedosporiosis [174]. In addition, adjunctive modalities such as surgery or use of interferon-γ have been reported to be useful in treating *S. apiospermum* infections [174]. *S. apiospermum* keratitis should be treated aggressively. Early detection and treatment likely improve visual outcome. Topical miconazole can be used, as well as other antifungals, such as natamycin and amphotericin B [150].

Scedosporium prolificans

Epidemiology and Pathogenesis

Scedosporium prolificans (formerly *Scedosporium inflatum*) is classified as an imperfect fungus, with a different teleomorph (*Petriella* species) than *S. apiospermum* (*P. boydii*) [140, 143]. The natural habitat of *S. prolificans* is the soil, although it is occasionally detected in the air of hospitals undergoing reconstruction [34]. Interestingly, *S. prolificans* is not distributed worldwide; most cases have been reported in the northern part of the Iberian Peninsula and Australia, and a few cases have been reported in the USA, especially in California and the southern USA [140, 145]. The cause of this limited geographic distribution is unknown [34].

S. prolificans can colonize the external ear or abnormal airways of patients with underlying lung disease, such as bronchiectasis, cystic fibrosis, or lung transplantation [175]. *S. prolificans* is an increasingly recognized human pathogen in both immunocompromised and normal hosts [36, 65, 140, 176]. Inhalation is the most likely the major route of acquisition, [34] but the organism also can enter the bloodstream through an indwelling central catheter [36]. Innate immune defenses play a critical role in host defense against *S. prolificans*. [158, 177] Human interleukin-15 also seems to play an important role in the immunomodulation of host response to *S. prolificans* infection by enhancing hyphal damage by neutrophils [44]. In vitro, interferon-γ and GM-CSF can enhance neutrophil superoxide production, increasing the damage of *S. prolificans* hyphae by neutrophils and enhancing the fungicidal activity of macrophages-monocytes [36, 138]. In murine models of *S. prolificans* infection, combined administration of liposomal amphotericin B and G-CSF has been reported to be effective [178].

Clinical Manifestations

Most reported cases of infection caused by *S. prolificans* have been localized infections complicating soil-contaminated wounds in immunocompetent individuals [34, 36]. *S. prolificans* has also been infrequently reported to cause posttraumatic osteomyelitis, septic arthritis, keratitis, keratouveitis, endocarditis, endophthalmitis, brain abscesses, meningoencephalitis, cerebritis, pneumonia, and peritonitis [143, 144, 179, 180]. This fungus has recently emerged as a cause of severe opportunistic infections, mainly in profoundly neutropenic patients, allogeneic HSCT recipients, and HIV-infected patients [158, 175, 179], in whom rapidly fatal pneumonia and disseminated disease can occur [36]. Among solid organ transplant recipients, the median time from transplantation to onset of *S. prolificans* infection was 2.6 months (range, 1–17 months) [158]. The lungs, brain, and kidneys are the organs most frequently involved in disseminated infections caused by *S. prolificans* [179]. These invasive infections generally mimic those produced by other moulds [34, 181]. For example, cutaneous lesions that mimic fusariosis can develop during fungemia and disseminated *S. prolificans* infection [182]. Because *S. prolificans* is resistant to currently used antifungals, it is a not uncommon cause of breakthrough infection occurring despite prophylactic, empiric, or targeted therapy with amphotericin B. Similar to infections caused by *Fusarium* species, disseminated *S. prolificans* infections are commonly diagnosed antemortem because of its ability to grow in blood cultures [36].

Compared with *S. apiospermum* and *S. aurantiacum, S. prolificans* seems to be more frequently associated with coincident hospital renovation, invasive disease, disseminated infection, fungemia, and isolation from other sterile sites [142]. For example, solid organ transplant recipients with *S. prolificans* infection were more likely to have fungemia (40%) than were those with *S. apiospermum* infection (4.7%) ($P = 0.009$) [158]. In patients with hematologic malignancies, neutropenia seems to be more common in patients with *S. prolificans* infection than in those with *S. apiospermum* infection [171]. Hints that infection may be due to disseminated *S. prolificans* infection include neutropenia, persistent fever, and central nervous system symptoms [180].

Laboratory Diagnosis

Blood cultures are positive for *S. prolificans* in 70–80% of cases, especially in patients with disseminated infection [179, 181]. *S. prolificans* is characterized by its inflated flask-shaped conidiogenous cells [183] and can be easily differentiated from *S. apiospermum* because the latter has cylindrical, free, or intercalary conidiogenous cells [34]. Recent data showed that PCR-based diagnostic methods allow quick and sensitive detection of *S. prolificans;* however, further studies are warranted [162].

Susceptibility In Vitro

S. prolificans is typically resistant to the currently available antifungal agents [184]. To date, there is no effective regimen with activity against *S. prolificans* infection [171]. Fluconazole and amphotericin B are inactive in vitro against this fungus [85], as are echinocandins [92, 185]. Itraconazole and voriconazole have variable activity against *S. prolificans* [34, 85, 87, 186, 187], and other broad-spectrum triazoles, such as ravuconazole and posaconazole, also show activity against this multiresistant fungus [34, 87, 163, 187]. In a recent study of 14 clinical isolates of *S. prolificans*, 13 (93%) had itraconazole MICs ≥ 1 μg/mL, all had amphotericin B MICs ≥ 4 μg/mL, and voriconazole was as active as, or more active than, either itraconazole or amphotericin B [164]. In several reports, the best in vitro activity has been found with voriconazole, with MICs ranging from 2.0 to 8.0 μg/mL; 9 of 11 isolates in one study had MICs ≥ 4 μg/mL [88, 140].

Synergistic in vitro activity has been demonstrated for amphotericin B and pentamidine in 85–100% of *S. prolificans* strains [188]. Other in vitro combination studies have demonstrated synergistic activity of itraconazole and terbinafine against 85–95% of *S. prolificans* isolates [189] and synergism when terbinafine was added to voriconazole [190]. A combination of voriconazole with micafungin was synergistic against 75% of *S. prolificans* isolates, [167] and amphotericin B and micafungin were synergistic for 82.4% of 17 *S. prolificans* isolates and 31.6% of 19 *S. apiospermum* isolates [168]. In another series, the most active combination was ravuconazole plus caspofungin, which was synergistic against 41.7% of 12 *S. prolificans* isolates [166]. In a murine model of systemic infection by *S. prolificans,* micafungin combined with voriconazole or amphotericin B was able to prolong survival and to reduce the fungal load in the kidneys and brain compared with monotherapies [191].

Treatment

Mortality rates have been reported to be as high as 100% for *S. prolificans* infection [171]. Patients with infection due to *S. prolificans* have significantly reduced survival times and were more likely to die from their fungal infection than were those with *S. apiospermum* infection [164]. The prognosis for solid organ transplant recipients with *S. prolificans* infection is similar to that for HSCT recipients with *S. prolificans* infection; in contrast, in *S. apiospermum*-infected patients, outcome is worse in HSCT recipients than in solid organ transplant recipients. [158] More specifically, the mortality rate among solid organ transplant recipients has been reported to be 78% for patients with *S. prolificans* infection and 55% for patients with *S. apiospermum* infection. Among HSCT recipients, the mortality rate was 78% for patients with *S. prolificans* infection and 62% for patients with *S. apiospermum* infection [158]. In a series of 18 solid organ transplant recipients with *S. prolificans* infection, 14 died [158]; fungemia and earlier onset of infection after transplantation statistically correlated with higher mortality rates [158]. Of 13 patients with *S. prolificans* infection treated with amphotericin B, 11 died, and 1 of 3 patients who received voriconazole died [158]. Failures of treatment in children with scedosporiosis occurred primarily in those with *S. prolificans* infection [192].

The voriconazole susceptibility range for *S. prolificans* is wide, which suggests that elevated higher dosages of voriconazole or combination therapy should be considered to treat these severe infections [88]. Recent data from a large multinational study showed successful responses to voriconazole therapy in 16 (44%) of 36 of *S. prolificans*-infected patients, many of whom were treated on a salvage protocol [164]. In this series, patients with *S. prolificans* infection were significantly less likely to achieve a successful clinical response to voriconazole therapy than those with *S. apiospermum* infection [164].

Cases of breakthrough *S. prolificans* infection have been reported in severely immunocompromised patients receiving voriconazole [193] or posaconazole prophylaxis [194].

The combination of voriconazole and terbinafine has been reported to be successful in some but not all immunocompromised patients with *S. prolificans* infection [194–196]. Adjunctive measures, such as aggressive surgical debridement and joint washout, were performed in most successfully treated patients [195, 196]. Combinations of voriconazole and caspofungin [197] or the antiparasitic drug hexadecylphospocholine (miltefosine) with terbinafine and voriconazole [198] have been successful in the treatment of *S. prolificans* osteomyelitis in immunocompetent children; other measures, such as surgical debridement or local irrigation, were undertaken in these patients.

The prognosis of patients with *S. prolificans* infection depends largely on the host's immune status, the extent of infection, and the feasibility of surgical removal [179, 194]. Recovery from neutropenia is considered critical in cases of *S. prolificans* infection [171]. Surgical removal of infected tissue, when possible, and immunorestoration are significantly associated with reduced risk of death from this devastating infection in patients with hematologic malignancies [144, 176, 180].

Acremonium Species

Epidemiology and Pathogenesis

Acremonium species (formerly *Cephalosporium* species) are ubiquitous fungi common in soil, plant debris, and rotting mushrooms [199]. These hyalohyphomycetes are distributed worldwide and found in Europe, Asia, Egypt, and North, Central, and South America [199–201]. *Acremonium* species are primarily pathogens of plants and insects and only rarely cause invasive disease in humans [202]. *Acremonium strictum*, *A. kiliense*, and *A. falciforme* are the most common human pathogens [200, 203]. Results of a recent phylogenetic analysis indicate that *A. falciforme* is a member of the *F. solani* clade [29].

The skin, lungs, and gastrointestinal tract are the apparent portals of entry [11]. Most infections are community acquired, but nosocomial transmission occurs sporadically. For example, an outbreak of *A. kiliense* endophthalmitis occurred in patients who had undergone cataract surgery; the reservoir was determined to be a contaminated humidifier within the heating, ventilation, and air-conditioning system of the ambulatory surgical center [200].

Clinical Manifestations

Following traumatic inoculation, *Acremonium* species cause infections ranging from posttraumatic or postsurgical keratitis to mycetoma in normal hosts [36, 204]. Indolent *Acremonium* skin infection has also been reported in immunocompetent patients [203]. In heavily immunocompromised patients, fungemia and disseminated infection can be seen [36, 65, 202, 205]. *Acremonium* species have also been reported to cause hypersensitivity pneumonitis, sinusitis, arthritis, hemodialysis access-graft infection, peritonitis, endocarditis, pyomyositis, cerebritis, and ocular infections [2, 199, 206–208]. Few cases of disseminated *Acremonium* infection have been encountered, most of them in patients with predisposing conditions, such as neutropenia due to HSCT or primary immunodeficiency, severe immunosuppression due to prolonged corticosteroid therapy, burns, solid organ transplantation, Addison's disease, intravenous drug abuse, and extreme prematurity [201, 209]. Disseminated cutaneous lesions may develop during fungemia and disseminated infection [11]. The failure rate of antifungal therapy is high (50%) [199].

Laboratory Diagnosis

When *Acremonium* species invade tissue, not only do they produce hyphae, like *Fusarium* species, but they also form adventitious structures within the infected tissue. Specifically, *Acremonium* species have been reported to form phialides, phialoconidia, and budding yeast-like cells in tissue [202]. These small conidia-like structures can disseminate widely through the bloodstream, permitting frequent premorten diagnosis based on the recovery of *Acremonium* species from blood cultures of patients with disseminated disease or fungemia [4, 7, 36]. The high frequency of fungemia during *Acremonium* infections is explained by angioinvasion with sustained release of fungal spores into the bloodstream [7]. The presence of adventitious forms has also been reported in infections with *Aspergillus terreus* and *Fusarium*, *Paecilomyces*, *Scedosporium*, and *Blastoschizomyces* species. [73, 202]

Acremonium species usually grow on Sabouraud agar within 5 days at 30°C [200]. When grown in culture, they produce small conidia on slender phialides, resembling the early growth of *Fusarium* species. Further incubation, however, does not reveal the characteristic canoe-shaped macroconidia observed in *Fusarium* species [11, 36].

Susceptibility In vitro

Acremonium species commonly lack susceptibility in vitro to current antifungal agents [36]. Using nonstandardized methods of susceptibility testing, some studies consistently found amphotericin B to be more active than ketoconazole, fluconazole, or itraconazole against *Acremonium* isolates [199, 206]. However, the susceptibility of this genus to amphotericin B, fluconazole, itraconazole, and voriconazole could be species-dependent. In support of this, the MICs of all these agents are much lower against *Acremonium alabamensis* than against *A. strictum* [85]. Promising in vitro data have recently been presented for posaconazole, ravuconazole, and voriconazole [84]. Echinocandins inhibited some of the 10 isolates of *Acremonium* species [95] and showed limited activity against *A. strictum* [210].

Treatment

The cure rate for patients with *Acremonium* infection has been reported to be 80% in pediatric patients and 63% in adults [207]. Optimal treatment of *Acremonium* infections is not well defined because of their rarity [207]. Amphotericin B, ketoconazole, itraconazole, fluconazole, flucytosine, voriconazole, and combinations of these antifungal drugs have been tried with inconsistent results [204].

Some infections due to *Acremonium* species are refractory to conventional dosages of amphotericin B [36]. Patients with infections that are unresponsive to amphotericin B deoxycholate therapy are candidates for treatment with lipid formulations of amphotericin B or triazoles [11, 36]. Amphotericin B lipid complex was successful in two of four immunocompromised patients with *Acremonium* infection [108]. The combination of surgery and azole derivatives has occasionally been successful [199]. Several reports note success with voriconazole when amphotericin B formulations had failed. [204, 211] Micafungin was ineffective against disseminated *Acremonium* infection in a HSCT recipient [210]. Several patients with endophthalmitis have been successfully treated with vitrectomy, repeated intravitreous administration of amphotericin B, and oral fluconazole [200, 212]. The outcome of severe *Acremonium* infection, like the outcome of severe *Fusarium* infections, depends on surgical intervention, when feasible, and the recovery of neutrophil counts [199, 207].

Scopulariopsis Species

Epidemiology and Pathogenesis

The genus *Scopulariopsis* has several species. Nine species have been reported to cause human infections: *Scopulariopsis acremonium*, *S. asperula*, *S. flava*, *S. fusca*, *S. carbonaria*, *S. koningii*, *S. brevicaulis*, *S. brumptii*, and *S. candida* [213, 214]. *S. brevicaulis* is the species most frequently associated with invasive disease [215, 216]. *Scopulariopsis* species are common soil saprobes with a wide geographic distribution [3, 213]. *Scopulariopsis* species are rare causes of localized invasive infections following traumatic or surgical injury and of serious infections in immunocompromised patients [36]. The organisms are identified by culture of involved tissue; *S. brevicaulis* can be isolated in blood cultures [214]. The detection of this mould by molecular testing is a promising diagnostic tool [217].

Clinical Manifestations

A variety of infections caused by *Scopulariopsis* species have been described: onychomycosis, mycetoma, keratitis, endophthalmitis, hypersensitivity pneumonitis, endocarditis, and, occasionally, localized invasive infections following traumatic inoculation [36, 215, 218]. More severe manifestations such as pneumonia, empyema, brain abscesses, head and neck abscesses, disseminated infection, and recurrent multiple subcutaneous or skin lesions have been described in immunocompromised hosts [214, 215, 219].

Susceptibility In vitro

Most antifungals have limited in vitro activity against *Scopulariopsis* species. As is the case for other hyalohyphomycetes, *Scopulariopsis* species appear to have inherent broad-spectrum resistance to different classes of antifungals. The MICs for amphotericin B, itraconazole, and voriconazole against *S. brumptii* have been shown to be>2 µg/mL [85], and flucytosine and itraconazole were inactive in vitro against all 32 clinical isolates of *S. brevicaulis* [220]. In 11 clinical isolates of *S. brevicaulis* obtained in patients with onychomycosis, MICs ranged from 1 to 16 to µg/mL for voriconazole and were >64 µg/mL for fluconazole [221]. In some studies, voriconazole showed activity superior to that of amphotericin B and itraconazole against *S. brevicaulis* [221], but in others, reduced susceptibility to itraconazole, voriconazole, posaconazole, and ravuconazole was observed [222, 223]. Terbinafine has been shown to have fungicidal activity against *S. brevicaulis,* but was not efficacious in treating nail infections [214]. Echinocandins are inactive in vitro against *S. brevicaulis* [95, 214, 216, 224]. Promising results against isolates of *S. brevicaulis* have been obtained with terbinafine combined with fluconazole, itraconazole, posaconazole, or voriconazole and with caspofungin combined with amphotericin B, posaconazole, or voriconazole [221, 222]. Amphotericin B in combination with azole agents did not exhibit synergy for most *S. brevicaulis* isolates [222].

Treatment

Most clinical experience with treatment of *Scopulariopsis* infection has involved treatment of onychomycosis [214]. To date, only a few cases of deep-seated *Scopulariopsis* infection have been reported; they have occurred in immunocompromised patients, and only the minority has responded to antifungal treatment [219, 225]. On the basis of very limited in vitro susceptibility data, therapeutic approaches have been designed to include amphotericin B or new triazoles. In one report, none of three patients with *Scopulariopsis* infection responded to treatment with amphotericin B lipid complex [108]. Combined surgery and long-term therapy with amphotericin B and itraconazole resulted in a favorable outcome in some patients with *Scopulariopsis* infections [226]. A patient with postoperative endophthalmitis caused by *Scopulariopsis* species was successfully treated with intraocular lens extraction, vitrectomy, and intravitreal voriconazole plus systemic voriconazole combined with caspofungin [216]. Success has not been consistently reported for *S. brevicaulis* infections in immunocompromised patients [219]. Combination therapy could be an alternative for treating severe *Scopulariopsis* infections; however, the effect of combinations is not predictable and depends on the strain tested and the adjunctive interventions, such as surgery [222]. Adequate immunoreconstitution appears to be essential to clinical success [214].

Paecilomyces Species

Epidemiology and Pathogenesis

Paecilomyces species are common environmental hyaline moulds that are seldom associated with severe invasive infections in immunocompromised patients [2, 11, 227–229]. These saprophytic fungi are found worldwide in soil and decaying vegetable matter and as airborne contaminants in clinical microbiology laboratories [230].

Most reported infections occurred in immunocompromised patients or those with foreign bodies in place [6, 231]. Acute leukemia, treatment with myeloablative chemotherapy or HSCT, and presence of neutropenia have been associated with *Paecilomyces lilacinus* infections [232]. Of all *Paecilomyces* species, only *P. lilacinus*, *P. variotii*, *P. marquandii*, and *P. javanicus* have been associated with human mycotic infections [233]. The apparent portals of entry for this organism are the respiratory tract, indwelling catheters, and the skin [11, 36, 233]. Outbreaks have occurred and have been associated with intraocular lens implants and contaminated hand lotion [234].

Clinical Manifestations

Most *Paecilomyces* infections are associated with the presence of biomedical devices, such as central venous catheters or peritoneal catheters, surgically implanted lenses, prosthetic cardiac valves, cerebrospinal fluid shunts, and breast implants [6]. Sinusitis, subcutaneous infection, cellulitis, bursitis, endocarditis, peritonitis, pyelonephritis, vaginitis, endophthalmitis, keratitis, and orbital granuloma caused by *Paecilomyces* species have been described in both immunocompetent and immunocompromised patients [2, 230, 233, 234]. Most infections involve the skin or ocular structures [176]. Skin lesions erupt insidiously and vary in appearance. They can appear as discrete erythematous papules or as molluscum contagiosum-like lesions similar to those seen in *Penicillium marneffei* infection [232]. Erythematous macules, vesicles, pustules, and nodular lesions are among the different cutaneous manifestations of *Paecilomyces* infection [228]. The lesions can be similar in appearance to the hemorrhagic necrotizing papulovesicular and ecthyma gangrenosum-like eruptions seen in *Fusarium* infections and in disseminated aspergillosis [232]. In immunocompromised hosts, invasive *Paecilomyces* infections may also manifest as fungemia, soft-tissue infections, pneumonia, or disseminated infection [11].

Laboratory Diagnosis

Similar to *Fusarium* species, *Scedosporium* species, and *Acremonium* species, *Paecilomyces* species can be recovered in blood cultures from patients with disseminated disease [235]. However, even in high-risk cancer patients, the significance of *Paecilomyces* isolation from blood is not always clear, and thus careful clinical assessment is recommended before antifungal treatment is begun [236]. Of note, *Paecilomyces* species in culture may be confused with *Penicillium* species owing to the similarity in the conidial structures of the two genera [229]. Molecular sequence analysis has been used successfully to identity *P. lilacinus* from an invasive infection [229].

Susceptibility In vitro

In vitro studies suggest that *P. variotii* is the most widely susceptible *Paecilomyces* species, whereas *P. lilacinus* and *P. marquandii* tend to be resistant to most antifungals [229]. For example, *P. lilacinus* is highly resistant in vitro to amphotericin B, flucytosine, and fluconazole, while *P. variotii* is usually susceptible to amphotericin B and flucytosine in vitro [235, 237]. *P. lilacinus* typically shows high MIC_{90} values for all antifungal agents tested. Amphotericin B, itraconazole, and ketoconazole show variable activity; fluconazole and flucytosine have poor efficacy; and posaconazole, voriconazole, and ravuconazole have better activity. [36, 80, 84, 85, 88, 184, 228, 232, 238] MICs of 0.25–8 μg/mL have been reported for terbinafine [233]. Echinocandins inhibited some isolates of *P. variotii* but were inactive against isolates of *P. lilacinus* [95, 233]. However, as is the case for mould infections in general, a correlation of susceptibility results for *Paecilomyces* species with clinical outcome has not been established [17, 36, 239]. A combination of terbinafine and voriconazole was the only combination that was synergistic against three strains of *P. lilacinus* [240]. In another study involving three isolates of *P. lilacinus*, although the interaction was generally indifferent, amphotericin B MICs of >16 μg/mL were reduced to 0.12 μg/mL when this drug was combined with voriconazole, ravuconazole, or terbinafine [233].

Treatment

The management of localized *Paecilomyces* infections relies on the surgical resection of infected foci when feasible. The optimal antifungal agent for treating systemic infections has not been defined [36]. Agents reported to be useful against *Paecilomyces* include miconazole, griseofulvin, amphotericin B, ketoconazole, itraconazole, and terbinafine [230, 231, 238]. The in vitro and in vivo multiresistance of *P. lilacinus* to amphotericin B, fluconazole, and itraconazole appears to correlate with poor outcome in HSCT recipients [11]. The results of clinical treatment with amphotericin B vary [109, 235, 237, 239, 241]. Less compromised patients have responded to amphotericin B followed by itraconazole [11].

The role of itraconazole, voriconazole, posaconazole, and ravuconazole in the primary treatment of invasive *Paecilomyces* infections is unclear, especially in the setting of persistent neutropenia or immunosuppression [36, 242]. On the basis of limited clinical experience, voriconazole seems to be the most effective agent for the treatment of *P. lilacinus* infection [233]. However, a case of disseminated *P. variotii* breakthrough infection in a patient on voriconazole prophylaxis has been reported [6]. Posaconazole may be a good alternative based on excellent activity in vitro [233]. Posaconazole salvage therapy resulted in a slow but persistent response in a highly immunosuppressed patient with *P. lilacinus* infection [243].

Triazoles in combination with either amphotericin B or flucytosine may also be effective in treating *Paecilomyces* infections; however, insufficient data are available to confirm this [239]. A nonneutropenic patient with progressive cutaneous infection due to *P. lilacinus* was treated successfully with a combination of caspofungin and itraconazole [228]. A patient with *P. lilacinus* peritonitis complicating peritoneal dialysis responded to combination therapy with voriconazole and terbinafine and another patient with splenic abscesses caused by *P. variotii* was cured by a partial splenectomy and long-term combination therapy with fluconazole and flucytosine [244]. A patient with *P. lilacinus* keratitis that did not respond to topical natamycin and oral itraconazole was successfully treated with topical voriconazole 1% and oral terbinafine in the absence of surgical intervention [245]. Recovery of neutropenia and removal of central venous catheters, if present, are essential to resolve the infection [233].

Less Common Agents of Hyalohyphomycosis

Localized infection, severe invasive infection, and disseminated infection caused by *Trichoderma* species and *Chrysosporium* species have been reported, mainly in the setting of profound immunosuppression [246–251]. Six species of the genus *Trichoderma* have been identified as human pathogens: *Trichoderma longibrachiatum, T. harzianum, T. koningii, T. pseudokoningii, T. viride*, and *T. citrinoviride* [252, 253]. *T. longibrachiatum* is the species most commonly encountered in patients with invasive infections [252].

Less common agents of hyalohyphomycosis, such as *Lecythophora mutabilis* (formerly *Phialophora mutabilis*), *Geotrichum candidum*, *Arthrographis kalrae*, *Colletotrichum gloeosporioides*, *Beauveria bassiana*, *Cephalotheca foveolata*, and *Myriodontium keratinophilum*, have been reported to cause infections in both immunocompetent and immunocompromised patients [2, 254–260].

Clinical Manifestations

Trichoderma infections have been sporadically reported in patients undergoing immunosuppressive therapies, including chemotherapy for solid tumors or hematologic malignancies or immunosuppression after HSCT or solid organ transplantation, and in patients receiving peritoneal dialysis [252]. Sinusitis, pneumonia, fungemia, brain abscess, hepatic abscess, soft tissue, and disseminated infections have been noted in immunocompromised patients [36, 252, 261]. In addition, *Trichoderma* species are frequently responsible for continuous ambulatory peritoneal dialysis-associated peritonitis. [261, 262] Most *Trichoderma* infections are due to *T. longibrachiatum* and, rarely, *T. citrinoviride* [249, 261–265]. *Chrysosporium* species have been reported to cause keratitis, osteomyelitis, and severe invasive infection, including dissemination, in immunosuppressed patients [246–248, 250, 251].

Laboratory Diagnosis

Trichoderma species appear as hyaline moulds indistinguishable from other hyalohyphomycetes in tissue [36]. *T. longibrachiatum* has been identified in blood cultures [252]. However, the clinical significance of *Trichoderma* isolation from blood is unclear, even in cancer patients [236]. DNA sequencing has been used to identify *T. longibrachiatum* [5].

Susceptibility In vitro

Most isolates of *Trichoderma* species show resistance to fluconazole and flucytosine in vitro and are either susceptible or intermediately resistant to amphotericin B, itraconazole, and ketoconazole [80, 249, 261]. In a study with 15 isolates of *T. longibrachiatum* and 1 isolate of *T. harzianum*, all strains showed reduced susceptibility to fluconazole (MICs $\geq$64 μg/mL) and amphotericin B (MICs 2 μg/mL), but lower MICs of 0.5–1 μg/mL were detected for voriconazole [266]. Posaconazole was inactive in vitro against most *Trichoderma* species [184]. Echinocandins were inactive in vitro against 5 isolates of *Trichoderma* species [95].

Treatment

Reported mortality rates for *Trichoderma* infections are as high as 50% [252]. A reasonable first-choice therapy in the rare case of *Trichoderma* infection is amphotericin B, either alone or in combination with itraconazole [108, 261]. However, there is mounting evidence that voriconazole can be used to successfully treat this infection. In a case of *Trichoderma* fungemia, infection resolved with a combination of amphotericin B deoxycholate and voriconazole along with central catheter removal [252]. In another patient, *T. longibrachiatum* pneumonia in a patient with acute leukemia was treated with a combination of voriconazole and caspofungin [5], and a combination of voriconazole and caspofungin was effective against *T. viride* pneumonia in another leukemia patient, in whom immune recovery occurred [267]. Treatment should be individualized according to the type and extent of the infection and the patient's underlying predisposing conditions [249]. The role of surgical resection is uncertain, but can be considered for patients who do not respond to medical therapy [249].

References

1. Ajello L. Hyalohyphomycosis and phaeohyphomycosis: two global disease entities of public health importance. Eur J Epidemiol. 1986;2:243–51.
2. Rippon J. Hyalohyphomycosis, pythiosis, miscellaneous and rare mycoses, and algoses. In: Rippon JW, editor. *Medical Mycology*. 3rd ed. Philadelphia: W. B. Saunders Company; 1988. p. 714–45.
3. Anaissie EJ, Bodey GP, Rinaldi MG. Emerging fungal pathogens. Eur J Clin Microbiol Infect Dis. 1989;8:323–30.
4. Liu K, Howell DN, Perfect JR, Schell WA. Morphologic criteria for the preliminary identification of *Fusarium*, *Paecilomyces*, and *Acremonium* species by histopathology. Am J Clin Pathol. 1998;109:45–54.
5. Alanio A, Brethon B. Feuilhade de Chauvin M, et al. Invasive pulmonary infection due to *Trichoderma longibrachiatum* mimicking invasive Aspergillosis in a neutropenic patient successfully treated with voriconazole combined with caspofungin Clin Infect Dis. 2008;46:e116–8.
6. Chamilos G, Kontoyiannis DP. Voriconazole-resistant disseminated *Paecilomyces variotii* infection in a neutropenic patient with leukaemia on voriconazole prophylaxis. J Infect. 2005;51:e225–8.
7. Mattei D, Mordini N, Lo Nigro C, et al. Successful treatment of *Acremonium* fungemia with voriconazole. Mycoses. 2003; 46:511–4.
8. Schinabeck MK, Ghannoum MA. Human hyalohyphomycoses: a review of human infections due to *Acremonium* spp., *Paecilomyces* spp., *Penicillium* spp., and *Scopulariopsis* spp. J Chemother. 2003;15 Suppl 2:5–15.
9. Young NA, Kwon-Chung KJ, Kubota TT, Jennings AE, Fisher RI. Disseminated infection by *Fusarium moniliforme* during treatment for malignant lymphoma. J Clin Microbiol. 1978;7:589–94.
10. Anaissie E, Kantarjian H, Ro J, et al. The emerging role of *Fusarium* infections in patients with cancer. Medicine (Baltimore). 1988;67:77–83.

11. Walsh TJ, Groll AH. Emerging fungal pathogens: evolving challenges to immunocompromised patients for the twenty-first century. Transpl Infect Dis. 1999;1:247–61.
12. Boutati EI, Anaissie EJ. *Fusarium*, a significant emerging pathogen in patients with hematologic malignancy: ten years' experience at a cancer center and implications for management. Blood. 1997;90:999–1008.
13. Marr KA, Carter RA, Crippa F, Wald A, Corey L. Epidemiology and outcome of mould infections in hematopoietic stem cell transplant recipients. Clin Infect Dis. 2002;34:909–17.
14. Girmenia C, Pagano L, Corvatta L, Mele L, del Favero A, Martino P. The epidemiology of fusariosis in patients with haematological diseases. Gimema Infection Programme. Br J Haematol. 2000;111:272–6.
15. Torres HA, Raad II, Kontoyiannis DP. Infections caused by *Fusarium* species. J Chemother. 2003;15 Suppl 2:28–35.
16. Guarro J, Gene J. Opportunistic fusarial infections in humans. Eur J Clin Microbiol Infect Dis. 1995;14:741–54.
17. Nir-Paz R, Strahilevitz J, Shapiro M, et al. Clinical and epidemiological aspects of infections caused by *Fusarium* species: a collaborative study from Israel. J Clin Microbiol. 2004;42:3456–61.
18. Azor M, Gene J, Cano J, et al. In vitro antifungal susceptibility and molecular characterization of clinical isolates of *Fusarium verticillioides* (*F. moniliforme*) and *Fusarium thapsinum*. Antimicrob Agents Chemother. 2008;52:2228–31.
19. Campos S, Caramori M, Teixeira R, et al. Bacterial and fungal pneumonias after lung transplantation. Transplant Proc. 2008;40:822–4.
20. Trabasso P, Vigorito A, De Souza C, et al. Invasive fungal infection in hematopoietic stem cell transplant recipients at a Brazilian university hospital. In: Abstracts of the 41st Interscience Conference on Antimicrobial Agents and Chemotherapy 2001 Chicago, IL; 2001.
21. Nucci M, Marr KA, Queiroz-Telles F, et al. *Fusarium* infection in hematopoietic stem cell transplant recipients. Clin Infect Dis. 2004;38:1237–42.
22. Fridkin SK, Jarvis WR. Epidemiology of nosocomial fungal infections. Clin Microbiol Rev. 1996;9:499–511.
23. Squier C, Yu VL, Stout JE. Waterborne nosocomial infections. Curr Infect Dis Rep. 2000;2:490–6.
24. Anaissie EJ, Kuchar RT, Rex JH, et al. Fusariosis associated with pathogenic fusarium species colonization of a hospital water system: a new paradigm for the epidemiology of opportunistic mold infections. Clin Infect Dis. 2001;33:1871–8.
25. Kivivuori SM, Hovi L, Vettenranta K, Saarinen-Pihkala UM. Invasive fusariosis in two transplanted children. Eur J Pediatr. 2004;163:692–3.
26. Raad I, Tarrand J, Hanna H, et al. Epidemiology, molecular mycology, and environmental sources of *Fusarium* infection in patients with cancer. Infect Control Hosp Epidemiol. 2002;23:532–7.
27. Alastruey-Izquierdo A, Cuenca-Estrella M, Monzon A, Mellado E, Rodriguez-Tudela JL. Antifungal susceptibility profile of clinical *Fusarium* spp. isolates identified by molecular methods. J Antimicrob Chemother. 2008;61:805–9.
28. Tortorano AM, Prigitano A, Dho G, et al. Species distribution and in vitro antifungal susceptibility patterns of 75 clinical isolates of *Fusarium* spp. from northern Italy. Antimicrob Agents Chemother. 2008;52:2683–5.
29. Summerbell RC, Schroers HJ. Analysis of phylogenetic relationship of *Cylindrocarpon lichenicola* and *Acremonium falciforme* to the *Fusarium solani* species complex and a review of similarities in the spectrum of opportunistic infections caused by these fungi. J Clin Microbiol. 2002;40:2866–75.
30. Guarro J, Rubio C, Gene J, et al. Case of keratitis caused by an uncommon *Fusarium* species. J Clin Microbiol. 2003;41:5823–6.
31. Cordoba S, Rodero L, Vivot W, Abrantes R, Davel G, Vitale RG. In vitro interactions of antifungal agents against clinical isolates of *Fusarium* spp. Int J Antimicrob Agents. 2008;31:171–4.
32. Mayayo E, Pujol I, Guarro J. Experimental pathogenicity of four opportunist *Fusarium* species in a murine model. J Med Microbiol. 1999;48:363–6.
33. Nelson PE, Dignani MC, Anaissie EJ. Taxonomy, biology, and clinical aspects of *Fusarium* species. Clin Microbiol Rev. 1994;7:479–504.
34. Ponton J, Ruchel R, Clemons KV, et al. Emerging pathogens. Med Mycol. 2000;38 Suppl 1:225–36.
35. Etzel RA. Mycotoxins. JAMA. 2002;287:425–7.
36. Groll AH, Walsh TJ. Uncommon opportunistic fungi: new nosocomial threats. Clin Microbiol Infect. 2001;7 Suppl 2:8–24.
37. Gong YY, Torres-Sanchez L, Lopez-Carrillo L, et al. Association between tortilla consumption and human urinary fumonisin B1 levels in a Mexican population. Cancer Epidemiol Biomark Prev. 2008;17:688–94.
38. Pitt JI. Toxigenic fungi: which are important? Med Mycol. 2000;38 Suppl 1:17–22.
39. Campo M, Lewis R, Kontoyiannis DP. Invasive fusariosis in patients with hematologic malignancy at MD Anderson Cancer Center: The last decade. In: Abstracts of the 47th Annual Meeting of the Infectious Diseases Society of America 2009; Philadelphia, Pennsylvania; 2009.
40. Girmenia C, Iori AP, Boecklin F, et al. *Fusarium* infections in patients with severe aplastic anemia: Review and implications for management. Haematologica. 1999;84:114–8.
41. Torres HA, Bodey GP, Rolston KV, Kantarjian HM, Raad II, Kontoyiannis DP. Infections in patients with aplastic anemia: experience at a tertiary care cancer center. Cancer. 2003;98:86–93.
42. Sagnelli C, Fumagalli L, Prigitano A, Baccari P, Magnani P, Lazzarin A. Successful voriconazole therapy of disseminated *Fusarium verticillioides* infection in an immunocompromised patient receiving chemotherapy. J Antimicrob Chemother. 2006;57:796–8.
43. Mansoory D, Roozbahany NA, Mazinany H, Samimagam A. Chronic *Fusarium* infection in an adult patient with undiagnosed chronic granulomatous disease. Clin Infect Dis. 2003;37:e107–8.
44. Winn RM, Gil-Lamaignere C, Roilides E, et al. Effects of interleukin-15 on antifungal responses of human polymorphonuclear leukocytes against *Fusarium* spp. and *Scedosporium* spp. Cytokine. 2005;31:1–8.
45. Lamaris GA, Chamilos G, Lewis RE, Kontoyiannis DP. Virulence studies of *Scedosporium* and *Fusarium* species in *Drosophila melanogaster*. J Infect Dis. 2007;196:1860–4.
46. Lionakis MS, Lewis RE, May GS, et al. Toll-deficient Drosophila flies as a fast, high-throughput model for the study of antifungal drug efficacy against invasive aspergillosis and Aspergillus virulence. J Infect Dis. 2005;191:1188–95.
47. Goldblum D, Frueh BE, Zimmerli S, Bohnke M. Treatment of postkeratitis *Fusarium* endophthalmitis with amphotericin B lipid complex. Cornea. 2000;19:853–6.
48. Chang DC, Grant GB, O'Donnell K, et al. Multistate outbreak of *Fusarium* keratitis associated with use of a contact lens solution. JAMA. 2006;296:953–63.
49. Girmenia C, Arcese W, Micozzi A, Martino P, Bianco P, Morace G. Onychomycosis as a possible origin of disseminated *Fusarium solani* infection in a patient with severe aplastic anemia. Clin Infect Dis. 1992;14:1167.
50. Kontoyiannis D. Mycetoma. In: Goldman L BJ, eds., ed. *Cecil Textbook of Medicine*. Philadelphia: W. B. Saunders; 2004:2067–8.
51. Wheeler MS, McGinnis MR, Schell WA, Walker DH. *Fusarium* infection in burned patients. Am J Clin Pathol. 1981;75:304–11.
52. Assaf C, Goerdt S, Seibold M, Orfanos C. Clinical picture. Cutaneous hyalohyphomycosis. Lancet. 2000;356:1185.
53. Marom EM, Holmes AM, Bruzzi JF, Truong MT, O'Sullivan PJ, Kontoyiannis DP. Imaging of pulmonary fusariosis in patients with hematologic malignancies. AJR Am J Roentgenol. 2008;190:1605–9.

54. Merz WG, Karp JE, Hoagland M, Jett-Goheen M, Junkins JM, Hood AF. Diagnosis and successful treatment of fusariosis in the compromised host. J Infect Dis. 1988;158:1046–55.
55. Richardson SE, Bannatyne RM, Summerbell RC, Milliken J, Gold R, Weitzman SS. Disseminated fusarial infection in the immunocompromised host. Rev Infect Dis. 1988;10:1171–81.
56. Minor Jr RL, Pfaller MA, Gingrich RD, Burns LJ. Disseminated *Fusarium* infections in patients following bone marrow transplantation. Bone Marrow Transplant. 1989;4:653–8.
57. el-Ani AS. Disseminated infection caused by *Fusarium solani* in a patient with aplastic anemia. NY State J Med. 1990;90:609–10.
58. Fang CT, Chang SC, Tang IL, et al. *Fusarium solani* fungemia in a bone marrow transplant recipient. J Formos Med Assoc. 1997; 96:129–33.
59. Segal BH, Walsh TJ, Liu JM, Wilson JD, Kwon-Chung KJ. Invasive infection with *Fusarium chlamydosporum* in a patient with aplastic anemia. J Clin Microbiol. 1998;36:1772–6.
60. Mattiuzzi GN, Kantarjian H, O'Brien S, et al. Intravenous itraconazole for prophylaxis of systemic fungal infections in patients with acute myelogenous leukemia and high-risk myelodysplastic syndrome undergoing induction chemotherapy. Cancer. 2004;100: 568–73.
61. Mattiuzzi GN, Alvarado G, Giles FJ, et al. Open-label, randomized comparison of itraconazole versus caspofungin for prophylaxis in patients with hematologic malignancies. Antimicrob Agents Chemother. 2006;50:143–7.
62. Cho CT, Vats TS, Lowman JT, Brandsberg JW, Tosh FE. *Fusarium* solani infection during treatment for acute leukemia. J Pediatr. 1973;83:1028–31.
63. Bodey GP, Boktour M, Mays S, et al. Skin lesions associated with *Fusarium* infection. J Am Acad Dermatol. 2002;47:659–66.
64. Nucci M, Anaissie E. Cutaneous infection by *Fusarium* species in healthy and immunocompromised hosts: implications for diagnosis and management. Clin Infect Dis. 2002;35:909–20.
65. Patel R, Paya CV. Infections in solid-organ transplant recipients. Clin Microbiol Rev. 1997;10:86–124.
66. Sampathkumar P, Paya CV. *Fusarium* infection after solid-organ transplantation. Clin Infect Dis. 2001;32:1237–40.
67. Lodato F, Tame MR, Montagnani M, et al. Systemic fungemia and hepatic localizations of *Fusarium solani* in a liver transplanted patient: an emerging fungal agent. Liver Transplant. 2006;12:1711–4.
68. Anandi V, Vishwanathan P, Sasikala S, Rangarajan M, Subramaniyan CS, Chidambaram N. *Fusarium solani* breast abscess. Indian J Med Microbiol. 2005;23:198–9.
69. Walsh TJ, Francesconi A, Kasai M, Chanock SJ. PCR and single-strand conformational polymorphism for recognition of medically important opportunistic fungi. J Clin Microbiol. 1995; 33:3216–20.
70. Hennequin C, Abachin E, Symoens F, et al. Identification of *Fusarium* species involved in human infections by 28S rRNA gene sequencing. J Clin Microbiol. 1999;37:3586–9.
71. Macedo DP, Neves RP, Fontan J, Souza-Motta CM, Lima D. A case of invasive rhinosinusitis by *Fusarium verticillioides* (Saccardo) Nirenberg in an apparently immunocompetent patient. Med Mycol. 2008;46:499–503.
72. Hayden RT, Isotalo PA, Parrett T, et al. In situ hybridization for the differentiation of *Aspergillus*, *Fusarium*, and *Pseudallescheria* species in tissue section. Diagn Mol Pathol. 2003;12:21–6.
73. Kontoyiannis DP, Sumoza D, Tarrand J, Bodey GP, Storey R, Raad II. Significance of aspergillemia in patients with cancer: a 10-year study. Clin Infect Dis. 2000;31:188–9.
74. Rex JH, Pfaller MA, Walsh TJ, et al. Antifungal susceptibility testing: practical aspects and current challenges. Clin Microbiol Rev. 2001;14:643–58.
75. Capilla J, Ortoneda M, Pastor FJ, Guarro J. In vitro antifungal activities of the new triazole UR-9825 against clinically important filamentous fungi. Antimicrob Agents Chemother. 2001;45:2635–7.
76. Kontoyiannis DP, Lewis RE. Antifungal drug resistance of pathogenic fungi. Lancet. 2002;359:1135–44.
77. Clinical and Laboratory Standards Institute. Reference Method for Broth Dilution Antifungal Susceptibility Testing of Filamentous Fungi: Approved Standard, 2nd ed. M38-A2. In: Clinical and Laboratory Standards Institute Wayne, PA, USA; 2008.
78. Speeleveld E, Gordts B, Van Landuyt HW, De Vroey C, Raes-Wuytack C. Susceptibility of clinical isolates of *Fusarium* to antifungal drugs. Mycoses. 1996;39:37–40.
79. Marco F, Pfaller MA, Messer SA, Jones RN. In vitro activity of a new triazole antifungal agent, Sch 56592, against clinical isolates of filamentous fungi. Mycopathologia. 1998;141:73–7.
80. Li RK, Rinaldi MG. In vitro antifungal activity of nikkomycin Z in combination with fluconazole or itraconazole. Antimicrob Agents Chemother. 1999;43:1401–5.
81. Arikan S, Lozano-Chiu M, Paetznick V, Rex JH. In vitro susceptibility testing methods for caspofungin against *Aspergillus* and *Fusarium* isolates. Antimicrob Agents Chemother. 2001;45:327–30.
82. Johnson EM, Szekely A, Warnock DW. In-vitro activity of voriconazole, itraconazole and amphotericin B against filamentous fungi. J Antimicrob Chemother. 1998;42:741–5.
83. Arikan S, Lozano-Chiu M, Paetznick V, Nangia S, Rex JH. Microdilution susceptibility testing of amphotericin B, itraconazole, and voriconazole against clinical isolates of *Aspergillus* and *Fusarium* species. J Clin Microbiol. 1999;37:3946–51.
84. Pfaller MA, Messer SA, Hollis RJ, Jones RN. Antifungal activities of posaconazole, ravuconazole, and voriconazole compared to those of itraconazole and amphotericin B against 239 clinical isolates of *Aspergillus* spp. and other filamentous fungi: report from SENTRY Antimicrobial Surveillance Program, 2000. Antimicrob Agents Chemother. 2002;46:1032–7.
85. Espinel-Ingroff A, Boyle K, Sheehan DJ. In vitro antifungal activities of voriconazole and reference agents as determined by NCCLS methods: review of the literature. Mycopathologia. 2001;150:101–15.
86. Paphitou NI, Ostrosky-Zeichner L, Paetznick VL, Rodriguez JR, Chen E, Rex JH. In vitro activities of investigational triazoles against *Fusarium* species: effects of inoculum size and incubation time on broth microdilution susceptibility test results. Antimicrob Agents Chemother. 2002;46:3298–300.
87. Minassian B, Huczko E, Washo T, Bonner D, Fung-Tomc J. In vitro activity of ravuconazole against Zygomycetes, *Scedosporium* and *Fusarium* isolates. Clin Microbiol Infect. 2003;9:1250–2.
88. Espinel-Ingroff A, Johnson E, Hockey H, Troke P. Activities of voriconazole, itraconazole and amphotericin B in vitro against 590 moulds from 323 patients in the voriconazole Phase III clinical studies. J Antimicrob Chemother. 2008;61:616–20.
89. Roilides E, Lyman CA, Armstrong D, Stergiopoulou T, Petraitiene R, Walsh TJ. Deoxycholate amphotericin B and amphotericin B lipid complex exert additive antifungal activity in combination with pulmonary alveolar macrophages against *Fusarium solani*. Mycoses. 2006;49:109–13.
90. Guinea J, Pelaez T, Recio S, Torres-Narbona M, Bouza E. In vitro antifungal activities of isavuconazole (BAL4815), voriconazole, and fluconazole against 1, 007 isolates of zygomycete, *Candida*, *Aspergillus*, *Fusarium*, and *Scedosporium* species. Antimicrob Agents Chemother. 2008;52:1396–400.
91. Ortoneda M, Capilla J, Pastor FJ, Pujol I, Guarro J. Efficacy of liposomal amphotericin B in treatment of systemic murine fusariosis. Antimicrob Agents Chemother. 2002;46:2273–5.
92. Espinel-Ingroff A. Comparison of In vitro activities of the new triazole SCH56592 and the echinocandins MK-0991 (L-743, 872) and LY303366 against opportunistic filamentous and dimorphic fungi and yeasts. J Clin Microbiol. 1998;36:2950–6.
93. Tawara S, Ikeda F, Maki K, et al. In vitro activities of a new lipopeptide antifungal agent, FK463, against a variety of clinically important fungi. Antimicrob Agents Chemother. 2000; 44:57–62.

94. Isham N, Ghannoum MA. Determination of MICs of aminocandin for *Candida* spp. and filamentous fungi. J Clin Microbiol. 2006;44:4342–4.
95. Cuenca-Estrella M, Gomez-Lopez A, Mellado E, Monzon A, Buitrago MJ, Rodriguez-Tudela JL. Activity profile in vitro of micafungin against Spanish clinical isolates of common and emerging species of yeasts and molds. Antimicrob Agents Chemother. 2009;53:2192–5.
96. Lamaris GA, Lewis RE, Chamilos G, et al. Caspofungin-mediated beta-glucan unmasking and enhancement of human polymorphonuclear neutrophil activity against *Aspergillus* and non-*Aspergillus* hyphae. J Infect Dis. 2008;198:186–92.
97. Lionakis MS, Lewis RE, Samonis G, Kontoyiannis DP. Pentamidine is active in vitro against *Fusarium* species. Antimicrob Agents Chemother. 2003;47:3252–9.
98. Li L, Wang Z, Li R, Luo S, Sun X. In vitro evaluation of combination antifungal activity against *Fusarium* species isolated from ocular tissues of keratomycosis patients. Am J Ophthalmol. 2008;146:724–8.
99. Ortoneda M, Capilla J, Javier Pastor F, Pujol I, Guarro J. In vitro interactions of licensed and novel antifungal drugs against *Fusarium* spp. Diagn Microbiol Infect Dis. 2004;48:69–71.
100. Arikan S, Lozano-Chiu M, Paetznick V, Rex JH. In vitro synergy of caspofungin and amphotericin B against *Aspergillus* and *Fusarium* spp. Antimicrob Agents Chemother. 2002;46:245–7.
101. Stern GA. In vitro antibiotic synergism against ocular fungal isolates. Am J Ophthalmol. 1978;86:359–67.
102. Clancy CJ, Nguyen MH. The combination of amphotericin B and azithromycin as a potential new therapeutic approach to fusariosis. J Antimicrob Chemother. 1998;41:127–30.
103. Gorman SR, Magiorakos AP, Zimmerman SK, Craven DE. *Fusarium oxysporum* pneumonia in an immunocompetent host. South Med J. 2006;99:613–6.
104. Kontoyiannis DP, Bodey GP, Hanna H, et al. Outcome determinants of fusariosis in a tertiary care cancer center: the impact of neutrophil recovery. Leuk Lymphoma. 2004;45:139–41.
105. Nucci M, Anaissie EJ, Queiroz-Telles F, et al. Outcome predictors of 84 patients with hematologic malignancies and *Fusarium* infection. Cancer. 2003;98:315–9.
106. Walsh TJ, Hiemenz JW, Seibel NL, et al. Amphotericin B lipid complex for invasive fungal infections: analysis of safety and efficacy in 556 cases. Clin Infect Dis. 1998;26:1383–96.
107. Cudillo L, Tendas A, Picardi A, et al. Successful treatment of disseminated fusariosis with high dose liposomal amphotericin-B in a patient with acute lymphoblastic leukemia. Ann Hematol. 2006;85:136–8.
108. Perfect JR. Treatment of non-*Aspergillus* moulds in immunocompromised patients, with amphotericin B lipid complex. Clin Infect Dis. 2005;40 Suppl 6:S401–8.
109. Torres HA, Hachem RY, Chemaly RF, Kontoyiannis DP, Raad II. Posaconazole: a broad-spectrum triazole antifungal. Lancet Infect Dis. 2005;5:775–85.
110. Consigny S, Dhedin N, Datry A, Choquet S, Leblond V, Chosidow O. Successsful voriconazole treatment of disseminated *Fusarium* infection in an immunocompromised patient. Clin Infect Dis. 2003;37:311–3.
111. Perfect JR, Marr KA, Walsh TJ, et al. Voriconazole treatment for less-common, emerging, or refractory fungal infections. Clin Infect Dis. 2003;36:1122–31.
112. Baden LR, Katz JT, Fishman JA, et al. Salvage therapy with voriconazole for invasive fungal infections in patients failing or intolerant to standard antifungal therapy. Transplantation. 2003;76:1632–7.
113. Cudillo L, Girmenia C, Santilli S, et al. Breakthrough fusariosis in a patient with acute lymphoblastic leukemia receiving voriconazole prophylaxis. Clin Infect Dis. 2005;40:1212–3.
114. Hachem R, Raad I, Afif C, al e. An open, non-comparative multicenter study to evaluate efficacy and safety of posaconazole (SCH 56592) in the treatment of invasive fungal infections refractory to or intolerant of standard therapy. In: Abstracts of the 40th Interscience Conference on Antimicrobial Agents and Chemotherapy; Toronto; 2000.
115. Raad II, Hachem RY, Herbrecht R, et al. Posaconazole as salvage treatment for invasive fusariosis in patients with underlying hematologic malignancy and other conditions. Clin Infect Dis. 2006;42:1398–403.
116. Alexander BD, Perfect JR, Daly JS, et al. Posaconazole as salvage therapy in patients with invasive fungal infections after solid organ transplant. Transplantation. 2008;86:791–6.
117. Ho DY, Lee JD, Rosso F, Montoya JG. Treating disseminated fusariosis: amphotericin B, voriconazole or both? Mycoses. 2007;50:227–31.
118. Durand-Joly I, Alfandari S, Benchikh Z, et al. Successful outcome of disseminated *Fusarium* infection with skin localization treated with voriconazole and amphotericin B-lipid complex in a patient with acute leukemia. J Clin Microbiol. 2003;41:4898–900.
119. Apostolidis J, Bouzani M, Platsouka E, et al. Resolution of fungemia due to *Fusarium* species in a patient with acute leukemia treated with caspofungin. Clin Infect Dis. 2003;36:1349–50.
120. Makowsky MJ, Warkentin DI, Savoie ML. Caspofungin and amphotericin B for disseminated *Fusarium verticillioides* in leukemia. Ann Pharmacother. 2005;39:1365–6.
121. Neuburger S, Massenkeil G, Seibold M, et al. Successful salvage treatment of disseminated cutaneous fusariosis with liposomal amphotericin B and terbinafine after allogeneic stem cell transplantation. Transpl Infect Dis. 2008;10:290–3.
122. Rothe A, Seibold M, Hoppe T, et al. Combination therapy of disseminated *Fusarium oxysporum* infection with terbinafine and amphotericin B. Ann Hematol. 2004;83:394–7.
123. Reuben A, Anaissie E, Nelson PE, et al. Antifungal susceptibility of 44 clinical isolates of *Fusarium* species determined by using a broth microdilution method. Antimicrob Agents Chemother. 1989;33:1647–9.
124. Hirose H, Terasaki H, Awaya S, Yasuma T. Treatment of fungal corneal ulcers with amphotericin B ointment. Am J Ophthalmol. 1997;124:836–8.
125. Sponsel WE, Graybill JR, Nevarez HL, Dang D. Ocular and systemic posaconazole(SCH-56592) treatment of invasive *Fusarium solani* keratitis and endophthalmitis. Br J Ophthalmol. 2002;86:829–30.
126. Rowsey JJ, Acers TE, Smith DL, Mohr JA, Newsom DL, Rodriguez J. *Fusarium oxysporum* endophthalmitis. Arch Ophthalmol. 1979;97:103–5.
127. Gabriele P, Hutchins RK. *Fusarium* endophthalmitis in an intravenous drug abuser. Am J Ophthalmol. 1996;122:119–21.
128. Glasgow BJ, Engstrom Jr RE, Holland GN, Kreiger AE, Wool MG. Bilateral endogenous *Fusarium* endophthalmitis associated with acquired immunodeficiency syndrome. Arch Ophthalmol. 1996;114:873–7.
129. Durand ML, Kim IK, D'Amico DJ, et al. Successful treatment of *Fusarium* endophthalmitis with voriconazole and *Aspergillus* endophthalmitis with voriconazole plus caspofungin. Am J Ophthalmol. 2005;140:552–4.
130. Restrepo A. Treatment of tropical mycoses. J Am Acad Dermatol. 1994;31:S91–102.
131. Barret JP, Ramzy PI, Heggers JP, Villareal C, Herndon DN, Desai MH. Topical nystatin powder in severe burns: a new treatment for angioinvasive fungal infections refractory to other topical and systemic agents. Burns. 1999;25:505–8.
132. Guzman-Cottrill JA, Zheng X, Chadwick EG. *Fusarium solani* endocarditis successfully treated with liposomal amphotericin B and voriconazole. Pediatr Infect Dis J. 2004;23:1059–61.
133. Gupta AK, Baran R, Summerbell RC. *Fusarium* infections of the skin. Curr Opin Infect Dis. 2000;13:121–8.
134. Dornbusch HJ, Buzina W, Summerbell RC, et al. *Fusarium verticillioides* abscess of the nasal septum in an immunosuppressed child: case report and identification of the morphologically atypical fungal strain. J Clin Microbiol. 2005;43:1998–2001.

135. Farmaki E, Roilides E. Immunotherapy in patients with systemic mycoses: a promising adjunct. BioDrugs. 2001;15:207–14.
136. Rodriguez-Adrian LJ, Grazziutti ML, Rex JH, Anaissie EJ. The potential role of cytokine therapy for fungal infections in patients with cancer: is recovery from neutropenia all that is needed? Clin Infect Dis. 1998;26:1270–8.
137. Winn R, Maloukou A, Gil-Lamaignere C, et al. The Eurofung Network. Interferon-gamma and granulocyte-macrophage colony stimulating factor enhance hyphal damage of *Aspergillus* and *Fusarium* spp by human neutrophils.. In: Abstracts of the 41st Interscience Conference on Antimicrobial Agents and Chemotherapy; Chicago; 2001.
138. Gil-Lamaignere C, Winn RM, Simitsopoulou M, Maloukou A, Walsh TJ, Roilides E. Inteferon gamma and granulocyte-macrophage colony-stimulating factor augment the antifungal activity of human polymorphonuclear leukocytes against *Scedosporium* spp.: comparison with *Aspergillus* spp. Med Mycol. 2005; 43:253–60.
139. Lewis R, Hogan H, Howell A, Safdar A. Progressive fusariosis: unpredictable posaconazole bioavailability, and feasibility of recombinant interferon-gamma plus granulocyte macrophage-colony stimulating factor for refractory disseminated infection. Leuk Lymphoma. 2008;49:163–5.
140. Cortez KJ, Roilides E, Quiroz-Telles F, et al. Infections caused by *Scedosporium* spp. Clin Microbiol Rev. 2008;21:157–97.
141. Gilgado F, Cano J, Gene J, Sutton DA, Guarro J. Molecular and phenotypic data supporting distinct species statuses for *Scedosporium apiospermum* and *Pseudallescheria boydii* and the proposed new species *Scedosporium dehoogii*. J Clin Microbiol. 2008;46:766–71.
142. Delhaes L, Harun A, Chen SC, et al. Molecular typing of Australian *Scedosporium* isolates showing genetic variability and numerous *S. aurantiacum*. Emerg Infect Dis. 2008;14:282–90.
143. Tadros TS, Workowski KA, Siegel RJ, Hunter S, Schwartz DA. Pathology of hyalohyphomycosis caused by *Scedosporium apiospermum* (*Pseudallescheria boydii*): an emerging mycosis. Hum Pathol. 1998;29:1266–72.
144. Rippon J. Pseudallescheriasis. In: Rippon JW, editor. *Medical Mycology*. 3rd ed. Philadelphia: W. B. Saunders Company; 1988. p. 651–80.
145. Malani AN, Kauffman CA. Changing epidemiology of rare mould infections: Implications for therapy. Drugs. 2007;67:1803–12.
146. Francis P, Walsh TJ. Approaches to management of fungal infections in cancer patients. Oncology (Williston Park). 1992;6:133–44. discussion 44, 47-8.
147. Corbel MJ, Eades SM. The relative susceptibility of New Zealand black and CBA mice to infection with opportunistic fungal pathogens. Sabouraudia. 1976;14:17–32.
148. Travis LB, Roberts GD, Wilson WR. Clinical significance of *Pseudallescheria boydii*: a review of 10 years' experience. Mayo Clin Proc. 1985;60:531–7.
149. Kiratli H, Uzun O, Kiraz N, Eldem B. *Scedosporium apiospermum* chorioretinitis. Acta Ophthalmol Scand. 2001;79:540–2.
150. Wu Z, Ying H, Yiu S, Irvine J, Smith R. Fungal keratitis caused by *Scedosporium apiospermum*: report of two cases and review of treatment. Cornea. 2002;21:519–23.
151. Mesfin FB, Tobin E, Adamo MA, Dirisio D. Fungal vertebral osteomyelitis due to *Scedosporium apiospermum* after near-drowning. J Neurosurg Spine. 2008;9:58–61.
152. Garzoni C, Emonet S, Legout L, et al. Atypical infections in tsunami survivors. Emerg Infect Dis. 2005;11:1591–3.
153. Kiraz N, Gulbas Z, Akgun Y, Uzun O. Lymphadenitis caused by *Scedosporium apiospermum* in an immunocompetent patient. Clin Infect Dis. 2001;32:E59–61.
154. Patterson TF, Andriole VT, Zervos MJ, Therasse D, Kauffman CA. The epidemiology of pseudallescheriasis complicating transplantation: nosocomial and community-acquired infection. Mycoses. 1990;33:297–302.
155. Armin AR, Reddy VB, Orfei E. Fungal endocarditis caused by *Pseudallescheria (Petriellidium) boydii* in an intravenous drug abuser. Tex Heart Inst J. 1987;14:321–4.
156. Patterson JE. Epidemiology of fungal infections in solid organ transplant patients. Transpl Infect Dis. 1999;1:229–36.
157. Nesky MA, McDougal EC, Peacock Jr JE. *Pseudallescheria boydii* brain abscess successfully treated with voriconazole and surgical drainage: case report and literature review of central nervous system pseudallescheriasis. Clin Infect Dis. 2000;31:673–7.
158. Husain S, Munoz P, Forrest G, et al. Infections due to *Scedosporium apiospermum* and *Scedosporium prolificans* in transplant recipients: clinical characteristics and impact of antifungal agent therapy on outcome. Clin Infect Dis. 2005;40:89–99.
159. Raj R, Frost AE. *Scedosporium apiospermum* fungemia in a lung transplant recipient. Chest. 2002;121:1714–6.
160. Jabado N, Casanova JL, Haddad E, et al. Invasive pulmonary infection due to *Scedosporium apiospermum* in two children with chronic granulomatous disease. Clin Infect Dis. 1998;27:1437–41.
161. Cimon B, Carrere J, Vinatier JF, Chazalette JP, Chabasse D, Bouchara JP. Clinical significance of *Scedosporium apiospermum* in patients with cystic fibrosis. Eur J Clin Microbiol Infect Dis. 2000;19:53–6.
162. Castelli MV, Buitrago MJ, Bernal-Martinez L, Gomez-Lopez A, Rodriguez-Tudela JL, Cuenca-Estrella M. Development and validation of a quantitative PCR assay for diagnosis of scedosporiosis. J Clin Microbiol. 2008;46:3412–6.
163. Meletiadis J, Meis JF, Mouton JW, Rodriquez-Tudela JL, Donnelly JP, Verweij PE. In vitro activities of new and conventional antifungal agents against clinical *Scedosporium* isolates. Antimicrob Agents Chemother. 2002;46:62–8.
164. Troke P, Aguirrebengoa K, Arteaga C, et al. Treatment of scedosporiosis with voriconazole: clinical experience with 107 patients. Antimicrob Agents Chemother. 2008;52:1743–50.
165. Gonzalez GM, Tijerina R, Najvar LK, et al. Activity of posaconazole against *Pseudallescheria boydii*: in vitro and in vivo assays. Antimicrob Agents Chemother. 2003;47:1436–8.
166. Cuenca-Estrella M, Alastruey-Izquierdo A, Alcazar-Fuoli L, et al. In vitro activities of 35 double combinations of antifungal agents against *Scedosporium apiospermum* and *Scedosporium prolificans*. Antimicrob Agents Chemother. 2008;52:1136–9.
167. Heyn K, Tredup A, Salvenmoser S, Muller FM. Effect of voriconazole combined with micafungin against *Candida*, *Aspergillus*, and *Scedosporium* spp. and *Fusarium solani*. Antimicrob Agents Chemother. 2005;49:5157–9.
168. Yustes C, Guarro J. In vitro synergistic interaction between amphotericin B and micafungin against *Scedosporium* spp. Antimicrob Agents Chemother. 2005;49:3498–500.
169. Caira M, Girmenia C, Valentini CG, et al. Scedosporiosis in patients with acute leukemia: a retrospective multicenter report. Haematologica. 2008;93:104–10.
170. Katragkou A, Dotis J, Kotsiou M, Tamiolaki M, Roilides E. *Scedosporium apiospermum* infection after near-drowning. Mycoses. 2007;50:412–21.
171. Lamaris GA, Chamilos G, Lewis RE, Safdar A, Raad II, Kontoyiannis DP. *Scedosporium* infection in a tertiary care cancer center: a review of 25 cases from 1989–2006. Clin Infect Dis. 2006;43:1580–4.
172. Nochez Y, Arsene S, Le Guellec C, et al. Unusual pharmacokinetics of intravitreal and systemic voriconazole in a patient with *Scedosporium apiospermum* endophthalmitis. J Ocul Pharmacol Ther. 2008;24:87–90.
173. Mellinghoff IK, Winston DJ, Mukwaya G, Schiller GJ. Treatment of *Scedosporium apiospermum* brain abscesses with posaconazole. Clin Infect Dis. 2002;34:1648–50.
174. Abzug MJ, Walsh TJ. Interferon-gamma and colony-stimulating factors as adjuvant therapy for refractory fungal infections in children. Pediatr Infect Dis J. 2004;23:769–73.

175. Cooley L, Spelman D, Thursky K, Slavin M. Infection with *Scedosporium apiospermum* and *S. prolificans*, Australia. Emerg Infect Dis. 2007;13:1170–7.
176. Perfect JR, Schell WA. The new fungal opportunists are coming. Clin Infect Dis. 1996;22 Suppl 2:S112–8.
177. Roilides E, Simitsopoulou M, Katragkou A, Walsh TJ. Host immune response against *Scedosporium* species. Med Mycol. 2009;47:433–40.
178. Ortoneda M, Capilla J, Pujol I, et al. Liposomal amphotericin B and granulocyte colony-stimulating factor therapy in a murine model of invasive infection by *Scedosporium prolificans*. J Antimicrob Chemother. 2002;49:525–9.
179. Berenguer J, Rodriguez-Tudela JL, Richard C, et al. Deep infections caused by *Scedosporium prolificans*. A report on 16 cases in Spain and a review of the literature. *Scedosporium prolificans* Spanish Study Group. Medicine (Baltimore). 1997;76:256–65.
180. Rodriguez-Tudela JL, Berenguer J, Guarro J, et al. Epidemiology and outcome of *Scedosporium prolifican*s infection, a review of 162 cases. Med Mycol. 2009;47:359–70.
181. Carreter de Granda ME, Richard C, Conde E, et al. Endocarditis caused by *Scedosporium prolificans* after autologous peripheral blood stem cell transplantation. Eur J Clin Microbiol Infect Dis. 2001;20:215–7.
182. Lopez L, Gaztelurrutia L, Cuenca-Estrella M, et al. Infection and colonization by *Scedosporium prolificans*. Enferm Infecc Microbiol Clín. 2001;19:308–13.
183. Salkin IF, McGinnis MR, Dykstra MJ, Rinaldi MG. *Scedosporium inflatum*, an emerging pathogen. J Clin Microbiol. 1988;26: 498–503.
184. Cuenca-Estrella M, Gomez-Lopez A, Mellado E, Buitrago MJ, Monzon A, Rodriguez-Tudela JL. Head-to-head comparison of the activities of currently available antifungal agents against 3, 378 Spanish clinical isolates of yeasts and filamentous fungi. Antimicrob Agents Chemother. 2006;50:917–21.
185. Del Poeta M, Schell WA, Perfect JR. In vitro antifungal activity of pneumocandin L-743, 872 against a variety of clinically important molds. Antimicrob Agents Chemother. 1997;41:1835–6.
186. McGinnis MR, Pasarell L, Sutton DA, Fothergill AW, Cooper Jr CR, Rinaldi MG. In vitro activity of voriconazole against selected fungi. Med Mycol. 1998;36:239–42.
187. Carrillo AJ, Guarro J. In vitro activities of four novel triazoles against *Scedosporium* spp. Antimicrob Agents Chemother. 2001;45:2151–3.
188. Afeltra J, Dannaoui E, Meis JF, Rodriguez-Tudela JL, Verweij PE. In vitro synergistic interaction between amphotericin B and pentamidine against *Scedosporium prolificans*. Antimicrob Agents Chemother. 2002;46:3323–6.
189. Meletiadis J, Mouton JW, Rodriguez-Tudela JL, Meis JF, Verweij PE. In vitro interaction of terbinafine with itraconazole against clinical isolates of *Scedosporium prolificans*. Antimicrob Agents Chemother. 2000;44:470–2.
190. Meletiadis J, Mouton JW, Meis JF, Verweij PE. In vitro drug interaction modeling of combinations of azoles with terbinafine against clinical *Scedosporium prolificans* isolates. Antimicrob Agents Chemother. 2003;47:106–17.
191. Rodriguez MM, Calvo E, Serena C, Marine M, Pastor FJ, Guarro J. Effects of double and triple combinations of antifungal drugs in a murine model of disseminated infection by *Scedosporium prolificans*. Antimicrob Agents Chemother. 2009;53:2153–5.
192. Walsh TJ, Lutsar I, Driscoll T, et al. Voriconazole in the treatment of aspergillosis, scedosporiosis and other invasive fungal infections in children. Pediatr Infect Dis J. 2002;21:240–8.
193. Tong SY, Peleg AY, Yoong J, Handke R, Szer J, Slavin M. Breakthrough *Scedosporium prolificans* infection while receiving voriconazole prophylaxis in an allogeneic stem cell transplant recipient. Transpl Infect Dis. 2007;9:241–3.
194. Ananda-Rajah MR, Grigg A, Slavin MA. Breakthrough disseminated *Scedosporium prolificans* infection in a patient with relapsed leukaemia on prolonged voriconazole followed by posaconazole prophylaxis. Mycopathologia. 2008;166:83–6.
195. Howden BP, Slavin MA, Schwarer AP, Mijch AM. Successful control of disseminated *Scedosporium prolificans* infection with a combination of voriconazole and terbinafine. Eur J Clin Microbiol Infect Dis. 2003;22:111–3.
196. Li JY, Yong TY, Grove DI, Coates PT. Successful control of *Scedosporium prolificans* septic arthritis and probable osteomyelitis without radical surgery in a long-term renal transplant recipient. Transpl Infect Dis. 2008;10:63–5.
197. Steinbach WJ, Schell WA, Miller JL, Perfect JR. *Scedosporium prolificans* osteomyelitis in an immunocompetent child treated with voriconazole and caspofungin, as well as locally applied polyhexamethylene biguanide. J Clin Microbiol. 2003;41:3981–5.
198. Kesson AM, Bellemore MC, O'Mara TJ, Ellis DH, Sorrell TC. *Scedosporium prolificans* osteomyelitis in an immunocompetent child treated with a novel agent, hexadecylphospocholine (miltefosine), in combination with terbinafine and voriconazole: a case report. Clin Infect Dis. 2009;48:1257–61.
199. Guarro J, Gams W, Pujol I, Gene J. *Acremonium* species: new emerging fungal opportunists–in vitro antifungal susceptibilities and review. Clin Infect Dis. 1997;25:1222–9.
200. Fridkin SK, Kremer FB, Bland LA, Padhye A, McNeil MM, Jarvis WR. *Acremonium kiliense* endophthalmitis that occurred after cataract extraction in an ambulatory surgical center and was traced to an environmental reservoir. Clin Infect Dis. 1996;22:222–7.
201. Pastorino AC, Menezes UP, Marques HH, et al. *Acremonium kiliense* infection in a child with chronic granulomatous disease. Braz J Infect Dis. 2005;9:529–34.
202. Schell WA, Perfect JR. Fatal, disseminated *Acremonium strictum* infection in a neutropenic host. J Clin Microbiol. 1996;34:1333–6.
203. Anadolu R, Hilmioglu S, Oskay T, Boyvat A, Peksari Y, Gurgey E. Indolent *Acremonium strictum* infection in an immunocompetent patient. Int J Dermatol. 2001;40:451–3.
204. Keynan Y, Sprecher H, Weber G. *Acremonium* vertebral osteomyelitis: molecular diagnosis and response to voriconazole. Clin Infect Dis. 2007;45:e5–6.
205. Roilides E, Bibashi E, Acritidou E, et al. *Acremonium* fungemia in two immunocompromised children. Pediatr Infect Dis J. 1995;14:548–50.
206. Fincher RM, Fisher JF, Lovell RD, Newman CL, Espinel-Ingroff A, Shadomy HJ. Infection due to the fungus *Acremonium (cephalosporium)*. Medicine (Baltimore). 1991;70:398–409.
207. Chang YH, Huang LM, Hsueh PR, et al. *Acremonium* pyomyositis in a pediatric patient with acute leukemia. Pediatr Blood Cancer. 2005;44:521–4.
208. Sener AG, Yucesoy M, Senturkun S, Afsar I, Yurtsever SG, Turk M. A case of *Acremonium strictum* peritonitis. Med Mycol. 2008;46:495–7.
209. Yalaz M, Hilmioglu S, Metin D, et al. Fatal disseminated *Acremonium strictum* infection in a preterm newborn: a very rare cause of neonatal septicaemia. J Med Microbiol. 2003;52:835–7.
210. Yamazaki R, Mori T, Aisa Y, et al. Systemic infection due to *Acremonium* after allogeneic peripheral blood stem cell transplantation. Intern Med. 2006;45:989–90.
211. Miyakis S, Velegraki A, Delikou S, et al. Invasive *Acremonium strictum* infection in a bone marrow transplant recipient. Pediatr Infect Dis J. 2006;25:273–5.
212. Weissgold DJ, Maguire AM, Brucker AJ. Management of postoperative *Acremonium* endophthalmitis. Ophthalmology. 1996; 103:749–56.
213. Filipello Marchisio V, Fusconi A. Morphological evidence for keratinolytic activity of *Scopulariopsis* spp. isolates from nail lesions and the air. Med Mycol. 2001;39:287–94.

214. Steinbach WJ, Schell WA, Miller JL, Perfect JR, Martin PL. Fatal *Scopulariopsis brevicaulis* infection in a paediatric stem-cell transplant patient treated with voriconazole and caspofungin and a review of *Scopulariopsis* infections in immunocompromised patients. J Infect. 2004;48:112–6.
215. Shankar EM, Vignesh R, Barton RC, et al. Hydrothorax in association with *Scopulariopsis brumptii* in an AIDS patient in Chennai, India. Trans R Soc Trop Med Hyg. 2007;101:1270–2.
216. Aydin S, Ertugrul B, Gultekin B, Uyar G, Kir E. Treatment of two postoperative endophthalmitis cases due to *Aspergillus flavus* and *Scopulariopsis* spp. with local and systemic antifungal therapy. BMC Infect Dis. 2007;7:87.
217. Vollmer T, Stormer M, Kleesiek K, Dreier J. Evaluation of novel broad-range real-time PCR assay for rapid detection of human pathogenic fungi in various clinical specimens. J Clin Microbiol. 2008;46:1919–26.
218. Isidro AM, Amorosa V, Stopyra GA, Rutenberg HL, Pentz WH, Bridges CR. Fungal prosthetic mitral valve endocarditis caused by *Scopulariopsis* species: case report and review of the literature. J Thorac Cardiovasc Surg. 2006;131:1181–3.
219. Sellier P, Monsuez JJ, Lacroix C, et al. Recurrent subcutaneous infection due to *Scopulariopsis brevicaulis* in a liver transplant recipient. Clin Infect Dis. 2000;30:820–3.
220. Cuenca-Estrella M, Gomez-Lopez A, Mellado E, Buitrago MJ, Monzon A, Rodriguez-Tudela JL. *Scopulariopsis brevicaulis,* a fungal pathogen resistant to broad-spectrum antifungal agents. Antimicrob Agents Chemother. 2003;47:2339–41.
221. Carrillo-Munoz AJ, Giusiano G, Guarro J, et al. In vitro activity of voriconazole against dermatophytes, *Scopulariopsis brevicaulis* and other opportunistic fungi as agents of onychomycosis. Int J Antimicrob Agents. 2007;30:157–61.
222. Cuenca-Estrella M, Gomez-Lopez A, Buitrago MJ, Mellado E, Garcia-Effron G, Rodriguez-Tudela JL. In vitro activities of 10 combinations of antifungal agents against the multiresistant pathogen *Scopulariopsis brevicaulis*. Antimicrob Agents Chemother. 2006;50:2248–50.
223. Cuenca-Estrella M, Gomez-Lopez A, Mellado E, Garcia-Effron G, Monzon A, Rodriguez-Tudela JL. In vitro activity of ravuconazole against 923 clinical isolates of nondermatophyte filamentous fungi. Antimicrob Agents Chemother. 2005;49:5136–8.
224. Wagner D, Sander A, Bertz H, Finke J, Kern WV. Breakthrough invasive infection due to Debaryomyces hansenii (teleomorph Candida famata) and *Scopulariopsis brevicaulis* in a stem cell transplant patient receiving liposomal amphotericin B and caspofungin for suspected aspergillosis. Infection. 2005;33:397–400.
225. Patel R, Gustaferro CA, Krom RA, Wiesner RH, Roberts GD, Paya CV. Phaeohyphomycosis due to *Scopulariopsis brumptii* in a liver transplant recipient. Clin Infect Dis. 1994;19:198–200.
226. Kriesel JD, Adderson EE, Gooch 3rd WM, Pavia AT. Invasive sinonasal disease due to *Scopulariopsis candida*: case report and review of scopulariopsosis. Clin Infect Dis. 1994;19:317–9.
227. Lovell RD, Moll M, Allen J, Cicci LG. Disseminated *Paecilomyces lilacinus* infection in a patient with AIDS. AIDS Read. 2002; 12:212–3. 8, 21.
228. Safdar A. Progressive cutaneous hyalohyphomycosis due to *Paecilomyces lilacinus*: rapid response to treatment with caspofungin and itraconazole. Clin Infect Dis. 2002;34:1415–7.
229. Van Schooneveld T, Freifeld A, Lesiak B, Kalil A, Sutton DA, Iwen PC. *Paecilomyces lilacinus* infection in a liver transplant patient: case report and review of the literature. Transpl Infect Dis. 2008;10:117–22.
230. Gutierrez-Rodero F, Moragon M, Ortiz de laTabla V, Mayol MJ, Martin C. Cutaneous hyalohyphomycosis caused by *Paecilomyces lilacinus* in an immunocompetent host successfully treated with itraconazole: case report and review. Eur J Clin Microbiol Infect Dis. 1999;18:814–8.
231. Clark NM. *Paecilomyces lilacinus* infection in a heart transplant recipient and successful treatment with terbinafine. Clin Infect Dis. 1999;28:1169–70.
232. Orth B, Frei R, Itin PH, et al. Outbreak of invasive mycoses caused by *Paecilomyces lilacinus* from a contaminated skin lotion. Ann Intern Med. 1996;125:799–806.
233. Pastor FJ, Guarro J. Clinical manifestations, treatment and outcome of *Paecilomyces lilacinus* infections. Clin Microbiol Infect. 2006;12:948–60.
234. Wessolossky M, Haran JP, Bagchi K. *Paecilomyces lilacinus* olecranon bursitis in an immunocompromised host: case report and review. Diagn Microbiol Infect Dis. 2008;61:354–7.
235. Shing MM, Ip M, Li CK, Chik KW, Yuen PM. *Paecilomyces varioti* fungemia in a bone marrow transplant patient. Bone Marrow Transplant. 1996;17:281–3.
236. Lionakis MS, Bodey GP, Tarrand JJ, Raad II, Kontoyiannis DP. The significance of blood cultures positive for emerging saprophytic moulds in cancer patients. Clin Microbiol Infect. 2004;10:922–5.
237. Aguilar C, Pujol I, Sala J, Guarro J. Antifungal susceptibilities of *Paecilomyces* species. Antimicrob Agents Chemother. 1998; 42:1601–4.
238. Gottlieb T, Atkins BL. Case report. Successful treatment of cutaneous *Paecilomyces lilacinus* infection with oral itraconazole in an immune competent host. Mycoses. 2001;44:513–5.
239. Das A, MacLaughlin EF, Ross LA, et al. *Paecilomyces variotii* in a pediatric patient with lung transplantation. Pediatr Transplant. 2000;4:328–32.
240. Ortoneda M, Capilla J, Pastor FJ, et al. In vitro interactions of approved and novel drugs against *Paecilomyces* spp. Antimicrob Agents Chemother. 2004;48:2727–9.
241. Chan-Tack KM, Thio CL, Miller NS, Karp CL, Ho C, Merz WG. *Paecilomyces lilacinus* fungemia in an adult bone marrow transplant recipient. Med Mycol. 1999;37:57–60.
242. Hilmarsdottir I, Thorsteinsson SB, Asmundsson P, Bodvarsson M, Arnadottir M. Cutaneous infection caused by *Paecilomyces lilacinus* in a renal transplant patient: treatment with voriconazole. Scand J Infect Dis. 2000;32:331–2.
243. Mullane K, Toor AA, Kalnicky C, Rodriguez T, Klein J, Stiff P. Posaconazole salvage therapy allows successful allogeneic hematopoietic stem cell transplantation in patients with refractory invasive mold infections. Transpl Infect Dis. 2007; 9:89–96.
244. Wang SM, Shieh CC, Liu CC. Successful treatment of *Paecilomyces variotii* splenic abscesses: a rare complication in a previously unrecognized chronic granulomatous disease child. Diagn Microbiol Infect Dis. 2005;53:149–52.
245. Ford JG, Agee S, Greenhaw ST. Successful medical treatment of a case of *Paecilomyces lilacinus* keratitis. Cornea. 2008; 27:1077–9.
246. Stillwell WT, Rubin BD, Axelrod JL. *Chrysosporium*, a new causative agent in osteomyelitis. A case report. Clin Orthop Relat Res 1984:184:190–2.
247. Levy FE, Larson JT, George E, Maisel RH. Invasive *Chrysosporium* infection of the nose and paranasal sinuses in an immunocompromised host. Otolaryngol Head Neck Surg. 1991;104:384–8.
248. Warwick A, Ferrieri P, Burke B, Blazar BR. Presumptive invasive *Chrysosporium* infection in a bone marrow transplant recipient. Bone Marrow Transplant. 1991;8:319–22.
249. Munoz FM, Demmler GJ, Travis WR, Ogden AK, Rossmann SN, Rinaldi MG. *Trichoderma longibrachiatum* infection in a pediatric patient with aplastic anemia. J Clin Microbiol. 1997; 35:499–503.
250. Roilides E, Sigler L, Bibashi E, Katsifa H, Flaris N, Panteliadis C. Disseminated infection due to *Chrysosporium zonatum* in a patient with chronic granulomatous disease and review of non-*Aspergillus*

fungal infections in patients with this disease. J Clin Microbiol. 1999;37:18–25.
251. Wagoner MD, Badr IA, Hidayat AA. *Chrysosporium* parvum keratomycosis. Cornea. 1999;18:616–20.
252. Lagrange-Xelot M, Schlemmer F, Gallien S, Lacroix C, Molina JM. *Trichoderma* fungaemia in a neutropenic patient with pulmonary cancer and human immunodeficiency virus infection. Clin Microbiol Infect. 2008;14:1190–2.
253. Kviliute R, Paskevicius A, Gulbinovic J, Stulpinas R, Griskevicius L. Nonfatal *Trichoderma citrinoviride* pneumonia in an acute myeloid leukemia patient. Ann Hematol. 2008;87:501–2.
254. Maran AG, Kwong K, Milne LJ, Lamb D. Frontal sinusitis caused by *Myriodontium keratinophilum*. Br Med J (Clin Res Ed). 1985;290:207.
255. Ahmad S, Johnson RJ, Hillier S, Shelton WR, Rinaldi MG. Fungal peritonitis caused by *Lecythophora* mutabilis. J Clin Microbiol. 1985;22:182–6.
256. Jacobs F, Byl B, Bourgeois N, et al. *Trichoderma viride* infection in a liver transplant recipient. Mycoses. 1992;35:301–3.
257. Farina C, Vailati F, Manisco A, Goglio A. Fungaemia survey: a 10-year experience in Bergamo, Italy. Mycoses. 1999;42:543–8.
258. Chin-Hong PV, Sutton DA, Roemer M, Jacobson MA, Aberg JA. Invasive fungal sinusitis and meningitis due to *Arthrographis kalrae* in a patient with AIDS. J Clin Microbiol. 2001;39:804–7.
259. Henke MO, De Hoog GS, Gross U, Zimmermann G, Kraemer D, Weig M. Human deep tissue infection with an entomopathogenic *Beauveria* species. J Clin Microbiol. 2002;40:2698–702.
260. Suh MK, Lim JW, Lee YH, et al. Subcutaneous hyalohyphomycosis due to *Cephalotheca foveolata* in an immunocompetent host. Br J Dermatol. 2006;154:1184–9.
261. Chouaki T, Lavarde V, Lachaud L, Raccurt CP, Hennequin C. Invasive infections due to T*richoderma* species: report of 2 cases, findings of in vitro susceptibility testing, and review of the literature. Clin Infect Dis. 2002;35:1360–7.
262. Loeppky CB, Sprouse RF, Carlson JV, Everett ED. *Trichoderma viride* peritonitis. South Med J. 1983;76:798–9.
263. Furukawa H, Kusne S, Sutton DA, et al. Acute invasive sinusitis due to *Trichoderma longibrachiatum* in a liver and small bowel transplant recipient. Clin Infect Dis. 1998;26:487–9.
264. Richter S, Cormican MG, Pfaller MA, et al. Fatal disseminated T*richoderma longibrachiatum* infection in an adult bone marrow transplant patient: species identification and review of the literature. J Clin Microbiol. 1999;37:1154–60.
265. Hennequin C, Chouaki T, Pichon JC, Strunski V, Raccurt C. Otitis externa due to *Trichoderma longibrachiatum*. Eur J Clin Microbiol Infect Dis. 2000;19:641–2.
266. Kratzer C, Tobudic S, Schmoll M, Graninger W, Georgopoulos A. In vitro activity and synergism of amphotericin B, azoles and cationic antimicrobials against the emerging pathogen *Trichoderma* spp. J Antimicrob Chemother. 2006;58:1058–61.
267. De Miguel D, Gomez P, Gonzalez R, et al. Nonfatal pulmonary T*richoderma viride* infection in an adult patient with acute myeloid leukemia: report of one case and review of the literature. Diagn Microbiol Infect Dis. 2005;53:33–7.

Phaeohyphomycoses (Brown-Black Moulds)

John R. Perfect, Barbara D. Alexander, and Wiley A. Schell

Phaeohyphomycosis, a term first introduced by Ajello and colleagues [1], is an encompassing clinical designation for a spectrum of infections caused by darkly pigmented moulds [2, 3]. In its simplest definition, phaeohyphomycosis is an infection caused by fungi that are characterized by a brown-to-black coloration of their vegetative or spore cell walls. Dark pigmentation of the moulds is caused by deposition within the cell wall of dihydroxynaphthalene melanin that is formed through pentaketide metabolism. These moulds collectively are known as dematiaceous fungi. In most cases the brown coloration of the fungus is apparent in host tissue, but at times it is revealed only when the fungus is grown in culture. The term phaeohyphomycosis (phaeo: dusky or brown; hypho: hyphal) is based on characteristics of the fungi as seen in infected tissue and thus includes many genera and species.

Taxonomy/Ecology

Within the broad definition of phaeohyphomycosis, more than 100 species of dematiaceous fungi have been reported to be associated with human colonization and disease [4–6]. These fungi belong to various taxonomic ranks, including Hyphomycetes, Ascomycota, Basidiomycota, and Zygomycota. As fungal taxonomy evolves in this era of molecular studies, reclassification of familiar fungi and name changes should be expected. There is variation in the numbers of infections caused by various dematiaceous fungi. Some species are rare causes of disease with only an occasional case report documented in the literature, and other species are associated with large series of reported human cases. The latter include *Exophiala jeanselmei* and *Wangiella dermatitidis* causing subcutaneous infection and *Cladophialophora bantiana* causing cerebral disease.

Infection in humans typically is preceded by traumatic inoculation with the fungus, although inhalation is the initiating event in some cases. Most dematiaceous fungi are ubiquitous, are cosmopolitan saprobes of soil and decaying matter, and are pathogens of plants. As a result, dematiaceous fungal infections occur worldwide. Although there has been no unique endemic area for most infections, cases can cluster in certain circumstances. For instance, there is some suggestion of a southern United States geographic bias in cases of allergic fungal sinusitis associated with dematiaceous fungi [7]. Similarly, chronic phaeohyphomycotic infections of the feet and legs are noted more frequently in tropical areas, where people commonly wear sandals or no shoes. In cases of localized skin and soft tissue infections, the mechanism for production of disease often is trauma from contaminated vegetation; medical instruments, including needles or catheters, have been implicated occasionally. Also, outbreaks of nosocomial dematiaceous fungal infections may be related to environmental contamination of fluids, drugs, or medical equipment [8, 9].

Increased numbers of cases of phaeohyphomycosis have been observed in medical centers that care for a large immunocompromised patient population. For instance, solid organ transplant recipients are at moderate risk for dematiaceous fungal infections, and phaeohyphomycoses have been seen at most transplant centers [10–13]. The transplant recipient, who is exposed to frequent invasive medical interventions and who has thinning of the skin due to corticosteroid use, is a particularly susceptible immunocompromised host for infection with these fungi. Phaeohyphomycosis is encountered increasingly in immunosuppressed cancer patients as well [14]. The most prevalent severe immunosuppressive event in the world today is HIV infection, and phaeohyphomycosis has been reported in this group [15–17]. However, these infections are uncommon events in this special group of immunocompromised patients compared to other opportunistic fungal infections, such as cryptococcosis, histoplasmosis, and penicilliosis.

J.R. Perfect (✉)
Duke Mycology Research Unit, Division of Infectious Diseases and International Health, Duke University Medical Center, Durham, NC, USA
e-mail: perfe001@mc.duke.edu;

C.A. Kauffman et al. (eds.), *Essentials of Clinical Mycology*,
DOI 10.1007/978-1-4419-6640-7_17, © Springer Science+Business Media, LLC 2011

Pathophysiology

As a descriptive term, phaeohyphomycosis encompasses a wide variety of phylogenetically diverse pathogenic fungal species. It is unlikely that there could be consistent unifying themes accounting for the virulence potential of all agents. However, several common aspects of fungal pathogenesis should be emphasized. The presence of melanin has been implicated by genetic studies to be a virulence factor. A mutant strain of *W. dermatitidis* that lacked melanin demonstrated reduced virulence by the measurement of survival in a mouse model of infection compared to the wild-type melanin-positive strain [18, 19]. Further studies used molecular biology methods to specifically disrupt a gene involved in dihydroxynaphthalene melanin biosynthesis. The null melanin-negative mutants were found to be less resistant to neutrophil killing and concordantly less virulent in acute infection animal models [20]. Another study confirmed that melanin can protect a fungus from oxidative host cells, such as neutrophils, and may bind hydrolytic enzymes [21]. However, it should be noted that nonmelanized fungal cells can persist in tissue and cause histopathology similar to that seen with the melanized cells [19]. Melanin also has been identified as a virulence factor in other fungi, such as the rice blast fungus, *Magnaporthe grisea*. In addition, melanin is a virulence factor for the basidiomycetous human pathogen, *Cryptococcus neoformans*.

Another area identified as likely to be important in virulence is chitin biosynthesis. Null mutants made in several of the chitin synthase genes of *W. dermatitidis* were less virulent than the wild-type strain in both immunocompetent and immunosuppressed murine models [22]. An additional virulence factor for many dematiaceous fungi is the ability to adapt locally to the harsh host tissue environment when introduced through trauma. This adaptive feature is seen in patients with fungal keratitis and those with subcutaneous nodules that likely represent direct inoculation into the skin and subcutaneous tissue.

Several of the dematiaceous fungi appear to have a tropism for brain tissue. For instance, brain abscesses are common clinical infections associated with *Cladophialophora bantiana*, *Ochroconis gallopava*, and *Rhinocladiella (Ramichloridium) mackenziei*. Finally, infections with dematiaceous fungi can occur in both immunocompetent and immunosuppressed patients, and thus some of these fungi are considered primary pathogens. However, the vast majority of disseminated infections with dematiaceous fungi, except those with brain infections, occur in immunosuppressed patients.

Understanding of the host immunology related to the phaeohyphomycoses remains rudimentary. The importance of both humoral and cell-mediated immunity has been demonstrated. For instance, humoral immunity studies have shown that purified rabbit IgG can inhibit the growth of *Fonsecaea pedrosoi* [23]. In the evaluation of cell-mediated immunity, a clinical study in patients with chromoblastomycosis demonstrated a normal response to bacterial antigens but a partial suppression of cell-mediated immune responses to fungal antigens at some time during infection [24]. Although risk factor analyses indicate that the host immune system plays an important role in phaeohyphomycotic infections, much work needs to be done to better characterize the components of the host responses to dematiaceous fungi.

Risk Factors

Dematiaceous fungi are not primarily equipped to invade the mammalian host as part of the fungal life-cycle; thus, in most cases the host presents with some risk factors that allow establishment and/or dissemination of fungal infection (Table 1). In an era of increasing numbers of immunocompromised hosts, phaeohyphomycoses are emerging diseases [14, 25, 26]. Bone marrow and solid organ transplant recipients are at major risk for infection [12, 13, 27]. The chronic use of corticosteroids predisposes to a myriad of immunodepressive actions and increases the risk of infection for patients who commonly are exposed to dematiaceous fungi in the environment. Patients with skin or soft tissue trauma from contaminated plant matter such as splinters, intravenous drug use, or cardiothoracic surgery that introduces fungi at the time of surgery [28–32] have been reported to develop phaeohyphomycosis. An occasional case of phaeohyphomycosis has been observed in AIDS patients and in those receiving chronic ambulatory peritoneal dialysis [15–17, 33]. These patient groups are at high risk for developing infections because of the combination of frequent exposures to dematiaceous fungi and their underlying immunosuppressive conditions.

Clinical Manifestations

Although the dematiaceous fungi represent a phylogenetically diverse group of fungi, there are several well-described clinical syndromes produced by these fungi.

Table 1 Risk factors for dematiaceous fungal infections

• Solid organ transplantation	• Long-term indwelling catheter
• Stem cell transplantation	• Continuous peritoneal dialysis
• Corticosteroid therapy	• Sinusitis
• Trauma	• HIV infection
• Intravenous drug use	• Cardiothoracic surgery
• Neutropenia	• Fresh-water immersion

Localized Infections

Superficial Phaeohyphomycosis

This category includes conditions known traditionally as *Tinea nigra* and black piedra [34]. *Tinea nigra* is a darkening of the skin due to growth in the stratum corneum of *Hortaea werneckii* (*Phaeoannellomyces werneckii*). Although the condition is harmless because only the stratum corneum is involved, *Tinea nigra* can be mistaken for melanoma. Black piedra is colonization of the hair shaft by *Piedraia hortae*, which results in very hard knots of discrete fungal growth along the shaft.

Cutaneous Phaeohyphomycosis

This condition represents both initial colonization and then proliferation of the fungus within keratinized tissue, resulting in a chronic inflammatory reaction from tissue invasion [35]. Examples include dermatomycosis secondary to dematiaceous fungi such as *Scytalidium* species and onychomycosis due to *Scytalidium* or *Phyllosticta* species. Furthermore, under certain skin conditions, the dematiaceous fungi may simply colonize devitalized skin without invading viable tissue. Treatment of the underlying condition or use of a simple antiseptic wash will remove these fungi from tissue. However, in severely immunosuppressed patients, some of these moulds may produce an aggressive soft tissue infection.

Mycotic Keratitis

Trauma to the cornea can provide a site for fungal organisms to lodge and grow. The fungus might be present on the instrument of trauma or as airborne spores that contact an injured eye. The frequent use of steroid ophthalmic drops for corneal injuries may aid in fungal invasion of the cornea. The dematiaceous fungi, as well as species of *Aspergillus*, *Fusarium*, and *Paecilomyces,* are the main causes of fungal keratitis. Corneal infections have the potential to progress to endophthalmitis by spreading into internal ocular structures. Multiple dematiaceous moulds have caused corneal disease, but *Curvularia*, *Exophiala*, and *Exserohilum* species are most commonly noted fungi in these infections [36–40].

Subcutaneous Phaeohyphomycosis

This form of phaeohyphomycosis is relatively common [12–14, 27, 35, 41]. Patients generally present with solitary, discrete, asymptomatic, subcutaneous lesions or cysts, which can be misdiagnosed as ganglion cysts, epidermal inclusion cysts, Baker's cysts, or foreign body granulomas (Fig. 1). Occasionally, deep subcutaneous ulcers develop, and satellite lesions rarely occur from autoinoculation. Cysts in the immunocompetent patient are often chronic and relatively asymptomatic; they can remain with little observable clinical change for years, but hyphae can be observed in tissue and mould will grow in culture from the cyst. Some of these resected cysts contain the original wood splinter that introduced the fungus into the tissue. Among immunosuppressed patients these cysts are most commonly seen in solid organ transplant recipients and patients receiving chronic corticosteroids. Even among immunosuppressed patients, the majority of these skin lesions represent direct or primary inoculation into tissue rather than skin lesions that result from dissemination from another site of infection. The most common dematiaceous fungi to produce these subcutaneous infections are *E. jeanselmei*, *W. dermatitidis*, and *Phialophora* species.

Foreign Body Phaeohyphomycosis

Indwelling catheters occasionally become colonized with dematiaceous fungi, and sometimes these moulds produce disease. This form of phaeohyphomycosis is most commonly seen as fungal peritonitis in patients receiving chronic ambulatory peritoneal dialysis [33]. Patients who have long-duration indwelling subcutaneous intravenous catheters can develop infection, which is likely related to a breech in sterile technique or to contaminated material introduced parenterally [9]. It is important to remove the foreign body in the treatment of these types of infections. It has not been established whether the dematiaceous fungi produce a biofilm that enhances attachment to catheters and protects the organism from host responses and antifungal drugs.

Fungal Sinusitis

Sinus infections with dematiaceous fungi can present in three forms. Allergic fungal sinusitis presents with histopathologic evidence of inflammatory mucin with eosinophils and hyphae present within the mucin [42]. A fungus ball or eumycetoma in the sinus cavity produces disease primarily by obstruction. There is no fungal invasion into local soft tissue or bone in either of these two forms[43]. Invasive fungal sinusitis is manifested by extension of infection into bone and, rarely, the brain [44]. *Aspergillus* species, zygomycetes, and dematiaceous moulds, such as *Bipolaris*, *Curvularia*, and *Alternaria* species, represent the primary etiologic agents in invasive fungal sinusitis [6, 42, 45–47].

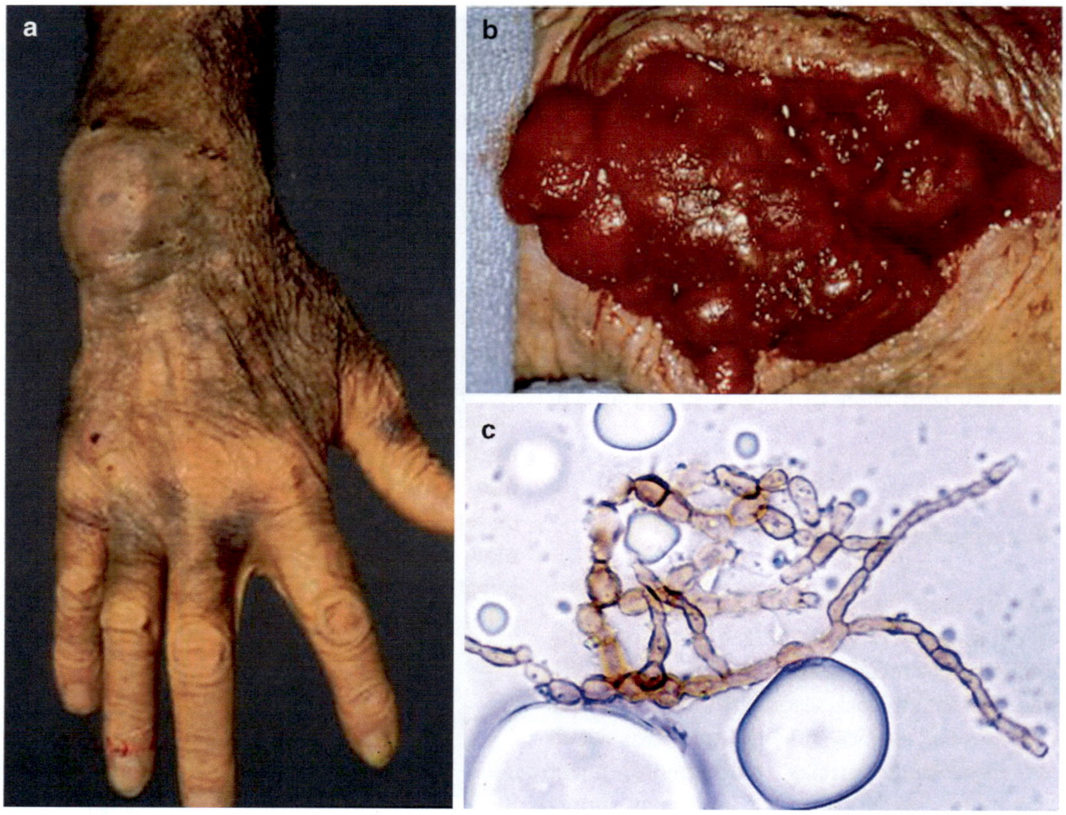

Fig. 1 (**a**) Cystic mass on the dorsum of the right wrist in a patient who had received long-term therapy with corticosteroids. (**b**) Exposure of the\ cystic structures within the mass. (**c**) Potassium hydroxide preparation of cyst contents showing pigmented hyphae of *Exophiala jeanselmei*

Disseminated Infection

Disseminated infection represents spread to distant organs from a colonized or infected site. The fungus may have gained entry to the host via surgery or trauma, or by inhalation from the environment. In certain circumstances, infection can spread to distant sites such as the heart or brain [30, 48, 49]. Cases of disseminated phaeohyphomycosis have increased significantly over the last decade. More than 85% of these cases are associated with some type of immunodeficiency, most commonly chemotherapy-induced neutropenia. However, there are occasional patients with disseminated phaeohyphomycosis who have no apparent risk factors [50–52]. Disseminated disease has been associated with peripheral eosinophilia, suggesting that certain patients with this infection have an ineffective TH2 immune response that allows dissemination [32]. Most patients with disseminated disease probably do not develop a proper immune response even when risk factors are not readily apparent.

The most commonly encountered dematiaceous fungi to produce disseminated disease include those that cause brain abscesses (Fig. 2) such as *C. bantiana*, *W. dermatitidis (Exophiala dermatitidis)*, *O. gallopava*, and *R. mackenziei*, and those that cause meningitis, such as *Scedosporium apiospermum* [49, 53]. *Scedosporium apiospermum* is a common cause of pneumonia or meningitis following near-drownings in fresh water, and is becoming a more common pathogen in severely immunosuppressed organ transplant recipients [54–57]. *Scedosporium prolificans*, which is the most common cause of blood culture-positive bloodstream infections due to dematiaceous fungi, was originally encountered in bone and joint infections. Fungemia has been documented frequently as a complication of neutropenia and in patients with prosthetic heart valves. *Scedosporium prolificans* presumably is able to invade blood vessels and sporulate in situ, releasing a series of unicellular spores into the bloodstream that eventually become lodged in other tissues where they subsequently germinate. This phenomenon of adventitious sporulation has been extensively documented for other opportunistic moulds [58–60]. After surgical trauma, prolonged neutropenia, or in the presence of contaminated catheters, *Scedosporium*, *Bipolaris*, and *Wangiella* species most commonly produce widely disseminated phaeohyphomycosis [32].

Disease Caused by Specific Agents

Table 2 matches the most common dematiaceous fungi with their primary clinical presentations. This list is not comprehensive;

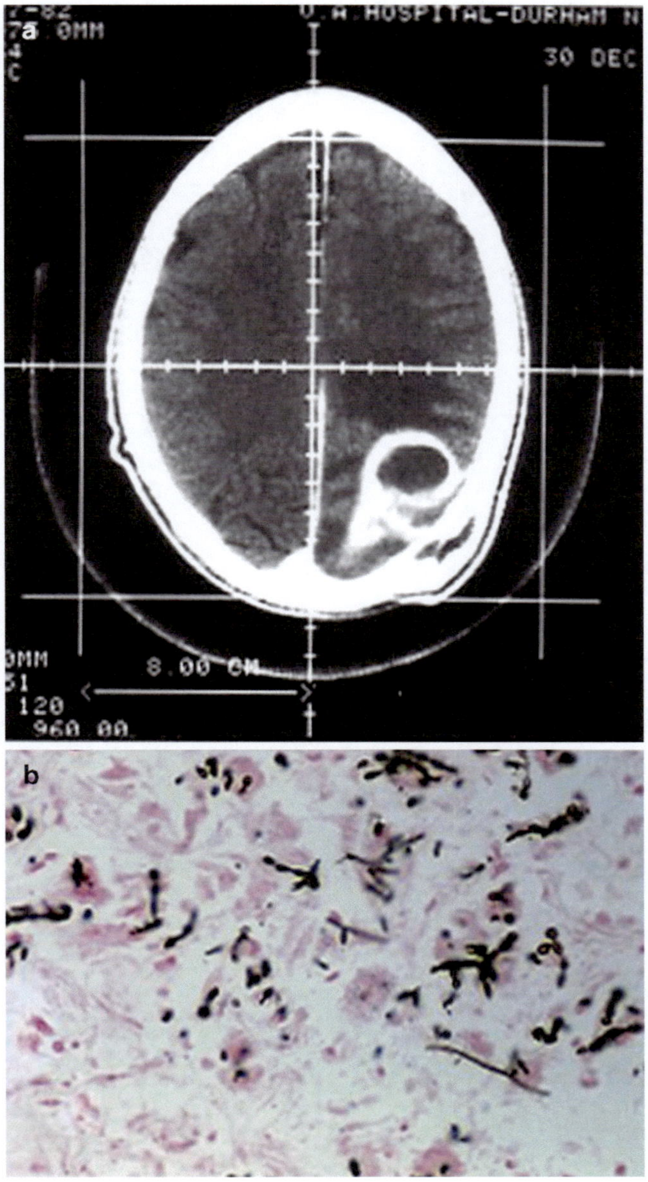

Fig. 2 (**a**) Large occipital brain abscess shown on CT scan. (**b**) Biopsy stained with hematoxylin and eosin showing pigmented hyphae and yeast-like forms

more than 100 species of dematiaceous moulds have been documented as etiologic agents of human disease, and the list continues to expand as the immunocompromised population grows. Also, this list emphasizes only the most common clinical presentations, but other manifestations may occur.

Several specific features about these selected dematiaceous fungal infections deserve mention. Virtually all cases of chromoblastomycosis are caused by four species: *Fonsecaea pedrosoi*, *F. monophora*, *Cladophialophora carrionii*, and *Phialophora verrucosa*. The most common group of dematiaceous fungi encountered in clinical practice is comprised of *Alternaria* spp., *Bipolaris* spp., *Curvularia* spp., *Exophiala* spp., and *W. dermatitidis*, which are associated with a variety of different clinical presentations. The group of fungi that typically produces CNS infections includes *C. bantiana*, *O. gallopava*, *W. dermatitidis*, and *R. mackenziei* [49, 53, 61, 62]. *Ochroconis gallopava* has shown its innate potential for CNS infectivity by causing outbreaks of fungal encephalitis in turkeys and occasional cases in humans [63, 64]. For this group of CNS pathogens, there is some geographic limitation of infection. For example, *R. mackenziei* infections have been limited to patients living in or originating from the Middle East [62, 65].

Along with the known potential of *S. apiospermum*, *S. aurantiacum*, and *Pseudallescheria boydii* to cause meningitis in diabetics, patients receiving steroid therapy, or victims of fresh water near-drownings, cases of meningitis have also been caused by species of *Bipolaris*, *Exophiala*, *Alternaria*, and *Sporothrix schenckii* [5, 6, 66–69]. Although many different dematiaceous fungi have caused disease, there is clearly a spectrum of virulence potential. For example, species of genera such as *Cladosporium* or *Rhinocladiella* are environmentally common and more frequent colonizers of skin and airways than the more pathogenic dematiaceous fungi, such as *F. pedrosoi*, *F. monophora*, *W. dermatitidis*, *O. gallopava*, and *C. bantiana*. *S. schenckii*, which is a dematiaceous mould in culture, is usually classified as a dimorphic fungus rather than under the dematiaceous mould group. However, the propensity of *S. schenckii* to produce soft tissue infections through traumatic inoculation does fit the common pattern of infection with dematiaceous fungi.

The clinical syndromes associated with several of the most common dematiaceous mould genera are summarized herein. For a more comprehensive description of the mycology of these dematiaceous fungi, the reader is referred to specific texts and atlases on dematiacious fungi [4–6].

Alternaria Species

The most common species is *Alternaria alternata*, but in the clinical laboratory, identification generally is left at the genus level. This mould often causes local cutaneous infections [70–72] (Fig. 3). In addition, it may cause a sinonasal infection characteristically seen in immunosuppressed patients, which is similar to zygomycosis, but which does not commonly disseminate [73, 74].

Bipolaris Species

Three species cause the majority of disease: *B. australiensis*, *B. hawaiiensis*, and *B. spicifera*. This genus of brown/black moulds may infect many different organs of the body and cause meningitis, sinusitis, keratitis, peritonitis, soft tissue infections, and endocarditis [31, 38, 51, 75–78].

Table 2 Dematiaceous fungi and their most common phaeohyphomycoses (Adapted from [5])

Etiologic agent	Clinical presentation	Frequency	References
Alternaria spp. (*alternata*)	Osteomyelitis, cutaneous, sinusitis	++	[5, 6, 71–74]
Aureobasidium spp. (*pullulans*)	Peritonitis, cutaneous, spleen infection	+	[5, 6, 14]
Bipolaris spp. (*australiensis, hawaiiensis, spicifera*)	Meningitis, sinusitis, keratitis, peritonitis, endocarditis, disseminated infection	+++	[5, 6, 38, 46, 51, 52, 75–78, 128]
Chaetomium spp. (*altrobrunneum*); *Achaetomium* spp. (*strumarium*)	Fungemia, cutaneous, brain abscess	+	[70]
Cladophialophora spp. (*bantiana, carrionii*)	Chromoblastomycosis, brain abscess	++	[5, 29, 48, 49, 61, 62, 129–131]
Cladosporium spp.	Colonizer, skin, keratitis	+	[5, 14, 61]
Coniothyrium spp. (*fuckelii*)	Cutaneous, liver infection	+	[6]
Curvularia spp. (*lunata*)	Sinusitis, keratitis, endocarditis, subcutaneous cyst, pneumonitis	+++	[5, 40, 50, 80–84]
Exophiala spp.(*jeanselmei*)	Subcutaneous cyst, eumycetoma, keratitis, meningitis/brain abscess, disseminated infection, peritonitis	++	[5, 8, 41, 85, 86, 98, 112]
Exserohilum spp. (*rostratum*)	Sinusitis, cutaneous, subcutaneous cyst, keratitis	+	[5, 38]
Fonsecaea spp. (*pedrosoi, monophora*)	Chromoblastomycosis, eumycetoma, pneumonitis	++	[5, 6, 87]
Lasiodiplodia spp. (*theobromae*)	Keratitis	+	[70]
Lecythophora spp. (*hoffmannii*)	Subcutaneous cyst, endocarditis, peritonitis	+	[17, 70]
Ochroconis spp. (*gallopava*)	Brain abscess, disseminated infection, pneumonitis	++	[5, 11, 49, 62, 64]
Phaeoacremonium spp. (*parasiticum*)	Cutaneous, subcutaneous cyst	+	[5]
Phaeoannellomyces spp. (*elegans, werneckii*)	Subcutaneous cyst	+	[70]
Phialemonium spp. (*curvatum, obovatum*)	Subcutaneous cyst, endocarditis, peritonitis	+	[9, 70]
Phialophora spp. (*verrucosa, richardsiae*)	Chromoblastomycosis, eumycetoma, keratitis, osteomyelitis, endocarditis	++	[5, 6]
Phoma spp.	Sinusitis, keratitis, subcutaneous cyst	+	[70]
Pseudallescheria spp. (*boydii*)	Eumycetoma, meningitis, pneumonitis, fungemia, disseminated infection		[56, 63, 68, 92]
Rhinocladiella spp. (*obovoidea, mackenziei*)	Brain abscess	+	[49, 62, 65, 68, 98]
Rhinocladiella spp. (*aquaspersa, atrovirens*)	Colonizer, chromoblastomycosis, meningitis	++	[6, 15, 89]
Scedosporium spp. (*apiospermum, aurantiacum, prolificans*)	Eumycetoma, meningitis, pneumonitis, fungemia, disseminated infection	+++	[55, 66–68, 92–94, 97, 114–118]
Scytalidium spp. (*dimidiatum*)	Cutaneous, nail, subcutaneous cyst	+	[17, 70]
Wangiella spp. (*dermatitidis*)	Cutaneous, subcutaneous cyst, keratitis, brain abscess, arthritis, disseminated infection	+++	[5, 28, 53, 62, 95, 96, 132]

+ Least common; +++ most common

Cladophialophora Species

Species of this genus have undergone several taxonomic changes over the last few decades, leading to confusion in the clinical literature. For instance, *Cladophialophora bantiana* had previously been named *Cladosporium trichoides*, *Cladosporium bantianum,* and *Xylohypha bantiana*. Despite controversy regarding the taxonomy, there is no clinical confusion about the ability of *C. bantiana* to cause central nervous system infection [49, 62]. Dozens of cases of cerebral phaeohyphomycosis have been reported, making *C. bantiana* the most common dematiaceous mould to cause central nervous system infection (Fig. 4). Occasionally, *C. bantiana* causes soft tissue infection. Another species, *C. carrioni*, is a leading cause of chromoblastomycosis in Africa and Australia [79].

Cladosporium Species

The vast majority of clinical isolates of this genus represent colonization of nonsterile body sites [5]. Furthermore, *C. cladosporioides* and *C. sphaerospermum* are among the most common dematiaceous mould contaminants in the clinical microbiology laboratory. In order to conclude with certainty

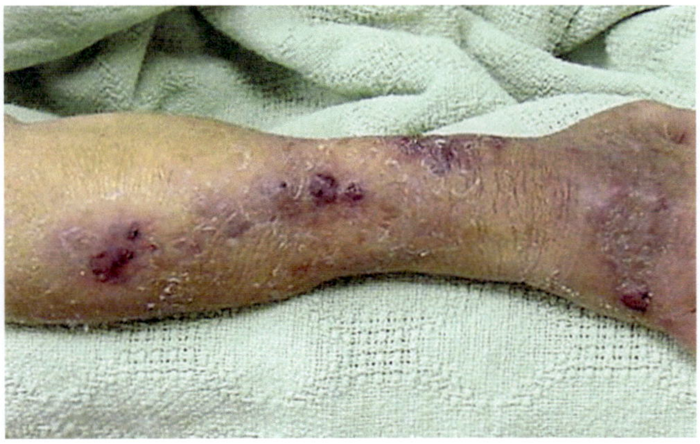

Fig. 3 *Alternaria alternata* skin and subcutaneous infection of the forearm in a renal transplant recipient

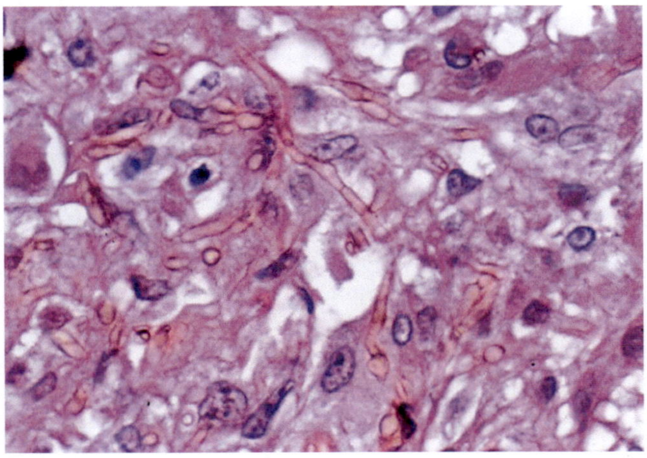

Fig. 4 Hematoxylin and eosin stain of brain tissue showing *Cladophialophora bantiana* showing light brown pigmented hyphae

that infection is attributable to *Cladosporium* species, there should be evidence of infection by direct microscopy, as well as a pure culture of the fungus, preferably obtained from a sterile body site.

Curvularia Species

Species of this genus are leading causes of dematiaceous fungal sinusitis and keratitis but, like *Bipolaris* species, they also can produce other infection, such as soft tissue infections, endocarditis, and disseminated disease [50, 80–84]. The most common species associated with clinical disease is *C. lunata*.

Exophiala Species

Species of this genus are a leading cause of subcutaneous phaeohyphomycosis, but they can also cause peritonitis in patients on chronic peritoneal dialysis, endocarditis, meningitis, and brain abscess [41, 85, 86]. *E. jeanselmei* is the major species producing clinical disease.

Fonsecaea Species

F. pedrosoi historically has been regarded is the most common cause worldwide of chromoblastomycosis [79]. Occasionally, this species can cause invasive infection in severely immunosuppressed patients [87]. Because of the pleomorphic structures of *F. pedrosoi*, it may be confused with *Rhinocladiella* and *Phialophora* species in culture; thus, specimens need careful mycologic evaluation [6]. Based on molecular methods, *F. pedrosoi* recently was determined to consist of three species: *F. pedrosoi, F. monophora,* and an as yet unnamed species. Clinically significant isolates appear to be evenly dispersed among the three species [88].

Phialophora Species

Species of this genus can produce a wide variety of infections ranging from chromoblastomycosis to opportunistic infections in AIDS patients and organ transplant recipients [5, 6]. Two of the most common species to infect humans are *P. verrucosa* and *P. richardsiae*.

Rhinocladiella Species

Species regularly identified in the clinical laboratory are *Rhinocladiella atrovirens* and *R. mackenziei*. Because it can colonize nonsterile sites or appear in cultures as a contaminant, *R. atrovirens* requires other confirmatory studies, such as histopathology, to support its significance when isolated from a nonsterile site. Although *R. atrovirens* has very little virulence potential, it has produced meningitis in severely immunosuppressed patients, and there is one reported case of eumycetoma caused by this organism [15, 89]. *Ramichloridium mackenziei* recently was reclassified as *Rhinocladiella mackenziei*. At least 19 brain infections have been reported due to *R.. mackenziei* [49, 62, 65].

Scedosporium Species and *Pseudallescheria boydii*

Historically, *Scedosporium apiospermum* and *Pseudallescheria boydii* have been regarded as having an anamorph–teleomorph connection. However, this has been disproved based on nucleic acid sequence analysis, primarily of the β-tubulin gene, and clinical isolates now have been recharacterized as belonging mainly to three distinct species, namely,

Pseudallescheria boydii, Scedosporium apiospermum, and *S. aurantiacum* [56, 90, 91]. Some mycologists have suggested these organisms be regarded as dematiaceous fungi because their colonies vary from smoky gray to dark brown in color. However, consensus places diseases caused by the species within the hyalohyphomycoses or hyaline moulds. Thus, for a detailed discussion of these infections, see the Chapter on hyaline moulds.

Clinical syndromes caused by these species incude disseminated disease, including central nervous system involvement, in patients with diabetes, those receiving corticosteroids, and near-drowning victims [92]. Eumycetoma are more common than disseminated infections. Relatively few clinical isolates have been reidentified using the combined approach of molecular and morphologic data analysis. Re-examination of 11 isolates from near-drowning victims found 8 were *S. apiospermum,* 2 were *S. aurantiacum,* and 1 was *P. boydii.* Antifungal susceptibility testing of these 11 isolates showed no species-specific pattern [56]. The common occurrence of *S. apiospermum* in the environment and the frequent use of empirical polyene drugs against which this fungus exhibits clinical resistance has enabled *S. apiospermum* to become an emerging pathogen in severely immunosuppressed patients. *Scedosporium prolificans* is another emerging pathogen [93, 94]. In addition to eumycetoma, it causes a range of infections similar to those of *S. apiospermum.* In patients with disseminated disease secondary to *S. prolificans*, blood cultures are likely to be positive, probably due to the ability of this species to form unicellular spores within the lumen of invaded blood vessels [58, 60]. Disseminated infection due to *S. prolificans* is frequently fatal, as this organism is resistant to most currently available antifungal agents.

Wangiella Species

Wangiella (*Exophiala*) dermatitidis can cause localized infection of skin, subcutaneous tissue, and also systemic infection involving the brain, joints, and eye [49, 53, 62, 95, 96]. Among the dematiaceous fungi, *W. dermatitidis* probably is the best-studied pathogen with respect to its molecular biology, animal model experimentation, and virulence factors.

Diagnosis

Unfortunately, there are no available serologic tests to diagnose infection with these fungi. Detection of infection due to dematiaceous fungi depends on direct microscopic examination of specimens as well as fungal culture. Tissue histopathology seen with phaeohyphomycosis is characteristic. The causative fungi can produce several morphologies in the tissue, including budding yeast-like forms, pseudohyphae, moniliform hyphae, true hyphae, enlarged subglobose cells, or various combinations of these forms. Routine stains, such as hematoxylin and eosin, are usually adequate for detecting dematiaceous fungi, as the intrinsic brown color of cells can be detected. However, not all dematiaceous fungal structures appear brown in tissue with the hematoxylin and eosin stain. Species of the genera *Alternaria*, *Bipolaris*, and *Curvularia* often appear to be hyaline in tissue due to a paucity of melanin formation in vivo: the dematiaceous nature of these species is evident when grown in culture. The methenamine silver stain can be more sensitive than the hematoxylin and eosin stain, but the silver stain also obscures the intrinsic color of the pathogen. The presence of melanin within the fungus in tissue specimens can be confirmed by use of the Fontana-Masson stain. Other fungi, such as *Aspergillus fumigatus* and *Coccidioides* species, occasionally stain with Fontana-Masson stain but less uniformly than dematiaceous moulds.

Dematiaceous fungi can occur as contaminants of body surfaces and/or clinical specimens. In order to document infection, material for culture and direct examination should be obtained from sterile body sites or from tissue in which histopathology confirms fungal invasion. The calcofluor-KOH procedure is relatively quick and extremely helpful in detecting the presence of fungi in specimens, although it should be noted it is not reliable for detecting the heavily melanized cells found in chromoblastomycosis. Specimens must not be allowed to become desiccated prior to processing for culture, and tissue specimens should be minced rather than homogenized and then placed onto media. Standard fungal media will support growth of these fungi. Some dematiaceous fungi will be inhibited by cycloheximide; therefore a culture plate without this inhibitor should also be used. Blood cultures may be positive in cases of disseminated disease with *Scedosporium* species, notably *S. prolificans* [97]. In addition, *Exophiala* and *Rhinocladiella* species have also been recovered from blood during nosocomial outbreaks characterized by fungemia [98].

The identification of dematiaceous fungi to genus and species levels traditionally is determined by macroscopic and microscopic morphology, supplemented by temperature tolerance testing in some cases [5, 6]. Increasingly, nucleic sequence analysis is being used, and the ideal approach is to combine molecular and morphocentric data in the identification process [56, 88–91, 99]. Though the details for identification of each specific dematiaceous fungus producing human disease are beyond the scope of this chapter, it is important to recognize that proper identification is important, and expert mycologic input may be necessary. Correct identification of genus and, in many cases, species can help establish the clinical significance of a given isolate, predict the extent of infection and the prognosis, and may help predict the drug susceptibility pattern and thus the choice of an appropriate antifungal agent. Unfortunately, correct identification can require expertise that often is not readily available. Though molecular methods hold promise for improving accuracy of laboratory identification of moulds, at this time, identifications in the great majority of clinical laboratories continue to be based almost exclusively on morphologic study of macroscopic and microscopic features.

Treatment

With regard to the treatment of phaeohyphomycosis, the majority of clinical experience represents isolated cases or small series of infections with multiple different fungi. While evidence-based algorithms for treatment are not robust, there are several surgical and medical strategies that should be considered.

Surgical Measures

Surgery is an integral part of any treatment strategy. In soft tissue infections, the surgical approach varies. Best results for an ulcerative lesion of the skin or soft tissue without a defined cyst are obtained with careful debridement and even use of Mohs-type micrographic surgery, a procedure in which infected tissues are excised at a 45-degree angle with subsequent identification of residual infection using light microscopy. This method provides histologic control of the surgical margins and helps achieve a low recurrence rate with maximal preservation of uninvolved tissue [100]. With surgery, lavage of residual tissue after surgery with an antiseptic agent is probably helpful, since fungal organisms might remain in the wound. For a subcutaneous cyst, complete removal of the encapsulated structure can be curative, but care must be taken not to leak contents into the wound. Simple aspiration of cyst fluid is not optimal.

For a single brain abscess, surgical debridement with adjunctive medical therapy is recommended for cure [101]. While complete surgical removal of a brain abscess may not be possible, even partial debulking of the brain mass is helpful. Occasionally, infection may be spread with surgery, but this is not a primary concern when patients are receiving antifungal agents [102]. Although medical treatment of brain abscesses alone occasionally has been successful, there are many reported failures without a combined medical–surgical therapeutic approach [11]. Medical treatment only should be reserved for patients with multiple abscesses and for patients in whom surgery is contraindicated.

In cases of sinus disease eumycetoma, removal of the fungal mass through endoscopy may be curative [103]. True eumycetoma in the extremities can be indolent and difficult to manage. Because of chronic scarring, fistula formation in soft tissue, and possible bone involvement, obtaining disease-free margins via surgery is difficult. In these circumstances, medical therapy may be the best option.

Antifungal Agents

Antifungal drugs have been used in the management of phaeohyphomycosis, based on in vitro and in vivo evidence for antifungal drug activity [104–107]. While it is beyond the scope of this chapter to detail the antifungal activity against each genus and species, several general comments on medical therapy are in order. Polyene drugs show modest antifungal activity in vitro against dematiaceous fungi and have been used in the treatment of some disseminated infections. However, polyenes are not consistently used as primary therapy for these infections. Flucytosine has in vitro antifungal activity against several dematiaceous fungi, but should be used in combination with other agents because of rapid development of drug resistance when used alone.

The azole drugs are commonly chosen in treatment strategies for phaeohyphomycosis because these agents exhibit moderate-to-excellent in vitro antifungal activity against dematiaceous fungi and can be given safely for prolonged periods. Among the older azoles, itraconazole has been best-studied, with a reported success rate of over 60% in one series [108]. The newer triazoles – voriconazole and posaconazole – have moderate to excellent in vitro activity against dematiaceous moulds and are thus promising drugs for treatment of phaeohyphomycoses [104–106, 109]. In fact, most dematiaceous fungal infections in single case reports or small series have responded to these triazoles [110–112]. In an animal model of cerebral *Rhinocladiella* infection, posaconazole was found to be more effective than itraconazole or amphotericin B [113].

Disease caused by *Scedosporium apiospermum, S. aurantiacum,* and *Pseudallescheria boydii*, which are resistant to amphotericin B, frequently responds to the newer triazoles such as voriconazole or posaconazole; in some cases these azoles have enabled dramatic clinical recoveries and have much better responses to treatment than *Scedosporium prolificans* [114–116]. On the other hand, *Scedosporium prolificans* appears to be resistant to most classes of available antifungal drugs and only occasionally responds to the extended-spectrum triazoles [116, 117]. The outcome in cases of disseminated disease is very poor, and this is particularly relevant among patients with hematologic malignancy [118]. Combinations of drugs have been tested for use against this fungus, but the clinical relevance of this approach remains unclear. It is likely that these extended-spectrum triazoles will become first-line therapy for phaeohyphomycosis.

Terbinafine, with or without an azole, remains an uncertain treatment for phaeohyphomycoses [13, 119], and the decision to use this agent should probably be guided by the results of in vitro susceptibility testing on a specific isolate. The echinocandins, which inhibit the synthesis of 1,3-beta-D-glucan that is crucial to fungal cell wall integrity, have inhibitory in vitro activity against many dematiaceous fungi [106, 120, 121], but there has been no significant clinical experience with these agents. If used, the echinocandins would probably be part of a combination antifungal drug strategy. Drug combinations in vitro commonly show additive or synergistic activity against these fungi [13, 107, 122]. However, there are no controlled clinical data to support the use of combination therapy. Until such studies are performed, two or three drug combinations, such as polyene, flucytosine, terbinafine, and/or a triazole, should be reserved for disseminated or intracranial disease with limited surgical options.

Adjunctive Measures

Immune modulation has been considered for treatment of some phaeohyphomycoses. In allergic fungal sinusitis, corticosteroids are used to decrease immune stimulation. Additionally, immunotherapy has been advocated by some experts in an attempt to decrease the allergic reaction to fungal antigens, but the precise value of this therapy remains unclear [123]. In patients with invasive dematiaceous fungal infections, control of the underlying disease and decreasing immunosuppression are important. Decreasing the dosage of corticosteroids and using agents to increase neutrophil counts should be a primary focus of management.

Another important aspect of treatment relates to the use of antifungal susceptibility tests. There is now an approved standardized method for performing in vitro antifungal susceptibility testing against the dematiaceous moulds, and work is ongoing to expand and refine its application [124–127]. In certain unique infections with dematiaceous fungi, an assessment of the in vitro antifungal activity of potentially useful antifungal agents may be useful.

References

1. Ajello L, Georg LK, Steigbigel RT. A case of phaeohyphomycosis caused by a new species of *Phialophora*. Mycologia. 1974;66:490–8.
2. Fader RC, McGinnis MR. Infections caused by dematiaceous fungi: chromoblastomycosis and phaeohyphomycosis. Infect Dis Clin North Am. 1988;2:925–38.
3. Rinaldi MG. Phaeohyphomycosis. Dermatol Clin. 1996;14:142–53.
4. de Hoog GS, Guarroe J, Gene J, Figueras MJ. Atlas of Clinical Fungi. 2nd ed. Utrecht: Centaalbureau voor Schimmelcultures; 2000.
5. Schell WA. Dematiaceous Hyphomycetes. In: Howard DH, editor. Fungi Pathogenic for Humans and Animals, revised and expanded. 2nd ed. New York: Marcel Dekker; 2003. p. 565–636.
6. Schell WA, Salkin IF, McGinnis JR. *Bipolaris*, *Exophiala*, *Scedosporium*, *Sporothrix* and other dematiaceous fungi. In: Murray PR, Baron EJ, Jorgensen JH, Pfaller MA, Yolken RH, editors. Manual of Clinical Microbiology. 8th ed. Washington: American Society for Microbiology; 2003. p. 1820–47.
7. Ferguson BJ, Barnes L, Bernstein JM, et al. Geographical variation in allergic fungal rhinosinusitis. Otolaryngol Clin North Am. 2000;33:441–9.
8. MMWR. *Exophiala* infection from contaminated injectable steroids prepared by a compounding pharmacy – United States, July–November, 2002. Morbidity and Mortality Weekly Report MMWR 2002;51:1109–1112.
9. Rao CY, Pachucki C, Cali S, et al. Contaminated product water as the source of *Phialemonium curvatum* bloodstream infection among patients undergoing hemodialysis. Infect Control Hosp Epidemiol. 2009;30:840–7.
10. Welty KE, Perfect JR. Cutaneous mycoses in solid organ transplants. Clin Adv Treat Fungal Infect. 1991;2:1–23.
11. Vukmir RB, Kusne S, Linden P, et al. Successful therapy for cerebral phaeohyphomycosis due to *Dactylaria gallopava* in a liver transplant recipient. Clin Infect Dis. 1994;19:714–9.
12. Singh N, Chang FY, Gayowski T, Marino IR. Infections due to dematiaceous fungi in organ transplant recipients: case report and review. Clin Infect Dis. 1997;24:369–74.
13. Clancy CJ, Wingard JR, Nguyen MH. Subcutaneous phaeohyphomycosis in transplant recipients: review of the literature and demonstration of in vitro synergy between antifungal agents. Med Mycol. 2000;38:169–75.
14. Ben-Ami R, Lewis RE, Raad II, Kontoyiannis DP. Phaeohyphomycosis in a tertiary care center. Clin Infect Dis. 2009;48:1033–41.
15. del Palacio-Hernanz A, Moore MK, Campbell CK, del Palacio-Perez-Medel A, del Castillo-Cantero R. Infection of the central nervous system by *Rhinocladiella atrovirens* in a patient with acquired immunodeficiency syndrome. J Med Vet Mycol. 1989;27:127–30.
16. Perfect JR, Schell WA, Rinaldi MG. Uncommon invasive fungal pathogens in the acquired immunodeficiency syndrome. J Med Vet Mycol. 1993;31:175–9.
17. Marriott DJ, Wong KH, Aznar E. *Scytalidium dimidiatum* and *Lecythophora hoffmannii*: unusual causes of fungal infections in a patient with AIDS. J Clin Microbiol. 1997;35:2949–52.
18. Dixon DM, Polak A, Conner GW. Mel-mutants of *Wangiella dermatitidis* in mice: evaluation of multiple mouse and fungal strains. J Med Vet Mycol. 1989;27:335–41.
19. Dixon DM, Migliozzi J, Cooper Jr CR, Solis O, Breslin B, Szaniszlo PJ. Melanized and non-melanized multicellular form mutants of *Wangiella dermatitidis* in mice: mortality and histopathology studies. Mycoses. 1992;35:17–21.
20. Feng B, Wang X, Hauser M, et al. Molecular cloning and characterization of WdPks1, a gene involved in dihydroxynaphthalene melanin biosynthesis and virulence in *Wangiella* (*Exophiala*) *dermatitidis*. Infect Immun. 2001;69:1781–94.
21. Schnitzler N, Peltroche-Llacsahuanga H, Bestier N, Zundorf J, Lutticken R, Haase G. Effect of melanin and carotenoids of *Exophiala* (*Wangiella*) *dermatitidis* on phagocytosis, oxidative burst, and killing by human neutrophils. Infect Immun. 1999;67:94–101.
22. Wang Z, Zheng L, Liu H, Wang Q, Hauser M, Kauffman S, et al. WdChs2p, a class I chitin synthase, together with WdChs3p class III contributes to virulence in *Wangiella* (*Exophiala*) dermatitidis. Infect Immun. 2001;69:7517–26.
23. Ibrahim-Granet O, de Bievre C, Jendoubi M. Immunochemical characterisation of antigens and growth inhibition of *Fonsecaea pedrosoi* by species-specific IgG. J Med Microbiol. 1988;26:217–22.

24. Fuchs J, Pecher S. Partial suppression of cell mediated immunity in chromoblastomycosis. Mycopathologia. 1992;119:73–6.
25. Perfect JR, Schell WA. The newer fungal opportunists are coming. Clin Infect Dis. 1996;22:112–8.
26. Silveira F, Nucci M. Emergence of black moulds in fungal disease: epidemiology and therapy. Curr Opin Infect Dis. 2001;14:679–84.
27. Benedict LA, Kusne S, Torre-Cisneros J, Hunt SJ. Primary cutaneous fungal infection after solid-organ transplantation. Clin Infect Dis. 1993;15:17–21.
28. Vartian CV, Shlaes DM, Padhye AA, Ajello L. *Wangiella dermatitidis* endocarditis in an intravenous drug user. Am J Med. 1985;78:703–7.
29. Walz R, Bianchin M, Chaves ML, Cerski MR, Severo LC, Londero AT. Cerebral phaeohyphomycosis caused by *Cladophialophora bantiana* in a Brazilian drug abuser. J Med Vet Mycol. 1997;35:427–31.
30. Kaufman SM. Curvularia endocarditis following cardiac surgery. Am J Clin Pathol. 1971;56:466–70.
31. Pauzner R, Goldschmied-Reouven A, Hay I, Vared Z, Ziskind Z, Hassin N, et al. Phaeohyphomycosis following cardiac surgery: case report and review of serious infection due to *Bipolaris* and *Exserohilum* species. Clin Infect Dis. 1997;25:921–3.
32. Revankar SG, Patterson JE, Sutton DA, Pullen R, Rinaldi MG. Disseminated phaeohyphomycosis: review of an emerging mycosis. Clin Infect Dis. 2002;34:467–76.
33. Kerr C, Perfect JR, Gallis HA, Craven PC, Drutz DJ, Shelburne J, et al. Fungal peritonitis in patients on chronic ambulatory peritoneal dialysis. Ann Intern Med. 1983;99:334–7.
34. Schwartz RA. Superficial fungal infections. Lancet. 2004; 364:1173–82.
35. Ronan SG, Vzoaru I, Nadimpalli V, Guitart J, Manaligod JR. Primary cutaneous phaeohyphomycosis: report of seven cases. J Cutan Pathol. 1993;20:223–8.
36. Forster RK, Rebell G, Wilson LA. Dematiaceous fungal keratitis: clinical isolates and management. Br J Ophthalmol. 1975;59:372–6.
37. Schell WA. Oculomycoses caused by dematiaceous fungi. Proceedings of the VI International Conference on the Mycoses. Pan American Health Organization, Washington: Scientific Publication No. 470. 1986, pp105–109.
38. McGinnis MR, Rinaldi MG, Winn RE. Emerging agents of phaeohyphomycosis: pathogenic species of *Bipolaris* and *Exserohilum*. J Clin Microbiol. 1986;24:250–9.
39. Thomas RA. Current perspectives on ophthalmic mycoses. Clin Microbiol Rev. 2003;16:730–97.
40. Wilhemus KR, Jones DB. *Curvularia* keratitis. Trans Am Ophthalmol Soc. 2001;99:111–30.
41. Sudduth EJ, Crumbley AJ, Farrar WE. Phaeohyphomycosis due to *Exophiala* species: clinical spectrum of disease in humans. Clin Infect Dis. 1992;15:639–44.
42. Schell WA. Histopathology of fungal rhinosinusitis. Otolaryngol Clin N Am. 2000;33:251–76.
43. Corey JR, Delsupeke KG, Ferguson BJ. Allergic fungal sinusitis: allergic, infectious or both? Otolaryngol Head Neck Surg. 1995;113:110–9.
44. Washburn RG, Kennedy DW, Begley MG, Henderson DK, Bennett JE. Chronic fungal sinusitis in apparently normal hosts. Medicine (Baltimore). 1988;67:231–47.
45. MacMillan III RH, Cooper PH, Body BA, Mills AS. Allergic fungal sinusitis due to *Curvularia lunata*. Hum Pathol. 1987;18:960–4.
46. Gourley DS, Whisman BA, Jorgensen NL, Martin ME, Reid MJ. Allergic *Bipolaris* sinusitis: clinical and immunopathologic characteristics. J Allergy Clin Immunol. 1990;85:583–91.
47. Schell WA. Unusual fungal pathogens in fungal sinusitis. Otolaryngol Clin North Am. 2000;33:367–73.
48. Palaoglu S, Sau A, Yalcinlar Y, Scheithauer BW. Cerebral phaeohyphomycosis. Neurosurgery. 1993;33:894–7.
49. Horre R, de Hoog GS. Primary cerebral infections by melanized fungi: a review. In: de Horre GS, editor. Studies in Mycology #43: Ecology and Evolution of Black Yeasts and Their Relatives. Baarn: Centralbureau Voor Schimmel; 1999. p. 176–93.
50. Rohwedder JJ, Simmons JL, Colfer H, Gatmaitan B. Disseminated *Curvularia lunata* infection in a football player. Arch Intern Med. 1979;139:940–1.
51. Flanagan KL, Bryceson AD. Disseminated infection due to *Bipolaris australiensis* in a young immunocompetent man: case report and review. Clin Infect Dis. 1997;25:311–3.
52. Khan JA, Hussain ST, Hasan S. Disseminated *Bipolaris* infection in an immunocompetent host: an atypical presentation. J Am Med Assoc. 2002;50:68–71.
53. Li DM, de Hoog GS. Cerebral phaeohyphomycosis: at cure at what lengths? Lancet Infect Dis. 2009;9:376–83.
54. Marr KA, Carter RA, Crippa RA, Wald A, Corey L. Epidemiology and outcome of mould infections in hematopoietic stem cell transplant recipients. Clin Infect Dis. 2002;34:909–17.
55. Marco de Lucas E, Sádaba P, Lastra García-Barón P, et al. Cerebral scedosporiosis: an emerging fungal infection in severe neutropenic patients: CT features and CT pathologic correlation. Eur Radiol. 2005;16:496–502.
56. Tintelnot K, Wagner N, Seibold M, de Hoog GS, Horré R. Re-identification of clinical isolates of the *Pseudallescheria boydii*-complex involved in near-drowning. Mycoses. 2008;51 Suppl 3:11–6.
57. Husain S, Alexander BD, Munoz P, et al. Opportunistic mycelial fungal infections in organ transplant recipients: emerging importance of non-*Aspergillus* mycelial fungi. Clin Infect Dis. 2003;37:221–9.
58. Schell WA. New aspects of emerging fungal pathogens. A multifaceted challenge. Clin Lab Med. 1995;15:365–87.
59. Schell WA, Perfect JR. Fatal, disseminated *Acremonium strictum* infection in a neutropenic host. J Clin Microbiol. 1996;34:1333–6.
60. Liu K, Howell DN, Perfect JR, Schell WA. Morphologic criteria for the preliminary identification of *Fusarium*, *Paecilomyces*, and *Acremonium* species by histopathology. Am J Clin Pathol. 1998;109:45–54.
61. Bennett JE, Bonner H, Jennings AE, Lopez RI. Chronic meningitis caused by *Cladosporium trichoides*. Am J Clin Pathol. 1973;59:398–407.
62. Kantarcioglu AS, de Hoog GS. Infections of the central nervous system by melanized fungi: a review of cases presented between 1999 and 2004. Mycoses. 2004;47:4–13.
63. Georg LK, Bierer BW, Cooke WB. Encephalitis in turkey poults due to a new fungus species. Sabouraudia. 1964;3:239–44.
64. Sides EH, Benson JD, Padhye AA. Phaeohyphomycotic brain abscess due to *Ochroconis gallopavum* in a patient with malignant lymphoma of a large cell type. J Med Vet Mycol. 1991;29:317–22.
65. Kanj SS, Amr SS, Roberts GD. *Ramichloridium mackenziei* brain abscess: report of two cases and review of the literature. Med Mycol. 2001;39:97–102.
66. Watanabe S, Hironaga M. An atypical isolate of *Scedoporium apiospermum* from a purulent meningitis in man. Sabouraudia. 1981;19:209–15.
67. Yoo D, Lee WHS, Kwon-Chung KJ. Brain abscess due to *Pseudallescheria boydii* associated with primary non-Hodgkin's lymphoma of the central nervous system: a case report and literature review. Rev Infect Dis. 1985;7:272–7.
68. Dworzack DL, Clark RB, Padgett PJ. New causes of pneumonia, meningitis, and disseminated infections associated with immersion. Infect Control Hosp Epidemiol. 1987;1:615–33.
69. Perfect JR, Durack DT. Pathogenesis and management of fungal infections in the central nervous system. In: Scheld WM, Whitley RJ, Durack DT, editors. Infections of the Central Nervous System. New York: Lippincott-Raven; 1997. p. pp 21–738.
70. Sigler L. Miscellaneous opportunistic fungi: microascaceae and other ascomycetes, hyphomycetes, coelomycetes and basidiomycetes. In: Howard DH, editor. Fungi Pathogenic for Humans and

Animals, revised and expanded. 2nd ed. New York: Marcel Dekker; 2003. p. 637–76.

71. Viviani MA, Tortorano AM, Laria G, Giannetti A, Bignotti G. Two new cases of cutaneous alternariosis with a review of the literature. Mycopathologia. 1986;96:3–12.
72. Wiest PM, Wiese K, Jacobs MR, et al. *Alternaria* infection in a patient with acquired immune deficiency syndrome: case report and review of invasive *Alternaria* infections. Rev Infect Dis. 1987;9:799–803.
73. Pastor FJ, Guarro J. *Alternaria* infections: laboratory diagnosis and relevant clinical features. Clin Microbiol Infect. 2008;14:734–46.
74. Morrison VA, Weisdorf DJ. *Alternaria*: a sinonasal pathogen of immunocompressed hosts. Clin Infect Dis. 1993;16:265–70.
75. Rolston KV, Hopfer RL, Larson DL. Infections caused by *Drechslera* species: case report and review of the literature. Rev Infect Dis. 1985;7:525–9.
76. Adam RD, Paquin ML, Peterson EA. Phaeohyphomycosis caused by the fungal genera *Bipolaris* and *Exserohilum*. A report of 9 cases and review of the literature. Medicine (Baltimore). 1986;65:203–17.
77. Karim M, Sheikh H, Alam M, Sheikh Y. Disseminated *Bipolaris* infection in an asthmatic patient: case report. Clin Infect Dis. 1993;17:248–53.
78. Latham RH. *Bipolaris spicifera* meningitis complicating a neurosurgical procedure. Scand J Infect Dis. 2000;32:102–3.
79. Schell WA, Esterre P. Chromoblastomycosis. In: Merz WG, Hay R, editors. Topley and Wilson's Microbiology and Microbial Infections, Medical Mycology. 10th ed. London: Edward Arnold; 2005. p. 356–66.
80. Monte SMD, Hutchens GM. Disseminated *Curvularia* infection. Arch Pathol Lab Med. 1985;109:872–4.
81. Yau YC, de Nanassy J, Summerbell RC, Matlow AG, Richardson SE. Fungal sternal wound infection due to *Curvularia lunata* in a neonate with congenital heart disease: case report and review. Clin Infect Dis. 1994;19:735–40.
82. Fernandez M, Noyola DE, Rosemann SN, Edwards MS. Cutaneous phaeohyphomycosis caused by *Curvularia lunata* and a review of *Curvularia* infections in pediatrics. Pediatr Infect Dis J. 1999; 18:727–31.
83. Janaki C, Sentamilselvi G, Janaki VR, Devesh S, Ajithados K. Eumycetoma due to *Curvularia lunata*. Mycoses. 1999;2:345–6.
84. Carter E, Boudreaux C. Fatal cerebral phaeohyphomycosis due to *Curvaularia lunata* in an immunocompetent host. J Clin Microbiol. 2004;42:5419–23.
85. Tintelnot K, de Hoog GS, Thomas E, Steudel WI, Huebner K, Seeliger HPR. Cerebral phaeohyphomycosis caused by an *Exophiala* species. Mycoses. 1991;34:239–44.
86. Gold WL, Vellend H, Salit IE, Campbell I, Summerbell R, Rinaldi M, et al. Successful treatment of systemic and local infections due to *Exophiala* species. Clin Infect Dis. 1994;19:339–41.
87. Morris A, Schell WA, McDonagh D, Chafee S, Perfect JR. *Fonsecaea pedrosoi* pneumonia and Emericella nidulans cerebral abscesses in a bone marrow transplant patient. Clin Infect Dis. 1995;21:1346–8.
88. Najafzadeh MJ, Gueidan C, Badali H, Gerrits van den Ende AHG, Lian X, de Hoog GS. Genetic diversity and species delimitation in the opportunistic genus *Fonsecaea*. Med Mycol. 2009;47:17–25.
89. Ndiaye B, Develoux M, Dieng MT, Kane A, Ndir O, Raphenon G, et al. Current report of eumycetoma in Senegal: report of 109 cases. J Mycol Med. 2000;10:140–4.
90. Gilgado F, Cano J, Gene J, Guarro J. Molecular phylogeny of the *Pseudallescheria boydii* species complex: proposal of two new species. J Clin Microbiol. 2005;43:4930–42.
91. Gilgado F, Cano J, Gene J, Sutton DA, Guarro J. Molecular and phenotypic data supporting distinct species statuses for *Scedosporium apiospermum* and *Pseudallescheria boydii* and the proposed new species *Scedosporium dehoogii*. J Clin Microbiol. 2008;46:766–71.
92. Berenguer J, Diaz-Mediavilla J, Urra D, Munoz P. Central nervous system infection caused by *Pseudallescheria boydii*: case report and review. Rev Infect Dis. 1989;11:890–6.
93. Berenguer J, Rodriquez-Tudela JL, Richard C. Deep infections caused by *Scedosporium prolificans*. A report on 16 cases in Spain and a review of the literature. Medicine (Baltimore). 1997;76:256–65.
94. Maertens J, Lagrou K, Deweerdt H. Disseminated infection by *Scedosporium profilicans*: An emerging fatality among haematology patients. Case report and review. Ann Hematol 2001; 79:340-344
95. Hiruma M, Kawada A, Ohata H, Ohnishi Y, Takahashi H, Yamazaki M, et al. Systemic phaeohyphomycosis caused by *Exophiala dermatitidis*. Mycoses. 1993;36:1–7.
96. Matsumoto T, Matsuda T, McGinnis MR, Ajello L. Clinical and mycological spectra of *Wangiella dermatitidis* infection. Mycoses. 1992;36:145–55.
97. Husain S, Munoz P, Forrest G, Alexander BD, Somani J, Brennan K, et al. Infections due to *Scedosporium apiospermum* and *Scedosporium prolificans* in transplant recipients: clinical characteristics and impact of antifungal agent therapy on outcome. Clin Infect Dis. 2005;40:89–99.
98. Nucci M, Akiti T, Barreiros G, Silveira F, Revankar SG, Sutton DA, et al. Nosocomial fungemia due to *Exophiala jeanselmei* var. *jeanselmei* and *Rhinocladiella* species newly described causes of bloodstream infection. J Clin Microbiol. 2001;39:514–8.
99. Gerrits van den Ende AHG, de Hoog GS. Variability and molecular diagnostics of the neyurotropic species *Cladophialophoraa bantiana.* Studies in Mycology 43: Ecology and Evolution of Black Yeasts and Their Relatives. Baarn/Delft, The Netherlands: Centralbureau Voor Schimmel. 1999, pp 151–162.
100. Heinz T, Serafin DB, Schell WA, Perfect JR. Soft tissue fungal infections: surgical management of 12 immunocompromised patients. Plast Reconstr Surg. 1996;97:1391–9.
101. Revankar SG, Sutton DA, Rinaldi MG. Primary central nervous system phaeohyphomycosis: a review of 101 cases. Clin Infect Dis. 2004;38:206–16.
102. Shimosaka S, Waga S. Cerebral chromoblastomycosis complicated by meningitis and multiple fungal aneurysms after resection of a granuloma. Case Report. J Neurosurg. 1983;59:158–61.
103. Ferguson BJ. Fungus balls of the paranasal sinuses. Otolaryngol Clin North Am. 2000;33:389–98.
104. McGinnis MR, Pasarell RL, Sutton DA. In vitro evaluation of voriconazole against some clinically important fungi. Antimicrob Agents Chemother. 1997;41:1821–34.
105. Espinel-Ingroff A. In vitro activity of the new triazole voriconazole UK 109, 496 against opportunistic filamentous and dimorphic fungi and common and emerging yeast pathogens. J Clin Microbiol. 1998;36:198–202.
106. Espinel-Ingroff A. A comparison of in vitro activities of the new triazole SCH56592 and the echinocandins MK 0991 L-743, 872 and LY303366 against opportunistic filamentous and dimorphic fungi and yeasts. J Clin Microbiol. 1998;36:2950–6.
107. McGinnis MR, Pasarell L. In vitro evaluation of terbinafine and itraconazole against dematiaceous fungi. Med Mycol. 1998;36:243–6.
108. Sharkey PK, Graybill JR, Rinaldi MG, et al. Itraconazole treatment of phaeohyphomycosis. J Am Acad Dermatol. 1990;23:577–86.
109. Fothergill AW, Rinaldi MG, Sutton DA. Antifungal susceptibility testing of *Exophiala* spp.: a head-to-head comparison of amphotericin B, itraconazole, posaconazole and voriconazole. Med Mycol. 2009;47:41–3.
110. Perfect JR, Marr KA, Walsh TJ, et al. Voriconazole treatment for less common, emerging or refractory fungal infections. Clin Infect Dis. 2003;36:112–1131.
111. Negroni R, Tobon A, Bustamante B, Shikanai-Yasuda MA, Patino H, Restrepo A. Posaconazole treatment of refractory eumycetoma

and chromoblastomycosis. Rev Inst Med Trop São Paulo. 2005; 47:339–46.

112. Negroni R, Helou SH, Petri N, Robles Am, Arechavala A, Bianchi MH. Case study: posaconazole treatment of disseminated phaeohyphomycosis due to *Exophiala spinifera*. Clin Infect Dis. 2004;38:e15–20.

113. Al-Abdely HM, Najvar L, Bocanegra R, et al. SCH 56592, amphotericin B, or itraconazole therapy of experimental murine cerebral phaeohyphomycosis due to *Ramichloridium obovoideum* (*Ramichloridium mackenziei*). Antimicrob Agents Chemother. 2000;44:1159–62.

114. Heath Ch, Slavin MA, Sorrell TC, et al. Population-based surveillance for scedosporiosis in Australia: epidemiology, disease manifestations and emergence of *Scedosporium aurantiacum* infection. Clin Microbiol Infect. 2009;15:689–93.

115. Walsh TJ, Lutsar I, Driscoll T, Dupont B, Rhoden M, Gharamani P, et al. Voriconazole in the treatment of aspergillosis, scedosporiosis and other invasive fungal infections in children. Pediatr Infect Dis J. 2002;21:240–8.

116. Troke P, Aquirrebengoak K, Arteaga C, Ellis D, Heath CH, Lutsar I, et al. Treatment of scedosporiosis with voriconazole: clinical experience with 107 patients. Antimicrob Agents Chemother. 2008;52:1743–50.

117. Rodriques-Tudela JL, Berenguer J, Guarro J, Kantarcioglu AS, Horre R, de Hoog GS, et al. Epidemiology and outcome of *Scedosporium prolificans* infection, a review of 162 cases. Med Mycol. 2009;47:359–70.

118. Caira M, Girmenia C, Valentini CG, et al. Scedosporiosis in patients with acute leukemia; a retrospective multicenter report. Haematologica. 2008;93:104–10.

119. Queiroz-Telles F, Esterre P, Perez-Blanco M, Vital RG, Salgado CG, Bonifaz A. Chromoblastomycosis: an overview of clinical manifestations, diagnosis and treatment. Med Mycol. 2009;47:3–15.

120. Del Poeta M, Schell WA, Perfect JR. In vitro antifungal activity of pneumocandin L-743, 872 against a variety of clinically important moulds. Antimicrob Agents Chemother. 1997;41:1835–6.

121. Espinel-Ingroff A. In vitro antifungal activities of anidulafungin and micafungin, licensed agents and the investigational triazole posaconazole as determined by NCCLS methods for 12, 052 fungal isolates: review of the literature. Rev Iberoam Micol. 2003; 20:121–36.

122. Meletiadis J, Mouton JW, Rodriquez-Tudela JL. In vitro interaction of terbinafine with itraconazole against clinical isolates of *Scedosporium prolificans*. Antimicrob Agents Chemother. 2000;44:470–2.

123. Ferguson BJ. What role do systemic corticosteroids, immunotherapy, and antifungal drugs play in the therapy of allergic fungal rhinosinusitis? Arch Otolaryngol Head Neck Surg. 1998;124:1174–8.

124. CLSI. Reference method for broth dilution antifungal susceptibility testing of filamentous fungi; Approved Standard-Second Edition. CLSI document M38-A2. Wayne: Clincal and Laboratory Standards Institute. 2008.

125. Espinel-Ingroff A, Fothergill A, Ghannoum M, et al. Quality control and reference guidelines for CLSI broth microdilution susceptibility method (M38 document) for amphotericin B, itraconazole, posaconazole, and voriconazole. J Clin Microbiol. 2005; 43:5243–6.

126. Espinel-Ingroff A, Fothergill A, Ghannoum M, Manavagthu E, Ostrosky-Zeichner L, Pfaller M, et al. Quality control and Reference Guidelines for CLSI Broth Microdilution Method (M38-A Document) for Susceptibility Testing of Anidulafungin against Molds. J Clin Microbiol. 2007;45:2180–2.

127. Espinel-Ingroff A, Arthington-Skaggs B, Iqbal N, Ellis D, Pfaller MA, Messer S, et al. Multicenter evaluation of a new disk agar diffusion method for susceptibility testing of filamentous fungi with voriconazole, posaconazole, itraconazole, amphotericin B, and caspofungin. J Clin Microbiol. 2007;45:1811–20.

128. Fuste FJ, Ajello L, Threlkeld R, Henry Jr JE. *Drechslera hawaiiensis*: causative agent of a fatal fungal meningo-encephalitis. Sabouraudia. 1973;11:59–63.

129. Seaworth BJ, Kwon-Chung CJ, Hamilton JD, Perfect JR. Brain abscess caused by a variety of *Cladosporium trichoides*. Am J Clin Pathol. 1983;79:747–52.

130. Dixon DM, Walsh TJ, Merz WG, McGinnis MR. Infections due to *Xylohypha bantiana* (*Cladosporium trichoides*). Rev Infect Dis. 1989;11:515–25.

131. Sekhon AS, Galbraith J, Mielke BW, Garg AK, Sheehan G. Cerebral phaeohyphomycosis caused by *Xylohypha bantiana*, with a review of the literature. Eur J Epidemiol. 1992;8:387–90.

132. Greer KE, Gross GP, Cooper PH, Harding SA. Cystic chromomycosis due to *Wangiella dermatitidis*. Arch Dermatol. 1979; 115:1433–4.

Part V
Mycoses Caused by Dimorphic Fungi

Histoplasmosis

Carol A. Kauffman

Histoplasmosis, the most common endemic mycosis in the United States, is caused by *Histoplasma capsulatum* var. *capsulatum*. *Histoplasma capsulatum* var. *duboisii* causes African histoplasmosis, which has different clinical manifestations. *Histoplasma capsulatum* is a thermally dimorphic fungus; in the environment and at temperatures below 35°C, it exists as a mould, and in tissues and at 35–37°C, as a yeast. In the highly endemic area, along the Mississippi and Ohio River valleys in the United States, most persons are infected in childhood. The primary site of infection is the lungs following inhalation of the conidia from the environment. The severity of disease is related to the number of conidia inhaled and the immune response of the host; the primary host defense mechanism against *H. capsulatum* is cell-mediated immunity. Pulmonary infection is asymptomatic or only mildly symptomatic in most persons who have been infected; acute severe pneumonia and chronic progressive pulmonary infection also can occur. Asymptomatic dissemination of *H. capsulatum* to the organs of the reticuloendothelial system occurs in most infected individuals; however, symptomatic acute or chronic disseminated histoplasmosis, which is a life-threatening infection, occurs almost entirely in persons who have deficient cell-mediated immunity. Antifungal therapy is highly effective. For patients with mild-to-moderate histoplasmosis, itraconazole is the treatment of choice; for patients with severe infection, amphotericin B is required.

Organism

Histoplasmosis was first described and the organism given its name in 1904 by Samuel Darling, a physician working at the Canal Zone Hospital in Panama. He erroneously thought the organism, which in tissues resembles *Leishmania*, was a parasite. Within a few years it became clear that this organism was indeed a fungus. Several decades later it was shown that *H. capsulatum* was a thermally dimorphic fungus, and by 1949, an environmental reservoir for *H. capsulatum* had been proved by Emmons.

Two varieties of *H. capsulatum* are pathogenic for humans: *H. capsulatum* var. *capsulatum* and *H. capsulatum* var. *duboisii*. These organisms mate in the laboratory and thus have been assigned varietal, rather than species, status. At 25–30°C, the organism exists in the mycelial form; the colony is white to tan in color. The aerial hyphae produce two types of conidia: Macroconidia (tuberculate conidia) are thick-walled, 8–15 μm in diameter, and have distinctive projections on their surfaces. Microconidia are smooth-walled, 2–4 μm in diameter, and are the infectious form (Fig. 1). *H. capsulatum* var. *capsulatum* and *H. capsulatum* var. *duboisii* are indistinguishable in the mycelial phase.

At 37°C in tissues and in vitro, the organism undergoes transformation to the yeast phase. In vitro, the colony is cream-colored and becomes gray with age. In tissues, the two varieties of *H. capsulatum* differ in their appearance. *H. capsulatum* var. *capsulatum* appears as tiny 2–4 μm oval budding yeasts often found inside macrophages (Fig. 2a and b). *Histoplasma capsulatum* var. *duboisii* is larger, 8–15 μm, thick-walled, may appear as short chains in tissues, and shows the "scar" from which its bud has been released at one end [1] (Fig. 2c).

In addition to the above two human pathogens, there is a third variety, *Histoplasma capsulatum* var. *farciminosum*, which is a pathogen of horses and mules. This organism causes lymphangitis in equines from the Middle East, northern Africa, central and southern Europe, Japan, the Philippines, and southern Asia [2]. The disease is characterized by multifocal suppurative lymphangitis and ulcerated cutaneous lesions that usually affect the head and forequarters; mucous membranes of the nares and oropharynx can also become ulcerated. Systemic infection does not occur.

In this chapter, *H. capsulatum* var. *capsulatum* is referred to simply as *H. capsulatum* and *H. capsulatum* var. *duboisii* as *H. duboisii*. Most of the chapter focuses on *H. capsulatum*, with additional comments, when relevant, regarding infection due to *H. duboisii*.

C.A. Kauffman (✉)
Division of Infectious Diseases, University of Michigan Medical School, VA Ann Arbor Healthcare System, Ann Arbor, MI, USA
e-mail: ckauff@umich.edu

C.A. Kauffman et al. (eds.), *Essentials of Clinical Mycology*,
DOI 10.1007/978-1-4419-6640-7_18, © Springer Science+Business Media, LLC 2011

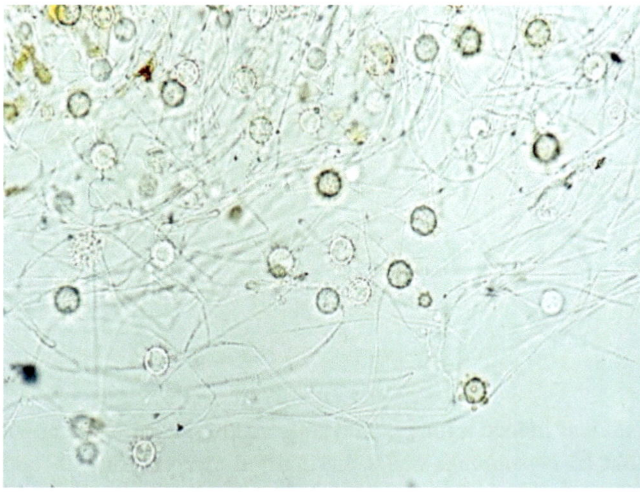

Fig. 1 Mycelial phase of *H. capsulatum* grown at 25°C showing mostly tuberculate macroconidia and a few smaller microconidia

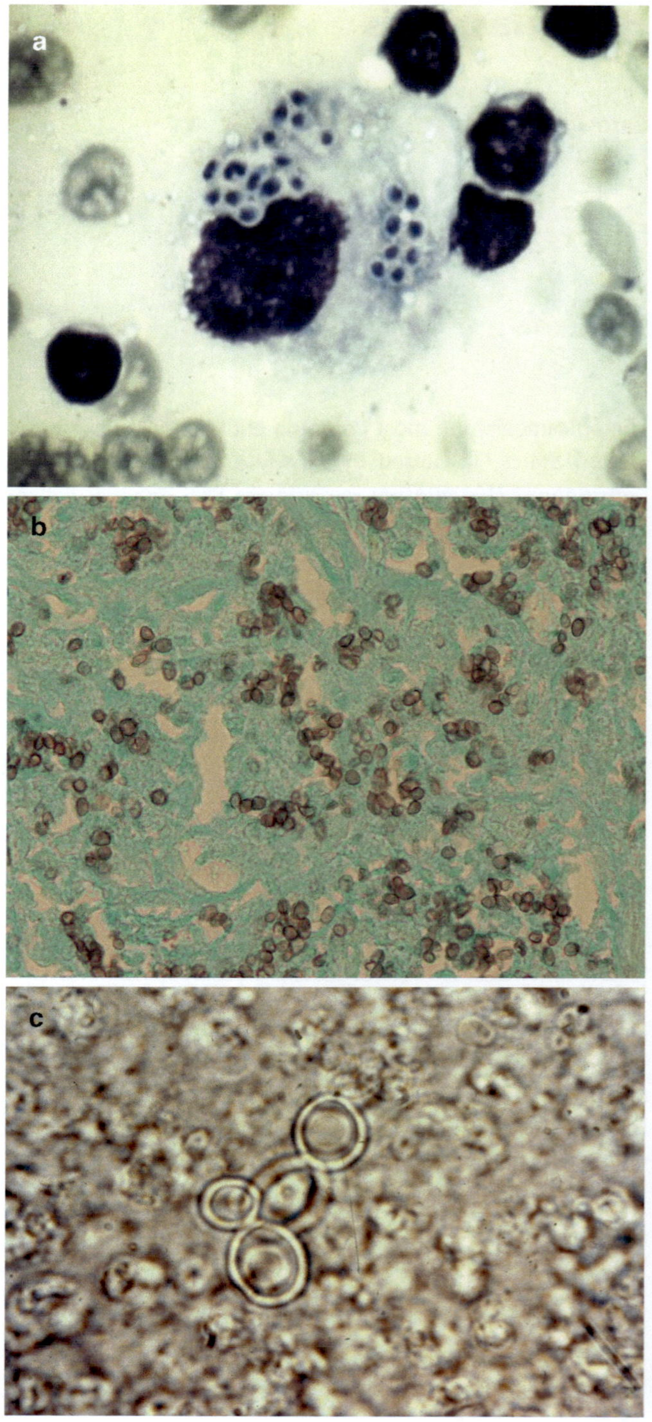

Fig. 2 Yeast phase of *Histoplasma*. (**a**) Smear of lung biopsy specimen stained with Giemsa stain showing 2–4 μm yeasts within an alveolar macrophage, typical of *Histoplasma capsulatum*; (**b**) Lung biopsy specimen stained with methenamine silver stain showing numerous budding yeasts of *H. capsulatum*; (**c**) KOH preparation of an aspirate taken from an abscess in bone showing thick-walled yeast forms typical of *H. duboisii* (Photo courtesy of Dr. Bertrand Dupont)

Ecology and Epidemiology

Histoplasmosis occurs throughout the world, but is most common in North and Central America. Isolated cases have been reported from Southeast Asia, Africa, and the Mediterranean Basin [3]. In the United States, *H. capsulatum* is endemic in the Mississippi and Ohio River valleys and in localized areas in several mideastern states (Fig. 3). In the environment, *H. capsulatum* appears to have precise growth requirements related to humidity, acidity, temperature, and nitrogen content, but all of the specific conditions needed for growth in the soil have not been completely elucidated. What is known, however, is that soil containing large amounts of droppings from birds or bats supports luxuriant mycelial growth [4]. The soil under blackbird roosts and around chicken coops is especially likely to harbor *H. capsulatum*. Birds themselves are not infected with *H. capsulatum,* but can transiently carry the organism on beaks and feet and contribute to its spread. Once contaminated, soil yields *H. capsulatum* for many years after birds no longer roost in the area. Bats, in contradistinction to birds, can become infected with *H. capsulatum* and excrete the organism in their feces [5]. Intestinal carriage by bats and their migratory patterns help to ensure expansion of geographic areas yielding *H. capsulatum.*

Infection with *H. capsulatum* results from passive exposure that occurs during typical day-to-day activities or from active exposure related to occupational or recreational activities. Most cases are sporadic, related to passive exposure, and not associated with a known source. Every year hundreds of thousands of individuals in the United States are infected with *H. capsulatum*; most of these individuals are not aware of this event. The two largest outbreaks ever reported were both associated with passive exposure of hundreds of thousands of people to *H. capsulatum* during urban construction projects in Indianapolis [6, 7]. In other outbreaks, workers became infected after involvement in specific activities, such as cleaning

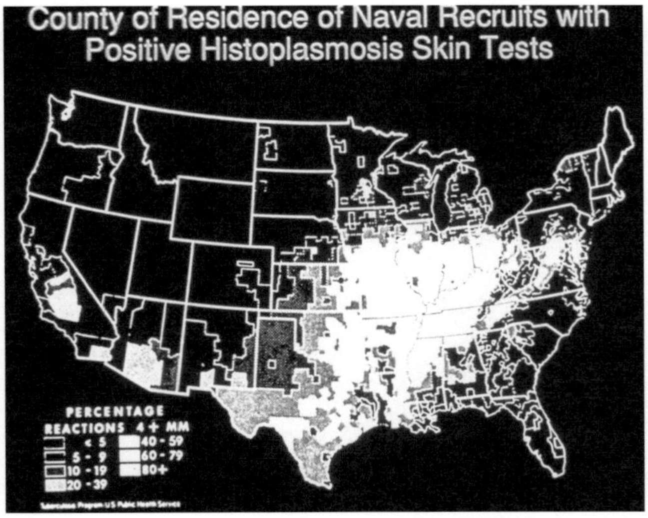

Fig. 3 Histoplasmin reactivity in the continental United States among 275,558 white male naval recruits, ages 17–21 years [112]

bird or bat guano from bridges or heavy equipment or tearing down or cleaning out old buildings, especially chicken coops [8, 9]. Other outbreaks have been associated with recreational pursuits, such as spelunking [10] and ecologic volunteer efforts [11].

AIDS has had a significant effect on the epidemiology of histoplasmosis in the highly endemic areas [12–14]. In the early 1990s, the rates of histoplasmosis in AIDS patients were as high as 12/100 patient-years in Kansas City, and 10/1,000 AIDS patients in Houston [12]. This has decreased markedly with antiretroviral therapy. Most cases of histoplasmosis in AIDS patients now are seen in those who are newly diagnosed with HIV infection [14]. Increasingly, histoplasmosis is reported among patients who have received solid organ transplants, corticosteroids, and tumor necrosis factor (TNF) antagonists [15–18].

Histoplasma duboisii is more restricted in its geography, and occurs only in Africa between the Tropic of Cancer and the Tropic of Capricorn. Within these boundaries, most cases occur in Nigeria, Mali, Senegal, and Zaire. The exact ecologic niche the organism occupies has not been determined, but cases have been described in association with bat guano [1, 19]. Cases of African histoplasmosis reported outside the endemic area have all been among travelers or immigrants from Africa [20]. *H. duboisii* has been reported to cause more severe disseminated infection in patients with HIV infection [20, 21].

Pathogenesis

The microcondia of the mycelial phase of *H. capsulatum* are 2–4 μm, a size that allows them to be easily aerosolized and inhaled into the alveoli of the host. At 37°C, the organism undergoes transformation to the yeast phase from the mycelial phase. Phagocytosis of either form (conidia or yeast) by alveolar macrophages and neutrophils occurs through binding of the organism to the CD18 family of adhesion promoting glycoproteins [22]. The yeast form of *H. capsulatum* is uniquely able to survive within the phagolysosome of macrophages through several mechanisms, including the ability to resist killing by toxic oxygen radicals and to modulate the intraphagosomal pH [23–25]. Iron and calcium acquisition by the yeast are important survival tools, allowing growth within the macrophage [25]. Surviving within the macrophage, *H. capsulatum* is transported to the hilar and mediastinal lymph nodes and subsequently disseminates hematogenously throughout the reticuloendothelial system in most cases of histoplasmosis.

After several weeks, specific T-cell immunity develops, macrophages become activated, and then killing of the organism ensues [24]. At this point, long-lasting immunity to *H. capsulatum* occurs. Experimental animal models show the importance of CD4 cells in developing specific immunity to *H. capsulatum* [26]. Interferon-gamma produced by CD4 cells is probably the most important factor for activation of macrophages, but TNF-alpha also plays a central role in immunity to *H. capsulatum* [27]. Other cytokines (IL-1, IL-12, GM-CSF) also aid in containing the organism [24, 28].

The clinical corollary in humans to the studies in the murine model is that most patients with severe infection with *H. capsulatum* are those with cellular immune deficiencies, especially those who have advanced HIV infection and low CD4 counts [29], transplant recipients [15, 18], those receiving TNF antagonists [16, 17], and rarely persons with genetic defects, such as interferon-gamma receptor deficiency [30]. Of all the human mycoses, histoplasmosis appears to be the most pure example of the pivotal importance of the cell-mediated immune system in limiting infection.

The extent of disease is determined both by the immune response of the host and the number of conidia that are inhaled. A healthy individual can develop severe life-threatening pulmonary infection if a large number of conidia are inhaled. This might occur during demolition of or renovations to old buildings or as a result of spelunking in a heavily infested cave. Conversely, a small inoculum can cause severe pulmonary infection or progress to acute symptomatic disseminated histoplasmosis in a host whose cell-mediated immune system is unable to contain the organism.

Most persons who have been infected have asymptomatic dissemination; only rarely will this lead to symptomatic disseminated histoplasmosis [5]. However, because dissemination is the rule, latent infection probably persists for a lifetime, and reactivation can result if the host becomes immunosuppressed. Presumably, this is the mechanism by which persons who were born in the endemic area and had not returned for years develop histoplasmosis years later [31, 32].

In immunosuppressed patients, histoplasmosis is most often acquired as a new infection from an environmental exposure, but also can result from reactivation of a latent infection that was acquired years before. In solid organ transplant recipients, *H. capsulatum* has rarely been transmitted with the donor organ [15].

Although uncommon, reinfection histoplasmosis can occur in persons who previously were infected and occurs most often after exposure to a heavily contaminated point source [33]. Reinfection histoplasmosis is usually less severe than primary infection because there is residual immunity induced by the initial episode.

Clinical Manifestations

Acute Pulmonary Histoplasmosis

The usual result of exposure of a normal host to *H. capsulatum* is asymptomatic infection (Table 1). In the highly endemic area, as many as 85% of adults have been infected with *H. capsulatum*, and most have not had symptoms that were attributed to histoplasmosis. Symptomatic acute pulmonary histoplasmosis is most often manifested as a self-limited illness characterized by dry cough, fever, and fatigue. Approximately 5% of patients will develop erythema nodosum [34], and 5–10% will develop myalgias and arthralgias/arthritis [35]. Joint involvement is usually polyarticular and symmetric. Chest radiographs show a patchy pneumonitis in one or more lobes, often accompanied by hilar or mediastinal lymphadenopathy [36] (Fig. 4). Some patients have only hilar lymphadenopathy; when this is accompanied by arthralgias and erythema nodosum, the clinical picture can mimic sarcoidosis and the two must be differentiated. Improvement within several weeks is typical, but in some individuals fatigue may linger for months. Joint symptoms usually resolve over several weeks in response to anti-inflammatory therapy.

When a person is exposed to a heavy inoculum of *H. capsulatum*, acute severe pulmonary infection, sometimes termed epidemic histoplasmosis, can ensue [36, 37]. Symptoms include high fever, chills, fatigue, dyspnea, cough, and chest pain. Acute respiratory failure and death can ensue. Chest radiographs show diffuse reticulonodular pulmonary infiltrates; mediastinal lymphadenopathy may or may not be present (Fig. 5). Over the ensuing months to years following resolution of the pneumonia, calcified nodules may develop throughout the lung fields [38] (Fig. 6).

If a physician sees several cases that appear to be similar and that share a possible exposure or if the patient recounts that several of his or her associates have a similar illness, then the possibility of a fungal etiology is more likely to be

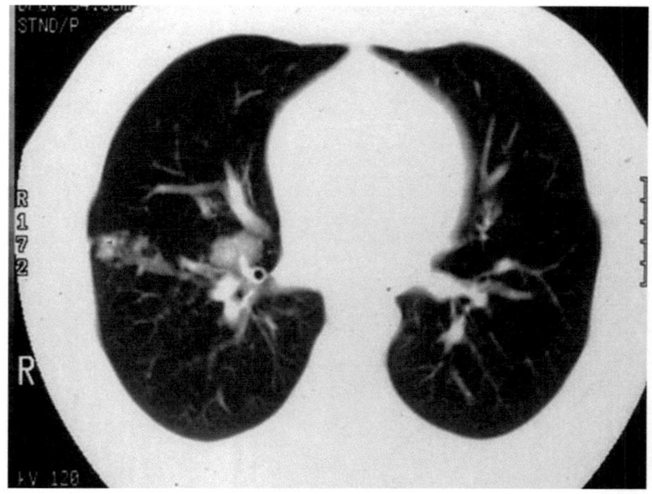

Fig. 4 CT scan of a patient with acute pulmonary histoplasmosis. Note hilar adenopathy and patchy pneumonitis

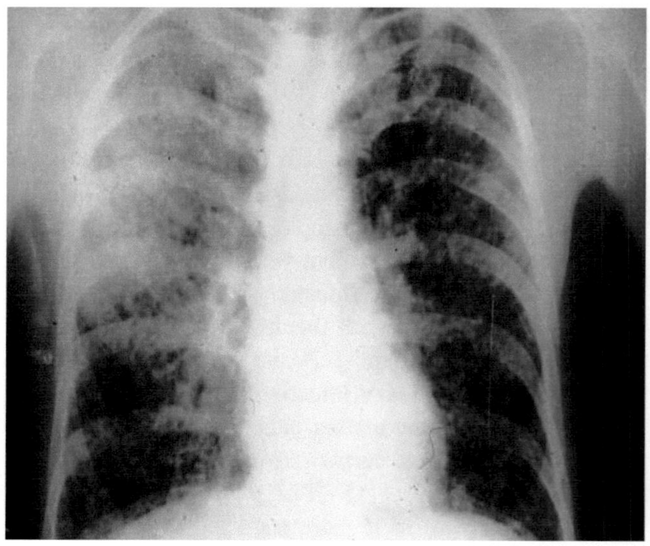

Fig. 5 Acute severe pulmonary histoplasmosis occurring in a construction worker who cleaned bird and bat guano from a bridge prior to painting the structure. The patient responded quickly to amphotericin B therapy

Table 1 Classification of clinical manifestations of histoplasmosis

Acute pulmonary
Chronic cavitary pulmonary
Complications of pulmonary histoplasmosis
Mediastinal granuloma
Fibrosing mediastinitis
Broncholithiasis
Pericarditis
Disseminated
Acute
Chronic progressive
Endocarditis
Central nervous system

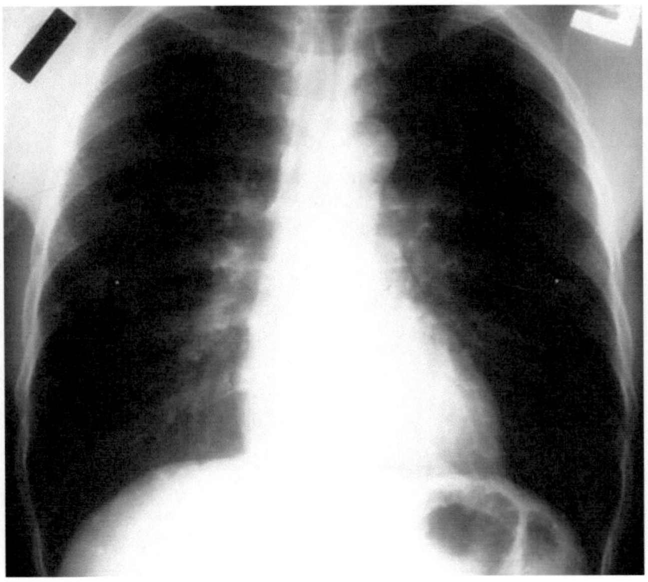

Fig. 6 Diffuse calcified nodules throughout the lung fields in a patient who had acute pulmonary histoplasmosis 20 years earlier

entertained. Sporadic cases almost always are initially thought to be due to one of the usual causes of community-acquired pneumonia. Only after the patient fails to respond to several courses of antibiotics is the possibility of a fungal pneumonia raised. A history of activities in an area endemic for *H. capsulatum* that are likely to lead to exposure to the organism several weeks prior to the onset of symptoms should lead to further diagnostic tests for histoplasmosis. Included in the differential diagnosis of acute pulmonary histoplasmosis are acute pulmonary blastomycosis and pneumonias due to *Mycoplasma*, *Legionella*, and *Chlamydia*. Hilar and mediastinal lymphadenopathy, common with histoplasmosis, are occasionally seen with blastomycosis but are rarely, if ever, noted with pneumonia due to the other organisms.

Acute pulmonary histoplasmosis in patients who have cell-mediated immune defects is more severe than in normal hosts. Prostration, fever, chills, and sweats are prominent; marked dyspnea and hypoxemia can progress quickly to acute respiratory distress syndrome (ARDS). Chest radiographs show diffuse bilateral infiltrates (Fig. 7). Dissemination to other organs is common.

Chronic Pulmonary Histoplasmosis

Chronic pulmonary histoplasmosis occurs almost entirely in older persons, predominantly men, with underlying chronic obstructive pulmonary disease (COPD) [39, 40]. The clinical manifestations include fatigue, fever, night sweats, chronic cough, sputum production, hemoptysis, dyspnea, and weight loss. This form of histoplasmosis is characterized by cavity

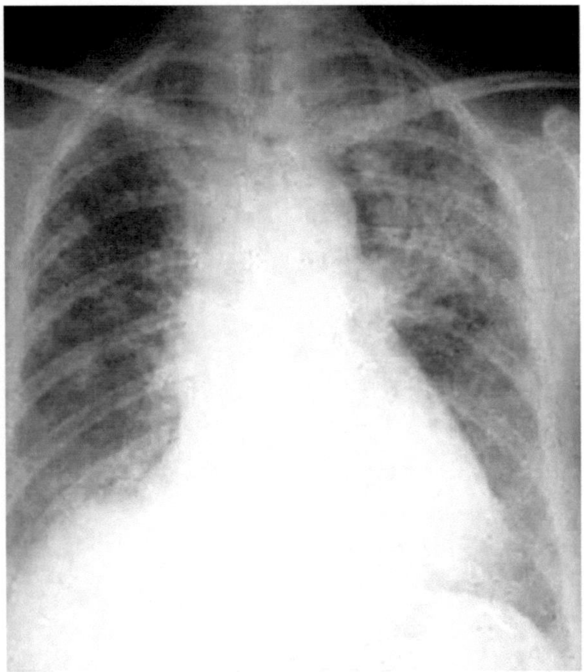

Fig. 7 Acute severe pulmonary histoplasmosis occurring in a kidney transplant recipient. Diffuse pulmonary infiltrates are present and the patient was markedly hypoxemic

formation in the upper lobes and progressive fibrosis in the lower lung fields (Fig. 8). The extensive scarring is thought to be related to the host's response to *H. capsulatum* antigens. Pleural involvement is uncommon. The disease is manifested by progressive respiratory insufficiency and if not treated is fatal in about 40% of patients [39, 41, 42]. A more recent study from the Mayo Clinic that was far less proscriptive in its definition of chronic pulmonary histoplasmosis, found that 48% of the cases were in women, and only 20% of patients had COPD [43]. In many aspects, chronic cavitary pulmonary histoplasmosis mimics reactivation tuberculosis. The differential diagnosis of chronic pulmonary histoplasmosis also includes nontuberculous mycobacterial infections, blastomycosis, sporotrichosis, and coccidioidomycosis.

Complications of Pulmonary Histoplasmosis

Mediastinal Granuloma. Involvement of mediastinal lymph nodes is common during the course of acute pulmonary histoplasmosis. However, mediastinal granuloma, characterized by massive enlargement of mediastinal lymph nodes that frequently undergo caseation necrosis, is distinctly uncommon. These nodes can remain enlarged for months to years and can lead to impingement on airways or major vessels, displacement of the esophagus, or formation of fistulae between the nodes and adjacent structures in the mediastinum [36, 44].

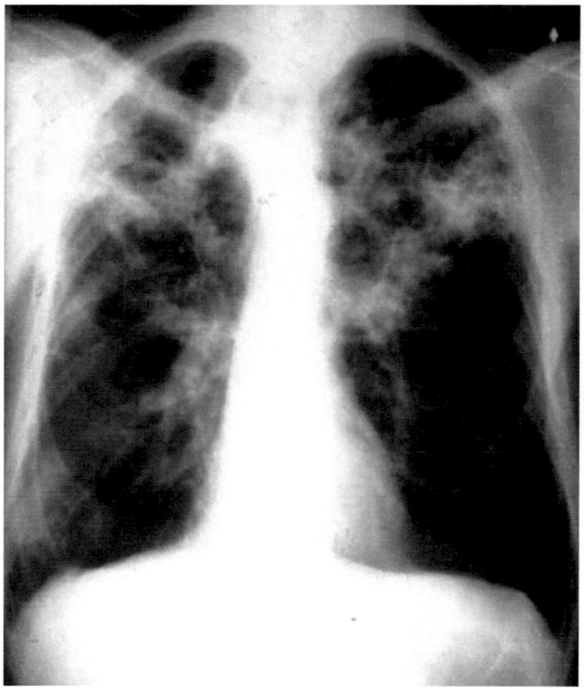

Fig. 8 Chronic cavitary pulmonary histoplasmosis in an elderly man with severe underlying emphysema

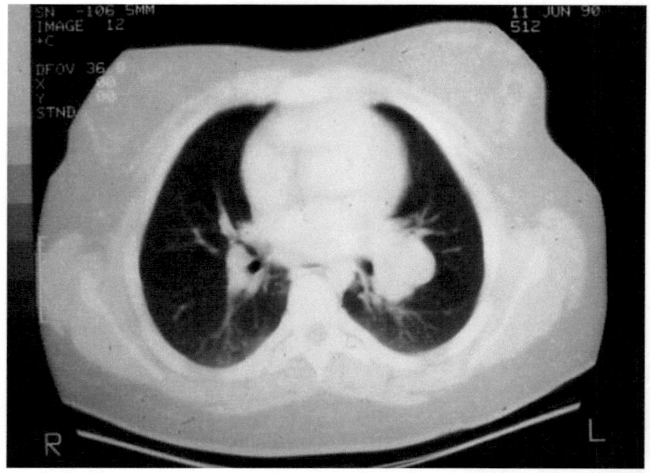

Fig. 9 CT scan of a young woman who developed mediastinal granuloma due to *Histoplasma capsulatum*. The multiple enlarged mediastinal and left hilar lymph nodes had been present for at least 1 year at the time this scan was performed

Compression of a bronchus can result in intermittent obstruction and pneumonia. In some cases, the nodes will spontaneously drain into adjacent soft tissues of the neck. Patients may be asymptomatic, have nonspecific systemic complaints of fatigue and not feeling well, or have symptoms such as dyspnea, cough, or odynophagia related to the effects of the nodes on adjacent structures. Although it was initially thought that mediastinal granuloma progressed to fibrosing mediastinitis, current thinking is that these are two separate complications of pulmonary histoplasmosis [37, 45].

Radiographs show only enlarged lymph nodes, sometimes with calcification noted. Computed tomography scans of the chest are more helpful, showing nodal enlargement, the presence of necrosis, and impingement on mediastinal structures [37, 38] (Fig. 9). Bronchoscopy or esophagoscopy can document extrinsic compression, traction diverticulae, or fistulae. Mediastinal granuloma as a complication of histoplasmosis must be differentiated from lymphoma and other tumors that cause mediastinal lymphadenopathy.

Fibrosing Mediastinitis. Fibrosing mediastinitis, an entity distinct from and much less common than mediastinal granuloma, is characterized by excessive fibrosis that progressively envelops the structures of the mediastinum [45–47]. The condition arises following infection with *H. capsulatum*, occurs mostly in young adults, and is caused by an abnormal fibrotic response to *H. capsulatum* in these individuals. When patients present with symptoms of fibrosing mediastinitis, there is rarely any sign of active histoplasmosis. The fibrosis can lead to obstruction of the superior vena cava or pulmonary arteries or veins; there may be occlusion of the bronchi. Rarely, the thoracic duct, recurrent laryngeal nerve, or right atrium are involved. Hemoptysis, dyspnea, and cough are common symptoms. Signs of superior vena cava syndrome or right heart failure may be prominent. Most patients have involvement of predominantly one side, but some have bilateral involvement, which is often fatal. Chest radiographs show subcarinal or superior mediastinal widening. Computed tomography scans and angiography are needed to reveal the extent of invasion of mediastinal structures and great vessels.

Broncholithiasis. Broncholithiasis occurs when calcified nodes or pulmonary granulomas erode into the bronchi. Ulceration into the bronchus with hemoptysis and expectoration of "stones" can ensue. Postobstructive pneumonia occurs if the node obstructs the bronchus. Computed tomography scans show the calcified node and its impingement on the bronchus, and bronchoscopy will usually confirm the diagnosis and rule out other endobronchial lesions [48].

Pericarditis. Pericarditis occurs in the setting of acute pulmonary histoplasmosis, is seen mostly in young persons, and is thought to be due to an inflammatory reaction to *H. capsulatum* in adjacent mediastinal nodes [49, 50] (Fig. 10). Pericardial fluid is often hemorrhagic with a predominance of lymphocytes, and *H. capsulatum* cannot be grown from the fluid. Pleural effusions are also common in this setting, and the fluid is exudative and frequently bloody. The majority of patients exhibit no hemodynamic consequences; however, tamponade can occur and requires immediate drainage. Outcome is excellent; only rarely does acute pericarditis progress to constriction requiring a surgical procedure for relief of symptoms.

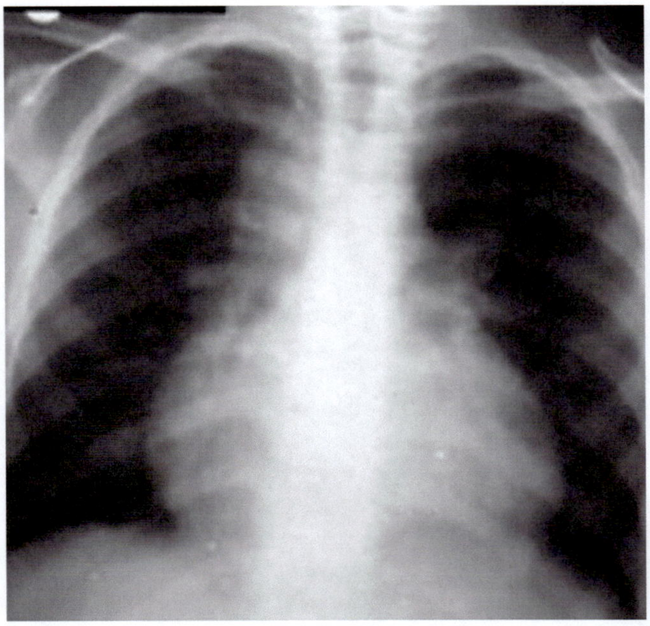

Fig. 10 Chest radiograph of a young girl with pericarditis complicating acute histoplasmosis. This resolved within a few weeks and she had no sequelae

Disseminated Histoplasmosis

Although dissemination is common during the course of most infections with *H. capsulatum,* symptomatic dissemination occurs primarily in immunosuppressed patients and infants [7, 51–53]. In persons with HIV-1 infection and histoplasmosis, a CD4 count <150/μL is associated with increased risk of disseminated histoplasmosis [29]. A rapidly fatal course with diffuse involvement of multiple organs characterizes the infection in most immunosuppressed patients [16, 18, 31, 53, 54]. Patients may present with dyspnea, renal failure, hepatic failure, coagulopathy, hypotension, and obtundation. Chest radiographs show diffuse interstitial or reticulonodular infiltrates, but may progress quickly to the findings associated with ARDS. Hemophagocytic syndrome has been associated with acute disseminated histoplasmosis [55, 56].

A chronic progressive course is typical of disseminated histoplasmosis in nonimmunocompromised middle-aged to older adults [51, 57]. This form of histoplasmosis is more common in men than women. A history of recent exposure often cannot be elicited, and overt defects in immune function have not been identified in these patients. However, because such patients are unable to eradicate the organism from their macrophages, it is presumed that they have a specific immune defect against *H. capsulatum* [51]. Fever, night sweats, anorexia, weight loss, and fatigue are prominent. Pulmonary symptoms may or may not be present, but usually are not prominent.

In both acute and chronic disseminated histoplasmosis, hepatosplenomegaly, lymphadenopathy, and skin and mucous membrane lesions are frequently noted. A variety of different skin lesions, including papules, pustules, ulcers, and subcutaneous nodules, have been noted in patients with disseminated histoplasmosis (Fig. 11a and b). Oropharyngeal ulcers or, less commonly, nodules can be found on the tongue, buccal and gingival mucosa, larynx, or lips in patients with either acute or chronic dissemination (Fig. 12). Patients with disseminated histoplasmosis can develop adrenal insufficiency as a result of destruction of the adrenal glands by infiltration with *H. capsulatum*. Addisonian crisis has been reported as the presenting manifestation of disseminated histoplasmosis.

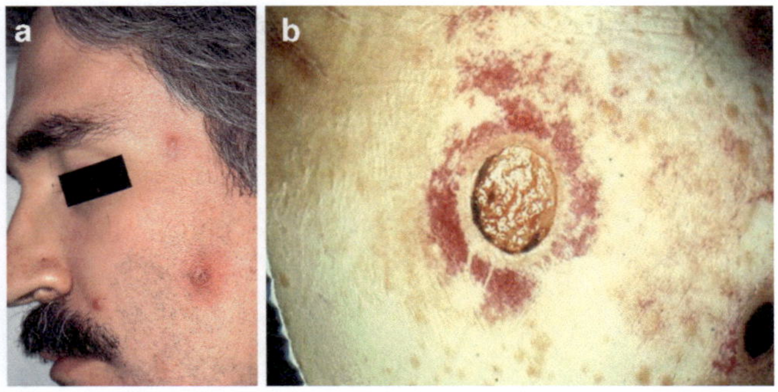

Fig. 11 Skin lesions noted in patients with disseminated histoplasmosis. (**a**) Multiple papulopustules which appeared on the face and chest in a patient with HIV infection; (**b**) chronic ulcer on the thigh of an elderly man with chronic progressive disseminated histoplasmosis

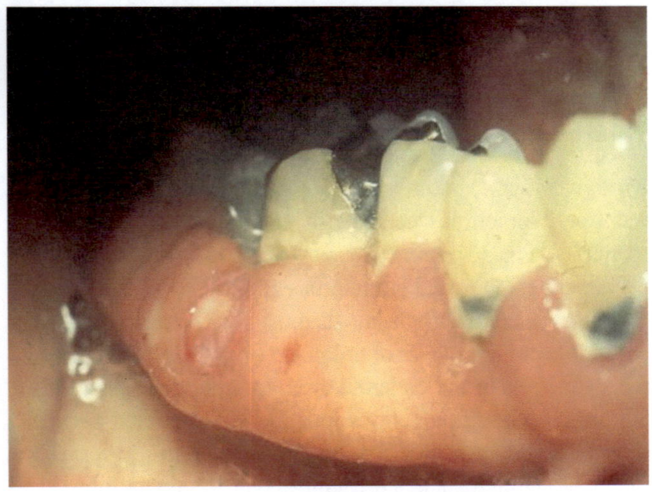

Fig. 12 Painful, slowly enlarging gingival ulcer that was present for 4 months in an elderly man who had chronic progressive histoplasmosis

Laboratory abnormalities noted with disseminated disease include an elevated erythrocyte sedimentation rate, pancytopenia, elevation of hepatic enzymes, especially alkaline phosphatase, and hyperbilirubinemia. Hypercalcemia has been associated with disseminated histoplasmosis, as it has with other granulomatous diseases, such as tuberculosis, coccidioidomycosis, and sarcoidosis. Patients with adrenal insufficiency may have hyponatremia, hyperkalemia, and

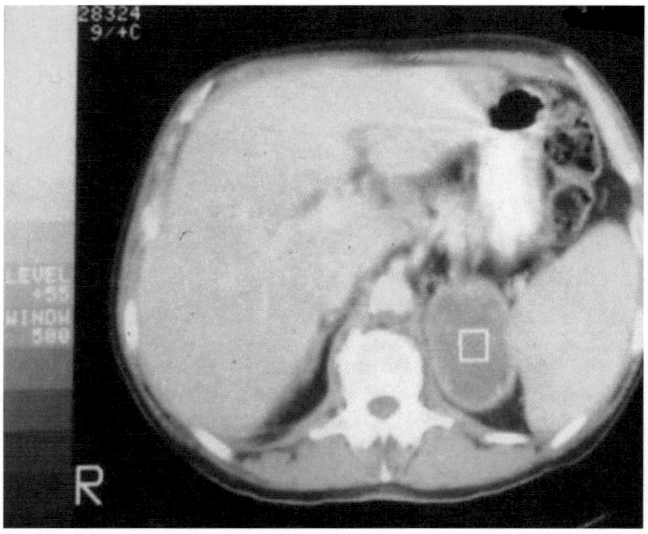

Fig. 13 Abdominal CT scan showing adrenal enlargement with central necrosis in a patient with chronic progressive histoplasmosis complicated by Addison's disease

hypoglycemia. Abdominal CT scans show adrenal enlargement and sometimes necrosis in those with adrenal involvement [58] (Fig. 13). Bone marrow, liver, and lymph node biopsy specimens often reveal granulomas and budding yeast.

Disseminated histoplasmosis must always be considered as a possible cause of fever of unknown origin in any person who has ever lived in the endemic area. Lymphomas, sarcoidosis, and mycobacterial infections must be differentiated from disseminated histoplasmosis. Whether the patient has histoplasmosis or sarcoidosis is a difficult diagnostic conundrum. The use of corticosteroids for presumed sarcoidosis without excluding active histoplasmosis can be risky. Although patients may initially appear to improve with corticosteroid treatment, they subsequently experience progressive illness and can die of overwhelming histoplasmosis [59].

Endocarditis is an uncommon manifestation of disseminated histoplasmosis. Both native and prosthetic valve endocarditis have been reported [60, 61], as well as an infected left atrial myxoma [62]. The disease is manifested by major embolic episodes and poor outcomes if the infected valve cannot be replaced. *H. capsulatum* has also been described as a cause of infection of an aortofemoral prosthetic graft [63].

Specific Organ System Involvement

Histoplasmosis of the central nervous system can be manifested as subacute or chronic meningitis or as an acute event that is just one manifestation of disseminated infection [64, 65]. Basilar meningeal involvement is typical and can lead to communicating hydrocephalus. Focal brain or spinal cord lesions can occur in those with meningitis, and in other

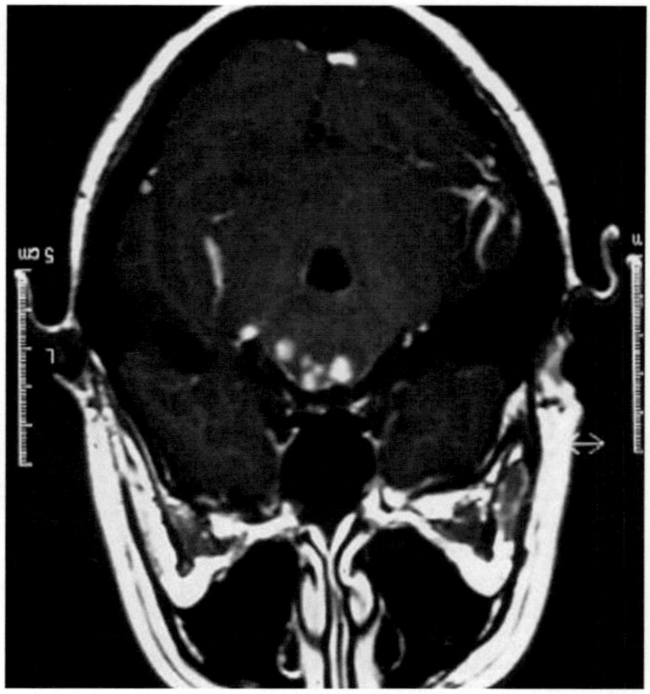

Fig. 14 MRI scan of a woman with isolated central nervous system histoplasmosis. The scan shows meningeal enhancement as well as several enhancing lesions in the midbrain

patients, they appear as isolated lesions without meningitis [65, 66]. In patients with meningitis, the typical CSF abnormalities include lymphocytic pleocytosis, elevated protein, and hypoglycorrachia; in those with focal lesions, the CSF findings are either within normal limits or show slight pleocytosis and elevated protein concentrations. Computed tomography or MRI scans show single or multiple enhancing brain lesions in those with focal infection and meningeal enhancement in those who have meningitis only (Fig. 14). *Histoplasma* meningitis must be differentiated from other causes of chronic lymphocytic meningitis, notably tuberculosis, coccidioidomycosis and, less commonly, blastomycosis, sporotrichosis, brucellosis, and sarcoidosis. Mass lesions must be differentiated from other infectious processes as well as tumors [66].

Osteoarticular histoplasmosis is not common. Typically, the manifestations are those of chronic tenosynovitis and, less commonly, osteomyelitis and septic arthritis of a native joint or, rarely, a prosthetic joint [67, 68]. Infection of osteoarticular structures must be differentiated from the self-limited arthralgias and arthritis that are noted during the course of acute histoplasmosis and that are presumed secondary to the immune response to *H. capsulatum* [35].

Isolated infection of the GI tract is an uncommon manifestation of histoplasmosis, but GI involvement as one manifestation of disseminated infection, especially among immunosuppressed patients, is common [69, 70]. Diffuse infiltration of the bowel wall is usually noted; abdominal pain and diarrhea are prominent, and malabsorption can result.

Genitourinary tract infection with *H. capsulatum* can be manifested as epididymal, testicular, or prostatic nodules [71–73]. Placental infection with spread to the fetus has been described rarely [74]. Other sites at which *H. capsulatum* has been reported to cause focal infection or in which involvement has been noted in association with widespread dissemination include kidneys, peritoneum, omentum, gallbladder, common bile duct, panniculus, breast, thymus, sinuses, optic nerve, eyes, and ears.

Presumed Ocular Histoplasmosis

Ocular histoplasmosis is a diagnosis based on ophthalmologic findings of discrete yellow-white lesions in the retina, so-called "histo spots"; these lesions are sight threatening when they occur in the macula [75]. However, there is little scientific evidence linking this syndrome to histoplasmosis [5]. The association is based primarily on residence in an area endemic for histoplasmosis and positive histoplasmin skin tests and not by demonstration of fungus in the eye. Similar ophthalmologic findings have been noted in patients who have never lived in the endemic area [76]. Rarely, *H. capsulatum* can be recovered from the eye in patients with disseminated histoplasmosis, but the clinical and ophthalmologic findings are not those described with ocular histoplasmosis [77].

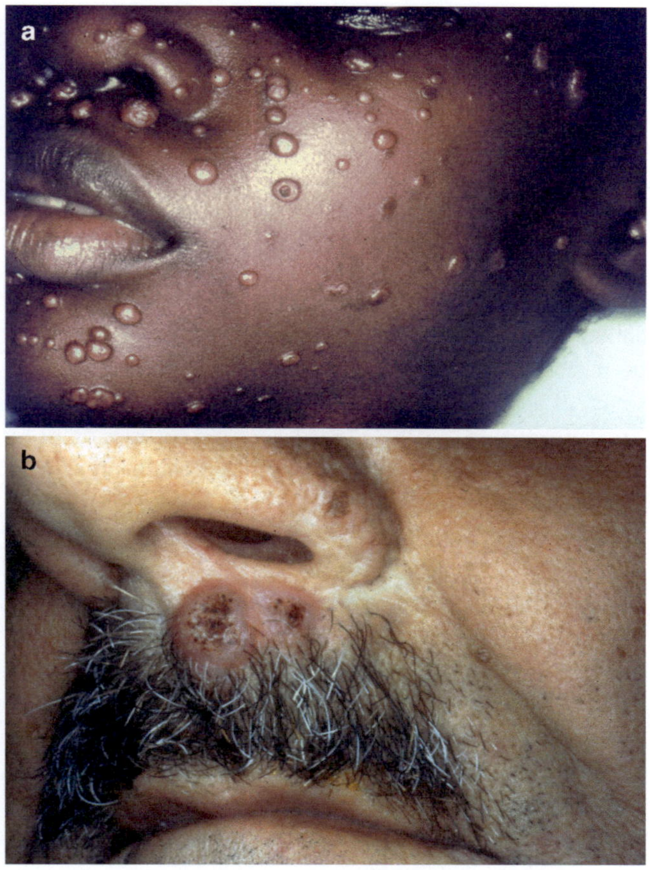

Fig. 15 (**a**) Numerous molluscum-type skin lesions that appeared on the face of an African child with disseminated infection due to *Histoplasma duboisii*; (**b**) solitary skin lesion typical of those seen with *H. duboisii* (Photos courtesy of Dr. Bertrand Dupont)

Histoplasmosis due to H. duboisii

Infection with *H. duboisii* differs from that due to *H. capsulatum* in that bones and skin are the two major organs affected [20, 21] (Figs. 15a and b). Osteolytic lesions are often found in association with subcutaneous nodules and abscesses; skin nodules can ulcerate and drain. Lung involvement is more common than previously thought, and lymphadenopathy is prominent in some cases. The infection is frequently indolent and not life threatening, but in the exceptional patient, widespread visceral dissemination occurs, and the disease resembles progressive disseminated histoplasmosis due to *H. capsulatum*; this is especially seen in patients who have HIV infection [20].

Diagnosis

Culture Methods

The definitive diagnostic test for histoplasmosis is growth of *H. capsulatum* from tissue or body fluids. For patients who have disseminated infection, samples taken from blood, bone marrow, liver, skin, or mucosal lesions often yield the organism. The lysis-centrifugation (Isolator tube) system is more sensitive than automated systems for growing *H. capsulatum* from blood [78]. When sputum or bronchoalveolar lavage fluid is sent for culture, the laboratory should be informed that histoplasmosis is a possibility; use of a selective medium that uses ammonium hydroxide decreases the growth of commensal fungi and increases the yield of *H. capsulatum* [79].

H. capsulatum may take as long as 6 weeks to grow at 30°C in the mould phase in vitro. Identifying tuberculate macroconidia allows a presumptive diagnosis of histoplasmosis, but a confirmatory test should always be performed. A chemiluminescent DNA probe specific for *H. capsulatum* is used to rapidly confirm the identification of the organism [80]. The laborious task of converting the mould phase to the yeast phase in vitro is no longer required for definitive identification of *H. capsulatum*. Cultures yield the organism in most cases of disseminated infection, in chronic pulmonary histoplasmosis, and in those cases of acute pulmonary histoplasmosis following a heavy-inoculum exposure. However, in many patients who have acute pulmonary histoplasmosis, and in most patients who have mediastinal granuloma or meningitis, cultures rarely yield *H. capsulatum*.

Antigen Detection

Detection of circulating *H. capsulatum* polysaccharide antigen in urine and serum has proved extremely useful in patients, especially those with AIDS, who have disseminated infection with a large burden of organisms [81, 82]. Originally developed as a radioimmunoassay, antigen detection is now performed by enzyme immunoassay with greater ease and equivalent sensitivity and specificity [83]. The sensitivity for antigen detection is higher in urine than in serum. Antigen can be detected in the urine of approximately 90% and in the serum of approximately 50% of AIDS patients with disseminated infection [82]. Antigen can be detected in urine or serum within the first few weeks of illness in approximately 65% of patients who have acute pulmonary histoplasmosis, especially in those who had been exposed to a high inoculum of organisms [84]. However, antigen is detected in only 10–20% of patients with less severe and chronic forms of pulmonary histoplasmosis and in patients who have complications of pulmonary histoplasmosis. Antigen detection has also proved useful in AIDS patients undergoing bronchoalveolar lavage for pneumonia due to histoplasmosis [85]. Antigen can be detected in CSF from some patients with *Histoplasma* meningitis [65].

False-positive reactions have been noted in a majority of samples of urine and serum taken from patients with blastomycosis, paracoccidioidomycosis, and penicilliosis [86], and have been described less commonly in patients with coccidioidomycosis [87]. The major diagnostic dilemma in the United States is obviously with blastomycosis. Samples from patients who have either histoplasmosis or blastomycosis show reactivity with antigen assays for both fungi [86, 88]. Antigen detection can be used to follow a patient's response to antifungal therapy. Levels should fall to below the level of detection with successful therapy, and a rise in antigen level may signal relapse [82].

PCR Assays

Several polymerase chain reaction (PCR) assays that might help with more rapid identification of *H. capsulatum* have been developed [89–92]. To date, there is no standardization, and none are commercially available. A real-time PCR assay correctly identified *H. capsulatum* from among a variety of culture extracts from different fungi grown in the laboratory [89]. This assay was used to identify *H. capsulatum* in tissue biopsies and bronchoalveolar lavage fluid from three patients who had documented histoplasmosis. Semi-nested PCR assays were shown to be very sensitive for detecting *H. capsulatum* in tissues from infected mice [90], and other similar assays have been used in a small number of samples of blood or tissues obtained from a few patients who had documented histoplasmosis [91, 92]. It is likely that PCR will assume an increasing role in the diagnosis of histoplasmosis in the future.

Serologic Tests

Although antigen detection has led to a less important role for antibody assays, these tests still play a role in the diagnosis of several forms of histoplasmosis [82]. The standard assays for antibodies to *H. capsulatum* are the complement fixation (CF) test that uses two separate antigens – yeast and mycelial (or histoplasmin) – and the immunodiffusion (ID) assay. A fourfold rise in CF antibody titer is considered indicative of active histoplasmosis. It is also frequently stated that a CF titer equal to 1:32 indicates active infection with *H. capsulatum*, but a diagnosis should never be based solely on such a titer. CF antibodies frequently persist for years after infection; thus, the presence of a single low CF titer means little other than that the patient was exposed to *H. capsulatum* at some time.

The ID assay tests for the presence of M and H precipitin bands. An M band develops with acute infection, is often present in chronic forms of histoplasmosis, and persists for months to years after the infection has resolved [93]. An H band is much less common, is rarely if ever found without an M band, and is indicative of chronic and progressive forms of histoplasmosis. The ID assay is more specific than the CF assay. Enzyme immunoassay methods are poorly standardized and are generally not recommended.

Serologic tests are most useful for patients with chronic pulmonary or disseminated histoplasmosis; in these forms of histoplasmosis, the chronicity of the infection ensures that sufficient time has elapsed for the patient to have developed antibodies. For acute pulmonary histoplasmosis, a rising antibody titer to *H. capsulatum* is diagnostic. Serologic tests are less definitive in patients who have mediastinal lymphadenopathy, and the diagnosis should always be confirmed by tissue biopsy. False-positive CF tests occur in patients with lymphoma, tuberculosis, sarcoidosis, and other fungal infections, all of which may present as a mediastinal mass. Because 2–4 weeks are required for appearance of antibodies, serologic assays are less helpful in establishing a diagnosis in patients who have severe acute infection, and they are rarely useful in immunosuppressed patients, who mount a poor antibody response. A special use for antibody detection is in patients who have *Histoplasma* meningitis. The presence of CF and/or ID antibodies against *H. capsulatum* in the CSF is adequate to make a diagnosis in the appropriate clinical setting, and frequently this is the only positive diagnostic test [65].

Histopathologic Examination

For the patient who is acutely ill, tissue biopsy should be done as soon as possible to look for *H. capsulatum*. Finding the distinctive 2–4 μm oval, budding yeasts allows a presumptive diagnosis of histoplasmosis. Routine hematoxylin and eosin stains rarely show the tiny yeasts; biopsy material

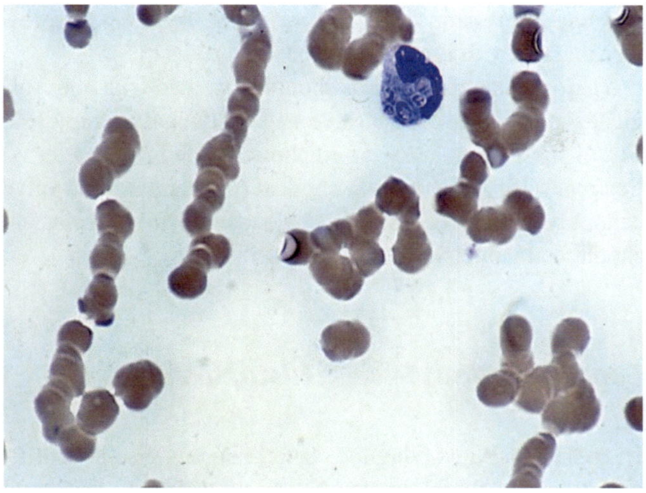

Fig. 16 Peripheral blood smear from an AIDS patient who was severely ill with disseminated histoplasmosis. Multiple tiny yeasts typical of *Histoplasma capsulatum* are seen within a monocyte

should be stained with methenamine silver or periodic acid–Schiff stains. Yeasts are typically found within macrophages, but also can be seen free in the tissues. In patients with disseminated infection, bone marrow, liver, skin, and mucocutaneous lesions usually reveal organisms, and in those with a large burden of organisms, routine peripheral blood smears may show yeasts within neutrophils (Fig. 16).

For patients with mediastinal granuloma, biopsy of nodes will often reveal caseous material, which may contain a few yeast-like organisms typical of *H. capsulatum.* It is unusual to find *H. capsulatum* on cytologic examination of sputum or bronchoalveolar lavage fluid unless there is a large organism burden.

In histopathology specimens, the yeast phase of *H. duboisii* is distinctly different from that of *H. capsulatum*. Yeast forms of *H. duboisii* are approximately fourfold larger than *H. capsulatum* and may be seen as short chains in tissues. The distinction between these two varieties of *Histoplasma* is clinically relevant only for a small number of patients who could have either infection because they live in areas of tropical Africa in which both organisms are found.

Treatment

Most patients infected with *H. capsulatum* are asymptomatic or have mild, self-limited disease and thus do not need treatment with an antifungal agent. However, patients who have severe acute pulmonary, chronic pulmonary, or disseminated histoplasmosis do require treatment with an antifungal agent. Guidelines for the treatment of histoplasmosis have been published recently by the Infectious Diseases Society of America [94].

Pulmonary Histoplasmosis

Acute pulmonary histoplasmosis. Most patients with acute pulmonary histoplasmosis do not require antifungal therapy; recovery usually occurs within a month. However, some patients remain symptomatic for longer periods of time and are likely to benefit from antifungal therapy. Oral itraconazole, 200 mg once or twice daily, for 6–12 weeks is recommended in such cases [94].

Patients who have moderately severe to severe acute pulmonary histoplasmosis should be treated initially with a lipid formulation of amphotericin B, 3–5 mg/kg daily, or with amphotericin B deoxycholate, 0.7–1 mg/kg daily. After the patient has shown improvement, usually in 1–2 weeks, therapy can be changed to oral itraconazole, 200 mg twice daily. Methylprednisolone, 0.5–1 mg/kg daily for the first 1–2 weeks is recommended for patients who are severely ill and for those with ARDS [94]. Antifungal treatment is usually given until the infiltrates resolve. For normal hosts, therapy may be as short as 12 weeks, but immunosuppressed hosts often require a longer course of therapy.

Chronic pulmonary histoplasmosis. Treatment is indicated for all patients with chronic pulmonary histoplasmosis [94]. Without therapy, inexorable progression to respiratory insufficiency is the usual course [39, 41, 42]. Most patients can be treated with itraconazole, 200 mg twice daily, and do not require therapy with amphotericin B [95]. Treatment should be given for at least 12 months, and some physicians recommend 18–24 months of azole therapy to decrease the risk of relapse. Fluconazole is less effective than itraconazole and is considered second-line therapy [96].

Complications of pulmonary histoplasmosis. It is not clear that antifungal agents alter the course of mediastinal granuloma. Most patients recover without treatment, but some continue to have symptoms, which usually leads to the use of antifungal agents. Reports of successful therapy with either azoles or amphotericin B remain anecdotal. Itraconazole, 200 mg once or twice daily for 6–12 weeks, is suggested for patients who are persistently symptomatic [94]. For some patients, surgical removal of the mass of obstructing nodes is necessary for symptomatic relief [37].

Antifungal therapy, corticosteroids, and anti-inflammatory agents are not useful for treating fibrosing mediastinitis. Surgery is considered to be risky and does not have a role in management of this condition [47, 94]. For some patients, placement of intravascular stents into obstructed pulmonary arteries or veins or the superior vena cava has been helpful [97]. Generally, stenting is performed in those patients who are more severely compromised with bilateral pulmonary vessel obstruction or superior vena cava syndrome [37, 97]. Unilateral occlusion of the pulmonary vessels is associated with a better prognosis, and stenting is generally not necessary.

Pericarditis is treated with nonsteroidal anti-inflammatory agents and, rarely, corticosteroids. Antifungal agents are not recommended unless corticosteroids are used, in which case itraconazole, 200 mg once or twice daily, is given for 6–12 weeks to prevent the possible occurrence of progressive infection with *H. capsulatum* [94]. In the exceptional case associated with tamponade, pericardiocentesis and creation of a pericardial window are important therapeutic measures.

Disseminated Histoplasmosis

All patients with disseminated histoplasmosis should be treated with an antifungal agent [94]. Patients with moderately severe to severe infection should be treated initially with liposomal amphotericin B, 3 mg/kg daily. Another lipid formulation at a dosage of 5 mg/kg daily or amphotericin B deoxycholate, 0.7–1 mg/kg daily, are alternatives. A randomized, blinded, controlled clinical trial in AIDS patients with moderately severe to severe disseminated histoplasmosis showed that liposomal amphotericin B, when compared with amphotericin B deoxycholate, resulted in faster resolution of fever and improved survival rates [98]. After clinical improvement is noted, which usually occurs within 2 weeks in most patients, therapy can be changed to oral itraconazole, 200 mg twice daily, to complete a course of 12 months of antifungal therapy [94]. Patients with mild-to-moderate disseminated histoplasmosis, including most patients who have the chronic progressive form of disseminated histoplasmosis, can be treated with oral itraconazole, 200 mg twice daily [94, 95, 99].

Fluconazole is less effective than itraconazole [96]; this has been most clearly shown in AIDS patients, in whom relapse rates while receiving fluconazole were noted to be unacceptably high [100]. Voriconazole and posaconazole have been reported to be effective for several different forms of histoplasmosis [18, 101–103]. However, there are no clinical trials to define the role of these newer agents in treating histoplasmosis, and most of these reports describe salvage therapy when other agents failed.

The length of therapy depends on the severity of the infection and the immune status of the host. The recommended treatment course is 12 months [94]. However, some patients with chronic progressive dissemination may respond slowly to antifungal therapy and require 18–24 months of therapy. For patients with AIDS, suppressive therapy with itraconazole, 200 mg daily, should continue beyond 12 months if the CD4 cell count remains <150 cells/μL [104]. For patients who are receiving effective antiretroviral therapy and whose CD4 cell counts are >150 cells/μL for at least 6 months, antifungal therapy can be stopped [105]. For patients whose immunosuppression cannot be reversed, life-long suppressive therapy with itraconazole may be prudent [94].

Histoplasma endocarditis should be treated with both surgical replacement of the valve and antifungal therapy [60, 61]. A lipid formulation of amphotericin B is the preferred treatment. If for any reason, surgical extirpation of the valve cannot be performed, lifelong suppression with itraconazole should be maintained.

Central Nervous System Histoplasmosis

Histoplasmosis involving the central nervous system is difficult to treat. Initial treatment should be with liposomal amphotericin B, 5 mg/kg daily for 4–6 weeks, and this is followed by oral azole therapy for at least 12 months. Itraconazole, 200 mg twice or three times daily, is the agent recommended in the IDSA guidelines [94]. Itraconazole does not achieve detectable CSF levels, but has been used successfully for *Histoplasma*, as well as other types of fungal meningitis [106, 107]. Conversely, fluconazole achieves higher CSF concentrations, but is less active against *H. capsulatum* than itraconazole. Fluconazole has been noted to be effective in a few case reports of *Histoplasma* meningitis [107, 108]. Anecdotal case reports show benefit for both voriconazole and posaconazole [101–103]. Antifungal therapy should continue for a total of at least 12 months and until all CSF abnormalities have resolved. Enhancing mass lesions in the brain or spinal cord appear to respond to antifungal agents and do not require excision in most patients. Magnetic resonance imaging scans should be followed to assure resolution.

Treatment of Infections Due to H. duboisii

Controlled trials have not been performed to determine the most efficacious treatment for *H. duboisii*. Anecdotal experience shows amphotericin B, ketoconazole, and itraconazole to be effective [21, 109]. There is no reason to doubt that the response to antifungal agents would be similar to that with *H. capsulatum*. However, osteoarticular involvement, which is common in this form of histoplasmosis, is slow to respond and requires long-term azole therapy.

Prevention

Persons who could be at risk for exposure to *H. capsulatum* through their occupation or leisure activities should be counseled to take appropriate precautions to prevent exposure [110].

Workers should wear a respirator when dismantling bird and bat roosts or chicken coops, refurbishing old structures that are found to have provided roosts for bats or birds, and moving large quantities of soil in areas known to be highly endemic for *H. capsulatum*. Soil or debris can be treated with formalin to inactivate the conidia prior to construction work, but this is rarely accomplished. Immunocompromised patients should be counseled to not undertake activities, such as spelunking or renovation projects, that might put them at risk for exposure to *H. capsulatum*.

Prophylactic use of antifungal agents has been studied only in persons with AIDS. In patients with CD4 counts <150 cells/μL, a placebo-controlled trial showed that prophylaxis with itraconazole, 200 mg daily, was effective at preventing histoplasmosis [111]. Prophylaxis should be considered only in highly endemic areas in which the rate of infection is at least ten cases/100 AIDS patient-years. There are no recommendations for the use of prophylaxis for other populations of immunosuppressed patients, such as those undergoing transplantation and those treated with TNF antagonists.

References

1. Schwarz J. African histoplasmosis, part 2. In: Baker RD, editor. Human Infection with Fungi, Actinomycetes, and Algae. New York: Springer; 1970. p. 139–46.
2. Gabal MA, Hassan FK, Siad AA, Karim KA. Study of equine histoplasmosis farciminosi and characterization of *Histoplasma farciminosum*. Sabouraudia. 1983;21:121–7.
3. Ashbee HR, Evans EGV, Viviani MA, et al. Histoplasmosis in Europe: report on an epidemiological survey from the European Confederation of Medical Mycology Working Group. Med Mycol. 2008;46:57–65.
4. Cano M, Hajjeh RA. The epidemiology of histoplasmosis: a review. Semin Respir Infect. 2001;16:109–18.
5. Schwarz J. Histoplasmosis. New York: Praeger Publishers; 1981.
6. Wheat LJ, Slama TG, Eitzen HE, Kohler RB, French MLV, Biesecker JL. A large urban outbreak of histoplasmosis: clinical features. Ann Intern Med. 1981;94:331–7.
7. Sathapatayavongs B, Batteiger BE, Wheat J, Slama TG, Wass JL. Clinical and laboratory features of disseminated histoplasmosis during two large urban outbreaks. Medicine (Baltimore). 1983;62:263–70.
8. Waldman RJ, England AC, Tauxe R, et al. A winter outbreak of acute histoplasmosis in northern Michigan. Am J Epidemiol. 1983;117:68–75.
9. Jones TF, Swinger GL, Craig AS, McNeil MM, Kaufman L, Schaffner W. Acute pulmonary histoplasmosis in bridge workers: a persistent problem. Am J Med. 1999;106:480–2.
10. Sacks JJ, Ajello L, Crockett LK. An outbreak and review of cave-associated *Histoplasmosis capsulati*. J Med Vet Mycol. 1986;24:313–27.
11. Brodsky AL, Gregg MB, Kaufman L, Mallison GF. Outbreak of histoplasmosis associated with the 1970 Earth Day activities. Am J Med. 1973;54:333–42.
12. Dupont B, Crewe Brown HH, et al. Mycoses in AIDS. Med Mycol. 2000;38 Suppl 1:259–67.
13. Mata-Essayag S, Colella MT, Rosello A, et al. Histoplasmosis. a study of 158 cases in Venezuela, 2000-2005. Medicine (Baltimore). 2008;87:193–202.
14. Baddley JW, Sankara IR, Rodriquez JM, Pappas PG, Wickliffe Jr JM. Histoplasmosis in HIV-infected patients in a southern regional medical center: poor prognosis in the era of highly active antiretroviral therapy. Diagn Microbiol Infect Dis. 2008;62:151–6.
15. Kauffman CA. Endemic mycoses after hematopoietic stem cell or solid organ transplantation. In: Bowden RA, Ljungman P, Paya CV, editors. Transplant Infections. 2nd ed. Lippincott: Williams & Wilkins; 2003. p. 524–34.
16. Smith JA, Kauffman CA. Endemic fungal infections in patients receiving tumor necrosis factor-alpha inhibitor therapy. Drugs. 2009;69(11):1403–15.
17. Tsiodras S, Samonis G, Boumpas DT, Kontoyiannis DP. Fungal infections complicating tumor necrosis factor-alpha blockade therapy. Mayo Clin Proc. 2008;83:181–94.
18. Freifeld AG, Iwen PC, Lesiak BL, Gilroy RK, Stevens RB, Kalil AC. Histoplasmosis in solid organ transplant recipients at a large Midwestern university transplant center. Transpl Infect Dis. 2005;7:109–15.
19. Gugnani HC, Muotoe-Okafar FA, Kaufman L, Dupont B. Natural focus of *Histoplasma capsulatum* var. *duboisii* in a bat cave. Mycopathologia. 1994;127:151–7.
20. Loulergue P, Bastides F, Baudouin V, et al. Literature review and case history of *Histoplasma capsulatum* var. *duboisii* infections in HIV-infected patients. Emerg Infect Dis. 2007;13:1647–52.
21. Manfredi R, Mazzoni A, Nanetti A, Chiodo F. *Histoplasmosis capsulati* and *duboisii* in Europe: the impact of the HIV pandemic, travel, and immigration. Eur J Epidemiol. 1994;10:675–81.
22. Bullock WE, Wright SD. Role of the adherence-promoting receptors, CR3, LFA-1, and p150,95 in binding of *H. capsulatum* by human macrophages. J Exp Med. 1987;165:195–210.
23. Eissenberg LG, Goldman WE, Schlesinger PH. *Histoplasma capsulatum* modulates the acidification of phagolysosomes. J Exp Med. 1993;177:1605–11.
24. Newman SL. Cell-mediated immunity to *Histoplasma capsulatum*. Semin Respir Infect. 2001;16:102–8.
25. Woods JP, Heinecke EL, Luecke JW, et al. Pathogenesis of *Histoplasma capsulatum*. Semin Respir Infect. 2001;16:91–101.
26. Deepe Jr GS. Protective immunity in murine histoplasmosis: functional comparison of adoptively transferred T-cell clones and splenic T cells. Infect Immun. 1988;56:2350–5.
27. Deepe Jr GS, Gibbons RS. T cells require tumor necrosis factor–alpha to provide protective immunity in mice infected with *Histoplasma capsulatum*. J Infect Dis. 2006;193:322–30.
28. Deepe Jr GS, McGuinness M. Interleukin-1 and host control of pulmonary histoplasmosis. J Infect Dis. 2006;194:855–64.
29. McKinsey DS, Spiegel RA, Hutwanger L, et al. Prospective study of histoplasmosis in patients infected with human immunodeficiency virus: incidence, risk factors, and pathophysiology. Clin Infect Dis. 1997;24:1195–203.
30. Zerbe CS, Holland SM. Disseminated histoplasmosis in persons with interferon–gamma receptor 1 deficiency. Clin Infect Dis. 2005;41:38–41.
31. Kauffman CA, Israel KS, Smith JW, White AC, Schwarz J, Brooks GF. Histoplasmosis in immunosuppressed patients. Am J Med. 1978;64:923–32.
32. Hajjeh RA. Disseminated histoplasmosis in persons infected with human immunodeficiency virus. Clin Infect Dis. 1995;21 Suppl 1:S108–10.
33. Dean AG, Bates JH, Sorrels C, et al. An outbreak of histoplasmosis at an Arkansas courthouse, with five cases of probable reinfection. Am J Epidemiol. 1978;108:36–46.
34. Ozols II, Wheat LJ. Erythema nodosum in an epidemic of histoplasmosis in Indianapolis. Arch Dermatol. 1981;117:709–12.

35. Rosenthal J, Brandt KD, Wheat LJ, Slama TG. Rheumatologic manifestations of histoplasmosis in the recent Indianapolis epidemic. Arthritis Rheum. 1983;26:1065–70.
36. Goodwin RA, Loyd JE, Des Prez RM. Histoplasmosis in normal hosts. Medicine (Baltimore). 1981;60:231–66.
37. Hage CA, Wheat JL, Loyd J, Allen SD, Blue D, Knox KS. Pulmonary histoplasmosis. Semin Respir Crit Care Med. 2008;29:151–65.
38. Gurney JW, Conces DJ. Pulmonary histoplasmosis. Radiology. 1996;199:297–306.
39. Goodwin Jr RA, Owens FT, Snell JD, et al. Chronic pulmonary histoplasmosis. Medicine (Baltimore). 1976;55:413–52.
40. Wheat LJ, Wass J, Norton J, Kohler RB, French MLV. Cavitary histoplasmosis occurring during two large urban outbreaks: analysis of clinical, epidemiologic, roentgenograghic, and laboratory features. Medicine (Baltimore). 1984;63:201–9.
41. Furcolow ML. Comparison of treated and untreated severe histoplasmosis. J Am Med Assoc. 1963;183:121–7.
42. Parker JD, Sarosi GA, Doto IL, Bailey RE, Tosh FE. Treatment of chronic pulmonary histoplasmosis. N Engl J Med. 1970;283:225–9.
43. Kennedy CC, Limper AH. Redefining the clinical spectrum of chronic pulmonary histoplasmosis. A retrospective case series of 46 patients. Medicine (Baltimore). 2007;86:252–8.
44. Parish JM, Rosenow EC. Mediastinal granuloma and mediastinal fibrosis. Semin Respir Crit Care Med. 2002;23:135–43.
45. Davis AM, Pierson RN, Loyd JE. Mediastinal fibrosis. Semin Respir Infect. 2001;16:119–30.
46. Goodwin RA, Nickell JA, des Prez RM. Mediastinal fibrosis complicating healed primary histoplasmosis and tuberculosis. Medicine (Baltimore). 1972;51:227–46.
47. Loyd JE, Tillman BF, Atkinson JB, Des Prez RM. Mediastinal fibrosis complicating histoplasmosis. Medicine (Baltimore). 1988;67:295–310.
48. Conces DJ, Tarver RD, Viz VA. Broncholithiasis: CT features in 15 patients. Am J Roentgenol. 1991;157:249–53.
49. Picardi JL, Kauffman CA, Schwarz J, Holmes JC, Phair JP, Fowler NO. Pericarditis caused by *Histoplasma capsulatum*. Am J Cardiol. 1976;37:82–8.
50. Wheat LJ, Stein L, Corya BC, et al. Pericarditis as a manifestation of histoplasmosis during two large urban outbreaks. Medicine (Baltimore). 1983;62:110–9.
51. Goodwin Jr RA, Shapiro JL, Thurman GH, Thurman SS, des Prez RM. Disseminated histoplasmosis: clinical and pathologic correlations. Medicine (Baltimore). 1980;59:1–33.
52. Wheat LJ, Connolly-Stringfield PA, Baker RL, et al. Disseminated histoplasmosis in the acquired immune deficiency syndrome: clinical findings, diagnosis and treatment, and review of the literature. Medicine (Baltimore). 1990;69:361–74.
53. Odio CM, Navarrete M, Carrillo JM, Mora L, Carranza A. Disseminated histoplasmosis in infants. Pediatr Infect Dis J. 1999;18:1065–8.
54. Davies SF, Khan M, Sarosi GA. Disseminated histoplasmosis in immunologically suppressed patients. Am J Med. 1978;64:94–100.
55. Koduri PR, Chundi V, DeMarais P, Mizock BA, Patel AR, Weinstein RA. Reactive hemophagocytic syndrome: a new presentation of disseminated histoplasmosis in patients with AIDS. Clin Infect Dis. 1995;21:1453–5.
56. Sanchez A, Celaya AK, Victorio A. Histoplasmosis-associated hemophagocytic syndrome: a case report. AIDS Read. 2007;17: 496–502.
57. Smith JW, Utz JP. Progressive disseminated histoplasmosis: a prospective study of 26 patients. Ann Intern Med. 1972;76:557–65.
58. Wilson DA, Muchmore HG, Tisda RG, Fahmy A, Pitha JV. Histoplasmosis of the adrenal glands studied by CT. Radiology. 1984;150:779–83.
59. Gulati M, Saint S, Tierney LM. Clinical problem-solving. Impatient inpatient care. N Engl J Med. 2000;342:37–40.
60. Gaynes RP, Gardner P, Causey W. Prosthetic value endocarditis caused by *Histoplasma capsulatum*. Arch Intern Med. 1981;141:1533–7.
61. Bradsher RW, Wickre CG, Savage AM, Harston WE, Alford RH. *Histoplasma capsulatum* endocarditis cured by amphotericin B combined with surgery. Chest. 1980;78:791–5.
62. Rogers EW, Weyman AE, Noble RJ, Bruins SC. Left artial myxoma infected with *Histoplasma capsulatum*. Am J Med. 1978;64:683–90.
63. Matthay RA, Levin DC, Wicks AB, Ellis JH. Disseminated histoplasmosis involving an aortofemoral prosthetic graft. J Am Med Assoc. 1976;235:1478–9.
64. Wheat LJ, Batteiger BE, Sathapatayavongs B. *Histoplasma capsulatum* infections of the central nervous system: a clinical review. Medicine (Baltimore). 1990;69:244–60.
65. Wheat LJ, Musial CE, Jenny-Avital E. Diagnosis and management of central nervous system histoplasmosis. Clin Infect Dis. 2005;40:844–52.
66. Klein CJ, Dinapoli RB, Temesgen Z, Meyer FB. Central nervous system histoplasmosis mimicking a brain tumor: difficulties in diagnosis and treatment. Mayo Clin Proc. 1999;74:803–7.
67. Darouiche RO, Cadle RM, Zenon GJ, Weinert MF, Hamill RJ, Lidsky MD. Articular histoplasmosis. J Rheumatol. 1992;19:1991–3.
68. Fowler Jr VG, Nacinovich FM, Alspaugh JA, Corey GR. Prosthetic joint infection due to *Histoplasma capsulatum*: case report and review. Clin Infect Dis. 1998;26:1017.
69. Lamps LW, Molina CP, West AB, Haggitt RC, Scott MA. The pathologic spectrum of gastrointestinal and hepatic histoplasmosis. Am J Clin Pathol. 2000;113:64–72.
70. Suh KN, Anekthananon T, Mariuz PR. Gastrointestinal histoplasmosis in patients with AIDS: case report and review. Clin Infect Dis. 2001;32:483–91.
71. Kauffman CA, Slama TG, Wheat LJ. *Histoplasma capsulatum* epididymitis. J Urol. 1981;125:434–5.
72. Schuster TG, Hollenbeck BK, Kauffman CA, Chensue SW, Wei JT. Testicular histoplasmosis. J Urol. 2000;164:1652.
73. Mawhorter SD, Curley GV, Kursh ED, Farver CE. Prostatic and central nervous system histoplasmosis in an immunocompetent host: case report and review of the prostatic histoplasmosis literature. Clin Infect Dis. 2000;30:595–8.
74. Whitt SP, Koch GA, Fender B, Ratnasamy N, Everett D. Histoplasmosis in pregnancy: case series and report of transplacental transmission. Arch Intern Med. 2004;164:454–8.
75. Oliver A, Ciulla TA, Comer GM. New and classic insights into presumed ocular histoplasmosis syndrome and its treatment. Curr Opin Ophthalmol. 2005;16:160–5.
76. Suttorp-Schulten MSA, Bollemeijer JG, Bos PJM, Rothova A. Presumed ocular histoplasmosis in the Netherlands – an area without histoplasmosis. Br J Ophthalmol. 1997;81:7–11.
77. Specht CS, Mitchell KT, Bauman AE, Gupta M. Ocular histoplasmosis with retinitis in a patient with acquired immune deficiency syndrome. Ophthalmology. 1991;98:1356–9.
78. Wilson ML, Davis TE, Mirrett S, et al. Controlled comparison of the BACTEC high-blood-volume fungal medium, BACTEC plus 26 aerobic blood culture bottle, and 10-milliliter isolator blood culture system for detection of fungemia and bacteremia. J Clin Microbiol. 1993;31:865–71.
79. Smith CD, Goodman L. Improved culture method for the isolation of *Histoplasma capsulatum* and *Blastomyces dermatitidis* from contaminated specimens. Am J Clin Pathol. 1975;63:276–80.
80. Stockman L, Clark KA, Hunt JM, Roberts GD. Evaluation of commercially available acridinium ester-labeled chemiluminescent DNA probes for culture identification of *Blastomyces dermatitidis, Coccidioides immitis, Cryptococcus neoformans,* and *Histoplasma capsulatum*. J Clin Microbiol. 1993;31:845–50.
81. Wheat LJ, Kohler RB, Tewari RP. Diagnosis of disseminated histoplasmosis by detection of *Histoplasma capsulatum* antigen in serum and urine specimens. N Engl J Med. 1986;314:83–8.

82. Wheat LJ. Improvements in diagnosis of histoplasmosis. Expert Opin Biol Ther. 2006;6:1207–21.
83. Connolly PA, Durkin MM, LeMonte AM, Hackett EJ, Wheat LJ. Detection of *Histoplasma* antigen by a quantitative enzyme immunoassay. Clin Vaccine Immunol. 2007;14:1587–91.
84. Swartzentruber S, Rhodes L, Kurkjian K, et al. Diagnosis of acute pulmonary histoplasmosis by antigen detection. Clin Infect Dis. 2009;49(6):928–30.
85. Wheat LJ, Connolly-Stringfield P, Williams B, et al. Diagnosis of histoplasmosis in patients with the acquired immunodeficiency syndrome by detection of *Histoplasma capsulatum* polysaccharide antigen in bronchoalveolar lavage fluid. Am Rev Respir Dis. 1992;145:1421–4.
86. Wheat J, Wheat H, Connolly P, et al. Cross-reactivity in *Histoplasma capsulatum* variety *capsulatum* antigen assays of urine samples from patients with endemic mycoses. Clin Infect Dis. 1997;24:1169–71.
87. Kuberski T, Myers R, Wheat LJ, Kubak BM, Bruckner D, Pegues D. Diagnosis of coccidioidomycosis by antigen detection using cross-reaction with a *Histoplasma* antigen. Clin Infect Dis. 2007;44:e50–4.
88. Durkin M, Witt J, LeMonte A, Wheat B, Connolly P. Antigen assay with the potential to aid in diagnosis of blastomycosis. J Clin Microbiol. 2004;42:4873–5.
89. Martagon-Villamil J, Shrestha N, Sholtis M, et al. Identification of *Histoplasma capsulatum* from culture extracts by real-time PCR. J Clin Microbiol. 2003;41:1295–8.
90. Bialek R, Ernst F, Dietz K, et al. Comparison of staining methods and a nested PCR assay to detect *Histoplasma capsulatum* in tissue sections. Am J Clin Pathol. 2002;117:597–603.
91. Bracca A, Tosello ME, Girardini JE, Amigot SL, Gomez C, Serra E. Molecular detection of *Histoplasma capsulatum* var. *capsulatum* in human clinical samples. J Clin Microbiol. 2003;41:1753–5.
92. Rickerts V, Bialek R, Tintelnot K, Jacobi V, Just-Nubling G. Rapid PCR-based diagnosis of disseminated histoplasmosis in an AIDS patient. Eur J Clin Microbiol Infect Dis. 2002;21:821–3.
93. Picardi JL, Kauffman CA, Schwarz J, Phair JP. Detection of precipitating antibodies to *Histoplasma capsulatum* by counterimmunoelectrophoresis. Am Rev Respir Dis. 1976;114:171–6.
94. Wheat LJ, Freifeld AG, Kleiman MG, et al. Clinical practice guidelines for the management of patients with histoplasmosis: 2007 update by the Infectious Diseases Society of America. Clin Infect Dis. 2007;45:807–27.
95. Dismukes WE, Bradsher Jr RW, Cloud GC, et al. Itraconazole therapy for blastomycosis and histoplasmosis. Am J Med. 1992;93:489–97.
96. McKinsey DS, Kauffman CA, Pappas PG, et al. Fluconazole therapy for histoplasmosis. Clin Infect Dis. 1996;23:996–1001.
97. Doyle TP, Loyd JE, Robbins IM. Percutaneous pulmonary artery and vein stenting: a novel treatment for mediastinal fibrosis. Am J Respir Crit Care Med. 2001;164:657–60.
98. Johnson PC, Wheat LJ, Cloud GA, et al. Safety and efficacy of liposomal amphotericin B compared with conventional amphotericin B for induction therapy of histoplasmosis in patients with AIDS. Ann Intern Med. 2002;137:105–9.
99. Wheat J, Hafner R, Korzun AH, et al. Itraconazole treatment of disseminated histoplasmosis in patients with the acquired immunodeficiency syndrome. Am J Med. 1995;98:336–42.
100. Wheat J, MaWhinney S, Hafner R, et al. Treatment of histoplasmosis with fluconazole in patients with acquired immunodeficiency syndrome. Am J Med. 1997;103:223–32.
101. Pitisuttithum P, Negroni R, Graybill JR, et al. Activity of posaconazole in the treatment of central nervous system fungal infections. J Antimicrob Chemother. 2005;6:745–55.
102. Restrepo A, Tobon A, Clark B, et al. Salvage treatment of histoplasmosis with posaconazole. J Infect. 2007;54:319–27.
103. Freifeld A, Proia L, Andes D, et al. Voriconazole use for endemic fungal infections. Antimicrob Agents Chemother. 2009;53:1648–51.
104. Wheat J, Hafner R, Wulfson M, et al. Prevention of relapse of histoplasmosis with itraconazole in patients with the acquired immunodeficiency syndrome. Ann Intern Med. 1993;118:610–6.
105. Goldman M, Zackin R, Fichtenbaum CJ, et al. Safety of discontinuation of maintenance therapy for disseminated histoplasmosis after immunologic response to antiretroviral therapy. Clin Infect Dis. 2004;38:1485–9.
106. Bamberger DM. Successful treatment of multiple cerebral histoplasmomas with itraconazole. Clin Infect Dis. 1999;28:915–6.
107. Schestatsky P, Chedid MF, Amaral OB, Unis G, Oliveira FM, Severo LC. Isolated central nervous system histoplasmosis in immunocompetent hosts: a series of 11 cases. Scand J Infect Dis. 2006;38:43–8.
108. Tiraboschi I, Casas Parera I, Pikielny R, Scattini G, Micheli F. Chronic *Histoplasma capsulatum* infection of the central nervous system successfully treated with fluconazole. Eur Neurol. 1992;32:70–3.
109. Lortholary O, Denning DW, Dupont B. Endemic mycoses: a treatment update. J Antimicrob Chemother. 1999;43:321–31.
110. Lenhart SW, Schafer MP, Singal M, Hajjeh RA. Histoplasmosis: Protecting Workers at Risk. Cincinnati: US Department of Health and Human Services; 1997.
111. McKinsey DS, Wheat LJ, Cloud GA, et al. Itraconazole prophylaxis for fungal infections in patients with advanced human immunodeficiency virus infection: randomized, placebo-controlled, double-blind study. Clin Infect Dis. 1999;28:1049–56.
112. Edwards LB, Acquaviva SA, Livesay VT, Cross FW, Palmer CE. An atlas of sensitivity to tuberculin, PPD-B, and histoplasmin in the United States. Am Rev Respir Dis. 1969;99:1–18.

Blastomycosis

Robert W. Bradsher and J. Ryan Bariola

Blastomycosis is caused by the dimorphic fungus *Blastomyces dermatitidis*. The organism exists in nature in the mould or mycelial phase and converts to the parasitic or yeast phase at body temperature. Epidemics of blastomycosis after a point-source exposure have been described, but most cases occur sporadically in the endemic areas. *B. dermatitidis* can cause an infection with a subclinical illness and subsequent protection against infection afforded by cellular immune mechanisms. Patients infected with *B. dermatitidis* can present with pneumonia or with extrapulmonary disease, or both. Lung involvement often mimics acute bacterial pneumonia, lung cancer, or tuberculosis. Skin lesions, presenting as either verrucous or ulcerative lesions, are the most common extrapulmonary manifestation, followed by bone, prostate, and central nervous system (CNS) disease. Diagnosis is usually confirmed by visualization of the yeast in smears or in tissue specimens, or by culture. Itraconazole has been shown to be the drug of choice for both pulmonary and extrapulmonary infection, except in cases of life-threatening infection, in which case, amphotericin B is recommended.

Organism

Gilchrist first described blastomycosis in Baltimore in the 1890s as a skin infection caused by what he thought was a protozoan organism [1], and the illness was known for a time as Gilchrist's disease. There were some errors in the initial description. Infection of the skin occurs secondarily rather than as a primary infection, and the organism is not a protozoan but a fungus. Gilchrist was the first to refute portions of his own description when he isolated and named the fungus *Blastomyces dermatitidis* [2]. Because skin manifestations of blastomycosis are often very striking, the initial cases were perceived to be a dermatologic condition. The concept of primary pulmonary blastomycosis was not recognized until pathologic descriptions allowed the pathophysiologic mechanisms to be delineated [3, 4]. There are rare cases of cutaneous inoculation of the fungus in laboratory workers and veterinarians, but almost all cases of blastomycosis are considered to originate from a pulmonary portal of entry [3].

B. dermatitidis is dimorphic, in that it exists as a mycelial form or mould in nature and as a yeast form in tissue. The mould is the infectious form, producing conidia that can be dispersed and subsequently inhaled. The perfect or sexual stage of the fungus is named *Ajellomyces dermatitidis*, with the imperfect or conidial stage named the familiar *B. dermatitidis*. In culture, *B. dermatitidis* grows at 25–28°C as a mould and at 37°C as a yeast. The physiologic mechanism for the dimorphism has been shown to be from hybrid histidine kinase sensing of host signals stimulating the conversion from mycelia to yeast [5].

This imperfect stage grows as a fluffy white mould on Sabouraud's agar at room temperature and as a brown, wrinkled, folded yeast at 37°C. In the yeast phase, the organism appears as a round, budding, thick-walled yeast cell with a daughter cell forming a single bud that has a broad base (Figs. 1 and 2). The yeast varies in size from 5 to 15 μm. Most are round and have a double cell wall appearance, which consists of the interior and exterior components of the thick cell surface. The yeast may be found inside or outside of macrophages in the pyogranulomatous tissue response.

Epidemiology

The endemic areas in North America for *B. dermatitidis* include the states bordering the Mississippi and Ohio Rivers, the Midwestern and Canadian provinces that border the Great Lakes, and a small area in New York and Canada along the St. Lawrence River [3]. The vast majority of patients with blastomycosis who were reported prior to the mid-1980s were from a fairly well defined geographic area of the South Central United States, comprising predominantly Mississippi,

R.W. Bradsher (✉)
University of Arkansas for Medical Sciences and Central Arkansas Veterans Health Care System,
Little Rock, AR, USA
e-mail: bradsherrobertw@uams.edu

C.A. Kauffman et al. (eds.), *Essentials of Clinical Mycology*,
DOI 10.1007/978-1-4419-6640-7_19, © Springer Science+Business Media, LLC 2011

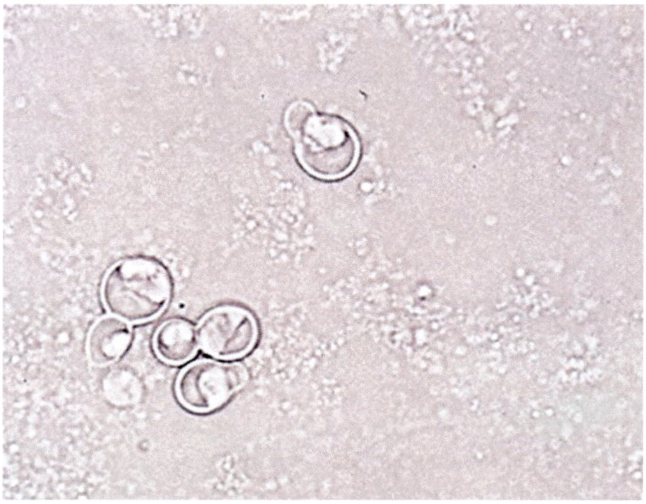

Fig. 1 Sputum sample showing the refractile thick walls and broad-based budding typical of *Blastomyces dermatitidis* (potassium hydroxide preparation, 40×)

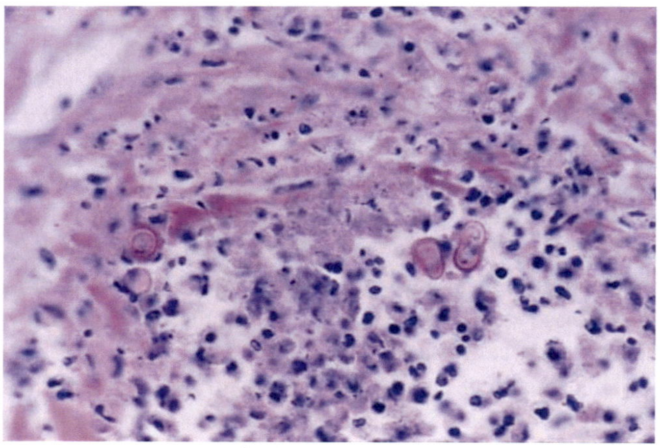

Fig. 2 Tissue obtained at lung biopsy showing broad-based budding yeast. Culture yielded *Blastomyces dermatitidis* (periodic acid – Schiff stain, 40×)

Arkansas, Kentucky, and Tennessee [6]. In the last 2 decades, there have been more cases reported from Illinois, Wisconsin, Ontario, and Manitoba [7–10]. There have been reports of cases of blastomycosis from Colorado, Hawaii, Israel, several areas of Africa, and South America. For the most part, the incidence of blastomycosis depends on the reporting of clinically diagnosed cases of infection because there are no simple and reliable markers of previous mild infection. Mandatory public health reporting of blastomycosis is required in only a few states or provinces, namely Illinois, Wisconsin, Mississippi, Manitoba, and Ontario, and thus cases are likely underreported.

The majority of reported cases of blastomycosis are sporadic and not related to outbreaks. Many patients with blastomycosis have a history of recreational or occupational exposure to wooded areas and often to bodies of water such as lakes or rivers. The stereotypical patient is a young to middle-aged man who either works in or visits outdoor areas in the endemic area. In sporadic cases, the male-to-female ratio has been reported to range from 4:1 to 15:1 in various series [11]. Some of these studies, however, were conducted in Veterans Affairs Medical Centers, which obviously adds bias to the ratio. However, in an outbreak, women and children are as likely as men to be infected. Aside from outbreaks, only rarely are children diagnosed with blastomycosis [12, 13].

Dogs in the same environment as humans also can become infected with *B. dermatitidis*. A clinical clue to the diagnosis of blastomycosis is a history of a pet dog having been found to have blastomycosis [14]. Blastomycosis is not transmitted from dogs to humans, but rather, both are infected as a result of similar exposure in the environment. However, there are very rare reports of a dog with oral lesions transmitting infection via a bite [15].

Outbreaks of blastomycosis have been well described [16–19]. Most have been associated with waterways [17–19]. It has yet to be determined whether water is the primary factor or simply an explanation for greater exposure potential because of recreational activities in areas with wildlife or water [20]. Investigation of these outbreaks has increased our knowledge of the spectrum of disease manifestations of infection with *B. dermatitidis* and allowed the recognition of subclinical infection due to this organism. The majority of cases associated with point-source outbreaks at Big Fork, Minnesota, and Eagle River, Wisconsin, recovered without antifungal therapy [16, 19]. In the Eagle River outbreak, only nine of the 44 patients with infection were treated with an antifungal agent, and none of the 35 untreated patients had relapse or progressive infection [16]. In the latter outbreak, further study revealed that not all of those who had immune markers of infection, such as positive serology or specific antigen-induced lymphocyte transformation, had signs and symptoms characteristic of blastomycosis [16].

In a study of specific immunity to *Blastomyces* antigens using cells from treated blastomycosis patients, two control persons who had no history of blastomycosis had evidence of immunity [21, 22]. Cells from these two control subjects displayed lymphocyte responses to a *Blastomyces* antigen and macrophage inhibition of intracellular growth of the fungus similar to those seen in patients who had culture-proven blastomycosis. Both of these control persons had potential exposure as long-term avid hunters in an endemic region for blastomycosis [22]. This observation prompted studies of other persons who had comparable environmental exposures to patients with clinical blastomycosis, specifically, forestry workers in areas endemic for blastomycosis, but not histoplasmosis, in northern Minnesota and Wisconsin [23]. Thirty percent of the workers had in vitro markers of immunity as evidence of subclinical infection with no question of cross-reactions due to prior infection with *Histoplasma capsulatum*.

Thus, it appears that blastomycosis has comparable patterns of subclinical infection with development of cellular immunity as the more extensively studied endemic mycoses, histoplasmosis and coccidioidomycosis.

It is thought that the ecologic niche for *B. dermatitidis* is the soil. However, the organism has been very difficult to isolate from soil. *B. dermatitidis* was recovered from soil and rotted wood in Georgia on three occasions [24]. The organism has been isolated from bird droppings on one occasion and from a dirt floor in Canada on another [25, 26]. The organism was recovered without animal inoculation from a woodpile from a hyperendemic region in Wisconsin in which several dogs in a nearby kennel had been found to have blastomycosis [27]. *B. dermatitidis* was isolated from soil in association with outbreaks in two separate reports [16, 17]. The isolations were from wet earth that was taken from near bodies of water and that contained animal droppings, showing that the fungus exists in microfoci in soil. However, many other investigators have been unsuccessful in recovering the organism from soil, including areas linked by epidemiologic information to a point-source exposure.

It has become clear that certain areas are hyperendemic for *B. dermatitidis* with unusually high rates of blastomycosis. In one report from Wisconsin, as many as 41.9 cases per 100,000 persons were reported with blastomycosis [28]. Factors that promote this hyperendemicity are being elucidated [29]. During a recent investigation of an outbreak in dogs, a polymerase chain reaction (PCR)–based technique successfully identified *B. dermatitidis* from environmental samples [30]. Additionally, molecular techniques are being used to look at genetic differences detected by PCR of components of the organisms recovered from patients and from the environment [31].

Pathogenesis

Infection with *B. dermatitidis* begins with inhalation of conidia into the alveoli, followed by clearing of the organism by bronchopulmonary phagocytes. Alveolar macrophages have been shown to kill conidia [32], which may explain why some persons are not infected even though they have the same exposure as an infected individual in an epidemic. As the fungus undergoes transition to the yeast phase, growth occurs in the lung, and the organisms can also spread hematogenously to other organs, especially the skin. With the development of immunity, inflammatory reactions occur, initially as a suppurative response with polymorphonuclear phagocytes and then with subsequent influx of monocyte-derived macrophages. This pyogranulomatous response is typical for blastomycosis, although necrosis or fibrosis can also be found. Typically, the granulomas of blastomycosis do not develop caseation necrosis, as found in tuberculosis. The host response leads to resolution of the initial infection. However, it is likely that foci of viable organisms remain, which can later reactivate and cause disease at either pulmonary or extrapulmonary sites [33]. Endogenous reactivation is the logical reason for patients with AIDS developing blastomycosis after leaving their initial residence in the endemic area many years before [34].

Clinical Manifestations

Blastomycosis is not a common diagnosis in most clinical practices, which often leads to a delay in diagnosis. The clinical presentations are protean and are similar to other more common conditions. Weight loss, fever, malaise, fatigue, and other nonspecific complaints are common but not helpful diagnostically. The stereotypical patient is a young to middle-aged man who either works in or visits outdoor areas in the endemic area, but in an outbreak, women and children are as likely as men to be infected. In an observational review of referrals of 135 patients over a 13-year period in Arkansas, 78 were male and 57 female [35]. Extrapulmonary manifestations were found in 47%, and 53% had only lung involvement. Women accounted for only 30% of the extrapulmonary cases, but 47% of the pneumonia cases were in women [35].

Pulmonary

The presentation of blastomycosis for most patients is pneumonia; radiography reveals an alveolar or mass-like infiltrate (Fig. 3). This was noted in 16 of 17 patients in one report [36]. In another series of 46 patients, 26 of whom had had only pulmonary disease, 8 had acute pneumonia and 16 had a chronic pneumonia picture; 32% of the radiographs revealed a mass-like lesion and 48% an alveolar infiltrate [21].

Acute pneumonia due to blastomycosis often presents the same as acute bacterial pneumonia, with fever, chills, and a productive cough with purulent sputum, with or without hemoptysis. Patients who have chronic pneumonia due to blastomycosis usually have weight loss, night sweats, fever, cough with sputum production, and chest pain. They are initially thought to have tuberculosis or lung cancer (Fig. 4). Although cavitary disease may occur, this pattern is not found as commonly as it is in chronic pulmonary histoplasmosis or tuberculosis. Miliary or reticulonodular types infiltrates can also be seen in patients with symptoms of pneumonia.

Patients may have no pulmonary symptoms, and the diagnosis is made following the discovery of pulmonary abnormalities on a chest radiograph obtained for another reason.

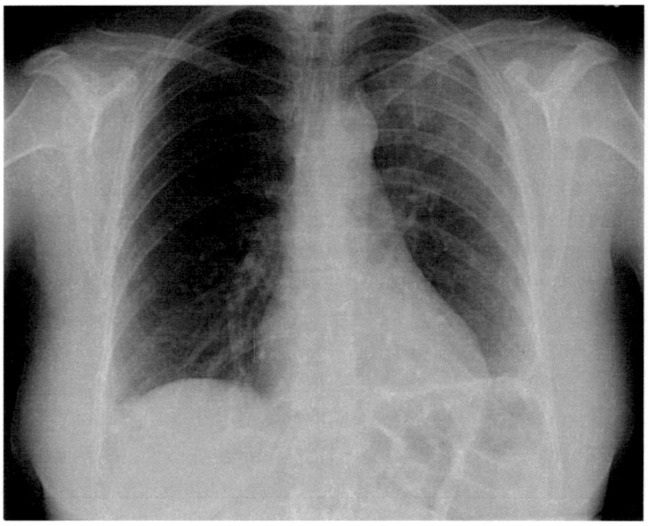

Fig. 3 Left upper and left lower lobe infiltrates in a 36-year-old woman with pulmonary blastomycosis (Courtesy of Dr. William Muth)

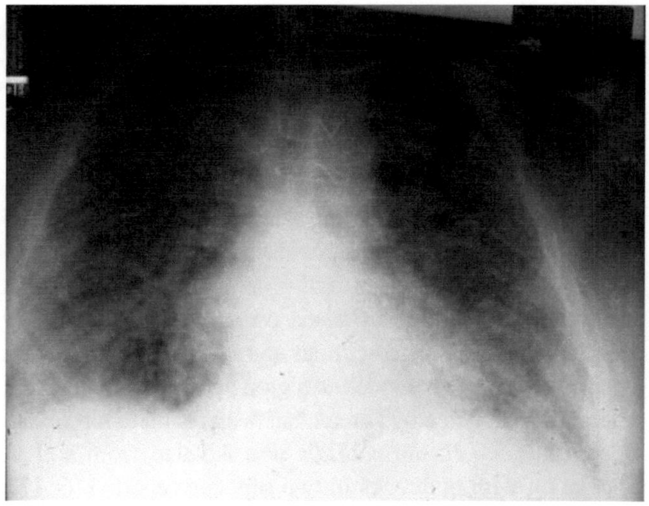

Fig. 5 Acute respiratory distress syndrome (*ARDS*) due to blastomycosis in a 60-year-old man who was previously healthy

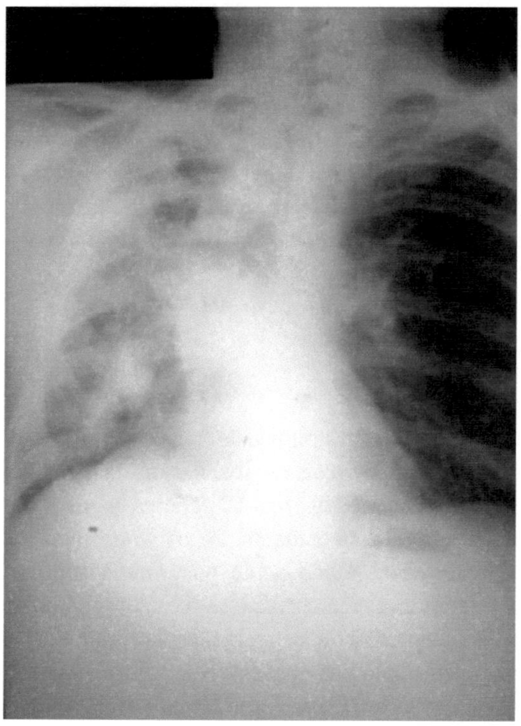

Fig. 4 Chronic destructive pneumonia due to *Blastomyces dermatitidis*

In a series of 46 patients, 26 of whom had had only pulmonary blastomycosis, two patients were found who were asymptomatic [21].

Uncommonly, patients with pulmonary blastomycosis develop the acute respiratory distress syndrome (ARDS) [37–40] (Fig. 5). These patients have diffuse pulmonary infiltrates and hypoxemia, and require ventilatory support. The mortality rate remains high, and often death ensues within a few days of the development of ARDS. For most patients it is unclear whether they have been infected with a huge burden of organisms or whether the host inflammatory response is responsible for the development of ARDS. One patient with this syndrome had a tracheal ulcer at the carina found on bronchoscopy, prompting speculation that a subcarinal lymph node ruptured into the trachea and spilled enough organisms into the lungs to precipitate this syndrome [37]. Early therapy may improve survival rates, and reports of the use of corticosteroids in patients who develop this complication need further study [40].

Cutaneous

Skin lesions are the most common manifestation of extrapulmonary blastomycosis [3, 4]; these lesions may be present with or without concomitant pulmonary lesions. Cutaneous lesions are either verrucous or ulcerative [11, 41]. The verrucous, or fungating, form has an irregular raised border, often with crusting and exudate above an abscess in the subcutaneous tissue (Figs. 6–8). Histologically, papillomatosis, downward proliferation of the epidermis with intraepidermal abscesses, and inflammatory cells in the dermis are features of the lesions [3, 41]. The cutaneous ulcerative form occurs when a subcutaneous abscess spontaneously drains; these demonstrate the same histologic changes as the verrucous form. The borders of the ulcer are usually raised and distinct (Fig. 9), and the base of the ulcer usually contains exudate. Polymorphonuclear leukocytes are typically present on the biopsy, even in those patients with little inflammation clinically apparent in the ulcer (Fig. 10). Subcutaneous lesions lacking either ulceration or the verrucous appearance also can be found (Fig. 11). These lesions are typically tender and may be confused with panniculitis or Weber-Christian disease [42]. The cutaneous lesions of

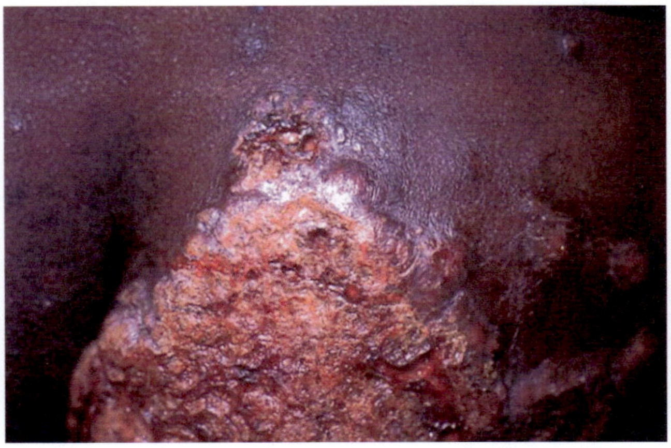

Fig. 6 Verrucous lesion with subcutaneous abscesses on the buttock caused by *Blastomyces dermatitidis*

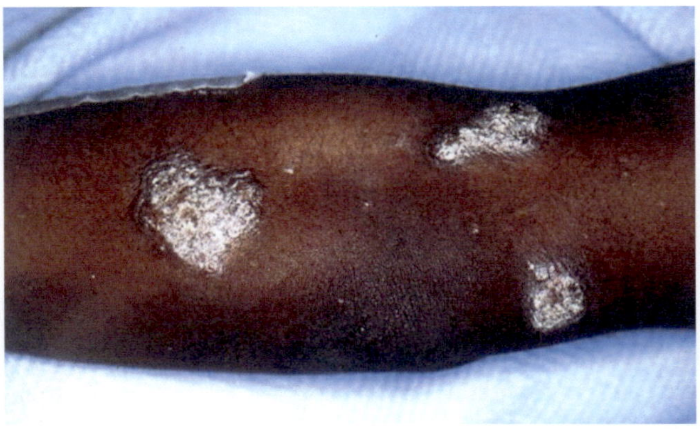

Fig. 7 Multiple verrrucous lesions on the forearm of a 20-year-old man with blastomycosis (Courtesy of Dr. Hector Bonilla)

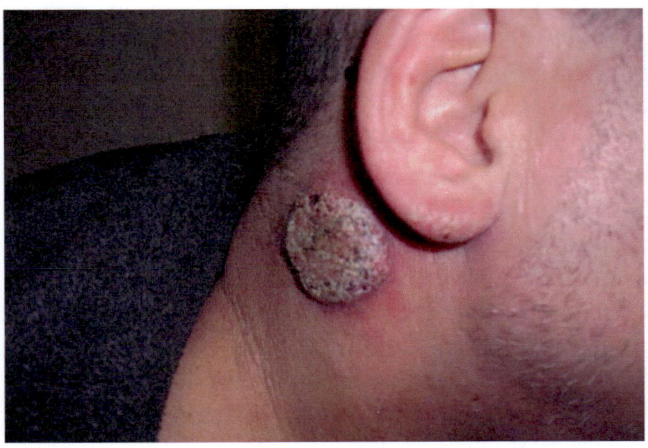

Fig. 8 Non-painful, heaped-up lesion due to *Blastomyces dermatitidis* behind the ear of a 35-year-old man

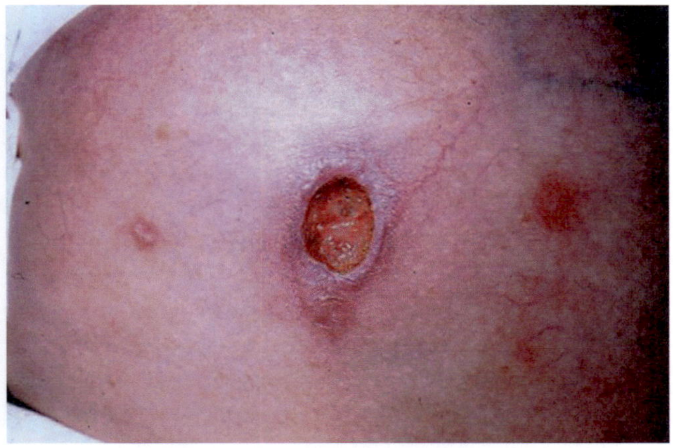

Fig. 9 Ulcerative lesion on the breast caused by *Blastomyces dermatitidis*. Note the distinct and raised borders

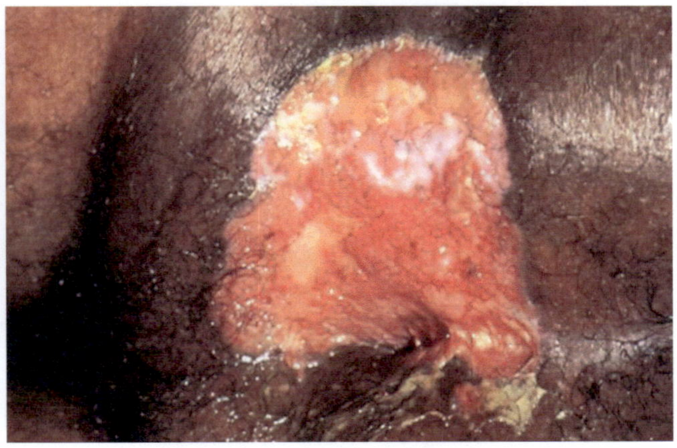

Fig. 10 Extensive perirectal ulcerative lesion with overlying exudate in a patient who had disseminated blastomycosis

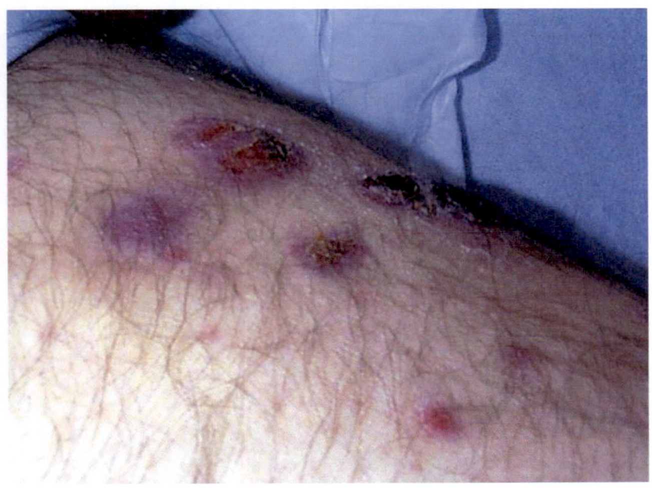

Fig. 11 Subcutaneous nodules with superficial crusts due to blastomycosis on the thigh of a young man

blastomycosis can be confused with a number of alternative diagnoses, including basal cell carcinoma, squamous cell carcinoma, pyoderma gangrenosum, or keratoacanthoma. One patient was reported with what appeared to be condyloma acuminatum surrounding the anus [43]. Only after postoperative suppurative drainage occurred was the histology re-reviewed, and *B. dermatitidis* found. Another similar case has been more recently reported [44].

Osteoarticular

Osteoarticular infection due to *B. dermatitidis* infection is reported in as many as one-fourth of extrapulmonary cases and may be the reason the patient seeks medical attention [45]. The symptoms of involvement of long bones are pain and swelling, with erythema, tenderness, and warmth noted on examination. Vertebral involvement manifests primarily as pain, but with epidural extension, neurologic signs can be seen. Granulomas, suppuration, or necrosis can be found in the bone biopsy. The vertebrae, pelvis, sacrum, skull, ribs, and long bones are the most frequently reported sites of infection, but essentially any bone may be involved [4]. The radiographic appearance of blastomycosis is not specific and cannot be discriminated from that of other fungal, bacterial, or neoplastic diseases. Debridement may be required for cure, but most blastomycosis bone lesions resolve with antimicrobial therapy alone.

Genitourinary

The genitourinary (GU) system follows lung, skin, and bone in frequency of involvement. Prostatitis and epididymo-orchitis have been the more commonly reported forms of genitourinary involvement [3, 4, 46]. Patients present with symptoms of prostatism or with a firm, nontender scrotal mass. In some patients, GU involvement is found incidentally on digital rectal examination. In most circumstances it is thought that the patient has cancer. Patients can have isolated GU disease or, as occurs more frequently, they have GU tract lesions concomitant with pulmonary disease. Chest radiographs should be performed in every case of GU tract blastomycosis, even in the patient without pulmonary complaints. GU infection can be detected when urine collected after prostatic massage yields the organism [46]. Endometrial infection acquired by sexual contact with a man who has blastomycosis on the penis and tubo-ovarian abscess following hematogenous disseminaton are examples of female genital tract infection, an uncommon manifestation of blastomycosis [47, 48]. Massive endometrial infection that caused uterine hemorrhage has been described in one patient [49].

Central Nervous System

Blastomycosis is reported to involve the CNS in 5–10% of cases of disseminated disease. Meningitis and/or cerebral or cerebellar abscesses are the most common manifestations of CNS blastomycosis [50–54]. Either can occur as isolated manifestations of blastomycosis, but more frequently CNS symptoms and signs occur in patients who have manifestations of widespread disease. MRI imaging is helpful in the diagnosis of mass lesions. For patients with meningitis, cerebrospinal fluid (CSF) analysis reveals high protein, slightly low glucose, and the presence of increased numbers of lymphocytes, but the organism is rarely grown from the fluid obtained by lumbar puncture. In one series of 22 patients with chronic meningitis, CSF from lumbar puncture provided the diagnosis in only two patients, whereas ventricular CSF was positive when cultured in six of seven cases [51]. A recent series noted that CSF obtained at lumbar puncture yielded the organism in a larger proportion of cases [54].

Other Organ Involvement

Lesions of blastomycosis can occur in virtually any organ. Abscesses are most common in the subcutaneous tissue, but they can be found in the brain, skeletal system, prostate, or any other organ, including the myocardium, pericardium, spleen, liver, lymph nodes, orbit, sinuses, pituitary, adrenal gland, and other organs [3, 4, 43, 55]. Blastomycosis can involve the mouth, oropharynx, and especially the larynx, where it mimics sqauamous cell carcinoma [56]. Laryngeal biopsy reveals histologic features similar to those seen in the skin and may initially be mistaken for carcinoma. In some cases, fixation of the vocal cords secondary to fibrosis has led to radiation therapy or total laryngectomy because of an incorrect diagnosis of cancer.

Ocular involvement may assume several forms. A patient with a mass on the iris prompted a review of the literature by Lopez and colleagues. A total of 11 cases of ocular blastomycosis, including cases with iritis, uveitis, endophthalmitis, and choroidal lesions, were found [57]. More cases of choroidal involvement have been reported [58, 59]. Eyelid involvement has been reported to occur in as many as 25% of patients with disseminated blastomycosis [60, 61], but this frequency appears to be higher than that noted in most experts' experiences. Ocular disease, endophthalmitis in particular, is very common in canine blastomycosis, but this type of involvement is rare in humans [62]. The reason for this discrepancy is not understood but may be due to later diagnosis in dogs, allowing more dissemination of the infection.

Two cases of otitis media with cranial extension due to *B. dermatitidis* have been reported [63]. One patient was described with infection in a presumed branchial cleft cyst [43]. Surgical removal demonstrated lymphadenopathy and suppurative and granulomatous inflammation with *B. dermatitidis* organisms. Peripheral lymphadenopathy is found in systemic blastomycosis; amyloid deposition in the node has rarely been reported [43].

Cases of blastomycosis involving the breast have been reported [64–66]. An abnormal mammogram may be the first sign, and the diagnosis is almost always thought to be carcinoma. In one patient, a CT scan which revealed partial destruction of a vertebral body consistent with metastatic disease almost led to treatment with cancer chemotherapy until a breast biopsy revealed *B. dermatitidis* on microscopy and subsequent culture [64].

Endocrine abnormalities have been reported in patients with blastomycosis [4]. Adrenal insufficiency from destruction of both adrenal glands is the most common. Thyroid involvement has been recently reported [67, 68]. Rarely, hypercalcemia, as seen with other granulomatous diseases, has been reported with blastomycosis. A single case of diabetes insipidus and another of hyperprolactinemia with galactorrhea and amenorrhea have been reported [69, 70].

Immunocompromised Patients

Blastomycosis causes infection in immunocompromised patients, including patients with AIDS, recipients of solid organ transplants, patients treated with tumor necrosis factor antagonists, and patients on corticosteroid therapy [71–77]. However, blastomycosis is seen much less commonly than infection with *Histoplasma capsulatum* or *Cryptococcus neoformans* in these groups. Immunosuppressed patients can develop infection following exposure in the environment or from reactivation of a latent focus of infection.

Pappas et al. reviewed the cases of immunosuppressed patients with blastomycosis who were seen in several tertiary care medical centers from 1956 to 1991. They found an increased proportion of cases from 1978 to 1991, as compared with 1956–1977 [76]. Although this could have been from a bias in referral patterns of patients, they speculated that this more likely reflected the continually enlarging population of patients who have complicated immune compromising illnesses and who have lived in the endemic area for this fungus. Tumor necrosis factor antagonist therapy is increasingly associated with disseminated infection with fungi and mycobacteria. A total of seven cases of blastomycosis had been reported to the FDA registry by the summer of 2008 [77].

Although not common in the immunosuppressed population, when blastomycosis is seen in a patient who is immunosuppresssed, it is usually widely disseminated and particularly severe. ARDS has developed in a number of cases, and CNS involvement is common [71, 74, 76]. The mortality rate in patients with AIDS who developed blastomycosis was 40% and most died within a few weeks [71]. With the use of current antiretroviral therapy, the occurrence of severe manifestations is less frequent, and the mortality rates are lower.

Other Patient Groups

Blastomycosis has been reported to occur with other infections or other illnesses, including tuberculosis, histoplasmosis, and coccidioidomycosis [78]. Blastomycosis has been reported in two patients, one of whom presented with idiopathic thrombocytopenic purpura and the other with hemolytic anemia [35]. Both patients were treated with corticosteroids for the hematologic conditions, and blastomycosis was treated with antifungal agents. Steroids were rapidly tapered, and the hematologic conditions did not recur after the blastomycosis was cured. Another patient with both sarcoidosis and blastomycosis was treated with both corticosteroids and itraconazole with cure of the fungal infection [43]. As long as effective antifungal chemotherapy is being given, steroid therapy may not have the deleterious result that has been described in untreated blastomycosis.

Several cases of blastomycosis have been reported during pregnancy [79–85]. In several well-documented cases, blastomycosis has been transmitted to the fetus via intrauterine transfer of the organisms [79, 82, 85].

Diagnosis

Culture

Growth of *B. dermatitidis* in culture is the definitive test to prove a diagnosis of blastomycosis. The organism is not particularly difficult to culture, but it may take 2–4 weeks for the organism to grow as a mould at 25–28°C. The appearance of the mould phase is not distinctive, and a confirmatory test must be performed. An exoantigen assay was developed to discriminate early cultures of *H. capsulatum* and *B. dermatitidis* [86], but currently, most laboratories use a rapid DNA probe test that is specific for *B. dermatitidis* [87]. With these rapid specific tests, it is no longer necessary to convert the mould phase to the yeast phase to confirm the organism as *B. dermatitidis*.

Histopathology

If suspected, a diagnosis of blastomycosis can be established quickly by seeing the characteristic yeasts in tissue, exudates, or body fluids. Exudates or sputum can be treated with potassium hydroxide or calcofluor white, which is more sensitive because the fluorescent dye allows easy visualization of the 8–15 μm thick-walled, broad-based, budding yeast cells [34]. Cytological preparations stained with Papanicolau stain also can be used for a dependable diagnosis [88]. Tissues stained with hematoxylin and eosin do not allow visualization of the yeasts in most circumstances; staining with periodic acid–Schiff or methenamine silver stains are preferred for visualization of the yeasts in tissues.

Serology

Serodiagnostic tests for blastomycosis started with complement fixation (CF) with yeast-phase antigens (blastomycin) to detect antibodies to *B. dermatitidis* and then proceeded to the use of an immunodiffusion (ID) assay and an enzyme immunoassay (EIA) [89–93]. The CF test had a low sensitivity (57%) and specificity (30%). In a large outbreak, only 9% of patients were found to have CF antibodies to blastomycin [90]. In another series, patients were as likely to have CF antibodies to *H. capsulatum* antigens as they were to *B. dermatitidis* antigens [3]. Given the overlapping endemic regions of these two fungi, this was obviously problematic.

Better results were obtained with the ID assay and with the EIA using a more specific antigen for *B. dermatitidis,* the A antigen. The ID assay resulted in reported sensitivity rates of 65–80% with 100% specificity. However, when applied to sera obtained from the previously mentioned outbreak in Wisconsin, antibodies were detected in only 28% of documented cases with the ID assay. The EIA using the A antigen proved more sensitive, detecting antibody in 77% of cases [91]. While better than CF antibody tests, ID and EIA tests were still plagued with cross-reactivity problems with other endemic mycoses, especially histoplasmosis, and the low sensitivity led to an unacceptable number of false-negative results, hindering its use as a diagnostic test, especially given the low prevalence in most areas.

Klein et al. described a 120 kD surface protein termed WI-1 and later renamed BAD-1 [92]. This protein was purer than A antigen and lacked the carbohydrate moieties that caused the majority of cross-reactions with *H. capsulatum* [92]. A radioimmunoassay (RIA) using this protein showed promise, identifying antibodies in 85% of patients with known blastomycosis. Only 3% of patients with other mycoses, and no healthy volunteers, tested positive using this assay [93]. This RIA, however, has not been adapted for clinical use.

Antigen Detection

There is now a commercially available assay for the detection of *B. dermatitidis* antigen in humans [94]. It has mostly been used in urine specimens and has a reported overall sensitivity in the urine of 92.9% and a reported specificity of 79.3%. Antigen was detected at levels considered positive in patients with both disseminated blastomycosis and isolated pulmonary blastomycosis. Cross-reactions were seen in subjects with other fungal infections, especially histoplasmosis, paracoccidioidomycosis, and penicilliosis. The cross-reactivity between *B. dermatitidis* and *H. capsulatum* is felt to be due to a shared polysaccharide [95]. The clinical pictures for these two infections can sometimes be similar, especially with isolated pulmonary disease, and the endemic areas for these fungi overlap. On the other hand, patients with either disseminated or pulmonary blastomycosis have had negative assays for *B. dermatitidis* antigen at the time of initial diagnosis. Thus, in the right clinical setting, a negative antigen should not be used to eliminate blastomycosis from the differential diagnosis.

The antigen assay has been shown to revert to a level considered negative in patients successfully treated for blastomycosis [96–98]. The time to resolution, however, remains undetermined, and there have been no large studies to evaluate the usefulness of repeated antigen testing during therapy to monitor for response. Antigen detection might prove helpful in less common presentations of blastomycosis, but this has not been studied. In clinical practice, the *Blastomyces* antigen assay can be a helpful tool, but should not supplant clinical evaluation and judgment.

Treatment

Spontaneous resolution of chronic blastomycosis is very uncommon, and untreated blastomycosis is associated with mortality rates approaching 60% [3, 4]. Thus, all patients with chronic pulmonary and extrapulmonary blastomycosis should receive antifungal therapy.

Controversy once existed concerning the need for antifungal therapy in all recognized cases of acute pulmonary blastomycosis. Experts agree that some of the cases of acute blastomycosis are self-limited [99, 100], but most advocate specific antifungal therapy for all cases of pulmonary blastomycosis, whether acute or chronic. Careful follow-up for several years is mandatory in patients with acute pneumonia who do not receive antifungal therapy to ensure that there is no recrudescence of infection.

The treatment of blastomycosis has evolved with the development of the azoles, ketoconazole, itraconazole and fluconazole. However, no randomized, blinded studies comparing different regimens have been performed, and there are only a few comparative trials for therapy of blastomycosis. Thus, the recently published treatment recommendations for blastomycosis are based on relatively small, open-label, controlled trials, case series, and anecdotal experience [101].

Ketoconazole was the first oral azole to be studied for the treatment of non-life-threatening, non-CNS blastomycosis. A single daily dose of 400 mg of ketoconazole for at least 6 months was recommended for patients with uncomplicated blastomycosis. Of note, there were multiple reports of CNS relapses following "successful" therapy of pulmonary blastomycosis with an appropriate course of ketoconazole [21, 102, 103], underscoring the poor penetration of this agent into the CNS and the need for careful monitoring during therapy and long-term follow-up after completion of therapy.

Itraconazole, an oral triazole with broad-spectrum antifungal activity, is now considered to be the drug of choice for patients with non-life-threatening, non-CNS blastomycosis. In a prospective, open-label, noncomparative multicenter study, 43 of 48 (90%) patients with mild-to-moderate disease were cured with itraconazole at doses ranging from 200 to 400 mg daily [104]. Of 40 patients who received at least 2 months of therapy, 39 (95%) were cured. Most patients responded to the lower dosage of itraconazole (200 mg), and the drug was better tolerated than ketoconazole based upon historic comparison. Another report suggested similar success among an additional 42 patients who received itraconazole at a daily dosage of 200 mg [105]. Based on these studies, the current recommendation for patients with non-life-threatening, non-CNS blastomycosis is to treat with itraconazole at an initial dosage of 200 mg daily for 6–12 months. For patients not responding to therapy, the dose should be increased to 200 mg twice daily [101]. Because absorption of the itraconazole capsule formulation is not reliable, measurement of drug levels is recommended, particularly if the infection does not respond quickly [101]. A minimum of 12 months of therapy is recommended for osteoarticular infection.

Fluconazole, another oral and parenteral triazole with broad-spectrum activity and superior pharmacokinetics compared with either itraconazole or ketoconazole, has also been studied for the treatment of non-life-threatening, non-CNS blastomycosis. To date, two multicenter trials have been conducted using fluconazole [106, 107]. In the pilot study comparing 200 and 400 mg of fluconazole daily, success was seen in only 65% of 23 patients who received therapy for at least 6 months [106]. The follow-up study using 400 and 800 mg daily showed improved efficacy with 34 (87%) of 39 patients successfully treated [107]. Average duration of therapy in this study was almost 9 months, and patients tolerated this therapy with few significant adverse events. The results of these studies suggest that fluconazole is comparable in efficacy to ketoconazole at similar doses, but it does not appear to be as efficacious as itraconazole. Therefore the role of fluconazole in the treatment of blastomycosis is limited and should be reserved for patients who are unable to tolerate itraconazole or ketoconazole because of adverse effects or specific drug-drug interactions. However, given the favorable pharmacokinetics of fluconazole, including its good penetration into the CNS, fluconazole could be considered in the treatment of patients with CNS blastomycosis who have had a favorable response to initial therapy with amphotericin B. Clinical experience with fluconazole in this setting is limited to a few patients [54].

Voriconazole has been used to treat patients with blastomycosis. Most have had CNS infection, and the response rate in this group of patients with severe disease has been excellent [54, 108, 109]. In additon, voriconazole has been used in solid organ transplant recipients with blastomycosis but the results have been mixed [74]. Posaconazole has potent activity against *B. dermatitidis* in vitro, but there are very limited anecdotal reports of patients with blastomycosis who have been treated with this agent.

For patients with severe, life-threatening blastomycosis, amphotericin B remains the drug of choice. Traditionally, a cumulative dose of 1.5–2.5 g of amphotericin B deoxycholate was advocated [110, 111], but this approach has been supplanted by current recommendations to treat with amphotericin B until the patient has improved and can take oral medications and then to step down to therapy with oral itraconazole, 200 mg twice daily [101]. Many institutions have eliminated amphotericin B deoxycholate in favor of lipid formulations of amphotericin because of the toxicity of the older agent. For CNS blastomycosis, the Infectious Diseases Society of America (IDSA) Guidelines recommend a lipid formulation of amphotericin B at a dosage of 5 mg/kg daily for the initial 4–6 weeks of therapy. These patients should then be treated with high doses of an oral azole (voriconazole, fluconazole, or itraconazole) for a minimum of a year [101].

Patients with blastomycosis who have AIDS, transplant recipients, those receiving chronic corticosteroids or tumor necrosis factor antagonists, and other significantly immunocompromised patients should receive initial therapy with amphotericin B. Blastomycosis among these patients is associated with significant complications, including ARDS, CNS, and multiorgan involvement, and with substantially higher mortality. Thus, early and aggressive therapy is essential in this population. Long-term suppressive therapy with oral itraconazole is generally advised in patients with significant ongoing immune dysfunction [101].

Pregnant women with blastomycosis constitute a special population in regards to therapy. Only a few cases of blastomycosis in pregnancy have been reported, and none have failed therapy with amphotericin B; lipid formulations are recommended [101]. There has been no evidence of adverse effects on the fetus from amphotericin B; thus it appears to be safe and effective in pregnant women. Azoles should specifically be avoided in this population due to potential teratogenicity.

Blastomycosis is uncommon in children, and therapeutic studies in this group are lacking. Current recommendations are based solely on anecdotal data. Some investigators suggest that children with blastomycosis have a less favorable response to initial therapy with an azole than do their adult counterparts and have advocated initial therapy with amphotericin B [12]. However, the IDSA Guidelines recommend therapy similar to that noted above for adults, with itraconazole as the agent of choice for mild-to-moderate infection and amphotericin B reserved for severely ill children [101].

References

1. Gilchrist TC. Protozoan dermatitis. J Cutan Gen Dis. 1894;12: 496–9.
2. Gilchrist TC, Stokes WR. Case of pseudo-lupus vulgaris caused by *Blastomyces*. J Exp Med. 1898;3:53–78.
3. Sarosi GA, Davies SF. Blastomycosis. State of the art. Am Rev Respir Dis. 1979;120:911–38.
4. Witorsch P, Utz JP. North American blastomycosis: a study of 40 patients. Medicine (Baltimore). 1968;47:169–200.
5. Nemecek JC, Wuthrich M, Klein BS. Global control of dimorphism and virulence in fungi. Science. 2006;312:583–8.
6. Cano MV, Ponce-de-Leon GF, Tippen S, Lindsley MD, Warwick M, Hajjeh RA. Blastomycosis in Missouri: epidemiology and risk factors for endemic disease. Epidemiol Infect. 2003;131:907–14.
7. Dworkin MS, Duckro AN, Proia L, Semel JD, Huhn G. The epidemiology of blastomycosis in Illinois and factors associated with death. Clin Infect Dis. 2005;41:e107–11.
8. Baumgardner Dj, Steber D, Glazier R. Geographic information system analysis of blastomycosis in northern Wisconsin, USA: waterways and soil. Med Mycol. 2005;43:117–25.
9. Morris SK, Brophy J, Richardson SE, et al. Blastomycosis in Ontario, 1994–2003. Emerg Infect Dis. 2006;12:274–9.
10. Crampton TL, Light RB, Berg GM, et al. Epidemiology and clinical spectrum of blastomycosis diagnosed at Manitoba hospitals. Clin Infect Dis. 2002;34:1310–6.
11. Bradsher RW. Blastomycosis. Infect Dis Clin North Am. 1988;2:877–98.
12. Steele RW, Abernathy RS. Systemic blastomycosis in children. Pediatr Infect Dis J. 1983;2:304–7.
13. Schutze GE, Hickerson SL, Fortin EM, et al. Blastomycosis in children. Clin Infect Dis. 1996;22:496–502.
14. Sarosi GA, Eckman MR, Davies SF, Laskey WK. Canine blastomycosis as a harbinger of human disease. Ann Intern Med. 1983;98:48–9.
15. Gnann JW, Bressler GS, Bodet CA, Avent KA. Human blastomycosis after a dog bite. Ann Intern Med. 1983;98:48–9.
16. Klein BS, Vergeront JM, Weeks RJ, et al. Isolation of *Blastomyces dermatitidis* in soil associated with a large outbreak of blastomycosis in Wisconsin. N Engl J Med. 1986;314:529–34.
17. Klein BS, Vergeront JM, DiSalvo AF, et al. Two outbreaks of blastomycosis along rivers in Wisconsin: isolation of *Blastomyces dermatitidis* from riverbank soil and evidence of its transmission along waterways. Am Rev Respir Dis. 1987;136:1333–8.
18. Baumgardner DJ, Buggy BP, Mattson BJ, Burdick JS, Ludwig D. Epidemiology of blastomycosis in a region of high endemicity in north central Wisconsin. Clin Infect Dis. 1993;15:629–35.
19. Tosh FE, Hammerman KJ, Weeks RJ, Sarosi GA. A common source epidemic of North American blastomycosis. Am Rev Respir Dis. 1974;109:525–9.
20. Bradsher RW. Water and blastomycosis: don't blame beaver. Am Rev Respir Dis. 1987;136:1324–6.
21. Bradsher RW, Rice DC, Abernathy RS. Ketoconazole therapy for endemic blastomycosis. Ann Intern Med. 1985;103:872–9.
22. Bradsher RW, Balk RA, Jacobs RF. Growth inhibition of *Blastomyces dermatitidis* in alveolar and peripheral macrophages from persons with blastomycosis. Am Rev Respir Dis. 1987;137:412–7.
23. Vaalar AK, Bradsher RW, Davies SF. Evidence of subclinical blastomycosis in forestry workers in northern Minnesota and northern Wisconsin. Am J Med. 1990;89:470–6.
24. Denton JF, Disalvo AF. Isolation of *Blastomyces dermatitidis* from natural sites in Augusta, Georgia. Am J Trop Med Hyg. 1964;13:716–22.
25. Sarosi GA, Serstock M. Isolation of *Blastomyces dermatitidis* from pigeon manure. Am Rev Respir Dis. 1976;114:1179–83.
26. Bakerspigel A, Kane J, Schaus D. Isolation of *Blastomyces dermatitidis* from an earthen floor in southwestern Ontario, Canada. J Clin Microbiol. 1986;24:890–1.
27. Baumgardner DJ, Paretsky DP. Identification of *Blastomyces dermatitidis* in the stool of a dog with acute pulmonary blastomycosis. J Med Vet Mycol. 1999;35:419–21.
28. The Centers for Disease Control and Prevention. Blastomycosis-Wisconsin, 1986–1995. MMWR Morb Mortal Wkly Rep. 1996;45:601–3.
29. Reed KD, Meece JK, Archer JR, et al. Ecologic niche modeling of *Blastomyces dermatitidis* in Wisconsin. PLoS ONE. 2008;3(4):e2034.
30. Burgess JW, Schwan WR, Volk TJ. PCR-based detection of DNA from the human pathogen *Blastomyces dermatitidis* from natural soil samples. Med Mycol. 2006;44:741–8.
31. Meece JK, Anderson JL, Klein BS, et al. Genetic diversity in *Blastomyces dermatitidis:* implications for PCR detection in clinical and environmental samples. Med Mycol. 2009:Jul;22:1–7. epub ahead of print.
32. Sugar AM, Picard M. Macrophage- and oxidant-mediated inhibition of the ability of live *Blastomyces dermatitidis* conidia to transform to the pathogenic yeast phase: Implications for the pathogenesis of dimorphic fungal infections. J Infect Dis. 1991;163:371–5.
33. Landis FB, Varkey B. Late relapse of pulmonary blastomycosis after adequate treatment with amphotericin B. Case report. Am Rev Respir Dis. 1976;113:77–81.
34. Bradsher RW, Chapman SW, Pappas PG. Blastomycosis. Infect Dis Clin North Am. 2003;17:21–40.
35. Bradsher RW. Clinical features of blastomycosis. Semin Respir Infect. 1997;12:229–34.
36. Halvorsen RA, Duncan JD, Merten DF, Gallis HA, Putman CE. Pulmonary blastomycosis. Radiology. 1984;150:1–5.
37. Evans ME, Haynes JB, Atkins JB, Atkinson JB, Delvaux Jr TC, Kaiser AB. *Blastomyces dermatitidis* and the adult respiratory distress syndrome. Am Rev Respir Dis. 1982;126:1099–102.
38. Meyer KC, McManus EJ, Maki DG. Overwhelming pulmonary blastomycosis associated with the adult respiratory distress syndrome. N Engl J Med. 1993;329:1231–6.
39. Skillrud DM, Douglas WW. Survival in ARDS caused by blastomycosis infection. Mayo Clin Proc. 1985;60:266–9.
40. Lahm T, Neese S, Thornburg AT, et al. Corticosteroids for blastomycosis-induced ARDS. Chest. 2008;133:1478–80.
41. Schwarz J, Salfelder K. Blastomycosis: a review of 152 cases. Curr Top Pathol. 1977;65:165–200.
42. Maioriello RP, Merwin CF. North American blastomycosis presenting as an acute panniculitis and arthritis. Arch Dermatol. 1970;102:92–6.
43. Bradsher RW, Martin MR, Wilkes TD, Waltman C, Bolyard K. Unusual presentations of blastomycosis: ten case summaries. Infect Med. 1990;7:10–9.
44. Ricciardi R, Alavi K, Filice GA, Heily SD, Spencer MP. *Blastomyces dermatitidis* of the perianal skin: report of a case. Dis Colon Rectum. 2007;50:118–21.

45. Moore RM, Green NE. Blastomycosis of bone. J Bone Joint Surg. 1982;64:1094–101.
46. Inoshita T, Youngberg GA, Boelen LJ, et al. Blastomycosis presenting with prostatic involvement: report of 2 cases and review of the literature. J Urol. 1983;130:160–2.
47. Farber ER, Leahy MS, Meadows TR. Endometrial blastomycosis acquired by sexual contact. Obstet Gynecol. 1968;32:195–9.
48. Murray JJ, Clark CA, Lands RH, Heim CR, Burnett LS. Reactivation blastomycosis presenting as a tuboovarian abscess. Obstet Gynecol. 1984;64:828–30.
49. Faro S, Pastorek JG, Collins J, Spencer R, Greer DL, Phillips LE. Severe uterine hemorrhage from blastomycosis of the endometrium. J Reprod Med. 1987;32:247–9.
50. Gonyea EF. The spectrium of primary blastomycotic meningitis: a review of central nervous system blastomycosis. Ann Neurol. 1979;3:26–39.
51. Kravitz GR, Davies SF, Eckman MR, Sarosi GA. Chronic blastomycotic meningitis. Am J Med. 1981;71:501–5.
52. Craig WM, Carmichael Jr FA. Blastomycoma of the cerebellum: report of a case. Mayo Clin Proc. 1938;13:347–51.
53. Wylen EL, Nanda A. *Blastomyces dermatitidis* occurring as an isolated cerebellar mass. Neurosurg Rev. 1999;22:152–4.
54. Bariola JR, Perry P, Pappas PG, et al. Blastomycosis of the central nervous system: a multicenter review of diagnosis and treatment in the modern era. Clin Infect Dis. 2010;50:797–804.
55. Dubuisson RL, Jones TB. Splenic abscess due to blastomycosis: scintigraphic, sonographic, and CT evaluation. Am JRadiol. 1983;140:66–8.
56. Suen JY, Wetmore SJ, Wetzel WJ. Blastomycosis of the larynx. Ann Otol Rhinol Laryngol. 1980;89:563–6.
57. Lopez R, Mason JO, Parker JS, Pappas PG. Intraocular blastomycosis: case report and review. Clin Infect Dis. 1994;18:805–7.
58. Gottlieb JL, McAllister IL, Guttman FA, Vine AK. Choroidal blastomycosis. Retina. 1995;15:248–52.
59. Almony A, Kraus CL, Ate RS. Successful treatment of choroidal blastomycosis with oral administration of voriconazole. Can J Ophthalmol. 2009;44:334–5.
60. Bartley GB. Blastomycosis of the eyelid. Ophthalmol. 1995; 102:2020–3.
61. Vida L, Moel SA. Systemic North American blastomycosis with orbital involvement. Am J Ophthalmol. 1974;77:240–2.
62. Pariseau B, Lucarelli MJ, Appen RE. A concise history of ophthalmic blastomycosis. Ophthalmology. 2007;114:e27–32.
63. Istorico LJ, Sanders M, Jacobs RF, Gillian S, Glasier C, Bradsher RW. Otitis media due to blastomycosis. Clin Infect Dis. 1992;14:335–8.
64. Farmer C, Stanley MW, Bardales RH, et al. Mycoses of the breast: diagnosis by fine needle aspiration. Diagn Cytopathol. 1995;12:51–5.
65. Seymour EQ. Blastomycosis of the breast. AJR. 1982;139:822–3.
66. Propeck PA, Scanlan KA. Blastomycosis of the breast. AJR. 1996;166:726.
67. Moinuddin S, Barazi H, Moinuddin M. Acute blastomycosis thyroiditis. Thyroid. 2008;18:659–61.
68. Wineland A, Siegel E, Franccis C, Chen C, Bodenner D, Satck Jr BC. Fine-needle aspiration diagnosis of thyroid blastomycosis. Endocr Pract. 2008;14:224–8.
69. Kelly PM. Systemic blastomycosis with associated diabetes insipidus. Ann Intern Med. 1982;96:66–7.
70. Arora NS, Oblinger MJ, Feldman PS. Chronic pleural blastomycosis with hyperprolactinemia, galactorrhea and ammenorrhea. Am Rev Respir Dis. 1989;120:451–5.
71. Pappas PG, Pottage JC, Powderly WG, et al. Blastomycosis in patients with the acquired immunodeficiency syndrome. Ann Intern Med. 1992;116:847–53.
72. Witzig RS, Hoadley DJ, Greer DL, Abriola KP, Hernandez RL. Blastomycosis and HIV. South Med J. 1994;87:715–9.
73. Guccion JG, Rohatgi PK, Saini NB, French A, Tavaloki S, Barr S. Disseminated blastomycosis and acquired immunodeficiency syndrome: a case report and ultrastructural study. Ultrastruct Pathol. 1996;20:429–35.
74. Gauthier GM, Safdar N, Klein BS, Andes DR. Blastomycosis in solid organ transplant recipients. Transpl Infect Dis. 2007;9:310–7.
75. Winquist EW, Walmsley SL, Berinstein NL. Reactivation and dissemination of blastomycosis complicating Hodgkin's disease. Am J Hematol. 1993;43:129–32.
76. Pappas PG, Threlkeld MG, Bedsole GD, Cleveland KO, Gelfand MS, Dismukes WE. Blastomycosis in immunocompromised patients. Medicine. 1993;72:311–25.
77. FDA Information for Healthcare Professionals: Cimzia (certolizumab pegol), Enbrel (etanercept), Humira (adalimumab), and Remicade (infliximab) 2008. http://www.fda.gov/Drugs/DrugSafety/PostmarketDrugSafetyInformationforPatientsandProviders/ucm124185.htm. Accessed 1 September 2009.
78. Causey WA, Campbell GD. Clinical aspects of blastomycosis. In: Al-Doory YA, DiSalvo AF, editors. Blastomycosis. New York: Plenum; 1992. p. 165–88.
79. Maxson S, Miller SF, Tryka F, Schutze GE. Perinatal blastomycosis: a review. Pediatr Infect Dis J. 1992;11:760–3.
80. Young L, Schutze GE. Perinatal blastomycosis: the rest of the story. Pediatr Infect Dis J. 1995;14:83.
81. Ismail MA, Lerner SA. Disseminated blastomycosis in a pregnant woman. Am Rev Respir Dis. 1982;126:350–3.
82. Tuthill SW. Disseminated blastomycosis with intrauterine transmission. South Med J. 1985;78:1526–7.
83. Daniel L, Salit IE. Blastomycosis during pregnancy. Can Med Assoc J. 1989;131:759–61.
84. MacDonald D, Alguire PC. Adult respiratory distress due to blastomycosis during pregnancy. Chest. 1990;98:1527–8.
85. Chakravarty A, Saliga R, Mason E, Rajendran R, Muthuswamy P. Pneumonia and infraorbital abscess in a 29 year old diabetic pregnant woman. Chest. 1995;107:1752–4.
86. Kaufman L, Standard PG, Weeks RJ, et al. Detection of two *Blastomyces dermatitidis* serotypes by exoantigen analysis. J Clin Microbiol. 1983;18:110–4.
87. Stockman L, Clark KA, Hunt JM, Roberts GD. Evaluation of commercially available acridinium ester-labeled chemiluminescent DNA probes for culture identification of *Blastomyces dermatitidis, Coccidioides immitis, Cryptococcus neoformans,* and *Histoplasma capsulatum.* J Clin Microbiol. 1993;31:845–50.
88. Sutliff WD, Cruthirds TP. *Blastomyces dermatitidis* in cytologic preparations. Am Rev Respir Dis. 1973;108:149–51.
89. Turner S, Kaufman L, Jalbert M. Diagnostic assessment of an enzyme-linked immunosorbent assay for human and canine blastomycosis. J Clin Microbiol. 1986;23:294–7.
90. Klein BS, Vergeront JM, Kaufman L, et al. Serologic tests for blastomycosis: assessment during a large point source outbreak in Wisconsin. J Infect Dis. 1987;155:262–8.
91. Klein BS, Kuritsky JN, Chappell WA, et al. Comparison of the enzyme immunoassay, immunodiffusion, and complement fixation tests in detecting antibody in human serum to the A antigen of *Blastomyces dermatitidis*. Am Rev Respir Dis. 1986;133:144–8.
92. Klein BS, Jones JM. Isolation, purification, and radiolabeling of a novel 120-kD surface protein on *Blastomyces dermatitidis* yeasts to detect antibody in infected patients. J Clin Invest. 1990;85:152–61.
93. Bradsher RW, Pappas PG. Detection of specific antibodies in human blastomycosis by enzyme imunoassay. South Med J. 1995;88:1256–9.
94. Durkin M, Witt J, Lemonte A, Wheat B, Connolly P. Antigen assay with the potential to aid in diagnosis of blastomycosis. J Clin Microbiol. 2004;42:4873–5.
95. Wheat J, Wheat H, Connolly P, et al. Cross-reactivity in *Histoplasma capsulatum* variety *capsulatum* antigen assays of

urine samples from patients with endemic mycoses. Clin Infect Dis. 1997;24:1169–71.
96. Bariola JR, Durkin M, Wheat LJ, et al. Persistent antigenuria during therapy for blastomycosis [abstract 564]. Presented at the 44th Annual Meeting of the Infectious Diseases Society of America. Toronto, Canada, October 12–15, 2006.
97. Mongkolrattanothai K, Peev M, Wheat LJ, Marcinak J. Urine antigen detection of blastomycosis in pediatric patients. Pediatr Infect Dis J. 2006;25:1076–8.
98. Tarr M, Marcinak J, Mongkolrattanothai K, et al. *Blastomyces* antigen detection for monitoring progression of blastomycosis in a pregnant adolescent. Infect Dis Obstet Gynecol. 2007;2007:e89059.
99. Sarosi GA, Davies SF, Phillips JR. Self-limited blastomycosis: a report of 39 cases. Semin Respir Infect. 1986;1:40–4.
100. Recht LD, Phillips JR, Eckman MR, Sarosi GA. Self-limited blastomycosis: a report of 13 cases. Am Rev Respir Dis. 1979;120: 1109–12.
101. Chapman SW, Dismukes WE, Proia LA, et al. Clinical practice guidelines for the management of blastomycosis: 2008 update by the Infectious Diseases Society of America. Clin Infect Dis. 2008;46:1801–12.
102. Pitrak DL, Andersen BR. Cerebral blastomycoma after ketoconazole therapy for respiratory blastomycosis. Am J Med. 1989;86:713–4.
103. Yancey Jr RW, Perlino CA, Kaufman L. Asymptomatic blastomycosis of the central nervous system with progression in patients given ketoconazole therapy: a report of two cases. J Infect Dis. 1991;164:807–10.
104. Dismukes WE, Bradsher RW, Cloud GC, et al. Itraconazole therapy for blastomycosis and histoplasmosis. Am J Med. 1992;93:489–97.
105. Bradsher RW. Blastomycosis. Clin Infect Dis. 1992;14 Suppl 1:S82–90.
106. Pappas PG, Bradsher RW, Chapman SW, et al. Treatment of blastomycosis with fluconazole: a pilot study. Clin Infect Dis. 1995;20:267–71.
107. Pappas PG, Bradsher RW, Kauffman CA, et al. Treatment of blastomycosis with higher doses of fluconazole. Clin Infect Dis. 1997;25:200–5.
108. Borgia SM, Fuller JD, Sarabia A, El-Helou P. Cerebral blastomycosis: a case series incorporating voriconazole in the treatment regimen. Med Mycol. 2006;44:659–64.
109. Bakleh M, Askamit AJ, Tieyjeh IM, Marshall WF. Successful treatment of cerebral blastomycosis with voriconazole. Clin Infect Dis. 2005;40:e69–71.
110. Busey JF. Blastomycosis: a comparative study of 2-hydroxystilbamidine and amphotericin B therapy. Am Rev Respir Dis. 1972;105:812–8.
111. Lockwood WR, Allison Jr F, Batson BE, Busey JF. The treatment of North American blastomycosis: ten years experience. Am Rev Respir Dis. 1969;100:314–20.

Coccidioidomycosis

Neil M. Ampel

Coccidioidomycosis is a disease of the Western hemisphere caused by dimorphic soil-dwelling fungi of the genus *Coccidioides*. First recognized as a clinical entity in Argentina in 1882, the first case associated with the San Joaquin Valley in California was reported soon after [1]. Early cases presented with inflammatory lesions of the skin, bones, and joints that progressed to death despite attempts at treatment. By the turn of the century, the causative organism was identified as a mould despite its resemblance in tissue to a protozoan [2]. For the first 40 years after its initial description, coccidioidomycosis was thought to be a relatively rare but disfiguring and usually fatal disease. However, more benign cases of pulmonary disease associated with erythema nodosum or erythema multiforme were linked with coccidioidal infection during the 1930s [3]. This form of illness, called Valley Fever, led to speculation that not all cases of coccidioidomycosis were fatal and that there was a wide spectrum of clinical manifestations after infection [4].

These observations ushered in a watershed period in the understanding of coccidioidomycosis led by Charles E. Smith and his colleagues. Smith developed the coccidioidin skin test, defined the incidence and prevalence of infection within the San Joaquin Valley, and described the relationship of skin-test reactivity to clinical disease [5]. He also developed the coccidioidal serum antibody tests [6], variations of which are still in use today. However, there was no treatment for coccidioidomycosis until 1957, when Fiese reported the first use of amphotericin B to manage a case of disseminated disease [7]. Further strides in the therapy of coccidioidomycosis using amphotericin B were pioneered and described by Winn [8].

Since those times, much more has been elucidated about coccidioidomycosis, particularly with regard to immunology, treatment, identification of hosts at risk, and fungal antigen expression. However, it is astounding how much of the basic epidemiology, pathology, clinical expression, and mycology of coccidioidomycosis was established within the first 60 years of its recognition. This initial progress is eloquently reviewed in the monograph by Fiese [9] and subsequently updated by Drutz and Catanzaro [10, 11]. Recently, Hirschmann has succinctly detailed the history of coccidioidomycosis from its first description until 1945 [12].

Organism

Life Cycle

Coccidioides is a soil-dwelling fungus in which humans are incidental and end-stage hosts. In the soil, the fungus exists as a mould with septate hyphae (Fig. 1). Intervening cells within the hyphal filaments degenerate. This arrangement allows for fragmentation of the hyphae with dislodgement of remaining intact cells, called arthroconidia. The barrel-shaped arthroconidia are approximately 2×5 μm, which makes airborne dispersal possible and increases the probability of reaching the small bronchi after inhalation into the lung of a susceptible host [13].

Once inside the host, the fungus undergoes a profound morphologic change in which the outer wall fractures, the inner wall thickens, and the entire structure rounds up. Increased temperature, a rise in CO_2 concentration [14], a decrease in pH, and an interaction with professional phagocytes [15] all facilitate this metamorphosis. The process can also be induced in vitro using a chemically defined medium [16]. The resulting structure, called a spherule and unique among pathogenic fungi, internally segments into multiple uninucleate compartments while growing to a size of up to 120 μm. These internal structures, called endospores, are 2–4 μm in diameter and are released into the surrounding tissue in packets if the spherule ruptures. After release, endospores can grow to become spherules themselves, repeating the cycle within the host [17]. Should the fungus subsequently encounter an environment outside the host, it returns to its mycelial morphology.

N.M. Ampel (✉)
Division of Infectious Diseases, Southern Arizona Veterans Affairs Health Care Center, University of Arizona, Tucson, AZ, USA
e-mail: nampel@email.arizona.edu

C.A. Kauffman et al. (eds.), *Essentials of Clinical Mycology*,
DOI 10.1007/978-1-4419-6640-7_20, © Springer Science+Business Media, LLC 2011

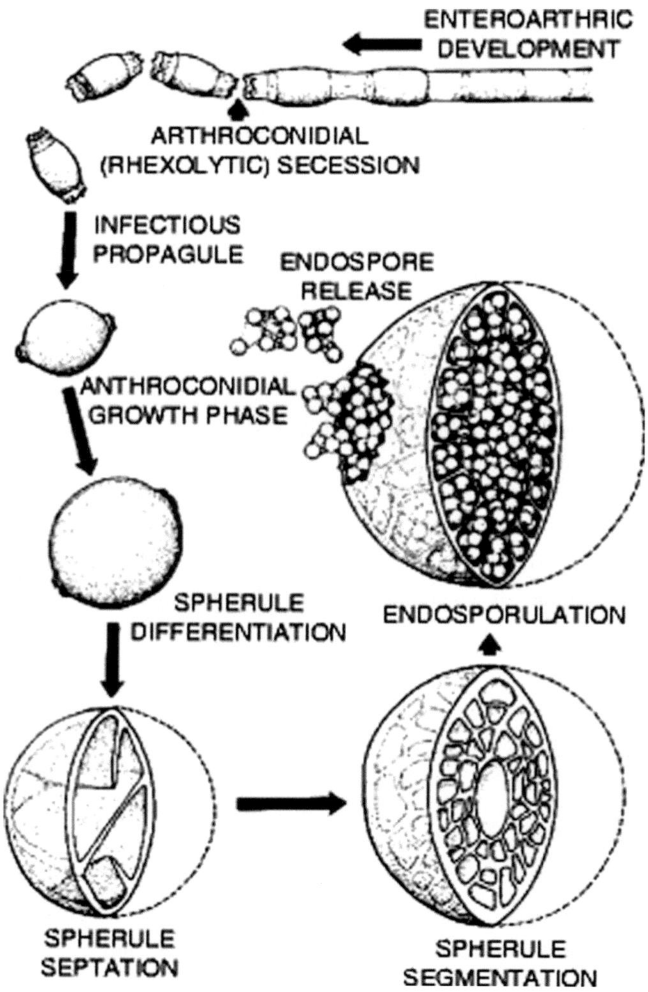

Fig. 1 Life cycle of *Coccidioides* (Based on Kirkland and Fierer [214])

Ecology

The observation that *Coccidioides* is a soil-dwelling organism was first made when it was isolated from the earth beneath a bunkhouse associated with an outbreak of coccidioidomycosis among farm workers [18]. Since then, several examples of organisms identified in the soil have been associated with human cases [19, 20]. Unfortunately, general soil sampling in the endemic area has not been very productive. Egeberg and Ely tested 500 soil samples obtained in and around animal burrows in the southern San Joaquin Valley and detected *Coccidioides* in only 35 [21]. More recently, Greene and colleagues isolated the organism only four times out of 720 samples from the San Joaquin Valley [22]. Overall, *Coccidioides* appears to prefer alkaline soils in relatively warm, dry climates [23], and it preferentially grows in soils of high salt content, including borates, at higher temperatures [24]. There are compelling data that it is not uniformly distributed in the soil but is concentrated in animal burrows [20, 21] or in other soils containing increased nitrogenous waste, such as Amerindian middens [25].

Fisher and coworkers have recently added to our knowledge by isolating *Coccidioides* from sites where human infection has repeatedly occurred. The index case was Swelter Shelter, an ancient Amerindian site located in Dinosaur National Monument in northeastern Utah, where an outbreak of coccidioidomycosis occurred in 2001 among workers building a retaining wall and sifting dirt. A similar outbreak of coccidioidomycosis may have occurred there in 1964–1965 [26]. At Swelter Shelter and at three other locations, Fisher and colleagues were able to isolate the fungus using mouse passage [27]. While no firm conclusions regarding soil type and vegetation could be made, the results demonstrate that *Coccidioides* resides for prolonged periods in certain environmental locations.

Taxonomy

The classification of *Coccidioides* remains uncertain but genetic analysis is clarifying this. Studies of 18 S ribosomal DNA confirms that *Coccidioides* is within the class Ascomycetes and is closely related to the pathogenic fungi *Histoplasma capsulatum* and *Blastomyces dermatiditis* [28]. Among all organisms, it is most closely related to the non-pathogenic soil-dwelling fungus *Uncinocarpus reesii.* [29] While no teleomorphic stage of *Coccidioides* has been observed, Burt and coworkers found molecular evidence for sexual recombination [30], and Mandel and colleagues have identified the genetic loci for mating [31]. Moreover, there is evidence of genetic variability between clinical isolates from California, Arizona, and Texas [32]. Isolates of *Coccidioides* from South America appear to have been derived from a single clade from Texas, arriving in the continent from 9,000 to 140,000 years ago, perhaps coincident with human migration into the area [33]. In addition, Fisher and colleagues have presented genetic evidence that *Coccidioides* consists of two distinct species, *C. immitis*, found only in California, and *C. posadasii*, found elsewhere [34]. Because to date there have been no clear microbiologic or clinical characteristics that distinguish these species, the genus term *Coccidioides* will be used throughout this chapter to refer to both species.

Epidemiology

The endemic regions of coccidioidomycosis lie between the latitudes of 40°N and 40°S in the Western Hemisphere. Within this general region, there is great variability in risk of infection. The endemic regions of coccidioidomycosis in North America have been associated with the Lower Sonoran Life Zone, a geoclimatic region characterized by hot summers, mild winters, rare freezes, and alkaline soil [10]. In Central and South America, there are several geographic pockets where individuals have acquired coccidioidal infection [13], including north-central Argentina, where the disease was first recognized. There are also reports of cases acquired in northeast Brazil [20, 35]. In general, these Central and South American areas are arid or semi-arid.

Smith and colleagues made the initial association of dust exposure and risk of coccidioidomycosis in a study of military personnel in the San Joaquin Valley [36]. They also found a strong inverse association in the frequency of cases and precipitation. That is, the number of cases waxed during the dry central California summers and waned during the relatively wet winters. Galgiani has noted a similar association in Arizona, except that there are two periods of increased frequency of cases. The first occurs in the spring, after the winter rains, and the second occurs during the autumn, after the summer monsoon [37].

Comrie has developed a predictive model of coccidioidal incidence in the endemic area using reports of symptomatic cases of coccidioidomycosis in Pima County, Arizona, in combination with monthly climate data for southeastern Arizona [38]. A striking relationship was that increased precipitation 1.5–2 years before the season of exposure was associated with an increased risk of coccidioidomycosis. Although this model is imperfect because of its reliance on reports of symptomatic cases rather than soil isolates of *Coccidioides*, it has gained validation after a similar model was applied to Maricopa County, Arizona, using data from 1998 to 2001 [39].

Epidemics of coccidioidomycosis may occur when geoclimatic patterns are exaggerated. For example, in December 1977, high-velocity winds over the lower San Joaquin Valley induced not only a local dust storm but also threw dust high into the atmosphere that blanketed regions to the north and west outside of the endemic zone, including the San Francisco Bay and Sacramento metropolitan regions. Within weeks of the storm, the number of cases of coccidioidomycosis in California was five times normal, with many cases being reported from outside the endemic region [40, 41]. Similarly, in January 1994, an earthquake-generated cloud of dust, emanating from the Santa Susana Mountains, dispersed over Ventura County, California, an area of low coccidioidal endemicity. Within 2 weeks, increasing numbers of cases of coccidioidomycosis occurred in Simi Valley, a city located at the base of the mountains and in the plume of the dust cloud [42]. In the early 1990s, a nearly tenfold increase in the number of cases of coccidioidomycosis was seen in the lower San Joaquin Valley. In this case, drought, followed by heavy rains and then another drought, was climatologically associated with the marked increase in cases [43]. Currently, both Arizona and the San Joaquin Valley of California have been experiencing increasing numbers of cases of symptomatic coccidioidomycosis [39, 44]. The reasons for this are not clear but probably are related to an influx of susceptible individuals into these areas and climatic changes.

There have also been many focal outbreaks of coccidioidomycosis associated with local conditions [19, 45–51]. These outbreaks share common traits. First, there was intense exposure to soil in a confined area, often in association with an archeological dig or other soil disturbance. In addition, those exposed were either young or not from the endemic region and so could be presumed to be nonimmune. These outbreaks are notable for their high attack rate and association with diffuse rash and extensive pulmonary infiltrates. When calculable, the incubation period between exposure and development of active disease was between 2 and 4 weeks. Because of this, the diagnosis was often established only after the individuals had returned to their homes outside the coccidioidal endemic area.

The prevalence and incidence of coccidioidomycosis in a region has been estimated using skin test studies measuring delayed-type dermal hypersensitivity. A study of the prevalence of coccidioidin skin test reactivity among naval recruits and others by Edwards and Palmer in 1957 did much to define the coccidioidal endemic area in the United States (Fig. 2) [52]. In this study, highest prevalence was found in the southern San Joaquin Valley, in south-central Arizona, and along the western portion of the lower Rio Grande Valley in Texas. Regions of lesser endemicity included most of southwestern Arizona, southern Nevada and southwestern Utah, southern New Mexico and far western Texas.

In the past, rates of skin test positivity were quite high in endemic regions. Among the few recent studies, that rate appears to be declining. In an analysis of skin test responses in high school students in the southern San Joaquin Valley, Larwood found that the incidence of new skin test reactions had decreased from greater than 10% each year in 1937–1939 to 2% in 1995 [53]. A study performed in 1985 in Tucson, Arizona, found a prevalence of positive skin test response of

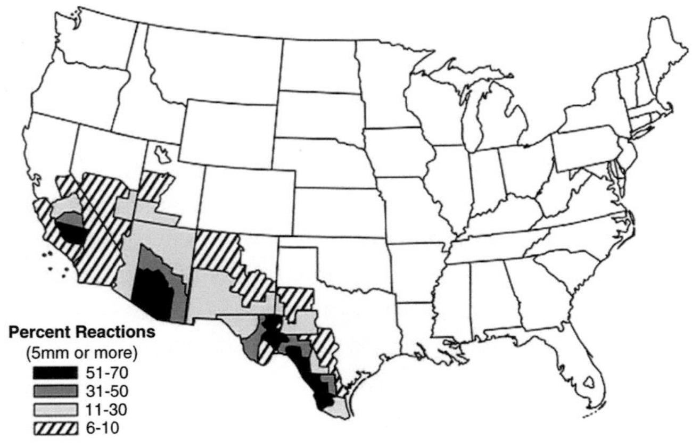

Fig. 2 Endemic regions for coccidioidomycosis in the United States based on response to dermal hypersensitivity testing. Increased intensity of shading indicates increased rates of positivity (Based on Edwards and Palmer [52])

approximately 30% [54], with an estimated yearly conversion rate of 3% each year. A recent study of Torreón, a city in northeastern Mexico in the state of Coahuila, found a prevalence of 40% [55]. These data indicate that even in the coccidioidal endemic regions, most individuals have not acquired coccidioidomycosis and remain susceptible to infection.

Given the ability of arthroconidia to become airborne, it is not surprising that most cases of coccidioidomycosis are due to inhalation, with the lung as the primary site of infection. A variety of occupations have been associated with an increased risk of acquiring coccidioidomycosis, and most of these are associated with working with soil or dust in endemic regions. These include agricultural workers, excavators, military personnel [56], and archeologists [45, 46].

In addition, there are numerous reports of laboratory-acquired coccidioidomycosis [9, 56–58]. *Coccidioides* grows readily as a mould on a variety of artificial laboratory media, and aerial mycelia begin to develop after 4 days. These can easily become dislodged and airborne. The concentrations of airborne arthroconidia from artificial media are undoubtedly far higher than might be encountered naturally and are presumed to result in a high-inoculum exposure. Recently, Stevens and colleagues have outlined an approach when accidental exposures to *Coccidioides* occur in the laboratory [59]. Initial advice includes having the clinician alert laboratory personnel whenever coccidioidomycosis is suspected and not opening any culture plate containing an unknown mould outside of a biologic safety cabinet. When a significant exposure has been deemed to have occurred, evacuation of the area with subsequent disinfection is recommended. All exposed personnel should have coccidioidal serologic tests performed at the time of exposure and after 6 weeks. Although not all experts would agree, Stevens et al. also recommend 6 weeks of prophylactic antifungal therapy [59]. In addition to airborne exposure, care should be taken to avoid percutaneous injury with cultures of *Coccidioides*, since laboratory instances of primary cutaneous coccidioidomycosis have also occurred [58]. In recognition of the potential of the mycelial phase for infectivity, *Coccidioides* is the only fungus listed by the United States government as a possible bioterrorist agent [60].

There is no evidence for person-to-person spread of coccidioidomycosis. However, interhuman transmission has been reported to occur via a contaminated fomite. In this case, pulmonary coccidioidomycosis occurred in six healthcare workers who changed the dressings and cast covering an area of draining osteomyelitis of a patient with disseminated coccidioidomycosis. Subsequent investigation revealed *Coccidioides* growing on the dressings and cast, which were dry at the time of removal. It was presumed that mycelial growth occurred on these objects and was the source of infection [61]. Fomite transmission of coccidioidomycosis has been reported under a variety of other circumstances. The handling of raw cotton grown in the endemic area has been noted in several instances [9, 62, 63]. Cleaning of dusty artifacts from an archeology site obtained from the coccidioidal endemic region has also resulted in infection [9]. Even a "dusty and dirty" suitcase from the endemic region has been the presumed source of infection in a child living outside the endemic region [64].

Pathogenesis

Necrotizing granulomata surrounding coccidioidal spherules are the classic pathologic manifestations of coccidioidomycosis and suggested to early investigators a similarity to the reaction seen in tuberculosis [9]. However, it was also recognized that an acute pyogenic response with polymorphonuclear leukocytes could occur, particularly in association with rapidly progressive lesions of disseminated disease. Some observers have suggested that this latter reaction is due to endospores and not to spherules. In many instances, the two reactions are in close proximity [65]. The concept proposed is that with unrestrained fungal growth, endospores are released from the spherule, and there is an intense but nonprotective polymorphonuclear response. Soluble extracts of both mycelia and spherules are chemotactic for polymorphonuclear leukocytes and may play a role in initiating inflammation [15]. This process may then evolve into a more protective granulomatous response surrounding the spherule in those individuals who are able to control their disease [9]. While in vitro data suggest that polymorphonuclear leukocytes can inhibit fungal growth [66], their role in controlling coccidioidal growth in vivo is unclear.

There have been numerous reports of tissue and peripheral blood eosinophilia in coccidioidomycosis. Peripheral blood eosinophilia during primary illness and eosinophils in cerebrospinal fluid in coccidioidal meningitis are common enough in coccidioidomycosis to suggest the respective diagnoses [67]. Pulmonary eosinophilia due to coccidioidomycosis may resemble idiopathic eosinophilic pneumonia histologically except for the finding of spherules in tissue [68]. Extreme peripheral blood eosinophilia (>20%) has been associated with disseminated disease [69, 70]. The pathologic finding of eosinophilic abscesses in coccidioidal-infected tissues has been associated with rupturing spherules with release of endospores.

The finding of the spherule in tissue is the sine qua non of coccidioidomycosis. The spherules seen are often of all sizes and sometimes can be shown to be rupturing and dislodging endospores. In addition, there have been reports of mycelia within pre-existing coccidioidal cavities [71, 72], a report of mycelia being found in a coccidioidal empyema [73], and another of mycelia identified in the CSF in a severe case of coccidioidal meningitis [74]. It is presumed that in these cases, local conditions allowed the fungus to revert to its saprophytic phase. There is no evidence that such patients are infectious.

Coccidioidomycosis may involve nearly any organ of the body. The most common symptomatic sites include the lungs, skin and subcutaneous soft tissue, bones and joints, and meninges. However, a variety of other organs may also be involved, often silently. These include the liver and spleen [9], peritoneum [75, 76], and female genital tract [77, 78]. While coccidioidomycosis of the male genital tract can present as symptomatic epididymitis, it also has been incidentally diagnosed during surgery or biopsy of the prostate [79, 80]. There have been numerous reports of pericarditis due to *Coccidioides* [81]. Unlike histoplasmosis and tuberculosis, direct involvement of the gastrointestinal mucosa is extremely rare [82], but there may be extension to the gastrointestinal tract from an adjacent site [83]. In addition, there are reports of direct infection of the tracheobronchial tree [84]. Eye involvement with coccidioidomycosis has been reported sparingly, mostly as asymptomatic chorioretinal scars [85] or as a scleritis or conjunctivitis associated with primary infection and erythema nodosum. Active iridocyclitis and chorioretinitis have been reported, usually as part of overtly disseminated disease [86].

While the most frequent pathologic response to central nervous system infection by *Coccidioides* is a basilar granulomatous meningitis, a variety of other processes are seen, including intracranial abscesses [87], parenchymal granulomata, and vasculitis [88]. Williams and colleagues have described the clinical presentation of vasculitis associated with CNS coccidioidomycosis in a small cohort [89]. Onset may occur early or late in the course of disease, and there are no clear predisposing factors. Patients usually present with a stroke-like syndrome, such as hemiparesis or aphasia, and the mortality rate is high.

A strong cellular immune response is critical to the control of coccidioidal infection. It is well-documented that patients with defects in such defenses, such as those with HIV infection [90], organ transplant recipients [91], and those on long-term corticosteroid therapy [92], are at increased risk for developing severe symptomatic coccidioidomycosis. In addition, there is an association between the strength and type of the coccidioidal-specific immune response and the severity of clinical infection. Persons with self-limited pulmonary illness usually express a strong cellular immune response, manifested as a positive coccidioidin skin test reaction, and transiently produce low-titer anticoccidioidal antibodies in their serum. On the other hand, those with disseminated coccidioidomycosis tend to lack a cellular immune response and have high and prolonged serum antibody titers [11].

Human in vitro immunologic studies have confirmed the importance of the cellular immune response in coccidioidomycosis. Peripheral blood mononuclear cells from subjects with disseminated coccidioidomycosis produce less interferon-gamma (IFN-γ) in response to coccidioidal antigen than do cells from healthy, immune donors, but the suppressive cytokines interleukin-4 (IL-4) and interleukin-10 (IL-10) are not demonstrated [93, 94]. However, secretion of IFN-γ by cells from immune donors can be increased in vitro by the addition of the stimulatory interleukin-12 and by addition of antibody directed against IL-10 in cells from anergic donors [95]. Pulmonary granulomata from patients with coccidioidomycosis contain both IFN-γ and IL-10 and are associated with peripheral clusters of lymphocytes containing B cells and well as CD4 and CD8 T cells [96].

Clinically, the expression of delayed-type hypersensitivity (DTH) after skin testing with a coccidioidal antigen has been associated with an intact cellular immune response. The lack of such expression, called anergy, has been clearly associated with more severe, disseminated disease [11, 97]. This has led to the speculation that agents that could reverse coccidioidal anergy might serve as potential treatments for disseminated coccidioidomycosis. A recent report on the use of dendritic cells in human coccidioidomycosis holds promise [98].

Vaccination of mice with whole, formalin-killed spherules protects them from subsequent lethal challenge with *Coccidioides* [99]. Unfortunately, the dose used proved to have a high incidence of local toxicity in humans [100]. A double-blind, placebo-controlled study inoculating a lower dose of formalin-killed spherules in nonimmune people living in the coccidioidal endemic area showed a trend toward disease reduction in the vaccine group, but the differences were not statistically significant [101]. Since this trial, several laboratories have shown that immunization with fungal subunits may be protective in mice and could serve as human vaccine candidates in future studies. These include the 27 K antigen preparation [102], recombinant Ag2/PRA [103, 104], and recombinant urease [105]. Recently, Xue and colleagues have successfully immunized mice using a live mutant of *Coccidioides* in which two chitinase genes were disrupted [106].

Clinical Manifestations

Primary Pulmonary Infection

Sixty percent of persons are completely asymptomatic at the time of initial pulmonary coccidioidal infection [5]. Their only indication of infection is a positive reaction to a coccidioidal skin test. The rest of those infected manifest a variety of symptoms, most commonly cough, usually dry but occasionally blood-tinged, fever, night sweats, pleuritic chest pain, and headache [107]. Fatigue may be prominent and profound [108]. In some cases, there is an evanescent, diffuse, pruritic rash over the trunk and extremities early in the course of illness that may be confused with contact dermatitis or measles [109, 110]. In up to one-quarter of cases, patients develop either erythema nodosum or erythema multiforme, usually a few days to weeks after the initial pulmonary symptoms. Erythema nodosum generally occurs as bright red, painful nodules on the lower extremities, while erythema multiforme tends to occur on the upper trunk and arms, often in a necklace distribution (Fig. 3). In about one-third of these cases, arthralgia may be present, most commonly of the ankles and knees and called desert rheumatism [9]. Primary pulmonary coccidioidomycosis with erythema nodosum or erythema multiforme has a predilection for white females and is rarely seen in African-American patients [97]. Smith correlated the onset of erythema nodosum with the development of coccidioidal skin test reactivity [4]. The development of either of these rashes during primary coccidioidomycosis is considered an indicator of a decreased risk for subsequent dissemination or chronic active infection [9, 111].

There is great variability in the radiographic findings of primary pulmonary coccidioidomycosis [112]. Most frequently, a unilateral parenchymal infiltrate is present. The appearance may range from a subsegmental patchy alveolar process to a dense lobar infiltrate with atelectasis (Fig. 4). Ipsilateral or bilateral hilar adenopathy or mediastinal adenopathy is often present [113]. A small pleural effusion ipsilateral to the pulmonary infiltrate occurs in about one-fifth of cases. Occasionally, large pleural effusions occur [114].

It is not uncommon for primary coccidioidal pneumonia to be confused with a community-acquired bacterial pneumonia. A recent study found that up to 29% of persons living in the coccidioidal endemic region diagnosed with a bacterial pneumonia had evidence of recent coccidioidal infection [115]. While at times difficult to distinguish, clues favoring a diagnosis of pulmonary coccidioidomycosis include persistent fatigue and headache, failure to improve with antibiotic therapy, hilar or mediastinal adenopathy on chest radiograph, and peripheral blood eosinophilia.

Pulmonary Sequelae of Primary Coccidioidal Pneumonia

In the vast majority of individuals with symptomatic primary coccidioidomycosis, the symptoms resolve spontaneously over a few weeks. However, radiographic abnormalities remain in about 5%. One of the most common is the coccidioidal nodule (Fig. 5). Nodules are benign residual lesions of coccidioidal pneumonia but are problematic because of their radiographic resemblance to pulmonary neoplasms. Although they appear as single lesions on plain chest radiograph, multiple lesions

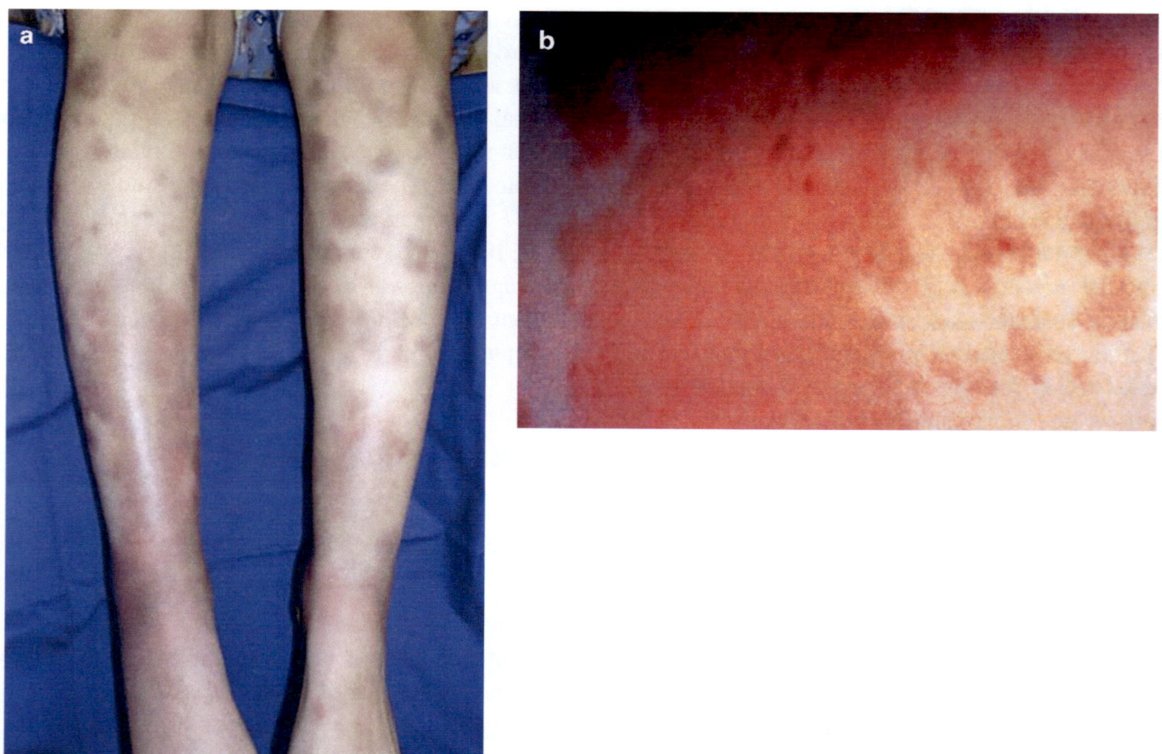

Fig. 3 Erythema nodosum (**a**) and erythema multiforme (**b**) in patients with primary coccidioidal pneumonia

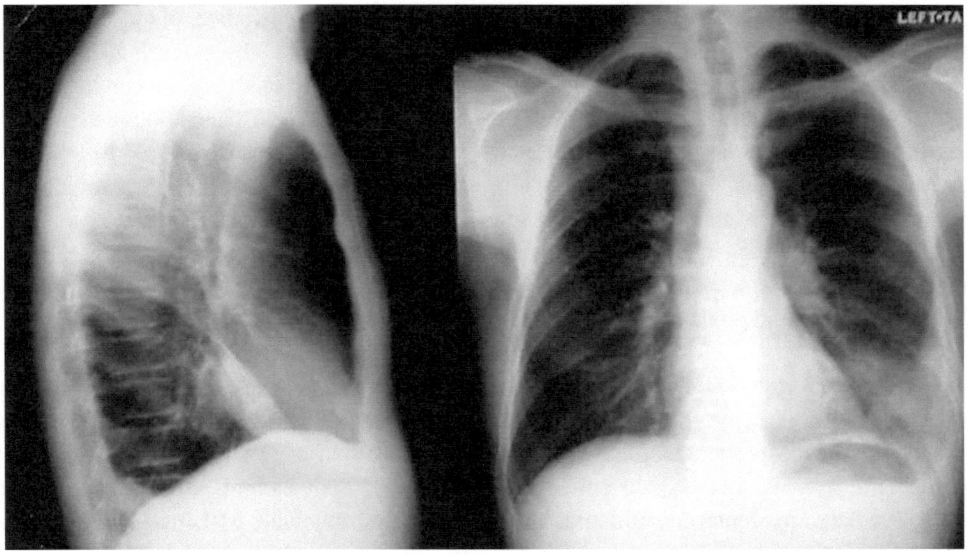

Fig. 4 Primary coccidioidal pneumonia. Note the dense infiltrate with evidence of atelectasis and ipsilateral small pleural effusion

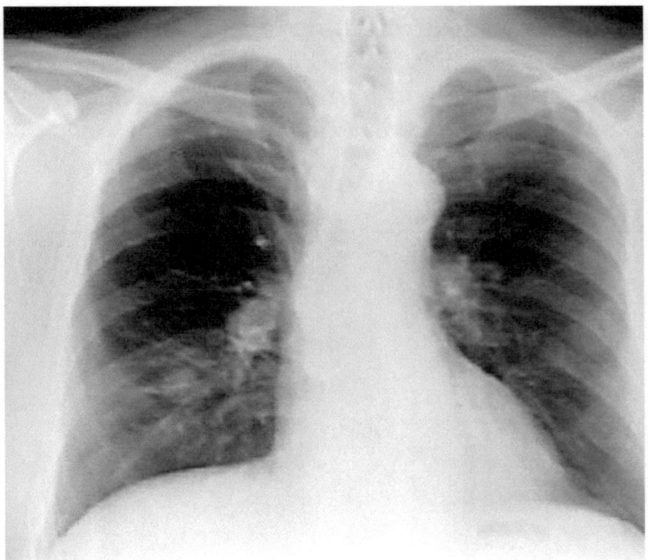

Fig. 5 Right lower lobe nodule due to coccidioidomycosis

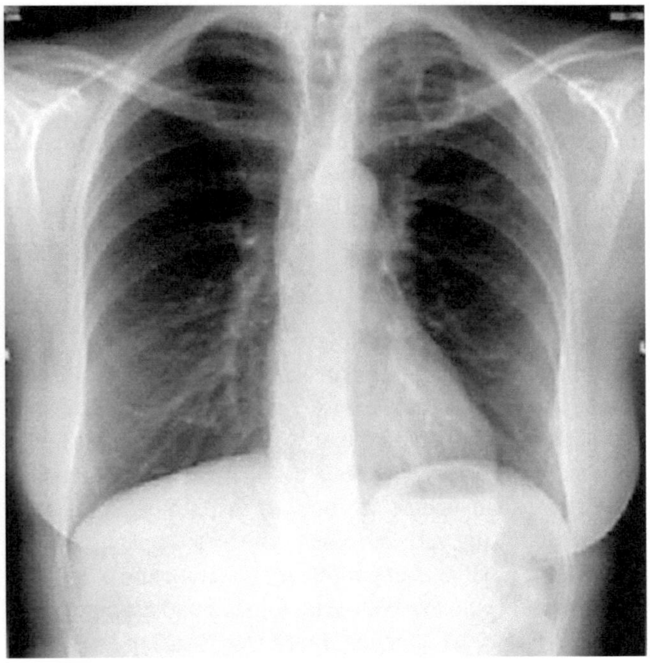

Fig. 6 Left upper lobe cavity. Patient acquired infection while working on an archeological site 2 years previously and complained of persistent cough and chest pain

are frequently seen on computed tomography (CT) of the chest, especially during primary pneumonia [116]. They range in size from a few millimeters to more than 5 cm in diameter and may be calcified. Currently, there is no radiographic way to clearly distinguish coccidioidal nodules from malignancies. Fine-needle percutaneous aspirate with histologic examination appears to be diagnostic in the majority of cases [117, 118].

Coccidioidal cavities occur when a pulmonary nodule excavates. In most cases, cavities are asymptomatic, between 2 and 4 cm in diameter, and their natural history is to close over time [119, 120]. Sputum cultures obtained from individuals with coccidioidal pulmonary cavities are frequently positive for *Coccidioides*. Radiographically, cavities are typically thin-walled but may have a surrounding area of infiltration (Fig. 6). Their course can be complicated. One syndrome is persistent chest pain and cough, often associated with an air-fluid level within the cavity. The symptoms may be due to coccidioidal infection per se or to secondary bacterial or fungal infection within the cavity. Even *Coccidioides* itself has been found to secondarily infect coccidioidal cavities [119]. Cavities have also occasionally been associated with significant hemoptysis. A unique complication is pyopneumothorax due to rupture of a cavity into the pleural space. Patients complain of abrupt dyspnea, and the chest radiograph reveals a collapsed lung with an ipsilateral pleural effusion that is inflammatory in nature [121].

Coccidioidomycosis may result in chronic progressive disease, often associated with bronchiectasis and fibrosis. The patient usually has persistent cough, fever, positive sputum cultures for *Coccidioides*, and persistently elevated coccidioidal serology. The chest radiograph may reveal biapical pulmonary fibrosis, similar to that seen in tuberculosis or histoplasmosis. Without therapy, the process is often chronic and progressive [122].

Finally, primary coccidioidomycosis may present as a diffuse pulmonary process, similar to miliary tuberculosis. There are two mechanisms. The first is overwhelming exposure among immunocompetent persons. Larsen and colleagues reported two such cases where apparent inhalation of a large inoculum of organisms resulted in a diffuse pneumonic process and respiratory failure [47]. Arsura and colleagues reported their experience among eight immunocompetent patients, who represented 1% of all patients hospitalized for coccidioidomycosis [123]. Diffuse pulmonary coccidioidomycosis may also be a manifestation of dissemination and is often associated with fungemia, usually occurring among immunocompromised patients. The mortality rate for this form of coccidioidomycosis is exceedingly high [92, 124].

Disseminated Coccidioidomycosis

Dissemination is defined as the spread of coccidioidal infection beyond the thoracic cavity. In most cases, it portends a poorer prognosis than pulmonary coccidioidomycosis and is associated with a less vigorous cellular immune response to the fungus than occurs in those with pulmonary disease. Dissemination usually becomes clinically apparent within the first few months after pulmonary infection and may occur in individuals who are both symptomatic and asymptomatic at the time of initial infection. Indeed, evidence of antecedent pulmonary infection is apparent in only about 60% of individuals [125]. It is estimated that disseminated coccidioidomycosis occurs in fewer than 1% of all those infected, and the risk is increased in those with underlying immunosuppression as well as in males of African-American or Filipino descent [125]. Patients may have single or multiple sites of dissemination. Hypercalcemia is an uncommon complication of coccidioidal dissemination. The process does not appear to be related to vitamin D metabolism and frequently responds to antifungal therapy and fluid resuscitation [126].

The skin is the most common site of extrathoracic dissemination. Reports of large, verrucous lesions, particularly of the face, were prominent in the earliest reports on coccidioidomycosis. However, skin lesions can take on a variety of forms, including papules, plaques, ulcers, draining sinuses, and subcutaneous abscesses [127]. Early in the course of disease, skin lesions may appear to be particularly benign. Punch biopsies of any suspicious cutaneous lesion in a patient with coccidioidomycosis should be performed with material sent both for histopathologic examination and for fungal culture.

Bones are also frequent sites of coccidioidal dissemination, and the vertebrae are most commonly affected [128]. The patient notes persistent back pain and, on examination, there is point tenderness and, in some cases, overlying soft tissue swelling. Plain radiography generally reveals a well-marginated lytic lesion [129]. When a vertebral body is involved, there are usually one or more erosive lesions within the body; body height is preserved, and the intervertebral disk is not involved. MR imaging reveals signal abnormalities within the vertebral body (Fig. 7) and, often, paravertebral and epidural soft tissue swelling [130]. This mixture of bony and soft tissue inflammation can be very destructive and result in nerve root and spinal cord compression. Because of this, neurosurgical consultation is imperative.

Joints may be infected with or without underlying bone involvement. The knee is the most common site of coccidioidal synovitis. Patients present with chronic pain and swelling of

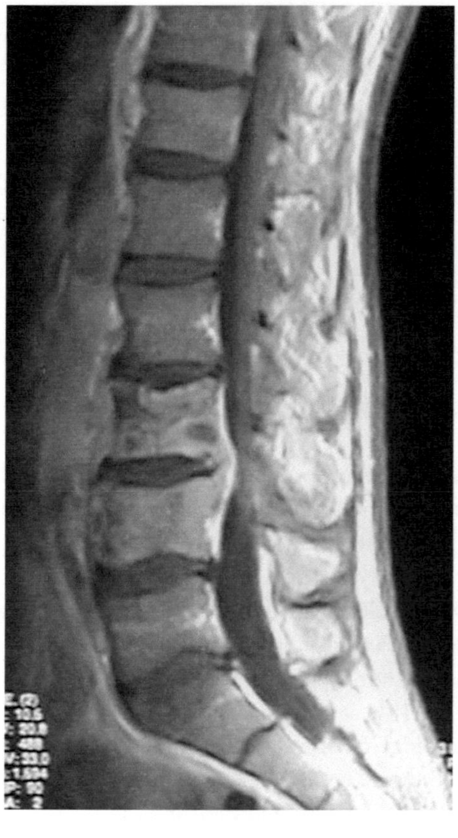

Fig. 7 Magnetic resonance image demonstrating coccidioidal vertebral osteomyelitis. Note nonhomogeneous enhancement in L3 and L4 with lack of involvement of disk space

the joint [131]. Magnetic resonance imaging (MRI) reveals a thickened and enhanced synovium and occasional underlying bone and cartilage loss [132]. Fluid from joint aspiration demonstrates an inflammatory process, but fungal culture is rarely positive. Synovial biopsy may be necessary to establish the diagnosis.

Meningitis presents with persistent headache and decreasing mental acuity. Lumbar puncture reveals a lymphocyte pleocytosis with an elevated protein and a markedly depressed CSF glucose concentration. A distinguishing characteristic is the presence of eosinophils in the CSF. Fungal culture is positive in only about one-third of cases [133]. Serum coccidioidal antibody tests are usually positive, and the specific diagnosis is most commonly established by the finding of anticoccidioidal antibodies in the CSF, although these may occasionally be negative [134]. Prior to the advent of antifungal therapy, coccidioidal meningitis was invariably fatal [135]. In one-half of patients, meningitis is the only clinically overt manifestation of disseminated coccidioidomycosis [133]. Coccidioidal meningitis should always be considered in the differential diagnosis of chronic lymphocytic meningitis, even outside the coccidioidal endemic region. A common complication is hydrocephalus, either communicating or noncommunicating. This may occur in the face of appropriate antifungal therapy. In all patients with coccidioidal meningitis, neuroradiography should be performed, with MRI the test of choice [136]. Some patients may develop encephalitis or stroke caused by cerebral vasculitis [137].

Special Hosts

Patients with conditions associated with depressed cellular immune function have been clearly identified as at increased risk for developing severe and disseminated coccidioidomycosis. Included are those with underlying lymphoma or cancer chemotherapy [138], those on chronic corticosteroids [92], and those with immunosuppression due to HIV infection [90]. Because of improved antiretroviral therapy and subsequent immune reconstitution, the severity of presentation and the number of cases of active coccidioidomycosis in association with HIV infection is declining [139]. The immune response inflammatory syndrome appears to occur very rarely in persons with concomitant HIV infection and coccidioidomycosis [139, 140].

There have been increasing reports of active coccidioidomycosis among those who have received solid organ transplants [141]. Most cases appear to be the result of a reactivated, previously acquired infection and emerge at a time of profound immunosuppression with resultant dissemination. Patients at risk usually have a history of prior active coccidioidomycosis or a positive coccidioidal serologic test just prior to transplantation. Antifungal prophylaxis with an azole appears to significantly reduce the risk of active coccidioidomycosis among such patients [142]. Four cases of donor-derived coccidioidomycosis have been reported [143–145]. However, a review of donors screened prior to transplantation within the endemic region found a low incidence of seropositivity and no instances of active coccidioidomycosis among the organ recipients, even when the donors had prior evidence of coccidioidomycosis [146].

Tissue necrosis factor-alpha (TNF-α) inhibitors have been associated with an increased risk of symptomatic illness with endemic fungi [147]. In a study performed among rheumatology clinics located in the coccidioidal endemic region [148], 13 cases of coccidioidomycosis were identified among patients receiving TNF-α inhibitors. Twelve cases occurred in those receiving the chimeric monoclonal antibody infliximab, and one occurred in a patient receiving the TNF-α receptor antagonist etanercept. All patients had pulmonary disease, and two had a history of prior coccidioidomycosis. While 10 patients had resolution of their pneumonia with antifungal therapy, 3 died after developing disseminated disease. In a cohort analysis, patients receiving infliximab had a fivefold higher risk of developing symptomatic coccidioidomycosis compared to patients on other rheumatologic medications. While it is unclear what proportion of cases in this group were due to acute infection compared to reactivation of previously acquired quiescent infection, there is a report of reactivation occurring outside the coccidioidal endemic region after the initiation of anti-TNF-α therapy [149]. Within the endemic area, it is reasonable to periodically obtain serology and chest radiographs for patients receiving monoclonal antibody TNF-α inhibitor therapy. Antifungal therapy should be considered for patients with evidence of active infection, and these patients must be closely monitored [150].

Male sex and increasing age, particularly over 60 years, have been associated with increased risk of developing symptomatic coccidioidomycosis but not necessarily disseminated disease [151–154]. Diabetics may have an increased risk of severe pulmonary disease with cavitation [13]. Numerous studies have found that African-American men are at markedly increased risk for the development of disseminated coccidioidomycosis when compared to other groups [41, 151, 153, 155, 156]. For these patients, the clinical presentation is often stereotypical, with widely disseminated disease typically involving the skin, subcutaneous tissue, and vertebrae (Fig. 8). Filipino men have also been suggested to be at similar risk [13].

Finally, women who acquire coccidioidomycosis during the second and third trimesters of pregnancy are at increased risk of developing severe, symptomatic, and often disseminated coccidioidomycosis, although morbidity and mortality appear to have declined markedly from the past [157]. Women

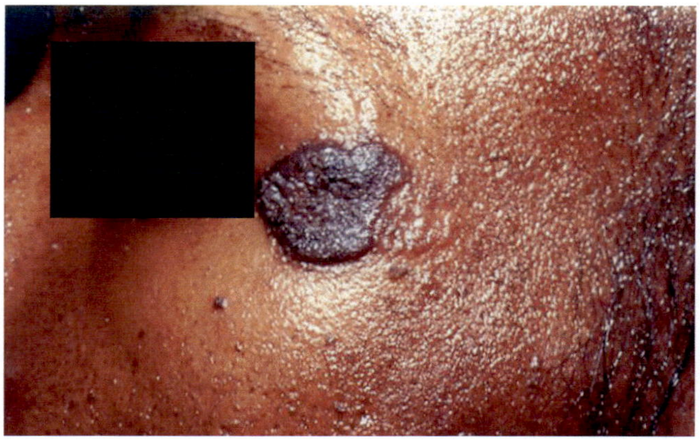

Fig. 8 Disseminated coccidioidomycosis in an African American man. Typical verrucous skin lesion on the face

who have stable or asymptomatic coccidioidomycosis prior to pregnancy do not appear to develop worsening disease as pregnancy advances. Congenital anomalies have been observed in the newborns of women who received high-dose fluconazole for coccidioidal meningitis during their pregnancy [158]. Although recent studies have not found a clear association [159], high-dose azole therapy during pregnancy should be avoided, particularly during the first trimester.

Diagnosis

There are three mainstays for the diagnosis of coccidioidomycosis: culture, histopathology, and serology. *Coccidioides* grows as a nonpigmented mould, usually after 3–7 days of incubation at 35 °C on a variety of artificial media, including blood agar. Any growth suspicious for *Coccidioides* can be formally identified using a commercially available chemiluminescent probe that hybridizes with coccidioidal-specific DNA sequences. It has a sensitivity and specificity of 99% and 100%, respectively [160]. Sputum or other respiratory secretions are frequently culture-positive in primary coccidioidomycosis, cavitary disease, and chronic or persistent pulmonary coccidioidomycosis. Biopsy specimens from disseminated sites are less likely to reveal growth. When coccidioidomycosis is suspected, cultures should always be obtained. If positive, they provide absolute confirmation of the diagnosis. As previously mentioned, the growth of *Coccidioides* on artificial media represents a laboratory hazard and suspected samples should be handled accordingly [161].

Histopathologic identification of spherules is another method for establishing the diagnosis of coccidioidomycosis (Fig. 9). In some instances, such as biopsy of pulmonary nodules, it appears to have greater sensitivity than culture [117, 118], while in other instances, such as respiratory secretions, it appears to be less sensitive [162, 163]. For routine biopsies, the Gomori methenamine silver (GMS) stain or the periodic acid–Schiff (PAS) stains are preferable to the hematoxylin-eosin method, because spherules stand out from tissue with these stains. Microscopic examination of specimens treated with 10% potassium hydroxide (KOH) has been used in the past to identify spherules in respiratory samples. However, it has a very low sensitivity. The Papanicolaou stain is more sensitive [163].

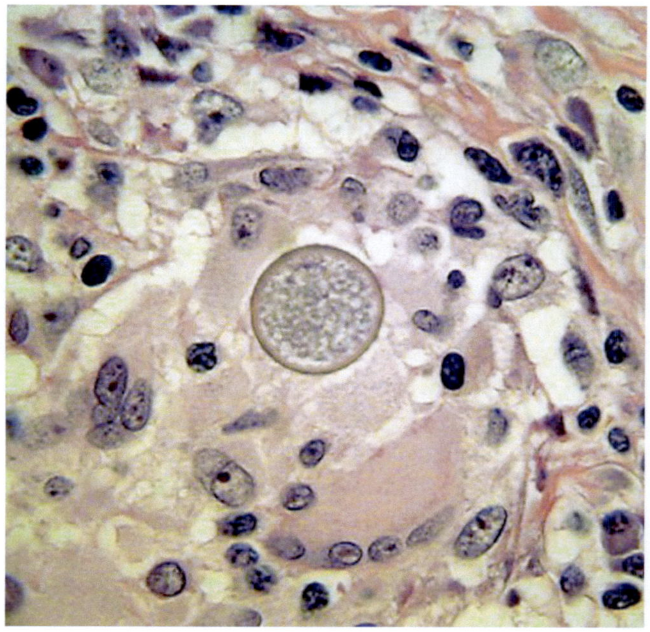

Fig. 9 Hematoxylin–eosin stain of lung tissue containing a coccidioidal spherule. Note surrounding inflammatory cells

Serologic tests identifying anticoccidioidal antibodies were initially developed by Smith and his colleagues nearly 50 years ago [164]. They remain important today both in the diagnosis and the management of coccidioidomycosis [165, 166]. Because of changes in nomenclature and methodology, coccidioidal serologic tests can be confusing. The tube precipitin (TP) assay employs a heat-stable antigen now known to be a β-glucosidase [167], detects IgM antibodies, and is generally positive very early during infection or during acute reactivation [166]. The complement fixation (CF) assay uses a heat-labile antigen that is a chitinase [168], detects IgG antibody, and is positive during early disease and remains positive in cases of severe illness and dissemination. Rising serum titers suggest more severe clinical disease, and detection in the CSF is usually diagnostic of coccidioidal meningitis. A modification of these assays employs immunodiffusion (ID) and the same antigen preparations to detect the presence of specific antibodies [169, 170]. The IDTP and IDCF are comparable to the standard assays [171] and have few or no false-positive results.

A commercial enzyme immunoassay (EIA) that detects IgM and IgG antibodies using proprietary antigens is also available. While it may be more sensitive than the TP and CF assays, its specificity has not been established, and there has been concern about false-positive results [172]. However, one report that examined the utility of an isolated IgM EIA result found it to be very specific after results were compared with clinical and laboratory follow-up [173].

Serologic tests are problematic in that they depend on host response, which may be dampened due to immunosuppression [174, 175]. Recently, assays that directly detect *Coccidioides* have become available. Following a report that some patients with coccidioidomycosis have *Histoplasma capsulatum* antigenuria [176], a specific assay that detects coccidioidal galactomannan was developed [177]. While not fully evaluated, it appears useful for patients with immunosuppression coexisting with severe and disseminated disease. Recently, there has been a series of reports on genomic detection of *Coccidioides* from a variety of samples [178–182]. While none are currently commercially available, they hold out the promise of a rapid, sensitive, and specific diagnostic tool for the future.

Treatment

Antifungal Options

Treatment alternatives for coccidioidomycosis must be tempered with the knowledge that there has never been a placebo-controlled trial of any antifungal agent in coccidioidomycosis and only one comparative trial. Amphotericin B, formulated with deoxycholate, has been used for the management of severe coccidioidomycosis for nearly 50 years [8]. While no formal study has ever been done, a review of published cases suggests that amphotericin B induces clinical improvement in up to 70% of patients treated [183]. Unfortunately, the well-known adverse events of amphotericin B have limited its usefulness. In addition, intravenous amphotericin is ineffective in coccidioidal meningitis, and intrathecal therapy is required. Because of these problems, the use of amphotericin B for the management of coccidioidomycosis has generally been supplanted by the oral azole antifungals. However, many clinicians still use intravenous amphotericin B as initial therapy for severely ill patients, and some patients will require amphotericin B if they fail to respond to azole antifungals. There are several lipid formulations of amphotericin B. To date, none has been shown to have superior efficacy to the deoxycholate formulation in the treatment of coccidioidomycosis, and at this time these newer formulations should be reserved for patients at risk for or with renal dysfunction.

Oral azoles have become the mainstay of therapy for most cases of coccidioidomycosis that require therapy. Because of reduced efficacy and toxicity, ketoconazole has been supplanted by the newer agents, particularly fluconazole and itraconazole. Initial studies performed by the Mycoses Study Group suggested that the minimum azole dose should be 400 mg daily and that relapses are frequent once therapy is discontinued [184, 185]. A landmark comparative trial of fluconazole and itraconazole completed among patients with pulmonary and nonmeningeal disseminated coccidioidomycosis demonstrated that the drugs were comparable in both efficacy and relapse rate, but the response rate was higher with itraconazole, particularly with bone disease [186]. Oral fluconazole and itraconazole have both demonstrated efficacy in the treatment of coccidioidal meningitis [187, 188].

The role of newer azole antifungals, such as posaconazole and voriconazole, has yet to be determined. Three small, nonrandomized clinical trials of posaconazole [189–191] suggest that it can be useful in patients who have failed previous azole therapy for coccidioidomycosis. For voriconazole, there are only individual case reports indicating efficacy in patients that have failed other treatments [192–194].

Other classes of antifungals hold promise for the future. The 1,3-β-D-glucan synthase inhibitor caspofungin, an echinocandin, was found to have efficacy in the treatment of murine coccidioidomycosis [195] and there are case reports of clinical use [196, 197], although efficacy remains unclear. Nikkomycin Z, a chitin synthase inhibitor, also may find a use in the future treatment of coccidioidomycosis [198]. Although it might be predicted that immune modulating agents would be useful adjuncts in the management of severe coccidioidomycosis, there is only a single report of possible efficacy using IFN-γ [199].

Antifungal susceptibility testing has gained credence as a useful technique for the management of some fungal infections, but there is no standardized method for performing such an assay with *Coccidioides*. While there are not enough data to advocate its general use, there are reports of consistency [200] and utility [201].

Although surgery plays a smaller role in the management of coccidioidomycosis than it did in the past, it still is vital as an adjunctive therapy in certain instances. It remains the major part of therapy in the management of pyopneumothorax and is occasionally required for extirpation of problematic pulmonary cavities. In addition, surgery is useful for drainage and debridement of extrapulmonary sites that fail to resolve with antifungal therapy [202] and in the placement of shunt catheters in patients with hydrocephalus due to coccidioidal meningitis [203]. Finally, many patients with coccidioidal vertebral osteomyelitis will require surgery in addition to chemotherapy [204].

Management of coccidioidomycosis is notoriously difficult because of the tremendous variability in the course of illness among patients with similar types of disease and because of the multifarious nature of the disease in any given patient. In spite of this, useful clinical guidelines have been recently updated [150].

Primary Pneumonia and Pulmonary Residuae

The goal of therapy for primary pneumonia is to ameliorate symptoms. There are no data that such therapy will prevent dissemination. It is clear that the vast majority of cases of primary pulmonary coccidioidomycosis will not require any therapy [205]. It is prudent to follow up with all such patients for at least 1 year to document resolution of the initial process and to ensure that dissemination has not occurred. Therapy should be considered in those patients with severe symptoms, including prostration, night sweats, and weight loss, in those with elevated serum CF titers (>1:16), or in those with underlying conditions that increase their risk of severe coccidioidomycosis, such as HIV infection with depressed peripheral blood CD4 cell counts, treatment with corticosteroids or TNF-α inhibitor therapy, Filipino or African-American race, and pregnant women who acquired infection during the second or third trimester. If treatment is initiated, it should be continued for at least 3–6 months [150]. An oral azole antifungal at a minimum daily dose of 400 mg is recommended.

Management of pulmonary residuae is more complex. Pulmonary nodules require no therapy. Most pulmonary cavities will also require no therapy, but antifungal therapy should be considered in those with persistent symptoms, including cough, chest pain, and hemoptysis. In cavities with an air-fluid level, treatment for a secondary bacterial infection is warranted. In rare cases, surgery may be required because of persistent hemoptysis or an enlarging cavity despite therapy. The mainstay of management of pyopneumothorax is surgical, but most clinicians would also use adjunctive antifungal therapy. For most cases where therapy is indicated, oral azole therapy similar to that for primary pneumonia is appropriate.

Diffuse Pneumonia and Chronic Pulmonary Disease

Diffuse pulmonary coccidioidomycosis, whether due to high inoculum exposures or to fungemia in an immunocompromised host, should always be treated. Because of the severity of this manifestation of coccidioidomycosis, most clinicians begin with intravenous amphotericin B with a concomitant azole antifungal as initial therapy and then change to an oral azole antifungal alone once the patient is clinically stable [150]. Antifungal therapy should be continued for at least 1 year, and many clinicians recommend life-long therapy, particularly for the immunocompromised patient.

Chronic persistent pneumonia, consisting of cough, fevers, inanition, and other symptoms for 6 weeks or more, also requires therapy. Treatment with an oral azole antifungal at 400 mg daily is usually adequate. Therapy for months to years is the rule. Monitoring symptoms, periodically rechecking sputum cultures for growth of *Coccidioides*, and repeated assessment of serum CF titers is helpful in determining response. Similar therapy is also recommended for those patients with fibrocavitary disease. However, many of these patients will have minimal pulmonary symptoms. In such cases, in the absence of a positive sputum culture and without elevated CF serologies, it may be appropriate to withhold antifungal therapy and observe the patient over time.

Disseminated Non-meningeal Coccidioidomycosis

With rare exceptions, all forms of extrathoracic disseminated coccidioidomycosis require antifungal therapy. For nonmeningeal disseminated coccidioidomycosis, the type of antifungal therapy will depend on the clinical severity of disease. In those hospitalized because of coccidioidomycosis, intravenous amphotericin B should be initiated. Many clinicians experienced in the management of coccidioidomycosis combine amphotericin B at the outset with an oral azole antifungal at 400 mg or more daily. While there is a theoretical risk of antagonism between these two classes of drugs [206], antagonism has not been observed clinically in coccidioidomycosis nor in other mycoses [207], and many patients have been observed to improve on such combined coverage. Once the patient has clinically stabilized, usually over 4–6 weeks, the amphotericin B can be tapered and stopped, leaving the patient on oral azole therapy alone. Some patients fail azole therapy after responding to amphotericin B. In such cases, reinstitution of amphotericin B will be required. Because relapse is frequent, particularly with oral azoles [184, 185], therapy should be continued for a prolonged period, often years. Patients should be periodically monitored for evidence of disease activity at the site of dissemination, either through direct clinical observation or through imaging. In addition, CF serology should be obtained at 3–6-month intervals. Assessment of coccidioidal-specific cellular immunity at similar time points is helpful. There are no strict guidelines for discontinuing therapy in patients with disseminated nonmeningeal coccidioidomycosis, and some patients may require life-long therapy. In a retrospective study, Oldfield and colleagues found that relapse was more frequent in those with a peak CF titer of ≥ 1:256 and in those who had persistently negative coccidioidal skin tests. End-of-therapy CF titer was not predictive [208]. The risk of relapse is between 15% and 30% after azole therapy is discontinued. Relapses usually occur at the site of initial disease and within 1 year of stopping therapy [184, 185, 209]. It is reasonable to taper and then stop antifungal therapy in a patient with disseminated nonmeningeal coccidioidomycosis if there is minimal or no evidence of clinical disease, if the CF titer is <1:2, and if there is evidence of return of cellular immune response. Such patients should be followed at 3-month intervals to ensure that relapse does not occur.

Coccidioidal Meningitis

Intrathecal amphotericin B was the first effective treatment for coccidioidal meningitis [210]. Unfortunately, it was associated with numerous adverse reactions, including discomfort due to repeated injections, arachnoiditis, myelitis, inadvertent brain stem puncture, and secondary bacterial infection. In 1993, a noncomparative study of oral fluconazole at 400 mg each day demonstrated a nearly 80% response rate to therapy, including in subjects previously on intrathecal amphotericin B [187]. In an earlier study, itraconazole also appeared to have efficacy [188]. Currently, the vast majority of patients receive oral azoles as their sole treatment for this form of disseminated coccidioidomycosis. Some clinicians will initiate therapy with doses higher than 400 mg daily and then reduce to this dose once the patient is stable [150]. Current data suggest that the risk of relapse is exceedingly high if azole therapy is discontinued in patients with coccidioidal meningitis [211]. Therefore, therapy should be life-long. If hydrocephalus occurs during treatment, a shunt is indicated, but no change in medication is required [150]. Some clinicians feel that clinical cure may be possible with the combination of intrathecal amphotericin B and oral azole therapy [212]. A recent report describes a novel approach to administering intrathecal amphotericin B by using a subcutaneous programmable pump [213].

Prevention

Because coccidioidomycosis is usually acquired environmentally, there are no established methods to prevent infection within the endemic area. Measures that reduce dust have been shown to be useful [36]. While it might be presumed that new construction might lead to an increase in risk, this has not been definitively proven [39]. Individuals who wish to reduce their risk of becoming infected should avoid activities that cause them to be exposed to soil or dust in endemic areas, since such activities have been shown to increase the risk of infection [49, 50]. In addition, efforts at predicting climatic conditions associated with the risk of symptomatic illness [38, 39] might prove useful in the future.

As noted above, several subunit antigens have been identified that have been demonstrated to protect animals from experimental coccidioidomycosis [102–105] and a live vaccine has shown promise in a murine model [106]. In the future, these efforts may lead to the development of a human vaccine.

References

1. Rixford E, Gilchrist TC. Two cases of protozoon (coccidioidal) infection of the skin and other organs. Johns Hopkins Hosp Rep. 1896;1:209–68.
2. Ophüls W. Further observations on a pathogenic mould formerly described as a protozoan (*Coccidioides immitis*; *Coccidioides pyogenes*). J Exp Med. 1905;6:443–85.
3. Dickson EC, Gifford MA. *Coccidioides* infection (coccidioidomycosis) II. The primary type of infection. Arch Intern Med. 1938;62:853–71.
4. Smith CE. Epidemiology of acute coccidioidomycosis with erythema nodosum ("San Joaquin" or "Valley Fever"). Am J Public Health. 1940;30:600–11.
5. Smith CE, Whiting EG, Baker EE, Rosenberger HG, Beard R, Saito MT. The use of coccidioidin. Am Rev Tuberc. 1948;57:330–60.
6. Smith CE, Saito MT, Beard RR, Kepp RM, Clark RW, Eddie BU. Serological tests in the diagnosis and prognosis of coccidioidomycosis. Am J Hyg. 1950;52:1–21.
7. Fiese MJ. Treatment of disseminated coccidioidomycosis with amphotericin B: report of a case. Calif Med. 1957;86:119–20.
8. Winn WA. The use of amphotericin B in the treatment of coccidioidal disease. Am J Med. 1959;27:617–35.
9. Fiese MJ. Treatment of disseminated coccidioidomycosis with amphotericin 8: report of a case calif Med 1951;86:119–20.
10. Drutz DJ, Catanzaro A. Coccidioidomycosis. Part I. Am Rev Respir Dis. 1978;117:559–85.
11. Drutz DJ, Catanzaro A. Coccidioidomycosis. Part II. Am Rev Respir Dis. 1978;117:727–71.
12. Hirschmann JV. The early history of coccidioidomycosis: 1892–1945. Clin Infect Dis. 2007;44:1202–7.
13. Pappagianis D. Epidemiology of coccidioidomycosis. Curr Top Med Mycol. 1988;2:199–238.
14. Klotz SA, Drutz DJ, Huppert M, Sun SH, DeMarsh PL. The critical role of CO_2 in the morphogenesis of *Coccidioides immitis* in cell-free subcutaneous chambers. J Infect Dis. 1984;150:127–34.
15. Galgiani JN, Isenberg RA, Stevens DA. Chemotaxigenic activity of extracts from the mycelial and spherule phases of *Coccidioides immitis* for human polymorphonuclear leukocytes. Infect Immun. 1978;21:862–5.
16. Converse JL. Effect of surface active agents on endosporulation of *Coccidioides immitis* in a chemically defined medium. J Bacteriol. 1957;74:106–7.
17. Sun SH, Huppert M. A cytological study of morphogenesis in *Coccidioides immitis*. Sabouraudia. 1976;14:185–98.

18. Stewart RA, Meyer KF. Isolation of *Coccidioides immitis* (Stiles) from the soil. Proc Soc Exp Biol Med. 1932;29:937–8.
19. Winn WA, Levine BE, Broderick JE, Crane RW. A localized epidemic of coccidioidal infection. N Engl J Med. 1963;268:867–70.
20. Wanke B, Lazera M, Monteiro PC, et al. Investigation of an outbreak of endemic coccidioidomycosis in Brazil's northeastern state of Piaui with a review of the occurrence and distribution of *Coccidioides immitis* in three other Brazilian states. Mycopathologia. 1999;148:57–67.
21. Egeberg RO, Ely AF. *Coccidioides immitis* in the soil of the southern San Joaquin Valley. Am J Med Sci. 1956;231:151–4.
22. Greene DR, Koenig G, Fisher MC, Taylor JW. Soil isolation and molecular identification of *Coccidioides immitis*. Mycologia. 2000;92:406–10.
23. Maddy KT. The geographic distribution of *Coccidioides immitis* and possible ecologic implications. Ariz Med. 1958;15:178–88.
24. Egeberg RO, Elconin AE, Egeberg MC. Effect of salinity and temperature on *Coccidioides immitis* and three antagonistic soil saphrophytes. J Bact. 1964;88:473–6.
25. Lacy GH, Swatek FE. Soil ecology of *Coccidioides immitis* at Amerindian middens in California. Appl Microbiol. 1974;27:379–88.
26. Petersen LR, Marshall SL, Barton-Dickson C, et al. Coccidioidomycosis among workers at an archeological site, northeastern Utah. Emerg Infect Dis. 2004;10:637–42.
27. Fisher FS, Bultman MW, Johnson SM, Pappagianis D, Zaborsky E. *Coccidioides* niches and habitat parameters in the southwestern United States: a matter of scale. Ann NY Acad Sci. 2007;1111:47–72.
28. Bowman BH, Taylor JW, White TJ. Molecular evolution of the fungi: human pathogens. Mol Biol Evol. 1992;9:893–904.
29. Pan S, Sigler L, Cole GT. Evidence for a phylogenetic connection between *Coccidioides immitis* and *Uncinocarpus reesii* (Onygenaceae). Microbiology. 1994;140(Pt 6):1481–94.
30. Burt A, Carter DA, Koenig GL, White TJ, Taylor JW. Molecular markers reveal cryptic sex in the human pathogen *Coccidioides immitis*. Proc Natl Acad Sci USA. 1996;93:770–3.
31. Mandel MA, Barker BM, Kroken S, Rounsley SD, Orbach MJ. Genomic and population analyses of the mating type Loci in *Coccidioides* species reveal evidence for sexual reproduction and gene acquisition. Eukaryot Cell. 2007;6:1189–99.
32. Burt A, Dechairo BM, Koenig GL, Carter DA, White TJ, Taylor JW. Molecular markers reveal differentiation among isolates of *Coccidioides immitis* from California, Arizona and Texas. Mol Ecol. 1997;6:781–6.
33. Fisher MC, Koenig GL, White TJ, et al. Biogeographic range expansion into South America by *Coccidioides immitis* mirrors New World patterns of human migration. Proc Natl Acad Sci USA. 2001;98:4558–62.
34. Fisher MC, Koenig GL, White TJ, Taylor JW. Molecular and phenotypic description of *Coccidioides posadasii* sp. nov., previously recognized as the non-California population of *Coccidioides immitis*. Mycologia. 2002;94:73–84.
35. de Aguiar Cordeiro R, Brilhante RS, Rocha MF, et al. Twelve years of coccidioidomycosis in Ceara State, Northeast Brazil: epidemiologic and diagnostic aspects. Diagn Microbiol Infect Dis. 2009;65(1):73–5.
36. Smith CE, Beard RR, Rosenberger HG, Whiting EG. Effect of season and dust control on coccidioidomycosis. JAMA. 1946;132:833–8.
37. Kerrick SS, Lundergan LL, Galgiani JN. Coccidioidomycosis at a university health service. Am Rev Respir Dis. 1985;131:100–2.
38. Comrie AC. Climate factors influencing coccidioidomycosis seasonality and outbreaks. Environ Health Perspect. 2005;113:688–92.
39. Park BJ, Sigel K, Vaz V, et al. An epidemic of coccidioidomycosis in Arizona associated with climatic changes, 1998–2001. J Infect Dis. 2005;191:1981–7.
40. Pappagianis D, Einstein H. Tempest from Tehachapi takes toll or *Coccidioides* conveyed aloft and afar. West J Med. 1978;129:527–30.
41. Flynn NM, Hoeprich PD, Kawachi MM, et al. An unusual outbreak of windborne coccidioidomycosis. N Engl J Med. 1979;301:358–61.
42. Schneider E, Hajjeh RA, Spiegel RA, et al. A coccidioidomycosis outbreak following the Northridge, Calif, earthquake. JAMA. 1997;277:904–8.
43. Pappagianis D. Marked increase in cases of coccidioidomycosis in California: 1991, 1992, and 1993. Clin Infect Dis. 1994;19 Suppl 1:S14–8.
44. CDC. Increase in Coccidioidomycosis – California, 2000–2007. MMWR Morb Mortal Wkly Rep. 2009;58:105–9.
45. Werner SB, Pappagianis D, Heindl I, Mickel A. An epidemic of coccidioidomycosis among archeology students in northern California. N Engl J Med. 1972;286:507–12.
46. Werner SB, Pappagianis D. Coccidioidomycosis in Northern California. An outbreak among archeology students near Red Bluff. Calif Med. 1973;119:10–20.
47. Larsen RA, Jacobson JA, Morris AH, Benowitz BA. Acute respiratory failure caused by primary pulmonary coccidioidomycosis. Two case reports and a review of the literature. Am Rev Respir Dis. 1985;131:797–9.
48. Standaert SM, Schaffner W, Galgiani JN, et al. Coccidioidomycosis among visitors to a *Coccidioides immitis*-endemic area: an outbreak in a military reserve unit. J Infect Dis. 1995;171:1672–5.
49. Cairns L, Blythe D, Kao A, et al. Outbreak of coccidioidomycosis in Washington state residents returning from Mexico. Clin Infect Dis. 2000;30:61–4.
50. CDC. Coccidioidomycosis in travelers returning from Mexico – Pennsylvania, 2000. MMWR Morb Mortal Wkly Rep. 2000;49:1004–6.
51. CDC. Coccidioidomycosis in workers at an archeologic site – Dinosaur National Monument, Utah, June–July 2001. MMWR Morb Mortal Wkly Rep. 2001;50:1005–8.
52. Edwards PQ, Palmer CE. Prevalence of sensitivity to coccidioidin, with special reference to specific and nonspecific reactions to coccidioidin and histoplasmin. Dis Chest. 1957;31:35–60.
53. Larwood TR. Coccidioidin skin testing in Kern County, California: decrease in infection rate over 58 years. Clin Infect Dis. 2000;30:612–3.
54. Dodge RR, Lebowitz MD, Barbee R, Burrows B. Estimates of *C. immitis* infection by skin test reactivity in an endemic community. Am J Public Health. 1985;75:863–5.
55. Padua y Gabriel A, Martinez-Ordaz VA, Velasco-Rodreguez VM, Lazo-Saenz JG, Cicero R. Prevalence of skin reactivity to coccidioidin and associated risks factors in subjects living in a northern city of Mexico. Arch Med Res. 1999;30:388–92.
56. Johnson WM. Occupational factors in coccidioidomycosis. J Occup Med. 1981;23:367–74.
57. Looney JM, Coccidioidomycosis ST. The hazard involved in diagnostic procedures, with report of a case. N Engl J Med. 1950;242:77–82.
58. Johnson III JE, Perry JE, Fekety FR, Kadull PJ, Cluff LE. Laboratory-acquired coccidioidomycosis. Ann Intern Med. 1964;60:941–56.
59. Stevens DA, Clemons KV, Levine HB, et al. Expert opinion: what to do when there is *Coccidioides* exposure in a laboratory. Clin Infect Dis. 2009;49:919–23.
60. Dixon DM. *Coccidioides immitis* as a select agent of bioterrorism. J Appl Microbiol. 2001;91:602–5.
61. Eckmann BH, Schaefer GL, Huppert M. Bedside interhuman transmission of coccidioidomycosis via growth on fomites. Am Rev Respir Dis. 1964;89:179–85.
62. Gehlbach SH, Hamilton JD, Conant NF. Coccidioidomycosis. An occupational disease in cotton mill workers. Arch Intern Med. 1973;131:254–5.

63. Ogiso A, Ito M, Koyama M, Yamaoka H, Hotchi M, McGinnis MR. Pulmonary coccidioidomycosis in Japan: case report and review. Clin Infect Dis. 1997;25:1260–1.
64. Stagliano D, Epstein J, Hickey P. Fomite-transmitted coccidioidomycosis in an immunocompromised child. Pediatr Infect Dis J. 2007;26:454–6.
65. Huntington RW. Pathology of coccidioidomycosis. In: Stevens DA, editor. Coccidioidomycosis a text. New York: Plenum Medical Book Company; 1980. p. 113–32.
66. Galgiani JN, Payne CM, Jones JF. Human polymorphonuclear-leukocyte inhibition of incorporation of chitin precursors into mycelia of *Coccidioides immitis*. J Infect Dis. 1984;149:404–12.
67. Ragland AS, Arsura E, Ismail Y, Johnson R. Eosinophilic pleocytosis in coccidioidal meningitis: frequency and significance. Am J Med. 1993;95:254–7.
68. Lombard CM, Tazelaar HD, Krasne DL. Pulmonary eosinophilia in coccidioidal infections. Chest. 1987;91:734–6.
69. Echols RM, Palmer DL, Long GW. Tissue eosinophilia in human coccidioidomycosis. Rev Infect Dis. 1982;4:656–64.
70. Harley WB, Blaser MJ. Disseminated coccidioidomycosis associated with extreme eosinophilia. Clin Infect Dis. 1994;18:627–9.
71. Putnam JS, Harper WK, Greene Jr JF, Nelson KG, Zurek RC. *Coccidioides immitis*. A rare cause of pulmonary mycetoma. Am Rev Respir Dis. 1975;112:733–8.
72. Rohatgi PK, Schmitt RG. Pulmonary coccidioidal mycetoma. Am J Med Sci. 1984;287:27–30.
73. Dolan MJ, Lattuada CP, Melcher GP, Zellmer R, Allendoerfer R, Rinaldi MG. *Coccidioides immitis* presenting as a mycelial pathogen with empyema and hydropneumothorax. J Med Vet Mycol. 1992;30:249–55.
74. Kleinschmidt-DeMasters BK, Mazowiecki M, Bonds LA, Cohn DL, Wilson ML. Coccidioidomycosis meningitis with massive dural and cerebral venous thrombosis and tissue arthroconidia. Arch Pathol Lab Med. 2000;124:310–4.
75. Chen KT. Coccidioidal peritonitis. Am J Clin Pathol. 1983;80:514–6.
76. Ampel NM, White JD, Varanasi UR, Larwood TR, Van Wyck DB, Galgiani JN. Coccidioidal peritonitis associated with continuous ambulatory peritoneal dialysis. Am J Kidney Dis. 1988;11:512–4.
77. Salgia K, Bhatia L, Rajashekaraiah KR, Zangan M, Hariharan S, Kallick CA. Coccidioidomycosis of the uterus. South Med J. 1982;75:614–6.
78. Bylund DJ, Nanfro JJ, Marsh Jr WL. Coccidioidomycosis of the female genital tract. Arch Pathol Lab Med. 1986;110:232–5.
79. Sohail MR, Andrews PE, Blair JE. Coccidioidomycosis of the male genital tract. J Urol. 2005;173:1978–82.
80. Yurkanin JP, Ahmann F, Dalkin BL. Coccidioidomycosis of the prostate: a determination of incidence, report of 4 cases, and treatment recommendations. J Infect. 2006;52:e19–25.
81. Crum-Cianflone NF, Truett AA, Teneza-Mora N, et al. Unusual presentations of coccidioidomycosis: a case series and review of the literature. Medicine (Baltimore). 2006;85:263–77.
82. Weisman IM, Moreno AJ, Parker AL, Sippo WC, Liles WJ. Gastrointestinal dissemination of coccidioidomycosis. Am J Gastroenterol. 1986;81:589–93.
83. Kuntze JR, Herman MH, Evans SG. Genitourinary coccidioidomycosis. J Urol. 1988;140:370–4.
84. Polesky A, Kirsch CM, Snyder LS, et al. Airway coccidioidomycosis – report of cases and review. Clin Infect Dis. 1999;28:1273–80.
85. Rodenbiker HT, Ganley JP, Galgiani JN, Axline SG. Prevalence of chorioretinal scars associated with coccidioidomycosis. Arch Ophthalmol. 1981;99:71–5.
86. Rodenbiker HT, Ganley JP. Ocular coccidioidomycosis. Surv Ophthalmol. 1980;24:263–90.
87. Banuelos AF, Williams PL, Johnson RH, et al. Central nervous system abscesses due to *Coccidioides* species. Clin Infect Dis. 1996;22:240–50.
88. Mischel PS, Vinters HV. Coccidioidomycosis of the central nervous system: neuropathological and vasculopathic manifestations and clinical correlates. Clin Infect Dis. 1995;20:400–5.
89. Williams PL, Johnson R, Pappagianis D, et al. Vasculitic and encephalitic complications associated with *Coccidioides immitis* infection of the central nervous system in humans: report of 10 cases and review. Clin Infect Dis. 1992;14:673–82.
90. Ampel NM, Dols CL, Galgiani JN. Coccidioidomycosis during human immunodeficiency virus infection: results of a prospective study in a coccidioidal endemic area. Am J Med. 1993;94:235–40.
91. Blair JE, Logan JL. Coccidioidomycosis in solid organ transplantation. Clin Infect Dis. 2001;33:1536–44.
92. Ampel NM, Ryan KJ, Carry PJ, Wieden MA, Schifman RB. Fungemia due to *Coccidioides immitis*. An analysis of 16 episodes in 15 patients and a review of the literature. Medicine (Baltimore). 1986;65:312–21.
93. Corry DB, Ampel NM, Christian L, Locksley RM, Galgiani JN. Cytokine production by peripheral blood mononuclear cells in human coccidioidomycosis. J Infect Dis. 1996;174:440–3.
94. Ampel NM, Kramer LA, Kerekes KM, Johnson SM, Pappagianis D. Assessment of the human cellular immune response to T27K, a coccidioidal antigen preparation, by flow cytometry of whole blood. Med Mycol. 2001;39:315–20.
95. Ampel NM, Kramer LA. In vitro modulation of cytokine production by lymphocytes in human coccidioidomycosis. Cell Immunol. 2003;221:115–21.
96. Li L, Dial SM, Schmelz M, Rennels MA, Ampel NM. Cellular immune suppressor activity resides in lymphocyte cell clusters adjacent to granulomata in human coccidioidomycosis. Infect Immun. 2005;73:3923–8.
97. Smith CE, Beard R. Varieties of coccidioidal infection in relation to the epidemiology and control of the diseases. Am J Public Health. 1946;36:1394–402.
98. Richards JO, Ampel NM, Galgiani JN, Lake DF. Dendritic cells pulsed with *Coccidioides immitis* lysate induce antigen-specific naive T cell activation. J Infect Dis. 2001;184:1220–4.
99. Levine BE, Cobb JM, Smith CE. Immunity to coccidioidomycosis induced mice by purified spherule, arthrospore, and mycelial vaccines. Trans NY Acad Sci. 1960;22:436–49.
100. Williams PL, Sable DL, Sorgen SP, et al. Immunologic responsiveness and safety associated with the *Coccidioides immitis* spherule vaccine in volunteers of white, black, and Filipino ancestry. Am J Epidemiol. 1984;119:591–602.
101. Pappagianis D. Evaluation of the protective efficacy of the killed *Coccidioides immitis* spherule vaccine in humans. The Valley Fever Vaccine Study Group. Am Rev Respir Dis. 1993;148:656–60.
102. Zimmermann CR, Johnson SM, Martens GW, White AG, Zimmer BL, Pappagianis D. Protection against lethal murine coccidioidomycosis by a soluble vaccine from spherules. Infect Immun. 1998;66:2342–5.
103. Jiang C, Magee DM, Quitugua TN, Cox RA. Genetic vaccination against *Coccidioides immitis*: comparison of vaccine efficacy of recombinant antigen 2 and antigen 2 cDNA. Infect Immun. 1999;67:630–5.
104. Abuodeh RO, Shubitz LF, Siegel E, et al. Resistance to *Coccidioides immitis* in mice after immunization with recombinant protein or a DNA vaccine of a proline-rich antigen. Infect Immun. 1999;67:2935–40.
105. Li K, Yu JJ, Hung CY, Lehmann PF, Cole GT. Recombinant urease and urease DNA of *Coccidioides immitis* elicit an immunoprotective response against coccidioidomycosis in mice. Infect Immun. 2001;69:2878–87.
106. Xue J, Chen X, Selby D, Hung CY, Yu JJ, Cole GT. A genetically engineered live attenuated vaccine of *Coccidioides posadasii*

protects BALB/c mice against coccidioidomycosis. Infect Immun. 2009;77:3196–208.
107. Smith CE. Diagnosis of pulmonary coccidioidal infections. Calif Med. 1951;75:385–91.
108. Muir Bowers J, Mourani JP, Ampel NM. Fatigue in coccidioidomycosis. Quantification and correlation with clinical, immunological, and nutritional factors. Med Mycol. 2006;44:585–90.
109. Werner SB. Coccidioidomycosis misdiagnosed as contact dermatitis. Calif Med. 1972;117:59–61.
110. DiCaudo DJ, Yiannias JA, Laman SD, Warschaw KE. The exanthem of acute pulmonary coccidioidomycosis: clinical and histopathologic features of 3 cases and review of the literature. Arch Dermatol. 2006;142:744–6.
111. Arsura EL, Kilgore WB, Ratnayake SN. Erythema nodosum in pregnant patients with coccidioidomycosis. Clin Infect Dis. 1998;27:1201–3.
112. McGahan JP, Graves DS, Palmer PE, Stadalnik RC, Dublin AB. Classic and contemporary imaging of coccidioidomycosis. AJR. 1981;136:393–404.
113. Greendyke WH, Resnick DL, Harvey WC. The varied roentgen manifestations of primary coccidioidomycosis. Am J Roentgenol Radium Ther Nucl Med. 1970;109:491–9.
114. Merchant M, Romero AO, Libke RD, Joseph J. Pleural effusion in hospitalized patients with coccidioidomycosis. Respir Med. 2008;102:537–40.
115. Valdivia L, Nix D, Wright M, et al. Coccidioidomycosis as a common cause of community-acquired pneumonia. Emerg Infect Dis. 2006;12:958–62.
116. Capone D, Marchiori E, Wanke B, et al. Acute pulmonary coccidioidomycosis: CT findings from 15 patients. Br J Radiol. 2008;81:721–4.
117. Forseth J, Rohwedder JJ, Levine BE, Saubolle MA. Experience with needle biopsy for coccidioidal lung nodules. Arch Intern Med. 1986;146:319–20.
118. Chitkara YK. Evaluation of cultures of percutaneous core needle biopsy specimens in the diagnosis of pulmonary nodules. Am J Clin Pathol. 1997;107:224–8.
119. Winn RE, Johnson R, Galgiani JN, Butler C, Pluss J. Cavitary coccidioidomycosis with fungus ball formation. Diagnosis by fiberoptic bronchoscopy with coexistence of hyphae and spherules. Chest. 1994;105:412–6.
120. Hyde L. Coccidioidal pulmonary cavitation. Dis Chest. 1968;54 Suppl 1:273–7.
121. Edelstein G, Levitt RG. Cavitary coccidioidomycosis presenting as spontaneous pneumothorax. AJR. 1983;141:533–4.
122. Sarosi GA, Parker JD, Doto IL, Tosh FE. Chronic pulmonary coccidioidomycosis. N Engl J Med. 1970;283:325–9.
123. Arsura EL, Kilgore WB. Miliary coccidioidomycosis in the immunocompetent. Chest. 2000;117:404–9.
124. Rempe S, Sachdev MS, Bhakta R, Pineda-Roman M, Vaz A, Carlson RW. *Coccidioides immitis* fungemia: clinical features and survival in 33 adult patients. Heart Lung. 2007;36:64–71.
125. Adam RD, Elliott SP, Taljanovic MS. The spectrum and presentation of disseminated coccidioidomycosis. Am J Med. 2009;122:770–7.
126. Caldwell JW, Arsura EL, Kilgore WB, Reddy CM, Johnson RH. Hypercalcemia in patients with disseminated coccidioidomycosis. Am J Med Sci. 2004;327:15–8.
127. Hobbs ER. Coccidioidomycosis. Dermatol Clin. 1989;7:227–39.
128. Kushwaha VP, Shaw BA, Gerardi JA, Oppenheim WL. Musculoskeletal coccidioidomycosis. A review of 25 cases. Clin Orthop Relat Res. 1996:190–9.
129. Zeppa MA, Laorr A, Greenspan A, McGahan JP, Steinbach LS. Skeletal coccidioidomycosis: imaging findings in 19 patients. Skeletal Radiol. 1996;25:337–43.
130. Olson EM, Duberg AC, Herron LD, Kissel P, Smilovitz D. Coccidioidal spondylitis: MR findings in 15 patients. AJR. 1998;171:785–9.
131. Bayer AS, Guze LB. Fungal arthritis. II. Coccidioidal synovitis: clinical, diagnostic, therapeutic, and prognostic considerations. Semin Arthritis Rheum. 1979;8:200–11.
132. Lund PJ, Chan KM, Unger EC, Galgiani TN, Pitt MJ. Magnetic resonance imaging in coccidioidal arthritis. Skeletal Radiol. 1996;25:661–5.
133. Bouza E, Dreyer JS, Hewitt WL, Meyer RD. Coccidioidal meningitis. An analysis of thirty-one cases and review of the literature. Medicine (Baltimore). 1981;60:139–72.
134. Johnson RH, Einstein HE. Coccidioidal meningitis. Clin Infect Dis. 2006;42:103–7.
135. Vincent T, Galgiani JN, Huppert M, Salkin D. The natural history of coccidioidal meningitis: VA-Armed Forces cooperative studies, 1955–1958. Clin Infect Dis. 1993;16:247–54.
136. Erly WK, Bellon RJ, Seeger JF, Carmody RF. MR imaging of acute coccidioidal meningitis. AJNR. 1999;20:509–14.
137. Williams PL. Vasculitic complications associated with coccidioidal meningitis. Semin Respir Infect. 2001;16:270–9.
138. Deresinski SC, Stevens DA. Coccidioidomycosis in compromised hosts. Experience at Stanford University Hospital. Medicine (Baltimore). 1975;54:377–95.
139. Masannat FY, Ampel NM. Coccidioidomycosis among patients with HIV-1 infection in the era of potent antiretroviral therapy. Clin Infect Dis. 2010;50:1–7.
140. Mortimer RB, Libke R, Eghbalieh B, Bilello JF. Immune reconstitution inflammatory syndrome presenting as superior vena cava syndrome secondary to *Coccidioides* lymphadenopathy in an HIV-infected patient. J Int Assoc Physicians AIDS Care (Chic Ill). 2008;7:283–5.
141. Blair JE. Approach to the solid organ transplant patient with latent infection and disease caused by *Coccidioides* species. Curr Opin Infect Dis. 2008;21:415–20.
142. Blair JE, Kusne S, Carey EJ, Heilman RL. The prevention of recrudescent coccidioidomycosis after solid organ transplantation. Transplantation. 2007;83:1182–7.
143. Wright P, Pappagianis D, Taylor J, et al. Transmission of *Coccidioides immitis* from donor organs: a description of two fatal cases of disseminated coccidioidomycosis [Abstract 619]. In: Annual Conference of the Infectious Diseases Society of America 2001, San Francisco, CA; 2001.
144. Tripathy U, Yung GL, Kriett JM, Thistlethwaite PA, Kapelanski DP, Jamieson SW. Donor transfer of pulmonary coccidioidomycosis in lung transplantation. Ann Thorac Surg. 2002;73:306–8.
145. Miller MB, Hendren R, Gilligan PH. Posttransplantation disseminated coccidioidomycosis acquired from donor lungs. J Clin Microbiol. 2004;42:2347–9.
146. Blair JE, Mulligan DC. Coccidioidomycosis in healthy persons evaluated for liver or kidney donation. Transpl Infect Dis. 2007;9:78–82.
147. Smith JA, Kauffman CA. Endemic fungal infections in patients receiving tumour necrosis factor-alpha inhibitor therapy. Drugs. 2009;69:1403–15.
148. Bergstrom L, Yocum DE, Ampel NM, et al. Increased risk of coccidioidomycosis in patients treated with tumor necrosis factor alpha antagonists. Arthritis Rheum. 2004;50:1959–66.
149. Dweik M, Baethge BA, Duarte AG. Coccidioidomycosis pneumonia in a nonendemic area associated with infliximab. South Med J. 2007;100:517–8.
150. Galgiani JN, Ampel NM, Blair JE, et al. Coccidioidomycosis. IDSA Guidelines. Clin Infect Dis. 2005;41:1217–23.
151. Gray GC, Fogle EF, Albright KL. Risk factors for primary pulmonary coccidioidomycosis hospitalizations among United

States Navy and Marine Corps personnel, 1981–1994. Am J Trop Med Hyg. 1998;58:309–12.
152. Arsura EL. The association of age and mortality in coccidioidomycosis. J Am Geriatr Soc. 1997;45:532–3.
153. Ampel NM, Mosley DG, England B, Vertz PD, Komatsu K, Hajjeh RA. Coccidioidomycosis in Arizona: increase in incidence from 1990 to 1995. Clin Infect Dis. 1998;27:1528–30.
154. Leake JA, Mosley DG, England B, et al. Risk factors for acute symptomatic coccidioidomycosis among elderly persons in Arizona, 1996–1997. J Infect Dis. 2000;181:1435–40.
155. Williams PL, Sable DL, Mendez P, Smyth LT. Symptomatic coccidioidomycosis following a severe natural dust storm. An outbreak at the Naval Air Station, Lemoore, California. Chest. 1979;76:566–70.
156. Rosenstein NE, Emery KW, Werner SB, et al. Risk factors for severe pulmonary and disseminated coccidioidomycosis: Kern County, California, 1995–1996. Clin Infect Dis. 2001;32:708–15.
157. Crum NF, Ballon-Landa G. Coccidioidomycosis in pregnancy: case report and review of the literature. Am J Med. 2006;119(993):e11–7.
158. Pursley TJ, Blomquist IK, Abraham J, Andersen HF, Bartley JA. Fluconazole-induced congenital anomalies in three infants. Clin Infect Dis. 1996;22:336–40.
159. De Santis M, Di Gianantonio E, Cesari E, Ambrosini G, Straface G, Clementi M. First-trimester itraconazole exposure and pregnancy outcome: a prospective cohort study of women contacting teratology information services in Italy. Drug Saf. 2009;32:239–44.
160. Stockman L, Clark KA, Hunt JM, Roberts GD. Evaluation of commercially available acridinium ester-labeled chemiluminescent DNA probes for culture identification of *Blastomyces dermatitidis*, *Coccidioides immitis*, *Cryptococcus neoformans*, and *Histoplasma capsulatum*. J Clin Microbiol. 1993;31:845–50.
161. Stevens DA, Clemons KV, Levine HB, et al. Expert opinion: what to do when there is *Coccidioides* exposure in a laboratory. Clin Infect Dis. 2009;49:919–23.
162. DiTomasso JP, Ampel NM, Sobonya RE, Bloom JW. Bronchoscopic diagnosis of pulmonary coccidioidomycosis. Comparison of cytology, culture, and transbronchial biopsy. Diagn Microbiol Infect Dis. 1994;18:83–7.
163. Sarosi GA, Lawrence JP, Smith DK, Thomas A, Hobohm DW, Kelley PC. Rapid diagnostic evaluation of bronchial washings in patients with suspected coccidioidomycosis. Semin Respir Infect. 2001;16:238–41.
164. Smith CE, Saito MT, Simons SA. Pattern of 39, 500 serologic tests in coccidioidomycosis. JAMA. 1956;160:546–52.
165. Pappagianis D, Zimmer BL. Serology of coccidioidomycosis. Clin Microbiol Rev. 1990;3:247–68.
166. Pappagianis D. Serologic studies in coccidioidomycosis. Semin Respir Infect. 2001;16:242–50.
167. Hung CY, Yu JJ, Lehmann PF, Cole GT. Cloning and expression of the gene which encodes a tube precipitin antigen and wall-associated beta-glucosidase of *Coccidioides immitis*. Infect Immun. 2001;69:2211–22.
168. Zimmermann CR, Johnson SM, Martens GW, White AG, Pappagianis D. Cloning and expression of the complement fixation antigen-chitinase of *Coccidioides immitis*. Infect Immun. 1996;64:4967–75.
169. Huppert M, Bailey JW. The use of immunodiffusion tests in coccidioidomycosis. I. The accuracy and reproducibility of the immunodiffusion test which correlates with complement fixation. Am J Clin Pathol. 1965;44:364–8.
170. Huppert M, Bailey JW. The use of immunodiffusion tests in coccidioidomycosis. II. An immunodiffusion test as a substitute for the tube precipitin test. Am J Clin Pathol. 1965;44:369–73.
171. Wieden MA, Galgiani JN, Pappagianis D. Comparison of immunodiffusion techniques with standard complement fixation assay for quantitation of coccidioidal antibodies. J Clin Microbiol. 1983;18:529–34.
172. Kaufman L, Sekhon AS, Moledina N, Jalbert M, Pappagianis D. Comparative evaluation of commercial Premier EIA and microimmunodiffusion and complement fixation tests for *Coccidioides immitis* antibodies. J Clin Microbiol. 1995;33:618–9.
173. Blair JE, Currier JT. Significance of isolated positive IgM serologic results by enzyme immunoassay for coccidioidomycosis. Mycopathologia. 2008;166:77–82.
174. Antoniskis D, Larsen RA, Akil B, Rarick MU, Leedom JM. Seronegative disseminated coccidioidomycosis in patients with HIV infection. AIDS. 1990;4:691–3.
175. Blair JE, Coakley B, Santelli AC, Hentz JG, Wengenack NL. Serologic testing for symptomatic coccidioidomycosis in immunocompetent and immunosuppressed hosts. Mycopathologia. 2006;162:317–24.
176. Kuberski T, Myers R, Wheat LJ, et al. Diagnosis of coccidioidomycosis by antigen detection using cross-reaction with a *Histoplasma* antigen. Clin Infect Dis. 2007;44:e50–4.
177. Durkin M, Connolly P, Kuberski T, et al. Diagnosis of coccidioidomycosis with use of the *Coccidioides* antigen enzyme immunoassay. Clin Infect Dis. 2008;47:e69–73.
178. Bialek R, Kern J, Herrmann T, et al. PCR assays for identification of *Coccidioides posadasii* based on the nucleotide sequence of the antigen 2/proline-rich antigen. J Clin Microbiol. 2004;42:778–83.
179. Johnson SM, Simmons KA, Pappagianis D. Amplification of coccidioidal DNA in clinical specimens by PCR. J Clin Microbiol. 2004;42:1982–5.
180. Brilhante RS, Cordeiro RA, Rocha MF, et al. Coccidioidal pericarditis: a rapid presumptive diagnosis by an in-house antigen confirmed by mycological and molecular methods. J Med Microbiol. 2008;57:1288–92.
181. Cordeiro RA, Brilhante RSN, Rocha MFG, Moura FEA, Camargo ZP, Sidrim JJC. Rapid diagnosis of coccidioidomycosis by nested PCR assay of sputum. Clin Microbiol Infect. 2007;13:449–51.
182. Binnicker MJ, Buckwalter SP, Eisberner JJ, et al. Detection of *Coccidioides* species in clinical specimens by real-time PCR. J Clin Microbiol. 2007;45:173–8.
183. Hardenbrook MH, Barriere SL. Coccidioidomycosis: evaluation of parameters used to predict outcome with amphotericin B therapy. Mycopathologia. 1982;78:65–71.
184. Graybill JR, Stevens DA, Galgiani JN, Dismukes WE, Cloud GA. Itraconazole treatment of coccidioidomycosis. NAIAD Mycoses Study Group. Am J Med. 1990;89:282–90.
185. Catanzaro A, Galgiani JN, Levine BE, et al. Fluconazole in the treatment of chronic pulmonary and nonmeningeal disseminated coccidioidomycosis. NIAID Mycoses Study Group. Am J Med. 1995;98:249–56.
186. Galgiani JN, Catanzaro A, Cloud GA, et al. Comparison of oral fluconazole and itraconazole for progressive, nonmeningeal coccidioidomycosis. A randomized, double-blind trial. The NIAID-Mycoses Study Group. Ann Intern Med. 2000;133:676–86.
187. Galgiani JN, Catanzaro A, Cloud GA, et al. Fluconazole therapy for coccidioidal meningitis. The NIAID-Mycoses Study Group. Ann Intern Med. 1993;119:28–35.
188. Tucker RM, Denning DW, Dupont B, Stevens DA. Itraconazole therapy for chronic coccidioidal meningitis. Ann Intern Med. 1990;112:108–12.
189. Anstead GM, Corcoran G, Lewis J, Berg D, Graybill JR. Refractory coccidioidomycosis treated with posaconazole. Clin Infect Dis. 2005;40:1770–6.
190. Stevens DA, Rendon A, Gaona-Flores V, et al. Posaconazole therapy for chronic refractory coccidioidomycosis. Chest. 2007;132:952–8.
191. Catanzaro A, Cloud GA, Stevens DA, et al. Safety, tolerance, and efficacy of posaconazole therapy in patients with nonmeningeal

disseminated or chronic pulmonary coccidioidomycosis. Clin Infect Dis. 2007;45:562–8.
192. Cortez KJ, Walsh TJ, Bennett JE. Successful treatment of coccidioidal meningitis with voriconazole. Clin Infect Dis. 2003;36:1619–22.
193. Prabhu RM, Bonnell M, Currier BL, Orenstein R. Successful treatment of disseminated nonmeningeal coccidioidomycosis with voriconazole. Clin Infect Dis. 2004;39:e74–7.
194. Proia LA, Tenorio AR. Successful use of voriconazole for treatment of *Coccidioides* meningitis. Antimicrob Agents Chemother. 2004;48:2341.
195. Gonzalez GM, Tijerina R, Najvar LK, et al. Correlation between antifungal susceptibilities of *Coccidioides immitis* in vitro and antifungal treatment with caspofungin in a mouse model. Antimicrob Agents Chemother. 2001;45:1854–9.
196. Park DW, Sohn JW, Cheong HJ, et al. Combination therapy of disseminated coccidioidomycosis with caspofungin and fluconazole. BMC Infect Dis. 2006;6:26.
197. Hsue G, Napier JT, Prince RA, Chi J, Hospenthal DR. Treatment of meningeal coccidioidomycosis with caspofungin. J Antimicrob Chemother. 2004;54:292–4.
198. Hector RF, Zimmer BL, Pappagianis D. Evaluation of nikkomycins X and Z in murine models of coccidioidomycosis, histoplasmosis, and blastomycosis. Antimicrob Agents Chemother. 1990;34:587–93.
199. Kuberski TT, Servi RJ, Rubin PJ. Successful treatment of a critically ill patient with disseminated coccidioidomycosis, using adjunctive interferon-gamma. Clin Infect Dis. 2004;38:910–2.
200. Ramani R, Chaturvedi V. Antifungal susceptibility profiles of *Coccidioides immitis* and *Coccidioides posadasii* from endemic and non-endemic areas. Mycopathologia. 2007;163:315–9.
201. Kriesel JD, Sutton DA, Schulman S, Fothergill AW, Rinaldi MG. Persistent pulmonary infection with an azole-resistant *Coccidioides* species. Med Mycol. 2008;46:607–10.
202. Baddley JW, Cobbs CS, Pappas PG. Surgical treatment of multiple skull abscesses associated with coccidioidomycosis. Mycoses. 2004;47:69–71.
203. Romeo JH, Rice LB, McQuarrie IG. Hydrocephalus in coccidioidal meningitis: case report and review of the literature. Neurosurgery. 2000;47:773–7.
204. Wrobel CJ, Chappell ET, Taylor W. Clinical presentation, radiological findings, and treatment results of coccidioidomycosis involving the spine: report on 23 cases. J Neurosurg. 2001;95:33–9.
205. Ampel NM, Giblin A, Mourani JP, Galgiani JN. Factors and outcomes associated with the decision to treat primary pulmonary coccidioidomycosis. Clin Infect Dis. 2009;48:172–8.
206. Sugar AM. Use of amphotericin B with azole antifungal drugs. What are we doing? Antimicrob Agents Chemother. 1995;39:1907–12.
207. Rex JH, Pappas PG, Karchmer AW, et al. A randomized and blinded multicenter trial of high-dose fluconazole plus placebo versus fluconazole plus amphotericin B as therapy for candidemia and its consequences in nonneutropenic subjects. Clin Infect Dis. 2003;36:1221–8.
208. Oldfield 3rd EC, Bone WD, Martin CR, Gray GC, Olson P, Schillaci RF. Prediction of relapse after treatment of coccidioidomycosis. Clin Infect Dis. 1997;25:1205–10.
209. Galgiani JN, Catanzaro A, Cloud GA, et al. Comparison of oral fluconazole and itraconazole for progressive, nonmeningeal coccidioidomycosis. A randomized, double-blind trial. Mycoses Study Group. Ann Intern Med. 2000;133:676–86.
210. Einstein H, Holeman CW, Sandidge LL, Holden DH. Coccidioidal meningitis. The use of amphotericin B in treatment. Calif Med. 1961;94:339–43.
211. Dewsnup DH, Galgiani JN, Graybill JR, et al. Is it ever safe to stop azole therapy for *Coccidioides immitis* meningitis? Ann Intern Med. 1996;124:305–10.
212. Stevens DA, Shatsky SA. Intrathecal amphotericin in the management of coccidioidal meningitis. Semin Respir Infect. 2001;16:263–9.
213. Berry CD, Stevens DA, Hassid EI, Pappagianis D, Happs EL, Sahrakar K. A new method for the treatment of chronic fungal meningitis: continuous infusion into the cerebrospinal fluid for coccidioidal meningitis. Am J Med Sci. 2009;338:79–82.
214. Kirkland TN, Fierer J. Coccidioidomycosis: a reemerging infectious disease. Emerg Infect Dis. 1996;2:192–9.

Paracoccidioidomycosis

Angela Restrepo, Angel Gonzalez, and Carlos A. Agudelo

Paracoccidioidomycosis is an endemic fungal infection of pulmonary origin that disseminates to different sites, notably oral mucous membranes, adrenal glands, reticuloendothelial system, and skin. The disease tends to run a chronic course with acute cases being rare; outbreaks have not been reported. Four clinical presentations are recognized: subclinical infection, progressive disease that can be either chronic (adult-type), or acute/subacute (juvenile-type), and the residual form. This mycosis is restricted to Latin America, and has a striking male predominance. The etiologic agent is a thermally dimorphic fungus, *Paracoccidioides brasiliensis,* which at 35–37°C assumes a yeast form characterized by a mother cell surrounded by multiple blastoconidia resembling a pilot's wheel. At lower temperatures the fungus grows as a mould that gives rise to conidia. The organism's microniche in nature has not yet been precisely defined. The disease can be successfully treated, but fibrotic sequelae are common.

Organism

Paracoccidioides brasiliensis is a thermally dimorphic fungus that in tissues and in cultures at 35–37°C grows as a yeast, whereas at temperatures <28°C, it develops as a mould [1, 2]. This morphogenetic process is reversible and implies the capacity to adapt to changing environmental conditions: the mould-to-yeast-form conversion occurs rapidly at the time of infection allowing fungal survival and host invasion. In the mould form the main cell wall component is a beta-1,3-glucan, and in the yeast form this compound is replaced by alpha-1,3-glucan [3]. This microorganism, recognized only in its asexual (anamorph) state [2] is now classified by molecular techniques in the phylum Ascomycota, order Onygenales, family Onygenacea, and is close in the phylogenetic tree to *Histoplasma capsulatum, Blastomyces dermatitidis,* and *Emmonsia parva,* which have teleomorphs in the genus *Ajellomyces* [3, 4]. At least three distinct phylogenetic species, or clades, are recognized within the genus (PS2, PS3, and S1) [5]. In addition and based on high polygenetic diversity and exclusive morphogenetic characteristics, a different species, designated as *P. lutzi,* has been proposed [6]. The BROAD Institute has now completed (2009, April 10) the data base for the *P. brasiliensis* genome, and this can be found at http://www.broad.mit.edu/annotation/genome/paracoccidioides_brasiliensis/.

Yeast colonies appear within a week of incubation at 36–37°C; they are soft, wrinkled and tan to cream in color. Microscopically, colonies reveal yeast cells varying in size from 4 to 40 μm with a predominance of round to oval structures. The most characteristic grouping is that of a mother cell surrounded by multiple buds of equal or different sizes resembling a pilot's wheel; the buds may present a connecting bridge with the mother cell. Sometimes single cells, with one bud or arranged in short chains can be observed; chalice-, balloon-shaped- or broken cells are not infrequent. The yeast has a thick, refractile cell wall and contains prominent intracytoplasmic lipid vacuoles. This is the form that is recognized in clinical samples and tissues (Figs. 1 and 2) [1, 2, 7].

At temperatures ranging from 19°C to 28°C, *P. brasiliensis* grows as a mould; growth takes 15–30 days. It produces white to tan, irregularly shaped colonies with short hairy-looking mycelia; some isolates produce a brown pigment. Microscopic preparations from the mould reveal only thin, septated hyphae with sparse terminal and intercalary chlamydospores. The latter are considered resistant structures and likely play a role in the mycelial to yeast transition by becoming yeast cells under the influence of temperature [1, 2]. When grown under nutritional deprivation, certain isolates produce conidia that can appear to be centrally bulging arthroconidia or single-celled to pear-shaped microconidia, all less than 5 μm. Conidia respond to temperature changes, transforming either into yeast cells at 36°C or producing hyphae at 20–24°C [7, 8]. Furthermore, conidia are infectious for mice and produce a chronic, disseminated process ending in fibrous changes of the lungs [9–11]. *P. brasiliensis* conidia and yeast cells have been shown to produce melanin-like

A. Restrepo (✉)
Medical and Experimental Mycology Unit, Corporacion para Investigaciones Biologicas, Medellin, Colombia
e-mail: angelares@une.net.co

C.A. Kauffman et al. (eds.), *Essentials of Clinical Mycology*,
DOI 10.1007/978-1-4419-6640-7_21, © Springer Science+Business Media, LLC 2011

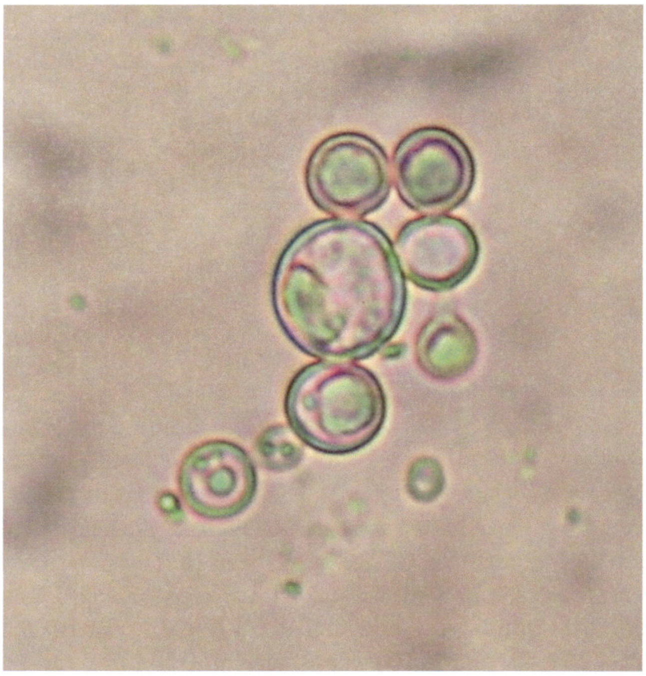

Fig. 1 *Paracoccidioides brasiliensis* yeast cells in an aspirate from a lesion. Note round shape, thick refractile cell wall, intracytoplasmic vacuoles, and differences in the size of the yeast cells (40×)

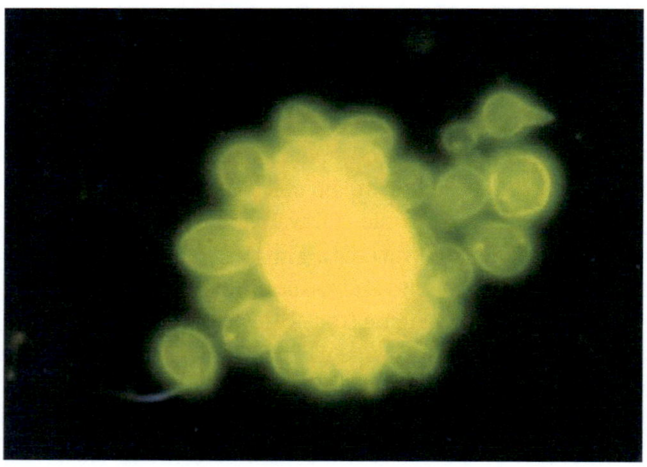

Fig. 2 Calcofluor white preparation showing *Paracoccidioides brasiliensis* yeast cell from a culture grown at 36°C. Note large mother cell with multiple buds attached (100×)

compounds, both in vitro and in vivo; melanin may play a role in pathogenesis [12, 13]. Both the mycelial and the yeast forms are aerobic and require ample oxygen supply for their growth; however, in residual lesions, yeast cells tolerate oxygen restriction and can be cultured only under microaerobic conditions [14].

Electron microscopy reveals a mycelial cell wall that has two layers, the outermost made of beta-1,3-glucan fibrils and the innermost, of rigid chitin fibrils; externally, there is accumulation of amorphous galactomannan. The cell wall constituent polysaccharides protect the fungus against the host's defense mechanisms [15]. The septum comes from a deep invagination of the internal layer and of the cytoplasmic membrane; growth toward the hyphal axis leaves a pore associated with Woronin bodies [16]. In the yeast form there is a thicker cell wall composed mainly of alpha-1,3-glucan, which has as its outermost layer a surface of complex mucopolysaccharides [15, 16]. Differences in cell wall glucose polymers in the two forms appear important in host-parasite interactions because macrophages do not have alpha glucanase and are unable to degrade the yeast cells [15].

P. brasiliensis isolates are not equally virulent, as shown by random amplified polymorphic DNA (RAPD) analysis that has demonstrated two different patterns, with some strains eliciting a localized infection and others giving rise to disseminated disease [17]. Thirty putative virulence genes have been categorized and related to genes encoding proteins connected with metabolism, cell wall structure, detoxification, and secretion of certain factors [18]. As an example, *P. brasiliensis* avoids toxic substances produced by macrophages by displaying antioxidant enzymes. Gene expression differs when yeast cells are in contact with human blood or have been rescued from infected mice [19–21].

The host's hormones influence *P. brasiliensis* mycelial to yeast transition. The original studies, which arose in response to the observed predominance of male over female patients (ratio 14:1), [7] revealed that in vitro *P. brasiliensis* secretes an estradiol-binding protein that attaches to the female hormone regulating protein expression. Estradiol hinders the mycelial to yeast transition [22]. Male and female mice infected with conidia behave differently. In normal male mice, conidia transformed promptly into yeast cells that multiplied readily, resulting in progressive infection. In normal female mice such transition was halted, fungal proliferation was inhibited, and the infection was controlled. These results support a role for 17 beta-estradiol in the innate resistance of females to paracoccidioidomycosis. This is in addition to the capacity of the hormone to modulate cytokine production, thus improving the immune response [23, 24]. *P. brasiliensis* isolates from diverse geographic regions studied by RAPD and restriction fragment length polymorphism (RFLP) methods allowed construction of a dendrogram that showed a high degree of similarity among strains with genetic differences expressed in clusters related to geographic origin. Five different groups were sorted, each of which was geographically distinct and corresponded to present country borders. The results support the concept that *P. brasiliensis* infections are acquired from exogenous sources and that this fungus occupies special niches within the natural environment [25].

Epidemiology

Geographic Distribution

Paracoccidioidomycosis is limited to Latin America, where it is regularly reported from Mexico (23°N) to Argentina (34°S), albeit not with the same frequency. Over 80% of all reports are from Brazil, followed by Venezuela, Colombia, Ecuador, and Argentina [1, 7, 26–28]. No cases have been reported in Chile, Surinam, Nicaragua, or Belize. With the exception of one case each in Trinidad, Granada, and Guadaloupe, the Caribbean Islands appear free of this mycosis [7, 27]. Cases are seen mostly in regions with significant rainfall, abundant forests, waterways, and temperature variation limited to 17–24°C [28]. In a large series of Colombian cases, several independent ecologic variables were found: altitude from 1,000 to 1,499 m above sea level, yearly rainfall from 2,000 to 2,999 mm, presence of humid forests, and coffee/tobacco crops [29].

Over 70 paracoccidioidomycosis cases have been published from countries outside of the recognized endemic areas; these are mostly from Europe, Japan, and the United States [7, 28, 30–33]. These patients had all lived or visited the Latin American endemic regions prior to the appearance of clinical manifestations. Those reports with sufficient data indicated that in 75% of cases, the disease was diagnosed an average of 14 years (range 4 months–60 years) after departure from the endemic zone [7, 28, 30–33].

Ecology

The precise microniche of *P. brasiliensis* has not been ascertained, and its isolation from nature has only been reported on six occasions [34]. Puzzling reports indicate isolation from bat guano and penguin feces [34]. The recognition of the particular site where the fungus has its habitat has been hindered by the long latency period, as well as by lack of epidemic outbreaks and scarcity of published reports on acute cases [1, 7, 28].

Search for the habitat of *P. brasiliensis* has been intense but unrewarding. It has been noticed that human-made changes in endemic areas are a constant feature [28]. Studies from Brazil have shown increased infection in children who live in areas in which intense human colonization resulted in gradual destruction of the originally abundant native forests [35–37]. Paracoccidoidin skin testing reagents, although not standardized, have been used to determine the incidence of infection with *P. brasiliensis* [38–40]. In Rio de Janeiro, Brazil, 34% of children who were tested reacted to paracoccidioidin, and 74% of them lived in the foothills around a particular sierra [36]. Other studies have shown that living in the vicinity of certain water sources, contact with armadillos, and work in orchards are associated with increased skin reactivity [37].

In the Amazon River basin, positive paracoccidioidin skin test reactions were significantly higher (43.3%) in a particular tribe that had adopted a novel agricultural practice of planting coffee, which required the felling of trees in the forest. This activity presumably increased the likelihood of exposure to *P. brasiliensis* [38]. Similar testing in residents of the Corrientes province, Argentina, where paracoccidioidomycosis had never been diagnosed, revealed 11.4% positive reactions. This province is close to the Brazilian Paraná River dam, where construction of a hydroelectric plant brought about great ecologic change [39]. The use of a more refined *P. brasiliensis* antigen (gp43) was studied in a cross-sectional study of asymptomatic school children in the Brazilian Amazon region. Reactivity to gp43 antigen was only 4.6%, suggesting that this antigen might provide a better estimate of exposure to *P. brasiliensis* than paracoccidioidin, which is known to cross-react with histoplasmin [40].

Simoes et al. [41] explored climatic influences on paracoccidioidomycosis by establishing ecologic correlates related to distribution of this infection in a hyperendemic area in southeastern Brazil. It was found that certain types of soils plus high annual precipitation rates (1,500 and 1,600 mm) were significantly associated with prevalence density. Barroso et al. further [42] analyzed the records of 91 acute/subacute patients in whom infection was calculated to have occurred 1–2 years previously, and found that absolute air humidity, soil water storage, and the Southern Oscillation Index enhanced human infection [42].

The existence of naturally infected animals had not been proven until 1986, when researchers working in the Brazilian jungles of Pará isolated *P. brasiliensis* from the organs of several nine-banded armadillos, *Dasypus novemcinctus* [43]. Presently, the existence of naturally occurring *P. brasiliensis* infections in armadillos (*D. novemcinctus, Cabassous centralis*) is widely accepted [43, 44]. *P. brasiliensis*–infected armadillos are preferentially found in humid and shady disturbed forests [45] Attempts to isolate *P. brasiliensis* from armadillo burrows and foraging places have failed, and the natural habitat remains undiscovered [28, 44, 45]. Paracoccidioidomycosis has also been diagnosed in a dog and various monkeys [46, 47]. Using molecular methods, the fungus has been detected in several road-killed wild animals [48]. These findings point toward a much broader range of infected hosts than previously considered.

Demographics

Paracoccidioidomycosis is infrequent in children, who comprise only 5–10% of all cases; adolescents and young adults represent 15–20% of cases. Overall, 60–70% of patients are over age 30 [1, 7, 26, 27, 35, 36]. Patients coinfected with HIV and paracoccidioidomycosis are reported to be younger than non-HIV-infected patients. [49]. One of the most peculiar aspects of paracoccidioidomycosis is its distribution by gender. Although the average male-to-female ratio in Brazil is l4:1, in Argentina, Colombia, and Venezuela this ratio can be as high as 70:1 [1, 7, 26, 50–54]. Interstingly in children gender differences in prevalence are not seen [1, 7, 26, 35, 36, 51].

There are no apparent effects of race on the distribution of paracoccidioidomycosis. According to a recent study, HLA antigens may influence the outcome of the host-parasite interaction by regulating the immune response to *P. brasiliensis* antigens [55]. Inadequate nutrition, smoking, and alcoholism are considered to be important predisposing conditions [1, 56, 57]. Approximately 70% of patients have or have had jobs centered in agriculture. In Uruguay, the disease is recognized as an occupational hazard, as most cases are reported in lumberjacks [1, 7, 26, 50–54]. Immigrants into endemic areas usually develop severe disease, indicative of their lack of immunity to *P. brasiliensis* [1].

Coutinho et al. [58] noted an annual incidence rate of 1–3 per 100,000 inhabitants and, based on 3,181 deaths, estimated a mean annual mortality rate of 1.45 per million inhabitants with a nonhomogenous spatial distribution among regions and States of Brazil. The majority of deaths, 85%, occurred in men in the older age groups. In Paraná State, Brazil, the average annual mortality rate was 3.48 per million inhabitants, which represented not only the fifth leading cause of death among chronic infectious diseases, but also the highest mortality rate among the systemic mycoses [59]. Santos reviewed 1,950 death certificates from patients in whom paracoccidioidomycosis was listed as a diagnosis. The main causes of death associated with this mycosis were pulmonary fibrosis, chronic lower respiratory tract diseases, and pneumonias with the largest number of deaths occurring in men in the older age groups and among rural workers [60].

Pathogenesis

In animal models of paracoccidioidomycosis, after the first 4 days, an inflammatory infiltrate composed mainly of neutrophils and macrophages becomes apparent [10, 61, 62]. These cells gradually begin to transform into epithelioid cells, and a week after challenge, granuloma formation is observed [9, 10]. Epithelioid cells and giant cells surround *P. brasiliensis* with limited phagocytosis taking place; granulomas increase in size and tend to coalesce. The epithelioid granuloma is the histologic hallmark of paracoccidioidomycosis [10, 63, 64]. Initially, granulomas are compact and contain only a few yeast cells. However, with progression of the infection, they become loose and the yeast cells begin to multiply. At this time, immunosuppression can be demonstrated in the animals [9, 63, 64].

It has been postulated that once the infective conidia reach the lung, their first interaction occurs with the extracellular matrix proteins and the lung epithelial cells. *P. brasiliensis* exhibits on its surface adhesin-type molecules that allow its binding to several extracellular matrix proteins and adherence to epithelial cells that have similar proteins on their surface. [65–67]. The conidia also interact with alveolar macrophages, initiating the inflammatory process through production of proinflammatory cytokines and chemokines that induce expression of adhesion molecules on leukocytes surface [61, 62].

In patients with paracoccidioidomycosis, bronchoalveolar lavage shows a predominance of neutrophils and macrophages; furthermore, the alveolar macrophages express both adhesion and costimulatory molecules, indicating that they had differentiated into activated macrophages in the lungs [68].

The initial infection in the alveoli can be exudative or granulomatous [9, 61]. In humans, observations reveal acute alveolitis, proliferation of reticulin fibers, and interstitial and peribronchial granulomatous inflammation surrounded by marked fibrosis [69, 70]. Fibrosis is prominent in the perihilar region, the main bronchi and their branches, and the large pulmonary vessels [69]. Human autopsies and experimental animal studies have revealed that fibrosis is the result of an active, progressive pulmonary infection characterized by strong inflammatory responses centered on the granuloma. Collagen I and reticulin-type fibers were visible and contributed to consolidation and fibrosis that interferes with proper gaseous exchange [10, 11, 69, 70]. In mice infected with *P. brasiliensis*, destruction of the lung's elastic system fibers takes place and this alteration leads to changes in the lung' s mechanical properties [71].

In lymph nodes, granulomas are initially formed in the cortex, but with time the inflammatory response encompasses the whole structure and fistula formation results. Involvement of the capsule facilitates coalescence of neighboring nodes with formation of large tumor-like masses. In the adrenal glands, lesions may be restricted or extensive; granulomas, necrosis, and fibrosis cause marked enlargement and damage to the glands. The mucosal and skin lesions reveal epithelioid granulomas and intraepithelial abscesses; in the skin, pseudoepitheliomatous hyperplasia is common. In ulcerated skin lesions or ruptured lymph nodes, granulomas are associated with a mixed pyogenic infiltration and central necrosis with caseation [69, 70, 72].

Two forms of active disease have been described: the acute/subacute form (juvenile type) and the chronic adult-type disease. The former is characterized by predominant dissemination to the reticuloendothelial system. Cell-mediated immune depression is a regular feature. As implied by its name, the chronic form has a prolonged course – months

Table 1 Paracoccidioidomycosis: characteristics of the clinical forms

Clinical forms	Definition	Special aspects	Host immune status	Immune response
Infection	No clinical manifestations	Defined by positive skin test	Normal	Average positive skin reactions: 12–20%
Disease divided into two broad categories	Presence of signs and symptoms	Male:female ratio 14:1	Variable	Imbalance of the two arms of the immune response
1. Regressive (residual)	Mild pulmonary symptoms not requiring medical intervention	Unnoticed but shown at autopsy in persons not known to have had disease	Normal and active	Host able to contain fungal infection
2. Progressive	Disseminated disease involving several organs/systems	Age and immune status influence clinical aspects	Abnormal	Humoral response intense; cellular immunity depressed
2a. Acute/subacute juvenile form	Significant involvement of reticuloendothelial system	Common in children, adolescents, and young adults; HIV + patients	Significant immuno-depression	High titers anti-idiotypic antibodies; abnormal CD4 cell response
2b. Chronic adult form	Systemic disease with pulmonary and extra-pulmonary manifestations	Lungs often involved, but respiratory symptoms may be minimal	Normal to depressed	Immune response varies from patient to patient

to years – and is manifested by lung damage, as well as by extrapulmonary manifestations. Cellular immune responses are variable [7, 72–74]. A residual form also exists and represents the sequelae from formerly active lesions [69, 71, 72] (Table 1). In paracoccidioidomycosis the host's immune response defines, to a great extent, the outcome of the infectious process with humoral and cellular immune responses playing prominent roles.

Humoral Response

Paracoccidioidomycosis is characterized by polyclonal activation of B cells, resulting in hypergammaglobulinemia [75]. Almost all patients produce specific antibodies against *P. brasiliensis* with high levels of specific IgA and IgG isotypes, as well as IgE antibodies [76–78]. Interestingly, the IgG2 isotype and IgA are found in patients presenting with chronic infection, while the IgG4 isotype and IgE are present in patients with the acute/subacute form [76, 77]. Anti-idiotypic antibodies are detected in a large proportion of patients with the acute/subacute form, but not in patients with the chronic form; thus, these antibodies may play a part in the modulation of the immune response [78]. In high and low antibody responder mice infected with *P. brasiliensis*, the highest mortality rates and the most extensive dissemination were found in the low responder group [79]. Additionally, mice develop specific antibody recognition patterns during infection, which suggests their active interaction during progressive infection [80]. Circulating immune complexes have been detected in patients with depressed T cell responses and are suspected to participate in cell-mediated immune depression [81].

Cell-Mediated Response

As in other infections caused by intracellular pathogens, the cellular immune response is crucial to control of *P. brasiliensis* infection. However, in paracoccidioidomycosis a dichotomy exists between humoral and cellular antigen-specific responses, manifested by high levels of antibodies and T-cell hypoproliferation [82], suggesting that a Th2 immunologic pattern plays a role in the patient's inability to control the infection [83]. Patients with the acute/subacute progressive form are incapable of responding to mitogens and/or skin tests [84–87]. A correlation between high antibody titers, lack of T cell lymphocyte responsiveness, and severity of disease has become apparent [83, 85, 87, 88]. Adult patients with progressive but less severe disease have low or undetectable anti-*P. brasiliensis* antibody titers and normal or slightly depressed cell-mediated immune responses [88]. This pattern is reversed in patients with more advanced, progressive disease in whom high antibody levels and important depression of cell mediated immune functions are recorded [86, 87].

Cytokines play an important role by modulating the immune response against *P. brasiliensis* infection [89, 90]. Increased production of Th-2 cytokines (IL-10, IL-4, and IL-5) occurs in severely ill patients, whereas Th-1 cytokines, especially IFN-γ and IL-2, decrease significantly [84, 86, 91]. Moreover, expression of mRNAs corresponding to Th-2 cytokines (IL-4, IL-10, IL-5, and TGF-β) was higher in patients with either the acute or chronic form than in asymptomatic infected individuals [92]. Additionally, serum levels of IL-18 and soluble tumor necrosis factor receptor-2 (TNF-RII) were significantly higher in patients with the acute form than in those with the chronic form, suggesting that determi-

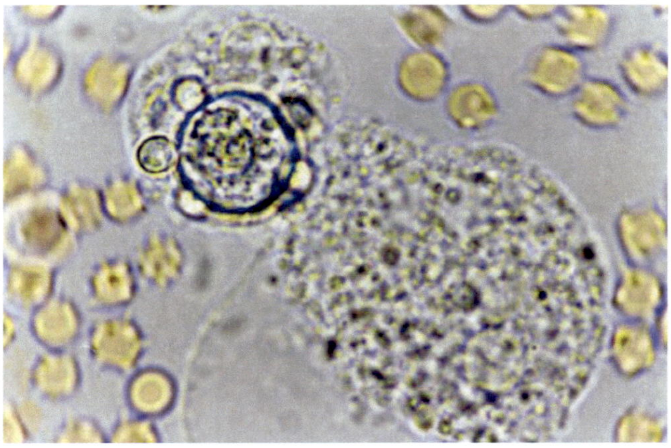

Fig. 3 Macrophage interaction with *Paracoccidioides brasiliensis*. Ingestion of a yeast cell with multiple buds by a pseudopod of the macrophage (100×)

nation of these molecules could represent a parameter for determining paracoccidioidomycosis severity [93].

The loss of immune balance observed in patients with the acute/subacute form of disease could also be influenced by *P. brasiliensis'* accelerated growth rate in tissues, as the resulting heavy fungal load may downregulate the Th-1 responses and favor Th-2 cytokine expression [88]. In support of the above, antifungal therapy that reduces fungal load is accompanied by restoration of the patient's immune capacity, including delayed hypersensitivity, lymphocyte proliferative responses, and production of Th-1 cytokines, especially INF-γ [87, 91].

The macrophage is the most important effector cell, but only if activated by interferon-γ or TNF-α; if not activated, they facilitate fungal multiplication (Fig. 3). Once activated, peritoneal murine macrophages inhibit the conidia to yeast transition resulting in destruction of conidia; they also are fungicidal to the yeast form [94, 95]. Killing is dependent on both reactive oxygen intermediates and reactive nitrogen intermediates, especially H_2O_2 and nitric oxide, respectively [94, 95]. Human monocytes activated with TNF-α are able to kill *P. brasiliensis* yeast cells through a reactive oxygen-dependent mechanism that uses H_2O_2 (118) [96].

Neutrophils also are important in the host-parasite interaction, especially during the initial stages of infection. Neutrophils are the first and most prominent cells in the inflammatory infiltrate and participate actively in phagocytosis of the infecting propagules [10, 62]. Similar to what was observed with human monocytes, human PMNs activated with several different cytokines exert antifungal mechanisms against *P. brasiliensis*, and such mechanisms depend, at least in part, on oxidative metabolism [97–100].

Development of fibrosis is an important facet of the host-parasite interaction. It appears to be mediated by fungal adherence to and increased production of extracellular matrix components. A tridimensional network of collagen, fibronectin, laminin, and proteoglycans, all of which surround fungal cells in active multiplication, is formed [71]. The ability of *P. brasiliensis* to bind to these molecules involves the activation of growth factors and cytokine production, thus reflecting the complexity of the host-parasite interactions [10, 65, 66, 71].

Clinical Manifestations

Paracoccidioidomycosis presents a wide range of clinical manifestations grouped according to the organs involved and the duration of the disease (Table 1 and Fig. 4) [72, 73, 101–104]. Inhalation of the conidia results in an asymptomatic primary infection that may give rise to several different forms of disease, depending on the age and immune status of the host and on the size of the infectious inoculum. Individuals who have an adequate cellular immune response usually overcome fungal invasion, the organism remains quiescent, and a latent infection is established, which can be detected by a reactive paracoccidioidin skin test. When an immunocompetent person is exposed to a large fungal inoculum, a subacute respiratory syndrome can occur that resolves spontaneously, leaving a residual lung lesion. The latter situation represents the so-called regressive form of paracoccidioidomycosis [104–108].

If progression from the original infectious focus takes place or if a latent infection becomes active years later, then the patient develops signs and symptoms of paracoccidioidomycosis that may manifest as two different forms. The acute/subacute progressive form is characterized by extensive involvement of the reticuloendothelial system and is seen mainly in undernourished children, adults less than 30 years of age, and immunosuppressed individuals, such as those who have HIV infection. The chronic progressive adult form of paracoccidioidomycosis is found in older patients, who often smoke and use alcohol and who usually exhibit extrapulmonary lesions and progressive lung damage [104–107].

A residual form is also recognized and represents the sequelae of prior infection. This form often follows the chronic progressive adult form of paracoccidioidomycosis. Patients presenting for medical care may already manifest this form of disease [1, 70, 72, 73, 101–107].

Initial (Latent or Regressive) Infection

For many patients, infection with *P. brasiliensis* causes no symptoms. The host is able to control the infection by producing granulomas around the fungal cells, some of which likely retain their viability [1, 70]. A reactive paracoccidioidin

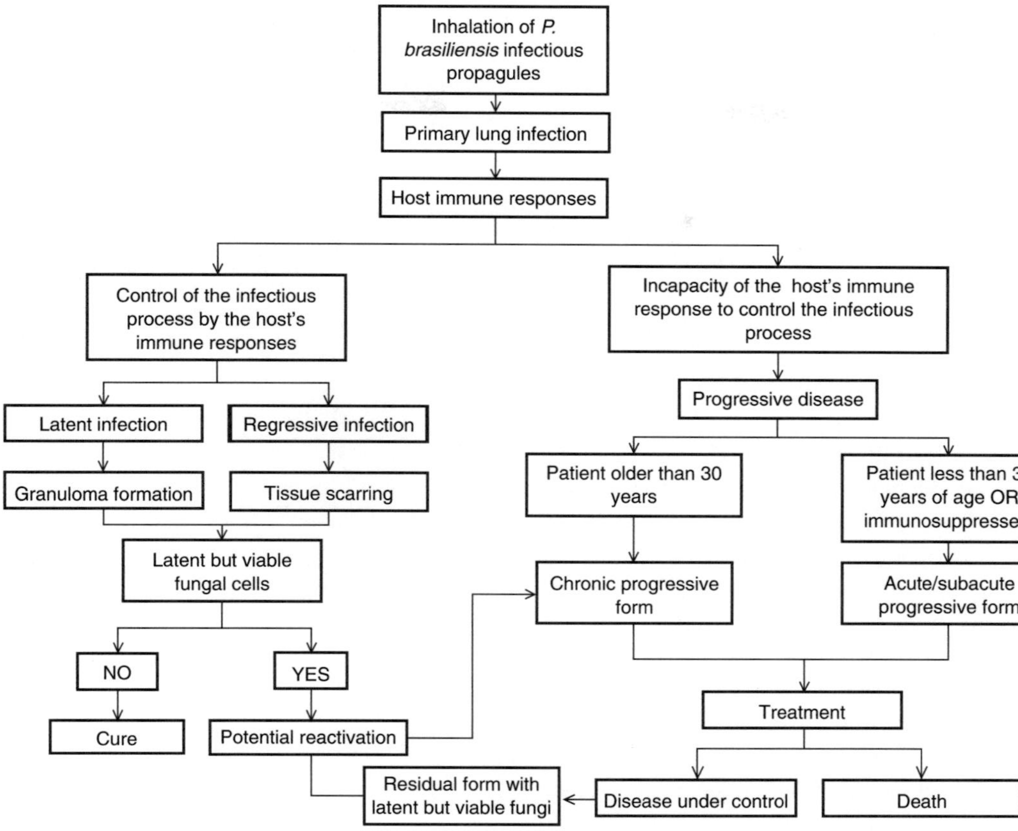

Fig. 4 Paracoccidioidomycosis: a model of pathogenesis and clinical manifestations

skin test can detect those who have been infected and has shown that up to 50% of the population in some endemic areas, such as Brazil, have been infected with *P. brasiliensis* some time in their life [13, 102, 108]. Some patients develop minor pulmonary symptoms that cannot be differentiated from those produced by other causes of pneumonia. The clinical manifestations often resolve spontaneously without medical intervention, but the persistence of viable *P. brasiliensis* yeast cells in infected foci may later allow endogenous reactivation of the disease, usually in connection with a depression of the host's cellular immunity [104].

Progressive Infection

This is a manifestation of the host's inability to control fungal invasion; it results in subsequent progression of lung lesions and extension of the infection to extrapulmonary organs. Progressive forms run a different course depending on the age of the patient and their immune response. Aggressive manifestations are observed in the acute/subacute juvenile form, and a more torpid progression occurs in patients with the chronic adult form, in whom lesions lead to residual scarring.

Acute/Subacute or Juvenile Form

This form is usually diagnosed in children and young adults who are not over 30 years of age, and also in patients with altered cellular immune responses. This form is characterized by predominant involvement of the reticuloendothelial system. The mean duration of symptoms at consultation is 60 days. Lymph nodes, especially those in the supraclavicular and axillary regions, are frequently involved; infected mesenteric lymph nodes can coalesce and present as an intra-abdominal mass. In other cases, lymph node involvement may go unnoticed and is detected incidentally by imaging studies [26, 51, 102, 106, 109–111].

In about half of the patients with this form, the liver and spleen are also involved, and liver function becomes abnormal [50, 106, 107, 109, 110]. Bone marrow invasion is almost exclusively noted in this clinical form; granulomas, fibrosis, and necrosis are seen [112, 113]. Skin lesions are also regularly observed in this form, and they are preferentially localized to the face, the perioral regions, the neck, and the trunk, although they may also appear on the extremities and male genitalia. The skin lesions can be ulcerated, ulcerovegetative, or nodular; in extensively disseminated cases, skin lesions may appear as papules or as an acneiform rash [52, 114].

In most cases, *P. brasiliensis* reaches the skin by hematogenous dissemination from the initial lung lesion, but in some patients, the skin can become involved by contiguous spread from a mucosal lesion or following rupture of an infected lymph node [50, 52–54, 69, 70, 72, 105, 114, 115]. Other organs that can be affected, albeit with lesser frequency, are stomach and small bowel, in which ulcerated mucosal lesions are found teeming with fungal organisms [116–118].

In children, paracoccidioidomycosis is characterized by fever, anemia, constitutional symptoms, lymph node hypertrophy, and hepatosplenomegaly. Bone and joint involvement is observed in about half of the patients. These lesions tend to be preferentially located in the upper limbs and rib cage, and the manifestations include pain and other inflammatory signs in the adjacent tissues [35, 51, 119]. In patients less than 30 years of age, paracoccidioidomycosis frequently involves the skin but does not involve the adrenal glands, in contrast with observations in older individuals with the chronic form of paracoccidiodomycosis [26, 51, 120].

Paracoccidioidomycosis patients coinfected by HIV tend to exhibit the acute/subacute form, with rapid progression of disease with fever, diffuse lymphadenopathy, hepatosplenomegaly, and disseminated skin lesions. Pulmonary symptoms are common even if the chest radiographs are normal; mucosal lesions associated with dysphonia have been seen, but are not common [49, 121].

Chronic Adult Form

This form of paracoccidioidomycosis has a prolonged course that lasts from months to years and is diagnosed mainly in patients aged 30–50 years of age. It is characterized by significant lung damage as well as extrapulmonary manifestations [122]. In this group of patients, the cellular immune response is variable.

Despite the fact that the lungs are the organs most frequently affected, respiratory symptoms are rather minimal; when present, they tend to be attributed to smoking, a habit common among the populations prone to paracoccidioidomycosis. Physical examination reveals few abnormalities, even in patients with extensive radiographic findings. The scarcity of respiratory symptoms explains why patients seek medical consultation based mainly on extrapulmonary manifestations, such as the presence of mucosal and skin lesions [26, 102, 107, 123–129].

As a rule, respiratory symptoms become apparent only after several years, and productive cough is seen in about half of the patients. Hemoptysis is recorded for about 10% of cases, and chest pain is unusual. Dyspnea is a frequent complaint and worsens as the disease progresses. Auscultation reveals rales, rhonchi, and diminished breath sounds. Chest radiographs show bilateral alveolar and interstitial infiltrates that are preferentially located in the lower and central lobes with sparing of the apices (Figs. 5 and 6). Over time, the infiltrates acquire a nodular or fibronodular

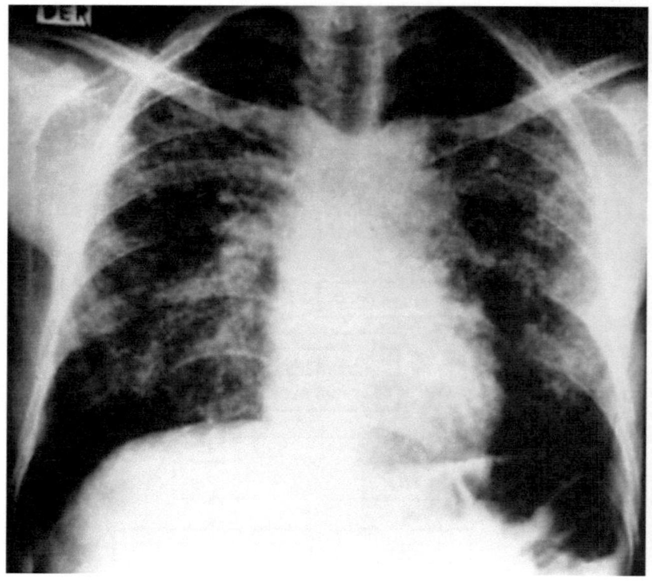

Fig. 5 Chest radiograph of a patient with the adult form of paracoccidioidomycosis. Note bilateral infiltrates in central and lower lobes with sparing of the apices and bullae at the lung bases

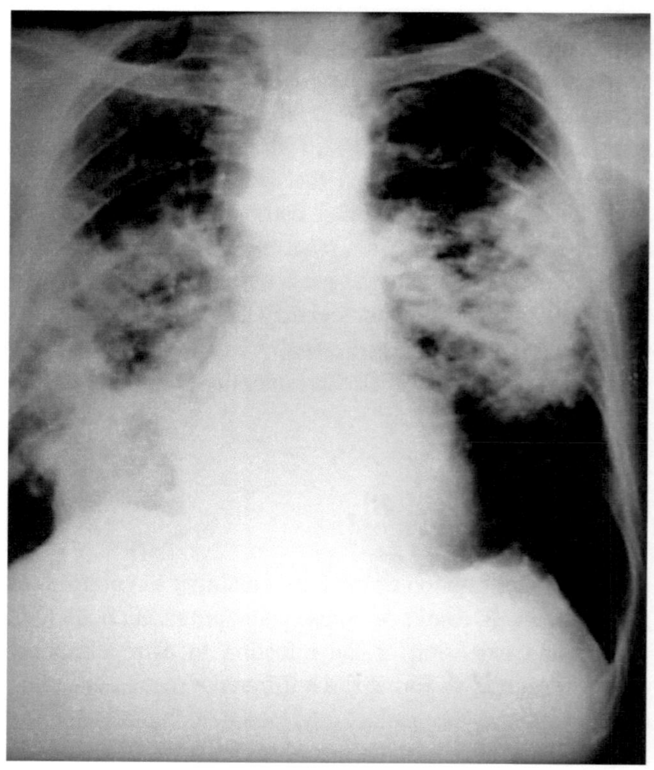

Fig. 6 Chest radiograph from a patient with more severe pulmonary involvement with paracoccidioidomycosis showing extensive infiltrates coalescing into nodules and sparing of the upper lobes

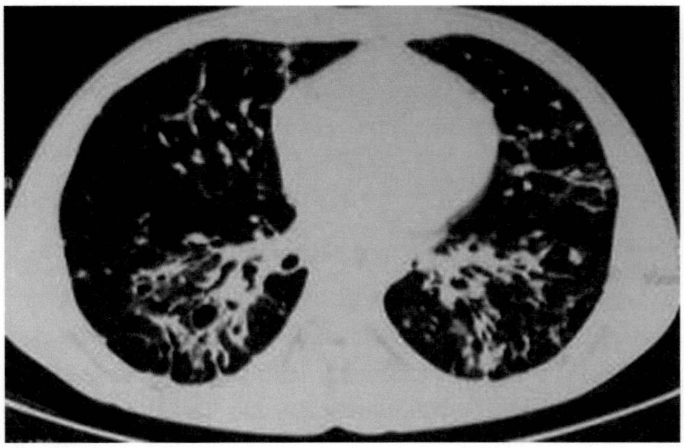

Fig. 7 CT scan showing bilateral alveolar and interstitial infiltrates, cavities, and fibrosis. Note predominance of lesions in the posterior aspects of the lower lobes

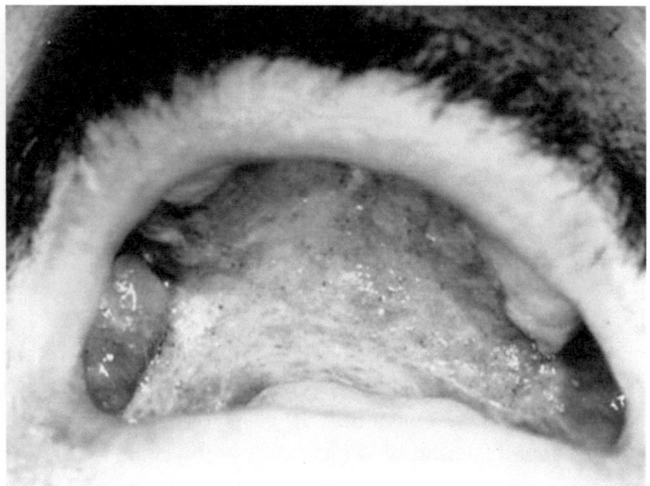

Fig. 8 Mucous membrane lesion showing multiple infiltrative lesions of the palate with hemorrhagic dots, so-called mulberry-like stomatitis

pattern and persist despite adequate antifungal treatment. Lung fibrosis is a prominent complication seen in 60% of patients and is accompanied by emphysematous changes, bullae, and cavities [73, 123, 126–128, 130–132]. Chest CT scans show preferential involvement of the lung periphery and posterior aspects; ground-glass changes, small centrilobular nodules, and large cavitating lesions can be seen. Septal bands with emphysematous areas and condensation zones leading to distortion of the pulmonary architecture may also be observed (Fig. 7). Enlarged hilar and mediastinal lymph nodes are seen, but calcification is rare [128, 131, 133]. Alterations of lung function are frequently noted and show mostly an obstructive pattern [126, 134, 135].

In half of the cases, oral mucosal lesions can be observed; the preferred sites are the gums and the hard palate, followed by oropharynx and larynx. Less frequently, the nasal and anal mucosa may present lesions. Lesions may be single or multiple; they are progressive and destructive and thus give rise to bleeding and pain. The mucosal lesions often present as tumor-like outgrowths covered by hemorrhagic dots (so-called mulberry-like stomatitis) and become ulcerated with surrounding edema (Fig. 8). Dysphonia, dysphagia, and sialorrhea are an aftermath of the above lesions, and gum lesions result in tooth loosening. Nearby lymph nodes are often enlarged and may spontaneously rupture, resulting in fistula formation (Fig. 9) Although patients with oral lesions tend to disregard the presence of respiratory symptoms, cultures and lung imaging reveal pulmonary involvement in most cases [1, 52–54, 73, 105, 107, 136–139].

In the chronic form, skin involvement occurs commonly, but in a smaller proportion (23%) than in patients with the acute/subacute form [73, 124, 130]. Lesions are polymorphic, extremely diverse, and may be single or multiple. They are found more frequently on the face, especially in the perioral region, but may also appear on the neck, trunk, extremities, and the male genitalia. Typically, the lesions are

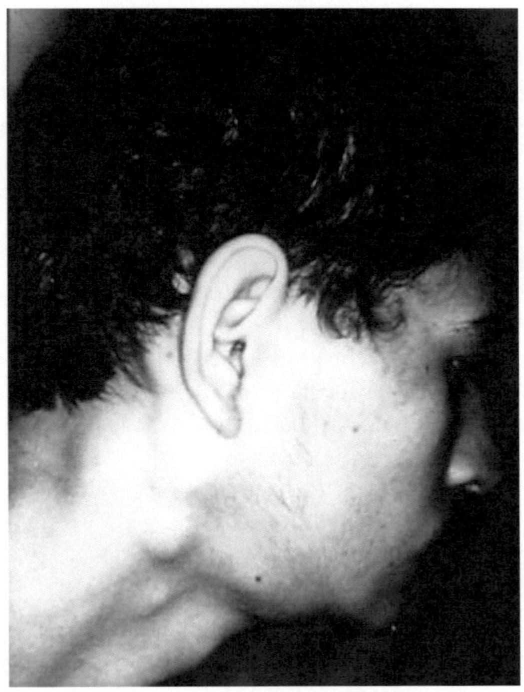

Fig. 9 Enlarged cervical lymph nodes in a patient with the juvenile form of paracoccidioidomycosis

ulcerative, but ulcerovegetative and nodular forms are also seen. Edema of the lips is frequent. In rare disseminated cases, multiple papulo-acneiform lesions may appear [50, 53, 54, 70, 72, 105, 114, 115]. Lung involvement is seen in about 90% of patients with skin lesions [138]. Recent studies have found a significant correlation with the simultaneous presence of skin lesions, dyspnea, and fibrotic sequelae that suggest a process of long duration. In contrast, those patients in whom mucosal lesions, lung infiltrates, and odynophagia/dysphagia coincided had a shorter disease course [139].

In adult patients, dissemination to the adrenal glands occurs commonly; nonetheless, the prevalence of such involvement varies according to the definition employed. For instance, 90% of autopsy cases have revealed direct fungal damage to the adrenals. However, adrenal insufficiency appears in only 48% of patients tested by adrenal stimulation tests. Adrenal function may normalize after completion of antifungal treatment, but some patients have complete destruction of the adrenal glands and require life-long hormonal supplementation [53, 140–143].

Central nervous system (CNS) involvement is observed in approximately 15% of the patients; the highest figures are reported for patients older than 30 years. CNS symptoms are the first manifestation of paracoccidioidomycosis in 20% of cases. *P. brasiliensis* invasion results in granulomatous lesions of the parenchyma, preferentially located in the cerebral hemispheres, although other localities, including the spinal cord, may be involved. In 17% of CNS cases, meningeal involvement can be demonstrated. The most frequently observed symptoms and signs of CNS involvement are convulsions, paresis, cerebellar signs, cephalalgia, and hydrocephalus. The spinal fluid may show increased protein values and a slight increase in leukocytes, represented by lymphocytes and mononuclear cells; the glucose usually is within normal limits. CT scans show single or multiple irregular hypodense lesions with ring enhancement and surrounding edema. The diagnosis is difficult, but is aided by epidemiologic data, typical lesions in other organs, and by findings on chest CT scan [144–147].

Genital involvement has been reported in patients older than 30 years and especially in males, in whom epididymitis, scrotal inflammation, penile ulceration, and prostatitis can occur [148].

Sequelae (Residual Form)

Pulmonary fibrosis occurs as a result of the host's response to the microorganism; granulomas and fibrosis develop around the bronchi, connecting them through fibrous septae to other bronchiolar structures and blood vessels. Residual lesions do not respond to antifungal treatment, partly because in a large proportion of the cases, they were already well formed when the diagnosis was established. The functional restriction imposed by fibrosis advances and evolves toward cor pulmonale, progressive lung incapacity, and finally death [1, 10, 70, 73, 123, 127, 132, 134, 135].

Residual damage resulting from the scarring of previous mucosal lesions located in the oral mucosa, the oropharynx, the nose, the larynx, and the trachea is manifested by microstomy, palate perforation, dysphonia, and loosening of the dental structures. In some cases, the anatomic deformities secondary to scarring do not produce functional alterations and the patient remains asymptomatic. However, other patients progress to the point of requiring tracheostomy due to extensive fibrous alterations of the larynx or trachea [149].

Association with Other Diseases

Paracoccidioidomycosis is known to occur simultaneously with other infections, especially with tuberculosis and HIV infection. The dual tuberculosis-paracoccidioidomycosis coinfection is of great importance on epidemiologic grounds, as well as in reference to clinical management, immune response, and treatment. This coinfection, which occurs in 5–10% of cases, is usually not diagnosed, and quite often only antituberculous treatment is prescribed, leaving the mycosis to progress. Even more important is the fact that paracoccidioidomycosis is often confused with tuberculosis and treated as if it were tuberculosis, even in the absence of microbiologic confirmation of this diagnosis. It is only when antituberculous treatment seems to be failing that other etiologies, including paracoccidioidomycosis, are considered. The preferred antifungal agent, itraconazole, is subject to induction of its metabolism by rifampin. When both medications are prescribed simultaneously, the itraconazole blood levels are strikingly decreased, hindering the antifungal activity [50, 115, 150, 151].

The association of paracoccidioidomycosis with neoplasia is controversial. It appears that up to 12% of patients with paracoccidioidomycosis may concomitantly present with cancer, usually involving organs previously invaded by *P. brasiliensis*. In the chronic adult form, solid tumors predominate over hematologic malignancies, while in the acute/subacute form the opposite occurs [50, 115, 152].

Differential Diagnosis

The differential diagnosis depends on the clinical form and the various organs involved. In the acute/subacute form, progressive disseminated tuberculosis, lymphoma, and disseminated histoplasmosis must be differentiated from paracoccidioidomycosis. When intestinal involvement is present, paracoccidioidomycosis can be confused with carcinoma or tuberculosis. Osteoarticular lesions may resemble tumors, and mucosal involvement may resemble carcinoma of the larynx or oropharynx. Skin lesions mimic histoplasmosis, sporotrichosis, leishmaniasis, and leprosy. Pulmonary manifestations in the chronic form are similar to those of tuberculosis or cancer. CNS involvement by *P. brasiliensis* must be differentiated from primary or metastatic brain tumors [49, 50, 53, 54, 73, 107, 118, 152].

Diagnosis

Direct Examination and Histopathology

In clinical specimens *P. brasiliensis* appears as an oval to round yeast cell, often displaying multiple peripheral buds in a pilot wheel configuration. The cells possess a thick refractile wall (0.2–1 μm) and intracytoplasmic vacuoles (Fig. 10). Yeast cells can appear in chains and have single buds, and bizarre yeast forms also can be observed [1–3, 74]. Several procedures are adequate to visualize fungal elements, including fresh or KOH wet preparations, calcofluor stains, and immunofluorescence methods [1, 2, 74]. Sensitivity of the direct examinations varies from 85% to 100% depending on the specimen, the clinical manifestations, and treatment status [7, 25, 31].

Histopathologic preparations stained with hematoxylin and eosin, Gomori methenamine-silver, Papanicolaou, or periodic acid–Schiff stains, as well as direct immunofluorescence stains, reveal the multiple budding yeast elements, especially within granulomatous foci (Fig. 11). When short chains and cells with single buds are seen, *P. brasiliensis* must be differentiated from *Cryptococcus neoformans*, *B. dermatitidis*, and *H. capsulatum* [1, 2, 69].

Culture

Isolation of *P. brasiliensis* from clinical specimens requires a battery of selective and nonselective culture media, including Sabouraud plus asparagine and thiamine, Mycocel, and BHI plus glucose. Repeated samples should be submitted for culture. The addition of antibacterial drugs and mould inhibitors to the media has improved recovery rates to about 80% [1, 7, 25]. The use of digestion and concentration procedures for mucus specimens is recommended. Modified Sabouraud's agar (Mycocel agar) and yeast extract agars incubated at room temperature (19–24°C) are the best media for isolation, but in specimens from sterile body sites, media without antibiotics incubated at 36°C can be used [1, 7]. At 18–24°C, growth is slow and takes 20–30 days. Microscopically, the mould shows only thin septate hyphae (3–4 μm in diameter) and intercalary chlamydospores (15–30 μm). On media with no carbohydrates and after prolonged incubation for 2 months, the mould may begin to produce conidia. The mycelial form is not distinctive; consequently, dimorphism must be demonstrated by subculturing at 36°C. At this temperature, *P. brasiliensis* grows in 8–10 days as a cream-colored colony with brain-like furrows. Microscopically, oval to spherical yeast cells, 4–40 μm in diameter can be observed. The large mother yeast cell bearing multiple buds (pilot's wheel) is characteristic (see Fig. 2) [1, 7].

Serology

Various highly sensitive serologic tests have been developed to measure antibodies. The frequency of positive tests varies from 70% to 95%, depending on the test used and the severity of the disease process [1, 7, 153–156]. The importance of immunodiffusion (ID), complement fixation (CF), counter-immunoelectrophoresis (CIE), indirect immunofluorescence (IFA), and enzyme-linked immunosorbent assay (ELISA) techniques for antibody detection in the diagnosis and follow-up of patients with paracoccidioidomycosis has been demonstrated [7, 154–157]. The most sensitive, but not always the most specific, tests include ELISA and, more

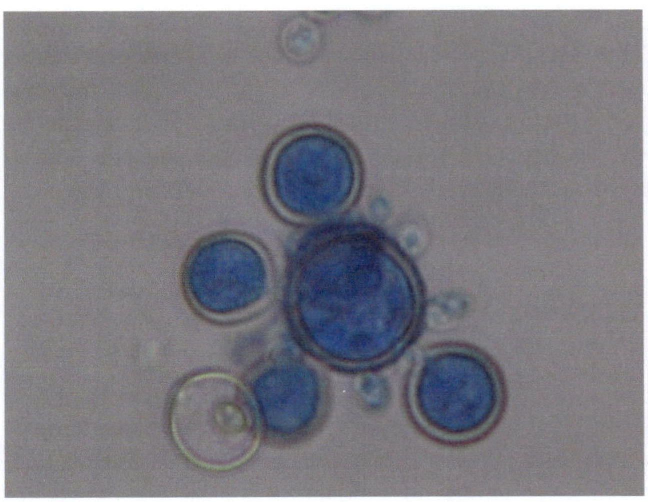

Fig. 10 Lactophenol cotton blue preparation showing a yeast cell of *Paracoccidioides brasiliensis* with multiple attached buds, so-called pilot's wheel configuration (Luctophenol cotton blue, 100×)

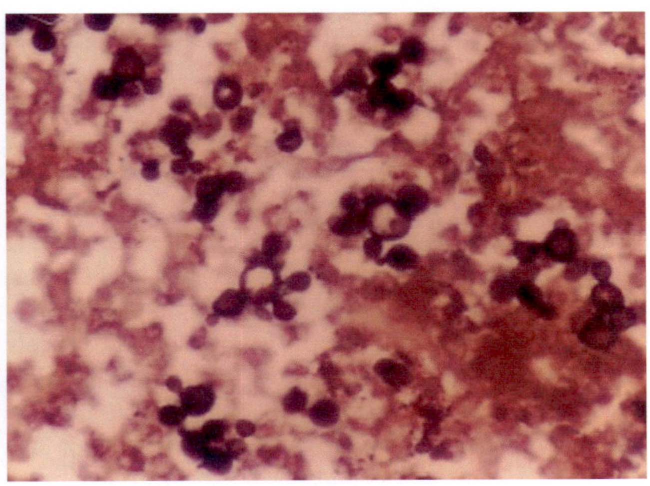

Fig. 11 Biopsy specimen showing *Paracoccidioides brasiliensis* yeast cells with multiple attached small buds (H & E plus methenamine silver stain, 40×)

recently, loop-mediated isothermal amplification (LAMP) methods [158].

In general, patients with severe forms of the disease, such as the acute juvenile and chronic adult forms, show significantly higher antibody levels than patients with less extensive disease [1, 7, 154–156]. Specificity of all tests is an issue because of cross-reactivity with other endemic mycoses [7, 154, 156]. For diagnosis, antibody detection by ID is the simplest of the tests and is highly sensitive and specific [7, 154, 156]. Antibodies may still be demonstrated after the first year of follow-up, even with successful therapy; consequently, quantitative techniques, rather than ID, are better to show changes in titers over time [7, 25, 154–156].

Antigens prepared from *P. brasiliensis* vary greatly in quality, depending on the strain used and the culture medium on which they have been grown. Efforts have been made to prepare purified exo-antigens or recombinant *P. brasiliensis* proteins capable of detecting specific antibodies [154, 157–160]. A specific gp43-kDa glycoprotein fraction, considered the immunodominant *P. brasiliensis* antigen, has been sequenced, cloned, and expressed in a yeast vector [159, 161]. Both a 7-day crude gp43 exoantigen and a 3-day gp43 antigen display sensitivity and specificity similar to that of the purified antigen [159, 161]. Various recombinant products have been prepared and assayed in patients, including gp43, [159, 162, 163] HSP60 and HSP70, HMM, 28 kDa, 70 kDa, and 78 kDa proteins, among others [162, 164–167]. Use of two different recombinant proteins (27 and 87 kDa) was found to be more sensitive than either one alone [168]. Recombinant antigens have been shown to react in 85–98% of proven cases [162, 167, 168].

Antigen Detection

Antigen detection is preferred for early diagnosis in immunocompromised individuals or when antibody detection is inconclusive. Monitoring circulating antigen could also be used to follow the course of the illness. An inhibition ELISA was developed with monoclonal antibodies against an 87-kDa antigenic fraction; test sensitivity was 80% and higher in severe forms of the disease [163, 169]. In patients with severe juvenile disease, follow-up studies during and after itraconazole therapy indicated that antigen titers dropped significantly after 20 weeks of therapy. In contrast, in those patients who had the same clinical form of disease but were also HIV positive, antigenemia persisted at elevated titers even after 68 weeks of treatment [163, 169]. Patients with chronic pulmonary and chronic disseminated disease had significant decreases in antigen titers after 28 and 40 weeks of treatment, respectively. Antigen decreases correlated with clinical improvement. Parallel testing of antibody titers in the same patients revealed that these were unpredictable [163, 169]. Similar studies in Brazil reached similar conclusions about the value of antigen monitoring [170].

Detection of 70- and 43-kDa circulating antigens in urine samples through the use of a polyclonal anti-*P. brasiliensis* antibody has also been tested. With this assay, 91% of patients had detectable urinary antigen by ELISA testing and 75% by immunoblot testing. Both tests appeared to be specific, as neither antigen was detected in control samples. In specimens collected during clinical recovery, reactivity decreased, and the 43-kDa antigen persisted or increased in those patients who relapsed [171]. Specimens other than sera, including urine, sputum, and saliva, have also been employed for the detection of circulating antigens [153, 160, 161, 168, 171].

Gene Probes

By 1997, diagnostic and research laboratories began to incorporate molecular methods, [172] with a preference for PCR and its various modifications. The purpose of such methods is to improve fungal identification and obtain better diagnostic accuracy. ITS and gp43 regions have served as templates for designing specific primers that allow recognition of *P. brasiliensis* in clinical specimens and in culture [172–176]. One of the advantages of these methods is their higher capacity to detect only a few gene copies [175]. A recent report found real-time PCR of great utility in detecting imported paracoccidioidomycosis cases [177]. Despite great potential, such methods still require standardization and wider use by more laboratories [3].

Treatment

Treatment of paracoccidioidomycosis includes antifungal agents, adequate nutrition, control of associated diseases, and smoking cessation. Antifungals presently available for the treatment of paracoccidioidomycosis include sulfonamides, amphotericin B, and azoles [178] (Table 2).

Sulfonamides

The combination of trimethoprim-sulfamethoxazole is recommended for the ambulatory treatment of minor and moderate forms of paracoccidioidomycosis. It is inexpensive, available as an oral formulation, and most side effects are minor. Up to 70% of patients respond initially, but the number of relapses during the long treatment course is as high as 25%, with 15% of isolates from relapsed cases having

Table 2 Paracoccidioidomycosis: treatment modalities

Antifungal (route of administration)	Minimal duration of treatment*	Dosing	Side effects	Recovery rate (%)	Relapse rate (%)
TMP-SMX (oral/IV)	Minor involvement: 6 months Moderate involvement: 12 months	Adults: TMP: 160–240 mg SMX: 800–1,200 mg twice daily Children: TMP: 8–10 mg/kg SMX: 40–50 mg/kg twice daily	Leukopenia Crystalluria Hypersensivity reactions	80	20–25
Amphotericin B (IV)	Total dose 2 g[a] OR until stable, then change to oral TMP-SMX or itraconazole	1 mg/kg daily	Nephrotoxicity Hypokalemia Fever Nausea/vomiting	70	15–25
Ketoconazole (oral)	6 months	200–400 mg daily	Hormonal alterations Elevated hepatic enzymes Nausea/vomiting	90	11
Itraconazole (oral/IV)	3 months	Adults: 200 mg tid for 3 days, then 200 mg daily Children <30 kg and <5 years of age: 5–10 mg/kg daily	Nausea/vomiting Altered tryglycerides Elevation hepatic enzymes	94–98	3–15
Voriconazole (oral/IV)	6 months	Initial dose: 400 mg every 12 h for 1 day; then 200 mg every12 h. Diminish dose by 50% if weight is <40 kg	Visual alterations Elevation liver enzymes Skin rash	88	Follow-up data not available
Posaconazole (oral)	6 months	400 mg twice daily with fatty food	Transitory elevation of liver enzymes Nausea/vomiting	Un-published	Data not available

*Presented only as a guide to proper therapy. Treatment duration should be guided by the clinical response and the indications furnished by laboratory tests

TMP-SMX trimethoprim-sulfamethoxazole

[a]Therapy should be continued and replaced by TMP-SMX or itraconazole once the patient is improving and oral antifungal agent is tolerated

becoming resistant to this medication. The recommended dose is 160–240 mg trimethoprim and 800–1,200 mg sulfamethoxazole, administered twice daily for 12 months for minor disease and from 18 to 24 months for moderate disease. Children should be given 8–10 mg/kg trimethoprim and 40–50 mg/kg sulfamethoxazole twice daily. Leukopenia, the most frequent side effect, can be prevented by the concomitant administration of folinic acid [178–180].

Amphotericin B

Despite being highly effective against *P. brasiliensis,* amphotericin B deoxycholate is reserved for the treatment of severely ill patients because of the need for intravenous administration and its well-known toxicities. The recommended dose is 1 mg/kg daily until the patient is capable of taking oral treatment with trimethoprim-sulfamethoxazole or itraconazole. With this regimen, relapses still occur in 15% of the cases. As for lipid formulations of amphotericin B, higher costs have limited the application of these new formulations in the endemic areas. Consequently, clinical experience is reduced to a few cases that do not allow determination of the therapeutic efficacy [73, 178–181].

Azoles

In vitro, ketoconazole, itraconazole, and fluconazole are all highly active against *P. brasiliensis*; minimum inhibitory concentrations (MICs) are 0.0009–0.015 μg/mL (ketoconazole), 0.0009–0.5 μg/mL (itraconazole), and 0.125–0.5 μg/mL (fluconazole). In patients, however, fluconazole has been ineffective; follow-up observations have shown that as many as 45% of patients relapse despite high doses and prolonged treatment periods. Ketoconazole is effective in 90% of the cases when administered at 200–400 mg daily for 6–18 months. However, it is now infrequently used due to a relatively high rate of failures (8%) and relapses (11%), a higher rate of adverse effects than noted with other azoles, and important drug-drug interactions [73, 178, 180–182].

Itraconazole has been used since 1982 for the treatment of paracoccidioidomycosis and continues as the best therapeutic option. It is effective in 98% of cases, irrespective of the clinical form, and has a low relapse rate (3%) [27, 73, 127, 180, 183]. It is administered at a loading dose of 200 mg three times daily for 3 days followed by 200 mg daily for 3–12 months, depending on the clinical and serologic response. In children less than 5 years old and weighing less than 30 kg, itraconazole is administered at 5–10 mg/kg daily. Adverse effects are usually minor and consist of elevated transaminases and gastrointestinal disturbances, but there are many drug-drug interactions that must be monitored. Absorption of the capsule formulation requires both gastric acid and food. Serum levels can be erratic because of the absorption issues and the drug-drug interactions.

Itraconazole is available as a suspension, which is the preferred formulation because absorption does not require gastric acid and is approximately 30% better than the capsule formulation. It is given on an empty stomach at the same doses listed above. Itraconazole intravenous formulation allows treatment of severely ill patients, but is not available in all countries. Despite the high costs and the problems indicated above, itraconazole is considered the agent of choice for most patients with paracoccidioidomycosis [27, 73, 127, 130, 180].

Voriconazole has proven effective for paracoccidioidomycosis. In a comparative pilot study with itraconazole done in 53 patients who were treated for 12 months, the response rate was 88% [183]. Posaconazole has been used as salvage therapy in only a few patients, and satisfactory results have been obtained (personal experience).

The goal of treatment is to control the infection in order to restore the patient's well-being. Attempts at eradicating the etiologic agent may not be possible, and the risk of endogenous reactivation persists. Treatment should continue until clinical manifestations are resolved, except for those due to residual fibrotic sequelae, and until antibody/antigen titers decrease or remain stationary at low titers for several months [27, 73, 127, 179, 180].

References

1. Lacaz C, Porto E, Martins J, et al. Paracoccidioidomicose. In: Lacaz C, Porto E, Martins J, et al., editors. Tratado de micologiamédica lacaz. 9th ed. Sao Paulo, Brazil: Sarvier; 2002. p. 639–729.
2. Lacaz CS. *Paracoccidioides brasiliensis*: morphology, evolutionary cycle, maintenance during saprophytic life, biology, virulence, taxonomy. In: Franco M, Lacaz CS, Restrepo A, del Negro G, editors. Paracoccidioidomycosis. Boca Raton, FL: CRC Press; 1994. p. 13–25.
3. San-Blas G, Nino-Vega G. *Paracoccidioides brasiliensis*: chemical and molecular tools for research on cell walls, antifungals, diagnosis, taxonomy. Mycopathologia. 2008;165:183–95.
4. Bialek R, Ibricevic A, Fothergill A, Begerow D. Small subunit ribosomal DNA sequence shows *Paracoccidioides brasiliensis* closely related to *Blastomyces dermatitidis*. J Clin Microbiol. 2000;38:3190–3.
5. Matute DR, McEwen JG, Puccia R, et al. Cryptic speciation and recombination in the fungus *Paracoccidioides brasiliensis* as revealed by gene genealogies. Mol Biol Evol. 2006;23: 65–73.
6. Teixeira MM, Theodoro RC, de Carvalho MJ, et al. Phylogenetic analysis reveals a high level of speciation in the *Paracoccidioides* genus. Mol Phylogenet Evol. 2009;52:273–83.
7. Brummer E, Castaneda E, Restrepo A. Paracoccidioidomycosis: an update. Clin Microbiol Rev. 1993;6:89–117.
8. Restrepo BI, McEwen JG, Salazar ME, Restrepo A. Morphological development of the conidia produced by *Paracoccidioides brasiliensis* mycelial form. J Med Vet Mycol. 1986;24:337–9.
9. McEwen JG, Bedoya V, Patino MM, Salazar ME, Restrepo A. Experimental murine paracoccidiodomycosis induced by the inhalation of conidia. J Med Vet Mycol. 1987;25:165–75.
10. Cock AM, Cano LE, Velez D, Aristizabal BH, Trujillo J, Restrepo A. Fibrotic sequelae in pulmonary paracoccidioidomycosis: histopathological aspects in BALB/c mice infected with viable and non-viable *Paracoccidioides brasiliensis* propagules. Rev Inst Med Trop São Paulo. 2000;42:59–66.
11. Gonzalez A, Restrepo A, Cano LE. Pulmonary immune responses induced in BALB/c mice by *Paracoccidioides brasiliensis* conidia. Mycopathologia. 2008;165:313–30.
12. Gomez BL, Nosanchuk JD, Diez S, et al. Detection of melanin-like pigments in the dimorphic fungal pathogen *Paracoccidioides brasiliensis* in vitro and during infection. Infect Immun. 2001;69:5760–7.
13. da Silva MB, Marques AF, Nosanchuk JD, Casadevall A, Travassos LR, Taborda CP. Melanin in the dimorphic fungal pathogen *Paracoccidioides brasiliensis*: effects on phagocytosis, intracellular resistance and drug susceptibility. Microbes Infect. 2006;8:197–205.
14. Restrepo A. Morphological aspects of *Paracoccidioides brasiliensis* in lymph nodes: implications for the prolonged latency of paracoccidioidomycosis? Med Mycol. 2000;38:317–22.
15. Queiroz Telles F. *Paracoccidioides brasiliensis*: ultrastructural findings. In: Franco M, CS L, Restrepo A, del Negro G, editors. Paracoccidioidomycosis. Boca Raton, FL: CRC Press; 1994. p. 27–48.
16. San Blas G, Niño-Vega G. *Paracoccidioides brasiliensis*: virulence and host response. In: Chilar R, Calderone R, editors. Fungal pathogenesis: principles and clinical applications. New York: Marcel Dekker Inc; 2001. p. 205–26.
17. Molinari-Madlum EE, Felipe MS, Soares CM. Virulence of *Paracoccidioides brasiliensis* isolates can be correlated to groups defined by random amplified polymorphic DNA analysis. Med Mycol. 1999;37:269–76.
18. Tavares AH, Silva SS, Bernardes VV, et al. Virulence insights from the *Paracoccidioides brasiliensis* transcriptome. Genet Mol Res. 2005;4:372–89.
19. Silva SS, Paes HC, Soares CM, Fernandes L, Felipe MS. Insights into the pathobiology of Paracoccidioides brasiliensis from transcriptome analysis–advances and perspectives. Mycopathologia. 2008;165:249–58.
20. Tavares AH, Silva SS, Dantas A, et al. Early transcriptional response of *Paracoccidioides brasiliensis* upon internalization by murine macrophages. Microbes Infect. 2007;9:583–90.

21. Bailao AM, Schrank A, Borges CL, et al. Differential gene expression by *Paracoccidioides brasiliensis* in host interaction conditions: representational difference analysis identifies candidate genes associated with fungal pathogenesis. Microbes Infect. 2006; 8:2686–97.
22. Restrepo A, Salazar M, Clemons Kea. Hormonal influences in the host-interplay with *Paracoccidioides brasiliensis*. In: Stevens D, Vanden Bosche H, Odds F, editors. Topics on fungal infections: national foundation for infectious diseases. 1997. p. 125–33.
23. Aristizabal BH, Clemons KV, Stevens DA, Restrepo A. Morphological transition of *Paracoccidioides brasiliensis* conidia to yeast cells: in vivo inhibition in females. Infect Immun. 1998;66:5587–91.
24. Aristizabal BH, Clemons KV, Cock AM, Restrepo A, Stevens DA. Experimental *Paracoccidioides brasiliensis* infection in mice: influence of the hormonal status of the host on tissue responses. Med Mycol. 2002;40:169–78.
25. Nino-Vega GA, Calcagno AM, San-Blas G, San-Blas F, Gooday GW, Gow NA. RFLP analysis reveals marked geographical isolation between strains of *Paracoccidioides brasiliensis*. Med Mycol. 2000;38:437–41.
26. Blotta MH, Mamoni RL, Oliveira SJ, et al. Endemic regions of paracoccidioidomycosis in Brazil: a clinical and epidemiologic study of 584 cases in the southeast region. Am J Trop Med Hyg. 1999;61:390–4.
27. Restrepo A, Tobón A, Agudelo C. Paracoccidioidomycosis. In: Hospenthal D, Rinaldi M, editors. Diagnosis and treatment of human mycoses. Totowa, NJ: Humana Press; 2008. p. 331–42.
28. Restrepo A, McEwen JG, Castaneda E. The habitat of *Paracoccidioides brasiliensis*: how far from solving the riddle? Med Mycol. 2001;39:233–41.
29. Calle D, Rosero DS, Orozco LC, Camargo D, Castaneda E, Restrepo A. Paracoccidioidomycosis in Colombia: an ecological study. Epidemiol Infect. 2001;126:309–15.
30. Manns BJ, Baylis BW, Urbanski SJ, Gibb AP, Rabin HR. Paracoccidioidomycosis: case report and review. Clin Infect Dis. 1996;23:1026–32.
31. Ginarte M, Pereiro Jr M, Toribio J. Imported paracoccidioidomycosis in Spain. Mycoses. 2003;46:407–11.
32. Kamei K, Sano A, Kikuchi K, et al. The trend of imported mycoses in Japan. J Infect Chemother. 2003;9:16–20.
33. Poisson M, Heitzmann A, Mille C, et al. *Paracoccidioides brasiliensis* in a brain abscess: first French case. J Mycol Med. 2007;17:114–8.
34. Franco M, Bagagli E, Scapolio S, da Silva Lacaz C. A critical analysis of isolation of *Paracoccidioides brasiliensis* from soil. Med Mycol. 2000;38:185–91.
35. Fonseca ER, Pardal PP, Severo LC. Paracoccidioidomycosis in children in Belem, Para. Rev Soc Bras Med Trop. 1999;32:31–3.
36. Goncalves AJ, Londero AT, Terra GM, Rozenbaum R, Abreu TF, Nogueira SA. Paracoccidioidomycosis in children in the state of Rio de Janeiro (Brazil). Geographic distribution and the study of a "reservarea". Rev Inst Med Trop São Paulo. 1998;40:11–3.
37. Cadavid D, Restrepo A. Factors associated with *Paracoccidiodes brasiliensis* infection among permanent residents of three endemic areas in Colombia. Epidemiol Infect. 1993;111:121–33.
38. Coimbra Junior CE, Wanke B, Santos RV, do Valle AC, Costa RL, Zancope-Oliveira RM. Paracoccidioidin and histoplasmin sensitivity in Tupi-Monde Amerindian populations from Brazilian Amazonia. Ann Trop Med Parasitol. 1994;88:197–207.
39. Mangiaterra ML, Giusiano GE, Alonso JM, Gorodner JO. *Paracoccidioides brasiliensis* infection in a subtropical region with important environmental changes. Bull Soc Pathol Exot. 1999;92:173–6.
40. Kalmar EM, Alencar FE, Alves FP, et al. Paracoccidioidomycosis: an epidemiologic survey in a pediatric population from the Brazilian Amazon using skin tests. Am J Trop Med Hyg. 2004;71:82–6.
41. Simoes LB, Marques SA, Bagagli E. Distribution of paracoccidioidomycosis: determination of ecologic correlates through spatial analyses. Med Mycol. 2004;42:517–23.
42. Barrozo LV, Mendes RP, Marques SA, Benard G, Silva ME, Bagagli E. Climate and acute/subacute paracoccidioidomycosis in a hyper-endemic area in Brazil. Int J Epidemiol. 2009;38(6):1642–9.
43. Naiff RD, Ferreira LC, Barrett TV, Naiff MF, Arias JR. Enzootic paracoccidioidomycosis in armadillos (Dasypus novemcinctus) in the State of Para. Rev Inst Med Trop São Paulo. 1986;28:19–27.
44. Bagagli E, Franco M, Bosco Sde M, Hebeler-Barbosa F, Trinca LA, Montenegro MR. Montenegro MR. High frequency of *Paracoccidioides brasiliensis* infection in armadillos (Dasypus novemcinctus): an ecological study. Med Mycol. 2003;41:217–23.
45. Bagagli E, Bosco SM, Theodoro RC, Franco M. Phylogenetic and evolutionary aspects of *Paracoccidioides brasiliensis* reveal a long coexistence with animal hosts that explain several biological features of the pathogen. Infect Genet Evol. 2006;6:344–51.
46. Ricci G, Mota FT, Wakamatsu A, Serafim RC, Borra RC, Franco M. Canine paracoccidioidomycosis. Med Mycol. 2004;42:379–83.
47. Corte AC, Svoboda WK, Navarro IT, et al. Paracoccidioidomycosis in wild monkeys from Parana State, Brazil. Mycopathologia. 2007;164:225–8.
48. Richini-Pereira VB, Bosco Sde M, Griese J, et al. Molecular detection of *Paracoccidioides brasiliensis* in road-killed wild animals. Med Mycol. 2008;46:35–40.
49. Morejon KM, Machado AA, Martinez R. Paracoccidioidomycosis in patients infected with and not infected with human immunodeficiency virus: a case-control study. Am J Trop Med Hyg. 2009;80:359–66.
50. Paniago AM, Aguiar JI, Aguiar ES, et al. Paracoccidioidomycosis: a clinical and epidemiological study of 422 cases observed in Mato Grosso do Sul. Rev Soc Bras Med Trop. 2003;36:455–9.
51. Pereira RM, Bucaretchi F, Barison Ede M, Hessel G, Tresoldi AT. Paracoccidioidomycosis in children: clinical presentation, follow-up and outcome. Rev Inst Med Trop São Paulo. 2004;46:127–31.
52. Verli FD, Marinho SA, Souza SC, Figueiredo MA, Yurgel LS. Clinical-epidemiologic profile of paracoccidioidomycosis at the Stomatology Department of Sao Lucas Hospital, Pontificia Universidade Catolica of Rio Grande do Sul. Rev Soc Bras Med Trop. 2005;38:234–7.
53. Ramos ESM, Saraiva Ldo E. Paracoccidioidomycosis. Dermatol Clin. 2008;26:257–69. vii.
54. Nucci M, Colombo A, Queiroz-Telles F. Paracoccidioidomycosis. Curr Fung Infect Rep. 2009;3:15–20.
55. Sadahiro A, Roque AC, Shikanai-Yasuda MA. Generic human leukocyte antigen class II (DRB1 and DQB1) alleles in patients with paracoccidioidomycosis. Med Mycol. 2007;45:35–40.
56. Martinez R, Moya MJ. The relationship between paracoccidioidomycosis and alcoholism. Rev Saúde Pública. 1992;26:12–6.
57. dos Santos WA, da Silva BM, Passos ED, Zandonade E, Falqueto A. Association between smoking and paracoccidioidomycosis: a case-control study in the State of Espirito Santo, Brazil. Cad Saúde Pública. 2003;19:245–53.
58. Coutinho ZF, Silva D, Lazera M, et al. Paracoccidioidomycosis mortality in Brazil (1980–1995). Cad Saúde Pública. 2002;18:1441–54.
59. Bittencourt JI, de Oliveira RM, Coutinho ZF. Paracoccidioidomycosis mortality in the State of Parana, Brazil, 1980/1998. Cad Saúde Pública. 2005;21:1856–64.
60. Santo AH. Paracoccidioidomycosis-related mortality trend, state of Sao Paulo, Brazil: a study using multiple causes of death. Rev Panam Salud Pública. 2008;23:313–24.
61. Gonzalez A, Lenzi HL, Motta EM, et al. Expression of adhesion molecules in lungs of mice infected with *Paracoccidioides brasiliensis* conidia. Microbes Infect. 2005;7:666–73.

62. Gonzalez A, Sahaza JH, Ortiz BL, Restrepo A, Cano LE. Production of pro-inflammatory cytokines during the early stages of experimental *Paracoccidioides brasiliensis* infection. Med Mycol. 2003;41:391–9.
63. Singer-Vermes LM, Caldeira CB, Burger E, Calich LG. Experimental murine paracoccidioidomycosis: relationship among the dissemination of the infection, humoral and cellular immune responses. Clin Exp Immunol. 1993;94:75–9.
64. Soares AM, Peracoli MT, Dos Santos RR. Correlation among immune response, morphogenesis of the granulomatous reaction and spleen lymphoid structure in murine experimental paracoccidioidomycosis. Med Mycol. 2000;38:371–7.
65. Gonzalez A, Gomez BL, Diez S, et al. Purification and partial characterization of a *Paracoccidioides brasiliensis* protein with capacity to bind to extracellular matrix proteins. Infect Immun. 2005;73:2486–95.
66. Mendes-Giannini MJ, Andreotti PF, Vincenzi LR, et al. Binding of extracellular matrix proteins to *Paracoccidioides brasiliensis*. Microbes Infect. 2006;8:1550–9.
67. Gonzalez A, Caro E, Munoz C, Restrepo A, Hamilton AJ, Cano LE. *Paracoccidioides brasiliensis* conidia recognize fibronectin and fibrinogen which subsequently participate in adherence to human type II alveolar cells: involvement of a specific adhesin. Microb Pathog. 2008;44:389–401.
68. Calvi SA, Soares AM, Peracoli MT, et al. Study of bronchoalveolar lavage fluid in paracoccidioidomycosis: cytopathology and alveolar macrophage function in response to gamma interferon; comparison with blood monocytes. Microbes Infect. 2003;5:1373–9.
69. Montenegro M, Franco M. Pathology. In: Franco M, Lacaz C, Restrepo A, del Negro G, editors. Paracoccidioidomycosis. Boca Raton, FL: CRC Press; 1994. p. 131–50.
70. Angulo A, Pollak L. Paracoccidioidomycosis. In: Baker R, editor. The pathologic anatomy of the mycoses: human infections with fungi, actinomycetes and algae. Berlin: Springer Verlag; 1971. p. 507–76.
71. Gonzalez A, Lenzi HL, Motta EM, Caputo L, Restrepo A, Cano LE. Expression and arrangement of extracellular matrix proteins in the lungs of mice infected with *Paracoccidioides brasiliensis* conidia. Int J Exp Pathol. 2008;89:106–16.
72. Franco M, Mendes RP, Moscardi-Bacchi MM, Rezkallah-Iwasso M, Montenegro MR. Paracoccidioidomycosis. Bailliere's Clin Trop Med Comm Dis. 1989;4:185–220.
73. Restrepo A, Benard G, de Castro CC, Agudelo CA, Tobon AM. Pulmonary paracoccidioidomycosis. Semin Respir Crit Care Med. 2008;29:182–97.
74. Bethlem EP, Capone D, Maranhao B, Carvalho CR, Wanke B. Paracoccidioidomycosis. Curr Opin Pulm Med. 1999;5:319–25.
75. Chequer-Bou-Habib D, Daniel-Ribeiro C, Banic DM, do Valle AC, Galvao-Castro B. Polyclonal B cell activation in paracoccidioidomycosis. Polyclonal activation in paracoccidioidomycosis. Mycopathologia. 1989;108:89–93.
76. Baida H, Biselli PJ, Juvenale M, et al. Differential antibody isotype expression to the major *Paracoccidioides brasiliensis* antigen in juvenile and adult form paracoccidioidomycosis. Microbes Infect. 1999;1:273–8.
77. Mamoni RL, Rossi CL, Camargo ZP, Blotta MH. Capture enzyme-linked immunosorbent assay to detect specific immunoglobulin E in sera of patients with paracoccidioidomycosis. Am J Trop Med Hyg. 2001;65:237–41.
78. Souza AR, Gesztesi JL, del Negro GM, et al. Anti-idiotypic antibodies in patients with different clinical forms of paracoccidioidomycosis. Clin Diagn Lab Immunol. 2000;7:175–81.
79. Soares AM, Rezkallah-Iwasso MT, Oliveira SL, Peracoli MT, Montenegro MR, Musatti CC. Experimental paracoccidioidomycosis in high and low antibody responder mice of selection IV-A. Med Mycol. 2000;38:309–15.
80. Vaz CA, Mackenzie DW, Hearn VM, et al. Specific recognition pattern of IgM and IgG antibodies produced in the course of experimental paracoccidioidomycosis. Clin Exp Immunol. 1992;88: 119–23.
81. Miura CS, Estevao D, Lopes JD, Itano EN. Levels of specific antigen (gp43), specific antibodies, and antigen-antibody complexes in saliva and serum of paracoccidioidomycosis patients. Med Mycol. 2001;39:423–8.
82. Cacere CR, Mendes-Giannini MJ, Fontes CJ, Kono A, Duarte AJ, Benard G. Altered expression of the costimulatory molecules CD80, CD86, CD152, PD-1 and ICOS on T-cells from paracoccidioidomycosis patients: lack of correlation with T-cell hyporesponsiveness. Clin Immunol. 2008;129:341–9.
83. Benard G, Mendes-Giannini MJ, Juvenale M, Miranda ET, Duarte AJ. Immunosuppression in paracoccidioidomycosis: T cell hyporesponsiveness to two *Paracoccidioides brasiliensis* glycoproteins that elicit strong humoral immune response. J Infect Dis. 1997;175:1263–7.
84. Benard G. An overview of the immunopathology of human paracoccidioidomycosis. Mycopathologia. 2008;165:209–21.
85. Oliveira SJ, Mamoni RL, Musatti CC, Papaiordanou PM, Blotta MH. Cytokines and lymphocyte proliferation in juvenile and adult forms of paracoccidioidomycosis: comparison with infected and non-infected controls. Microbes Infect. 2002;4:139–44.
86. Benard G, Romano CC, Cacere CR, Juvenale M, Mendes-Giannini MJ, Duarte AJ. Imbalance of IL-2, IFN-gamma and IL-10 secretion in the immunosuppression associated with human paracoccidioidomycosis. Cytokine. 2001;13:248–52.
87. Karhawi AS, Colombo AL, Salomao R. Production of IFN-gamma is impaired in patients with paracoccidioidomycosis during active disease and is restored after clinical remission. Med Mycol. 2000;38:225–9.
88. Sugizaki MF, Peracoli MT, Mendes-Giannini MJ, et al. Correlation between antigenemia of *Paracoccidioides brasiliensis* and inhibiting effects of plasma in patients with paracoccidioidomycosis. Med Mycol. 1999;37:277–84.
89. Kashino SS, Fazioli RA, Cafalli-Favati C, et al. Resistance to *Paracoccidioides brasiliensis* infection is linked to a preferential Th1 immune response, whereas susceptibility is associated with absence of IFN-gamma production. J Interferon Cytokine Res. 2000;20:89–97.
90. Calich VL, Kashino SS. Cytokines produced by susceptible and resistant mice in the course of *Paracoccidioides brasiliensis* infection. Braz J Med Biol Res. 1998;31:615–23.
91. Bozzi A, Reis BS, Goulart MI, Pereira MC, Pedroso EP, Goes AM. Analysis of memory T cells in the human paracoccidioidomycosis before and during chemotherapy treatment. Immunol Lett. 2007;114:23–30.
92. Mamoni RL, Blotta MH. Kinetics of cytokines and chemokines gene expression distinguishes *Paracoccidioides brasiliensis* infection from disease. Cytokine. 2005;32:20–9.
93. Corvino CL, Mamoni RL, Fagundes GZ, Blotta MH. Serum interleukin-18 and soluble tumour necrosis factor receptor 2 are associated with disease severity in patients with paracoccidioidomycosis. Clin Exp Immunol. 2007;147:483–90.
94. Gonzalez A, de Gregori W, Velez D, Restrepo A, Cano LE. Nitric oxide participation in the fungicidal mechanism of gamma interferon-activated murine macrophages against *Paracoccidioides brasiliensis* conidia. Infect Immun. 2000;68:2546–52.
95. Moreira AP, Dias-Melicio LA, Peracoli MT, Calvi SA, de Campos V, Soares AM. Killing of *Paracoccidioides brasiliensis* yeast cells by IFN-gamma and TNF-alpha activated murine peritoneal macrophages: evidence of H(2)O (2) and NO effector mechanisms. Mycopathologia. 2008;166:17–23.
96. Carmo JP, Dias-Melicio LA, Calvi SA, Peracoli MT, Soares AM. TNF-alpha activates human monocytes for *Paracoccidioides*

brasiliensis killing by an H2O2-dependent mechanism. Med Mycol. 2006;44:363–8.
97. Kurita N, Oarada M, Brummer E. Fungicidal activity of human peripheral blood leukocytes against *Paracoccidioides brasiliensis* yeast cells. Med Mycol. 2005;43:417–22.
98. Rodrigues DR, Dias-Melicio LA, Calvi SA, Peracoli MT, Soares AM. *Paracoccidioides brasiliensis* killing by IFN-gamma, TNF-alpha and GM-CSF activated human neutrophils: role for oxygen metabolites. Med Mycol. 2007;45:27–33.
99. Tavian EG, Dias-Melicio LA, Acorci MJ, Graciani AP, Peracoli MT, Soares AM. Interleukin-15 increases *Paracoccidioides brasiliensis* killing by human neutrophils. Cytokine. 2008;41:48–53.
100. Kurita N, Oarada M, Miyaji M, Ito E. Effect of cytokines on antifungal activity of human polymorphonuclear leucocytes against yeast cells of *Paracoccidioides brasiliensis*. Med Mycol. 2000; 38:177–82.
101. Severo LC, Geyer GR, Londero AT, Porto NS, Rizzon CF. The primary pulmonary lymph node complex in paracoccidioidomycosis. Mycopathologia. 1979;67:115–8.
102. Londero AT. Paracoccidioidomicose: patogenia, formas clinicas, manifestacões pulmonares e diagnostico. J Pneumol (Brazil). 1986;12:41–57.
103. Franco M, Montenegro MR, Mendes RP, Marques SA, Dillon NL, Mota NG. Paracoccidioidomycosis: a recently proposed classification of its clinical forms. Rev Soc Bras Med Trop. 1987;20:129–32.
104. Benard G, Kavakama J, Mendes-Giannini MJ, Kono A, Duarte AJ, Shikanai-Yasuda MA. Contribution to the natural history of paracoccidioidomycosis: identification of the primary pulmonary infection in the severe acute form of the disease–a case report. Clin Infect Dis. 2005;40:e1–4.
105. Negroni R. Paracoccidioidomycosis (South American blastomycosis, Lutz's mycosis). Int J Dermatol. 1993;32:847–59.
106. Benard G, Orii NM, Marques HH, et al. Severe acute paracoccidioidomycosis in children. Pediatr Infect Dis J. 1994;13:510–5.
107. Mendes RP. The gamut of clinical manifestations. In: Franco M, Lacaz C, Restrepo A, del Negro G, editors. Paracoccidioidomycosis. Boca Raton, FL: CRC Press; 1994. p. 233–58.
108. Maluf ML, Pereira SR, Takahachi G, Svidzinski TI. Prevalence of paracoccidioidomycosis infection determined by sorologic test in donors' blood in the Northwest of Parana, Brazil. Rev Soc Bras Med Trop. 2003;36:11–6.
109. Londero AT, Rios-Gonçalves AJ, Terra GM, Nogueira SA. Paracoccidioidomycosis in Brazilian children. A critical review (1911–1994). Arq Bras Med. 1996;70:197–203.
110. Calegaro JU, Gomes EF, Rodah JE. Paracoccidioidomicose infantil. Relato de dos casos estudados por galio67 (67 Ga). Radiol Bras. 1997;30:343–6.
111. de Castro CC, Benard G, Ygaki Y, Shikanai-Yasuda M, Cerri GG. MRI of head and neck paracoccidioidomycosis. Br J Radiol. 1999;72:717–22.
112. Resende LS, Mendes RP, Bacchi MM, et al. Infiltrative myelopathy by paracoccidioidomycosis. A review and report of nine cases with emphasis on bone marrow morphology. Histopathology. 2006;48:377–86.
113. Resende LS, Mendes RP, Bacchi MM, et al. Bone marrow necrosis related to paracoccidioidomycosis: the first eight cases identified at autopsy. Histopathology. 2009;54:486–9.
114. Marques SA. Cutaneous lesions. In: Franco M, Lacaz CS, Restrepo A, del Negro G, editors. Paracoccidioidomycosis. Boca Raton, FL: CRC Press; 1994. p. 259–80.
115. Campos MV, Penna GO, Castro CN, Moraes MA, Ferreira MS, Santos JB. Paracoccidioidomycosis at Brasilias university hospital. Rev Soc Bras Med Trop. 2008;41:169–72.
116. Gabellini Gde C, Martinez R, Ejima FH, et al. Gastric paracoccidioidomycosis. A case report and considerations on the pathogenesis of this disease. Arq Gastroenterol. 1992;29:147–52.
117. Martinez R, Modena JL, Barbieri-Neto J, Fiorillo AM. Endoscopic evaluation of the involvement of the esophagus, stomach and duodenum in human paracoccidioidomycosis. Arq Gastroenterol. 1986;23:21–5.
118. Chojniak R, Vieira RA, Lopes A, Silva JC, Godoy CE. Intestinal paracoccidioidomycosis simulating colon cancer. Rev Soc Bras Med Trop. 2000;33:309–12.
119. Amstalden EM, Xavier R, Kattapuram SV, Bertolo MB, Swartz MN, Rosenberg AE. Paracoccidioidomycosis of bones and joints. A clinical, radiologic, and pathologic study of 9 cases. Medicine (Baltimore). 1996;75:213–25.
120. Pereira RM, Guerra-Junior G, Tresoldi AT. Adrenal function in 23 children with paracoccidioidomycosis. Rev Inst Med Trop São Paulo. 2006;48:333–6.
121. Paniago AM, de Freitas AC, Aguiar ES, et al. Paracoccidioidomycosis in patients with human immunodeficiency virus: review of 12 cases observed in an endemic region in Brazil. J Infect. 2005;51:248–52.
122. Yamaga LY, Benard G, Hironaka FH, et al. The role of gallium-67 scan in defining the extent of disease in an endemic deep mycosis, paracoccidioidomycosis: a predominantly multifocal disease. Eur J Nucl Med Mol Imaging. 2003;30:888–94.
123. Tuder RM, el Ibrahim R, Godoy CE, De Brito T. Pathology of the human pulmonary paracoccidioidomycosis. Mycopathologia. 1985;92:179–88.
124. Londero AT, Melo IS. Paracoccidioidomicose. J Bras Med. 1988;55:96–111.
125. Restrepo A, Trujillo M, Gomez I. Inapparent lung involvement in patients with the subacute juvenile type of paracoccidioidomycosis. Rev Inst Med Trop São Paulo. 1989;31:18–22.
126. do Valle AC, Guimaraes RR, Lopes DJ, Capone D. Thoracic radiologic aspects in paracoccidioidomycosis. Rev Inst Med Trop São Paulo. 1992;34:107–15.
127. Tobon AM, Gómez I, Franco L, Restrepo A. Seguimiento postterapia en pacientes con paraoccidioidomicosis tratados con itraconazol. Rev Colomb Neumol. 1995;7:74–8.
128. Marchiori E, Valiante PM, Mano CM, et al. Paracoccidioidomycosis: high-resolution computed tomography-pathologic correlation. Eur J Radiol. 2009.
129. Gomes E, Wingeter MA, Svidzinski TI. Clinical-radiological dissociation in lung manifestations of paracoccidioidomycosis. Rev Soc Bras Med Trop. 2008;41:454–8.
130. Naranjo MS, Trujillo M, Munera MI, Restrepo P, Gomez I, Restrepo A. Treatment of paracoccidioidomycosis with itraconazole. J Med Vet Mycol. 1990;28:67–76.
131. Funari M, Kavakama J, Shikanai-Yasuda MA, et al. Chronic pulmonary paracoccidioidomycosis (South American blastomycosis): high-resolution CT findings in 41 patients. AJR Am J Roentgenol. 1999;173:59–64.
132. Tobon AM, Agudelo CA, Osorio ML, et al. Residual pulmonary abnormalities in adult patients with chronic paracoccidioidomycosis: prolonged follow-up after itraconazole therapy. Clin Infect Dis. 2003;37:898–904.
133. Souza Jr AS, Gasparetto EL, Davaus T, Escuissato DL, Marchiori E. High-resolution CT findings of 77 patients with untreated pulmonary paracoccidioidomycosis. AJR Am J Roentgenol. 2006;187:1248–52.
134. Lemle A, Wanke B, Miranda JL, Kropf GL, Mandel MB, Mandel S. Pulmonary function in paracoccidioidomycosis (South American blastomycosis). An analysis of the obstructive defect. Chest. 1983;83:827–8.
135. Campos EP, Padovani CR, Cataneo AM. Paracoccidioidomycosis: radiologic and pulmonary study in 58 cases. Rev Inst Med Trop São Paulo. 1991;33:267–76.
136. Sant'Anna GD, Mauri M, Arrarte JL, Camargo Jr H. Laryngeal manifestations of paracoccidioidomycosis (South American

blastomycosis). Arch Otolaryngol Head Neck Surg. 1999;125: 1375–8.
137. Migliari DA, Sugaya NN, Mimura MA, Cuce LC. Periodontal aspects of the juvenile form of paracoccidioidomycosis. Rev Inst Med Trop São Paulo. 1998;40:15–8.
138. Correa AL, Franco L, Restrepo A. Paracoccidioidomicosis: coexistencia de lesiones pulmonares y patología pulmonar silente. Descripción de 64 pacientes. Acta Med Coll. 1991;16:304–8.
139. Restrepo A, Tobon AM, Agudelo CA, et al. Co-existence of integumentary lesions and lung x-ray abnormalities in patients with paracoccidioidomycosis (PCM). Am J Trop Med Hyg. 2008;79:159–63.
140. Agudelo CA, Munoz C, Ramirez A, et al. Identification of *Paracoccidioides brasiliensis* in adrenal glands biopsies of two patients with paracoccidioidomycosis and adrenal insufficiency. Rev Inst Med Trop São Paulo. 2009;51:45–8.
141. Faical S, Borri ML, Hauache OM, Ajzen S. Addison's disease caused by *Paracoccidioides brasiliensis*: diagnosis by needle aspiration biopsy of the adrenal gland. AJR Am J Roentgenol. 1996;166:461–2.
142. Moreira AC, Martinez R, Castro M, Elias LL. Adrenocortical dysfunction in paracoccidioidomycosis: comparison between plasma beta-lipotrophin/adrenocorticotrophin levels and adrenocortical tests. Clin Endocrinol (Oxf). 1992;36:545–51.
143. Tendrich M, Wanke B, del Negro G, Wajchenberg BL. Adrenocortical involvement. In: Franco M, Lacaz CS, Restrepo A, del Negro G, editors. Paracoccidioidomycosis. Boca Raton, FL: CRC Press; 1994. p. 303–12.
144. de Almeida SM, Queiroz-Telles F, Teive HA, Ribeiro CE, Werneck LC. Central nervous system paracoccidioidomycosis: clinical features and laboratorial findings. J Infect. 2004;48:193–8.
145. Tristano AG, Chollet ME, Willson M, Perez J, Troccoli M. Central nervous system paracoccidioidomycosis: case report and review. Invest Clin. 2004;45:277–88.
146. Rodacki MA, De Toni G, Borba LA, Oliveira GG. Paracoccidioidomycosis of the central nervous system: CT findings. Neuroradiology. 1995;37:636–41.
147. Gasparetto EL, Liu CB, de Carvalho Neto A, Rogacheski E. Central nervous system paracoccidioidomycosis: imaging findings in 17 cases. J Comput Assist Tomogr. 2003;27:12–7.
148. Severo LC, Kauer CL, Oliveira F, Rigatti RA, Hartmann AA, Londero AT. Paracoccidioidomycosis of the male genital tract. Report of eleven cases and a review of Brazilian literature. Rev Inst Med Trop São Paulo. 2000;42:38–40.
149. do Valle AC, Aprigliano Filho F, Moreira JS, Wanke B. Clinical and endoscopic findings in the mucosae of the upper respiratory and digestive tracts in post-treatment follow-up of paracoccidioidomycosis patients. Rev Inst Med Trop São Paulo. 1995;37:407–13.
150. Quagliato Junior R, Grangeia Tde A, Massucio RA, De Capitani EM, Rezende Sde M, Balthazar AB. Association between paracoccidioidomycosis and tuberculosis: reality and misdiagnosis. J Bras Pneumol. 2007;33:295–300.
151. Jaruratanasirikul S, Sriwiriyajan S. Effect of rifampicin on the pharmacokinetics of itraconazole in normal volunteers and AIDS patients. Eur J Clin Pharmacol. 1998;54:155–8.
152. Shikanai-Yasuda MA, Conceicao YM, Kono A, Rivitti E, Campos AF, Campos SV. Neoplasia and paracoccidioidomycosis. Mycopathologia. 2008;165:303–12.
153. de Camargo ZP, de Franco MF. Current knowledge on pathogenesis and immunodiagnosis of paracoccidioidomycosis. Rev Iberoam Micol. 2000;17:41–8.
154. de Camargo ZP. Serology of paracoccidioidomycosis. Mycopathologia. 2008;165:289–302.
155. Del Negro GM, Pereira CN, Andrade HF, et al. Evaluation of tests for antibody response in the follow-up of patients with acute and chronic forms of paracoccidioidomycosis. J Med Microbiol. 2000;49:37–46.
156. Do Valle AC, Costa RL, Fialho Monteiro PC, Von Helder J, Muniz MM, Zancope-Oliveira RM. Interpretation and clinical correlation of serological tests in paracoccidioidomycosis. Med Mycol. 2001;39:373–7.
157. Blotta MH, Camargo ZP. Immunological response to cell-free antigens of Paracoccidioides brasiliensis: relationship with clinical forms of paracoccidioidomycosis. J Clin Microbiol. 1993;31:671–6.
158. Tatibana BT, Sano A, Uno J, et al. Detection of *Paracoccidioides brasiliensis* gp43 gene in sputa by loop-mediated isothermal amplification method. J Clin Lab Anal. 2009;23:139–43.
159. Puccia R, McEwen JG, Cisalpino PS. Diversity in *Paracoccidioides brasiliensis*. The PbGP43 gene as a genetic marker. Mycopathologia. 2008;165:275–87.
160. Marques da Silva SH, Colombo AL, Blotta MH, Lopes JD, Queiroz-Telles F, Pires de Camargo Z. Detection of circulating gp43 antigen in serum, cerebrospinal fluid, and bronchoalveolar lavage fluid of patients with paracoccidioidomycosis. J Clin Microbiol. 2003;41:3675–80.
161. da Silva SH, Colombo AL, Blotta MH, Queiroz-Telles F, Lopes JD, de Camargo ZP. Diagnosis of neuroparacoccidioidomycosis by detection of circulating antigen and antibody in cerebrospinal fluid. J Clin Microbiol. 2005;43:4680–3.
162. Carvalho KC, Vallejo MC, Camargo ZP, Puccia R. Use of recombinant gp43 isoforms expressed in *Pichia pastoris* for diagnosis of paracoccidioidomycosis. Clin Vaccine Immunol. 2008;15:622–9.
163. Gomez BL, Figueroa JI, Hamilton AJ, et al. Antigenemia in patients with paracoccidioidomycosis: detection of the 87-kilodalton determinant during and after antifungal therapy. J Clin Microbiol. 1998;36:3309–16.
164. Cunha DA, Zancope-Oliveira RM, Sueli M, et al. Heterologous expression, purification, and immunological reactivity of a recombinant HSP60 from *Paracoccidioides brasiliensis*. Clin Diagn Lab Immunol. 2002;9:374–7.
165. Marquez AS, Vicentini AP, Ono MA, Watanabe MA, de Camargo ZP, Itano EN. Reactivity of antibodies from patients with acute and chronic paracoccidioidomycosis to a high molecular mass antigen from *Paracoccidioides brasiliensis*. J Clin Lab Anal. 2005;19:199–204.
166. Reis BS, Bozzi A, Prado FL, et al. Membrane and extracellular antigens of *Paracoccidioides brasiliensis* (Mexo): identification of a 28-kDa protein suitable for immunodiagnosis of paracoccidioidomycosis. J Immunol Methods. 2005;307:118–26.
167. Bisio LC, Silva SP, Pereira IS, et al. A new *Paracoccidioides brasiliensis* 70-kDa heat shock protein reacts with sera from paracoccidioidomycosis patients. Med Mycol. 2005;43:495–503.
168. Diez S, Gomez BL, McEwen JG, Restrepo A, Hay RJ, Hamilton AJ. Combined use of *Paracoccidioides brasiliensis* recombinant 27-kilodalton and purified 87-kilodalton antigens in an enzyme-linked immunosorbent assay for serodiagnosis of paracoccidioidomycosis. J Clin Microbiol. 2003;41:1536–42.
169. Gomez BL, Figueroa JI, Hamilton AJ, et al. Use of monoclonal antibodies in diagnosis of paracoccidioidomycosis: new strategies for detection of circulating antigens. J Clin Microbiol. 1997;35:3278–83.
170. da Silva SH. Grosso Dde M, Lopes JD, et al. Detection of *Paracoccidioides brasiliensis* gp70 circulating antigen and follow-up of patients undergoing antimycotic therapy. J Clin Microbiol. 2004;42:4480–6.
171. Salina MA, Shikanai-Yasuda MA, Mendes RP, Barraviera B, Mendes Giannini MJ. Detection of circulating *Paracoccidioides brasiliensis* antigen in urine of paracoccidioidomycosis patients before and during treatment. J Clin Microbiol. 1998;36:1723–8.
172. Sandhu GS, Aleff RA, Kline BC, da Silva Lacaz C. Molecular detection and identification of *Paracoccidioides brasiliensis*. J Clin Microbiol. 1997;35:1894–6.

173. Gomes GM, Cisalpino PS, Taborda CP, de Camargo ZP. PCR for diagnosis of paracoccidioidomycosis. J Clin Microbiol. 2000;38:3478–80.
174. Bialek R, Ibricevic A, Aepinus C, et al. Detection of *Paracoccidioides brasiliensis* in tissue samples by a nested PCR assay. J Clin Microbiol. 2000;38:2940–2.
175. Semighini CP, de Camargo ZP, Puccia R, Goldman MH, Goldman GH. Molecular identification of *Paracoccidioides brasiliensis* by 5' nuclease assay. Diagn Microbiol Infect Dis. 2002;44:383–6.
176. San-Blas G, Nino-Vega G, Barreto L, et al. Primers for clinical detection of *Paracoccidioides brasiliensis*. J Clin Microbiol. 2005;43:4255–7.
177. Buitrago MJ, Merino P, Puente S, et al. Utility of real-time PCR for the detection of *Paracoccidioides brasiliensis* DNA in the diagnosis of imported paracoccidioidomycosis. Med Mycol. 2009;31:1–4.
178. Mendes RP, Negroni R, Arechavala A. Treatmente and control of cure. In: Franco M, Lacaz C, Restrepo A, del Negro G, editors. Paracoccidioidomycosis. Boca Raton, FL: CRC Press; 1994. p. 373–92.
179. Shikanai-Yasuda MA, Benard G, Higaki Y, et al. Randomized trial with itraconazole, ketoconazole and sulfadiazine in paracoccidioidomycosis. Med Mycol. 2002;40:411–7.
180. Shikanai-Yasuda MA, Telles Filho Fde Q, Mendes RP, Colombo AL, Moretti ML. Guidelines in paracoccidioidomycosis. Rev Soc Bras Med Trop. 2006;39:297–310.
181. Dietze R, Fowler Jr VG, Steiner TS, Pecanha PM, Corey GR. Failure of amphotericin B colloidal dispersion in the treatment of paracoccidioidomycosis. Am J Trop Med Hyg. 1999;60: 837–9.
182. Hahn RC, Hamdan JS. Effects of amphotericin B and three azole derivatives on the lipids of yeast cells of *Paracoccidioides brasiliensis*. Antimicrob Agents Chemother. 2000;44:1997–2000.
183. Queiroz-Telles F, Goldani LZ, Schlamm HT, Goodrich JM, Espinel-Ingroff A, Shikanai-Yasuda MA. An open-label comparative pilot study of oral voriconazole and itraconazole for long-term treatment of paracoccidioidomycosis. Clin Infect Dis. 2007;45:1462–9.

Sporotrichosis

Peter G. Pappas

Sporotrichosis is a chronic pyogranulomatous infection caused by the thermally dimorphic fungus *Sporothrix schenckii*. Infection is usually limited to the skin and subcutaneous tissues, but can involve virtually any organ in its disseminated form. Less common localized forms of sporotrichosis include arthritis, osteomyelitis, meningitis, chronic pneumonitis, and laryngeal and ocular disease.

Schenck originally described sporotrichosis in 1898 in a 36-year-old man who presented with several discrete indurated lesions extending along the lymphatics from the index finger proximally to the forearm. The organism obtained from cultures of the purulent drainage from one of these lesions revealed heavy growth of a moderately rapidly growing fungus that he designated as possibly related to *Sporotrichum* species [1]. Subsequently, investigators reported a second case of sporotrichosis in a 5-year-old boy with chronic ulceration of the index finger and associated nodular lymphangitis of the forearm [2]. Treatment entailed serial incision and drainage of each subcutaneous nodule followed by local wound care resulting in eventual full recovery. The fungus isolated from this young patient was referred to as *Sporothrix schenckii*. However, the more common designation, *Sporotrichum schenckii*, was used through the 1960s until Carmichael's observation that the organism had a different manner of sporulation when compared to *Sporotrichum* species. The name *Sporothrix schenckii* was officially readopted thereafter [3].

After the initial description of sporotrichosis, most early cases were reported from France. One of the earliest case series from France involved approximately 250 patients with sporotrichosis, and remains one of the largest reports of this condition to date [4]. As knowledge of the disease became more widespread, fewer cases were identified in Europe, and cases of sporotrichosis began to be reported worldwide, with the abundance of cases emerging from the USA, Japan, Mexico, and South America.

P.G. Pappas (✉)
Division of Infectious, Diseases, University of Alabama at Birmingham School of Medicine, Birmingham, AL, USA
e-mail: pappas@uab.edu

Since its original description, sporotrichosis was perceived to be a sporadic infection, although clusters of cases and larger epidemics were occasionally observed. In the largest of these outbreaks, almost 3,000 cases of sporotrichosis were reported among South African gold miners between 1941 and 1944. The cause of the outbreak was discovered to be infected mine timbers, and the epidemic was brought under control by spraying these timbers with fungicidal agents [5]. Since the report of the large South African outbreak, many smaller epidemics have been reported, mostly occurring in the Americas and Japan [6–17].

Organism

Sporothrix schenckii demonstrates thermal dimorphism, growing as a mould at room temperature (25–28°C), and as a yeast at 35–37°C [12]. There is evidence to suggest that isolates from fixed dermatologic lesions are less tolerant to higher temperatures, growing well at 35°C, but either failing to grow or growing only very slowly at 37°C. In contrast, isolates from lung, synovial tissue, or lymphocutaneous lesions and other deep tissues usually grow well at body temperature. Most recently, several investigators have demonstrated genetic differences among geographically diverse *Sporothrix* isolates, and these observations have led to the concept that *Sporothrix schenckii* is actually a complex of phylogenetically distinct species [18, 19]. It has been proposed that these variants be recognized as *S. mexicana*, *S. globosa*, *S. luriei*, and *S. brasiliensis* [20, 21]. With the exception of *S.luriei*, these organisms are morphologically indistinguishable on artificial media, and it is unclear whether there are differences in the clinical manifestations of disease caused by these organisms.

Colonies grow within a few days to 2 weeks when incubated on Sabouraud's dextrose agar at 25–28°C. The initial colony is moist and whitish. Within 10–14 days, most colonies develop a black or brown pigmentation around the periphery of the colony [12]. The identification of *S. schenckii* is based on its colonial and microscopic morphology in the

C.A. Kauffman et al. (eds.), *Essentials of Clinical Mycology*,
DOI 10.1007/978-1-4419-6640-7_22,

mould phase and its conversion to yeast phase at 35–37°C. The yeast phase of *S. schenckii*, while rarely seen in clinical specimens, is acapsular and has a distinctive oval to cigar-shaped appearance. Morphologic distinction between *S. schenckii* and a much less common pathogen, *S. cyanescens*, can be difficult, although the colonies of *S. cyanescens* produce a water-soluble purplish pigment and thermal dimorphism is less readily demonstrated in this species [12]. *Sporothrix luriei* has a distinctive morphologic appearance, with a yeast form that is large, thick-walled, and demonstrates budding. In addition, the organism can survive as a yeast at 25°C [21, 22].

Pathogenesis

Virulence factors for *S. schenckii* have not been elucidated completely. It is clear that the organism is not very virulent in many animal models, including the guinea pig, rabbit, mouse, and hamster [23–25]. The organism produces melanin, which is a virulence factor for other yeasts, including *Cryptococcus neoformans* [26]. The organism also produces extracellular proteins, which could possibly play a role in virulence. In addition, *S. schenckii* contains the unique substance L-rhamnose, which complexes with other glycoproteins to form rhamnomannans, which are not found in other fungal cell walls. The potential role of the rhamnomannans as a virulence factor is poorly understood [27].

Conditions of growth may also play an important role in virulence. In experimental models, conidia grown for 4 days demonstrate more virulence than conidia grown for 10–12 days [28]. Thermotolerance is also probably an important virulence factor among selected strains of *S. schenckii* causing visceral or lymphonodular disease, as these organisms tend to multiply at 37°C, whereas organisms that are less thermotolerant tend to be less invasive and cause chronic fixed cutaneous lesions [12, 23, 29, 30]. It is unclear whether the reclassification of *Sporothrix* species as a phylogenetic complex will improve our understanding of the various clinical patterns associated with sporotrichosis, but it is likely that differences exist in virulence potential and tissue tropisms among this family of pathogens that are clinically relevant [20, 31, 32].

Epidemiology

In recent decades, most cases of sporotrichosis have been reported from the USA, Central and South America, Africa, and Japan [6–11, 13–15, 33–35]. The majority of cases are sporadic, occurring after direct inoculation through the skin from an infectious source. There is a predominance of males among reported cases of sporotrichosis, possibly reflecting occupational exposure. Occupational risk groups include gardeners, farmers, forestry and nursery workers, veterinarians, outdoor laborers, and those involved in other activities that involve exposure to *S. schenckii*-contaminated material, such as sphagnum moss, roses, farm crops, hay, and other vegetation [8, 10, 36, 37].

The incidence of sporotrichosis varies widely from country to country based on observational data and case reports. Few countries have national surveillance or reporting systems for the deep mycoses; consequently only crude estimates of disease incidence are generally available. Surveillance data notwithstanding, the disease appears to have become extremely rare in Western Europe, with the exception of Italy, where sporadic cases are still reported [13]. In the USA, the incidence is less than 1 case per 100,000 and probably more accurately approximates one case per million persons [14]. Data from Japan suggest a similar incidence [9, 11]. Currently, the countries of Central and South America appear to have the heaviest burden of disease based on scattered reports and a few prospective studies. In a large epidemiologic investigation from urban areas in Brazil, over 800 cases have been reported since 1997 [15]. Studies suggest an important role for feline transmission in the genesis of this ongoing outbreak. Observations from hyperendemic regions in the Andean highlands of South America, where sporotrichosis has been recognized commonly, suggest that the incidence of disease is highest among children and adolescents living in rural villages, and approximates 1 case per 1,000 in these regions [35, 38]. Among these and other reports of children with sporotrichosis, there appears to be no male predominance in disease [35, 38–40].

Transmission of *S. schenckii* usually occurs through a traumatic break in the skin and exposure to infectious material. A primary lesion usually occurs at the site of inoculation, and this may be followed by local lymphangitic spread or the development of a fixed cutaneous lesion. Extracutaneous sporotrichosis may occur as a result of direct inoculation such as penetrating trauma into a joint or the eye, or through dissemination from another site such as the skin or lungs. Most patients with pulmonary sporotrichosis provide no history consistent with cutaneous disease; thus, it is hypothesized that these patients acquire infection through inhalation of airborne spores [41].

Sporotrichosis as result of zoonotic exposure to domestic and wild animals is well described [15, 42–47]. Clinical sporotrichosis may occur in birds, dogs, squirrels, horses, rats, and cats; thus, veterinarians and pet owners are at relatively increased risk for acquiring infection. Fish exposure is an uncommon risk for sporotrichosis, but there are reports of cutaneous sporotrichosis following a puncture wound from the dorsal fin of commercially raised tilapia [48]. There have been several well-documented cases of feline-transmitted sporotrichosis reported in the USA and Brazil [42, 44, 45, 49]. In many of these cases, the cats had facial ulcerations that contained a large number of organisms. A recent case-control analysis in Brazil demonstrated that cat exposure was significantly associated with the development of sporotrichosis in this region [15]. A smaller epidemiologic study in Peru suggested a similar relationship between cat exposure and disease, although these findings were not as dramatic as those demonstrated in the Brazilian studies [50].

Several cases of laboratory-acquired sporotrichosis have been reported [51, 52]. These cases have occurred typically among persons working with infected laboratory animals or other contaminated material, with direct inoculation to the upper extremities. In two cases, direct inoculation into the conjunctivae occurred when a suspension of *S. schenckii* mycelial elements was spattered into the eyes [51]. Person-to-person transmission, if it occurs, is exceedingly rare. There are, however, several reports of sporotrichosis occurring in family members or persons living in the same household [53–55]. In most of these instances, disease was felt to be due to a common source rather than person-to-person spread.

There are several well-described point-source outbreaks of sporotrichosis. Most outbreaks have been traced to occupational exposure such as workers handling plants, contaminated sphagnum moss, or soil. Forrester was among the first to suggest an occupational predisposition to sporotrichosis in his review of 14 tree nursery workers with sporotrichosis from Wisconsin in 1926 [56]. More recent epidemics in the USA in Wisconsin, Florida, Vermont, Mississippi, and a large multistate outbreak have been reported following exposure to seedlings, other plants, and sphagnum moss [6–8, 36]. In the largest of these epidemics, 84 cases of cutaneous sporotrichosis occurred in persons handling conifer seedlings that had been packed with sphagnum moss harvested in Wisconsin [10, 37]. Cases were confirmed in 14 states in this multistate outbreak.

The most recently documented outbreak of sporotrichosis in the USA occurred among nine tree nursery workers from a theme park in Florida in 1994 [14]. A case-control study conducted in parallel with this epidemic suggested that occupational inexperience and handling sphagnum moss were independently associated with an increased risk, whereas longer work experience and wearing gloves were associated with decreased risk of sporotrichosis [14].

Clinical Manifestations

Lymphocutaneous

Lymphocutaneous lesions are the clinical hallmark of sporotrichosis. Disease typically arises at a site of minor trauma and may begin as a erythematous papule that enlarges over days or weeks. The lesion may become a fixed subcutaneous nodule or plaque, or may develop into a chronic nonhealing ulcerative lesion (Figs. 1 and 2). These lesions are usually painless, and systemic symptoms of fever, malaise, weight loss, and chills are usually absent. Classically, a "sporotrichoid" eruption of similar-appearing subcutaneous nodules develops along the lymphatic system of the involved anatomic site (Figs. 3 and 4).

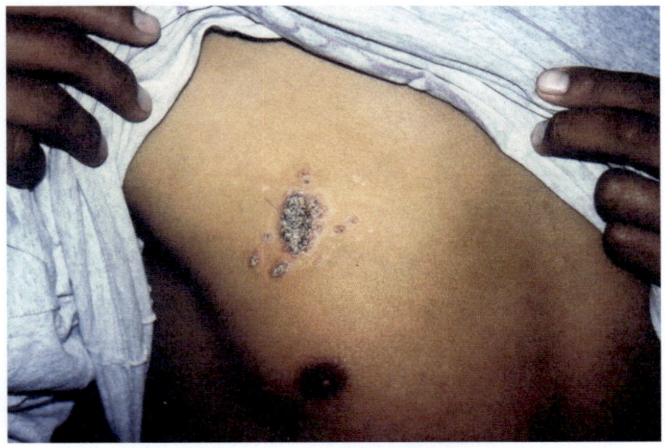

Fig. 1 Plaque-like lesion due to *S. schenckii* on the anterior chest wall of an 18-year-old man

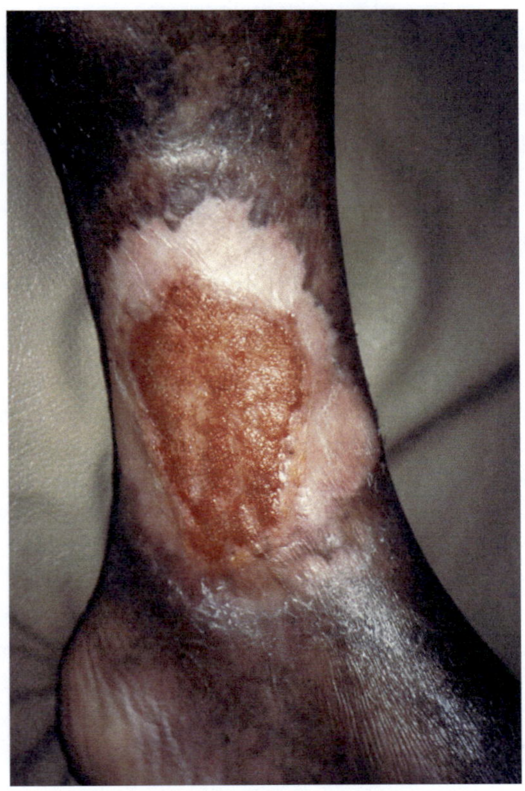

Fig. 2 Fixed chronic ulcerative lesion of sporotrichosis in a 58-year-old woman. The lesion had been present for 18 months

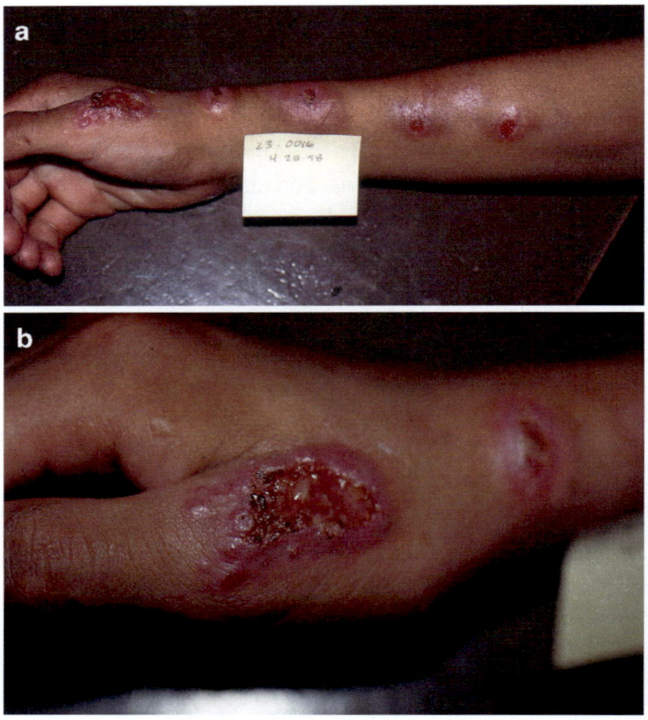

Fig. 3 (**a**) Characteristic lesions of lymphocutaneous sporotrichosis of the forearm in a 45-year-old landscaper. (**b**) Primary lesion, which has ulcerated, in the same patient

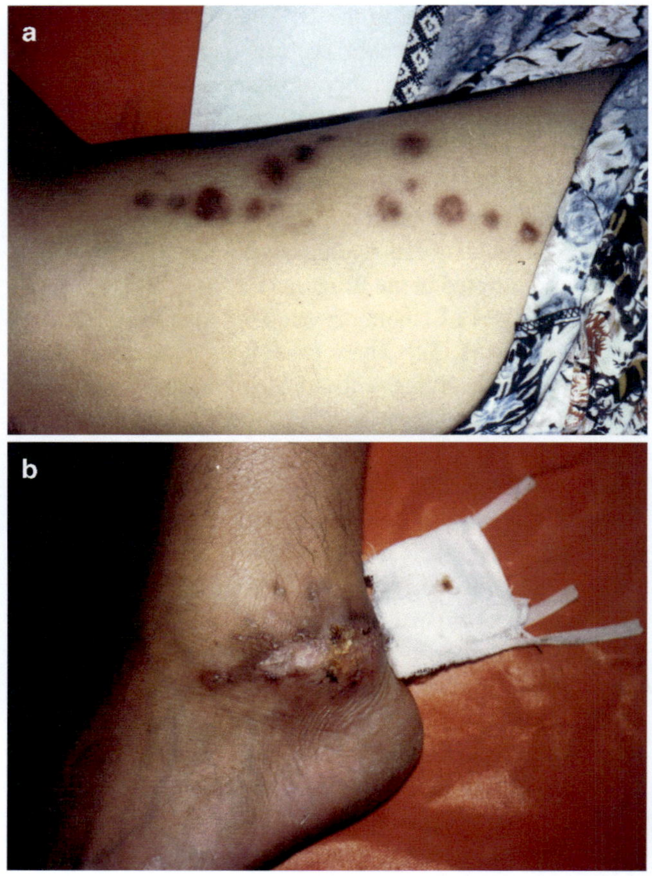

Fig. 4 (**a**) Hyperpigmented lymphocutaneous sporotrichosis on the leg of a 28-year-old Peruvian woman. (**b**) Primary ulcerative lesion overlying the lateral malleolus in the same patient

Lesions are typically erythematous or violaceous, and the intervening skin is usually normal. Untreated, these nodules may undergo suppuration, drainage, and ulcer formation, similar to the primary lesion. Secondary lymphadenopathy may occur, although lymph nodes are not usually involved directly with *S. schenckii* infection, and most cases of enlarged nodes represent reactive lymphadenopathy.

Some patients present with a fixed ulceration or a proliferative, plaque-like lesion. These lesions can be chronic for many months or years, remaining more or less unchanged [27]. Persistent lesions for as long as 10 years have been reported [57]. The propensity for these lesions to evolve into progressive nodular lymphangitis or disseminated disease is very low, and may relate to the observation that many of these organisms are less thermotolerant than more invasive strains [13].

Disseminated cutaneous lesions involving multiple extremities, the face, trunk, and abdomen may occur in normal individuals after either intense exposure to the organism, significant autoinoculation, or rarely, hematogenous dissemination. Patients with disseminated skin lesions secondary to hematogenous spread are virtually all severely immunocompromised as a consequence of advanced HIV disease, organ transplantation, or another significant underlying disorder [58–61].

Osteoarticular

Osteoarticular sporotrichosis usually manifests as a slowly progressive, indolent process involving a major peripheral joint, typically the knee, elbow, ankle, or wrist [62–67]. Occasionally, metacarpal or metatarsal joints may be involved, either as a manifestation of dissemination or direct extension from a cutaneous lesion. Arthritis has also been reported to follow a penetrating joint injury. Frank bony involvement is a frequent concomitant of sporotrichoid arthritis, usually at a contiguous periarticular site [62, 65]. Patients with osteoarticular sporotrichosis often present with localized pain and swelling without significant fever or other systemic symptoms. Untreated, the process inevitably progresses until the joint is destroyed and/or function significantly impaired.

Sporothrix schenckii is also a cause of granulomatous tenosynovitis, usually presenting in the wrist with painless swelling and limited range of motion. In severe cases, neurologic or musculoskeletal symptoms due to entrapment of the median nerve or tendon rupture can be seen [68, 69]. Surgical intervention is necessary for decompression, debridement, and repair of damaged tendons. At surgery, the finding of "rice bodies" in the synovial space is a nonspecific finding consistent with sporotrichosis, but can also be seen in cases of granulomatous tenosynovitis due to other organisms, such as mycobacteria.

Pulmonary

Pulmonary sporotrichosis is a rare disorder. In the largest review of this topic, Pluss and Opal reviewed 51 cases, of which the vast majority were middle-aged white males presenting with cough, low-grade fever, weight loss, and upper lobe cavitary disease [41]. Preexisting lung disease was common. Hemoptysis occurred in fewer than 20%, but could be significant if present. Chest roentgenographic findings associated with pulmonary sporotrichosis are nonspecific. Cavitary lung lesions, which are common with pulmonary sporotrichosis, are usually single and often involve the upper lobes [41, 67]. There may be extensive surrounding fibrosis, which is indistinguishable from the fibrosis associated with other causes of chronic necrotizing pneumonia (Fig. 5). The classic single thin-walled cavity associated with pulmonary sporotrichosis and coccidioidomycosis is relatively uncommon [41]. Among patients with pulmonary sporotrichosis, disease is usually limited to the lungs, although multiple organ involvement can occur. Untreated, pulmonary sporotrichosis leads to slow and inexorable clinical deterioration; spontaneous remission is rare. Laryngeal sporotrichosis is also a rare manifestation of this infection, likely reflecting the same manner of disease acquisition as those with pulmonary sporotrichosis [70–72]. The disease can be easily misdiagnosed as larygeal carcinoma [70].

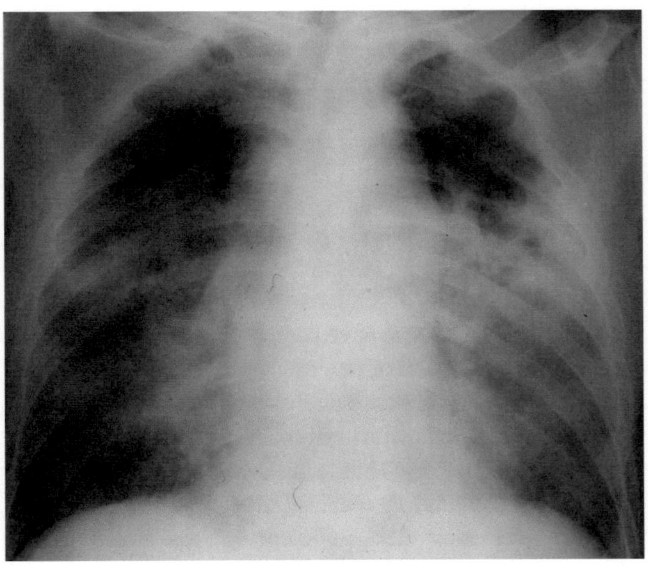

Fig. 5 Chest radiograph of a patient who had chronuc fibrocavitary pulmonary sporotrichosis

Disseminated

Sporotrichosis can involve virtually any organ, manifesting as disseminated disease in either of two forms: (1) disseminated cutaneous disease and (2) disseminated visceral disease [67, 73–75]. Both of these disease presentations result from hematogenous dissemination. In the first form, multiple skin lesions may occur spontaneously on the extremities, trunk, abdomen, and head and neck. These lesions are often small pustules on an erythematous base and not particularly distinctive. They can be mistaken for the skin lesions of varicella, disseminated bacterial infection, or another disseminated fungal infection. In the second form, the central nervous system (CNS) and peripheral joints are probably the most common sites for disseminated visceral disease [67, 76]. Clinically, CNS disease is usually associated with chronic indolent meningitis, focal cranial nerve abnormalities, and hydrocephalus. Cerebrospinal fluid analysis usually reveals evidence of chronic inflammation with hypoglycorrhachia, elevated CSF protein, and mononuclear cell pleocytosis [67, 75]. Endophthalmitis due to *S. schenckii* may occur either as an extension of a CNS infection, or independently as a consequence of hematogenous dissemination or directly from penetrating trauma [77, 78].

Special Populations

Children

Unlike cryptococcosis and blastomycosis, sporotrichosis is not uncommon in children [39, 40, 79–82]. Indeed, in some populations the highest incidence of disease is among preadolescent children [35, 38]. Disease manifestations are similar to those in adults, although multiple cutaneous sites and facial lesions are more common in children with sporotrichosis, possibly due in part to autoinoculation [35, 79–82]. For unclear reasons, extracutaneous and hematogenously disseminated cutaneous disease are particularly uncommon among children.

Immunocompromised Patients

A growing number of patients with sporotrichosis and HIV/AIDS or another significant underlying immune disorder have been reported [58, 59, 61, 75, 76, 78, 83–88]. Patients with these disorders are much more likely to present with hematogenously disseminated disease, and a disproportionate number of these patients develop complicated *S. schenckii* infections, including fungemia, meningitis, endophthalmitis, and disseminated cutaneous and multiorgan disease. Whereas the mortality rate associated with sporotrichosis among non-immunocompromised patients is very low, disseminated disease in the immunocompromised patient can be rapidly fatal if unrecognized and untreated.

Diagnosis

The clinical diagnosis of lymphocutaneous sporotrichosis can be misleading because sporotrichosis is clinically indistinguishable from other common causes of nodular lymphangitis [89]. Lymphonodular sporotrichosis may appear identical to cutaneous nocardiosis, mycobacterial infections (especially due to *Mycobacterium marinum* and *Mycobacterium chelonae)*, tularemia resulting from direct cutaneous inoculation, and cutaneous leishmaniasis [89]. Less common causes of a lymphonodular sporotrichoid eruption include *Mycobacterium avium* complex, other mycobacteria, *C. neoformans*, *B. dermatitidis*, and rarely, *C. immitis.*

The diagnosis of sporotrichosis is confirmed by a positive culture for *S. schenckii* from an involved site (tissue or body fluid). The organism is not considered a colonizer; thus, isolation from a clinical specimen is virtually always considered diagnostic. Optimally, clinical specimens for culture should be collected from purulent cutaneous lesions. Alternatively, a skin biopsy from a suspicious area is usually sufficient. For patients with suspected pulmonary sporotrichosis, expectorated purulent sputum can be a helpful source for culture, although bronchoalveolar lavage or a transbronchial biopsy specimen are frequently necessary [41, 90]. Patients with laryngeal sporotrichosis usually require a biospy of involved tissue for a definitive diagnosis. For patients with osteoarticular disease, the organism is readily recovered from synovial fluid or involved bone or synovial tissue. Isolation of *S. schenckii* from blood and other body fluids, including cerebrospinal fluid, is unusual even among patients with disseminated disease [91].

Direct examination of clinical specimens is usually unsuccessful in a search for specific histopathologic evidence of sporotrichosis. Owing to the relative paucity of organisms, yeast forms are seen uncommonly on biopsy specimens using Gram stain, KOH, or other special stains. The fungal cell may have a very pleomorphic appearance ranging from spherical to elongated. The typical ovoid cigar-shaped yeast forms, which are most suggestive of the diagnosis, are uncommonly seen. Similarly, the classic finding of asteroid bodies in tissue specimens is uncommon (Fig. 6). Serologic assays for the detection of antibodies to *S. schenckii* are neither readily available nor appropriately standardized; thus, this method of diagnosis is not generally useful [92–94]. An assay of CSF for antibody to *S. schenckii* was advocated for patients with suspected meningitis, but this test is not available [91].

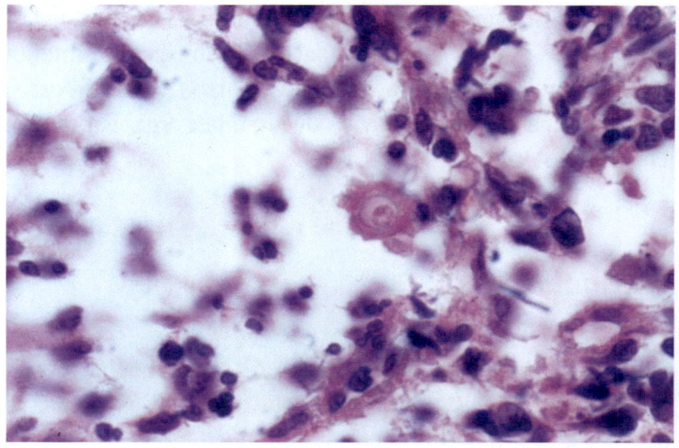

Fig. 6 Asteroid body seen on H&E stain of tissue from a patient with cutaneous sporotrichosis

In many countries, a skin test (sporotrichin test) is available to detect exposure to *S. schenckii*. The skin test antigen, which consists of an extract from laboratory-cultured strains of *S. schenckii,* is not standardized. The test is used as an adjunct to the diagnosis of cutaneous sporotrichosis among patients with clinically compatible lesions before culture data are available or in whom cultures are negative. Although a positive skin test is generally regarded as evidence of recent exposure to *S. schenckii,* this diagnostic modality remains of questionable value, even in areas of the world where it is readily available. At present, the sporotrichin skin test is not available commercially within the USA.

Treatment

There are a variety of effective treatment modalities for sporotrichosis, and these have been reviewed and updated in the most recent version of the Infectious Diseases Society of America clinical practice guidelines [95]. For all forms of sporotrichosis, spontaneous resolution without specific therapy is uncommon [96]. Thus, a fundamental principle in the approach to the management of this disorder is that all patients require some therapeutic intrevention. Notably, there are no comparative trials between different agents for the treatment of sporotrichosis. The largest trials involve pilot studies or dose-ranging studies to determine a range of efficacy and optimal dosing of a single agent. Furthermore, there are no studies of combinations of antifungal agents. The main limitation to the study of the treatment of sporotrichosis pertains to its rarity compared to other invasive mycoses. Specific appraoches to therapy are discussed below.

Supersaturated Solution of Potassium Iodide (SSKI)

Effective therapy for cutaneous sporotrichosis has been available for almost a century. In the early 1900s, deBeurmann noted that iodides were effective in the treatment of this form of sporotrichosis, though the mechanism by which iodides act is still not understood over 100 years later [97–99]. Supersaturated solution of potassium iodide (SSKI) does not inhibit or kill *S. schenckii* directly, nor does it enhance killing of the organism when combined with neutrophils [100]. Nonetheless, a large amount of clinical experience and published data indicate that SSKI is an acceptable and very effective treatment for uncomplicated cutaneous sporotrichosis.

For patients undergoing treatment with SSKI, it is recommended to begin with five drops SSKI in water or juice three times daily, gradually increasing each dose by five drops weekly to a maximum of 40 or 50 drops SSKI three times daily as tolerated. Administration usually continues until active lesions have disappeared, which is usually for at least 4 weeks at a minimum. Therapy is rarely continued beyond 6 months, in part because of poor patient tolerance and difficulty in administration. Recognizing these problems, Cabezas and colleagues, studying a group of Andean natives in Peru, found that once daily dosing with SSKI was equivalent to standard dosing at two to three times daily, thereby demonstrating that this was an effective approach to treatment for many patients with cutaneous sporotrichosis [101]. SSKI has also been used successfully in combination with terbinafine among patients with lymphocutaneous disease [102].

Adverse effects, which are common with SSKI, especially at higher doses, include anorexia, nausea, a metallic taste, swelling of the salivary glands, rash, and fever [98]. Despite these obvious obstacles to good compliance, SSKI remains the least expensive and widely used therapy for sporotrichosis [95]. Given that sporotrichosis primarily occurs in regions of the world where antifungal therapy with azole drugs is generally not affordable, SSKI remains the treatment of choice for individuals in these regions with uncomplicated lymphocutaneous sporotrichosis. Response to therapy among compliant patients with uncomplicated disease is in excess of 90% [95]. SSKI is not effective for visceral sporotrichosis.

Hyperthermia

Hyperthermia has been used successfully in the treatment of lymphocutaneous sporotrichosis based on an observation made originally in 1951 [103]. Most of the recent work on hyperthermic therapy for sporotrichosis has been conducted in Japan, utilizing hot baths, hot compresses, and hand-held heating devices [98]. Hiruma and colleagues reported that 18 of 21 patients were cured when using pocket warmers directly applied over a fixed lesion for 40–60 min daily for an average of 8 weeks [104]. Other recent scattered anecdotes report success with hyperthermia. Additional studies evaluating infrared therapy have been done, but have been limited due to the potential for phototoxicity [105].

The mechanism by which hyperthermia leads to improvement in sporotrichosis remains unknown, but probably relates to the limited thermotolerance of *S. schenckii*. Over two decades ago, Kwon Chung demonstrated the inability of *S. schenckii* obtained from fixed cutaneous lesions to survive at temperatures of 37°C or higher [12]. Additionally, Hiruma and Kagawa demonstrated that *S. schenckii* germination was markedly decreased when organisms were heated to 40°C [104]. Despite clinical evidence to support its use, the role of hyperthermia as therapy for sporotrichosis remains very limited, and probably should be restricted to patients with fixed cutaneous lesions who cannot afford or tolerate existing oral therapies [95].

Azoles

The azole antifungal drugs have become the mainstay of therapy for most patients with lymphocutaneous sporotrichosis. Of the three available oral azoles, itraconazole is the drug of choice with a success rate exceeding 90% [95, 106, 107]. Itraconazole should be administered orally at doses of 100–200 mg daily for at least 1 month beyond resolution of symptoms and signs [95]. Recent experience with "pulse dose" itraconazole, 400 mg daily for 1 week each month for at least 3 months, has been successful in a small number of patients with uncomplicated lymphocutaneous disease, but this approach has not been studied on a large scale [108]. Fluconazole is less effective than itraconazole at similar doses and should be considered a second-line therapy for sporotrichosis among patients who either have no access to or cannot tolerate itraconazole, or for whom itraconazole is contraindicated due to drug–drug interactions [95, 109]. Fluconazole should be administered orally starting at doses of 400 mg daily, and higher doses may be needed. Ketoconazole is the least effective of the available oral azoles and should only be used when access to the other two agents is limited [95, 110]. If therapy with ketoconazole is necessary, initial dosing is 400 mg daily, increasing to 600 and 800 mg daily as clinically indicated for unresponsive cases. All of the azole drugs are better tolerated than SSKI.

For patients with extracutaneous disease, especially those with osteoarticular disease, itraconazole 200 mg twice daily provides a reasonably effective oral alternative to amphotericin B [95, 106]. Fluconazole has been disappointing [95], and ketoconazole is not recommended for the treatment of patients with extracutaneous sporotrichosis. Among patients with non-life-threatening pulmonary disease, itraconazole provides an effective alternative to amphotericin B. For central nervous system and other forms of disseminated sporotrichosis, there is little role for initial therapy with any of the azoles, although they may play a role as chronic suppressive therapy among those who demonstrate a favorable initial response to amphotericin B [95].

There is very limited clinical experience with the expanded-spectrum triazoles, including voriconazole and posaconazole, for treatment of sporotrichosis. Voriconazole demonstrates poor in vitro activity versus *S. schenckii* and should not be used for this disorder [111, 112]. In contrast, posaconazole demonstrates excellent in vitro activity and is a potentially effective agent for patients with lymphocutaneous, osteoarticular, and pulmonary disease [111, 112]. Unfortunately, there are only a few clinical anecdotes describing a response to posaconazole among patients with sporotrichosis.

Terbinafine

Terbinafine, an allylamine antifungal agent, has good activity against *S. schenckii* in vitro and in vivo, and there is a moderate amount of clinical data supporting its usefulness for the treatment of lymphocutaneous sporotrichosis [113–116]. In a randomized, double-blinded study involving 63 patients, two different regimens of terbinafine were compared among patients with uncomplicated lymphocutaneous sporotrichosis. Patients received either terbinafine 500 or 1,000 mg daily for up to 24 weeks. A much better response was noted among the group receiving higher-dose terbinafine (87% vs 52%), and the percent success rate in the higher-dose group was similar to that seen in patients treated with itraconazole [116]. In a more recent study, as little as 250 mg terbinafine daily has led to a successful outcome among patients with uncomplicated lymphocutaneous disease [117]. While not approved for this purpose, terbinafine appears to be safe, well-tolerated, and a reasonable alternative to itraconazole for patients with lymphocutaneous disease. Because there are few data concerning the use of terbinafine in the treatment of extracutaneous sporotrichosis, it is not recommended in this setting.

Amphotericin B

Amphotericin B, preferably in a lipid formulation, remains the mainstay of therapy for patients with disseminated or life-threatening sporotrichosis, including those patients with CNS disease, moderate-to-severe pulmonary sporotrichosis, and disseminated cutaneous and/or visceral disease [95]. It is also the most appropriate initial therapy for immunocompromised patients with disseminated disease. There are few data comparing amphotericin B to other forms of therapy, especially for more serious complications of sporotrichosis, such as pulmonary and CNS disease; however, the seriousness of these manifestations generally merit a more aggressive therapeutic approach. Thus, the recently published treatment guidelines for sporotrichosis suggest amphotericin B be used as initial therapy for patients with either meningeal or life-threatening disease until the condition has been clinically stabilized [95].

Surgery

The role of surgery in the treatment of sporotrichosis is limited to a few specific and uncommon conditions. Among patients with pulmonary sporotrichosis involving a well-defined anatomic area and no more than one lobe, surgery may be a reasonable option provided there are no contraindications to surgery and there is no evidence of sporotrichosis involving the other lung or other extracutaneous sites [12, 41]. Another potential role for surgery is its use in the debridement of involved synovial spaces, particularly for synovitis involving the wrist [68, 69]. The role of synovectomy in this setting is difficult to assess since most of these patients have received concomitant antifungal therapy. However, in many instances surgery is performed to preserve or improve function that has been lost due to progressive destruction of bones and joints. There are scattered reports of successful prosthetic joint replacement in the face of active articular sporotrichosis [118]. In each of these instances, patients were treated with chronic suppressive antifungal therapy to prevent relapsing disease.

Prevention

There is no vaccine for sporotrichosis; thus, prevention of the disease involves avoidance of exposure to the organism among individuals involved in high-risk activities. In particular, gardeners, nursery workers, foresters, veterinarians, cat owners in certain geographic areas, and construction workers are at increased risk of developing sporotrichosis as a consequence of direct cutaneous inoculation. Avoidance of exposure requires the wearing of gloves. There is no evidence that wearing a mask prevents airborne transmission of the organism. Perhaps the greatest potential role for prevention is in developing countries in which sporotrichosis remains a significant regional public health threat. In those settings where lack of sanitation, poverty, and poor personal hygiene are common problems, efforts to expand awareness of the disease, limit exposure to potential vectors such as cats, and improve personal hygiene might lessen morbidity associated with *S. schenckii* infection.

References

1. Schenck BR. Refractory subcutaneous abscesses caused by a fungus possibly related to the sporotricha. Johns Hopkins Hosp Bull. 1898;9:286–90.
2. Hektoen L, Perkins CF. Refractory subcutaneous abscesses caused by *Sporothrix schenckii*. A new pathogenic fungus. J Exp Med. 1900;5:77–89.
3. Carmichael JW. *Chrysosporium* and some other aleuriosporic hyphomycetes. Can J Bot. 1962;40:1137–73.
4. de Beurmann L, Gougerot H. Les Sporotrichoses. Paris: Felix Alcan; 1912.
5. Transvaal Mine Medical Officers' Association. Sporotrichosis infection in mines of the Witwatersrand: a symposium. Johannesburg, Transvaal Chamber of Mines, 1947.
6. Ellner PD. An outbreak of sporotrichosis in Florida. JAMA. 1960;173:113–7.
7. D'Alessio DJ, Leavens LJ, Strumpf GB, Smith CD. An outbreak of sporotrichosis in Vermont associated with sphagnum moss as the source of infection. N Engl J Med. 1965;272:1054–8.
8. Powell KE, Taylor A, Phillips BJ, et al. Cutaneous sporotrichosis in forestry workers: epidemic due to contaminated sphagnum moss. JAMA. 1978;240:232–5.
9. Itoh M, Okamoto S, Kariya H. Survey of 200 cases of sporotrichosis. Dermatologica. 1986;172:209–13.
10. Centers for Disease Control. Multistate outbreak of sporotrichosis in seedling handlers. MMWR. 1988;37:652–3.
11. Kushuhara M, Hachisuka H, Sasai Yoichiro. Statistical survey of 150 cases with sporotrichosis. Mycopathologia. 1988;102:129–33.
12. Kwon-Chung KJ, Bennett JE. Sporotrichosis. In: Kwon-Chung KJ, Bennett JE, editors. Medical Mycology. Philadelphia: Lea & Febiger; 707. p. 729–1992.
13. Barile F, Mastrolonardo M, Loconsole F, Rantuccio F. Cutaneous sporotrichosis in the period 1978–1992 in the province of Bari, Apulia, Southern Italy. Mycoses. 1993;36:182–5.
14. Hajjeh R, McDonnell S, Reef S, et al. Outbreak of sporotrichosis among tree nursery workers. J Infect Dis. 1997;176:499–504.
15. Barros MB, Schubach AO, Schubach TM, Wanke B, Lambert-Passos SR. An epidemic of sporotrichosis in Rio de Janeiro, Brazil: epidemiological aspects of a series of cases. Epidemiol Infect. 2008;136:1192–6.
16. da Rosa AC, Scroferneker ML, Vettorato R, Gervini RL, Vettorato G, Weber A. Epidemiology of sporotrichosis: a study of 304 cases in Brazil. J Am Acad Dermatol. 2005;52:451–9.
17. Agarwal S, Gopal K, Umesh Kumar B. Sporotrichosis in Uttarakhand (India): a report of nine cases. Int J Dermatol. 2008; 47:367–71.
18. de Meyer EM, de Beer ZW, Summerbell RC, et al. Taxonomy and phylogeny of new wood-and soil-inhabiling *Sporothrix* species in the *Ophiostoma stenoceras-Sporothrix schenckii* complex. Mycologia. 2008;100:647–61.
19. Marimon R, Gené J, Cano J, Trilles L, Lazéra M, Guarro J. Molecular phylogeny of *Sporothrix schenckii*. J Clin Microbiol. 2006;44:3251–6.
20. Marimon R, Cano J, Gené J, Sutton D, Kawasaki M, Guarro J. *Sporothrix brasiliensis*, *S. globosa*, and *S. mexicana*, three new *Sporothrix* species of clinical interest. J Clin Microbiol. 2007; 45:3198–206.
21. Marimon R, Gené J, Cano J, Guarro J. *Sporothrix luriei*: a rare fungus from clinical origin. Med Mycol. 2008;46:621–5.
22. Alberici F, Paties CT, Lombardi G, Ajello L, Daufman L, Chandler F. *Sporothrix schenckii var luriei* as the cause of sporotrichosis in Italy. Eur J Epidemiol. 1989;5:173–7.
23. Mackinnon JE, Conti-Diaz IA, Yarzabal LA. Experimental sporotrichosis, ambient temperature and amphotericin B. Sabouraudia. 1964;3:192–4.
24. Dixon DM, Duncan RA, Hurn NJ. Use of a mouse model to evaluate clinical and environmental isolates of *Sporothrix* spp. from the largest U.S. outbreak of sporotrichosis. J Clin Microbiol. 1992;30:951–4.
25. Tachibani T, Matsuyama T, Ito M, Mitsuyama M. *Sporothrix schenckii* thermo-intolerant mutants losing fatal visceral infectivity but retaining high cutaneous infectivity. Med Mycol. 2001;39:295–8.
26. Romero-Martinez R, Wheeler M, Guerreo-Plata A, Rico G, Torres-Guerrero H. Biosynthesis and functions of melanin in *Sporothrix schenckii*. Infect Immun. 2000;68:3696–703.
27. Kauffman CA. Sporotrichosis. Clin Infect Dis. 1999;29:231–7.
28. Fernandes KS, Mathews HL, Lopes Bezerra LM. Differences in virulence of *Sporothrix schenckii* conidia related to culture conditions and cell-wall components. J Med Microbiol. 1999;48:195–203.
29. Mackinnon JE, Conti-Diaz IA. The effect of temperature on sporotrichosis. Sabouraudia. 1962;2:56–9.
30. Mackinnon JE, Conti-Diaz IA, Gezuele E, Civila E, DaLuz S. Isolation of *Sporothrix schenckii* from nature and considerations on its pathogenicity and ecology. Sabouraudia. 1969 ;7:38–45.
31. Arenas R, Miller D, Campos-Macias P. Epidemiological data and molecular characterization (mtDNA) of *Sporothrix schenckii* in 13 cases from Mexico. Int J Dermatol. 2007;46:177–9.
32. Mesa-Arango AC, Reyes-Montes M, Pérez-Mejía A, et al. Phenotyping and genotyping of *Sporothrix schenckii* isolates according to geographic origin and clinical form of sporotrichosis. J Clin Microbiol. 2002;40:3004–11.
33. Ochoa AG, Ricoy E, Velasco O, Lopez R, Navarrete F. Valoracion comparativa de los antigenos polisacarido y cellar de *Sporothrix schenckii*. Rev Invest Salud Publ Mex. 1970;30:303–15.
34. Velasco-Castrejón O, Gonzalez-Ochoa YA. La esporotricosis en un peque o poblado de la Sierra de Puebla. Rev Invest Salud Publ Mex. 1976;36:133–7.
35. Pappas PG, Tellez I, Deep AA, Nolasco D, Holgado W, Bustamante B. Sporotrichosis in Peru: description of a hyperendemic area. Clin Infect Dis. 2000;30:65–70.
36. Centers for Disease Control. Sporotrichosis associated with Wisconsin sphagnum moss. MMWR. 1982;31:542–4.
37. Coles FB, Schuchat A, Hibbs JR, et al. A multistate outbreak of sporotrichosis associated with sphagnum moss. Am J Epidemiol. 1992;136:475–87.
38. Lyon GM, Zurita S, Casquero J, et al. Population-based surveillance and a case-control study of risk factors for endemic lymphocutaneous sporotrichosis in Peru. Clin Infect Dis. 2003; 36:34–9.
39. Barros MB, Costa KL, Schubach TM, et al. Endemic of zoonotic sporotrichosis: profile of cases in children. Pediatr Infect Dis J. 2008;27:246–50.

40. Bonifaz A, Saúl A, Paredes-Solis V, Fierro L, Rosales A, Palacios C, et al. Sporotrichosis in childhood: clinical and therapeutic experience in 25 patients. Pediatr Dermatol. 2007;24:369–72.
41. Pluss JL, Opal SM. Pulmonary sporotrichosis: review of treatment and outcome. Medicine (Baltimore). 1986;65:143–53.
42. Carvalho J, Caldwell JB, Radford BL, Feldman AR. Feline-transmitted sporotrichosis in the Southwestern United States. West J Med. 1991;154:462–5.
43. de Lima Barros MB, Schubach TM, Galhardo MC, et al. Sporotrichosis: an emergent zoonosis in Rio de Janeiro. Mem Inst Oswaldo Cruz. 2001;96:777–9.
44. Fleury RN, Taborda PR, Gupta AK, et al. Zoonotic sporotrichosis. Transmission to humans by infected domestic cat scratching: report of four cases in Sao Paulo, Brazil. Int J Dermatol. 2001;40:318.
45. Reed KD, Moore FM, Geiger GE, Stemper ME. Zoonotic transmission of sporotrichosis: case report and review. Clin Infect Dis. 1993;16:384–7.
46. Saravanakumar PS, Eslami P, Zar FA. Lymphocutaneous sporotrichosis associated with a squirrel bite: case report and review. Clin Infect Dis. 1996;23:647–8.
47. de Lima Barros MB, de Oliveira Schubach A, Galhardo MC, Schubach TM, do Valle AC. Sporotrichosis with widespread cutaneous lesions: report of 24 cases related to transmission by domestic cats in Rio de Janeiro, Brazil. Int J Dermatol. 2003;42:677–81.
48. Haddad VJ, Miot HA, Bartoli LD, Cardoso AC, de Camargo RM. Localized lymphatic sporotrichosis after fish-induced injury. Med Mycol. 2002;40:425–7.
49. Schubach A, de Lima Barros M, Wanke B. Epidemic sporotrichosis. Curr Opin Infect Dis. 2008;21:129–33.
50. Kovarik CL, Neyra E, Bustamante B. Evaluation of cats as the source of endemic sporotrichosis in Peru. Med Mycol. 2008;46:53–6.
51. Thompson DW, Kaplan AW. Laboratory-acquired sporotrichosis. Sabouraudia. 1977;15:167–70.
52. Cooper DR, Dixon DM, Salkin IF. Laboratory-acquired sporotrichosis. J Med Vet Mycol. 1992;30:169–91.
53. Garrett HD, Robbins JB. An unusual occurrence of sporotrichosis: eight cases in one residence. Arch Dermatol. 1960;82:570–1.
54. Yamada Y, Dekio S, Jidoi J, Ozasa S, Tohgi K. A familial occurrence of sporotrichosis. J Dermatol. 1990;17:255–9.
55. Umemoto N, Demitsu T, Osawa M, Toda A, Kawasaki M, Mochizuki T. Sporotrichosis in a husband and wife. J Dermatol. 2005;32:569–73.
56. Forrester HR. Sporotrichosis, an occupational dermatosis. JAMA. 1926;87:1605–9.
57. Rathi SK, Raman M, Rajendran C. Localized cutaneous sporotrichosis lasting for 10 years. Indian J Dermatol Venereol Leprol. 2003;69:239–40.
58. Ware AJ, Cockrell CJ, Skiest DJ, Kussman HM. Disseminated sporotrichosis with extensive cutaneous involvement in a patient with AIDS. J Am Acad Dermatol. 1999;40:350–5.
59. Carvalho MTM, de Castro AP, Baby C, Werner B, Neto JF, Queiroz-Telles F. Disseminated cutaneous sporotrichosis in a patient with AIDS: report of a case. Rev Soc Bras Med Trop. 2002;35:655–9.
60. Yelverton CB, Stetson CL, Bang RH, Clark JW, Butler DF. Fatal sporotrichosis. Cutis. 2006;78:253–6.
61. Hardman S, Stephenson I, Jenkins DR, Wiselka MJ, Johnson EM. Disseminated *Sporothrix schenckii* in a patient with AIDS. J Infect. 2005;51:e73–7.
62. Altner PC, Turner RR. Sporotrichosis of bones and joints: review of the literature and report of six cases. Clin Orthop. 1970;68:138–48.
63. Crout JE, Brewer NS, Tompkins RB. Sporotrichosis arthritis: clinical features in seven patients. Ann Intern Med. 1977;86:294–7.
64. Chowdhary G, Weinstein A, Klein R, Mascarenhas BR. Sporotrichal arthritis. Ann Rheum Dis. 1991;50:112–4.
65. Yao J, Penn RG, Ray S. Articular sporotrichosis. Clin Orthop. 1986;204:207–14.
66. Appenzeller S, Amaral TN, Amstalden EMI, et al. *Sporothrix schenckii* infection presented as monoarthritis: report of two cases and review of the literature. Clin Rheumatol. 2006;25:926–8.
67. Wilson DE, Mann J, Bennett JE, Utz JP. Clinical features of extra-cutaneous sporotrichosis. Medicine (Baltimore). 1967;46:265–79.
68. Stratton CW, Lichtenstein KA, Lowenstein SR, Phelps DB, Reller LB. Granulomatous tenosynovitis and carpal tunnel syndrome caused by *Sporothrix schenckii*. Am J Med. 1981;71:161–4.
69. Schwartz DA. *Sporothrix* tenosynovitis – differential diagnosis of granulomatous inflammatory disease of the joints. J Rheumatol. 1989;16:550–3.
70. Henry LR, Danaher PJ, Boseley ME. Laryngeal sporotrichosis mimicking merkel cell carcinoma recurrence. Otolaryngol Head Neck Surg. 2005;132:336–8.
71. Khabie N, Boyce TG, Roberts GD, Thompson DM. Laryngeal sporotrichosis causing stridor in a young child. Int J Pediatr Otorhinolaryngol. 2003;67:819–23.
72. Torrealba JR, Carvalho J, Corliss R, England D. Laryngeal granulomatous infection by *Sporothrix schenckii*. Otolaryngol Head Neck Surg. 2005;132:339–40.
73. Lurie HI. Five unusual cases of sporotrichosis from South Africa showing lesions in muscles, bones, and viscera. Br J Surg. 1963; 50:585–91.
74. Castrejon OV, Robles M, Zubieta Arroyo OE. Fatal fungaemia due to *Sporothrix schenckii*. Mycoses. 1995;38:373–6.
75. Donabedian H, O'Donnell E, Olszewski C, MacArthur RD, Budd N. Disseminated cutaneous and meningeal sporotrichosis in an AIDS patient. Diagn Microbiol Infect Dis. 1994;18:111–5.
76. Edwards C, Reuther WL, Greer DL. Disseminated osteoarticular sporotrichosis: treatment in a patient with acquired immunodeficiency syndrome. South Med J. 2000;93:803–6.
77. Cartwright MJ, Promersberger M, Stevens GA. *Sporothrix schenckii* endophthalmitis presenting as granulomatous uveitis. Br J Ophthalmol. 1993;77:61–2.
78. Kurosawa A, Pollock SC, Collins MP, Kraff CR, Tso MO. *Sporothrix schenckii* endophthalmitis in a patient with human immunodeficiency virus infection. Arch Ophthalmol. 1988; 106:376–80.
79. Burch JM, Morelli JG, Weston WL. Unsuspected sporotrichosis in childhood. Pediatr Infect Dis J. 2001;20:442–5.
80. Chandler JW, Kriel RL, Tosh FE. Childhood sporotrichosis. Am J Dis Child. 1968;115:368–72.
81. Gluckman I. Sporotrichosis in children. S Afr Med J. 1965; 39:991–1002.
82. Orr ER, Riley HD. Sporotrichosis in childhood: report of ten cases. J Pediatr. 1971;78:951–7.
83. al-Tawfiq JA, Wools KK. Disseminated sporotrichosis and *Sporothrix schenckii* fungemia as the initial presentation of human immunodeficiency virus infection. Clin Infect Dis. 1998;26: 1403–6.
84. Fontes PC, Kitakawa D, Carvalho YR, Brandão AA, Cabral LA, Almeida JD. Sporotrichosis in an HIV-positive man with oral lesions: a case report. Acta Cytol. 2007;51:648–50.
85. Fonseca-Reyes S, Maldonado F, Miranda-Ackerman R, et al. Extracutaneous sporotrichosis in a patient with liver cirrhosis. Rev Iberoam Micol. 2007;24:41–3.
86. Keiser P, Whittle D. Sporotrichosis in human immunodeficiency virus-infected patients: report of a case. Rev Infect Dis. 1991; 13:1027–8.
87. Silva-Vergara ML, Maneira FR, De Oliveira RM, Santos CT, Etchebehere RM, Adad SJ. Multifocal sporotrichosis with meningial involvement in a patient with AIDS. Med Mycol. 2005; 43:187–90.
88. Vilela R, Souza GF, Cota GF, Mendoza L. Cutaneous and meningeal sporotrichosis in a HIV patient. Rev Iberoam Micol. 2007; 24:161–3.

89. Kostman JR, DiNubile MJ. Nodular lymphangitis: a distinctive but often unrecognized syndrome. Ann Intern Med. 1993; 118:883–8.
90. Farley ML, Fagan MF, Mabry LC, Wallace RJ. Presentation of *Sporothrix schenckii* in pulmonary cytology specimens. Acta Cytol. 1991;35:389–95.
91. Scott EN, Kaufman L, Brown AC, Muchmore HG. Serologic studies in the diagnosis and management of meningitis due to *Sporothrix schenckii*. N Engl J Med. 1987;317:935–8.
92. Almeida-Paes R, Pimenta MA, Monteiro PC, Nosanchuk JD, Zancopé-Oliveira RM. Immunoglobulins G, M, and A against *Sporothrix schenckii* exoantigens in patients with sporotrichosis before and during treatment with itraconazole. Clin Vaccine Immunol. 2007;14:1149–57.
93. Bernardes-Engemann AR, Costa RC, Miguens BR, et al. Development of an enzyme-linked immunosorbent assay for the serodiagnosis of several clinical forms of sporotrichosis. Med Mycol. 2005;43:487–93.
94. Costa RO, de Mesquita KC, Damasco PS, et al. Infectious arthritis as the single manifestation of sporotrichosis: serology from serum and synovial fluid samples as an aid to diagnosis. Rev Iberoam Micol. 2008;25:54–6.
95. Kauffman CA, Bustamante B, Chapman SW, Pappas PG. Clinical practice guidelines for the management of sporotrichosis: 2007 update by the Infectious Diseases Society of America. Clin Infect Dis. 2007;45:1255–65.
96. de Almeida HL, Lettnin CB, Barbosa JL, Dias MC. Spontaneous resolution of zoonotic sporotrichosis during pregnancy. Rev Inst Med Trop S Paulo. 2009;51:237–8.
97. Urabe H, Nagasthima T. Mechanism of antifungal action of potassium iodide on sporotrichosis. Dermatol Int. 1969;1:36–8.
98. Sterling JB, Heymann WR. Potassium iodide in dermatology: a 19th century drug for the 21st century-users, pharmacology, adverse effects, and contraindications. J Am Acad Dermatol. 2000; 43:691–7.
99. Kauffman CA. Old and new therapies for sporotrichosis. Clin Infect Dis. 1995;21:981–5.
100. Rex JH, Bennett JE. Administration of potassium iodide to normal volunteers does not increase killing of *Sporothrix schenckii* by their neutrophils or monocytes. J Med Vet Mycol. 1990; 28:158–89.
101. Cabezas C, Bustamante B, Holgado W, Begue RE. Treatment of cutaneous sporotrichosis with one daily dose of potassium iodide. Pediatr Infect Dis J. 1996;15:352–4.
102. Coskun B, Saral Y, Akpolat N, Ataseven A, Çiçek D. Sporotrichosis successfully treated with terbinafine and potassium iodide: Case report and review of the literature. Mycopathologia. 2004; 158:53–6.
103. Thomas CL, Pierce HE, Babiner GW. Sporotrichosis responding to fever therapy. JAMA. 1951;147:1342–3.
104. Hiruma M, Kagawa S. The effects of heat on *Sporothrix schenckii in vitro* and *in vivo*. Mycopathologica. 1983;84:21–30.
105. Hiruma M, Kawada A, Noguchi H, Ishibashi A, Conti Diaz IA. Hyperthermic treatment of sporotrichosis: experimental use of infrared and far infrared rays. Mycoses. 1992;35:293–9.
106. Sharkey-Mathis PK, Kauffman CA, Graybill JR, et al. Treatment of sporotrichosis with itraconazole. Am J Med. 1993;95:279–85.
107. Restrepo A, Robledo J, Gomez I, Tabares AM, Gutiérrez R. Itraconazole therapy in lymphangitic and cutaneous sporotrichosis. Arch Dermatol. 1986;122:413–7.
108. Bonifaz A, Fierro L, Saúl A, Ponce RM. Cutaneous sporotrichosis. Intermittent treatment (pulses) with itraconazole. Eur J Dermatol. 2008;18:61–4.
109. Kauffman CA, Pappas PG, McKinsey DS, et al. Treatment of lymphocutaneous and visceral sporotrichosis with fluconazole. Clin Infect Dis. 1996;22:46–50.
110. Calhoun DL, Waskin H, White MP, et al. Treatment of systemic sporotrichosis with ketoconazole. Rev Infect Dis. 1991;13:47–51.
111. Alvarado-Ramírez E, Torrez-Rodríguez JM. In vitro susceptibility of *Sporothrix schenckii* to six antifungal agents determined using three differrent methods. Antimicrob Agents Chemother. 2007; 51:2420–3.
112. Marimon R, Serena C, Gené J, Cano J, Guarro J. In vitro antifungal susceptibilities of five species of *Sporothrix*. Antimicrob Agents Chemother. 2008;2:732–4.
113. Hull PR, Vismer HF. Treatment of cutaneous sporotrichosis with terbinafine. Br J Dermatol. 1992;39:51–5.
114. Hull PR, Vismer HF. Potential use of terbinafine in the treatment of cutaneous sporotrichosis. Rev Contemp Pharmacother. 1997; 8:343–7.
115. Kohler LM, Monteiro PC, Hahn RC, Hamdan JS. In vitro susceptibilities of isolates of *Sporothrix schenckii* to itraconazole and terbinafine. J Clin Microbiol. 2004;42:4319–20.
116. Chapman SW, Pappas P, Kauffman C, et al. Comparative evaluation of the efficacy and safety of two doses of terbinafine (500 and 100 mg day(−1)) in the treatment of cutaneous or lymphocutaneous sporotrichosis. Mycoses. 2004;47:62–8.
117. Francesconi G, Valle A, Passos S, Reis R, Galhardo M. Terbinafine (250 mg/day): an effective and safe treatment of cutaneous sporotrichosis. J Eur Acad Dermatol Venereol. 2009;23:1273–6.
118. Koëter S, Jackson RW. Successful total knee arthroplasty in the presence of sporotrichal arthritis. Knee. 2006;13:236–7.

Penicilliosis

Kenrad E. Nelson, Khuanchai Supparatpinyo, and Nongnuch Vanittanakom

More than 200 species of the *Penicillium* genus have been described. *Penicillium* organisms are abundant in nature and are common laboratory contaminants. However, *Penicillium marneffei* is the only dimorphic species. The organism is commonly responsible for disseminated invasive infections in humans with HIV infection or AIDS in the endemic areas of Southeast Asia and southern China. *Penicillium marneffei* has also been found to cause natural infections in several species of rodents in the endemic areas, and rodents can be infected experimentally.

History

Penicillium marneffei was originally isolated from the liver of a bamboo rat (*Rhizomys sinensis*) at the Pasteur Institute in Dalat, Viet Nam, in 1956. Capponi and colleagues observed the death of bamboo rats due to disseminated infections with *Penicillium* involving their reticuloendothelial system [1]. These investigators inoculated mice with the newly discovered organism, and it was sent to the Pasteur Institute. The fungus was characterized by Segretain and named *Penicillium marneffei* in honor of Dr. Hubert Marneffe, the Director of the Pasteur Institute of Indochina [2]. Subsequently, Segretain became the first known human to be infected with the organism in 1959 when he accidentally stuck his finger with a needle he was using to inoculate a hamster. The clinical manifestations of his infection were a subcutaneous nodule at the site of the inoculation and lymphadenitis involving the draining axillary lymph nodes. The infection responded to treatment with high doses of oral nystatin.

The first natural human infection with *P. marneffei* was reported in 1973 in a 61-year-old US missionary who was suffering from Hodgkin's disease. His infection was discovered when he underwent a staging splenectomy for Hodgkin's disease [3]. The missionary had visited Southeast Asia after Hodgkin's disease had been diagnosed 1 year prior to the splenectomy. At surgery the excised spleen contained a tan nodular mass, 9 cm in diameter with a necrotic center, which grew *P. marneffei* when cultured on Sabouraud dextrose agar at 25°C. The patient survived after being treated with amphotericin B.

The second case of penicilliosis was reported in 1984 in a 59-year-old man who had traveled in Southeast Asia [4]. He had recurrent episodes of hemoptysis, and *P. marneffei* organisms were isolated from his sputum. Also in 1984, five additional cases involving individuals who had been seen at Ramathibodi Hospital in Bangkok, Thailand, between 1974 and 1982 were reported [5]. Eight cases of *P. marneffei* infection were reported from Guangxi province in southern China that had occurred between 1964 and 1983 [6]. Additional cases were recognized from 1985 to 1991 in southern China [7–9]. These patients were not immunocompromised. All cases had occurred prior to the AIDS epidemic in Southeast Asia.

In the late 1980s and early 1990s several reports of disseminated penicilliosis in HIV-infected patients were published; these included patients who were infected in Southeast Asia but whose infections were diagnosed after they returned to the USA or Europe [10–17]. An HIV-positive Congolese physician developed disseminated penicilliosis while he was working at the Pasteur Institute in Paris [18]. The organism had not been handled directly by the physician, but organisms were being cultured in the building where he was attending a course. This case illustrates the potential hazard of laboratory-acquired infection and suggests an airborne route of infection.

As the HIV/AIDS pandemic has spread in Southeast Asia, *P. marneffei* infection has become a very common opportunistic infection in HIV-infected patients in the region [19–21]. Infection with this organism is now the fourth most common opportunistic infection in AIDS patients in northern Thailand, exceeded only by tuberculosis, *Pneumocystis jiroveci* pneumonia, and cryptococcosis [21]. A total of 550 cases of penicilliosis and 743 cases of cryptococcosis were diagnosed at

K.E. Nelson (✉)
Departments of Epidemiology, Bloomberg School of Public Health, International Health and Medicine, Johns Hopkins University, Baltimore, MD, USA
e-mail: kenelson@jhsph.edu

C.A. Kauffman, et al. (eds.), *Essentials of Clinical Mycology*,
DOI 10.1007/978-1-4419-6640-7_23, © Springer Science+Business Media, LLC 2011

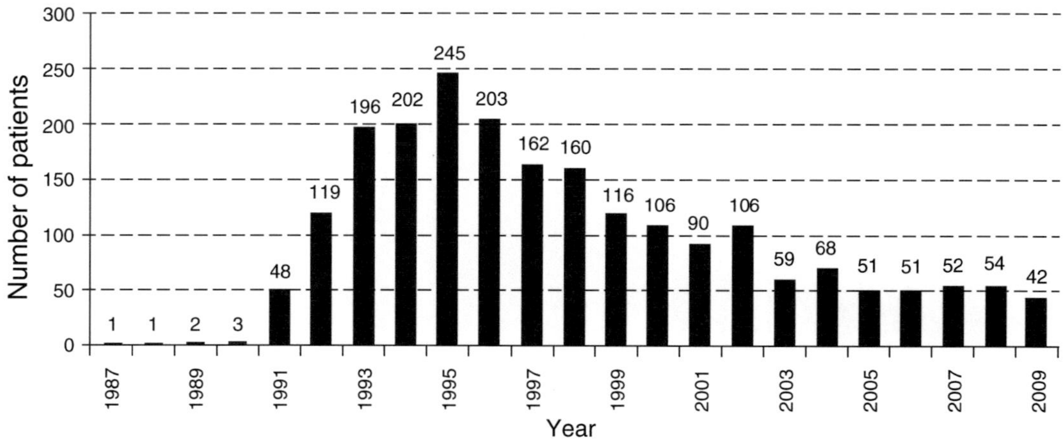

Fig. 1 Number of patients with HIV and *Penicillium marneffei* infection at Chiang Mai Hospital from 1987 to 2009

Chiang Mai University Hospital in northern Thailand between 1991 and 1994. Nearly all of these patients were HIV positive [22]. The number of patients with proven *P. marneffei* infection has declined in the last few years because of a decreased incidence of HIV and widespread availability of antiretroviral treatment (Fig. 1). The endemic area includes Thailand, southern China, Hong Kong, Taiwan, Burma, Laos, Vietnam, Malaysia, and northeast India.

Epidemiology

The natural reservoir of *P. marneffei* is almost certainly the soil. However, the organism was first isolated from Chinese bamboo rats, *Rhizomys sinensis*, in Vietnam in 1956 [1]. Since the original isolation, several investigators in China and Southeast Asia have cultured rodents and environmental samples in order to better understand the reservoir. The organism has been isolated from the internal organs of four species of bamboo rats in Asia (Table 1). Two investigators reported data from bamboo rats collected from Guangxi province in China. Deng and colleagues isolated *P. marneffei* from the internal organs of 18 of 19 *R. pruinosus* rats [24], and Li and colleagues found the organism in 15 of 16 *R. pruinosus* rats [8]. These infected animals showed no signs of illness. However, fatal infections had been observed in bamboo rats that were experimentally infected in Vietnam in 1956 [1, 29]. In another survey in Guangxi province in China, workers isolated *P. marneffei* from 39 of 43 bamboo rats (37 of 41 *R. pruinosus* and 2 of 2 *R. sinensis* [23]. They were also able to isolate *P. marneffei* from soil samples taken from three burrows of *R. pruinosus* rats and from the feces of three animals. Another survey in southern China isolated *P. marneffei* from 114 of 179 (63.7%) *R.* pruinosus rats [25]. A study of the prevalence of *P. marneffei* infections in bamboo rats in central Thailand was done in 1987, and *P. marneffei* was isolated from 6 of 8 (75%) *R. pruinosus* rats and 6 of 31 (19%) *Cannomys badius* rats [26]. Organisms were cultured from the lungs (83%), liver (33%), and pancreas (33%) of these animals.

The prevalence of *P. marneffei* in bamboo rats from northern Thailand was studied in 75 bamboo rats; *P. marneffei* was isolated from the internal organs of 13 of 14 (92.8%) large bamboo rats, *R. sumatrensis*, and 3 of 10 (30%) reddish-brown small bay bamboo rats, *Cannomys badius* [27]. All 51 grayish black *C. badius* rats were negative on culture. Among the *R. sumatrensis* rats, the fungus was most commonly isolated from lungs (86%), spleen (50%), and liver (29%). The investigators also studied 28 soil samples and 67 environmental samples, which had been collected from the residential areas of patients with clinical *P. marneffei* infection. These samples were evaluated using a modified flotation method combined with mouse inoculation to isolate the fungus from the environmental samples [30]. *Penicillium marneffei* was isolated from one soil sample obtained from a burrow of *R. sumatrensis* rats using this method [27]. The other environmental samples were negative.

It is somewhat curious that the prevalence of *P. marneffei* infection among bamboo rats is very high in the numerous surveys that have been reported in the literature, yet the fungus has not been isolated from any other animal in nature. This observation might reflect the animals that are selected for study, since other species have not been extensively studied. However, in part this finding might also reflect the fact that the range of the two genera of bamboo rats, *Rhizomys* and *Cannomys*, coincides with the environmental soil reservoir of *P. marneffei* [31] (Fig. 2). Furthermore, bamboo rats inhabit remote mountainous areas and have extensive soil contact when they burrow. The common isolation of *P. marneffei* from the lungs of infected animals and the rarity of recovery of the organism from the gastrointestinal tract suggests that *P. marneffei* infection is commonly acquired by these animals by inhaling conidia rather than by ingestion.

Table 1 Prevalence of *Penicillium marneffei* infection in trapped bamboo rats in Asia

Species	Positive/tested (%)	Country	References
Rhizomys sinenis	1/1 (100)	Vietnam	Capponi et al. [1]
(Chinese bamboo rat)	2/2(100)	China	Deng et al. [23]
Rhizomys pruinosus	37/41 (90)	China	Deng et al. [24]
(Hoary bamboo rat)	15/16 (94)	China	Li et al. [8]
	114/179 (64)	China	Wei et al. [25]
	6/8 (75)	Thailand	Ajello et al. [26]
Cannomys badius	6/31 (19)	Thailand	Ajello et al. [26]
(Bay bamboo rat or lesser bamboo rat)	3/61 (5)	Thailand	Chariyalertsak et al. [27]
	10/110 (9)	India	Gugnani et al. [28]
Rhizomys sumatrensis	13/14 (93)	Thailand	Chariyalertsak et al. [27]
(Sumatran bamboo rat)			

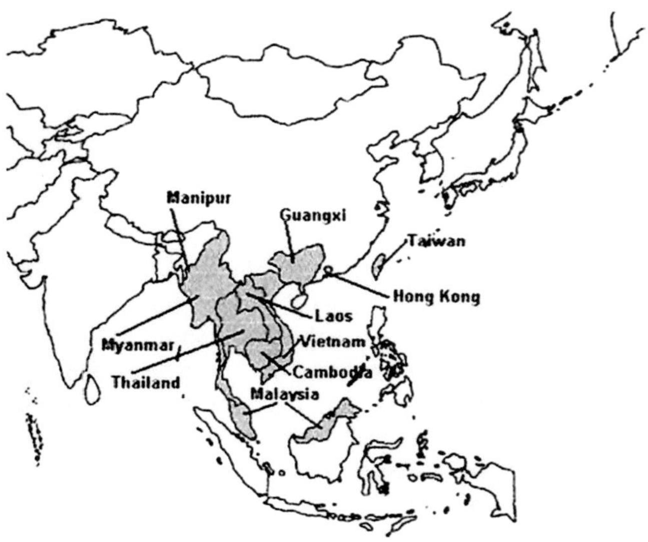

Fig. 2 Endemic areas for *Penicillium marneffei*

In a recent report from India 10 (9.1%) of 110 *C. badius* bamboo rats from Manipur were infected with *P. marneffei*, whereas 72 rodents of other species, including *Bandicota bengalensis*, *Rattus norvegicus*, *Rattus rattus*, *Rattus nitidus*, and *Mus musculus* were all negative. Since these rats were all collected from the same geographic area, and were studied with similar methods, the data suggest that bamboo rats may have increased susceptibility to infection. One bamboo rat isolate had an identical multilocus microsatellite typing pattern to a human isolate from this area [28].

A case-control study compared patients with AIDS who had *P. marneffei* infections to AIDS patients with negative *P. marneffei* cultures in order to help understand the risk factors associated with infection [32]. This study included 80 patients with penicilliosis and 160 control AIDS patients who were admitted to Chiang Mai University Hospital in northern Thailand between December 1993 and October 1995. The main risk factor was occupational soil exposures, especially during the rainy season. Both cases and controls often were familiar with and had seen bamboo rats; 31.3% of cases and 28.1% of controls had eaten bamboo rats but these differences were not significant. The most tenable hypothesis at present is that *P. marneffei* infections, both in humans and bamboo rats, are acquired from a common soil reservoir.

Disseminated *P. marneffei* infections in northern Thailand have been markedly seasonal with a doubling of cases during the rainy season [22]. This seasonality contrasts with *C. neoformans* infection in AIDS patients, which has shown a steady increase during the 1990s as the number of AIDS cases has increased but is not associated with seasonality. This seasonality suggests that many *P. marneffei* infections in AIDS patients may be acquired recently. Also, the environmental reservoir for *P. marneffei* appears to expand during the rainy season. Penicilliosis, while occurring in AIDS patients throughout Thailand, is much more common in the upper northern areas of the country [33]. Whereas penicilliosis accounted for nearly 7.0% of AIDS-defining illnesses in northern Thailand, penicilliosis was seen in only 0.4–1.0% of AIDS patients in other regions of the country. A total of 8,393 patients (2.4%) with disseminated *P. marneffei* infections were reported to the Ministry of Health of Thailand among 358,260 HIV/AIDS cases reported between September 1984 and October 2009 (website, Department of Disease Control, Ministry of Public Health, Thailand).

Organism

Penicillium marneffei grows as a mould on Sabouraud's dextrose agar at 25°C. The mycelial form of the organism is quite variable with green/yellow color with a reddish center. The reverse side of the colony becomes red-brown, and a soluble red pigment diffuses into the agar (Fig. 3). Microscopic examination of the mycelial colony reveals hyaline, septate, branched hyphae with branched conidiophores, or penicilli (Fig. 4). The conidiophores consist of basal stripes with terminal verticils of 3–5 metulae. Each metula has 3–16 phialides. The conidia are oval, smooth-walled, and are 3 μm×2 μm. They are formed basipetally in chains from each phialide. When the organism is transferred to brain–heart infusion agar

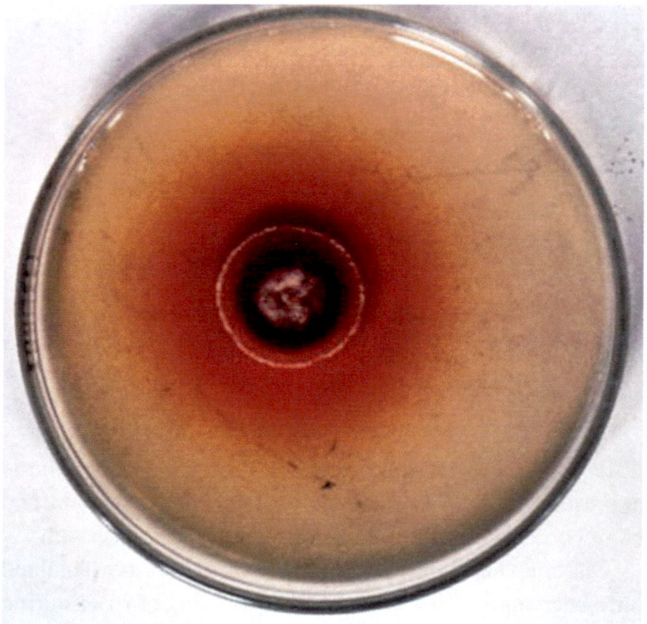

Fig. 3 Mould form of *Penicillium marneffei* plated on Sabouraud's dextrose agar after incubation at 25°C for 5 days, showing the characteristic soluble red pigment that has diffused into the medium

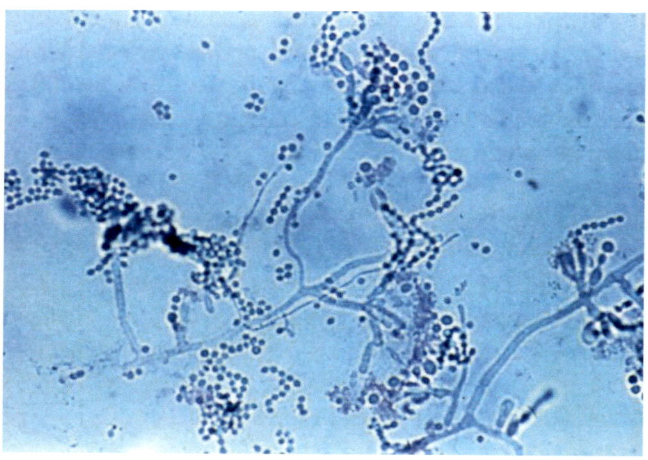

Fig. 4 Mould form of *Penicillium marneffei* grown on Sabouraud's dextrose agar at 25°C. Note the hyaline septate branching hyphae with branched conidiophores, or penicilli, and terminal conidia (600×)

and incubated at 37°C, white to tan-colored colonies of the yeast form develop; no diffusible pigment is produced. Under the microscope the yeasts are unicellular, pleomorphic, elliptical to rectangular cells, which are approximately 2 μm×6 μm in diameter and divide by fission. One or occasionally two septae are seen in the yeast cells.

The organism was first studied in 1959 [2]. *Penicillium marneffei* was originally classified among *Penicillium* species in the section Asymmetrica, subsection of Divaricata in Raper and Thom's taxonomic classification of *Penicillium* species [34]. Pitt later placed *P. marneffei* in the subgenus *Biverticillium* [35]. Recent phylogenetic analysis of nucleotide sequences of nuclear and mitochondrial ribosomal DNA has found that *P. marneffei* is closely related to species of *Penicillium* subgenus *Biverticillium* and sexual *Talaromyces* species with asexual biverticillate states [36]. This genetic analysis allowed the design of unique oligonucleatide primers for the specific amplification of *P. marneffei* DNA.

Penicillium marneffei requires an organic source of nitrogen for mycelial growth. Casein hydrolysate, peptone, and asparagine are utilized, whereas $NaNO_3$ and $(NH_4)_2\ PO_4$ are not. Glucose, lactose, xylose, maltose, laevulose, and mannitol are used as carbon sources. The organism is sensitive to cycloheximide [37]. Investigators have biotyped 32 clinical isolates of *P. marneffei* and found 17 different biotypes [38]. However, none of the biotypes correlated with the clinical characteristics of the infection.

Pathogenesis

Penicillium marneffei infection results from the inhalation of infectious spores or hyphal fragments from the mould form of the organism. At body temperatures (35–37°C), the fungus converts to the yeast form which is disseminated by hematogenous means. The organism primarily infects the reticuloendothelial system, commonly involving liver, spleen, lymph nodes, bone marrow, bone, skin, and lungs. *Penicillium marneffei* conidia bind to the extracellular matrix protein laminin via a sialic acid-dependent process [39]. Also, *P. marneffei* conidia bind to fibronectin, but the binding is less than that to laminin. This binding is also sialic acid-dependent [40]. Similar to other pathogenic dimorphic fungi, the initial host response to *P. marneffei* is histiocytic in nature. The infected histiocytes contain anywhere from a few to many globose to oval yeast cells of *P. marneffei* of fairly uniform size. In the immunocompetent host, the immune response leads to the formation of granulomas that include histiocytes, lymphocytes, plasma cells, and multinucleated giant cells. In patients whose cellular immunity is compromised, tissue necrosis occurs with little or no granuloma formation. Necrotic lesions are surrounded by histiocytes containing yeast cells. Many extracellular yeasts are also present, which are longer and may be irregular in shape compared to intracellular organisms. This histopathologic appearance is common in patients with disseminated penicilliosis. As the infection progresses, the intracellular fungi are released after cellular disruption, and abscess formation and necrosis may occur.

In histologic specimens, neither the cell wall nor the cytoplasm of *P. marneffei* cells takes up hematoxylin eosin stain well. Thus, in routine stained sections, the organisms may appear to be encapsulated. However, the cell walls and septae are readily stained with Gomori methenamine-silver or periodic acid-Schiff stains. The *P. marneffei* organisms in histiocytes resemble *H. capsulatum* var. *capsulatum*. However, when found extracellularly, *P. marneffei* is usually considerably larger than *H. capsulatum*. The extracellular *P. marneffei* organisms are elongated, sometimes curved, and measure up to 8–13 μm in length. In contrast, yeast cells of *H. capsulatum* var. *capsulatum* are smaller in size, measuring 2–4 μm. By contrast, *H. capsulatum* var. *duboisii* cells are larger, measuring 6–17 μm. *P. marneffei* organisms characteristically contain a single transverse septum and divide by schizogony (fission), whereas *Histoplasma* divide by budding (Table 2).

Chronic latent infections with *P. marneffei* are likely to be common among persons exposed in areas where the organism is endemic. This hypothesis is supported in part by analogy with histoplasmosis pathogenesis and by the long latent periods in some patients between exposure in an endemic area and the onset of clinical infection subsequent to immunosuppression from HIV infection [12, 47]. However, no laboratory methods have been reported to detect latently infected individuals. The development of a skin test or other methods to detect delayed-type hypersensitivity has not been reported for *P. marneffei*. The normal host develops a cell-mediated immune response to *P. marneffei* [23]. The role of T lymphocytes in host defenses against *P. marneffei* has been evaluated in mice experimentally depleted of CD4+ T lymphocytes [48]. These mice developed disseminated infections similar to those seen in AIDS patients. In addition, the in vitro interaction of *P. marneffei* with human leukocytes demonstrated that monocyte-derived macrophages recognize and phagocytose *P. marneffei* even in the absence of opsonization [49]. However, serum factors are required to stimulate TNF-α production. The organisms are able to survive as intracellular pathogens within macrophages. One mechanism of survival is by inhibiting the production of reactive oxygen metabolites or by neutralizing inhibitory host metabolites [50]. The production of acid phosphatase is one of the virulence factors which protects the intracellular *P. marneffei* from the respiratory burst. *Histoplasma capsulatum* has three catalase genes which detoxify hydrogen peroxide [51]. Also, an antigenic catalase-peroxidase protein encoding gene (*cpeA*) in *P. marneffei* was recently isolated by antibody screening of a cDNA yeast-phase library of this organism [52]. The high expression of this *cpeA* gene at 37°C may contribute to the survival of this fungus within host cells. Recently a copper-zinc superoxide dismutase encoding gene has been described and characterized in *P. marneffei* [53]. This polypeptide enzyme has the ability to neutralize toxic levels of reactive oxygen species within the macrophage, thereby allowing the intracellular survival of the organism. Additional research on the sequence of phagocytosis and killing or persistence of *P. marneffei* is needed in order to better understand the natural history and pathogenesis of this infection.

Studies of fungal pathogenesis have included heat shock responses during phase transition as an adaptation response to a higher incubation temperature or to the presence of other noxious stimuli [54, 55]. Recently, *hsp70*, the gene encoding heat shock protein 70 (Hsp70), was cloned and characterized from *P. marneffei* [56]. Expression of *hsp70* is upregulated during temperature-induced and heat shock condition. Moreover, protein profiling of both mould and yeast phases of *P. marneffei* demonstrated the same Hsp70 expression pattern [57, 58]. Expression of a small heat shock protein gene, *P. marneffei* Hsp30, in response to temperature increase was recently reported [59]. A high level of *hsp30* transcript was detected in yeast cells grown at 37°C, whereas a very low or undetectable transcript level was observed in mycelial cells at 25°C. A recombinant Hsp30 protein was produced and tested preliminarily for its immunoreactivity with sera from *P. marneffei*-infected AIDS patients using Western blot analysis. The positive immunoblot result with some serum samples confirmed the antigenic property of the Hsp30. Collectively, the high response of *hsp70* and *hsp30* to temperature increase could indicate that they may play a role in heat stress response and cell adaptation, thereby enabling the parasitic growth of *P. marneffei* in host cells.

Table 2 Microbiologic characteristics of *Penicillium marneffei* and *Histoplasma capsulatum*

Characteristic	*P. marneffei*	*H. capsulatum*
Morphologic features	Biphasic (mould form at 25–30°C, yeast form at 35–37°C)	Biphasic (mould form at 25–30°C, yeast form at 35–37°C)
Distribution	Southern China and Southeast Asia	Worldwide (N. America, S. America, Asia, Africa (*H. duboisii*))
Tissue form	Yeast	Yeast
Size; intracellular (Macrophages)	2–3 × 2–6 μm	2–3 × 2–3 μm
Extracellular	2–3 × 8–13 μm, elongated, curved	Smaller 3–4 μm, diameter
	Septae visible with GMS stain	(*H. duboisii* larger, 6–17 μm diameter)
		No septae
Cell division	Schizogony (fission)	Budding
Specific exoantigen	Positive	Positive

Another possible host-pathogen factor that may play a role in virulence is pigment production. The red pigment of *P. marneffei*, which is synthesized only by the mould phase and is similar to that produced by the nonpathogenic species *Penicillium herquei* [60], is not considered a virulence factor. However, melanins are known virulence factors for many pathogenic fungi [61]. Most fungal melanins are synthesized by either the 3,4-dihydroxy-L-phenylalanine (L-DOPA) or dihydroxynapthalene pathways. Collectively, these dark pigments appear to function in a variety of protective roles, including the inhibition of killing by phagocytes. Like other fungal pathogens, yeast cells of *P. marneffei* have been shown to produce L-DOPA melanin in vivo [62]. Further experimentation will be needed to assess whether melanin may be involved in the virulence of *P. marneffei*.

The collective data described above reveal some insights into the pathogenesis of *P. marneffei* that will need more investigation for the functions of those reported genes or factors involved in phase transition and virulence. Such knowledge may lead to better chemotherapeutic interventions of *P. marneffei* infection.

Clinical Manifestations

Clinically apparent infection with *P. marneffei* occurs most frequently in patients who are severely immunocompromised from an HIV infection. However, infections may also occur in healthy persons or in those immunocompromised for reasons other than HIV/AIDS [63, 64]. Serologic evidence of subclinical infection in a laboratory technician working with the organism has been demonstrated [65]. It is likely that subclinical infections may occur commonly in persons living in endemic areas who are exposed to the organism in nature; however, there is no method to document subclinical infections at present. Disseminated infections have been documented among individuals who have not had contact with areas where the organism is endemic for more than a decade [12].

Typical symptoms and signs of disseminated penicilliosis include fever, malaise, marked weight loss, generalized lymphadenopathy, hepatosplenomegaly, and cough [19, 21]. These nonspecific symptoms are commonly experienced by patients with other chronic infections, such as tuberculosis and other disseminated mycoses. In addition, over 70% of HIV-infected patients with disseminated *P. marneffei* infections present with skin lesions, which are typically symmetrical lesions on the face, chest, and extremities. They appear originally as papules and subsequently become umbilicated, and may become necrotic (Figs. 5–7). Some patients may have smaller, nearly confluent papules, which resemble acne vulgaris or seborrhea. Although skin lesions are more common in patients with *P. marneffei* infection than in those with histoplasmosis or cryptococcosis, the appearance of these lesions is not sufficiently characteristic to be diagnostic. However, a diagnosis can be made by examining a Wright's stain of a skin biopsy or skin smear.

Patients with HIV infection who have disseminated penicilliosis are usually severely immunosuppressed with CD4+ cell counts below 100 cells/μL; the mean CD4+ cell count in one series of cases was 63.8 cells/μL [64]. Disseminated penicilliosis infections have been reported in children with AIDS who lived in an endemic area [66]; however, the incidence appears to be lower in pediatric than in adult AIDS cases, probably because of less frequent exposure to an environmental reservoir among children. One study reported 5 cases of penicilliosis among 157 pediatric AIDS cases diagnosed in northern Thailand [66].

Unusual Clinical Manifestations

As the pandemic of HIV/AIDS spread in Asia and penicilliosis was more widely recognized, an increasing number of patients have been reported with unusual manifestations of *P. marneffei* infections. Patients with chronic lymphadenopathy resembling tuberculous lymphadenopathy have been reported from Hong Kong [67]. Osteomyelitis has been reported in infected adults and may be more common in pediatric patients infected with *P. marneffei* [66, 68]. Some patients have prominent pulmonary symptoms, including localized bronchopulmonary disease, bronchopneumonia,

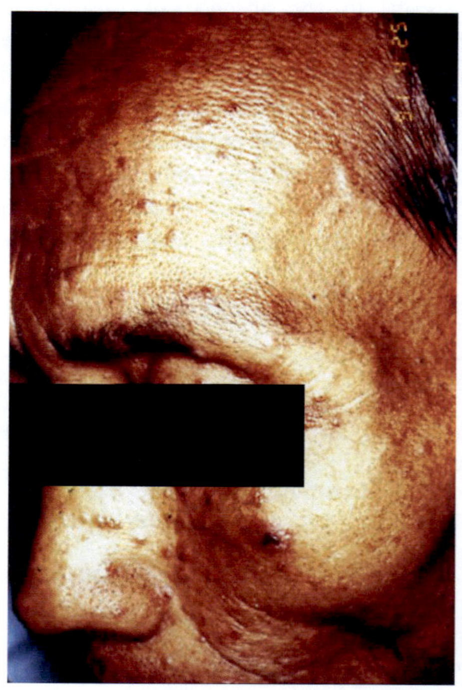

Fig. 5 Patient with disseminated penicilliosis and small papular skin lesions with umbilication and early central necrosis

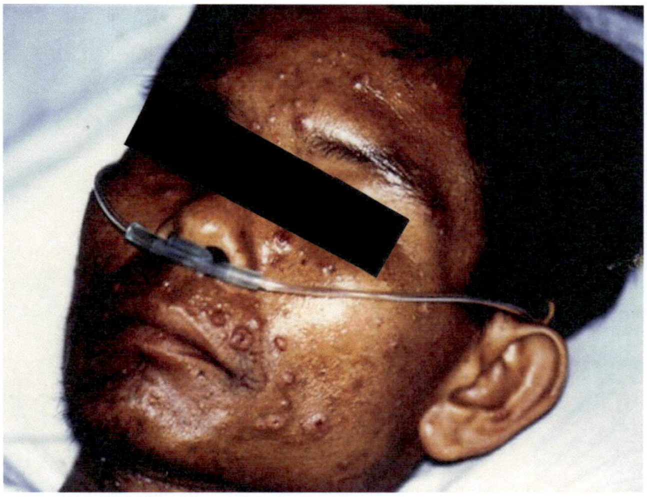

Fig. 6 Young man with disseminated penicilliosis and papulo-umbilicated skin lesions of varying sizes

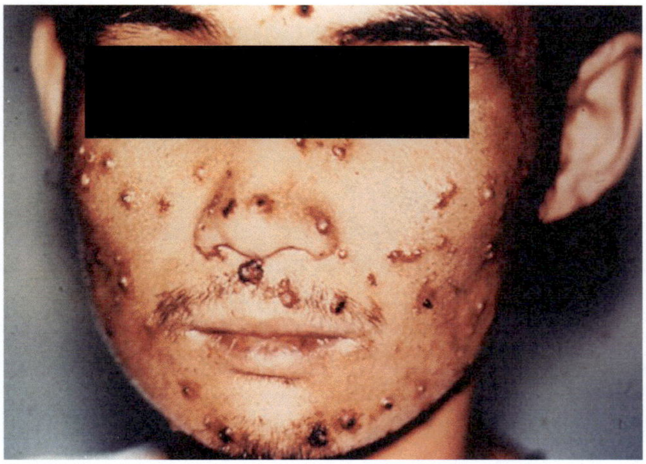

Fig. 7 Papulonecrotic skin lesions seen in a patient with disseminated penicilliosis

cavitary lung disease, and pleural effusions [69, 70]. A retropharyngeal abscess with upper airway obstruction has also been observed [71]. One patient had reactive hemophagocytic syndrome characterized by the proliferation of activated histiocytes throughout the reticuloendothelial system [72]. Rarely, *P. marneffei* has been noted to cause oral [73] and genital ulceration [74].

Penicilliosis in HIV-negative Patients

Although most patients with disseminated penicilliosis infection are severely immunocompromised due to AIDS, some patients are HIV negative. Cooper and Haycocks reviewed 63 penicilliosis cases that had been reported in HIV-negative patients. Twenty-four of the 63 patients (38%) had other conditions predisposing them to a systemic fungal infection. The response to antifungal therapy did not differ substantially whether or not the patients were HIV infected; patients who were untreated had very high mortality rates irrespective of their HIV status [75].

Investigators from Hong Kong compared the clinical and laboratory features of eight HIV-positive and seven HIV-negative patients with penicilliosis [76]. Most of the HIV-negative patients (85.2%) had underlying diseases, including hematologic malignancies, or had received corticosteroids or cytotoxic drugs. The clinical features were not greatly different in the two groups of patients. However, HIV-infected patients had a higher prevalence of fungemia. The investigators, utilizing a *P. marneffei*-specific mannoprotein, Mp1p EIA, found that serum antigen titers were higher in HIV-positive patients, whereas serum antibody levels were higher in HIV-negative patients.

Diagnosis

The diagnosis of penicilliosis rests on the demonstration of the organism in the tissues or the isolation of the organism in cultures from infected patients.

Cultures

The organism grows readily on routine mycologic media, such as Sabouraud dextrose agar or inhibitory mould agar. When cultures are incubated at 25–30°C, *P. marneffei* grows as a mould with typical filamentous reproductive structures of the genus *Penicillium*. The mould form produces a pink or rose-red pigment that diffuses into the medium (Fig. 3). Other *Penicillium* species may also produce a pigment [77]. Therefore, conversion of an organism to the yeast form is required before concluding the isolate is *P. marneffei*. The organism grows as a yeast when incubated at 35–37°C. This form does not produce a red pigment. When incubated at this temperature, the organism undergoes transition into the yeast phase after 12–24 h or so of incubation. The conidia swell and develop into septate hyphae. These hyphae fragment and develop single cells that divide by schizogony (fission). The conversion of the mycelial phase of the organism into the fission yeast phase at higher incubation temperatures is diagnostic of *P. marneffei*. No other *Penicillium* converts to the yeast phase when incubated at 35–37°C. In addition, an exoantigen test for *P. marneffei* has been described, which can also be used to identify cultures of the organism [37].

The organism can be isolated from several sites, including skin, blood, bone marrow, lymph nodes, and sputum. In a population of patients in northern Thailand with disseminated penicilliosis, the organism was isolated from the blood cultures of 76% of 78 patients [20]. However, the blood cultures were positive for gram-negative bacilli (*Salmonella choleraesuis*, *S. enteritidis*, and *Shigella flexneri*) in 9 of the 19 patients whose cultures did not yield *P. marneffei*. Since these gram-negative organisms grow more rapidly, they could have outgrown the fungus and been responsible for a false-negative culture for *P. marneffei*.

Histopathology

Detection of the organism in biopsies or touch smears of skin lesions or bone marrow aspirates is often possible. A presumptive diagnosis can be made if microscopic examination of a Wright or Giemsa-stained specimen discloses intracellular or extracellular basophilic, spherical, oval, and elliptical yeast-like organisms that are 3–8 μm in diameter, and if the organisms have a clear central septation and are dividing by schizogony (fission) (Fig. 8). *Histoplasma capsulatum* can resemble *P. marneffei*, but *H. capsulatum* divides by budding and is usually smaller. Occasionally *P. marneffei* can be detected in stained smears of peripheral blood [70]. Recently several investigators have reported the identification of *P. marneffei* nucleic acids in clinical specimens as a diagnostic method [78–81].

The use of an exoantigen test has been described for the identification of *P. marneffei* and its differentiation from other species of *Penicillium* [37, 82]; however, the test is not widely used because commercial reagents are not available. Investigators have described the use of a monoclonal antibody in formalin-fixed tissues to detect a specific galactomannan that has an epitope common to *P. marneffei* and *Aspergillus* species [83]. The two invasive fungi must then be differentiated using morphologic criteria. Workers have also reported the use of a specific fluorescent antibody that will differentiate *P. marneffei* from other dimorphic fungi in tissue sections [84].

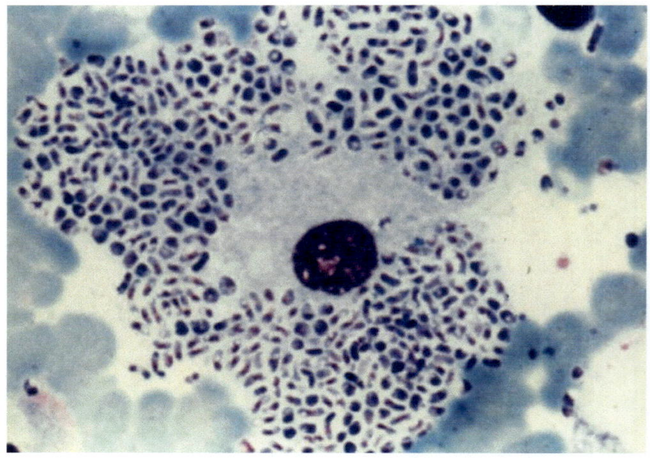

Fig. 8 Bone marrow aspirate showing numerous basophilic bipolar intracellular and extracellular *Penicillium marneffei* organisms in the yeast form. The organisms divide by fission (schizogony) and are 3–8 μm in diameter (Wright's stain, 400×)

Serology

Several investigators using different methodologies have reported the detection of antibodies to *P. marneffei* antigens in infected patients. A study in an HIV-infected patient found *P. marneffei* antibodies in serum specimens using immunodiffusion methods with a mycelial phase culture filtrate as antigen [48]. Similar antibodies were found in immunocompetent patients infected with *P. marneffei* [85]. Immunodiffusion has been used to detect antibodies to specific fission arthroconidial filtrate antigens; however, only 2 of 17 *P. marneffei*-infected patients had antibody responses with this assay [86]. An indirect fluorescent antibody test for *P. marneffei* successfully detected antibodies in eight infected patients and was negative in uninfected controls [87]. Serum antibodies were detected by ELISA to a purified recombinant mannoprotein of *P. marneffei* in 14 of 17 (82%) HIV-infected patients with documented infection [88]. No false-positive results were found in 90 healthy blood donors, 20 patients with typhoid fever, or 55 patients with tuberculosis.

The protein antigens of yeast and mould phases of *P. marneffei* have been studied by gel electrophoresis and immunoblot assays [89]. More than 20 yeast phase proteins were detected, of which 10 reacted with IgG in the pooled sera of 28 AIDS patients with *P. marneffei* infection. Four immunogenic proteins of 200, 88, 54, and 50 kDa size were produced in large quantity by cultures in the early stationary growth phase. Antibodies to two of these proteins, 54 and 50 kDa, were detected by immunoblot in about 60% of *P. marneffe*-infected AIDS patients but rarely (<5–10%) in AIDS patients without penicilliosis or other controls. One patient's serum was strongly positive 2 months prior to a clinical *P. marneffei* infection, and one asymptomatic laboratory worker working with *P. marneffei* cultures was antibody positive. Further studies of these proteins and a 61-kDa antigen after purification found that 86% of sera from 21 *P. marneffei*-infected patients recognized the 61-kDa, and 71% and 48% recognized the 54-kDa and 50-kDa antigens, respectively [90]. Other investigators have identified a 38-kDa antigen from *P. marneffei* that was recognized by 45% of sera from AIDS patients with penicilliosis [91].

Antigen Detection

Several investigators have described methods to detect *P. marneffei* antigens in serum or urine of infected patients as a method to confirm the diagnosis prior to the isolation of the organism in culture. Evaluation of immunodiffusion and latex agglutination tests to detect antigenemia in 17 *P. marneffei*-infected patients yielded positive results in 58.8% of infected patients with the immunodiffusion test and 76.5% of patients with the latex agglutination test [86]. Fifteen controls and six patients with cryptococcosis and histoplasmosis were nonreactive. A solid-phase enzyme immunoassay utilizing antibody to *H. capsulatum* var. *capsulatum* to detect *H. capsulatum* antigen in the urine of actively infected patients was cross-reactive with *P. marneffei* in 17 of 18 patients [92]. This assay also was commonly positive in patients with *Blastomyces dermatitidis* and *Paracoccidioides brasiliensis* infections.

Desakorn and colleagues reported the development of a method for quantifying *P. marneffei* antigen in the urine using fluorescein isothiocyanate-labeled purified rabbit hyperimmune immunoglobulin G in an enzyme immunoassay [93]. These investigators studied 33 patients with culture-proven *P. marneffei* infection and 300 controls, including 52 healthy subjects and 248 hospitalized patients in northeast Thailand with a variety of other infections, including melioidosis (N=168), other septicemias (N = 12), other fungal infections (N=34), and miscellaneous conditions (N = 34). All of the patients with penicilliosis had measureable antigen in the urine, and in all but two patients, the titers were over 1:40; the median titer was 1:20,480. Whereas 27% of the hospitalized controls and 6% of healthy subjects were positive, the titers were usually below 1:40 in these control groups, leading the investigators to propose a diagnostic cutoff titer of 1:40, which yielded an assay that was 97% sensitive and 98% specific and had a positive predictive value of 84.2% and a negative predictive value of 99.7%.

A follow-up study using this antigen assay in 37 *P. marneffei*-infected patients and 300 controls using ELISA, dot-blot ELISA, or latex agglutination (LA) to detect *P. marneffei* antigen in the urine found sensitivities of 94.6% (dot-ELISA), 97.3% (ELISA), and 100% (LA) and specificities of 97.3–99.3%) [94]. Huang et al. reported that a Platelia *Aspergillus* enzyme immunoassay kit (BioRad) to detect serum galactomannan in patients with *P. marneffei* had a sensitivity of 73.3% [95].

Molecular Diagnosis

Molecular diagnosis in *P. marneffei* is based on specific oligonucleotide primers designed from the internally transcribed spacer and 5.8 S rRNA gene (ITS1-5.8 S-ITS2) of *P. marneffei*. The specificity of these *P. marneffei* primers was tested in a nested PCR [36], and the method was used successfully to identify *P. marneffei* from a skin biopsy [96]. An oligonucleotide probe, based on the 18 S rDNA of *P. marneffei*, has been designed and has proved specific for *P. marneffei* in a PCR-hybridization reaction, regardless of whether the fungus was isolated from humans or natural habitats [97]. This technique could be used to detect *P. marneffei* DNA in EDTA-blood samples collected from AIDS patients with *P. marneffei* infection. Although the method was shown to be highly sensitive and specific, the hybridization technique as described is labor intensive and requires a high level of competence in the laboratory.

To address these concerns, single and nested PCR methods for the rapid identification of *P. marneffei* were then developed using newly designed specific primers, also based on the 18 S rDNA sequence of *P. marneffei* [98]. The sensitivities of single and nested PCR were 1.0 pg/μL and 1.8 fg/μL, respectively, and successful discrimination of a very young culture of *P. marneffei* (2-day-old filamentous colony, 2 mm in diameter) could be performed by the use of this assay. The test has been applied to detect the DNA of *P. marneffei* in patients' serum samples [79, 80] and also in paraffin-embedded tissues [81] from patients and bamboo rats. This PCR method appears to be a valuable, rapid, and complementary technique for the diagnosis of *P. marneffei* infection.

Finally, several investigators have reported methods using restriction enzymes to subtype *P. marneffei* isolates. The use of *Hae*III restriction enzymes to digest *P. marneffei* DNA yielded two DNA profiles (RFLP types I and II) [99]. More recently, the use of *Not*I and pulsed-field gel electrophoresis (PFGE) was used to study the genomic DNA of 64 *P. marneffei* isolates from patients in Thailand [100]. A total of 54 distinct macrorestriction profiles were identified in these patients. Antifungal sensitivity tests, restriction fragment-length polymorphism, and randomly amplified polymorphic DNA patterns in combination have been utilized to subtype 24 strains isolated between 1987 and 1998 from patients in Taiwan [101]. The investigators identified eight highly related patterns and found increased numbers and diversity of strains isolated between 1996 and 1998 compared to those isolated prior to 1996.

Treatment

Disseminated penicilliosis is usually fatal if not treated with appropriate antifungal drugs. However, with early diagnosis and institution of appropriate therapy the mortality rate can be reduced to 10–20% or lower, even among patients with AIDS. Relapse is commonly seen after clinical response among immunocompromised patients unless suppressive doses of antifungal agents are continued.

The in vitro susceptibility of *P. marneffei* to antifungal agents has been evaluated by several investigators (Table 3). A study of 30 clinical isolates from Thailand found that all

Table 3 In vitro drug susceptibility (MIC, range) of *Penicillium marneffei*

References	Number of isolates	Amb	Flu	Itra	Keto	Vor
Jayanetra et al. [5]	3	0.78–3.12	ND	ND	ND	
Sekhon et al. [41]	10	<0.195–1.56	0.195–100	<0.195	0.195–0.39	
Drouhet [42]	10	0.04–1.6	50	≤0.04	≤0.04	
Supparatpinyo et al. [43]	30	0.25–4.0	≤0.313–20	≤0.02–0.078	0.002–0.078	
Imwidthaya et al. [44]	30	0.125–0.5	4.0–8.0	<0.032	<0.125	
Radford et al. [45]	7			≤0.03		≤0.03
Sar et al. [46]	29	0.002–2.0	1.50–256.0	0.002–0.23	0.002–0.19	

Amb amphotericin B, *Flu* fluconazole, *Itra* itraconazole, *Keto* ketoconazole, *Vor* voriconazole

were susceptible to itraconazole, ketoconazole, and miconazole [43]. The organisms were intermediately susceptible to amphotericin B and least susceptible to fluconazole. Some strains were resistant to fluconazole. A study of 29 isolates from AIDS patients in Cambodia and 10 isolates from the lungs of bamboo rats found similar sensitivities to antifungal drugs to the report from Thailand [46]. The in vitro sensitivity of *P. marneffei* to voriconazole is similar to that of itraconazole [45]. Clinical responses to therapy correlate with in vitro susceptibility. Amphotericin B has been shown to be effective in the treatment of disseminated penicilliosis [102]; however, the drug needs to be continued for at least 6–8 weeks. Itraconazole is also effective clinically, but clearance of positive fungal cultures is often delayed for 8 weeks or more [103].

Therapy with voriconazole given intravenously at 6 mg/kg on day 1, 4 mg/kg the next 2 days, and then orally at 200–400 mg twice daily yielded good treatment results in nine of ten evaluable patients [104]. However, the reported experience with voriconazole therapy of *P. marneffei* is limited.

Based upon these clinical results and in vitro data on the antifungal susceptibility of *P. marneffei*, an open-label noncomparative study was done to evaluate the regimen of amphotericin B given intravenously for 2 weeks at 0.6 mg/kg/day followed by itraconazole 400 mg/day taken orally for 10 weeks. This regimen was evaluated in the hope of minimizing the duration and toxicity associated with parenteral amphotericin B while concurrently clearing the fungal cultures more rapidly than with oral itraconazole alone [102]. Of 74 HIV-positive patients with disseminated pencilliosis treated with this regimen, 72 (97.3%) responded. No serious adverse drug effects were observed. After 2 weeks of therapy, 12 patients remained febrile and 11 patients still had skin lesions. By the fourth week of therapy, all patients were afebrile and had resolved their skin lesions. Fungemia was cleared after 2 weeks of treatment in the 65 patients who had a positive blood culture at baseline [102].

Since most patients who present with *P. marneffei* have advanced immunosuppression at the time of diagnosis, initiation of antiretroviral therapy (ART) is recommended in all patients unless there is clear contraindication. The appropriate time for initiation of ART in HIV patients with active opportunistic infection is still controversial. However, ART should be initiated within approximately 2–8 weeks of antifungal therapy in order to match the benefit seen with earlier ART in other opportunistic infections [105].

The immune restoration inflammatory syndrome (IRIS) has been reported uncommonly in HIV patients with *P. marneffei* infection. [106–108] It usually occurs within a few weeks or months after starting ART, suggesting a possibility of immune reconstitution unmasking active disease. Antiretroviral therapy should be continued even if the IRIS occurs. In patients with severe symptomatic IRIS, short-course glucocorticosteroids may be useful [105].

Despite the favorable initial responses to therapy with amphotericin B and itraconazole, relapses are common after antifungal therapy is discontinued in patients with AIDS who have low CD4 counts [43]. Therefore, continued suppressive therapy is required to prevent relapse in patients with disseminated penicilliosis who respond to initial therapy. Suppressive therapy is probably required in AIDS patients for as long as significant immunocompromise persists. In a controlled trial of 71 HIV-infected patients with penicilliosis in Thailand who were not receiving retroviral therapy, 20 (57%) of 35 patients assigned to the placebo group relapsed, whereas none of 36 patients given suppressive itraconazole 200 mg once daily relapsed ($p<0.001$) [109]. The therapy was well tolerated, and the patients in this trial were very compliant with treatment. Suppressive antifungal therapy may be discontinued safely in HIV-infected patients who are treated with ART drugs and respond with clinically significant increases in their CD4 counts [110].

In areas where systemic fungal infections such as *P. marneffei*, *H. capsulatum*, *C. neoformans*, and other fungal infections are common AIDS-associated opportunistic infections, primary prophylaxis against these infections should be considered. In northern Thailand HIV infections are common, involving 2–3% of the general population. Moreover, disseminated fungal infections, especially these due to *P. marneffei*, *C. neoformans*, and *H. capsulatum*, are also common, accounting for over a third of the reported AIDS-defining illnesses in this population [33]. In order to evaluate the efficacy of primary prophylaxis to prevent systemic fungal infection in this population, a clinical trial was done in 129 patients who were HIV positive, had CD4 cell counts <200 cells/μL, and had not experienced a systemic fungal infection. Patients were randomized to receive oral itraconazole (200 mg/day) or a matched placebo [63]. Systemic fungal infections developed in 1 (1.6%) of 63 patients assigned to itraconazole and 11 (16.7%) of 66 patients assigned to placebo ($p = .003$). In the placebo group, 7 patients developed cryptococcosis and 4 had penicilliosis. The one patient in the itraconazole group who became infected developed penicilliosis. Clearly, prophylaxis to prevent systemic fungal infections is only necessary in AIDS patients whose HIV infection is not effectively treated with ART. Several clinical trials have clearly shown that patients with systemic pneumocystis [111], cryptococcosis [112], or histoplasmosis [113] are not at risk of relapse of their infection if they have a satisfactory response to HIV therapy.

References

1. Capponi M, Segretain G, Sureau P. Penicillosis from *Rhizomys sinensis*. Bull Soc Pathol Exot Filiales. 1956;49:418–21.
2. Segretain G. Description d'une nouvelle espiece de pencillium: *Penicillium marneffei* n. sp. Bull Soc Mycol France. 1959;75:412–6.
3. DiSalvo AF, Fickling AM, Ajello L. Infection caused by *Penicillium marneffei*: description of first natural infection in man. Am J Clin Pathol. 1973;60:259–63.
4. Pautler KB, Padhye AA, Ajello L. Imported *penicilliosis marneffei* in the United States: report of a second human infection. Sabouraudia. 1984;22:433–8.
5. Jayanetra P, Nitiyanant P, Ajello L, et al. *Penicilliosis marneffei* in Thailand: report of five human cases. Am J Trop Med Hyg. 1984;33:637–44.
6. Deng ZL, Connor DH. Progressive disseminated penicilliosis caused by *Penicillium marneffei*. Report of eight cases and differentiation of the causative organism from *Histoplasma capsulatum*. Am J Clin Pathol. 1985;84:323–7.
7. Li JS, Pan LQ, Deng ZL, Yoo CL. A case report on *Penicillium marneffei*. J Clin Dermatol (China). 1985;14:24–6.
8. Li JS, Pan LQ, Wu SX. Mycologic investigation on *Rhizomys pruinosus* senex in Guangxi as natural carrier with *Penicillium marneffei*. Clin Med J. 1989;102:477–85.
9. Li JS, Pan Q, Wu SX, Su SX, Su B, Shan JH. Diseminated *Penicilliosis marneffei* in China: report of three cases. Clin Med J. 1991;104:247–51.
10. Hilmarsdottir I, Meynard JL, Rogeaux O, Gentilini M. Disseminated *Penicillium marneffei* infection associated with human immunodeficiency virus: a report of two cases and a review of 35 published cases. J Acquir Immune Defic Syndr. 1993;6:466–71.
11. Hulshof CM, van Zanten RA, Sluiters JF, et al. *Penicillium marneffei* infection in an AIDS patient. Eur J Clin Microbiol Infect Dis. 1990;9:370.
12. Jones PD, See J. *Penicillium marneffei* infection in patients infected with human immunodeficiency virus: late presentation in an area of nonendemicity. Clin Infect Dis. 1992;15:744.
13. Kronauer CM, Schar G, Barben M, Buhler H. HIV-associated *Penicillium marneffei* infection. Schweiz Med Wochenschr. 1993; 123:385–90.
14. Peto TE, Bull R, Millard PR, et al. Systemic mycosis due to *Penicillium marneffei* in a patient with antibody to human immunodeficiency virus. J Infect. 1988;16:285–90.
15. Piehl MR, Kaplan RL, Haber MH. Disseminated penicilliosis in a patient with acquired immunodeficiency syndrome. Arch Pathol Lab Med. 1988;112:1262–4.
16. Sobottka I, Albrecht H, Mack D, et al. Systemic *Penicillium marneffei* infection in a German AIDS patient. Eur J Clin Microbiol Infect Dis. 1996;15:256–9.
17. Viviani MA, Tortoranto AM, Rizzardini G, et al. Treatment and serological studies of an Italian case of *Penicilliosis marneffei* contracted in Thailand by a drug addict infected with the human immunodeficiency virus. Eur J Epidemiol. 1993;9:79–85.
18. Hilmarsdottir I, Coutellier A, Elbaz J, et al. A French case of laboratory-acquired disseminated *Penicillium marneffei* infection in a patient with AIDS (letter). Clin Infec Dis. 1994;19:357–8.
19. Nelson KE, Kaufman L, Cooper CR, Merz WG. *Penicillium marneffei:* an AIDS-related illness from Southeast Asia. Infect Med. 1999;16:118–21.
20. Supparatpinyo K, Chiewchanvit S, Hirunsri P, Uthammachai C, Nelson KE, Sirisanthana T. *Penicillium marneffei* infection in patients infected with human immunodeficiency virus. Clin Infect Dis. 1992; 14:871–4.
21. Supparatpinyo K, Khamwan C, Baosoung V, Nelson KE, Sirisanthana T. Disseminated *Penicillium marneffei* infection in southeast Asia. Lancet. 1994;344:110–3.
22. Chariyalertsak S, Sirisanthana T, Supparatpinyo K, Nelson KE. Seasonal variation of disseminated *Penicillium marneffei* infections in northern Thailand: a clue to the reservoir? J Infect Dis. 1996;173:1490–3.
23. Deng Z, Ribas JL, Gibson DW, Connor DH. Infections caused by *Penicillium marneffei* in China and Southeast Asia: review of eighteen published cases and report of four more Chinese cases. Rev Infect Dis. 1988;10:640–52.
24. Deng ZL, Yun M, Ajello L. Human *penicilliosis marneffei* and its relation to the bamboo rat *(Rhizomys pruinosus)*. J Med Vet Mycol. 1986;24:383–9.
25. Wei XG, Ling YM, Li C, Zhang FS. Study of 179 bamboo rats carrying *Penicillium marneffei* (in Chinese). China J Zoonoses. 1987;3:34–5.
26. Ajello L, Padhye AA, Sukroongreung S, Nilakul CH, Tantimavanic S. Occurrence of *Penicillium marneffei* infections among wild bamboo rats in Thailand. Mycopathologia. 1995;131:1–8.
27. Chariyalertsak S, Vanittanakom P, Nelson KE, Sirisanthana T, Vanittanakom N. *Rhizomys sumatrensis* and *Cannomys badius*, new natural animal hosts of *Penicillium marneffei*. J Med Vet Mycol. 1996;34:105–10.
28. Gugnani H, Fisher MC, Paliwal-Johsi A, Vanittanakom N, Singh I, Yadav PS. Role of *Cannomys badius* as a natural animal host of *Penicillium marneffei* in India. J Clin Microbiol. 2004; 42:5070–5.
29. Segretain G. *Penicillium marneffei* n.sp.agent d'une mycose du système reticuloendothelial. Mycopath Mycolgia Appl. 1959; 11:327–53.
30. Vanittanakom N, Mekaprateep M, Sriburee P, Vanittanakom P, Khanjanasthiti P. Efficiency of the flotation method in the isolation of *Penicillium marneffei* from seeded soil. J Med Vet Mycol. 1995; 33:271–3.
31. Corbet GB, Hill JE. Subfamily *Rhizomyinae*: bamboo rats. In: The mammals of the Indo Malaya region: a systemic review. New York: Oxford University Press; 1992. p. 404–7.
32. Chariyalertsak S, Sirisanthana T, Supparatpinyo K, Praparattanapan J, Nelson KE. Case-control study of risk factors for *Penicillium marneffei* infection in human immunodeficiency virus-infected patients in northern Thailand. Clin Infect Dis. 1997;24:1080–6.
33. Chariyalertsak S, Sirisanthana T, Saengwonloey O, Nelson KE. Clinical presentation and risk behaviors of patients with acquired immunodeficiency syndrome in Thailand, 1994–1998: regional variation and temporal trends. Clin Infect Dis. 2001;32:955–62.

34. Raper KB, Thom CA. A manual of the penicillia. Baltimore: The Williams and Wilkins Co; 1949.
35. Pitt JI. The genus *Penicillium* and its teleomorphic states *Eupenicillium* and *Talaromyces*. New York: Academic Press Inc; 1979.
36. LoBuglio KF, Taylor JW. Phylogeny and PCR identification of the human pathogenic fungus *Penicillium marneffei*. J Clin Microbiol. 1995;33:85–9.
37. Sekhon AS, Li JS, Garg AK. *Penicillosis marneffei*: serological and exoantigen studies. Mycopathologia. 1982;77:51–7.
38. Wong SS, Ho TY, Ngan AH, Woo PC, Que TL, Yuen KY. Biotyping of *Penicillium marneffei* reveals concentration-dependent growth inhibition by galactose. J Clin Microbiol. 2001;39:1416–21.
39. Hamilton AJ, Jeavons L, Youngchim S, Vanittanakom N, Hay RJ. Sialic acid-dependent recognition of laminin by *Penicillium marneffei* conidia. Infect Immun. 1998;66:6024–6.
40. Hamilton AJ, Jeavons L, Youngchim S, Vanittanakom N. Recognition of fibronectin by *Penicillium marneffei* conidia via a sialic acid-dependent process and its relationship to the interaction between conidia and laminin. Infect Immun. 1999;67:5200–5.
41. Sekhon AS, Padhye AA, Garg AK. In vitro sensitivity of *Penicillium marneffei* and *Pythium insidiosum* to various antifungal agents. Eur J Epidemiology. 1992;8:427–32.
42. Drouhet E. Penicilliosis due to *Penicillium marneffei*: a new emerging sysemic mycosis in AIDS patients traveling or living in Southeast Asia, Review of 44 cases reported in HIV infected patients during the last 5 years compared to 44 cases of non AIDS patients reported over 20 years. J Mycol Med (Paris). 1993;4:195–224.
43. Supparatpinyo K, Nelson KE, Merz WG, et al. Response to antifungal therapy by human immunodeficiency virus-infected patients with disseminated *Penicillium marneffei* infections and in vitro susceptibilities of isolates from clinical specimens. Antimicrob Agents Chemother. 1993;37:2407–11.
44. Imwidthaya P, Thipsuvan K, Chaiprasert A, Danchaivijitra S, Suthent R, Jearanaisilavong J. *Penicillium marneffei*: types and drug susceptibility. Mycopathologia. 2001;149:109–15.
45. Radford SA, Johnson EM, Warnock DW. In vitro studies of activity of voriconazole (UK-109, 496), a new triazole antifungal agent, against emerging and less-common mold pathogens. Antimicrob Agents Chemother. 1997;41:841–3.
46. Sar B, Boy S, Keo C, et al. In vitro antifungal-drug susceptibilities of mycelial and yeast forms of *Penicillium marneffei* isolates in Cambodia. J Clin Microbiol. 2006;44:4208–10.
47. Hilmarsdottir I, Meynard JL, Rogeaux O, et al. Disseminated *Penicillium marneffei* infection associated with human immunodeficiency virus: a report of two cases and a review of 35 published cases. J Acquir Immune Defic Syndr. 1993;6:466–71.
48. Viviani MA, Tortorano AM, Rizzardini G, et al. Treatment and serological studies of an Italian case of *Penicilliosis marneffei* contracted in Thailand by a drug addict infected with the human immunodeficiency virus. Eur J Epidemiol. 1993;9:79–85.
49. Rongruagruang Y, Levitz SM. Interaction of *Penicillium marneffei* with human leukocytes in vitro. Infect Immun. 1999;67:4732–6.
50. Vanittanakom N, Cooper Jr CR, Fisher MC, Sirisanthana T. *Penicillium marneffei* infection and recent advances in the epidemiology and molecular biology aspects. Clin Microbiol Rev. 2006;19:95–110.
51. Woods JP. *Histoplasma capsulatum* molecular genetics, pathogenesis, and responsiveness to its environment. Fungal Genet Biol. 2002;35:81–97.
52. Pongpom P, Cooper Jr CR, Vanittanakom N. Isolation and characterization of a catalase-peroxidase gene from the pathogenic fungus, *Penicillium marneffei*. Med Mycol. 2005;43:403–11.
53. Thirach S, Cooper Jr CR, Vanittanakom P, Vanittanakom N. The copper, zinc superoxide dismutase gene of *Penicillium marneffei*: cloning, characterization, and differential expression during phase transition and macrophage infection. Med Mycol. 2007;45:409–17.
54. Bastos KP, Bailao AM, Borges CL, et al. The transcriptome analysis of early morphogenesis in *Paracoccidioides brasiliensis* mycelium reveals novel and induced genes potentially associated to the dimorphic process. BMC Microbiol. 2007;7:29.
55. Burnie JP, Carter TL, Hodgetts SJ, Matthews RC. Fungal heat-shock proteins in human disease. FEMS Microbiol Rev. 2006;30:53–88.
56. Kummasook A, Pongpom P, Vanittanakom N. Cloning, characterization and differential expression of an hsp70 gene from the pathogenic dimorphic fungus, *Penicillium marneffei*. DNA Seq. 2007;18:385–94.
57. Chandler JM, Treece ER, Trenary HR, et al. Protein profiling of the dimorphic, pathogenic fungus *Penicillium marneffei*. Proteome Sci. 2008;6:17.
58. Cooper CR, Vanittanakom N. Insights into the pathogenicity of *Penicillium marneffei*. Future Microbiol. 2008;3:43–55.
59. Vanittanakom N, Pongpom M, Praparattanapan J, Cooper Jr CR, Sirisanthana T. Isolation and expression of heat shock protein 30 gene from *Penicillium marneffei*. Med Mycol. 2009;47:521–6.
60. Bhardwaj S, Shukla A, Mukherjee S, et al. Putative structure and characteristics of a red water-soluble pigment secreted by *Penicillium marneffei*. Med Mycol. 2007;45:419–27.
61. Nosanchuk JD, Casadevall A. Impact of melanin on microbial virulence and clinical resistance to antimicrobial compounds. Antimicrob Agents Chemother. 2006;50:3519–28.
62. Youngchim S, Hay RJ, Hamilton AJ. Melanization of *Penicillium marneffei* in vitro and in vivo. Microbiology. 2005;151:291–9.
63. Chariyalertsak S, Supparatpinyo K, Sirisanthana T, Nelson KE. A controlled trial of itraconazole as primary prophylaxis for systemic fungal infections in patients with advanced human immunodeficiency virus infection in Thailand. Clin Infect Dis. 2002;34:277–84.
64. Vanittanakom N, Sirisanthana T. *Penicillium marneffei* infection in patients infected with human immunodeficiency virus. Curr Top Med Mycol. 1997;8:35–42.
65. Vanittanakom N, Merz WG, Nelson KE, Sirisanthana T. Rapid detection of *Penicillium marneffei* by polymerase chain reaction/hybridization technique. 13th Congress of International Society for Human and Animal Mycology, Parma, Italy, 8–13 June 1997.
66. Sirisanthana V, Sirisanthana T. Disseminated *Penicillium marneffei* infection in human immunodeficiency virus-infected children. Pediatr Infect Dis J. 1995;14:935–40.
67. Yuen WC, Chan YF, Loke SL, Seto WH, Poon GP, Wong KK. Chronic lymphadenopathy caused by *Penicillium marneffei*: a condition mimicking tuberculous lympadenopathy. Br J Surg. 1986;73:1007–8.
68. Chan YF, Woo KC. *Penicillium marneffei* osteomyelitis. J Bone Joint Surg Br. 1990;72:500–3.
69. Chan JK, Tsang DN, Wong DK. *Penicillium marneffei* in bronchoalveolar lavage fluid. Acta Cytol. 1989;33:523–6.
70. Supparatpinyo K, Sirisanthana T. Disseminated *Penicillium marneffei* infection diagnosed on examination of a peripheral blood smear of a patient with human immunodeficiency virus infection. Clin Infect Dis. 1994;18:246–7.
71. Ko KF. Retropharyngeal abscess caused by *Penicillium marneffei*: an unusual cause of upper airway obstruction. Otolaryngol Head Neck Surg. 1994;110:445–6.
72. Chim CS, Fong CY, Ma SK, Wong SS, Yuen KY. Reactive hemophagocytic syndrome associated with *Penicillium marneffei* infection. Am J Med. 1998;104:196–7.
73. Tong AC, Wong M, Smith NJ. *Penicillium marneffei* infection presenting as oral ulcerations in a patient infected with human immunodeficiency virus. J Oral Maxillofac Surg. 2001;59:953–6.
74. Annam V, Inamadar AC, Palit A, Koppad M, Peerapur BV, Yelikar BR. Genital ulcer caused by *Penicillium marneffei* in an HIV-infected patient. Sex Transm Infect. 2007;83:249–50.
75. Cooper Jr CR, Haycocks NG. *Penicillium marneffei*: an insurgent species among the penicillia. J Eukaryot Microbiol. 2000;47:24–8.
76. Wong SSY, Wong KH, Hui WT, et al. Differences in clinical and laboratory diagnostics characteristics of *Penicilliosis marneffei* in human immunodeficiency virus (HIV) and non-HIV infected patients. J Clin Microbiol. 2001;39:4534–40.

77. Viviani MA, Tortoranto AM. *Penicillium marneffei*. In: Ajello L, Hay RJ, editors. Topley and Wilson's microbiology and microbial infections. 9th ed. London, UK: Arnold Press; 1998. p. 409–19.
78. Hsiue HC, Huang YT, Kuo YL, Liao CH, Chang TC, Hsueh PR. Rapid identification of fungal pathogens in positive blood cultures using oligonucleotide array hybridization. Clin Microbiol Infect. 2010;16(5):493–500. 15 July 2009 (Epub ahead of print).
79. Pongpom M, Sirisanthana T, Vanittanakom N. Application of nested PCR to detect *Penicillium marneffei* in serum samples. Med Mycol. 2009;47:549–53.
80. Pornprasert S, Praparattanapan J, Khamwan C, et al. Development of TaqMan real-time polymerase chain reaction for the detection and identification of *Penicillium marneffei*. Mycoses. 2009;52:487–92.
81. Zeng H, Li X, Chen X, et al. Identification of *Penicillium marneffei* in paraffin-embedded tissue using nested PCR. Mycopathologia. 2009;168:31–5.
82. Sekhon AS, Garg AK, Padhye AA, Standard PG, Kaufman L, Ajello L. Antigenic relationship of *Penicillium marneffei* to *P. primulinum*. J Med Vet Mycol. 1989;27:105–12.
83. Estrada JA, Stynen D, Cutsem JV, Pierar-Franchimont C, Pierard GE. Immunohistochemical identification of *Penicillium marneffei* by monoclonal antibody. Dermatol. 1992;31:410–2.
84. Kaufman L, Standard PG, Anderson SA, Jalbert M, Swisher BL. Development of specific fluorescent-antibody test for tissue form of *Penicillium marneffei*. J Clin Microbiol. 1995;33:2136–8.
85. Sekhon AS, Stein L, Garg AK, Black WA, Glezos JD, Wong C. Pulmonary *penicillosis marneffei*: report of the first imported case in Canada. Mycopathologia. 1994;128:3–7.
86. Kaufman L, Standard PG, Jalbert M, Kantipong P, Limpakarnjanarat K, Mastro TD. Diagnostic antigenemia tests for *Penicilliosis marneffei*. J Clin Microbiol. 1996;34:2503–5.
87. Yuen K, Wong SS, Tsang DN, Cau PY. Serodiagnosis of *Penicillium marneffei* infection. Lancet. 1994;344:444–5.
88. Cao L, Chen DL, Lee C, et al. Detection of specific antibodies to an antigenic mannoprotein for diagnosis of *Penicillium marneffei* penicilliosis. J Clin Microbiol. 1998;36:3028–31.
89. Vanittanakom N, Mekaprateep M, Sittisombut N, et al. Western immunoblot analysis of protein antigens of *Penicillium marneffei*. J Med Vet Mycol. 1997;35:123–31.
90. Jeavons L, Hamilton AJ, Vanittanakom N, et al. Identification and purification of specific *Penicillium marneffei* antigens and their recognition by human immune sera. J Clin Microbiol. 1998;36:949–54.
91. Chongtrakool P, Chaiyaroj SC, Vithayasai V, et al. Immunoreactivity of a 38-kilodalton *Penicillium marneffei* antigen with human immunodeficiency virus-positive sera. J Clin Microbiol. 1997;35:2220–3.
92. Wheat J, Wheat H, Connolly P, et al. Cross-reactivity in *Histoplasma capsulatum* variety *capsulatum* antigen assays of urine samples from patients with endemic mycoses. Clin Infect Dis. 1997;24:1169–71.
93. Desakorn V, Smith MD, Walsh AL, et al. Diagnosis of *Penicillium marneffei* infection by quantitation of urinary antigen by using an enzyme immunoassay. J Clin Microbiol. 1999;37:117–21.
94. Desakorn V, Simpson AJ, Wuthiekanun V, et al. Development and evaluation of rapid urinary antigen detection tests for diagnosis of *Penicilliosis marneffei*. J Clin Microbiol. 2002;40:3179–83.
95. Huang YT, Hung CC, Liao CH, Sun HY, Chang SC, Chen YC. Detection of circulating galactomannan in serum samples for diagnosis of *Penicillium marneffei* infection and cryptococcosis among patients infected with human immunodeficiency virus. J Clin Microbiol. 2007;45:2858–62.
96. Tsunemi Y, Takahashi T, Tamaki T. *Penicillium marneffei* infection diagnosed by polymerase chain reaction from the skin specimen. J Am Acad Dermatol. 2003;49:344–6.
97. Vanittanakom N, Merz WG, Sittisombut N, Khamwan C, Nelson KE, Sirisanthana T. Specific identification of *Penicillium marneffei* by a polymerase chain reaction/hybridization technique. Med Mycol. 1998;36:169–75.
98. Vanittanakom N, Vanittanakom P, Hay RJ. Rapid identification of *Penicillium marneffei* by PCR-based detection of specific sequences on the rRNA gene. J Clin Microbiol. 2002; 40:1739–42.
99. Vanittanakom N, Cooper Jr CR, Chariyalertsak S, Youngchim S, Nelson KE, Sirisanthana T. Restriction endonuclease analysis of *Penicillium marneffei*. J Clin Microbiol. 1996;34:1834–6.
100. Trewatcharegon S, Sirisinha S, Romsai A, Eampokalap B, Teanpaisan R, Chaiyaroj SC. Molecular typing of *Penicillium marneffei* isolates from Thailand by NotI macrorestriction and pulsed-field gel electrophoresis. J Clin Microbiol. 2001; 39:4544–8.
101. Hsueh PR, Teng LJ, Hung CC, et al. Molecular evidence for strain dissemination of *Penicillium marneffei*: an emerging pathogen in Taiwan. J Infect Dis. 2000;181:1706–12.
102. Sirisanthana T, Supparatpinyo K, Perriens J, Nelson KE. Amphotericin B and itraconazole for treatment of disseminated *Penicillium marneffei* infection in human immunodeficiency virus-infected patients. Clin Infect Dis. 1998;26:1107–10.
103. Supparatpinyo K, Chiewchanvit S, Hirunsri P, et al. An efficacy study of itraconazole in the treatment of *Penicillium marneffei* infection. J Med Assoc Thailand. 1992;75:688–91.
104. Supparatpinyo K, Schlamm HT. Voriconazole as therapy for systemic *Penicillium marneffei* infections in AIDS patients. Am J Trop Med Hyg. 2007;77:350–3.
105. Kaplan JE, Benson C, Holmes KH, Brooks JT, Pau A, Masur H. Guidelines for prevention and treatment of opportunistic infections in HIV-infected adults and adolescents: recommendations from CDC, the National Institutes of Health, and the HIV Medicine Association of the Infectious Diseases Society of America. MMWR Recomm Rep. 2009;58:1–207.
106. Gupta S, Mathur P, Maskey D, Wig N, Singh S. Immune restoration syndrome with disseminated *Penicillium marneffei* and cytomegalovirus co-infections in an AIDS patient. AIDS Res Ther. 2007;4:21.
107. Manosuthi W, Chaovavanich A, Tansuphaswadikul S, et al. Incidence and risk factors of major opportunistic infections after initiation of antiretroviral therapy among advanced HIV-infected patients in a resource-limited setting. J Infect. 2007;55:464–9.
108. Saikia L, Nath R, Biswanath P, Hazarika D, Mahanta J. *Penicillium marneffei* infection in HIV infected patients in Nagaland & immune reconstitution after treatment. Indian J Med Res. 2009;129:333–4.
109. Supparatpinyo K, Perriens J, Nelson KE, Sirisanthana T. A controlled trial of itraconazole to prevent relapse of *Penicillium marneffei* infection in patients infected with the human immunodeficiency virus. N Engl J Med. 1998;339:1739–43.
110. Chaiwarith R, Charoenyos N, Sirisanthana T, Supparatpinyo K. Discontinuation of secondary prophylaxis against *Penicilliosis marneffei* in AIDS patients after HAART. AIDS. 2007;21:365–7.
111. Lopez Bernaldo de Quiros JC, Miro JM, Pena JM, et al. A randomized trial of the discontinuation of primary and secondary prophylaxis against *Pneumocystis carinii* pneumonia after highly active antiretroviral therapy in patients with HIV infection. Grupo de Estudio del SIDA 04/98. N Engl J Med. 2001;344:159–67.
112. Rollot F, Bossi P, Tubiana R, et al. Discontinuation of secondary prophylaxis against cryptococcosis in patients with AIDS receiving highly active antiretroviral therapy. AIDS. 2001; 15:1448–9.
113. Goldman M, Zackin R, Fichtenbaum CJ, et al. Safety of discontinuation of maintenance therapy for disseminated histoplasmosis after immunologic response to antiretroviral therapy. Clin Infect Dis. 2004;38:1485–9.

Part VI
Mycoses Involving Skin and Subcutaneous Tissues

Eumycetoma

Beatriz Bustamante and Pablo E. Campos

Mycetoma is a chronic subcutaneous infection that develops after one of the multiple etiologic microorganisms is inoculated into a site of skin trauma. Although mycetoma is primarily a subcutaneous disease, it can involve bone and lymph nodes by contiguous spread. Mycetoma shows three clinical characteristics: tumor, sinuses, and grains. The tumor results as a consequence of a progressive and relatively painless swelling. Sinuses are a characteristic of the disorder; they can be absent in early stages, but later develop and drain purulent material and grains. Grains are colonies of the causative agent and can be black, white, or red. Mycetoma can be caused by a variety of fungal agents (eumycetoma), or filamentous gram-positive branching bacteria belonging to the aerobic Actinomycetales (actinomycetoma).

Gill first described mycetoma while working in Madura, India, in 1842, and this was subsequently documented by Godfrey in Madras [1]. Gill reported this entity as "foot tumor," and Colenbrook introduced the term "Madura foot" in 1846. Ballingal described the microscopic details of the disease for the first time in 1855; however, he did not define its etiology. In 1860, Carter described a disease principally affecting the foot and assigned a fungal origin to this disease in 1861 [2]. He also introduced the term mycetoma, meaning "fungus tumor," and extended the concept to include infections with grains that had colors other than black. During the second half of the nineteenth century, mycetomas were reported throughout the world: in Europe in 1888, in Africa in 1894, and in the USA in 1896.

The hyphomycete isolated from a black grain was given the generic name *Madurella* by Brumpt [3]. In 1913, Pinoy subclassified this disease into two categories: "actinomycosis" and "true mycetoma" according to the type of etiologic agent [4]. In 1916, Chalmers and colleagues coined the term maduromycoses for the first time to refer to mycetomas of fungal etiology, rejecting the term "Madura foot" to include extrapedal forms of this disease [5,6]. Even though distinction between eumycetomas and actinomycetomas was achieved at this time, the term mycetoma is still used to refer to both entities, and most of the published literature has mixed these terms, making it difficult to draw clear conclusions about these distinct disorders.

Despite the acquisition of considerable new knowledge concerning this disease during the last century, including the identification of new agents by the use of novel molecular techniques, there are still important gaps in information regarding eumycetoma, mainly related to pathogenesis and management. The goal of this chapter is to review the epidemiologica and clinical aspects of eumycetoma, also known as eumycotic mycetoma.

Organisms and Epidemiology

More than 20 hyaline and pigmented moulds can cause eumycetomas (Table 1). *Madurella mycetomatis* is the predominant pathogen worldwide, followed by *Pseudallescheria boydii/Scedesporium apiospermum, Leptosphaeria senegalensis*, and *Madurella grisea* [7]. These four fungi account for approximately 95% of eumycetoma cases. *S. apiospermum* has been considered the anamorph (the asexual state) of *P. boydii*; but new molecular studies indicate they are two different species, and that *P. boydii* is a complex that includes at least eight phylogenetic species [8,9]. However, most of the existing literature does not differentiate between the species, and their individual involvement in human infections has not been determined. Hereafter, we will use the name *P. boydii* complex when referring to *P. boydii* or to *S. apiospermum*.

Although eumycetoma has been reported worldwide, most of the cases come from tropical and subtropical regions around the Tropic of Cancer, between 15° south and 30° north [10], with sporadic cases occurring in temperate zones. Over 60% of all cases are reported from India, Sudan, and Senegal [11–18]. Endemic regions are characteristically arid

B. Bustamante (✉)
Instituto de Medicina Tropical; "Alexander von Humboldt," Universidad Peruana Cayetano Heredia; Departamento de Enfermedades Transmisibles y Dermatológicas, Hospital Nacional Cayetano Heredia, Lima, Peru
e-mail: ana.bustamante@upch.pe

C.A. Kauffman et al. (eds.), *Essentials of Clinical Mycology*,
DOI 10.1007/978-1-4419-6640-7_24,

Table 1 Eumycetoma etiologic agents and their geographic distribution

Etiologic agents	Geographic distribution
Black Grain Eumycetomas	
Cladophialophora bantiana	Central America
Corynespora cassiicola	Africa
Curvularia lunata	Africa, Asia
Exophiala jeanselmei	North, Central and South America, Europe
Leptosphaeria senegalensis	Africa, Asia
Leptosphaeria tompkinsii	Africa, Asia
Madurella grisea	North, Central and South America, Africa, Asia
Madurella mycetomatis	North, Central and South America, Caribbean, Africa, Europe, Middle East, Asia
Phialophora verrucosa	Asia[a]
Pyrenochaeta mackinnonii	South America
Pyrenochaeta romeroi	Central and South America, Africa, Asia
White to Yellow Grain Eumycetomas	
Acremonium falciforme	North, Central and South America, Asia, Europe, Oceania
Acremonium kiliense	Asia
Acremonium recifei	South America, Asia
Arthrographis kalrae	Europe
Aspergillus nidulans	Africa
Aspergillus flavus	North America
Cylindrocarpon cyanescens	Asia
Cylindrocarpon destructans	Caribbean, West Africa
Cylindrocarpon lichenicola	Asia
Fusarium moniliforme (syn: *Fusarium verticilloides*)	Europe
Fusarium solani	South America, Caribbean, Africa, Asia
Neotestudina rosatii	West Africa
Phaeoacremonium krajdenii	Asia
Polycytella hominis	Asia
Pseudallescheria boydii complex	North, Central and South America, Africa, Oceania, Europe, Asia

[a]Thai patients who traveled in Europe, Asia, and North America

with a moderate rainy season (4–6 months), a rainfall of 50–1,000 mm per year, and daytime temperatures from 30°C to 37°C, with small variations between day and night [19].

Temperature, rainfall, type of soil, and prevalent vegetation influence the prevalence of specific eumycetoma agents in a particular region [20], with rainfall being the most influential factor. Black grain fungi cause eumycetomas in arid regions, whereas white grain fungi cause eumycetomas in regions with higher rainfall and without a significant dry season [21]. *M. mycetomatis* prevails in hot and dry areas with low rainfall and can be found in temperate zones, but it is rare in the equatorial zone [11]. *P. boydii* complex prevails in areas with hyperprecipitation (~2,000 mm per year) [10,22] and has been reported sporadically in the northern temperate zone among sewage workers [23].

Most eumycetoma agents such as *M. mycetomatis*, *M. grisea*, *P. boydii* complex, and *Neotestudina rosatii* have been isolated from soil samples [24–27], and *M. mycetomatis* and *P. boydii* complex have also been isolated from termite mounds. *L. senegalensis* and *L. tompkinsii* are recovered from 50% of acacia dry thorns in the Senegal River region, but not from green thorns [25,27,28], suggesting that thorns may play a role as mechanical vectors. Recently, the use of molecular techniques has facilitated the study of natural reservoirs of *M. mycetomatis*. Polymerase chain reaction (PCR) detection followed by restriction fragment length polymorphism (RFLP) analysis have demonstrated the presence of the organism in 23% of soil samples from endemic areas of Sudan and have successfully linked environmental and clinical isolates [29].

Reports of eumycetoma affecting animals are unusual. Equine and canine cases due to *M. mycetomatis* have been reported [30,31]. Cases due to *Curvularia lunata* and *Cladophialophora bantiana* in dogs and an unspecified organism in buffalo have been reported [32–34].

Pathogenesis

Disease usually develops as a result of minor trauma that inoculates contaminated material, usually soil, into the skin or subcutaneous tissue. A history of any trauma at the site of eumycetoma is uncommon, ranging from 0% to 34% of cases, with the higher figures reported from endemic areas of Sudan and India [35,36]. This observation suggests that either these fungi do not need deep inoculation, or that disease occurs after a prolonged incubation period [37].

After inoculation, a poorly defined host response precludes the development of free fungal filaments in the infected tissue, and instead leads to the development of the characteristic grain. Neutrophil-mediated tissue reaction leads to partial grain disintegration, but most of the grain remains and perpetuates a chronic inflammatory response. Macrophages and multinucleated giant cells clear dead neutrophils and grain fragments, and an epithelioid granuloma develops [38]. Results of immunologic studies performed among patients affected by mycetomas are scarce and conflicting. Mahgoub and co-workers found a moderately decreased cell-mediated immune response [39], while Bendl et al. were not able to demonstrate any immunologic alterations in 15 patients [40].

The role of genetic predisposition to develop mycetoma has not been established. Although many residents of endemic areas have antibodies to *M. mycetomatis*, very few develop eumycetoma. It has been postulated that those who develop eumycetoma have inadequate neutrophil function resulting from polymorphisms in the functional expression of those genes that direct neutrophil function [41].

The role of melanin that is present in variable amounts in grains from certain organisms, such as *M. mycetomatis*, is not completely understood. Melanin has been linked to virulence and pathogenicity, and it is considered the most important component of the grain cement. Melanin strengthens the grain and protects fungal cells from antibodies, hydrolytic enzymes, strong oxidants, and azole antifungal agents [42,43].

Clinical Aspects

Clinical Manifestations

Eumycetoma principally affects otherwise normal men living and working in rural areas. The male-to-female ratio ranges between 3:1 and 5:1; the age at the time of diagnosis ranges from 3 to 77 years (mean 32.6 years). The average duration of symptoms ranges between 7.7 and 9.8 years, ranging from 1 month to 25 years [44–50]. Most patients with eumycetoma are not classically immunocompromised, although diabetes is a frequent comorbidity. Indeed, 9 of 26 mycetoma patients diagnosed over a 9-year period in the UK had diabetes as an underlying disease [10]. Eumycetoma has been reported in patients receiving chronic immunosuppressive therapy for renal and heart transplantation, leukemia, and idiopathic CD4 lymphopenia [51–56]. Eumycetoma has not been reported in an HIV-infected patient.

Male predominance among eumycetoma patients can be explained by higher rates of exposure to etiologic agents related to occupational cutaneous injury, such as might occur in farming. This is similar to the acquisition of other subcutaneous mycoses, such as sporotrichosis and chromoblastomycosis. Male predominance could also be a consequence of higher susceptibility to this disease, an explanation based on an inhibitory effect of progesterone on the growth of *M. mycetomatis* and *Pyrenochaeta romeroi* in the laboratory [57].

The incubation period of eumycetoma is not well established, as most patients seek care after long periods of disease and without recall of the inoculation event. Clinical characteristics and evolution of eumycetoma lesions are independent of the etiologic fungus; the clinical course depends on the anatomic location, duration of lesions, and medical intervention. Lesions begin as small, firm, painless, indurated subcutaneous nodules or plaques that gradually increase in size. The clinical course is somewhat slower for eumycetoma than for actinomycetoma. Initially, the lesion is well demarcated and may be encapsulated, especially when *M. mycetomatis* is the etiologic agent. The disease usually runs a chronic course from several years to decades, with lesions spreading slowly to adjacent structures by contiguous spread, and virtually never by hematogenous dissemination.

The tumor develops as a result of the enlargement of existing nodules and formation of new nodules. Generally it is firm and round but may be soft and lobulated. Enlarged nodules open to the skin through sinus tracts, discharging sanguineous, seropurulent or purulent exudate that contains grains (Figs. 1, 2, and 3). A history of sinus tracts discharging grains is present in up to 60% of the cases [14].

Sinus tracts develop relatively early in the course of disease; at least one-third of patients develop sinuses between 3 and 6 months, and almost all patients have sinus tracts within 1 year of the development of skin lesions [58]. Established sinuses heal and recur as new sinuses continue to develop. Sinus tracts are very characteristic of both eumycetoma and

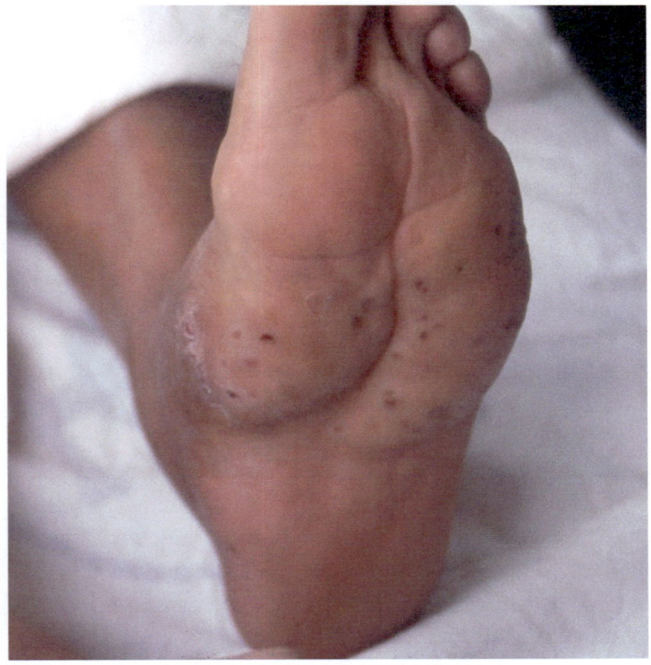

Fig. 1 Eumycetoma on the plantar surface of the foot showing tumor and fistulae

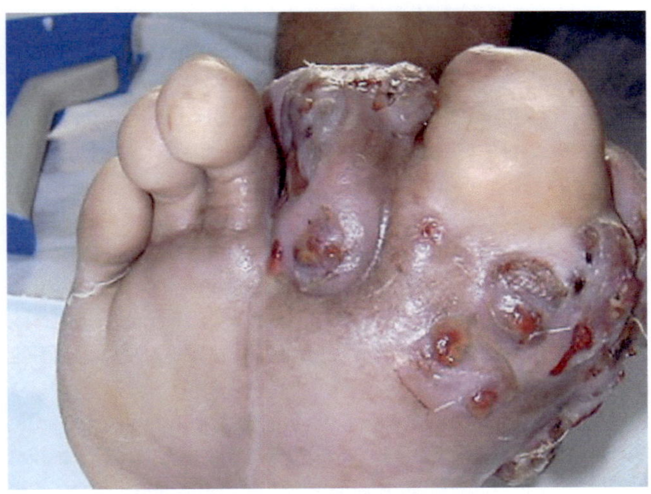

Fig. 2 Eumycetoma due to *Madurella mycetomatis* showing multiple sinus tracts

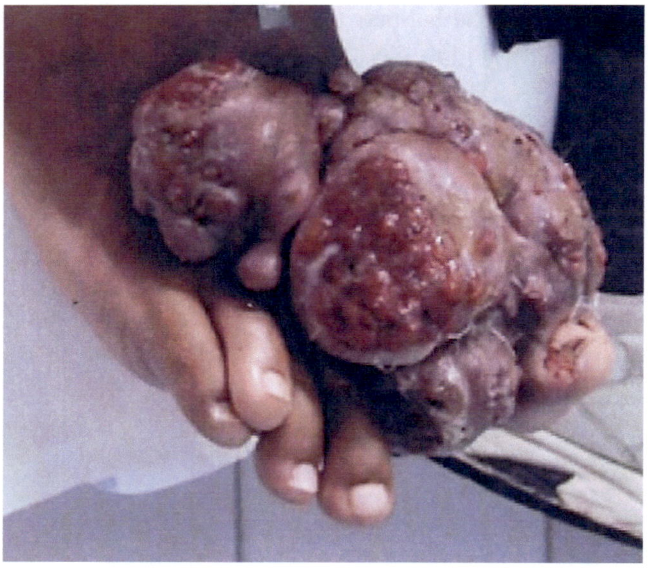

Fig. 3 Large tumor from eumycetoma due to *Madurella mycetomatis*

actinomycetoma and help support the clinical diagnosis, but also occur in other diseases and are not specific.

Destruction of adjacent structures can be dramatic and is especially characteristic late in the course of the disease. Destructive lesions are relatively painless. Pain, fever, and other systemic symptoms are not characteristic of eumycetoma, and when present, suggest a secondary bacterial infection. Bacterial cellulitis should be ruled out when pain is present, especially when edema and increasing discharge are evident. Massive fibrosis occurs after healing of involved tissue, contributing to the tumor-like appearance and woody texture of the affected area.

Eumycetoma lesions are located most frequently in areas with a high frequency of repeated trauma, especially the lower limbs. Feet, legs, and hands account for approximately 90% of black grain eumycetomas and 95% of *M. mycetomatis* eumycetomas [35,59]. Involvement of the foot is more common in eumycetomas than in actinomycetomas, occurring in 75–85% of cases [35,59]; legs and hands are involved in 7% and 6% of eumycetoma cases, respectively [60].

Extrapedal eumycetomas appear when repeated trauma occurs to other parts of the body. For example, lesions can occur on the abdominal wall in patients who do not wear a shirt and who carry organic products, such as vegetables or straw [61,62]. Rare anatomic sites described for eumycetoma include intraspinal [63], scalp [35], neck [13], mandible [64], eyelid [65], cheek [50], perineum [10], testicle [35], buttock [66,67], and thigh [10].

Multiple eumycetomas involving more than one anatomic site are rare. Most of these "double eumycetomas" described in the literature represent two lesions in the same anatomic region [68]. One report from Argentina of double eumycetoma described a patient with lesions on the foot and wrist, both lesions caused by *M. grisea* [69]. Eumycetoma caused by more than one fungus is also a rare clinical occurrence, but the occurrence of *M. mycetomatis* and *M. grisea* in a foot lesion has been reported [70].

Lymphatic spread is uncommon with eumycetomas, occurring in fewer than 3% of the cases [71]. It appears to be more frequent in actinomycetomas, possibly because the grains are smaller in this condition [72]. Among the agents of eumycetomas, *M. mycetomatis* has the lowest frequency of lymph node involvement, possibly because of the extensive fibrotic reaction that often accompanies this agent. Only 3 of 578 (0.5%) patients in one series experienced this complication [73].

In both eumycetoma and actinomycetoma, bone involvement occurs by contiguous spread, with changes occurring first in cortical bone [74]. Bone involvement occurs in up to 76% of cases and is more extensive with longer duration of disease [35,46]. In addition, bone lesions are more frequent and occur sooner when they are located in areas with thin subcutaneous tissue, such as the feet, hands, and skull.

Radiologic Findings

The most frequent radiologic findings in patients with eumycetomas are soft tissue swelling and osteolytic changes (Fig. 4). Loss of the cortical border and external erosion of the bone is the earliest osteolytic manifestation [7,75]. Later, the medullary canal and epiphysis are affected, resulting in bone destruction followed by bone remodeling [76]. Bone lesions can be manifested radiographically as demineralization, periosteal reaction, osteolysis, endosteal bone cavitation, sclerosis, and frank osteomyelitis [46]. Osteolytic lesions associated with eumycetoma are usually large and few in number, often with well-defined margins. Grossly, these lesions are filled with necrotic material and grains [20,76,77]. No particular pattern of bone involvement is associated with a specific eumycetoma agent. Moreover, it is not possible to differentiate between eumycetoma and actinomycetoma using radiologic studies [77,78].

Computerized tomography (CT) and MRI typically demonstrate bone lesions earlier than x-rays. CT should be used to evaluate pedal mycetomas, whereas MRI is preferred for extrapedal lesions. In addition, CT has greater sensitivity to detect early bone involvement, while MRI easily detects late manifestations as a coarse trabecular pattern, bone destruction, marrow infiltration, and sequestra [74]. MRI is also helpful for determining the extent of soft tissue involvement and for monitoring the response to treatment [74,78]. A "dot-in-circle sign" demonstrated by MRI is considered as a specific sign of both eumycetoma and actinomycetoma. It represents inflammatory granulomata containing grains and surrounded by a fibrous matrix [79].

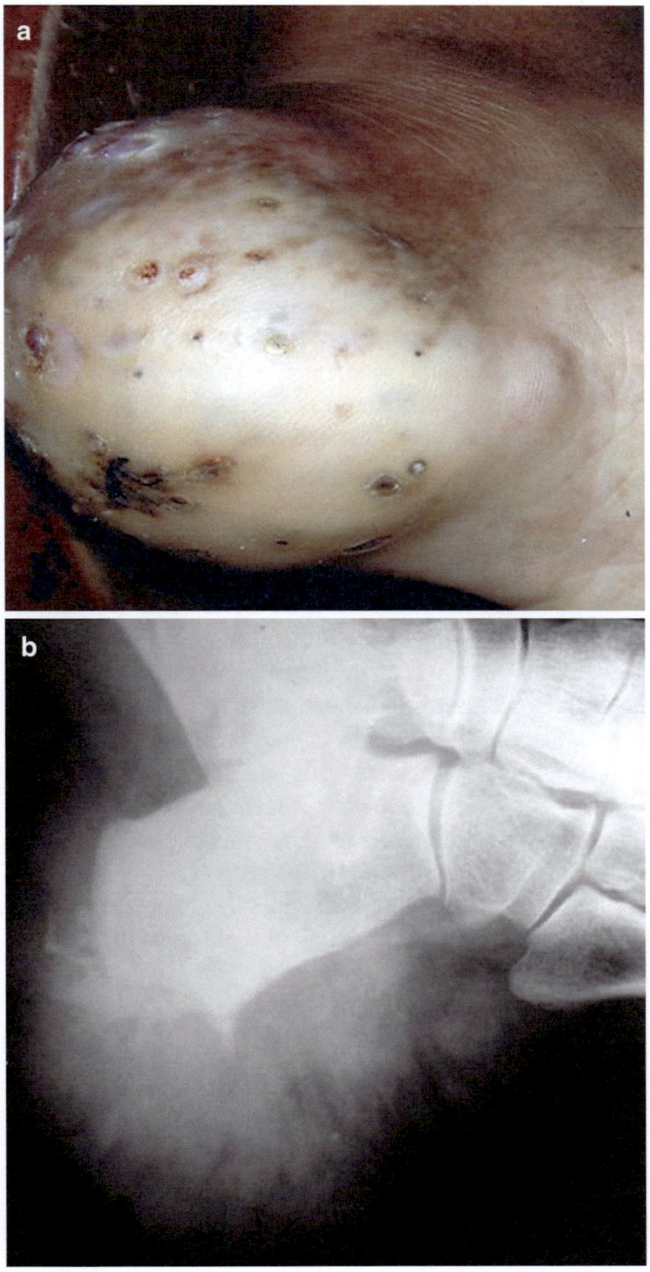

Fig. 4 (**a**) Tumorous swelling on the heel from *Madurella mycetomatis* showing sinus tracts. (**b**) Radiograph of the same heel showing soft tissue swelling and osteolytic changes of the calcaneus

Complications

The most common complication is secondary bacterial infection, which occurs in up to 66% of patients with black grain eumycetomas [80]. Massive bone destruction induced by eumycetomas can produce pathologic fractures [81]. Other complications are related to the site of disease, e.g., deformity of the foot in tumoral pedal eumycetoma. Rare complications include bronchopleural-cutaneous fistulae [82] and palatal deformity and dysfunction [83].

Differential Diagnosis

The differential diagnosis of eumycetoma lesions at any stage of their evolution should always include actinomycetoma due to aerobic filamentous actinomycetes and botryomycosis, due to gram-positive and gram-negative bacteria.

Small eumycetoma lesions may be confused with folliculitis, soft tissue tumors. or cystic lesions [84], while exophytic verrucous eumycetoma lesions of the foot can mimic verrucous tuberculosis, blastomycosis, chromoblastomycosis, and sporotrichosis. More extensive tumoral pedal lesions without sinus tracts should be differentiated from elephantiasis of the foot, as well as benign and malignant tumors. When bone involvement is present, the differential diagnosis includes bacterial osteomyelitis, osseous tuberculosis, osteosarcoma, and other malignant bone tumors. Extrapedal lesions should be differentiated from dermatophytic pseudomycetoma when the scalp is affected. In addition, cutaneous tuberculosis, endemic fungal diseases, such as blastomycosis and coccidioidomycosis, and cutaneous nocardiosis should be excluded.

Diagnosis

When draining sinus tracts are present, these provide the optimum material for microscopic examination and culture. Grains in discharged fluid are visible to the naked eye and can be collected from dressings covering a draining sinus tract. If discharged grains are not available, a deep skin biopsy taken from a small abscess or around a sinus tract is necessary for both culture and histopathologic studies. Fine-needle aspiration also can be useful for the diagnosis of eumycetoma [85]. Specimens should be submitted for macroscopic and microscopic examination and cultured appropriately.

Evaluation of Grains

Grain color, size, shape, and consistency should be noted because these characteristics help to guide identification of the causative fungus. For example, *M. mycetomatis* grains are large, black, and hard; *L. senegalensis* grains are large, black, and firm to hard; *M. grisea* and *P. romeroi* grains are small, black, and soft to firm; and *P. boydii* complex and *Aspergillus nidulans* grains are large, white, and soft. After macroscopic examination, grains should be placed in a drop of 10–20% KOH on a slide, compressed between two slides, and examined under microscopy. This direct examination

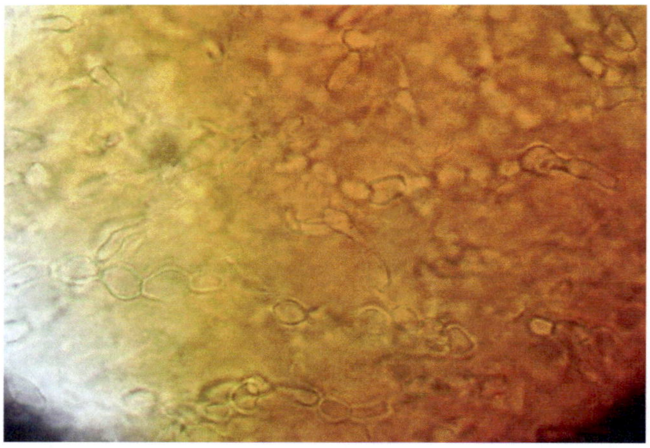

Fig. 5 Direct examination of a black grain from a eumycetoma showing intertwined broad hyphae and swollen cells (potassium hydroxide preparation, 1,000×)

will differentiate the grains of eumycetomas from the grains of actinomycetomas. Eumycetoma grains contain intertwined, broad hyphae (2–5 μm), and may contain large swollen cells (15 μm or more) at the periphery (Fig. 5).

Culture

Culture is essential for an etiologic diagnosis; however, performing cultures with eumycetoma specimens is laborious and complicated by a high rate of bacterial contamination. Prior to culture, grains should be washed several times with sterile saline solution to reduce bacterial and mould contamination, then crushed using sterile technique and plated on Sabouraud's dextrose agar containing chloramphenicol. Medium containing cycloheximide should be avoided because it inhibits the growth of some eumycetoma agents, such as some *Fusarium* spp. and *Aspergillus* spp. Specimens should be incubated at both room temperature and at 37°C for 6–8 weeks.

Species identification is based on both macroscopic and microscopic examination of colonies. Other tests may be helpful. For example, patterns of sugar assimilation and optimal growth temperature differentiate *M. mycetomatis* from *M. grisea*. The former can utilize glucose, galactose, lactose, and maltose, but not sucrose, and grows well at 37°C. By comparison, *M. grisea* can utilize glucose, galactose, maltose, and sucrose, but not lactose, and grows well at 30°C [55]. More recently, molecular techniques, such as the random amplification of polymorphic DNA (RAPD), RFLP, and DNA sequencing are being used for identification of various fungal species. These techniques are particularly useful when routine fungal isolation has failed [86–88].

Histopathology

The basic histopathologic picture of eumycetoma is chronic nonspecific granulomatous inflammation, with a central focus of acute inflammatory reaction surrounding one or more grains. Grains can be difficult to visualize in tissue sections, making it necessary to examine numerous sections of the biopsy. A zone formed by histiocytes surrounds the central and abscessed focus; this is surrounded by an outer zone consisting of new capillaries, isolated histiocytes, plasma cells, mast cells, and eosinophils. Lymphocytes characteristically are found infiltrating the fibrous tissue of the outer zone [19,36]. The fungal hyphae, which constitute the main element of the grain, are more easily observed with the use of periodic acid–Schiff (PAS) or methenamine silver stains.

As shown in Table 2, histopathologic characteristics on hematoxylin-eosin stain of black grain eumycetomas can be quite distinctive, and may allow for a presumptive diagnosis [89,90]. For example, *M. mycetomatis* grains, vesicular type, show a dense brown cement-like substance with hyphae and large chlamydospores in the periphery (Fig. 6). By contrast, *Exophiala jeanselmei* grains do not have cement-like substance. On the other hand, pale grain eumycetomas have similar histopathologic findings, making their differentiation uncertain [89]. The use of immunofluorescent antibodies facilitates the identification of the etiologic agent in tissue sections. A specific fluorescent antibody conjugate for identification of *P. boydii* is available in some areas [91,92], and monoclonal antibodies against *Aspergillus* galactomannan have been used to identify *Aspergillus* species without cross-reactivity with other fungi [93,94].

Serology

There is no reliable serologic test available for diagnosis of eumycetoma. Lack of standardized preparation of antigens has hampered development of such a test. In addition, many etiologic agents of eumycetoma require independent testing with several antigens or the use of a polyvalent antigen preparation. Immunodiffusion (ID) and counterimmunoelectrophoresis (CIE) have been the most widely used tests for detecting antibodies in eumycetoma patients, but both have shown inconsistent results [95–97]. Enzyme-linked immunosorbent assay (ELISA) is more sensitive and reproducible than ID and CIE [98]; its limitation is that asymptomatic patients from endemic areas may also show elevated antibody titers by ELISA.

Serologic assays may play a role in the follow-up of patients on antifungal treatment after the specific etiology is established.

Table 2 Appearance in tissue sections of eumycetoma grains for selected agents

Causative fungus	Grain shape	Cement characteristics	Hyphal arrangement	Chlamydoconidia characteristics
Black Grain Eumycetomas				
Exophiala jeanselmei	Round or oval with a hollow in the center	Cement absent	Hyphae located in the periphery	Located in the periphery
Leptosphaeria senegalensis	Round or lobulated	Black cement in periphery	Irregular network of hyphae in the center	Large and located in the periphery
Madurella grisea	Variable	Presence variable	Homogeneous network of hyphae in the center and dense network in the periphery	Located in the periphery
Madurella mycetomatis	Variable	Compact type: Homogeneous brown-cement throughout the grain	Hyphae throughout the grain	
		Vesicular type: Dense brown-cement in periphery	Hyphae located in the periphery	Large and located in the periphery
Pyrenochaeta romeroi	Variable	Presence variable	Central dense network of hyphae	Absent
White to Yellow Grain Eumycetomas				
Acremonium falciforme	Variable	Absent	Dense pattern of hyphae	Present
Fusarium spp.	Oval or lobulated	Absent	Dense pattern of interlaced hyphae	Rare
Neotestudina rosatii	Variable	Located in the periphery	Hyphae in the center and in the periphery; presence of oval or rounded hyphal fragments	Located in the center
Pseudallescheria boydii complex	Polylobulated or oval	Absent	Dense network of interwoven hyphae	Large

Treatment

Antifungal Agents

No evidence-based treatment recommendations are available for eumycetoma, as no large randomized clinical trials have been conducted. Moreover, the few clinical reports of the use of antifungal agents in the treatment of eumycetomas often involve a limited number of patients, do not differentiate by presence of bone involvement, and fail to establish a definitive response status due to the limited follow-up period. Even though new triazole drugs have been shown to be effective in treating eumycetomas, current options remain limited because of insufficient clinical data.

The in vitro activity of various antifungal agents against the organisms causing eumycetoma does not reliably predict clinical response. For example, amphotericin B has good in vitro activity against *M. mycetomatis*, *M. grisea*, and *E. jeanselmei*, but in vivo responses are poor, and clinical data do not support an important role for amphotericin B in the treatment of eumycetomas [99,100]. Liposomal amphotericin B has been used to treat eumycetomas caused by *M. grisea* and *Fusarium* species, producing temporary remission followed by clinical relapses 6 months after therapy was stopped [101]. Based on these limited anecdotal data, most experts believe that there is little role for amphotericin B in the treatment of eumycetoma.

Black grain eumycetoma agents are sensitive in vitro to the older azoles, with itraconazole demonstrating the most activity, followed by ketoconazole and miconazole [102]. Among the new triazoles, posaconazole is highly active in vitro against *Aspergillus* species and *P. boydii* complex [103,104], and voriconazole is active in vitro against *M. mycetomatis*, *M. grisea*, and *E. jeanselmei*. Voriconazole also has in vitro fungicidal activity against *Aspergillus* species and is more active than itraconazole against *P. boydii* complex isolates [105–107].

In general, itraconazole and ketoconazole appear to perform better against black grain than white grain eumycetomas [108]. Fluconazole 400 mg per day is not effective for eumycetoma caused by *M. mycetomatis*, *M. grisea*, or *P. boydii* complex [109].

For eumycetomas due to *M. mycetomatis* or *M. grisea*, itraconazole 100 mg twice daily is the regimen of choice. Preliminary results from the evaluation of posaconazole as salvage therapy of patients with various fungal infections resistant or refractory to standard treatment, including a small number of eumycetomas due to a variety of agents, are encouraging. Based on these data, posaconazole administered 200 mg orally four times daily or 400 mg twice daily is an acceptable alternative treatment for eumycetomas caused

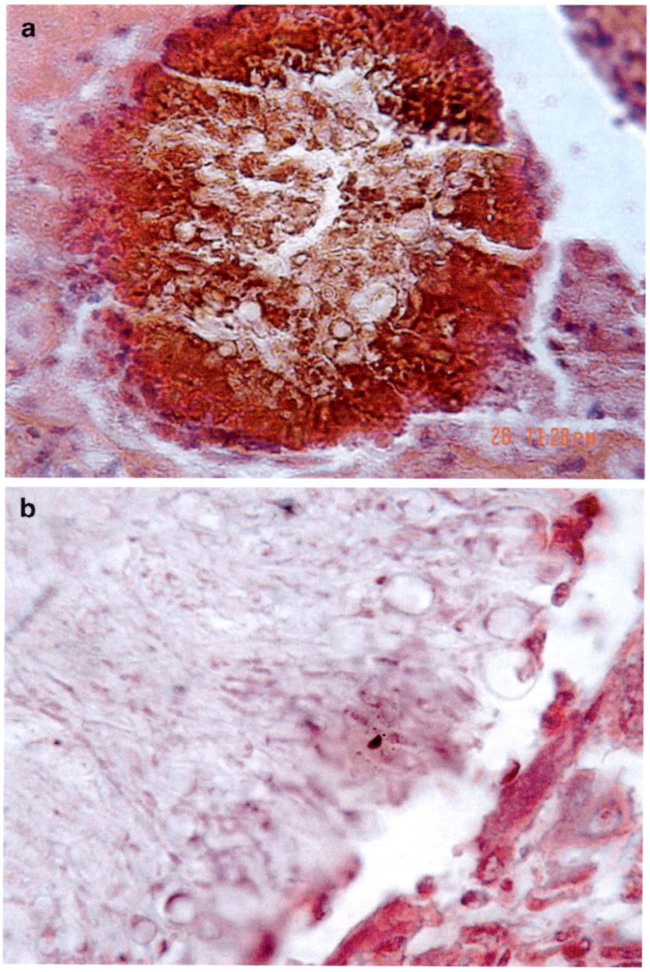

Fig. 6 (**a**) Histopathologic preparation of a grain from eumycetoma caused by *Madurella mycetomatis* (H&E stain, 400×). (**b**) Higher magnification showing hyphae and peripheral chlamydoconidia at the edge of a grain (H&E, 1,000×)

by *M. mycetomatis* or *M. grisea* [110]. Ketoconazole is also an effective agent for eumycetoma due to *M. mycetomatis* with reported rates of success greater than 70% when 400 mg or more daily is given for more than 6 months [99,101,108,111]. Ketoconazole at doses of 400 mg or more daily should be the first treatment option in areas in which the cost of itraconazole is prohibitive. Periodic evaluations of liver enzymes are mandatory, especially when ketoconazole is administered for prolonged periods.

Management of *P. boydii* complex infections is challenging because this fungus has intrinsic resistance to some antifungal agents, including fluconazole and amphotericin B. Ketoconazole alone or combined with surgery has been tried with varied outcomes [112–114]. Voriconazole demonstrates good in vitro fungicidal activity against *P. boydii* complex [106], and has been approved by the Food and Drug Administration (FDA) and the European Medicines Agency (EMEA) as salvage therapy for refractory scedosporiosis. Voriconazole has been successfully used to treat patients with severe *P. boydii* complex infections, including CNS and disseminated disease [115–119]. There are very limited data on the use of voriconazole specifically for the treatment of eumycetoma caused by *P. boydii* complex. However, based on the results noted above, voriconazole, 200 mg twice daily, could be considered a preferred regimen in areas in which the cost is not prohibitive [120,121]. Similarly, itraconazole alone or combined with surgery has been effective in some cases [120,122] and is considered an alternative therapy.

The optimal therapeutic regimen for *Acremonium* eumycetoma is unknown due to the scarcity of reports concerning therapy of this condition. Ketoconazole is not an effective treatment [114]; some eumycetomas caused by *Acremonium* species have been treated successfully with itraconazole. One patient with eumycetoma caused by *A. falciforme* responded satisfactorily to itraconazole 200 mg daily for 10 weeks [37], and a patient with *A. kiliense* eumycetoma, who had failed 3 years of ketoconazole 400 mg daily, rapidly improved when treated with itraconazole 300 mg daily [99]. Similarly, treatment of eumycetomas caused by *Aspergillus* species, *Arthrographis kalrae*, or *L. senegalensis* has not been established. Based on anecdotal reports and in vitro results, itraconazole 100 mg twice daily is considered the treatment of choice, and voriconazole is a promising alternative [105–107,123].

An unsatisfactory response to antifungal therapy correlates with the duration and extent of disease, susceptibility of the causative organism, and drug concentrations in the affected tissues. The latter is influenced by the pharmacokinetics of the agent used, the amount of fibrosis, and the local blood supply [124]. The absence of ischemic changes and necrosis in mycetoma lesions indicates that blood supply probably does not contribute significantly to the failure of medical treatment. However, it is likely that antifungal agents cannot reach adequate concentrations in grains surrounded by fibrotic and abscessed tissue.

Surgery

Early surgery can be curative for small and well-defined eumycetoma lesions, and is used to remove the greater bulk of the lesion when used as an adjunct to antifungal treatment. Antifungal therapy reduces the size of lesions when administered prior to surgery, and reduces recurrences when used following surgical debridement [99,111]. Additional indications for surgery in the management of eumycetoma are less well defined. Use of surgery to drain sinuses and remove grains or as a measure to reduce pain and swelling caused by inflammation is generally discouraged. Most experts advocate delaying surgery until patients have completed several months of antifungal chemotherapy [99]. Radical surgical procedures should generally be avoided [76].

Outcomes

An accepted time of follow-up to define cure for eumycetoma has not been firmly established. Many experts require 2 years of relapse-free survival, while others consider a patient cured only after 3 years have passed without evidence of relapse [40]. Assessment of stability, improvement, cure, or relapse is based on clinical and mycologic parameters, including the amount of discharge, degree of swelling, evolution of fistulae, radiographic findings, the results of histopathologic studies, and culture results.

References

1. Godfrey J. Disease of the foot not hitherto described. Lancet. 1846;1:593–4.
2. Carter HV. On a new and striking form of fungus disease, principally affecting the foot, and prevailing endemically in many parts of India. Trans Med Phys Soc Bombay. 1860;6:104–42.
3. Brumpt E. Les mycétomes. Arch Parasitol. 1906;10:489–564.
4. Pinoy E. Actinomycoses and mycetomas. Bull Inst Pasteur. 1913;11:929–38.
5. Chalmers AJ, Christopherson JB. A Sudanese actinomycosis. Ann Trop Med Parasitol. 1916;10:223–82.
6. Chalmers AJ, Archibald RG. A Sudanese maduromycosis. Ann Trop Med Parasitol. 1916;10:169–222.
7. McGinnis MR, Fader RC. Mycetoma: A contemporary concept. Infect Dis Clin N Am. 1988;2:939–54.
8. Gilgado F, Cano J, Gene J, Sutton DA, Guarro J. Molecular and phenotypic data supporting distinct species statuses for *Scedosporium apiospermum* and *Pseudallescheria boydii* and the proposed new species *Scedosporium dehoogii*. J Clin Microbiol. 2008;46:766–71.
9. Harun A, Perdomo H, Gilgado F, Chen SC, Cano J, Guarro J, et al. Genotyping of *Scedosporium* species: a review of molecular approaches. Med Mycol. 2009;47:406–14.
10. Hay RJ, Mahgoub ES, Leon G, Al-Sogair S, Welsh O. Mycetoma. J Med Vet Mycol. 1992;30 suppl 1:41–9.
11. Mariat F. On the geographic distribution and incidence of mycetoma agents. Bull Soc Pathol Exot Filiales. 1963;56:35–45.
12. Klokke AH, Swamidasan G, Anguli R, Verghese A. The causal agents of mycetoma in South India. Trans R Soc Trop Med Hyg. 1968;62:509–16.
13. Gumaa SA, Mahgoub ES, El Sid MA. Mycetoma of the head and neck. Am J Trop Med Hyg. 1986;35:594–600.
14. Hazra B, Bandyopadhyay S, Saha SK, Banerjee DP, Dutta G. A study of mycetoma in eastern India. J Commun Dis. 1988;30:7–11.
15. Venugopal PV, Venugopal TV. Treatment of eumycetoma with ketoconazole. Australas J Dermatol. 1993;34:27–9.
16. Maiti PK, Ray A, Bandyopadhyay S. Epidemiological aspects of mycetoma from a retrospective study of 264 cases in West Bengal. Trop Med Int Health. 2002;7:788–92.
17. Dieng MT, Sy MH, Diop BM, Niang SO, Ndiaye B. Mycetoma: 130 cases. Ann Dermatol Vénéréol. 2003;130:16–9.
18. Bakshi R, Mathur DR. Incidence and changing pattern of mycetoma in western Rajasthan. Indian J Pathol Microbiol. 2008;51:154–5.
19. Lavalle P. Mycetoma. In: Canizares O, Harman RRM, editors. Clinical Tropical Dermatology. 2nd ed. Boston: Blackwell Scientific Publication; 1992. p. 41–60.
20. Boiron P, Locci R, Goodfellow M, et al. Nocardia, nocardiosis and mycetoma. Med Mycol. 1998;36 Suppl 1:26–37.
21. Buot G, Lavalle P, Mariat F, Suchil P. Étude épidémiologique des mycétomes au Mexique. Bull Soc Pathol Exot. 1987;80:329–39.
22. Mahgoub ES. Mycetoma. In: Mahgoub ES, editor. Tropical mycoses. Beerse, Belgium: Janssen Research Council; 1989. p. 57–74.
23. Cooke WB, Kahler PW. Isolation of potentially pathogenic fungi from polluted water and sewage. Public Health Rep. 1955;70: 689–94.
24. Borelli D. *Madurella mycetomi* y *Madurella grisea*. Arch Venez Med Trop Parasit Med. 1962;4:195–211.
25. Segretain G, Mariat F. Recherche sur la presence d'agents de mycètomes dans le sol et sur les épineux du Sénégal et de la Mauritanie. Bull Soc Pathol Exot. 1968;61:194–201.
26. Thirumalachar MJ, Padhye AA. Isolation of *Madurella mycetomi* from soil in India. Hindustan Antibiot Bull. 1968;10:314–8.
27. Segretain G, Mariat F. Recherche sur l´écologie des agents de mycètomes fungiques au Sénégal. *5th Congress International Society Human and Animal Mycology*, Paris, France. pp. 153–154, 1971.
28. Segretain G. Epidémiologie des mycétomes. Ann Soc Belge Méd Trop. 1972;52:277–86.
29. Ahmed A, Adelmann D, Fahal A, Verbrugh H, van Belkum A, de Hoog S. Environmental occurrence of *Madurella mycetomatis*, the major agent of human eumycetoma in Sudan. J Clin Microbiol. 2002;40:1031–6.
30. Van Amstel SR, Ross M, Van Den Berg SS. Maduromycosis (*Madurella mycetomatis*) in a horse. J South Afr Vet Assoc. 1984;55:81–3.
31. Lambrechts N, Collett MG, Henton M. Black grain eumycetoma (*Madurella mycetomatis*) in the abdominal cavity of a dog. J Med Vet Mycol. 1991;29:211–4.
32. Elad D, Orgal U, Yakobson B, et al. Eumycetoma caused by *Curvularia lunata* in a dog. Mycopathologia. 1991;116:113–8.
33. Guillot J, Garcia-Hermoso D, Degorce F, et al. Eumycetoma caused by *Cladophialophora bantiana* in a dog. J Clin Microbiol. 2004;42:4901–3.
34. Ramachandran PK. Mycetoma caused by an unknown fungus in Indian buffaloes (*Bos bubalis*). Ceylon Vet J. 1968;16:77–80.
35. Abbott P. Mycetoma in the Sudan. Trans R Soc Trop Med Hyg. 1956;50:11–24.
36. Yu AM, Zhao S, Nie LY. Mycetomas in northern Yemen: identification of causative organisms and epidemiologic considerations. Am J Trop Med Hyg. 1993;48:812–7.
37. Lee MW, Kim JC, Choi JS, Kim KH, Greer DL. Mycetoma caused by *Acremonium falciforme*: successful treatment with itraconazole. J Am Acad Dermatol. 1995;32:897–900.
38. Fahal AH, el Toum EA, el Hassan AM, Mahgoub ES, Gumaa SA. The host tissue reaction to *Madurella mycetomatis*: new classification. J Med Vet Mycol. 1995;33:15–7.
39. Mahgoub ES, Gumma SA, El Hassan AM. Immunological status of mycetoma patients. Bull Soc Pathol Exot Filiales. 1977; 70:48–54.
40. Bendl BJ, Mackey D, Al-Saati F, Sheth KV, Ofole SN, Bailey TM. Mycetoma in Saudi Arabia. J Trop Med Hyg. 1987;90:51–9.
41. van de Sande WW, Fahal A, Verbrugh H, van Belkum A. Polymorphisms in genes involved in innate immunity predispose toward mycetoma susceptibility. J Immunol. 2007;179:3065.
42. Findlay GH, Vismer HF. Black grain mycetoma. A study of the chemistry, formation and significance of the tissue grain in *Madurella mycetomi* infection. Br J Dermatol. 1974;91:297–303.
43. van de Sande WW, de Kat J, Coppens J, et al. Melanin biosynthesis in *Madurella mycetomatis* and its effect on susceptibility to itraconazole and ketoconazole. Microbes Infect. 2007;9:1114–23.
44. Green Jr WO, Adams TE. Mycetoma in the United States: a review and report of seven additional cases. Am J Clin Pathol. 1964; 42:75–91.

45. Develoux M, Audoin J, Treguer J, Vetter JM, Warter A, Cenac A. Mycetoma in the Republic of Niger: clinical features and epidemiology. Am J Trop Med Hyg. 1985;38:386–90.
46. Castro LG, Belda Junior W, Salebian A, Cuce LC. Mycetoma: a retrospective study of 41 cases seen in Sao Paulo, Brazil, from 1978 to 1989. Mycoses. 1993;36:89–95.
47. Queiroz-Telles F, McGinnis MR, Salkin I, Graybill JR. Subcutaneous mycoses. Infect Dis Clin North Am. 2003;17:59–85.
48. Daoud M, Ezzine Sebai N, Badri T, Mokhtar I, Fazza B, Kamoun MR. Mycetoma: retrospective study of 13 cases in Tunisia. Acta Dermatoven APA. 2005;14:153–6.
49. N'diaye B, Dieng MT, Perez A, Stockmeyer M, Bakshi R. Clinical efficacy and safety of oral terbinafine in fungal mycetoma. Int J Dermatol. 2006;45:154–7.
50. Mirza SH, Gardezi AH, Khan Y, Wiqar MA. Subcutaneous facial mycosis in a child due to *Madurella mycetomatis*. J Pak Med Assoc. 2007;57:466–8.
51. Van Etta LL, Peterson LR, Gerding DN. *Acremonium falciforme* (*Cephalosporium falciforme*) mycetoma in a renal transplant patient. Arch Dermatol. 1983;119:707–8.
52. Meis JF, Schouten RA, Verweij PE, Dolmans W, Wetzels JF. Atypical presentation of *Madurella mycetomatis* mycetoma in a renal transplant patient. Transpl Infect Dis. 2000;2:96–8.
53. O'Riordan E, Denton J, Taylor PM, Kerr J, Short CD. Madura foot in the U.K.: fungal osteomyelitis after renal transplantation. Transplantation. 2002;73:151–3.
54. Geyer AS, Fox LP, Husain S, et al. *Acremonium* mycetoma in a heart transplant recipient. J Am Acad Dermatol. 2006;55:1095–100.
55. Satta R, Sanna S, Cottoni F. *Madurella* infection in an immunocompromised host. Int J Dermatol. 2000;39:939–41.
56. Neumeister B, Zollner TM, Krieger D, Sterry W, Marre R. Mycetoma due to *Exophiala jeanselmei* and *Mycobacterium chelonae* in a 73-year-old man with idiopathic CD4+ T lymphocytopenia. Mycoses. 1995;38:271–6.
57. Mendez-Tovar LJ, de Bièvre C, Lopez-Martinez R. Effets des hormones sexuelles humaines sur le development in vitro des agents d´eumycetomes. J Mycol Med. 1991;1:141–3.
58. Lynch JB. Mycetoma in the Sudan. Ann R Coll Surg. 1964;35:319–40.
59. Destombes P, Mariat L, Rosati G, Segretain G. Les mycétomes en Somalie – conclusions d´une enquête menée de 1959 à 1964. Acta Trop. 1977;34:335–73.
60. Bustamante B, Campos PE. Eumycetoma. In: Kauffman CA, editor. Atlas of fungal infections. 2nd ed. Philadelphia: Current Medicine; 2007. p. 203.
61. Lopez-Martinez R, Mendez-Tovar LJ, Lavalle P, Welsh O, Saul A, Macotela Ruiz E. Epidemiology of mycetoma in Mexico: study of 2105 cases. Gac Méd Méx. 1992;128:477–81.
62. Elhardello OA, Adam ES, Adam I. Abdominal wall mycetoma presented as obstructed incisional hernia of cesarean section in Eastern Sudan. Infect Dis Obstet Gynecol. 2007, on-line publication (Article ID 74643, doi:10.1155/2007/74643).
63. Arbab MA, el Hag IA, Abdul Gadir AF, Siddik H el-R. Intraspinal mycetoma: report of two cases. Am J Trop Med Hyg. 1997;56:27–9.
64. Gumma SA, Satir AA, Shehata AH, Mahgoub ES. Tumor of the mandible caused by *Madurella mycetomii*. Am J Trop Med Hyg. 1975;24:471–4.
65. Aldrige J, Kirk R. Mycetoma of the eyelid. Br J Ophthalmol. 1940;24:211–2.
66. Soni N, Gupta A, Shekhawat NS. Mycetoma - an unusual site. Surgery. 2000;127:709–10.
67. Ly F, Develoux M, Deme A, Dangou JM, Kane A, Ndiaye B, et al. Tumoral mycetoma of the buttock. Ann Dermatol Vénéréol. 2000;127:67–9.
68. Ravisse P, Huerre M, De Bièvre C, et al. Les mycétomes en Mauritanie: Étude histologique de 150 cas. J Mycol Med. 1992;2:154–9.
69. Negroni R, Lopez-Daneri G, Arechavala A, Bianchi MH, Robles AM. Clinical and microbiological study of mycetomas at the Muniz hospital of Buenos Aires between 1989 and 2004. Rev Argent Microbiol. 2006;38:13–8.
70. Niño FL. Coexistencia de *Madurella mycetomi* y de *M. grisea* en una misma observacion de maduromicosis podal negra. Mycopathologia. 1962;16:323–32.
71. Mahgoub ES. Mycetoma. Semin Dermatol. 1985;4:230–9.
72. Camain R. Processus d´extension et de limitation des mycétomes africains. Bull Soc Pathol Exot. 1968;61:517–23.
73. El Hassan AM, Mahgoub ES. Lymph node involvement in mycetoma. Trans R Soc Trop Med Hyg. 1972;66:165–9.
74. Sharif HS, Clark DC, Aabed MY, et al. Mycetoma: comparison of MR imaging with CT. Radiology. 1991;178:865–70.
75. Tomimori-Yamashita J, Ogawa MM, Hirata SH, Fischman O, Michalany NS, Yamashita HK, et al. Mycetoma caused by *Fusarium solani* with osteolytic lesions on the hand: case report. Mycopathologia. 2001;153:11–4.
76. McGinnis MR. Mycetoma. Dermatol Clin. 1996;14:97–104.
77. Abd El-Bagi ME, Fahal AH. Mycetoma revisited: Incidence of various radiographic signs. Saudi Med J. 2009;30:529–33.
78. Czechowski J, Nork M, Haas D, Lestringant G, Ekelund L. MR and other imaging methods in the investigation of mycetomas. Acta Radiol. 2001;42:24–6.
79. Sarris I, Berendt AR, Athanasous N, Ostlere SJ. MRI of mycetoma of the foot: two cases demonstrating the dot-in-circle sign. Skeletal Radiol. 2003;32:179–83.
80. Ahmed AO, Abugroun ES. Unexpected high prevalence of secondary bacterial infection in patients with mycetoma. J Clin Microbiol. 1998;36:850–1.
81. Fahal AH, Sheik HE, El Hassan AM. Pathological fractures in mycetoma. Trans R Soc Trop Med Hyg. 1996;90:675–67.
82. Fahal AH, Sharfi AR, Sheik HE, El Hassan AM, Mahgoub ES. Internal fistula formation: An unusual complication of mycetoma. Trans R Soc Trop Med Hyg. 1996;90:550–2.
83. Fahal AH, Yagi HI, El Hassan AM. Mycetoma-induced palatal deficiency and pharyngeal plexus dysfunction. Trans R Soc Trop Med Hyg. 1996;90:676–7.
84. Lopez-Cepeda LD, Mora-Ruiz S, Padilla-Desgarennes M del C, Ramos-Garibay JA. Small eumycetic mycetoma due to black grain. Arch Dermatol. 2005;141:783–4.
85. Gabhane SK, Gangane N, Anshu. Cytodiagnosis of eumycotic mycetoma: a case report. Acta Cytol. 2008;52:354–6.
86. Ahmed A, van de Sande W, Verbrugh H, et al. *Madurella mycetomatis* strains from mycetoma lesions in Sudanese patients are clonal. J Clin Microbiol. 2003;41:4537–41.
87. Hemashettar BM, Siddaramappa B, Munjunathaswamy BS, et al. *Phaeoacremonium krajdenii*, a cause of white grain eumycetoma. J Clin Microbiol. 2006;44:4619–22.
88. Desnos-Ollivier M, Bretagne S, Dromer F, et al. Molecular identification of black-grain mycetoma agents. J Clin Microbiol. 2006;44:3517–23.
89. Hay RJ, Mackenzie DWR. The histopathological features of pale grain eumycetoma. Trans R Soc Trop Med Hyg. 1982;76:839–44.
90. Hay RJ. Mycetoma (Maduromycosis). In: Strickland GT, editor. Hunter`s Tropical Medicine and Emerging Infectious Diseases. 8th ed. Philadelphia: W.B. Saunders; 2000. p. 537–41.
91. Chandler FW, Kaplan W, Ajello L. A Colour Atlas and Textbook of the Histopathology of Mycotic Diseases. London: Wolfe Medical Publication; 1980. p. 76–83. and 222–239.
92. Jackson JA, Kaplan W, Kaufman L, Standard P. Development of fluorescent-antibody reagents for demonstration of *Pseudallescheria boydii* in tissues. J Clin Microbiol. 1983;18:668–73.
93. Fenelon LE, Hamilton AJ, Figueroa JI, et al. Production of specific monoclonal antibodies to *Aspergillus* species and their use in

immunohistochemical identification of aspergillosis. J Clin Microbiol. 1999;37:1221–3.
94. Choi JK, Mauger J, McGowan KL. Immunohistochemical detection of *Aspergillus* species in pediatric tissue samples. Am J Clin Pathol. 2004;121:18–25.
95. Murray IG, Mahgoub ES. Further studies on the diagnosis of mycetoma by double diffusion in agar. Sabouraudia. 1968;6:106–10.
96. Gumma SA, Mahgoub ES. Counterimmunoelectrophoresis in the diagnosis of mycetoma and its sensitivity as compared to immunodiffusion. Sabouraudia. 1975;13:309–15.
97. Hay RJ, Mackenzie DWR. Mycetoma (madura foot) in the United Kingdom - a survey of forty-four cases. Clin Exp Dermatol. 1983;8:553–62.
98. Wethered DB, Markey MA, Hay RJ, Mahgoub ES, Gumma SA. Humoral immune responses to mycetoma organisms: characterization of specific antibodies by the use of enzyme-linked immunosorbent assay and immunoblotting. Trans R Soc Trop Med Hyg. 1988;82:918–23.
99. Welsh O. Mycetoma: current concepts in treatment. Int J Dermatol. 1991;30:387–98.
100. Restrepo A. Treatment of tropical mycoses. J Am Acad Dermatol. 1994;31:S91–102.
101. Welsh O, Salinas MC, Rodriguez MA. Treatment of eumycetoma and actinomycetoma. Curr Topics Med Mycol. 1995;6:47–71.
102. Venugopal PV, Venugopal TV, Ramakrishna ES, Ilavarasi S. Antimycotic susceptibility testing of agents of black grain eumycetoma. J Med Vet Mycol. 1993;31:161–4.
103. Marco F, Pfaller MA, Messer SA, Jones RN. *In vitro* activity of a new triazole antifungal agent, Sch 56592, against clinical isolates of filamentous fungi. Mycopathologia. 1998;141:73–7.
104. Sabatelli F, Patel R, Mann PA, et al. *In vitro* activities of posaconazole, fluconazole, itraconazole, voriconazole, and amphotericin B against a large collection of clinically important molds and yeasts. Antimicrob Agents Chemother. 2006;50:2009–15.
105. Clancy CJ, Nguyen MH. *In vitro* efficacy and fungicidal activity of voriconazole against *Aspergillus* and *Fusarium* species. Eur J Clin Microbiol Infect Dis. 1998;17:573–5.
106. McGinnis MR, Pasarell L. *In vitro* testing of susceptibilities of filamentous ascomycetes to voriconazole, itraconazole, and amphotericin B, with consideration of phylogenetic implications. J Clin Microbiol. 1998;36:2353–5.
107. Cuenca-Estrella M, Ruiz-Díez B, Martínez-Suárez JV, Monzón A, Rodríguez-Tudela JL. Comparative in-vitro activity of voriconazole (UK-109, 496) and six other antifungal agents against clinical isolates of *Scedosporium prolificans* and *Scedosporium apiospermum*. J Antimicrob Chemother. 1999;43:149–51.
108. Poncio-Mendes R, Negroni R, Bonifaz A, Pappagianis D. New aspects of some endemic mycoses. Med Mycol. 2000;38 suppl 1:237–41.
109. Diaz M, Negroni R, Montero-Gei F, et al. A Pan-American 5-year study of fluconazole therapy for deep mycoses in the immunocompetent host. Clin Infect Dis. 1992;14 Suppl 1:S68–76.
110. Pitisuttithum P, Negroni R, Graybill JR, et al. Activity of posaconazole in the treatment of central nervous system fungal infections. J Antimicrob Chemother. 2005;56:745–55.
111. Mahgoub ES, Gumma SA. Ketoconazole in the treatment of eumycetoma due to *Madurella mycetomii*. Trans R Soc Trop Med Hyg. 1984;78:376–9.
112. Symoens J, Moens M, Dom J, et al. An evaluation of two years of clinical experience with ketoconazole. Rev Infect Dis. 1980;2: 674–87.
113. Drohuet E, Dupont B. Laboratory and clinical assessment of ketoconazole in deep-seated mycosis. Am J Med. 1983;74:30.
114. Hay RJ. Ketoconazole in the treatment of fungal infection. Clinical and laboratory studies. Am J Med. 1983;74:16–9.
115. Poza G, Montoya J, Redondo C, et al. Meningitis caused by *Pseudallescheria boydii* treated with voriconazole. Clin Infect Dis. 2000;30:981–2.
116. Muñoz P, Marín M, Tornero P, Martín-Rabadán P, Rodríguez-Creixems M, Bouza E. Successful outcome of *Scedesporiun apiospermum* disseminated infection treated with voriconazole in a patient receiving corticosteroid therapy. Clin Infect Dis. 2000;31:1499–501.
117. Nesky MA, McDougal EC, Peacock JE. *Pseudallesheria boydii* brain abscess successfully treated with voriconazole and surgical drainage: case report and literature review of central nervous system pseudallesheriasis. Clin Infect Dis. 2000;31:673–7.
118. Porte L, Khatibi S, Hajj LE, et al. *Scedosporium apiospermum* mycetoma with bone involvement successfully treated with voriconazole. Trans R Soc Trop Med Hyg. 2006;100:891–4.
119. Troke P, Aguirrebengoa K, Arteaga C, et al. Treatment of scedosporiosis with voriconazole: clinical experience with 107 patients. Antimicrob Agents Chemother. 2008;52:1743–50.
120. Lexier R, Walmsley SL. Successful treatment of Madura foot caused by *Pseudallescheria boydii* with *Escherichia coli* superinfection: a case report. Can J Surg. 1999;42:307–9.
121. Turner PG. Madura foot or plantar fibromatosis. J Bone Joint Surg Br. 1989;71:531.
122. Queiroz-Telles F, Queiroz-Telles JE. Treatment of paracoccidiodomycosis and *Pseudallescheria boydii* mycetoma with itraconazole: a preliminary report of two cases. Rev Iberica Micología. 1988;5 Suppl 1:72.
123. Degavre B, Joujoux JM, Dandurand M, Guillot B. First report of mycetoma caused by *Arthrographis kalrae*: successful treatment with itraconazole. J Am Acad Dermatol. 1997;37:318–20.
124. Fahal AH, el Hag IA, Gadir AF, el Lider AR, el Hassan AM, Baraka OZ, et al. Blood supply and vasculature of mycetoma. J Med Vet Mycol. 1997;35:101–6.

Chromoblastomycosis

John W. Baddley and William E. Dismukes

Chromoblastomycosis is a chronic fungal infection of the skin and subcutaneous tissues characterized by the presence of nodular, verrucous lesions, often of the lower extremities. Upon histopathologic examination of infected tissues, the characteristic finding is single or multiple muriform cells, also called sclerotic bodies. The term muriform designates the presence of vertical and horizontal septa of the cells. These muriform cells are dark brown, septate fungal cells that resemble yeast forms (Fig. 1). Chromoblastomycosis is caused by several species of dematiaceous, or pigmented, fungi, of which the most common causative organism is *Fonsecaea pedrosoi*. The disease is usually chronic, localized, and is rarely life-threatening. Surgical resection and cryotherapy are effective for small lesions, while antifungal agents, including itraconazole and terbinafine, are sometimes effective in more extensive disease.

For the purposes of this chapter, chromoblastomycosis is defined as a chronic infection of the skin or subcutaneous tissues caused by dematiaceous fungi and characterized by the presence of muriform cells on histopathologic examination. Chromoblastomycosis has been referred to as chromomycosis, although these terms are not synonymous. The term chromomycosis has come to represent not only the classic definition of chromoblastomycosis, but also additional non-skin and subcutaneous infections due to dematiaceous fungi [1, 2]. Phaeohyphomycoses represent the broad group of fungal infections caused by dematiaceous fungi and are defined by the presence of yeast-like cells, hyphal forms, or pseudohyphae-like elements in tissue, but without the presence of muriform cells as seen in chromoblastomycosis [1]. Phaeohyphomycoses are addressed in a separate chapter.

Organisms

The organisms causing chromoblastomycosis are saprophytic fungi found in soil, wood, vegetation, pulp, and paper [3, 4]. Several species of dematiaceous fungi cause chromoblastomycosis, and the similarity between organisms lies in the tissue appearance of muriform cells (Fig. 1). The agents of chromoblastomycosis belong to a single order of ascomycetous fungi, the Chaetothyriales [5]. Common etiologic agents include *F. pedrosoi*, *F. compacta*, *Phialophora verrucosa*, *Cladosporium carrionii* and *Rhinocladiella aquaspersa* [5]. Additional organisms reported less commonly as etiologic agents include *Exophiala spinifera*, *E. jeanselmei*, *E. dermatitidis*, and *Aureobasidium pullulans* [6–8]. More recently, other cases presented have been caused by *Rhytidhysteron* species, *Chaetomium funicola*, *Catenulostroma chromoblastomycosum* and *F. monophora* [9–11]. A list of reported causative agents is provided in Table 1.

Fungi causing chromoblastomycosis are slow growing and usually need to be incubated at least 4 weeks on standard fungal media, such as Sabouraud's dextrose agar. Most species form dark brown, green, or black velvety colonies upon incubation. Morphologic differences on media and microscopy are variable, and have led to placement of the causative organisms in many different genera. The mycology and nomenclature of organisms that cause chromoblastomycosis have been reviewed extensively elsewhere [1, 2, 12].

Epidemiology

Chromoblastomycosis occurs worldwide, although the majority of reported cases are from tropical and subtropical regions of the Americas and Africa. The mode of acquisition of infection is traumatic inoculation of the fungus into exposed skin, usually the lower extremities. Affected patients are frequently outdoor laborers or those who do not routinely wear shoes [13]. Most patients do not recall a specific injury, but in a series of patients who remembered a traumatic inciting event, inoculation resulted from thorns, wood splinters, or minor cuts from tools [14].

J.W. Baddley (✉)
Division of Infectious Diseases, Birmingham VA Medical Center, University of Alabama at Birmingham School of Medicine, Birmingham, AL, USA
e-mail: jbaddley@uab.edu

C.A. Kauffman et al. (eds.), *Essentials of Clinical Mycology*,
DOI 10.1007/978-1-4419-6640-7_25,

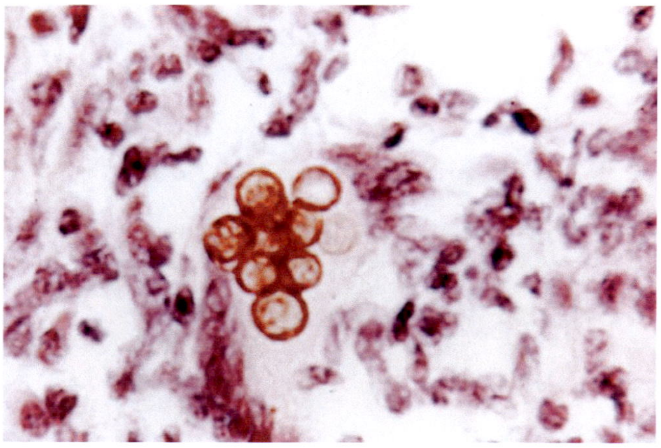

Fig. 1 H&E-stained tissue section showing sclerotic bodies typical of chromoblastomycosis (Courtesy of David W. Warnock)

Table 1 Causative agents of chromoblastomycosis

Organism
Fonsecea pedrosoi
Fonsecea compacta
Cladosporium carrionii
Rhinocladiella aquaspersa
Phialophora verrucosa
Botryomyces caespitosus
Exophiala dermatitidis
Exophiala jeanselmei
Exophiala spinifera
Aureobasidium pullulans
Fonsecaea monophora
Rhytidhysteron spp.
Chaetomium funicola
Catenulostroma chromoblastomycosum

Epidemiology of chromoblastomycosis often depends on geographic region. For example, in Brazil, Colombia, Japan, and humid parts of Venezuela, *F. pedrosoi* is the predominant causative agent [15, 16], while in arid parts of Australia, China, Mexico, Cuba, and Venezuela, *C. carrionii* is the most common cause [13, 17]. Site of involvement also seems to differ in patients from various geographic locations. In most countries, the lower extremities are the most frequently affected sites; the exceptions are Japan and Australia, where upper body sites predominate [15, 17, 18].

Most cases of chromoblastomycosis occur among males aged 30–60 [18]; children are rarely affected. The male predominance probably represents increased exposure due to a preponderance of male outdoor workers in some countries. By contrast, in Japan, among a large series of cases the ratio of males to females was equal [15].

Clinical Manifestations

The cutaneous lesions of chromoblastomycosis are highly variable, and typically begin at the site of a traumatic inoculation of the fungal organism [5, 12]. Lesions grow slowly, and are asymptomatic in the majority of cases [14]. Symptoms, when present, include pruritus and, rarely, pain. Lesions are usually present months to years before patients seek medical attention and are diagnosed [5, 14, 18–21]. In one series of 100 patients, the mean interval between first symptoms and diagnosis was 14 years [14].

The most commonly involved anatomic sites are the lower extremities, particularly the foot, ankle, and lower leg. However, skin lesions can be present on virtually any part of the body, including the abdomen, chest, back, upper extremities, neck, face, buttocks and rarely, mucous membranes such as the nasal septum [5, 14, 22–24]. Most skin lesions are localized, but disseminated disease has been reported in a small percentage of patients [14, 15]. Spread of lesions may occur by autoinoculation resulting from scratching or by lymphatic spread [5, 25]. Hematogenous dissemination is extremely rare, even among immunosuppressed patients, but has resulted in brain abscess and death in several cases [15, 26, 27].

The initial lesions of chromoblastomycosis are small papules or nodules that become confluent to form irregular, verrucous plaques. In 1950, Carrion reported a series of agricultural workers with chromoblastomycosis and described five types of lesions seen during the progression of disease: nodular, tumorous, verrucous, plaque, and cicatricial [28]. Nodular lesions are soft, pink growths that can be smooth, verrucous, or scaly. These lesions may continue to enlarge and form tumorous growths that appear papillomatous, lobulated, or may enlarge and resemble cauliflower (Fig. 2). Verrucous lesions, the most common type, have a wart-like, dry appearance and are frequently present on the borders of the foot [1]. Plaque lesions are slightly raised, pink to reddish in color, and are scaly (Fig. 3). Cicatricial lesions, often large and serpiginous, expand centrifugally while healing; atrophic scarring occurs in the center of the lesions (Fig. 4).

A grading system has been developed for clinical forms of chromoblastomycosis lesions. This system may be useful for determining therapeutic options and stratifying treatment groups for therapeutic trials [5, 13, 20]. With this system, *mild* disease is defined as a solitary plaque or nodule measuring less than 5 cm in diameter. *Moderate* disease comprises solitary or multiple lesions: verruciform, nodular, or plaque types, covering one or two adjacent cutaneous regions and measuring less than 15 cm in diameter. The *severe* form is defined as any type of lesion, either single or multiple, covering extensive cutaneous regions [13].

Complications of chromoblastomycosis include secondary bacterial infection, which may present with fever, pain, edema,

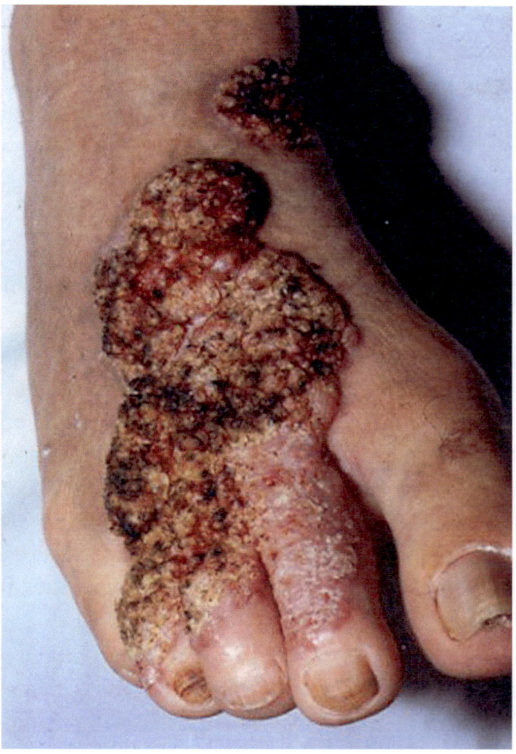

Fig. 2 Nodular, cauliflower-like lesions of chromoblastomycosis (Courtesy of Flavio Queiroz-Telles)

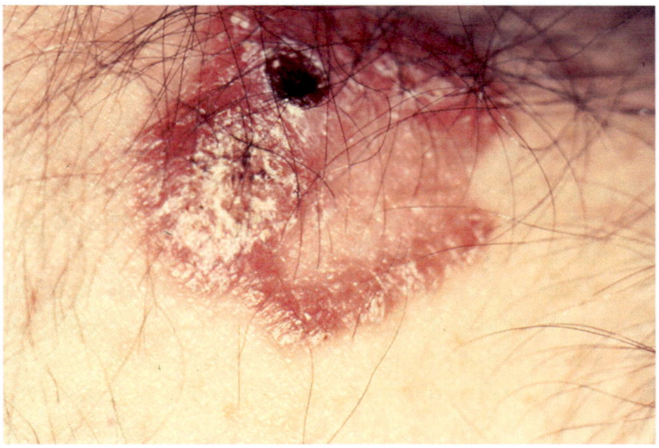

Fig. 3 Plaque lesion of chromoblastomycosis

localized lymphadenopathy, and chronic lymphedema. For long-standing lesions, carcinomatous transformation, particularly to squamous cell cancer, has been described [14, 29].

Diagnosis

The diagnosis of chromoblastomycosis is made on the basis of typical skin lesions and the presence of muriform cells on histopathologic examination. Tissues, including skin

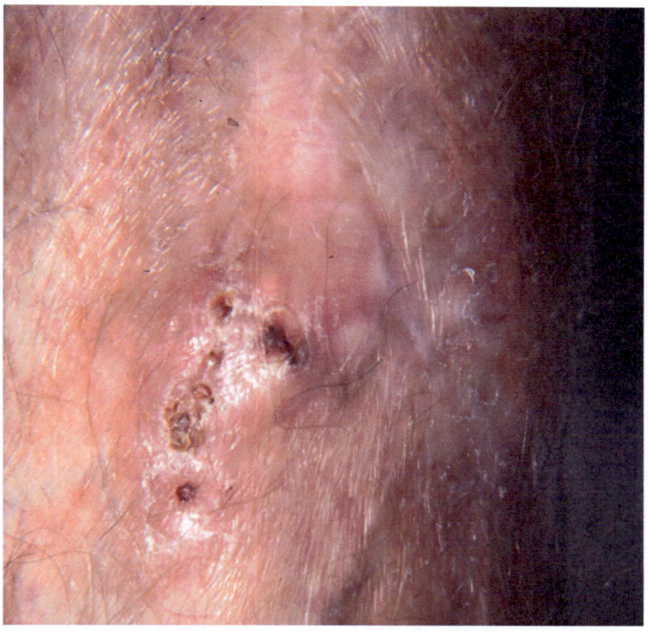

Fig. 4 Cicatricial lesion with atrophic scarring

scrapings, aspirated exudates, or biopsy specimens, can be visualized under the microscope and may demonstrate muriform cells without special staining. Muriform cells are seen in the dermis, while hyphal elements, when present, are confined to epidermal layers. Culture of the causative organism must be performed on fungal media containing antibiotics, such as Sabouraud's dextrose agar with chloramphenicol and cycloheximide, as bacterial contamination is common. Cultures should be incubated at 25–30°C and kept for 4–6 weeks [1, 2, 12]. Non-culture-based methods using PCR for diagnosis of chromoblastomycosis have been reported recently [30, 31].

Histopathologic examination of lesions of chromoblastomycosis reveals hyperkeratosis and pseudoepitheliomatous hyperplasia in the stratum corneum and epidermis. In the dermis, a mixed pyogenic and granulomatous inflammatory process comprised of neutrophils, plasma cells, eosinophils, lymphocytes, and multinucleated giant cells is seen. Fibrosis may be evident, particularly in older lesions [32]. Muriform cells, also referred to as sclerotic bodies, Medlar cells, or "copper pennies," are found in dermal tissue, and range in size from 5 to 15 μm in diameter (Fig. 1). They are dark brown in color, have thick walls, are septate, and may be single, in pairs, or in clusters. Muriform cells may be found extracellularly among inflammatory cells, intracellularly in giant cells, and rarely, in macrophages.

Transepithelial migration, or transepithelial elimination, is a pathologic finding in chromoblastomycosis. In this process, foreign matter, blood, damaged tissue, and muriform cells are expelled through the epidermis as a healing process [1, 5]. Accordingly, transepithelial migration will manifest as "black dots" on the surface of lesions, which, upon slide microscopy with 10% or 20% KOH, reveal clotted blood and muriform cells [1, 5, 33, 34].

Treatment

Chromoblastomycosis is a chronic disease that is difficult to treat. Therapy is usually sought for aesthetic or functional reasons, but therapy is also necessary to prevent associated complications. Clinical response may range from 10% to 80%, but is often related to the stage of disease [5, 35, 36]. In patients with extensive disease, cure rates are low and relapse is not uncommon. No single therapy is uniformly effective, and treatment modalities for chromoblastomycosis have been difficult to evaluate because of the small number of cases, variability in extent of disease, and lack of randomized treatment trials. In a large retrospective review, Minotto and colleagues reported that disease was eradicated with therapy in 57% of patients [14]. Over the period of this 30-year study, numerous therapies were used for different lengths of time, and therefore an optimal therapy could not be determined. In another retrospective review of 51 cases, 31% of patients were cured, and 57% improved with various treatments [22]. Multiple therapeutic strategies, including surgical intervention; topical therapies (cryotherapy, applied heat); systemic antifungal agents; or a combination of therapies are employed and described below (Table 2).

Systemic Antifungal Therapy

In general, antifungal therapy for chromoblastomycosis has been minimally successful, and prolonged therapy is required.

Table 2 Treatment of chromoblastomycosis

Chemotherapy		
Drug	Dosage	Selected References
Itraconazole (po)	200–400 mg/day	[20, 22, 37–40]
Flucytosine (po)	50–150 mg/kg/day	[41–43]
Terbinafine (po)	500 mg/day	[44–46]
Amphotericin B(IV)	0.5–1.0 mg/kg/day	[41, 47, 48]
Fluconazole (po)	200–800 mg/day	[49]
Ketoconazole (po)	200–400 mg/day	[50, 51]
Posaconazole (po)	800 mg/day	[52]
Other Therapies		
Surgical resection		[53–55]
Cryotherapy		[22, 38, 56, 57]
CO_2 laser therapy		[58–60]
Heat therapy		[59, 61–63]
Electrosurgery and curettage		[48, 64]

Systemic antifungal agents are usually needed in cases of moderate or extensive disease, or when surgery is not possible. Antifungal therapy may also be required for lesions in areas of flexion where cryosurgery is not indicated. The most commonly used drugs are itraconazole, terbinafine, flucytosine, and amphotericin B, although there is experience with numerous antimicrobial agents (Table 2).

Itraconazole appears to be the most promising chemotherapeutic agent for the treatment of chromoblastomycosis and is usually given at a daily dose of 200–400 mg. Antifungal susceptibility testing of itraconazole against *Fonsecaea* species and other agents of chromoblastomycosis shows good activity, although it does not appear that the minimal inhibitory concentration (MIC) predicts clinical response [65–68]. Clinical results with itraconazole have been variable, depending upon extent of disease and length and dosage of therapy [20, 22, 37–40, 68–70]. In an early open-label study of 14 patients with chromoblastomycosis, itraconazole was given at dosages of 100–400 mg daily for 4–8 months [38]. Among nine patients with *C. carrionii* infection, cure was achieved in eight, and one improved; among five patients infected with *F. pedrosoi*, two were cured, and three improved. In the two cases of infection due to *F. pedrosoi* that were cured, itraconazole was given in combination with either flucytosine or local heat.

In a noncomparative open-label trial of 19 Brazilian patients with chromoblastomycosis due to *F. pedrosoi*, itraconazole at doses of 200–400 mg daily for 3–30.5 months was effective [20]. Among ten patients with mild-to-moderate disease, eight achieved complete clinical and biologic cure. Among the remaining patients who had moderate or severe disease, all had clinical healing or improvement. Itraconazole was well tolerated, and no adverse events were reported that warranted discontinuation of therapy.

Another trial evaluated combination therapy with itraconazole and cryosurgery, itraconazole alone, and cryosurgery alone in 12 patients with chromoblastomycosis due to *F. pedrosoi* [37]. Among patients with small lesions, cryotherapy appeared more effective than itraconazole alone at a dose of 300 mg daily. One group, comprised of patients with extensive disease, was treated with itraconazole until lesions maximally improved, followed by cryosurgery. Among these four patients, two were cured, and two improved. The authors suggest that cryosurgery may be a useful adjunct to chemotherapy for patients with extensive disease.

Recent reports outline the use of pulse therapy with itraconazole, either alone or in combination with cryotherapy [39, 40, 70]. While success was seen in several cases, the potential impact of pulse therapy with itraconazole needs further study.

Other azole agents, including fluconazole and ketoconazole, have been used as single-agent therapy to treat chromoblastomycosis in a small number of patients but have not been very effective [49–51, 71]. The newer broad-spectrum triazoles, posaconazole and voriconazole, appear to have good in vitro activity against *Cladosporium* species [68, 72]. Posaconazole at a dose of 800 mg daily for up to 34 months was used to successfully treat five of six patients with refractory chromoblastomycosis [52].

Oral flucytosine, 50–150 mg/kg per day divided in four doses, has been used for up to 1 year with associated clinical improvement [17, 41–43, 73]. However, when used as a single therapy, only partial response with progression of disease or relapse has occurred, suggesting clinical and microbiologic resistance [74]. Subsequently, combination therapy with flucytosine is preferred. Flucytosine in combination with amphotericin B, itraconazole, ketoconazole, or thiabendazole is sometimes effective [41, 47, 48, 75–77].

Terbinafine, an allylamine antifungal, has been effective in the treatment of patients with chromoblastomycosis [44–46, 78]. In an open-label pilot study of 43 patients, oral terbinafine at doses of 500 mg daily for 12 months gave very promising results, namely, mycologic cure in 82.5% of patients and total cure in 47% of patients with lesions present longer than 10 years [46].

Intravenous amphotericin B as single therapy appears to be minimally effective, and is often associated with adverse events after prolonged use [1, 41, 47, 48]. Amphotericin B, when used, is often given in combination with flucytosine for moderate or severe chromoblastomycosis [1, 41, 47, 48].

Surgical Therapy

For small or few lesions, surgical intervention may be effective, although adequate comparative studies are not available [53, 54]. Wide and deep resection to healthy tissue is necessary in order to prevent relapse, but as a result, skin grafting may be required. For larger, more extensive lesions, surgical resection is less effective and is often not possible for functional reasons [53]. Moh's micrographic surgery has been used successfully for treatment in one reported case [55]. Procedures such as curettage and desiccation are discouraged because of associated high recurrence rates and the potential for lymphatic dissemination [1, 48, 64].

Topical Therapy

Alternative procedures to surgical resection include minor interventions such as cryosurgery with liquid nitrogen; thermotherapy; and carbon dioxide laser therapy, all of which have been used with varying degrees of success [37, 56–59, 61, 62]. The best results have been observed with a combination of antifungal agents and cryotherapy [22, 37, 38, 57, 79, 80]. For smaller lesions, cryotherapy is effective, but this method cannot be used for lesions in flexion areas or skin folds because of the risk of fibrosis and scarring. Important side effects of cryotherapy include pain at the site, local edema, formation of blisters, and bacterial superinfection. Because of risk of dissemination of infection with cryosurgery alone, some experts recommend that antifungal therapy and cryotherapy always be given in combination [5, 22].

Because organisms such *F. pedrosoi* are unable to grow at temperatures greater than 40°C, applying heat to skin lesions may theoretically lead to fungal death. Local heat therapy, which may be applied several times daily with pocket warmers, has been effective as single therapy in several cases but may be more appropriate as an adjunct to antifungal agents or cryotherapy [38, 59, 61–63].

Carbon dioxide laser therapy has been used as a treatment modality in only a small number of cases, and its place in the treatment hierarchy is unclear [58–60].

Although promising agents are available for the treatment of chromoblastomycosis, appropriate comparative trials to evaluate therapies remain difficult to perform due to the rarity of cases, variability of disease, and the need for prolonged therapy. Combination therapy with an antifungal drug plus surgical therapy or cryotherapy represents a potential advance in treatment and an important area for further study.

References

1. Fader RC, McGinnis MR. Infections caused by dematiaceous fungi: chromoblastomycosis and phaeohyphomycosis. Infect Dis Clin N Am. 1988;2:925–38.
2. Kwon-Chung KJ, Bennett JE. Medical Mycology. Philadelphia: Lea & Febiger; 1992.
3. Ridley MF. The natural habitat of *Cladosporium carrionii*, a cause of chromoblastomycosis in man. Aust J Dermatol. 1957;4:23–7.
4. Gezuele E, Mackinnon JE, Conti-Diaz IA. The frequent isolation of *Phialophora verrucosa* and *Phialophora pedrosoi* from natural sources. Sabouraudia. 1972;10:266–73.
5. Queiroz-Telles F, Esterre P, Perez-Blanco M, et al. Chromoblastomycosis: an overview of clinical manifestations, diagnosis and treatment. Med Mycol. 2009;47:3–15.
6. Padhye AA, Hampton MT, Hutton NW, Proevost-Smith E, Davis MS. Chromoblastomycosis caused by *Exophiala spinifera*. Clin Infect Dis. 1996;22:331–5.
7. Naka W, Harada T, Nishikawa T, Fukushiro R. A case of chromoblastomycosis: with special reference to the mycology of the isolated *Exophiala jeanselmei*. Mykosen. 1986;29:445–52.
8. Redondo-Bellon P, Idoate M, Rubio M, Ignacio HJ. Chromoblastomycosis produced by *Aureobasidium pullulans* in an immunosuppressed patient. Arch Dermatol. 1997;133:663–4.
9. Chowdarry A, Guarro J, Randhawa HS, et al. A rare case of chromoblastomycosis in a renal transplant recipient caused by a non-sporulating species of *Rhytidhysteron*. Med Mycol. 2008;46:163–6.
10. Piepenbring M, Caceres Mendez OA, Espino Espinoza AA, et al. Chromoblastomycosis caused by *Chaetomium funicola*: a case report from Western Panama. Br J Dermatol. 2007;157:1025–9.

11. Xi L, Changming L, Jiufeng S, et al. Chromoblastomycosis caused by a meristemic mutant of *Fonsecaea monophora*. Med Mycol. 2009;l47:77–80.
12. McGinnis MR. Chromoblastomycosis and phaeohyphomycosis: new concepts, diagnosis and mycology. J Am Acad Dermatol. 1983; 8:1–16.
13. Queiroz-Telles F, McGinnis MR, Salkin I, et al. Subcutaneous mycoses. Infect Dis Clin N Am. 2003;17:59–85.
14. Minotto R, Bernardi CDV, Mallmann LF, Edelweiss MIA, Scroferneker ML. Chromoblastomycosis: A review of 100 cases in the state of Rio Grande do Sul, Brazil. J Am Acad Dermatol. 2001;44:585–92.
15. Fukushiro R. Chromomycosis in Japan. Int J Dermatol. 1983; 22:221–9.
16. Velasquez LF, Restrepo A, Calle G. Cromomicosis: experiencia de doce anos. Acta Med Colombiana. 1976;1:165–71.
17. Leslie DF, Beardmore GL. Chromoblastomycosis in Queensland: a retrospective study of 13 cases at the Royal Brisbane Hospital. Aust J Dermatol. 1979;20:23–30.
18. Silva JP, De Souza W, Rozental S. Chromoblastomycosis: a retrospective study of 325 cases on Amazonic region (Brazil). Mycopathologica. 1998;143:171–5.
19. Londero AT, Ramos CD. Chromomycosis: a clinical and mycological study of thirty-five cases observed in the hinterland of Rio Grande do Sul, Brazil. Am J Trop Med Hyg. 1976;25:132–5.
20. Queiroz-Telles F, Purim KS, Fillus JN, et al. Itraconazole in the treatment of chromoblastomycosis due to *Fonsecaea pedrosoi*. Int J Dermatol. 1992;31:805–12.
21. Rajendran C, Ramesh V, Misra RS, Kandhari S, Upreti HB, Datta KK. Chromoblastomycosis in India. Int J Dermatol. 1997;36:29–33.
22. Bonifaz A, Carrasco-Gerard E, Saul A. Chromoblastomycosis: clinical and mycologic experience of 51 cases. Mycoses. 2001;44:1–7.
23. Nakamura T, Grant JA, Threlkeld R, Wible L. Primary chromoblastomycosis of the nasal septum. Am J Clin Pathol. 1972;58:365–70.
24. Zaror L, Fischman O, Pereira CA, Felipe RG, Gregorio LC, Castelo A. A case of primary nasal chromoblastomycosis. Mykosen. 1987; 30:468–71.
25. Ogawa MM, Alchorne MM Barbieri A, et al. Lymphoscintigraphic analysis in chromoblastomycosis. Int J Dermatol. 2003;42:622–5.
26. Takase T, Baba T, Ueno K. Chromomycosis. A case with a widespread rash, lymph node metastasis and multiple subcutaneous nodules. Mycoses. 1988;31:343–52.
27. Wackym PA. Cutaneous chromomycosis in renal transplant recipients. Arch Intern Med. 1985;145:1036–7.
28. Carrion A. Chromoblastomycosis. Ann NY Acad Sci. 1950; 50:1255–81.
29. Foster HM, Harris TJ. Malignant change (squamous carcinoma) in chronic chromoblastomycosis. Aust N Z Surg. 1987;57:775–7.
30. Abliz P, Fukushima K, Takizawa K, et al. Specific oligonucleotide primers for identification of *Cladophialophora carrionii*, a causative agent of chromoblastomycosis. J Clin Microbiol. 2004; 42:404–7.
31. de Andrade TS, Cury AE, de Castro LG, et al. Rapid identification of *Fonsecaea* by duplex polymerase chain reaction in isolates from patients with chromoblastomycosis. Diagn Microbiol Infect Dis. 2007;57:267–72.
32. Uribe F, Zuluga AI, Leon W, Restrepo A. Histopathology of chromoblastomycosis. Mycopathologia. 1989;105:1–6.
33. Banks IS, Palmier JR, Lanoie L, Connor DH, Meyers WM. Chromomycosis in Zaire. Int J Dermatol. 1985;24:302–7.
34. Goette DK, Robertson D. Transepithelial elimination in chromomycosis. Arch Dermatol. 1984;120:400–1.
35. Bonifaz A, Paredes-Solis V, Saul A. Treating chromoblastomycosis with systemic antifungals. Expert Opin Pharmacother. 2004; 4:247–54.
36. Esterre P, Querioz-Telles F. Management of chromoblastomycosis: novel perspectives. Curr Opin Infect Dis. 2006;19:148–52.
37. Bonifaz A, Martínez-Soto E, Carrasco-Gerard E, Peniche J. Treatment of chromoblastomycosis with itraconazole, cryosurgery, and a combination of both. Int J Dermatol. 1997;35:542–7.
38. Borelli D. A clinical trial of itraconazole in the treatment of deep mycoses and leishmaniasis. Rev Infect Dis. 1987;9 Suppl 1: S57–63.
39. Ranawaka RR, Amarainghe N, Hewage D. Chromoblastomycosis: combined treatment with pulsed itraconazole therapy and liquid nitrogen cryotherapy. Int J Dermatol. 2009;48:397–400.
40. Restrepo A, Gonzalez A, Gomez I, Arango M, DeBedout C. Treatment of chromoblastomycosis with itraconazole. Ann NY Acad Sci. 1988;544:504–16.
41. Bopp CC. De cromobladtomicose por novo tratamiento. Med Cut ILA. 1976;4:285–92.
42. Lopes CF, Alvarenga RJ, Cisalpino EO, Resende MA, Oliveira LG. Six years' experience in treatment of chromomycosis with 5-fluorocytosine. Int J Dermatol. 1978;17:414–8.
43. Lopes CF. Recent developments in the therapy of chromoblastomycosis. Bull Pan Am Health Organ. 1981;15:58–64.
44. Tanuma H, Hiramatsu M, Mukai H, et al. Case report. A case of chromoblastomycosis effectively treated with terbinafine. Characteristics of chromoblastomycosis in the Kitasato region, Japan. (Review). Mycoses. 2000;43:79–83.
45. Bonifaz A, Saul A, Paredes-Solis V, et al. Treatment of chromoblastomycosis with terbinafine: experience with four cases. J Dermatol Treat. 2005;16:47–51.
46. Esterre P, Inzan CK, Ramarcel ER, et al. Treatment of chromomycosis with terbinafine: preliminary results of an open pilot study. Br J Dermatol. 1996;134 Suppl 46:33–6. discussion 40.
47. Astorga B, Bonilla E, Martínez C, Mora W. Tratamiento de la cromomicosis con anfortericina B y 5-fluorocitosina. Med Cut ILA. 1981;9:125–8.
48. Restrepo A. Treatment of tropical mycoses. J Am Acad Dermatol. 1994;31:S91–102.
49. Diaz M, Negroni R, Montero-Gei F, et al. A Pan-American 5-year study of fluconazole therapy for deep mycosis in the immunocompetent host. Clin Infect Dis. 1992;14(Suppl):S568–76.
50. Drouhet E, Dupont B. Laboratory and clinical assessment of ketoconazole in deep-seated mycoses. Am J Med. 1983;74:30–47.
51. McBurney EI. Chromoblastomycosis treatment with ketoconazole. Cutis. 1982;30:746–8.
52. Negroni R, Tobin A, Bustamante B, et al. Posaconazole treatment of refractory eumycetoma and chromoblastomycosis. Rev Inst Med Trop São Paulo. 2005;47:339–46.
53. Bansal AS, Prabhakar P. Chromomycosis: a twenty-year-analysis of histologically confirmed cases in Jamaica. Trop Geogr Med. 1989;41:222–6.
54. Conway H, Berkeley W. Chromoblastomycosis (mycetoma form) treated by surgical excision. AMA Arch Dermatol Syphil. 1952;66:695–702.
55. Pavlidakey GP, Snow SN, Mohs FE. Chromoblastomycosis treated by Mohs micrographic surgery. J Dermatol Surg Oncol. 1986;12:1073–5.
56. Pimentel ER, Castro LG, Cuce LC, Sampaio SA. Treatment of chromomycosis by cryosurgery with liquid nitrogen: a report of seven cases. J Dermatol Sur Oncol. 1989;15:72–9.
57. Castro LG, Pimentel ER, Lacaz CS. Treatment of chromomycosis by cryosurgery with liquid nitrogen: 15 year's experience. Int J Dermatol. 2003;42:408–12.
58. Kuttner BJ, Siegle RJ. Treatment of chromomycosis with CO_2 laser. J Dermatol Surg Oncol. 1986;12:965–8.
59. Hira K, Yamada H, Takahashi Y, et al. Successful treatment of chromomycosis using carbon dioxide laser associated with topical heat applications. J Eur Acad Dermatol Venereol. 2002;16:273–5.

60. Tsianakas A, Pappai D, Basoglu Y, et al. Chromomycosis-successful CO_2 laser vaporization. J Eur Acad Dermatol Venereol. 2008; 22:1385–6.
61. Hiruma M, Kawada A, Yoshida M, Kouya M. Hyperthermic treatment of chromomycosis with disposable chemical pocket warmers. Mycopathologia. 1993;122:107–14.
62. Tagami H, Ginoza M, Imaizumi S, Urano-Suehisa S. Successful treatment of chromoblastomycosis with topical heat therapy. J Am Acad Dermatol. 1984;10:615–9.
63. Kinbara T, Fukushiro R, Eryu Y. Chromomycosis – report of two cases successfully treated with local heat therapy. Mykosen. 1982;25:689–94.
64. Bayles MAH. Tropical mycoses. Chemotherapy. 1992;38 Suppl 1:27–34.
65. Andrade TS, Castro LG, Nunes RS, et al. Susceptibility of sequential *Fonsecaea pedrosoi* isolates from chromoblastomycosis patients to antifungal agents. Mycoses. 2004;47:216–21.
66. Radford SA, Johnson EM, Warnock DW. In vitro studies of activity of voriconazole (UK-109, 496), a new triazole antifungal agent, against emerging and less-common mold pathogens. Antimicrob Agents Chemother. 1997;41:841–3.
67. Johnson EM, Szekely A, Warnock DW. In-vitro activity of voriconazole, itraconazole and amphotericin B against filamentous fungi. J Antimicrob Chemother. 1998;42:741–5.
68. McGinnis MR, Pasarell L. In vitro testing of susceptibilities of filamentous ascomycetes to voriconazole, intraconazole, and amphotericin B, with consideration of phylogenetic implications. J Clin Microbiol. 1998;36:2353–5.
69. Lavalle P, Suchil P, De Ovando F, Reynoso S. Itraconazole for deep mycoses: Preliminary experience in Mexico. Rev Infect Dis. 1987;9:S64–70.
70. Ungpakorn R, Reangchainam S. Pulse itraconazole 400 mg daily in the treatment of chromoblastomycosis. Clin Exp Dermatol. 2006; 31:245–7.
71. Cucé LC, Wroclawski EL, Sampaio SAP. Treatment of paracoccidioidomycosis, candidiasis, chromomycosis, lobomycosis, and mycetoma with ketoconazole. Int J Dermatol. 1980;19:405–8.
72. Vitale RG, Perez-Blanco M, De Hoog GS. In vitro activity of antifungal drugs against *Cladophialophora* species associated with human chromoblastomycosis. Med Mycol. 2009;47:35–40.
73. Uitto J, Santa-Cruz DJ. Chromomycosis. J Cutan Pathol. 1979; 6:77–84.
74. Oliveira LG, Resende MA, Cisalpino EO, Figueiredo YP, Lopes CF. *In vitro* sensitivity to 5-fluorocytosine of strains isolated from patients under treatment for chromomycosis. Int J Dermatol. 1975;141:141–3.
75. Atukorala DN, Pothupitiya GM. Treatment of chromomycosis with a combination of ketoconazole and 5-fluorocytosine. Ceylon Med J. 1985;30:193.
76. Silber JG, Gombert ME, Green K, Shalita AR. Treatment of chromomycosis with ketoconazole and 5-fluorocytosine. J Am Acad Dermatol. 1983;8:236–8.
77. Solano A, Hildago H, Castro C, Montero-Gei F. Cromomicosis. Tratamiento con la asociacion thiabendazole y 5-fluorocitosina, seis anos de seguimiento. Med Cut ILA Lat Am. 1983;11:413.
78. Xibao Z, Changxing L, Quan L, et al. Treatment of chromoblastomycosis with terbinafine: a report of four cases. J Dermatol Treat. 2005;16:121–4.
79. Kullavanijaya P, Rojanavanich V. Successful treatment of chromoblastomycosis due to *Fonsecaea pedrosoi* by the combination of itraconazole and cryotherapy. Int J Dermatol. 1995;34:804–7.
80. Lubritz RR, Spence JE. Chromoblastomycosis: cure by cryosurgery. Int J Dermatol. 1978;17:830–2.

Part VII
Other Mycoses

Pneumocystosis

Catherine F. Decker and Henry Masur

Although considered an organism of low virulence, *Pneumocystis jiroveci* is an important cause of pneumonia in immunocompromised hosts, especially those with hematologic malignancies, organ transplants, HIV infection, certain congenital immunodeficiencies, and those receiving potent immunosuppressive drugs [1–8]. As the population of immunosuppressed patients has grown, and as our ability to detect organisms in respiratory specimens has improved, more and more cases have been recognized in the period 1970–2000 [1–3]. *Pneumocystis* infections continue to cause morbidity and mortality among susceptible patients who do not receive chemoprophylaxis.

Organism

Pneumocystis was traditionally considered a protozoan, based on its morphology, since its original identification by Chagas in 1906. Inability to culture *Pneumocystis* had hindered the clarification of its taxonomy until application of molecular techniques demonstrated that the organism shares with fungi many characteristics, such as cell wall and enzyme structure [4–7]. *P. jiroveci* is now considered to be a fungus, but is unusual among fungi in that the organism lacks ergosterol in its plasma membranes and is insensitive to antifungal drugs that target ergosterol biosynthesis.

Based on its morphology, which is more characteristic of a protozoon, the life cycle of *P. jiroveci* has been divided into three stages: the trophozoite, found outside the cyst and believed to be intermediate between the sporozoite and the cyst; the cyst, a spherical or crescent-shaped form which contains two to eight sporozoites; and the sporozoite or intracystic bodies, found within the cysts [7]. The life cycle has not been fully elucidated, though it has been suggested that the mode of replication occurs through binary fission of sporozoites and excystment with subsequent attachment to pneumocytes.

Several enzymes have been isolated from *Pneumocystis*, including dihydropteroate synthase (DHPS) and dihydrofolate reductase (DHFR), which are the targets of sulfamethoxazole and trimethoprim, respectively [9, 10]. Genes encoding these enzymes and the cytochrome B locus, which is the site of action of atovaquone, have been identified and sequenced, and mutations in these genes have been identified [11–16]. The organism that infects humans is distinct from that infecting rodents and other animals [17, 18]. *Pneumocystis* found in rats is named *P. carinii* after its discoverer, Dr. Carini. The species that infects humans has been named after Dr. Jirovec, one of the earliest scientists to recognize pneumocystosis in humans.

P. jiroveci pneumonia is still abbreviated PCP. For the sake of consistency this abbreviation now stands for "Pneumo" "Cystis" "Pneumonia" instead of *Pneumocystis carinii* Pneumonia [18].

Epidemiology

Serologic data in the USA indicate that most humans become subclinically infected with *P. jiroveci* during childhood, and that this infection is usually well contained by an intact immune system [19–25]. Serologic studies also have shown that *P. jiroveci* has a worldwide distribution. The frequency of PCP among HIV-infected patients in tropical and developing countries, including Africa, appears lower than in industrialized countries. However, more contemporary studies suggest that this may reflect an underreporting secondary to a failure to establish a diagnosis [22, 26–29]. The mode of transmission in humans is likely through the respiratory route [30].

Disease may occur in association with primary infection, recent reinfection, or reactivation of organisms acquired in the distant past. Serologic studies in infants and observational studies documenting the frequency of PCP in very young

H. Masur (✉)
Critical Care Medicine, National Institutes of Health,
Bethesda, MD, USA
e-mail: hmasur@nih.gov

C.A. Kauffman et al. (eds.), *Essentials of Clinical Mycology*,
DOI 10.1007/978-1-4419-6640-7_26, © Springer Science+Business Media, LLC 2011

infants have led to considerable speculation about the route of transmission to infants. While this organism could be an environmental contaminant, it seems more likely that infants acquire this by person-to-person spread from healthy, asymptomatic parents or other adults [31].

In the older literature, it was suggested that PCP usually occurs through reactivation of latent infection that occurs if the host becomes immunosuppressed. However, recent data have demonstrated that in some patients, disease is caused by a recently acquired strain; these observations are based on typing of organisms and the presence of DHPS mutations in organisms recovered from patients with no history of sulfonamide exposure [32–35]. Some patients have had serial episodes of PCP due to genotypically distinct organisms, which supports the concept that PCP episodes can be caused by recently acquired organisms.

The incubation period for PCP after acquisition of the organism is unknown [36–39].

Pathogenesis

Pneumocystis pneumonia is a disease that occurs exclusively in patients who have substantial immunosuppression. Acute pneumonia has not been documented in patients who are immunologically normal as assessed by conventional laboratory parameters and clinical history.

As more serologic studies have been done, and as molecular probes have been used more widely in research studies, there has been intriguing speculation linking *Pneumocystis* to either mild respiratory illnesses in immunocompetent individuals or to specific pathologic syndromes. Some prominent investigators have published preliminary data linking *Pneumocystis* to sudden infant death syndrome, but subsequent well-designed studies have not substantiated this association [40, 41].

Pneumocystis has been identified by molecular probes in patients with chronic obstructive lung disease. An expanding body of data suggests that *Pneumocystis* may be related to exacerbations of chronic obstructive pulmonary disease, especially when present with specific cofactors such as tobacco [42, 43]. As more longitudinal studies are done in patients with obstructive lung disease, the role of *Pneumocystis* should be clarified. It is intriguing to consider the possibility that primary *Pneumocystis* infection could cause mild symptomatic disease, and that primary or recurrent disease could cause pathology in some persons who have largely intact immune systems.

P. jiroveci has been well described as the cause of acute or subacute pneumonia in patients with B cell defects, severe combined immunodeficiency disease, prematurity, and HIV, as well as patients receiving certain potent immunosuppressive drugs, especially high-dose corticosteroids and immunomodulating monoclonal antibodies, cyclosporine, tacrolimus, and certain antineoplastic chemotherapeutic regimens, such as cladribine and fludarabine [42–57]. These clinical observations suggest that both humoral and cell-mediated immunity are important host defenses against this infection [58]. Neutropenia does not appear to be a risk factor for developing PCP.

The literature on specific drugs has been difficult to interpret in terms of what dose and what duration of therapy is sufficient to cause susceptibility to PCP. Corticosteroids are a prime example: administration of a 21-day course of corticosteroids used in tapering doses to treat allergic reactions or asthma have not been shown to be associated with a risk of PCP. However, a corticosteroid dose equivalent to 16 mg of prednisone or more for at least 2 weeks was associated with a significant risk for PCP in patients who did not have AIDS [59]. Defining an exact threshold of susceptibility with any more precision has not been possible. When patients are receiving multiple doses of immunosuppressive therapy during overlapping time periods, it has been particularly difficult to determine exactly when PCP should be considered a risk.

CD4 T lymphocytes are pivotal in the host's defense against *Pneumocystis* among patients with HIV/AIDS. For patients with HIV infection, the degree of depletion of CD4 cells strongly correlates with the likelihood of developing *P. jiroveci* pneumonia [60–62]. About 90% of cases of *P. jiroveci* pneumonia in patients with HIV infection occur when recent CD4 cell counts have been <200 cells/μL. The majority of these cases occur at CD4 cell counts <100 cells/μL. However, it should be noted that not all cases of HIV-associated PCP occur at CD4 counts below 200 cells/μL. About 10–15% of patients develop *P. jiroveci* pneumonia at CD4 cell counts >200 cells/μL [63]. Clinicians must be aware that at CD4 counts >200 cells/μL, PCP is unlikely to occur, but "unlikely" events do occur on occasion.

For patients who have benefited from therapy with antiretroviral drugs (ART) in terms of a rise in CD4 cell count, considerable evidence supports the concept that CD4 counts continue to be an accurate indicator of susceptibility to *P. jiroveci* [64–67]. The nadir of the CD4 count prior to the institution of ART does not influence the predictive value of subsequent counts in any clinically important manner [65–67]. For patients with immunosuppressive disorders other than HIV, CD4 cell counts are less helpful [68]. There is no reliable laboratory marker for susceptibility in these patients. Non-HIV-infected patients with CD4 counts <200 cells/μL have a higher likelihood of PCP than patients with higher counts, but this test is not nearly as sensitive or specific as it is in HIV-infected patients [68]. CD4 cell counts should not be used to determine which non-HIV-infected patients are susceptible to PCP and which patients need prophylaxis.

For non-HIV-infected patients, decisions about prophylaxis should be based on clinical parameters, such as the dose and duration of corticosteroid administration, exposure to other immunosuppressive drugs, and time since transplantation, all of which require clinical judgment and observational experience with specific patient populations. Recent guidelines on stem cell transplants have provided only general guidance on the precise time and conditions for which PCP prophylaxis is indicated [56]. Many different factors must be taken into account in making such a determination, including the drugs used in conditioning regimens, drugs used for immunosuppression of graft-versus-host response, and immunosuppression associated with the underlying disease.

Pneumocystis is very likely inhaled, bypasses the defenses of the upper respiratory tract, and is deposited into the alveolar space. The organism has a unique tropism for the lungs, where it exists primarily as an alveolar pathogen. Individuals with intact immunity control this primary infection. There are no apparent clinical manifestations of primary infection in immunocompetent individuals, and the organism likely remains latent in the lungs for long periods of time. Clinically apparent pneumonia occurs when cellular or humoral immunity becomes severely deficient. Organisms proliferate, evoking a mononuclear cell response. Alveoli become filled with proteinaceous material and intact and degenerating organisms. The principal histologic finding is the formation of a foamy vacuolated eosinophilic alveolar exudate. Alveolar-capillary permeability decreases, leading to impairment of gas exchange, not unlike that seen with adult respiratory distress syndrome. Physiologically, hypoxemia occurs with an increased alveolar-arterial oxygen gradient and respiratory alkalosis, impaired diffusion capacity, and alterations in lung compliance and total lung capacity. As the disease progresses in severity, there may also be hyaline membrane formation along with interstitial fibrosis and edema. Without treatment, the disease will progress to respiratory failure and death. Organisms are largely confined to the lungs, although occasional evidence of dissemination to other organs has been well documented.

Clinical Manifestations

Presenting symptoms in patients with *P. jiroveci* pneumonia are usually acute or subacute, nonspecific, and include fever, nonproductive cough, dyspnea, substernal chest tightness, and shortness of breath [69, 70]. Cough may be similar to that seen with a viral infection, and the shortness of breath may initially be noticed only with exertion. Constitutional symptoms and prolonged prodromal illness may be present for days, weeks, or months before presentation to healthcare providers. There is nothing unique about the presentation of PCP compared to other diffuse pulmonary processes, which would allow it to be diagnosed without a specific microbiologic test identifying the organism in pulmonary secretions or tissue. AIDS patients tend to have a more indolent course with a longer duration of symptoms and less hypoxia than patients treated with cytotoxic chemotherapy or corticosteroids [71]. HIV-infected patients typically present after 1–4 weeks of symptoms, while non-HIV-infected immunosuppressed patients present within a few days of the onset of symptoms with a more acute and rapidly progressive infection.

Physical examination is often unrevealing, except for fever and tachypnea. Patients often have a chest examination that is normal early in their course. However, diffuse rales and, eventually, signs of consolidation are usually present as the disease progresses.

Routine laboratory testing is also unremarkable except for nonspecific elevations of serum lactate dehydrogenase (LDH), which is a reflection of tissue damage (lung), rather than a specific marker for PCP. The total white blood count may rise modestly. In patients with HIV infection, this rise may not be noted by clinicians unless they are aware of the pre-PCP baseline, which is often below the normal range. Hypoxemia is characteristic of patients with PCP. Normal arterial blood gases can be seen in up to 20% of patients who present with very mild disease, and this finding should not dissuade the clinician from initiating an evaluation in patients with compatible symptoms especially if the CD4 cell count is <200 cells/μL.

Radiographic Findings

The radiographic findings (Figs. 1 and 2) are dictated by the stage of illness at the time the patient presents for evaluation. Early in the course of disease, especially for patients with HIV disease, the chest radiograph may be normal despite substantial hypoxemia [71–73]. In patients with a normal chest radiograph, a high-resolution computed tomography (CT) scan of the thorax will usually demonstrate a characteristic ground-glass appearance [74]. As the disease worsens, diffuse interstitial infiltrates develop which progress to dense alveolar filling. The typical chest radiograph is one of diffuse and symmetrical increased interstitial markings. However, a substantial number of patients have atypical chest radiographs. Almost all types of infiltrates have been described with *P. jiroveci* pneumonia, including the classic diffuse interstitial and alveolar infiltrates, upper lobe predominance, asymmetrical involvement, lobar patterns, nodules, and cavities.

Clinicians should be aware that the finding of a pneumothorax in an HIV-infected patient with interstitial infiltrates should raise the possibility of *P. jiroveci* pneumonia, although other destructive pulmonary processes can also cause lung collapse [75, 76]. Patients may present with pneumothorax as the predominant reason to come to medical attention. In these cases, the contralateral lung usually has diffuse infiltrates that may not have produced enough symptoms for the patient to seek medical attention prior to the pneumothorax.

Images of the liver, spleen, kidneys, or even the brain may reveal inflammatory masses due to *P. jiroveci*. These lesions probably represent subclinical lesions of disseminated pneumocystosis, which occur predominately in patients with advanced HIV infection, especially those who are receiving aerosolized pentamidine. These extrapulmonary lesions rarely cause symptomatic disease, and appear to resolve with therapy [77, 78].

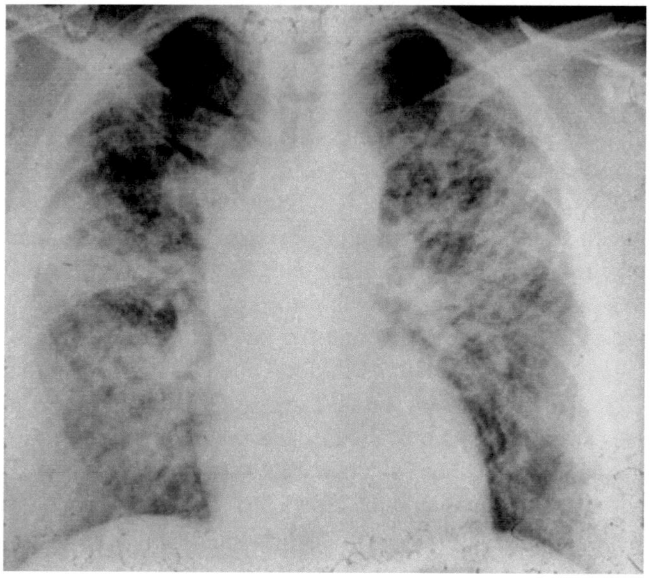

Fig. 1 Chest radiograph showing symmetrical interstitial infiltrates typical of severe *Pneumocystis* pneumonia

Diagnosis

The definitive diagnosis of *P. jiroveci* disease requires the demonstration of cysts or trophozoites within tissue or body fluids (Fig. 3) [79–87]. In most clinical laboratories, organisms are recognized via colorimetric or immunofluorescent stains since the human organism cannot be cultured in laboratory animals or in vitro.

Before the AIDS epidemic, the diagnosis of *P. jiroveci* pneumonia typically required an open lung biopsy. With the development of improved diagnostic techniques, diagnoses are now established by less invasive methods. PCP in virtually all patients, HIV-infected or uninfected, can be diagnosed by careful analysis of bronchoalveolar lavage (BAL) fluid [79, 80]. Induced sputum has been shown in some studies to be a sensitive, simple, and noninvasive means to diagnose *P. jiroveci* pneumonia and may preclude the need for bronchoscopy. [81–86] Reported yields for recovery of the organism range from 70% to 95% [81, 83, 85]. On rare occasions in the current era, tissue will be necessary to establish the diagnosis; a video-assisted transthoracic (VATS) biopsy, a transbronchial biopsy, or an open lung biopsy can be performed. Most often, when BAL has failed to reveal *Pneumocystis*, a biopsy will reveal a pathologic process other than PCP.

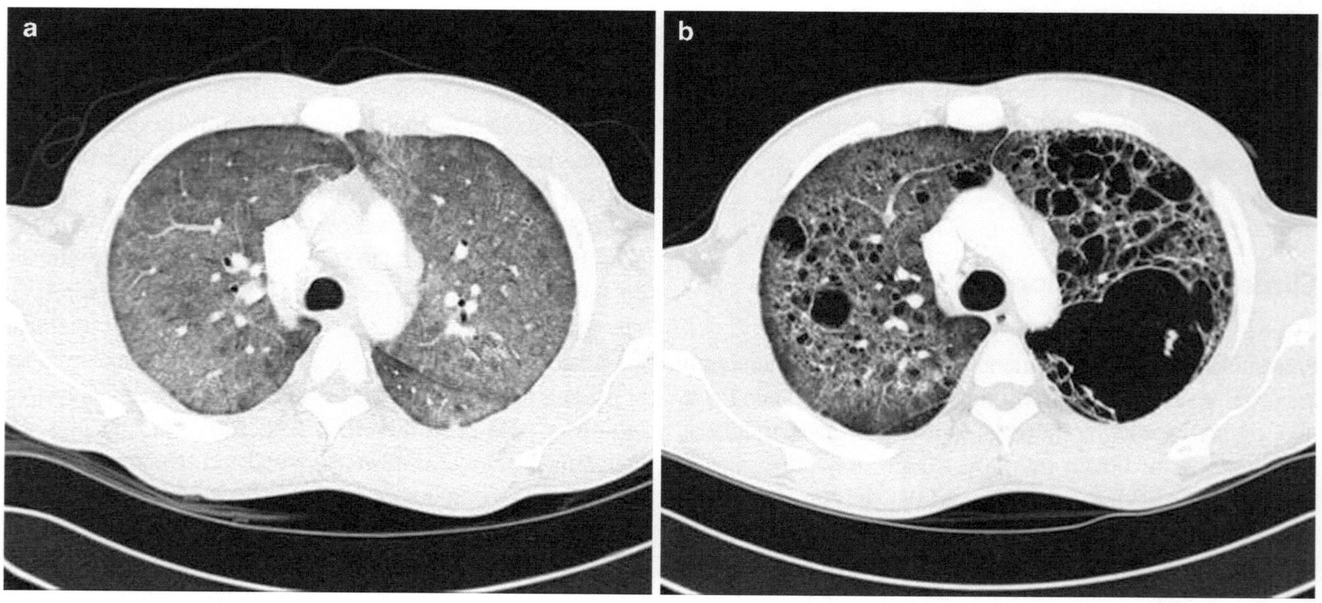

Fig. 2 CT scan of patient with PCP who developed pneumatoceles despite TMP-SMX therapy

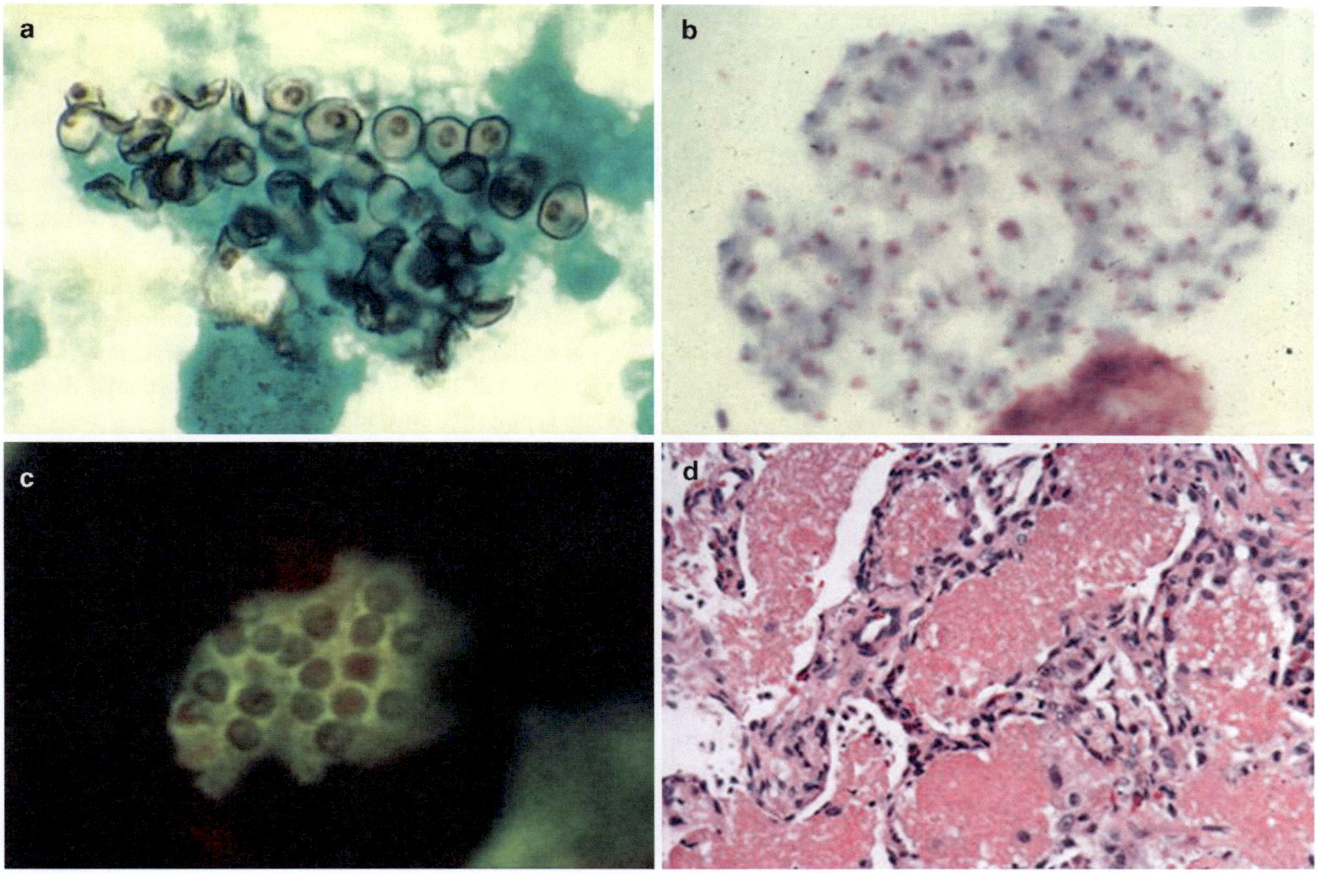

Fig. 3 Morphology of *Pneumocystis jiroveci*. (**a**) Methenamine silver stain of bronchoalveolar lavage; (**b**) Diff Quik stain of bronchoalveolar lavage; (**c**) immunofluorescence stain of bronchoalveolar lavage; (**d**) hematoxylin and eosin stain of lung biopsy

The development of monoclonal antibodies against *P. jiroveci* has resulted in a rapid, sensitive, and easy method to detect *P. jiroveci* in smears of respiratory specimens [82–84, 87]. The gold standard for diagnosis is the demonstration of two or more organisms in a respiratory specimen by direct smear and staining by immunofluorescence, Giemsa stain, or Diff Quik stain.

More recently, molecular detection assays have been developed for detecting *P. jiroveci* in BAL or induced sputum samples. PCR methods have used a variety of gene targets, but those with the highest sensitivity use either a multicopy gene target, such as mitochondrial rRNA, a major surface glycoprotein [88, 89], or a nested PCR assay requiring two amplification rounds [90–92]. The nested assay is too labor intensive to be practical for most clinical laboratories. PCR has also allowed the detection of *P. jiroveci* in more easily obtained specimens, such as oral washes or gargles [93–95].

Quantitative PCR assays provide a very sensitive test for detecting *Pneumocystis*. A variety of copy number thresholds have been proposed to provide specificity. No commercial test is available. As PCR becomes more widely available, there will need to be standardization and a systematic approach to understanding the meaning of positive or negative results. Respiratory secretions may contain low copy numbers of *Pneumocystis* in individuals who are free of pulmonary dysfunction and who are either immunologically normal or abnormal. Thus, a positive PCR test does not necessarily imply the *Pneumocystis* is the cause of pulmonary dysfunction. Copy number is probably helpful, although the quality of the specimen and the type of specimen (sputum vs BAL) will influence the copy number. It is plausible to believe that high copy numbers correlate with *Pneumocystis* as a cause of pulmonary dysfunction and that negative PCR has a high negative predictive value. However, these likely scenarios need to be confirmed in clinical investigations under standardized protocols for specimen collection and PCR performance.

There is no sensitive or specific serologic test to diagnose PCP. IgG antibody is present in asymptomatic adults and thus is not useful. Even a negative test would not be helpful since heavily immunosuppressed patients may be unable to produce IgG antibody, even if assessed weeks after the acute event [96, 97].

One group of investigators reported that *Pneumocystis* cannot synthesize S-adenosylmethionine synthetase, an essential growth factor for PCP. This group has proposed that the presence of PCP in the lung correlates with a depletion of

S-adenosylmethionine synthetase in the serum [98]. These results have not been confirmed in other laboratories [99].

C-reactive protein, LDH, and beta-D-glucan assays are also not sufficiently sensitive and specific to be useful [100–104]. There are several useful investigations that have evaluated these tests for PCP. However, given their sensitivity and specificity characteristics, they are not clinically helpful.

Treatment

The efficacy of antimicrobials in the treatment of PCP depends on several factors: the degree of hypoxia at the time therapy is started; the degree of immunosuppression; comorbid conditions; and the ability of the patient to tolerate the most effective agents [105–108]. The earlier therapy is started, the better the prognosis is likely to be.

Table 1 lists the options available for treatment of PCP [56, 109–122]. Once the diagnosis of *P. jiroveci* is made, outpatient therapy with an oral agent, preferably TMP-SMX, is recommended for mild to moderately severe disease (PaO_2 > 70 mmHg). Other alternatives for oral outpatient therapy include TMP-dapsone, clindamycin-primaquine, and atovaquone. Patients who are more severely ill with moderate-to-severe disease or who cannot tolerate oral medications should be hospitalized and given intravenous TMP-SMX. In sulfonamide-intolerant patients, intravenous pentamidine should be administered.

Anti-Pneumocystis Agents

Trimethoprim-sulfamethoxazole (TMP-SMX) is the agent of choice for initial therapy for any severity of acute PCP [107].

Table 1 Drug regimens for treatment of *Pneumocystis* pneumonia

Agent	Dose	Interval	Route
Specific therapy			
Trimethoprim/	5 mg/kg	6–8 h	i.v. or p.o
Sulfamethoxazole	25 mg/kg		
Pentamidine isethionate	4 mg/kg	24 h	i.v.
Trimethoprim plus	5 mg/kg	8 h	p.o
Dapsone	100 mg	24 h	p.o
Clindamycin plus	600–900 mg	8 h	p.o/i.v.
Primaquine	15–30 mg	24 h	p.o
Atovaquone	750 mg	12 h	p.o
Adjunctive therapy			
Prednisone (if room air PaO_2 < 70 mmHg within 72 h of initiating therapy)	40 mg q 12 h for 5 days then 40 mg q d for 5 days then 20 mg q d for 11 days		p.o. or i.v.

TMP-SMX is the most effective agent. If a patient has mild disease (PaO_2 greater than 70 mmHg), and is able to tolerate oral medications, TMP-SMX may be given in the dosage of two double-strength tablets (160 mg TMP and 800 mg SMX) every 6–8 h. The 8-h regimen is preferred by many clinicians because toxicity would be expected to be less with a lower daily dosage, and there is no evidence that efficacy is improved with the higher dose. With more severe disease or if the patient is unable to tolerate oral medication, intravenous TMP-SMX (5 mg/kg TMP and 25 mg/kg sulfamethoxazole every 8 h) should be given. Total duration of therapy is usually 21 days, but there is no concrete evidence that 21 days of therapy is more effective than 14 days [123].

TMP-SMX is associated with many toxicities, including fever, rash, headache, nausea, vomiting, pancytopenia, hepatitis, aseptic meningitis, and nephrotoxicity. Trimethoprim can cause hyperkalemia. Patients with suppressed bone marrow function have predictable difficulty tolerating TMP-SMX. Some toxicities of TMP-SMX can be life threatening, including Stevens-Johnson syndrome and a distributive shock syndrome that appears to be anaphylactoid. Treatment-limiting toxicities usually occur between day 6 and day 10 of therapy. For AIDS patients, trials suggest that approximately 25% of patients are unable to tolerate a full course of TMP-SMX. Minor laboratory abnormalities should not be an indication to switch to a less effective alternative therapy.

Intravenous pentamidine is the most potent alternative agent to TMP-SMX as initial therapy in patients who are sulfonamide intolerant. It has been shown to have equivalent efficacy to TMP-SMX in trials of patients with HIV infection or with cancer [105, 109]. However, pentamidine is not preferred because of the high incidence of substantial toxicities, and it can only be administered parenterally. The standard dose of pentamidine is 4 mg/kg/day, given intravenously over at least 1 h for a minimum of 14–21 days. Small studies suggest that a lower dose of 3 mg/kg/day may be less toxic but equally effective [110–113]. Toxicities include renal dysfunction, dysglycemias, pancreatitis, and torsades de pointes. Renal function must be monitored closely. If there is renal dysfunction, dosages do not need to be adjusted for pentamidine. However, patients with renal dysfunction are more likely to develop dysglycemias. Pentamidine can cause initial islet cell destruction that causes insulin release and hypoglycemia, followed subsequently by an inability to produce insulin and hyperglycemia. This may occur during therapy or weeks to months after the completion of therapy. Some patients may subsequently develop insulin-requiring diabetes mellitus. Patients need to be carefully assessed to determine what other drugs they are receiving that prolong the QT interval in order to reduce the likelihood that torsades will occur. The latter has been reported only rarely.

Other regimens that have clinical efficacy but are usually used in mild-to-moderate disease and in those who are sulfa intolerant include trimethoprim-dapsone [107, 117–119], primaquine-clindamycin [106–108], and atovaquone [116]. None of these is as effective as either TMP-SMX or intravenous pentamidine [105, 107, 116].

Dapsone, as a single agent, is not as effective as other alternatives in the treatment of PCP. Failure rates are approximately 40% in patients with HIV infection [117, 118]. In combination with trimethoprim (20 mg/kg/day), however, its efficacy is comparable to TMP-SMX [119]. TMP-dapsone is used as an alternative oral regimen in mild-to-moderate disease for patients intolerant of TMP-SMX. Approximately 50% of sulfonamide-intolerant patients tolerate dapsone. This regimen can only be given orally and is, therefore, not suitable for patients with severe disease or gastrointestinal dysfunction. Trimethoprim and dapsone are not formulated into one pill.

The combination of clindamycin plus primaquine is another reasonable alternative for the treatment of PCP [106, 108, 120]. Investigators report success rates of 75–80% in open, noncomparative trials with patients who are intolerant of or failed standard treatment [106, 108]. A randomized trial found the combination to be comparable in efficacy to TMP-SMX or TMP-dapsone in mild-to-moderate disease [107]. Clindamycin-primaquine has also been used as a salvage regimen in patients with *Pneumocystis* induced respiratory failure [121], although many authorities are reluctant to use an oral agent (i.e., primaquine) in this setting. A primaquine base of 30 mg is the usual dose. Clindamycin is given either orally (300–450 mg every 6–8 h) or intravenously (600–900 mg every 6–8 h).

Oral atovaquone, another approved agent for treating PCP, demonstrated a higher rate of treatment failures and was less effective than TMP-SMX in mild-to-moderate disease [116, 120]. Oral atovaquone and intravenous pentamidine were found to have similar success rates in mild and moderate PCP in AIDS patients who were intolerant of TMP-SMX. Atovaquone was better tolerated, but patients receiving atovaquone more frequently failed to respond to therapy, and patients receiving pentamidine had more treatment-limiting adverse drug toxicities [122]. Low plasma atovaquone levels are associated with a poor response [116]. Low plasma levels have been in part due to the poor bioavailability of the drug. Even with the liquid formulation of the drug, absorption can be unpredictable, and steady-state may not be reached for several days. Atovaquone absorption is improved by ingestion of a fatty meal. Atovaquone has a role as therapy for patients with mild, stable disease who have no evidence of gastrointestinal dysfunction. If neither TMP-SMX nor TMP-dapsone is tolerable, atovaquone is a reasonable option.

Other agents under investigation include analogs of primaquine, analogs of pentamidine, albendazole, and echinocandins or pneumocandins. There is interest in the activity of caspofungin against the cyst form of *Pneumocystis*, but there is scant clinical evidence that this drug is useful for treating or preventing human disease [124–127].

Corticosteroid Adjunctive Therapy

The use of corticosteroids in conjunction with antimicrobial agents has become the standard of care in the treatment of moderate-severe PCP in AIDS patients. Three randomized controlled studies revealed that corticosteroids significantly decreased the frequency of early deterioration in oxygenation and improved survival in patients who had an initial room air $PO_2 < 70$ mmHg [60, 128, 129]. Corticosteroid therapy is not recommended unless the diagnosis of *P. jiroveci* is confirmed before or immediately after starting therapy since corticosteroids could have a deleterious effect on other pathogenic processes, such as cytomegalovirus pneumonia.

Corticosteroids hasten the symptomatic resolution of mild PCP, and prevent the early deterioration in oxygenation (often subclinical) in this population as well. However, for patients with mild disease, corticosteroids are rarely used because of concern regarding the metabolic complications of corticosteroids, including osteonecrosis [130]. Corticosteroid therapy is logical to use in patients with underlying immunodeficiency disorders other than HIV and in those with a slow response to therapy, although no prospective trials have documented this efficacy [130, 131].

It is unclear how to manage corticosteroids in patients who were receiving these drugs when they developed PCP. There are potential benefits from raising the dose to reduce lung inflammation, but this has not been studied.

Monitoring Therapy

Respiratory rate, arterial oxygenation, ventilation, temperature, and chest radiographs should be assessed to determine initial clinical status and then reassessed serially to determine response to therapy. Arterial blood gases provide more precise measurement of oxygenation than percutaneous oxygen saturation monitoring, but the latter can be used, especially with mild disease. The median time to show improvement with therapy is 4–10 days. Laboratory tests should be done to check for bone marrow, liver, pancreatic, or renal toxicity due to therapy or concurrent morbidities. Immediately after initiation of therapy, many patients appear to have a paradoxical response. Many HIV-infected patients will get worse with a decline in partial pressure of oxygen by 10–30 mmHg during the initial 2–5 days after initiation of therapy before clinical improvement is observed [132]. This decline has been attributed to dying organisms, which elicit an intense inflammatory response. The benefit of corticosteroids appears to have the ability to blunt this inflammatory response.

For patients who do not demonstrate a well-defined improvement in clinical status, the initial anti-*Pneumocystis* regimen should probably be continued for at least 5–10 days before considering a change in therapy. Fluid status should be monitored carefully because patients with PCP may have unsuspected cardiac disease due to age, accelerated atherosclerosis, or drug-induced cardiomyopathy. Congestive heart failure may not be evident until the patient is challenged with large volumes of fluids. Intravenous TMP-SMX is often mixed with considerable volumes of fluid.

Survival from an episode of PCP correlates most closely with the pretreatment arterial-alveolar gradient [72, 133] as well as with pre-existing co-morbidities. Other factors that influence outcome include number of tachyzoites in bronchoalveolar lavage, degree of chest radiograph abnormality, level of LDH elevation and, for patients with HIV infection, low CD4 cell counts [71, 72, 134–137].

For a patient with an initial PaO_2 >70 mmHg while breathing room air, expected survival rates are 60–80% in non-AIDS patients and 80–95% in patients with AIDS [8, 72, 105]. Evaluation of response to therapy should be based on clinical parameters, including temperature, respiratory rate, oxygenation, and radiographic examination. The use of bronchoscopy to assess response to drug therapy by quantitating organisms is not helpful in the clinical setting since cysts and trophozoites are difficult to quantitate, and *P. jiroveci* will be present in bronchoscopy specimens for many weeks after initiation of therapy, even in patients who rapidly improve [135].

In recent years, survival from an episode of PCP appears to be about 90%, although there is considerable variation depending on the underlying disease and how severe the disease is when the patient presents and the diagnosis of PCP is made [136–138].

In a patient who appears to be failing therapy after 4–6 days, clinicians need to assess for other concurrent pulmonary processes. Up to 20% of HIV-infected patients with PCP will have another concurrent pulmonary process, such as tuberculosis, Kaposi's sarcoma, or bacterial pneumonia [139]. Most clinicians perform BAL if patients are not responding promptly, especially if the initial diagnosis was established by sputum examination. It is not common to find a second treatable infectious process, but cases have been described in which pneumococcus, *Legionella*, *Cryptococcus*, or cytomegalovirus were found to be concurrent pathogenic microorganisms. For some microorganisms that can either colonize or cause disease, it is often difficult to know whether treatment is indicated. *Aspergillus*, atypical mycobacteria, respiratory syncytial virus, and parainfluenza virus are examples of organisms that may or may not be contributing to lung dysfunction. In refractory cases, open biopsy or VATS procedures are warranted to determine if a treatable cause of deterioration had been missed by BAL or to determine which of the various potential pathogens that have been recovered is the causative agent. Noninfectious causes such as congestive heart failure, embolic disease, or alveolar hemorrhage should also be considered as causes or contributors to lung dysfunction.

Patients with PCP, especially HIV-related PCP, develop pneumatocoeles that can rupture, causing pneumothorax. For patients with PCP who experience a sudden deterioration, one of the first diagnostic tests should be physical examination followed by chest imaging to look for this reversible cause of sudden clinical deterioration.

For patients with HIV-related PCP who are not receiving ART, clinicians often consider starting such therapy soon after the PCP is improving. In the past, one of the multiple reasons to be cautious about such a change in therapy was the possibility that ART could augment immune response and cause immune reconstitution inflammatory syndrome (IRIS) [140–144]. As the viral load declines and CD4 cell counts increase, a more robust inflammatory and immunologic response can occur at sites of an existing opportunistic infection, a recent infection, or latent infection. Risk for IRIS is greatest in patients who experience rapid increases in CD4 cells, especially in those who had CD4 counts < 50 cells/μL and high viral loads > 100,000 copies/mL. IRIS can occur within days or weeks of instituting antiretroviral therapy. With PCP, the syndrome can manifest as deteriorating oxygenation, worsening symptoms of cough and fever and shortness of breath, and worsening chest imaging. In one small case series, patients with PCP who initially improved on conventional *Pneumocystis* therapy began ART within 15–18 days of PCP diagnosis. Within 1 week of beginning ART, the patients developed respiratory failure. No other etiology aside from PCP could be documented. How often this occurs when ART is initiated soon after PCP is unknown. Initially, there were enough cases to make concern over IRIS one reason to delay ART for many weeks following PCP treatment [141, 144]. However, completed clinical trials suggest that in the absence of compelling contraindications, early initiation of ART near the time of initiating opportunistic infection therapy should be considered for most patients with an acute opportunistic infection [109, 145].

There is no diagnostic test for IRIS. Patients must be reevaluated to determine which process is causing their deterioration, i.e., IRIS, another infection, or another noninfectious syndrome. IRIS is a diagnosis of exclusion based on temporal relationship and absence of another plausible cause [146].

Optimal management of IRIS has not been clearly defined. Treatment of IRIS ranges from watchful waiting to nonsteroidal agents or corticosteroids and can include changing or intensifying the regimen used to treat the opportunistic infection. Clinical judgment must direct management because there are no concrete data-driven guidelines.

When evaluating a patient who is deteriorating, an echocardiogram is useful to assess congestive heart failure. Empirical therapy for community-acquired pneumonia may also be a reasonable strategy. Prednisone should be added to the regimen if not already instituted. There are no randomized trials to help determine when specific anti-*Pneumocystis* therapy should be modified because of inadequate response. A change in therapy to a different agent is usually reserved until the patient has had 4–8 days of first-line therapy and other pulmonary processes have been investigated. Most authorities recommend a switch from TMP-SMX to intravenous pentamidine. If IV pentamidine cannot be used, then clindamycin-primaquine is a reasonable alternative, although primaquine is only available as an oral drug. Whether combining two regimens, such as TMP-SMX plus pentamidine or atovaquone, produces synergy or antagonism has not been determined If a patient is deteriorating or failing to improve on a regimen other than TMP-SMX, strong consideration should be given to using TMP-SMX, even if desensitization is required in the intensive care unit.

Prevention

PCP can largely be prevented by administering chemoprophylaxis to susceptible individuals (Table 2). Chemoprophylaxis against PCP is indicated for the period of time when patients are at risk for developing PCP. The challenge for clinicians is to define the magnitude and duration of risk and then to determine if the toxicities of the chemotherapeutic agent are warranted compared to the risk of PCP. For patients with HIV infection, there are considerable data and many prospective trials to help the clinician develop a management strategy for patients. For most other diseases, there are only observational data, especially in areas in which immunosuppressive regimens have changed dramatically in recent years. In situations such as solid organ or stem cell transplantation, clinicians and guideline committees make recommendations based on expert opinion guided by limited data.

Table 2 Drug regimens for prophylaxis for *Pneumocystis* pneumonia

Agent	Total daily dose	Route	Interval
First Choice			
Trimethoprim/	160/800 mg (DS)	Oral	Daily
Sulfamethoxazole	160/800 mg (DS)	Oral	Twice daily
	80/400 mg (SS)	Oral	Daily
Alternatives			
Pentamidine	300 mg	Aerosol	Monthly
Dapsone	100 mg	Oral	Daily
Pyrimethamine plus	75 mg	Oral	Weekly
Dapsone plus	200 mg	Oral	Weekly
Leucovorin	25 mg	Oral	Weekly
Atovaquone	1,500 mg	Oral	Daily

Historically, the successful use of TMP-SMX in controlled trials for primary prevention of *P. jiroveci* pneumonia in pediatric oncology patients [8] has been the model for the development of prophylactic strategies. Prophylaxis for *P. jiroveci* pneumonia has been shown most convincingly to decrease morbidity and mortality in children with acute leukemia and patients with HIV infection. Most authorities believe that it is prudent to institute primary prophylaxis for groups of patients felt to be at high risk, including patients with organ transplants, especially lung or heart-lung transplants, lymphoreticular malignancies, HIV with CD4 cell counts < 200 cells/μL, and patients with primary immunodeficiencies [56, 57, 109, 147–151]. It is generally recommended that prophylaxis should be continued for as long as the immunosuppressive condition continues.

For patients with HIV infection, the CD4 counts are a good marker for determining risk, as mentioned above, and can be monitored to help define the period of risk. For immunosuppressive conditions other than HIV infection, CD4 cell counts are not reliable, nor is any other clinical or laboratory marker a reliable indicator for risk for PCP [68]. Thus, factors such as the temporal relationship to immunosuppressive drugs, time since transplantation, and time since the occurrence of graft-versus-host disease are used to estimate the period of risk [56, 152].

Most clinicians provide chemoprophylaxis during periods of heavy immunosuppression for allogeneic stem cell transplant recipients, solid organ transplant recipients, and patients receiving antineoplastic chemotherapy, high-dose corticosteroids (≥20 mg prednisone daily for >1 month), or certain other immunosuppressive agents [56, 152]. Fludarabine and 2-chlorodeoxyadenosine are two drugs with a strong association with PCP.

In patients with malignant neoplasms or organ transplants, observational databases provide data about when to initiate prophylaxis and how long to continue. The use of TMP-SMX for PCP prophylaxis in stem cell transplant patients has greatly reduced this infection in this population [56, 152–154]. Current guidelines for prophylaxis include all allogeneic hematopoietic stem cell transplant recipients and autologous recipients who have lymphoma or leukemia and who are receiving intense conditioning regimens or graft manipulations and those who have recently received fludarabine or 2-chlorodeoxyadenosine. Prophylaxis should be administered from the time of engraftment for at least 6 months after transplantation for all recipients [56, 152]. Prophylaxis should be continued for more than 6 months after transplantation for all persons who are receiving immunosuppressive therapy, such as prednisone or cyclosporine, or those who have chronic graft-versus-host disease or rejection. Prophylaxis is usually begun 1–2 weeks before transplantation [154]. Cases of PCP in stem cell transplant recipients usually occur when prophylaxis is stopped despite high levels of ongoing immunosuppression [155].

Recommendations formulated to prevent *P. jiroveci* pneumonia in HIV-infected patients are based on large databases, which demonstrated that prophylactic agents should be initiated when an HIV-infected patient's absolute CD4 cell count falls to <200 cells/μL [109, 149], as well as for patients who have oropharyngeal candidiasis, regardless of CD4 cell count. Persons who have a CD4 cell percentage <14% or a history of an AIDS-defining illness should also be considered for prophylaxis, regardless of their current CD4 cell count.

Prior to the era of potent ART, prophylaxis was recommended to be lifelong, once the patient's CD4 count fell to <200 cells/μL, the patient had oral candidiasis, or the patient had an episode of PCP [62, 109, 149, 156, 157]. However, since the introduction of ART, there have been convincing data that primary or secondary chemoprophylaxis can be discontinued in patients whose CD4 cell counts rise to >200 cells/μL for 3 months on ART [158–163]. However, for some patients who have CD4 counts >200 cells/μL, it may be prudent to continue prophylaxis if they have high viral loads>50,000–100,000 copies/mL, rapidly declining CD4 cell counts, wasting, oral candidiasis, or a prior episode of an opportunistic infection with CD4 counts >200 cell/μL. Prophylaxis should be reinstituted if the CD4 cell count decreases to <200 cells/μL. The risk of PCP is reduced by viral suppression, regardless of the CD4 count, but CD4 counts continue to be the accepted parameter for determining the need for PCP prophylaxis in HIV infected patients [109, 164].

TMP-SMX is the preferred chemoprophylactic agent for patients who can tolerate it and is more effective than any other regimen (Table 2) [56, 109–111, 120, 165–169]. This drug has a long history of consistent efficacy in a wide variety of patients. Cytopenias, skin rashes, hepatitis, pancreatitis, and nephritis have been reported as toxicities when prophylactic doses are used. Hematologists and transplant providers are often reluctant to use this agent as prophylaxis because of its potential effects on bone marrow.

True breakthroughs of PCP are unusual for patients who are adherent to the recommended regimens of TMP-SMX. There are data in patients with HIV infection to suggest that intermittent regimens (one DS tablet thrice weekly) may be slightly less effective than daily regimens, although lower doses of TMP-SMX are better tolerated than higher doses [170]. In children with malignant neoplasms, such differences were not observed [171].

Aerosolized pentamidine, dapsone, dapsone-trimethoprim, dapsone-pyrimethamine, and atovaquone also have a high degree of efficacy. Each of these regimens has some disadvantages, and none is as effective as TMP-SMX.

In a large trial (ACTG 081), 843 patients with HIV infection were randomized to TMP-SMX (1 DS tablet twice daily), dapsone (50 mg twice daily) or aerosolized pentamidine (300 mg once monthly). Fewer episodes of PCP occurred among patients receiving TMP-SMX than in the other two arms when patients with CD4 counts <100 cells/μL were considered, but not when patients with higher CD4 counts were assessed. In this trial, the efficacy of dapsone appeared to be better than aerosolized pentamidine. Dapsone given at doses of 50 mg daily or less was not as effective as 50 mg twice daily [120].

A secondary prophylaxis study was carried out in the USA involving 310 patients with HIV infection who were randomly assigned either to administration of aerosolized pentamidine by a Respirgard II nebulizer or to one TMP-SMX DS tablet daily [110]. When analyzed by the intention-to-treat, the recurrence rate of PCP was significantly higher among the patients assigned to aerosolized pentamidine (18%) than among those that received TMP-SMX (4%). As expected, patients that received TMP-SMX experienced frequent toxicity, resulting in discontinuation of the agent.

TMP-SMX has advantages not provided by aerosolized pentamidine, which include low cost, oral preparation, and probable protective effect against toxoplasmosis, enteric bacterial infections, respiratory infections, and disseminated *Pneumocystis* infection [110, 172].

Aerosolized pentamidine is usually well tolerated when delivered by the Respirgard II at a dose of 300 mg monthly. Other delivery systems have not been as extensively evaluated and cannot be recommended. Coughing or wheezing occurs in 30–40% of patients, but this reaction can be diminished or prevented by the administration of a beta-adrenergic agonist such as albuterol [114, 132, 173–175]. Bronchospasm rarely necessitates discontinuation of prophylaxis with aerosolized pentamidine Patients with reactive airway disease or bullous lung disease may not distribute aerosolized pentamidine effectively to all lung segments and thus may not obtain optimal protection. There have been reports of disseminated pneumocystosis in patients receiving aerosolized pentamidine for prophylaxis [131, 166]. Some human stem cell transplant programs use aerosolized pentamidine prophylaxis in preference to TMP-SMX in order to avoid potential bone marrow suppression.

Before administering aerosolized pentamidine, all patients should be screened for active tuberculosis. Because the treatment induces coughing, patients with pulmonary tuberculosis who receive aerosolized pentamidine could transmit tuberculosis to others [175, 176]. Ideally, aerosolized pentamidine should be administered in individual booths or rooms with negative pressure ventilation and direct exhaust to the outside. After the administration of aerosolized pentamidine, patients should not return to common waiting areas until coughing has subsided.

Dapsone is an attractive alternative to aerosolized pentamidine because it is oral, convenient, and inexpensive. Dapsone is considered by some experts to be the best alternative for patients who cannot tolerate TMP-SMX [120, 167]. It is estimated that only 20–50% of patients who are TMP-SMX intolerant will be able to tolerate dapsone [177]. Dose reduction to improve tolerability is not recommended because doses less than 100 mg daily are considerably less effective than the full dose regimen. A case control study in stem cell transplant recipients showed the efficacy of daily dapsone to be similar to that of TMP-SMX. Dapsone has been well tolerated among TMP-SMX allergic stem cell transplant recipients [178].

Weekly doses of dapsone (200 mg) and pyrimethamine (75 mg) are well tolerated, but less effective than TMP-SMX [179]. Dapsone-pyrimethamine has efficacy as a prophylactic regimen against PCP pneumonia that is similar to aerosol pentamidine but less than TMP-SMX. This regimen can be given as a daily regimen (dapsone 50 mg daily plus pyrimethamine 75 mg weekly) or as a weekly regimen (dapsone 200 mg plus pyrimethamine 75 mg) [165, 180]. It is not clear if pyrimethamine truly adds potency against PCP [120]. Dapsone alone has no antibacterial activity. It is not clear if it has adequate anti-*Toxoplasma* activity when used without pyrimethamine.

Daily atovaquone (1,500 mg of the liquid suspension) has comparable efficacy to aerosolized pentamidine or oral dapsone [181, 182]. Atovaquone does have activity against *Toxoplasma*, but the relative efficacy of this regimen for preventing toxoplasmosis has not been adequately studied. Atovaquone has no antibacterial activity. This regimen is also much more expensive than other drug regimens.

Other potential prophylactic agents that have been used empirically or evaluated in small clinical trials include pyrimethamine-sulfadoxine (Fansidar), trimethoprim-dapsone, parenteral pentamidine, and primaquine-clindamycin. Pyrimethamine-sulfadoxine is effective, but its high rate of adverse reactions and long half-life make this an unattractive option and one that has little benefit over TMP-SMX. Small trials with parenteral pentamidine and clindamycin-primaquine have been surprisingly disappointing in terms of efficacy and cannot be recommended.

Recent Advances

Sulfonamide Resistance/DHPS Mutations

Since *Pneumocystis* has been widely exposed to sulfonamide during the past 25 years, it is reasonable to expect that this organism might develop sulfonamide resistance. Both dapsone and SMX act by inhibiting the folate biosynthesis enzyme, dihydropteroate synthase (DHPS). Sulfonamide resistance results from point mutations in the DHPS gene. Because human *P. jiroveci* cannot be cultured and hence no sensitivities can be directly performed, resistance is elucidated by the indirect method of sequencing the organism's DHPS gene and looking for characteristic mutations [183, 184]. It is unclear if the identified DHPS mutations affect the response to therapeutic doses of TMP-SMX. A Danish study reported that patients with mutant DHPS were less likely to survive PCP, but other trials have found that there was no effect on survival or response to therapy in those who had mutant DHPS [32, 33, 185–187]. Whether the presence of these mutations does in fact predict failure of prophylaxis or treatment remains controversial. There is currently no compelling evidence to date that suggests a change is warranted in the approach to the treatment or prevention of PCP based on these studies.

Association of Pneumocystis with Chronic Obstructive Lung Disease

There are intriguing studies linking *Pneumocystis* to the occurrence and exacerbation of chronic bronchitis and chronic obstructive lung disease [42]. At this point it is not clear whether this association is causal. It would be intriguing to consider the possibility that primary *Pneumocystis* infection, or *Pneumocystis* reinfection, could be related to short-term or long-term exacerbations of lung disease. This association is being actively investigated.

Diagnosis of PCP by PCR

As detailed above, more and more laboratories are using locally developed PCR assays to detect *Pneumocystis* in respiratory secretions [88–95]. These assays appear to be highly sensitive and highly specific at many laboratories. However, they are so sensitive that they are likely to recognize small quantities of *Pneumocystis* that may be unrelated to the cause of pulmonary dysfunction and unrelated to the need for chemoprophylaxis. Before these assays can be used to make clinical decisions, they need to be correlated with clinical outcomes. Quantitation may improve their specificity. At this point, their major use may be to confirm negative smears; in other words, these assays probably have a very high negative predictive value when performed in rigorous laboratory settings.

References

1. Kaplan JE, Hanson D, Dworkin MS, et al. Epidemiology of human immunodeficiency virus-associated opportunistic infections in the United States in the era of highly active antiretroviral therapy. Clin Infect Dis. 2000;30 Suppl 1:S5–14.

2. Thomas Jr CF, Limper AH. Pneumocystis pneumonia. N Engl J Med. 2004;350:2487–98.
3. Brooks JT, Kaplan JE, Holmes KK, Benson C, Pau A, Masur H. HIV-associated opportunistic infections–going, going, but not gone: the continued need for prevention and treatment guidelines. Clin Infect Dis. 2009;48:609–11.
4. Cailliez JC, Seguy N, Denis CM, et al. *Pneumocystis carinii*: an atypical fungal micro-organism. J Med Vet Mycol. 1996;34: 227–39.
5. Edman JC, Kovacs JA, Masur H, Santi DV, Elwood HJ, Sogin ML. Ribosomal RNA sequence shows *Pneumocystis carinii* to be a member of the fungi. Nature. 1988;334:519–22.
6. Stringer SL, Hudson K, Blase MA, Walzer PD, Cushion MT, Stringer JR. Sequence from ribosomal RNA of *Pneumocystis carinii* compared to those of four fungi suggests an ascomycetous affinity. J Protozool. 1989;36:14S–6S.
7. Barton E, Campbell WGJ. *Pneumocystis carinii* in lungs of rats treated with cortisone acetate: Ultrastructural observations relating to the life cycle. Am J Pathol. 1969;54:209–36.
8. Hughes WT, Kuhn S, Chaudhary S, et al. Successful chemoprophylaxis for *Pneumocystis carinii* pneumonitis. N Engl J Med. 1977;297:1419–26.
9. Edman JC, Edman U, Cao M, Lundgren B, Kovacs JA, Santi DV. Isolation and expression of the *Pneumocystis* carinii dihydrofolate reductase gene. Proc Natl Acad Sci USA. 1989;86:8625–9.
10. Volpe F, Ballantine SP, Delves CJ. The multifunctional folic acid synthesis fas gene of *Pneumocystis carinii* encodes dihydroneopterin aldolase, hydroxymethyldihydropterin pyrophosphokinase and dihydropteroate synthase. Eur J Biochem. 1993;216:449–58.
11. Basselin M, Hunt SM, Abdala-Valencia H, Kaneshiro ES. Ubiquinone synthesis in mitochondrial and microsomal subcellular fractions of *Pneumocystis* spp.: differential sensitivities to atovaquone. Eukaryot Cell. 2005;4:1483–92.
12. Huang L, Crothers K, Atzori C, et al. Dihydropteroate synthase gene mutations in *Pneumocystis* and sulfa resistance. Emerg Infect Dis. 2004;10:1721–8.
13. Iliades P, Meshnick SR, Macreadie IG. Mutations in the *Pneumocystis jiroveci* DHPS gene confer cross-resistance to sulfa drugs. Antimicrob Agents Chemother. 2005;49:741–8.
14. Kessl JJ, Hill P, Lange BB, Meshnick SR, Meunier B, Trumpower BL. Molecular basis for atovaquone resistance in *Pneumocystis jiroveci* modeled in the cytochrome bc(1) complex of *Saccharomyces cerevisiae*. J Biol Chem. 2004;279:2817–24.
15. Nahimana A, Rabodonirina M, Bille J, Francioli P, Hauser PM. Mutations of *Pneumocystis jiroveci* dihydrofolate reductase associated with failure of prophylaxis. Antimicrob Agents Chemother. 2004;48:4301–5.
16. Stein CR, Poole C, Kazanjian P, Meshnick SR. Sulfa use, dihydropteroate synthase mutations, and *Pneumocystis jiroveci* pneumonia. Emerg Infect Dis. 2004;10:1760–5.
17. Gigliotti F. *Pneumocystis carinii*: has the name really been changed? Clin Infect Dis. 2005;41:1752–5.
18. Stringer JR, Beard CB, Miller RF, Wakefield AE. A new name (*Pneumocystis jiroveci*) for Pneumocystis from humans. Emerg Infect Dis. 2002;8:891–6.
19. Kovacs JA, Halpern JL, Swan JC, Moss J, Parrillo JE, Masur H. Identification of antigens and antibodies specific for *Pneumocystis carinii*. J Immunol. 1988;140:2023–31.
20. Peglow SL, Smulian AG, Linke MJ, et al. Serologic responses to *Pneumocystis carinii* antigens in health and disease. J Infect Dis. 1990;161:296–306.
21. Pifer LL, Hughes WT, Stagno S, Woods D. *Pneumocystis carinii* infection: evidence for high prevalence in normal and immunosuppressed children. Pediatrics. 1978;61:35–41.
22. Morris A, Lundgren JD, Masur H, et al. Current epidemiology of *Pneumocystis* pneumonia. Emerg Infect Dis. 2004;10:1713–20.
23. Spencer L, Ukwu M, Alexander T, et al. Epidemiology of *Pneumocystis* colonization in families. Clin Infect Dis. 2008;46: 1237–40.
24. Walzer PD, Djawe K, Levin L, et al. Long-term serologic responses to the *Pneumocystis jiroveci* major surface glycoprotein in HIV-positive individuals with and without *P. jiroveci* infection. J Infect Dis. 2009;199:1335–44.
25. Davis JL, Welsh DA, Beard CB, et al. *Pneumocystis* colonisation is common among hospitalised HIV infected patients with non-Pneumocystis pneumonia. Thorax. 2008;63:329–34.
26. Bakeera-Kitaka S, Musoke P, Downing R, Tumwine JK. *Pneumocystis carinii* in children with severe pneumonia at Mulago Hospital, Uganda. Ann Trop Paediatr. 2004;24:227–35.
27. Fisk DT, Meshnick S, Kazanjian PH. *Pneumocystis carinii* pneumonia in patients in the developing world who have acquired immunodeficiency syndrome. Clin Infect Dis. 2003;36:70–8.
28. Tudor-Williams G. HIV infection in children in developing countries. Trans R Soc Trop Med Hyg. 2000;94:3–4.
29. Worodria W, Okot-Nwang M, Yoo SD, Aisu T. Causes of lower respiratory infection in HIV-infected Ugandan adults who are sputum AFB smear-negative. Int J Tuberc Lung Dis. 2003;7:117–23.
30. Hughes WT. Natural mode of acquisition for de novo infection with *Pneumocystis carinii*. J Infect Dis. 1982;145:842–8.
31. Beard CB, Fox MR, Lawrence GG, et al. Genetic differences in *Pneumocystis* isolates recovered from immunocompetent infants and from adults with AIDS: epidemiological implications. J Infect Dis. 2005;192:1815–8.
32. Huang L, Beard CB, Creasman J, et al. Sulfa or sulfone prophylaxis and geographic region predict mutations in the *Pneumocystis carinii* dihydropteroate synthase gene. J Infect Dis. 2000;182:1192–8.
33. Kazanjian P, Armstrong W, Hossler PA, et al. *Pneumocystis carinii* mutations are associated with duration of sulfa or sulfone prophylaxis exposure in AIDS patients. J Infect Dis. 2000;182:551–7.
34. Kovacs JA, Masur H. Evolving health effects of *Pneumocystis*: one hundred years of progress in diagnosis and treatment. JAMA. 2009;301:2578–85.
35. Ripamonti C, Orenstein A, Kutty G, et al. Restriction fragment length polymorphism typing demonstrates substantial diversity among *Pneumocystis jiroveci* isolates. J Infect Dis. 2009;200:1616–22.
36. Helweg-Larsen J, Tsolaki AG, Miller RF, Lundgren B, Wakefield AE. Clusters of *Pneumocystis carinii* pneumonia: analysis of person-to-person transmission by genotyping. Q J Med. 1998;91: 813–20.
37. Keely SP, Stringer JR. Sequences of *Pneumocystis carinii* f. sp. hominis strains associated with recurrent pneumonia vary at multiple loci. J Clin Microbiol. 1997;35:2745–7.
38. Keely SP, Stringer JR, Baughman RP, Linke MJ, Walzer PD, Smulian AG. Genetic variation among *Pneumocystis carinii* hominis isolates in recurrent pneumocystosis. J Infect Dis. 1995;172: 595–8.
39. Rabodonirina M, Vanhems P, Couray-Targe S, et al. Molecular evidence of interhuman transmission of *Pneumocystis* pneumonia among renal transplant recipients hospitalized with HIV-infected patients. Emerg Infect Dis. 2004;10:1766–73.
40. Vargas SL, Ponce CA, Galvez P, et al. *Pneumocystis* is not a direct cause of sudden infant death syndrome. Pediatr Infect Dis J. 2007;26:81–3.
41. Vargas SL, Ponce CA, Hughes WT, et al. Association of primary *Pneumocystis carinii* infection and sudden infant death syndrome. Clin Infect Dis. 1999;29:1489–93.
42. Morris A, Sciurba FC, Lebedeva IP, et al. Association of chronic obstructive pulmonary disease severity and *Pneumocystis* colonization. Am J Respir Crit Care Med. 2004;170:408–13.
43. Morris A, Netravali M, Kling HM, et al. Relationship of *Pneumocystis* antibody response to severity of chronic obstructive pulmonary disease. Clin Infect Dis. 2008;47:e64–8.

44. Browne MJ, Hubbard SM, Longo DL, et al. Excess prevalence of *Pneumocystis carinii* pneumonia in patients treated for lymphoma with combination chemotherapy. Ann Intern Med. 1986;104:338–44.
45. Byrd JC, Hargis JB, Kester KE, Hospenthal DR, Knutson SW, Diehl LF. Opportunistic pulmonary infections with fludarabine in previously treated patients with low-grade lymphoid malignancies: a role for *Pneumocystis carinii* pneumonia prophylaxis. Am J Hematol. 1995;49:135–42.
46. Hughes WT, Feldman S, Aur RJ, Verzosa MS, Hustu HO, Simone JV. Intensity of immunosuppressive therapy and the incidence of *Pneumocystis carinii* pneumonitis. Cancer. 1975;36:2004–9.
47. Kolstad A, Holte H, Fossa A, Lauritzsen GF, Gaustad P, Torfoss D. *Pneumocystis jiroveci* pneumonia in B-cell lymphoma patients treated with the rituximab-CHOEP-14 regimen. Haematologica. 2007;92:139–40.
48. Komano Y, Harigai M, Koike R, et al. *Pneumocystis jiroveci* pneumonia in patients with rheumatoid arthritis treated with infliximab: a retrospective review and case-control study of 21 patients. Arthritis Rheum. 2009;61:305–12.
49. Peters SG, Prakash UB. *Pneumocystis carinii* pneumonia. Review of 53 cases. Am J Med. 1987;82:73–8.
50. Sepkowitz KA, Brown AE, Telzak EE, Gottlieb S, Armstrong D. *Pneumocystis carinii* pneumonia among patients without AIDS at a cancer hospital. JAMA. 1992;267:832–7.
51. Sugimoto H, Uchida H, Akiyama N, et al. Improved survival of renal allograft recipients with *Pneumocystis carinii* pneumonia by early diagnosis and treatment. Transplant Proc. 1992;24:1556–8.
52. Tuan IZ, Dennison D, Weisdorf DJ. *Pneumocystis carinii* pneumonitis following bone marrow transplantation. Bone Marrow Transplant. 1992;10:267–72.
53. Sowden E, Carmichael AJ. Autoimmune inflammatory disorders, systemic corticosteroids and pneumocystis pneumonia: a strategy for prevention. BMC Infect Dis. 2004;4:42.
54. Kadoya A, Okada J, Iikuni Y, Kondo H. Risk factors for *Pneumocystis carinii* pneumonia in patients with polymyositis/dermatomyositis or systemic lupus erythematosus. J Rheumatol. 1996;23:1186–8.
55. Sepkowitz KA. *Pneumocystis carinii* pneumonia among patients with neoplastic disease. Semin Respir Infect. 1992;7:114–21.
56. Tomblyn M, Chiller T, Einsele H, et al. Guidelines for preventing infectious complications among hematopoietic cell transplantation recipients: a global perspective. Biol Blood Marrow Transplant. 2009;15:1143–238.
57. Rizzo JD, Wingard JR, Tichelli A, et al. Recommended screening and preventive practices for long-term survivors after hematopoietic cell transplantation: joint recommendations of the European Group for Blood and Marrow Transplantation, the Center for International Blood and Marrow Transplant Research, and the American Society of Blood and Marrow Transplantation. Biol Blood Marrow Transplant. 2006;12:138–51.
58. Roths JB, Sidman CL. Single and combined humoral and cell-mediated immunotherapy of *Pneumocystis carinii* pneumonia in immunodeficient scid mice. Infect Immun. 1993;61:1641–9.
59. Yale SH, Limper AH. *Pneumocystis carinii* pneumonia in patients without acquired immunodeficiency syndrome: associated illness and prior corticosteroid therapy. Mayo Clin Proc. 1996; 71:5–13.
60. Bozzette SA, Sattler FR, Chiu J, et al. A controlled trial of early adjunctive treatment with corticosteroids for *Pneumocystis carinii* pneumonia in the acquired immunodeficiency syndrome. California Collaborative Treatment Group. N Engl J Med. 1990;323:1451–7.
61. Masur H, Ognibene FP, Yarchoan R, et al. CD4 counts as predictors of opportunistic pneumonias in human immunodeficiency virus (HIV) infection. Ann Intern Med. 1989;111:223–31.
62. Phair J, Munoz A, Detels R, Kaslow R, Rinaldo C, Saah A. The risk of *Pneumocystis carinii* pneumonia among men infected with human immunodeficiency virus type 1. Multicenter AIDS Cohort Study Group. N Engl J Med. 1990;322:161–5.
63. Chu SY, Hanson DL, Ciesielski C, Ward JW. Prophylaxis against *Pneumocystis carinii* pneumonia at higher CD4+ T-cell counts. JAMA. 1995;273:848.
64. Dworkin MS, Hanson DL, Navin TR. Survival of patients with AIDS, after diagnosis of *Pneumocystis carinii* pneumonia, in the United States. J Infect Dis. 2001;183:1409–12.
65. Dworkin MS, Hanson DL, Kaplan JE, Jones JL, Ward JW. Risk for preventable opportunistic infections in persons with AIDS after antiretroviral therapy increases CD4+ T lymphocyte counts above prophylaxis thresholds. J Infect Dis. 2000;182:611–5.
66. Lyles RH, Munoz A, Yamashita TE, et al. Natural history of human immunodeficiency virus type 1 viremia after seroconversion and proximal to AIDS in a large cohort of homosexual men. Multicenter AIDS Cohort Study. J Infect Dis. 2000;181:872–80.
67. Miller V, Mocroft A, Reiss P, et al. Relations among CD4 lymphocyte count nadir, antiretroviral therapy, and HIV-1 disease progression: results from the EuroSIDA study. Ann Intern Med. 1999;130:570–7.
68. Mansharamani NG, Balachandran D, Vernovsky I, Garland R, Koziel H. Peripheral blood CD4+T-lymphocyte counts during Pneumocystis carinii pneumonia in immunocompromised patients without HIV infection. Chest. 2000;118:712–20.
69. Engelberg LA, Lerner CW, Tapper ML. Clinical features of Pneumocystis pneumonia in the acquired immune deficiency syndrome. Am Rev Respir Dis. 1984;130:689–94.
70. Walzer PD, Perl DP, Krogstad DJ, Rawson PG, Schultz MG. *Pneumocystis carinii* pneumonia in the United States. Epidemiologic, diagnostic, and clinical features. Ann Intern Med. 1974;80:83–93.
71. Kovacs JA, Hiemenz JW, Macher AM, et al. *Pneumocystis carinii* pneumonia: a comparison between patients with the acquired immunodeficiency syndrome and patients with other immunodeficiencies. Ann Intern Med. 1984;100:663–71.
72. Brenner M, Ognibene FP, Lack EE, et al. Prognostic factors and life expectancy of patients with acquired immunodeficiency syndrome and *Pneumocystis carinii* pneumonia. Am Rev Respir Dis. 1987;136:1199–206.
73. DeLorenzo LJ, Huang CT, Maguire GP, Stone DJ. Roentgenographic patterns of *Pneumocystis carinii* pneumonia in 104 patients with AIDS. Chest. 1987;91:323–7.
74. Gruden JF, Huang L, Turner J, et al. High-resolution CT in the evaluation of clinically suspected *Pneumocystis carinii* pneumonia in AIDS patients with normal, equivocal, or nonspecific radiographic findings. AJR. 1997;169:967–75.
75. Metersky ML, Colt HG, Olson LK, Shanks TG. AIDS-related spontaneous pneumothorax. Risk factors and treatment. Chest. 1995;108:946–51.
76. Sepkowitz KA, Telzak EE, Gold JW, et al. Pneumothorax in AIDS. Ann Intern Med. 1991;114:455–9.
77. Raviglione MC. Extrapulmonary pneumocystosis: the first 50 cases. Rev Infect Dis. 1990;12:1127–38.
78. Telzak EE, Cote RJ, Gold JW, Campbell SW, Armstrong D. Extrapulmonary *Pneumocystis carinii* infections. Rev Infect Dis. 1990;12:380–6.
79. Baughman R. Current methods in diagnosis. In: Walzer P, editor. *Pneumocystis carinii* pneumonia. New York: Marcel Dekker; 1994.
80. Meduri GU, Stover DE, Greeno RA, Nash T, Zaman MB. Bilateral bronchoalveolar lavage in the diagnosis of opportunistic pulmonary infections. Chest. 1991;100:1272–6.
81. Bigby TD, Margolskee D, Curtis JL, et al. The usefulness of induced sputum in the diagnosis of *Pneumocystis carinii* pneumonia

in patients with the acquired immunodeficiency syndrome. Am Rev Respir Dis. 1986;133:515–8.
82. Kovacs JA, Halpern JL, Lundgren B, Swan JC, Parrillo JE, Masur H. Monoclonal antibodies to *Pneumocystis carinii*: identification of specific antigens and characterization of antigenic differences between rat and human isolates. J Infect Dis. 1989;159:60–70.
83. Kovacs JA, Ng VL, Masur H, et al. Diagnosis of *Pneumocystis carinii* pneumonia: improved detection in sputum with use of monoclonal antibodies. N Engl J Med. 1988;318:589–93.
84. Ng VL, Virani NA, Chaisson RE, et al. Rapid detection of *Pneumocystis carinii* using a direct fluorescent monoclonal antibody stain. J Clin Microbiol. 1990;28:2228–33.
85. Pitchenik AE, Ganjei P, Torres A, Evans DA, Rubin E, Baier H. Sputum examination for the diagnosis of *Pneumocystis carinii* pneumonia in the acquired immunodeficiency syndrome. Am Rev Respir Dis. 1986;133:226–9.
86. Kirsch CM, Jensen WA, Kagawa FT, Azzi RL. Analysis of induced sputum for the diagnosis of recurrent *Pneumocystis carinii* pneumonia. Chest. 1992;102:1152–4.
87. Gill VJ, Evans G, Stock F, Parrillo JE, Masur H, Kovacs JA. Detection of *Pneumocystis carinii* by fluorescent-antibody stain using a combination of three monoclonal antibodies. J Clin Microbiol. 1987;25:1837–40.
88. Huang SN, Fischer SH, O'Shaughnessy E, Gill VJ, Masur H, Kovacs JA. Development of a PCR assay for diagnosis of *Pneumocystis carinii* pneumonia based on amplification of the multicopy major surface glycoprotein gene family. Diagn Microbiol Infect Dis. 1999;35:27–32.
89. Wakefield AE, Pixley FJ, Banerji S, et al. Amplification of mitochondrial ribosomal RNA sequences from *Pneumocystis carinii* DNA of rat and human origin. Mol Biochem Parasitol. 1990;43:69–76.
90. Lipschik GY, Gill VJ, Lundgren JD, et al. Improved diagnosis of *Pneumocystis carinii* infection by polymerase chain reaction on induced sputum and blood. Lancet. 1992;340:203–6.
91. Lu JJ, Chen CH, Bartlett MS, Smith JW, Lee CH. Comparison of six different PCR methods for detection of *Pneumocystis carinii*. J Clin Microbiol. 1995;33:2785–8.
92. Gupta R, Mirdha BR, Guleria R, et al. Diagnostic significance of nested polymerase chain reaction for sensitive detection of *Pneumocystis jiroveci* in respiratory clinical specimens. Diagn Microbiol Infect Dis. 2009;64:381–8.
93. Helweg-Larsen J, Jensen JS, Benfield T, Svendsen UG, Lundgren JD, Lundgren B. Diagnostic use of PCR for detection of *Pneumocystis carinii* in oral wash samples. J Clin Microbiol. 1998;36:2068–72.
94. Larsen HH, Masur H, Kovacs JA, et al. Development and evaluation of a quantitative, touch-down, real-time PCR assay for diagnosing *Pneumocystis carinii* pneumonia. J Clin Microbiol. 2002;40: 490–4.
95. Fischer S, Gill VJ, Kovacs J, et al. The use of oral washes to diagnose *Pneumocystis carinii* pneumonia: a blinded prospective study using a polymerase chain reaction-based detection system. J Infect Dis. 2001;184:1485–8.
96. Bishop LR, Kovacs JA. Quantitation of anti-*Pneumocystis jiroveci* antibodies in healthy persons and immunocompromised patients. J Infect Dis. 2003;187:1844–8.
97. Daly KR, Huang L, Morris A, et al. Antibody response to *Pneumocystis jiroveci* major surface glycoprotein. Emerg Infect Dis. 2006;12:1231–7.
98. Skelly M, Hoffman J, Fabbri M, Holzman RS, Clarkson Jr AB, Merali S. S-adenosylmethionine concentrations in diagnosis of *Pneumocystis carinii* pneumonia. Lancet. 2003;361:1267–8.
99. Wang P, Huang L, Davis JL, et al. A hydrophilic-interaction chromatography tandem mass spectrometry method for quantitation of serum S-adenosylmethionine in patients infected with human immunodeficiency virus. Clin Chim Acta. 2008;396:86–8.
100. Shimizu Y, Sunaga N, Dobashi K, et al. Serum markers in interstitial pneumonia with and without *Pneumocystis jiroveci* colonization: a prospective study. BMC Infect Dis. 2009;9:47.
101. Tasaka S, Hasegawa N, Kobayashi S, et al. Serum indicators for the diagnosis of Pneumocystis pneumonia. Chest. 2007;131:1173–80.
102. Watanabe T, Yasuoka A, Tanuma J, et al. Serum (1->3) beta-D-glucan as a noninvasive adjunct marker for the diagnosis of Pneumocystis pneumonia in patients with AIDS. Clin Infect Dis. 2009;49:1128–31.
103. Del Bono V, Mularoni A, Furfaro E, et al. Clinical evaluation of a (1, 3)-beta-D-glucan assay for presumptive diagnosis of *Pneumocystis jiroveci* pneumonia in immunocompromised patients. Clin Vaccine Immunol. 2009;16:1524–6.
104. Desmet S, Van Wijngaerden E, Maertens J, et al. Serum (1-3)-{beta}-D-glucan as a diagnostic tool for *Pneumocystis jiroveci* pneumonia in patients with HIV infection or hematological malignancy. J Clin Microbiol. 2009;47:3871–4.
105. Sattler FR, Cowan R, Nielsen DM, Ruskin J. Trimethoprim-sulfamethoxazole compared with pentamidine for treatment of *Pneumocystis carinii* pneumonia in the acquired immunodeficiency syndrome. A prospective, noncrossover study. Ann Intern Med. 1988;109:280–7.
106. Ruf B, Rohde I, Pohle HD. Efficacy of clindamycin/primaquine versus trimethoprim/sulfamethoxazole in primary treatment of *Pneumocystis carinii* pneumonia. Eur J Clin Microbiol Infect Dis. 1991;10:207–10.
107. Safrin S, Finkelstein DM, Feinberg J, et al. Comparison of three regimens for treatment of mild to moderate *Pneumocystis carinii* pneumonia in patients with AIDS. A double-blind, randomized, trial of oral trimethoprim-sulfamethoxazole, dapsone-trimethoprim, and clindamycin-primaquine. ACTG 108 Study Group. Ann Intern Med. 1996;124:792–802.
108. Toma E. Clindamycin/primaquine for treatment of *Pneumocystis carinii* pneumonia in AIDS. Eur J Clin Microbiol Infect Dis. 1991;10:210–3.
109. Kaplan JE, Benson C, Holmes KH, Brooks JT, Pau A, Masur H. Guidelines for prevention and treatment of opportunistic infections in HIV-infected adults and adolescents: recommendations from CDC, the National Institutes of Health, and the HIV Medicine Association of the Infectious Diseases Society of America. MMWR Recomm Rep. 2009;58:1–207. quiz CE1-4.
110. Hardy WD, Feinberg J, Finkelstein DM, et al. A controlled trial of trimethoprim-sulfamethoxazole or aerosolized pentamidine for secondary prophylaxis of *Pneumocystis carinii* pneumonia in patients with the acquired immunodeficiency syndrome. AIDS Clinical Trials Group Protocol 021. N Engl J Med. 1992;327: 1842–8.
111. Schneider MM, Hoepelman AI, Eeftinck Schattenkerk JK, et al. A controlled trial of aerosolized pentamidine or trimethoprim-sulfamethoxazole as primary prophylaxis against *Pneumocystis carinii* pneumonia in patients with human immunodeficiency virus infection. The Dutch AIDS Treatment Group. N Engl J Med. 1992;327:1836–41.
112. Conte Jr JE, Chernoff D, Feigal Jr DW, Joseph P, McDonald C, Golden JA. Intravenous or inhaled pentamidine for treating *Pneumocystis carinii* pneumonia in AIDS. A randomized trial. Ann Intern Med. 1990;113:203–9.
113. Conte Jr JE, Hollander H, Golden JA. Inhaled or reduced-dose intravenous pentamidine for *Pneumocystis carinii* pneumonia. A pilot study. Ann Intern Med. 1987;107:495–8.
114. Leoung GS, Feigal Jr DW, Montgomery AB, et al. Aerosolized pentamidine for prophylaxis against *Pneumocystis carinii* pneumonia. The San Francisco community prophylaxis trial. N Engl J Med. 1990;323:769–75.
115. Medina I, Mills J, Leoung G, et al. Oral therapy for *Pneumocystis carinii* pneumonia in the acquired immunodeficiency syndrome.

A controlled trial of trimethoprim-sulfamethoxazole versus trimethoprim-dapsone. N Engl J Med. 1990;323:776–82.
116. Hughes W, Leoung G, Kramer F, et al. Comparison of atovaquone (566C80) with trimethoprim-sulfamethoxazole to treat *Pneumocystis carinii* pneumonia in patients with AIDS. N Engl J Med. 1993;328:1521–7.
117. Mills J, Leoung G, Medina I, Hopewell PC, Hughes WT, Wofsy C. Dapsone treatment of *Pneumocystis carinii* pneumonia in the acquired immunodeficiency syndrome. Antimicrob Agents Chemother. 1988;32:1057–60.
118. Safrin S, Sattler FR, Lee BL, et al. Dapsone as a single agent is suboptimal therapy for *Pneumocystis carinii* pneumonia. J Acquir Immune Defic Syndr. 1991;4:244–9.
119. Leoung GS, Mills J, Hopewell PC, Hughes W, Wofsy C. Dapsone-trimethoprim for *Pneumocystis carinii* pneumonia in the acquired immunodeficiency syndrome. Ann Intern Med. 1986;105:45–8.
120. Bozzette SA, Finkelstein DM, Spector SA, et al. A randomized trial of three antipneumocystis agents in patients with advanced human immunodeficiency virus infection. NIAID AIDS Clinical Trials Group. N Engl J Med. 1995;332:693–9.
121. Noskin GA, Murphy RL, Black JR, Phair JP. Salvage therapy with clindamycin/primaquine for *Pneumocystis carinii* pneumonia. Clin Infect Dis. 1992;14:183–8.
122. Dohn MN, Weinberg WG, Torres RA, et al. Oral atovaquone compared with intravenous pentamidine for *Pneumocystis carinii* pneumonia in patients with AIDS. Atovaquone Study Group. Ann Intern Med. 1994;121:174–80.
123. Catterall JR, Potasman I, Remington JS. *Pneumocystis carinii* pneumonia in the patient with AIDS. Chest. 1985;88:758–62.
124. Annaloro C, Della Volpe A, Usardi P, Lambertenghi Deliliers G. Caspofungin treatment of *Pneumocystis* pneumonia during conditioning for bone marrow transplantation. Eur J Clin Microbiol Infect Dis. 2006;25:52–4.
125. Deresinski SC, Stevens DA. Caspofungin. Clin Infect Dis. 2003;36: 1445–57.
126. Kamboj M, Weinstock D, Sepkowitz KA. Progression of *Pneumocystis jiroveci* pneumonia in patients receiving echinocandin therapy. Clin Infect Dis. 2006;43:e92–4.
127. Utili R, Durante-Mangoni E, Basilico C, Mattei A, Ragone E, Grossi P. Efficacy of caspofungin addition to trimethoprim-sulfamethoxazole treatment for severe *Pneumocystis* pneumonia in solid organ transplant recipients. Transplantation. 2007;84: 685–8.
128. Gagnon S, Boota AM, Fischl MA, Baier H, Kirksey OW, La Voie L. Corticosteroids as adjunctive therapy for severe *Pneumocystis carinii* pneumonia in the acquired immunodeficiency syndrome. A double-blind, placebo-controlled trial. N Engl J Med. 1990;323: 1444–50.
129. Briel M, Bucher HC, Boscacci R, Furrer H. Adjunctive corticosteroids for *Pneumocystis jiroveci* pneumonia in patients with HIV-infection. Cochrane Database Syst Rev. 2006;3:CD006150.
130. Delclaux C, Zahar JR, Amraoui G, et al. Corticosteroids as adjunctive therapy for severe *Pneumocystis carinii* pneumonia in non-human immunodeficiency virus-infected patients: retrospective study of 31 patients. Clin Infect Dis. 1999;29:670–2.
131. Pareja JG, Garland R, Koziel H. Use of adjunctive corticosteroids in severe adult non-HIV *Pneumocystis carinii* pneumonia. Chest. 1998;113:1215–24.
132. Montaner JS, Lawson LM, Gervais A, et al. Aerosol pentamidine for secondary prophylaxis of AIDS-related *Pneumocystis carinii* pneumonia. A randomized, placebo-controlled study. Ann Intern Med. 1991;114:948–53.
133. Dohn MN, Baughman RP, Vigdorth EM, Frame DL. Equal survival rates for first, second, and third episodes of *Pneumocystis carinii* pneumonia in patients with acquired immunodeficiency syndrome. Arch Intern Med. 1992;152:2465–70.
134. Kales CP, Murren JR, Torres RA, Crocco JA. Early predictors of in-hospital mortality for *Pneumocystis carinii* pneumonia in the acquired immunodeficiency syndrome. Arch Intern Med. 1987;147:1413–7.
135. Shelhamer JH, Ognibene FP, Macher AM, et al. Persistence of *Pneumocystis carinii* in lung tissue of acquired immunodeficiency syndrome patients treated for Pneumocystis pneumonia. Am Rev Respir Dis. 1984;130:1161–5.
136. Radhi S, Alexander T, Ukwu M, Saleh S, Morris A. Outcome of HIV-associated *Pneumocystis* pneumonia in hospitalized patients from 2000 through 2003. BMC Infect Dis. 2008;8:118.
137. Morris A. Is there anything new in Pneumocystis jirovecii pneumonia? Changes in *P. jiroveci* pneumonia over the course of the AIDS epidemic. Clin Infect Dis. 2008;46:634–6.
138. Powell K, Davis JL, Morris AM, Chi A, Bensley MR, Huang L. Survival for patients With HIV admitted to the ICU continues to improve in the current era of combination antiretroviral therapy. Chest. 2009;135:11–7.
139. Stover DE, Zaman MB, Hajdu SI, Lange M, Gold J, Armstrong D. Bronchoalveolar lavage in the diagnosis of diffuse pulmonary infiltrates in the immunosuppressed host. Ann Intern Med. 1984;101:1–7.
140. Barry SM, Lipman MC, Deery AR, Johnson MA, Janossy G. Immune reconstitution pneumonitis following *Pneumocystis carinii* pneumonia in HIV-infected subjects. HIV Med. 2002;3:207–11.
141. Dean GL, Williams DI, Churchill DR, Fisher MJ. Transient clinical deterioration in HIV patients with *Pneumocystis carinii* pneumonia after starting highly active antiretroviral therapy: another case of immune restoration inflammatory syndrome. Am J Respir Crit Care Med. 2002;165(Dean GL, Williams DI, Churchill DR, Fisher MJ):1670. author reply.
142. Koval CE, Gigliotti F, Nevins D, Demeter LM. Immune reconstitution syndrome after successful treatment of *Pneumocystis carinii* pneumonia in a man with human immunodeficiency virus type 1 infection. Clin Infect Dis. 2002;35:491–3.
143. Ratnam I, Chiu C, Kandala NB, Easterbrook PJ. Incidence and risk factors for immune reconstitution inflammatory syndrome in an ethnically diverse HIV type 1-infected cohort. Clin Infect Dis. 2006;42:418–27.
144. Wislez M, Bergot E, Antoine M, et al. Acute respiratory failure following HAART introduction in patients treated for *Pneumocystis carinii* pneumonia. Am J Respir Crit Care Med. 2001;164:847–51.
145. Zolopa A, Andersen J, Powderly W, et al. Early antiretroviral therapy reduces AIDS progression/death in individuals with acute opportunistic infections: a multicenter randomized strategy trial. PLoS ONE. 2009;4:e5575.
146. Hirsch HH, Kaufmann G, Sendi P, Battegay M. Immune reconstitution in HIV-infected patients. Clin Infect Dis. 2004;38:1159–66.
147. Gryzan S, Paradis IL, Zeevi A, et al. Unexpectedly high incidence of *Pneumocystis carinii* infection after lung-heart transplantation. Implications for lung defense and allograft survival. Am Rev Respir Dis. 1988;137:1268–74.
148. Henson JW, Jalaj JK, Walker RW, Stover DE, Fels AO. *Pneumocystis carinii* pneumonia in patients with primary brain tumors. Arch Neurol. 1991;48:406–9.
149. Masur H. Prevention and treatment of *Pneumocystis* pneumonia. N Engl J Med. 1992;327:1853–60.
150. Rodriguez M, Fishman JA. Prevention of infection due to *Pneumocystis* spp. in human immunodeficiency virus-negative immunocompromised patients. Clin Microbiol Rev. 2004;17: 770–82.
151. Fischl MA, Dickinson GM, La Voie L. Safety and efficacy of sulfamethoxazole and trimethoprim chemoprophylaxis for *Pneumocystis carinii* pneumonia in AIDS. JAMA. 1988;259: 1185–9.

152. Tomblyn M, Chiller T, Einsele H, et al. Guidelines for preventing infectious complications among hematopoietic cell transplant recipients: a global perspective. Bone Marrow Transplant. 2009;44: 453–5.
153. Winston DJ. Prophylaxis and treatment of infection in the bone marrow transplant recipient. Curr Clin Topics Infect Dis. 1993;13:293–321.
154. Guidelines for preventing opportunistic infections among hematopoietic stem cell transplant recipients. MMWR Recomm Rep 2000;49:1–125, CE1-7.
155. De Castro N, Neuville S, Sarfati C, et al. Occurrence of *Pneumocystis jiroveci* pneumonia after allogeneic stem cell transplantation: a 6-year retrospective study. Bone Marrow Transplant. 2005;36:879–83.
156. Kovacs JA, Masur H. Prophylaxis for *Pneumocystis carinii* pneumonia in patients infected with human immunodeficiency virus. Clin Infect Dis. 1992;14:1005–9.
157. Mofenson LM, Brady MT, Danner SP, et al. Guidelines for the Prevention and Treatment of Opportunistic Infections among HIV-exposed and HIV-infected children: recommendations from CDC, the National Institutes of Health, the HIV Medicine Association of the Infectious Diseases Society of America, the Pediatric Infectious Diseases Society, and the American Academy of Pediatrics. MMWR Recomm Rep. 2009;58:1–166.
158. Furrer H, Egger M, Opravil M, et al. Discontinuation of primary prophylaxis against *Pneumocystis carinii* pneumonia in HIV-1-infected adults treated with combination antiretroviral therapy. Swiss HIV Cohort Study. N Engl J Med. 1999;340:1301–6.
159. Furrer H, Opravil M, Rossi M, et al. Discontinuation of primary prophylaxis in HIV-infected patients at high risk of *Pneumocystis carinii* pneumonia: prospective multicentre study. AIDS. 2001;15:501–7.
160. Green H, Hay P, Dunn DT, McCormack S. A prospective multicentre study of discontinuing prophylaxis for opportunistic infections after effective antiretroviral therapy. HIV Med. 2004;5:278–83.
161. Kirk O, Lundgren JD, Pedersen C, Nielsen H, Gerstoft J. Can chemoprophylaxis against opportunistic infections be discontinued after an increase in CD4 cells induced by highly active antiretroviral therapy? AIDS. 1999;13:1647–51.
162. Ledergerber B, Mocroft A, Reiss P, et al. Discontinuation of secondary prophylaxis against *Pneumocystis carinii* pneumonia in patients with HIV infection who have a response to antiretroviral therapy. Eight European Study Groups. N Engl J Med. 2001;344:168–74.
163. de Quiros JC Lopez Bernaldo, Miro JM, Pena JM, et al. A randomized trial of the discontinuation of primary and secondary prophylaxis against *Pneumocystis carinii* pneumonia after highly active antiretroviral therapy in patients with HIV infection. Grupo de Estudio del SIDA 04/98. N Engl J Med. 2001;344:159–67.
164. D'Egidio GE, Kravcik S, Cooper CL, Cameron DW, Fergusson DA, Angel JB. *Pneumocystis jiroveci* pneumonia prophylaxis is not required with a CD4+ T-cell count<200 cells/microl when viral replication is suppressed. AIDS. 2007;21:1711–5.
165. Girard PM, Landman R, Gaudebout C, et al. Dapsone-pyrimethamine compared with aerosolized pentamidine as primary prophylaxis against *Pneumocystis carinii* pneumonia and toxoplasmosis in HIV infection. The PRIO Study Group. N Engl J Med. 1993;328:1514–20.
166. Hardy WD, Northfelt DW, Drake TA. Fatal, disseminated pneumocystosis in a patient with acquired immunodeficiency syndrome receiving prophylactic aerosolized pentamidine. Am J Med. 1989;87:329–31.
167. Ioannidis JP, Cappelleri JC, Skolnik PR, Lau J, Sacks HS. A meta-analysis of the relative efficacy and toxicity of *Pneumocystis carinii* prophylactic regimens. Arch Intern Med. 1996;156:177–88.
168. Podzamczer D, Salazar A, Jimenez J, et al. Intermittent trimethoprim-sulfamethoxazole compared with dapsone-pyrimethamine for the simultaneous primary prophylaxis of *Pneumocystis* pneumonia and toxoplasmosis in patients infected with HIV. Ann Intern Med. 1995;122:755–61.
169. Saah AJ, Hoover DR, Peng Y, et al. Predictors for failure of *Pneumocystis carinii* pneumonia prophylaxis. Multicenter AIDS Cohort Study. JAMA. 1995;273:1197–202.
170. El-Sadr WM, Luskin-Hawk R, Yurik TM, et al. A randomized trial of daily and thrice-weekly trimethoprim-sulfamethoxazole for the prevention of *Pneumocystis carinii* pneumonia in human immunodeficiency virus-infected persons. Terry Beirn Community Programs for Clinical Research on AIDS (CPCRA). Clin Infect Dis. 1999;29:775–83.
171. Hughes WT, Rivera GK, Schell MJ, Thornton D, Lott L. Successful intermittent chemoprophylaxis for *Pneumocystis carinii pneumonitis*. N Engl J Med. 1987;316:1627–32.
172. Carr A, Tindall B, Brew BJ, et al. Low-dose trimethoprim-sulfamethoxazole prophylaxis for toxoplasmic encephalitis in patients with AIDS. Ann Intern Med. 1992;117:106–11.
173. Conte Jr JE, Upton RA, Phelps RT, Wofsy CB, Zurlinden E, Lin ET. Use of a specific and sensitive assay to determine pentamidine pharmacokinetics in patients with AIDS. J Infect Dis. 1986;154:923–9.
174. Murphy RL, Lavelle JP, Allan JD, et al. Aerosol pentamidine prophylaxis following *Pneumocystis carinii* pneumonia in AIDS patients: results of a blinded dose-comparison study using an ultrasonic nebulizer. Am J Med. 1991;90:418–26.
175. Consensus statement on the use of corticosteroids as adjunctive therapy for *Pneumocystis* pneumonia in the acquired immunodeficiency syndrome. The National Institutes of Health-University of California Expert Panel for Corticosteroids as Adjunctive Therapy for Pneumocystis Pneumonia. N Engl J Med. 1990;323: 1500–4.
176. Blumberg HM, Watkins DL, Berschling JD, et al. Preventing the nosocomial transmission of tuberculosis. Ann Intern Med. 1995;122:658–63.
177. Holtzer CD, Flaherty Jr JF, Coleman RL. Cross-reactivity in HIV-infected patients switched from trimethoprim-sulfamethoxazole to dapsone. Pharmacotherapy. 1998;18:831–5.
178. Sangiolo D, Storer B, Nash R, et al. Toxicity and efficacy of daily dapsone as *Pneumocystis jiroveci* prophylaxis after hematopoietic stem cell transplantation: a case-control study. Biol Blood Marrow Transplant. 2005;11:521–9.
179. Lavelle J, Falloon J, Morgan A, et al. Weekly dapsone and dapson/pyrimethamine for *Pneumocystis* pneumonia prophylaxis. In: VII International Conference on AIDS 1991;7:233. Florence; 1991.
180. Opravil M, Hirschel B, Lazzarin A, et al. Once-weekly administration of dapsone/pyrimethamine vs. aerosolized pentamidine as combined prophylaxis for *Pneumocystis carinii* pneumonia and toxoplasmic encephalitis in human immunodeficiency virus-infected patients. Clin Infect Dis. 1995;20:531–41.
181. Chan C, Montaner J, Lefebvre EA, et al. Atovaquone suspension compared with aerosolized pentamidine for prevention of *Pneumocystis carinii* pneumonia in human immunodeficiency virus-infected subjects intolerant of trimethoprim or sulfonamides. J Infect Dis. 1999;180:369–76.
182. El-Sadr WM, Murphy RL, Yurik TM, et al. Atovaquone compared with dapsone for the prevention of *Pneumocystis carinii* pneumonia in patients with HIV infection who cannot tolerate trimethoprim, sulfonamides, or both. Community Program for Clinical Research on AIDS and the AIDS Clinical Trials Group. N Engl J Med. 1998;339:1889–95.
183. Kazanjian P, Locke AB, Hossler PA, et al. *Pneumocystis carinii* mutations associated with sulfa and sulfone prophylaxis failures in AIDS patients. AIDS. 1998;12:873–8.
184. Mei Q, Gurunathan S, Masur H, Kovacs JA. Failure of co-trimoxazole in *Pneumocystis carinii* infection and mutations in dihydropteroate synthase gene. Lancet. 1998;351:1631–2.

185. Crothers K, Beard CB, Turner J, et al. Severity and outcome of HIV-associated *Pneumocystis* pneumonia containing *Pneumocystis jiroveci* dihydropteroate synthase gene mutations. AIDS. 2005;19:801–5.
186. Helweg-Larsen J, Benfield TL, Eugen-Olsen J, Lundgren JD, Lundgren B. Effects of mutations in *Pneumocystis carinii* dihydropteroate synthase gene on outcome of AIDS-associated *P. carinii* pneumonia. Lancet. 1999;354:1347–51.
187. Navin TR, Beard CB, Huang L, et al. Effect of mutations in *Pneumocystis carinii* dihydropteroate synthase gene on outcome of *P. carinii* pneumonia in patients with HIV-1: a prospective study. Lancet. 2001;358:545–9.

Infections due to Miscellaneous Fungi

John W. Baddley and William E. Dismukes

Over the past 2 decades, rare and unusual fungi, often common soil saprophytes, have been reported increasingly as causing invasive infections in humans. Possible reasons for an increased frequency of unusual fungal infections include increasing numbers of patients with immunosuppression and increasing chance for environmental exposure. This chapter will focus on unusual and rare yeast and mould organisms and their disease manifestations. Lobomycosis, a chronic skin infection caused by the yeast-like organism *Lacazia loboi*, will be described, followed by infections due to basidiomycetes, and *Emmonsia crescens,* the agent of adiaspiromycosis. Finally, rhinosporidiosis and pythiosis will be discussed, although evidence indicates that these infections are not due to true fungi.

Infections due to Yeast-Like Organisms

Lobomycosis

Lobomycosis is a chronic skin infection characterized by nodules, plaques, and verrucoid or ulcerated lesions. The agent of lobomycosis, *L. loboi* (order Onygenales), is a yeast-like organism in tissues, and an obligate human pathogen [1, 2]. Dolphins (*Tursiops truncatus* and *Sotalia fluviatilis*) are the only nonhuman hosts that acquire natural infection [2–6]. Lobomycosis occurs in tropical and subtropical forests, and has been reported in South, Central, and North America and in Europe [7, 8]. The majority of cases are from the Brazilian and Colombian Amazonian regions; only recently have cases from North America been described [9, 10].

The natural habitat of *L. loboi* is unknown and is difficult to investigate because the organism has never been isolated and cultured in vitro [11]. Most infections occur on the skin in areas exposed to trauma, suggesting that the organism is present in soil or on vegetation [7]. An aquatic source is also likely, based on reported infections among dolphins [2–4]. Lobomycosis was described initially in 1931 by the dermatologist Jorge Lobo [12], who described a native of the Amazon Valley with numerous plaques and nodules in the lumbosacral region. His disease had progressed slowly for 19 years. Based on clinical and histologic findings of the case, Lobo believed that the etiologic fungus was similar to *Paracoccidioides brasiliensis*, and referred to the infection as "keloidal blastomycosis" [12].

Since the initial description of lobomycosis, more than 300 human cases have been confirmed [7, 9, 13]. Most reported cases have been in males, and the occupations of those infected often are related to mining, agricultural activities, fishing, or hunting [8]. Lesions occur on cool, exposed areas such as the feet, legs, ears, arms, elbows, and less frequently the face. Lesions can be localized or disseminated throughout the skin, resulting from contiguous extension, autoinoculation, or lymphatic spread. A single case has been described which suggests visceral involvement [14]. A patient who had had lobomycosis of the leg and knee for 47 years was found to have a presumed testicular tumor; however histopathology results showed granulomas with giant cells and fungi consistent with lobomycosis.

Lobomycosis usually begins as a well-circumscribed, indurated papule, and as the cutaneous disease progresses, the lesions enlarge and new lesions appear. Nodular lesions are most frequent, although macules, papules, plaques, ulcers, and verrucous lesions may be present [7] (Fig. 1). Generally, the disease is insidious, and may progress over a period of many years [15].

Diagnosis of lobomycosis is based on clinical features of the skin lesions and histologic examination with special stains of tissues; the organism has not yet been cultured in vitro. Microscopically, the dermis contains granulomas with foamy macrophages and multinucleated giant cells, without the presence of necrosis. Both macrophages and giant cells may ingest the fungi [7, 16]. The fungus, between 5 and 12 μm in diameter, is yeast-like, lemon-shaped, and forms beads joined together by thin bridges (Fig. 2). Cells

J.W. Baddley (✉)
Division of Infectious Diseases, Birmingham VA Medical Center, University of Alabama at Birmingham School of Medicine, Birmingham, AL, USA
e-mail: jbaddley@uab.edu

C.A. Kauffman et al. (eds.), *Essentials of Clinical Mycology*,
DOI 10.1007/978-1-4419-6640-7_27, © Springer Science+Business Media, LLC 2011

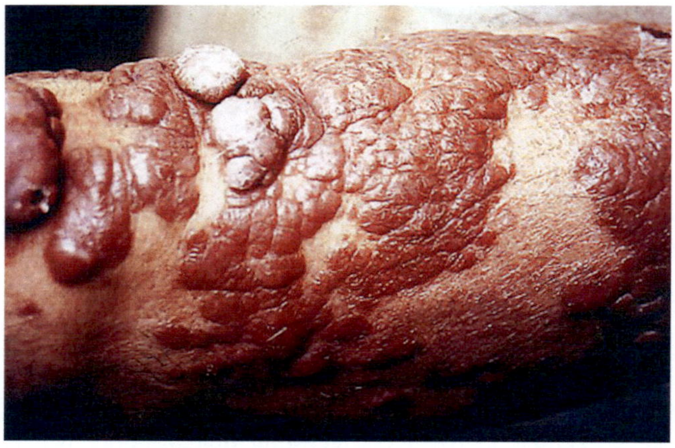

Fig. 1 Multiple nodular, plaque-like lesions of the leg in a Peruvian patient with lobomycosis (Courtesy of Beatriz Bustamante)

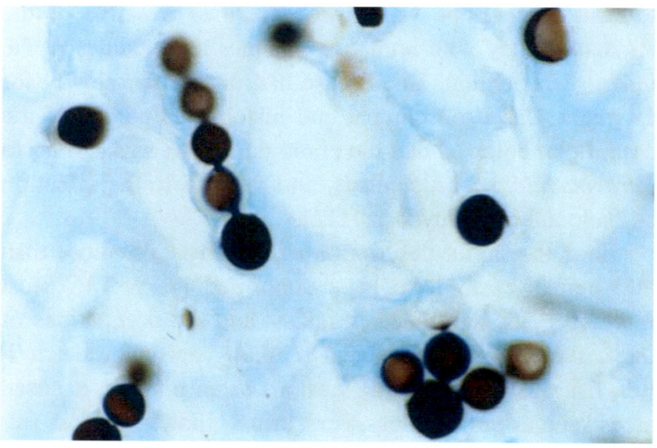

Fig. 2 Gomori-methenamine silver stain showing chains of *Lacazia loboi* cells and multiple buds (Courtesy of David W. Warnock)

with multiple budding are frequently seen, and may resemble budding seen with *P. brasiliensis* [16].

Therapy of lobomycosis is difficult, and treatment with amphotericin B, itraconazole, ketoconazole, miconazole, trimethoprim, and flucytosine has been tried but is often of little benefit [17–19]. For small skin lesions, cryosurgery or electrosurgery may be curative. Clofazimine has been used with some success in addition to surgery [9, 20]. For early lesions, surgical removal may be effective, but in chronic cases relapse after surgery is frequent [9, 13, 21].

Infections due to Miscellaneous Moulds

Basidiomycosis

The basidiomycetes, comprising mushrooms and toadstools, are distributed widely in nature, with over 16,000 recognized species [22]. Basidiomycetes are common plant pathogens or soil saprophytes, but rarely cause invasive disease in humans [23]. Although basidiomycetes are recognized increasingly as pathogens, their identification is problematic. On examination of infected tissues, septate, hyaline hyphae are seen, and may be confused with those of *Aspergillus* species. Frequently, tissue specimens show initial growth of hyphae in culture but are difficult to identify to the genus or species level. Among basidiomycetes causing human infection, the most recognized species is *Filobasidiella neoformans*, the teleomorph (sexual state) of *Cryptococcus neoformans*. Less common, but emerging, pathogens include *Schizophyllum commune*, *Coprinus* species, *Hormographiella aspergillata*, and *Ustilago* species.

Few cases of confirmed invasive infection due to basidiomycetes, other than those of *Filobasidiella neoformans*, exist in the literature, but cases and identification of isolates as basidiomycetes appear to be increasing [24]. *S. commune*, one of the more common pathogens, has been reported as causing a palatal ulcer that was treated successfully with amphotericin B [25]. Other reports include several cases of invasive or allergic sinusitis [26–31], pulmonary nodules after cardiac transplantation [32], pneumonia [33], a case of allergic bronchopulmonary mycosis [34], and infection associated with a bronchogenous cyst [35]. In 1996, a case of *S. commune* causing pulmonary disease and brain abscess was described in a patient receiving corticosteroid therapy for presumptive lymphoma [24]. The patient improved with amphotericin B and itraconazole, but later died of bacterial pneumonia and sepsis.

Infection with *Coprinus cinereus* is less common, and was the causative agent in a well-documented case of aortic valve endocarditis [36]. No obvious source of infection was identified. Aortic valve tissue grew *C. cinereus*, but the patient died during valve replacement surgery and was not treated. An additional case of *Coprinus* pulmonary infection was described in a patient with non-Hodgkin's lymphoma who responded to treatment with amphotericin B [37]. Several cases of fatal pneumonia in leukemic patients due to *H. aspergillata*, the anamorph of *C. cinereus*, have also been described [38, 39]. Only a few cases of *Ustilago* species infection have been reported. The organism was implicated as the cause of skin infections and a brain lesion [23, 40].

The ideal treatment for basidiomycete infections is unknown, and the paucity of cases does not allow for comparisons of outcomes with different antifungal agents. Amphotericin B has been effective in several cases, either as single therapy or in combination with itraconazole [24, 25, 37]. Azole agents, particularly itraconazole and fluconazole, as single therapy have achieved mixed results [34, 41]. In four cases of sinusitis, surgical therapy alone was curative [26, 28, 29]. Recently, susceptibility data have been reported for several different antifungal drugs against a large number of basidiomycetes, several of which caused invasive infection [42]. For the species tested, 96-h minimum inhibitory concentrations (MICs) for amphotericin B, itraconazole, voriconazole, and posaconazole were low (0.125–1 μg/mL), while the MICs were somewhat higher for 5-flucytosine and fluconazole. Correlation between in vitro data and clinical efficacy is as yet unknown, but may become important if the emergence of basidiomycete infections continues.

Adiaspiromycosis

Adiaspiromycosis is an unusual pulmonary mycosis that affects humans and animals, but is most common in rodents [43, 44]. The organisms that cause adiaspiromycosis are *Emmonsia crescens* (formerly *Chrysosporium parvum* var. *crescens*), which causes disease in humans and animals, and *Emmonsia parva* (formerly *Chrysosporium parvum* var. *parvum*), which is responsible for disease in animals.

In humans, adiaspiromycosis occurs after inhalation of dust-borne asexual conidia of the saprophytic mould. Adiaspiromycosis is a unique mycosis because the inhaled conidia enlarge, but do not germinate or reproduce in the host tissues. The conidia form adiaspores, also known as adiaconidia, which resemble spherules in tissue. Adiaspiromycosis is diagnosed by the characteristic finding of adiaspores, ranging in size from 50 to 500 μm, surrounded by granulomatous inflammation in tissue (Fig. 3). Recently, a case of disseminated adiaspiromycosis was diagnosed by polymerase chain reaction (PCR) and sequencing, in addition to histopathology [45].

The first human case of adiaspiromycosis, in which an adiaspore was found incidentally in a lung nodule from a patient with aspergillosis, was described in France [46]. Since the initial description, more than 40 human cases have been reported worldwide [43]. Pulmonary disease is most common, although adiaspiromycosis involving other organs, including peritoneum, skin, bone, and eyes has been described [47–51].

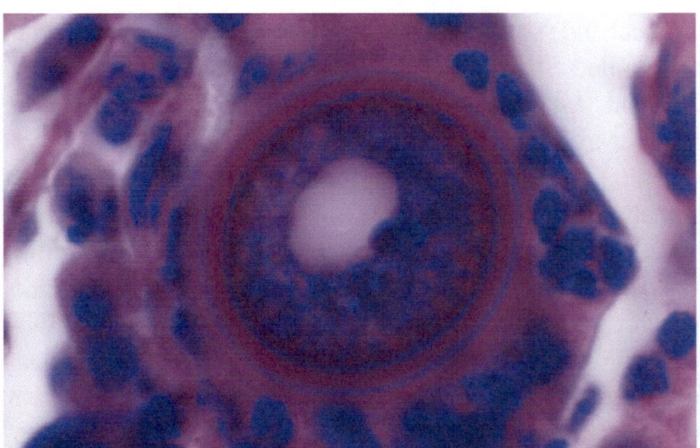

Fig. 3 A section of lung tissue showing an adiaspore of *Emmonsia crescens* (Courtesy of David W. Warnock)

A recent review describes the common features of infection in 11 cases of pulmonary adiaspiromycosis [43]. Lung infection can be localized (few adiaspores limited to a segment or lobe of lung) or disseminated (bilateral disease with multiple adiaspores). Because the inhaled conidia do not multiply, but only enlarge in tissues, severity of disease and extent of infection may be related to the initial inoculum of inhaled conidia [43, 52].

In patients with localized lung disease, adiaspiromycosis is often an incidental finding and patients are asymptomatic. In patients with disseminated lung disease, cough, dyspnea, asthenia, and fever are frequently seen, and respiratory failure can occur [43, 53]. Physical examination is often normal, but may reveal basilar crackles on auscultation. In patients with disseminated disease, radiographic studies may reveal a reticulonodular pattern similar to that seen with miliary tuberculosis [43].

Diagnosis of adiaspiromycosis is based on histopathologic examination of lung tissue. Culture of the organism is difficult, and sputum or bronchoalveolar lavage specimens are rarely culture positive in patients with disease [49, 53]. On gross examination of lung tissue, nodules, usually white to various shades of gray, can be seen. On microscopic exam, adiaspores are found within the nodules (Fig. 3). In some instances the adiaspores may be confused with parasites, such as *Dirofilaria* or *Strongyloides*, but can be easily distinguished from the characteristic spherules of *Coccidioides* species, which contain numerous endospores, and *Rhinosporidium seeberi* [43, 44].

Adiaspiromycosis often regresses, and patients improve without any therapy. In contrast, some patients have progressive disease that may contribute to a fatal outcome [43, 52]. Given the few reported cases of adiaspiromycosis, the utility of antifungal treatment in altering the disease course is unknown. However, patients have improved when treated with various antimicrobial agents, including amphotericin B plus flucytosine, itraconazole, ketoconazole, and thiabendazole [45, 47, 49, 53, 54]. In the rare cases of clinical progression, persistence of disease, or involvement of organs other than lung, surgical intervention may be required for cure [43, 51].

Other Organisms Resembling Fungi

Rhinosporidiosis

Rhinosporidiosis is a chronic granulomatous infection of the mucous membranes characterized by the formation of friable, polypoid masses that most often involve the nose, nasopharynx, or conjunctiva. The etiologic agent, *R. seeberi*, has traditionally been regarded as a fungus on the basis of morphologic and histochemical characteristics. However, it is now most appropriately classified as an aquatic protistan parasite, a Mesomycetozoa [55, 56]. Animal infections have occurred, as evidenced by recent descriptions of rhinosporidiosis in a domestic cat and dog [57, 58]. Rhinosporidiosis has a worldwide distribution, but most of the reported cases have occurred in India or Sri Lanka [59–61]. Other geographic regions with a significant number of reported cases include areas of South America, Europe, and Africa [62–64].

The first description of rhinosporidiosis was by Malbran in 1892, after examination of a nasal polyp revealed the presence of an organism. In 1900, Guillermo Seeber, for whom the organism is named, described the causative organism in a nasal polyp [65]. Since the initial description, approximately 2,000 cases of rhinosporidiosis have been reported worldwide. Disease favors a male predominance (4:1), and usually affects those between the ages of 15 and 40. Nasal infection is twice as common as ocular infection. The precise mode of transmission and extent of habitat of rhinosporidiosis is unknown, but trauma of the mucous membranes is probably necessary for most infections to occur. Water is most likely involved in the transmission of the organism [44, 66].

Rhinosporidiosis typically involves the mucous membranes, with formation of red or purple pedunculated, polypoid masses. Lesions may range in size from small, discrete nodules to extensive, lobulated masses. Lesions are friable, irregular, and frequently bleed. White dots are found on the outside of the lesions, which may give a strawberry-like appearance. The nasal mucosa is most frequently affected, but infection may also involve the ocular mucosa, nasopharynx, genital tract, and skin [64, 67, 68]. Disseminated disease is rare [67, 69, 70]. Patients with nasal mucosal involvement typically present with nasal obstruction or epistaxis. These symptoms may be accompanied by nasal drainage and pruritus, but seldom is there nasal pain. Ocular infection usually presents with tearing, bleeding, or foreign-body sensation [71]. The palpebral conjunctiva is most commonly affected, followed by the bulbar conjunctiva, corneal limbus, and lacrimal sac.

R. seeberi has not been cultured in the laboratory, so the diagnosis of rhinosporidiosis is based on typical clinical features and histologic examination with special stains. Diagnosis of rhinosporidiosis can be made on histopathologic analysis of the excised lesion, but it can also be made after microscopic analysis of nasal drainage [72]. Examination of tissue reveals a variety of inflammatory cells, including neutrophils, multinucleated giant cells, plasma cells, and lymphocytes. Vascularity of the tissue is prominent. On the epithelial surface of the lesion and in the submucosa, numerous sporangia are seen, ranging up to 300 μm in diameter (Fig. 4). Fungal stains, such as Gomori-methenamine silver, and periodic acid–Schiff, are useful to highlight the walls of the sporangia and the spores.

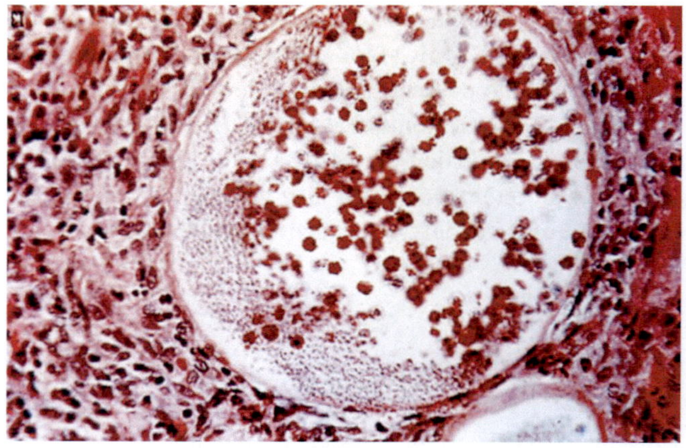

Fig. 4 Nasal tissue demonstrating a sporangium of *Rhinosporidium seeberi*. The sporangium contains numerous spores (Courtesy of David W. Warnock)

The most effective therapy for rhinosporidiosis is surgical excision of the lesions. Electrosurgery has been successful in many cases; however, recurrence of the lesions is common [73]. Response to medications such as dapsone, amphotericin B, and griseofulvin is reported, although the effectiveness of medical therapy is unknown [74–76].

Pythiosis

Pythiosis is a life-threatening pseudofungal infection of humans and animals caused by *Pythium insidiosum*. The organism was originally thought to be a fungus, but it is now known that it is an aquatic oomycete, belonging to the Kingdom Stramenopila, phylum Oomycota, class Oomycetes [44]. The oomycetes differ from fungi in several ways: They do not have chitin in their cell walls, several metabolic pathways differ, and part of their life cycle involves production of motile flagellated zoospores. *P. insidiosum* is found in tropical aquatic climates, and the disease occurs primarily in tropical and subtropical areas. Pythiosis has been reported in the United States, Thailand, Australia, India, Brazil, New Zealand, Malaysia, and Haiti, and was first described in humans by De Cock in 1987 [77–81].

Human pythiosis is characterized by several clinical presentations: subcutaneous or cutaneous lesions, ocular disease, vascular disease, and disseminated disease [44, 81]. Lesions, typically painful pustules, nodules, ulcers, or cellulitis, develop on the limbs, face, or periorbital area. Keratitis with corneal ulceration can also occur. Vascular pythiosis is characterized by an arterial insufficiency syndrome of the lower extremities [81]. Clinical findings may include claudication, fever, leg or groin swelling, painful masses, or ulcers. Vascular disease develops more often in patients with thalassemia [81]. Disseminated disease has been reported rarely and occurs typically in patients with underlying comorbidities, such as malignancy or thalassemia [81].

P. insidiosum is acquired through traumatic implantation. Zoospores, the infectious stage of the organism's life cycle, have a tropism for damaged skin, hair, and plant tissues, and are able to encyst and form germ tubes that produce hyphae in the tissues [44]. Invasive disease can result from local, lymphatic, or vascular spread.

The organism can be isolated from clinical material plated onto mycologic media. *P. insidiosum* grows in culture as white colonies, and hyaline hyphae that have sparse septae can be demonstrated on histopathology. The hyphae resemble those of the agents of zygomycosis, but in contrast, the hyphae of *P. insidiosum* stain weakly with Gomori-methenamine silver or other fungal stains [44]. Immunofluorescence or molecular assays have been useful to diagnose pythiosis in the absence of cultures [82, 83].

Treatment of pythiosis usually requires surgical debridement and systemic antifungal agents. For ocular disease, topical miconazole, amphotericin B, natamycin, and ketoconazole, in addition to systemic antifungals, have been used with success [78]. For cutaneous or subcutaneous disease, itraconazole, amphotericin B, supersaturated solution of potassium iodide, and terbinafine may be effective [77, 78, 81]. Because of the morbidity associated with arterial disease, prompt recognition, early surgical intervention, and systemic antifungals are necessary. However, only marginal success has been achieved with amphotericin B, terbinafine, or itraconazole [81, 84].

References

1. Taborda PR, Taborda VA, McGinnis MR. *Lacazia loboi* gen. nov., comb. nov., the etiologic agent of lobomycosis. J Clin Microbiol. 1999;37:2031–3.
2. Rotstein DS, Burdett LG, McLellan W, et al. Lobomycosis in offshore bottlenose dolphins (*Tursiops truncatus*), North Carolina. Emerg Infect Dis. 2009;15:588–90.
3. Cowan DF. Lobo's disease in a bottlenose dolphin (*Tursiops truncatus*) from Matagorda Bay, Texas. J Wildlife Dis. 1993;29:488–9.
4. Migaki G, Valerio MG, Irvine B, Garner FM. Lobo's disease in an Atlantic bottle-nosed dolphin. J Am Vet Med Assoc. 1971; 159:578–82.
5. Paniz-Mondolfi AE, Sander-Hoffmann L. Lobomycosis in inshore and estuarine dolphins. Emerg Infect Dis. 2009;15:672–3.
6. Murdoch ME, Reif JS, Mazzoil M, McCulloch SD, Fair PA, Bossart GD. Lobomycosis in bottlenose dolphins (*Tursiops truncatus*) from the Indian River Lagoon, Florida: estimation of prevalence, temporal trends, and spatial distribution. EcoHealth. 2008;5:289–97.
7. Rodriguez-Toro G. Lobomycosis. Int J Dermatol. 1993;32:324–32.
8. Paniz-Mondolfi AE, Reyes Jaimes O, Davila Jones L. Lobomycosis in Venezuela. Int J Dermatol. 2007;46:180–5.
9. Burns RA, Roy JS, Woods C, Padhye AA, Warnock DW. Report of the first human case of lobomycosis in the United States. J Clin Microbiol. 2000;38:1283–5.
10. Elsayed S, Kuhn SM, Barber D, Church DL, Adams S, Kasper R. Human case of lobomycosis. Emerg Infect Dis. 2004;10:715–8.
11. Herr RA, Tarcha EJ, Taborda PR, Taylor JW, Ajello L, Mendoza L. Phylogenetic analysis of *Lacazia loboi* places this previously uncharacterized pathogen within the dimorphic Onygenales. J Clin Microbiol. 2001;39:309–14.
12. Lobo J. Um caso de lastomycose produzido por uma especie nova encontrado em Recife. Rev Med (Pernambuco). 1931;1:763–5.
13. Fuchs J, Milbradt R, Pecher SA. Lobomycosis (keloidal blastomycosis): case reports and overview. Cutis. 1990;46:227–34.
14. Montero-Gei. Blastomicosis queloidiana. In: Memorias VII Congreso Iberolatinoamericano de Dermatologia. Caracas: Sintesis Dosmil; 1971. p. 165.
15. Al-Daraji WI. Cutaneous lobomycosis: a delayed diagnosis. Am J Dermatopathol. 2008;30:575–7.
16. Kwon-Chung KJ, Bennett JE. Medical mycology. Philadelphia: Lea & Febiger; 1992.
17. Lawrence DN, Ajello L. Lobomycosis in western Brazil: report of a clinical trial with ketoconazole. Am J Trop Med Hyg. 1986;35:162–6.
18. Carneiro FP, Maia LB, Moraes MA, et al. Lobomycosis: diagnosis and management of relapsed and multifocal lesions. Diagn Microbiol Infect Dis. 2009;65:62–4.
19. Cuce LC, Wroclawski EL, Sampaio SA. Treatment of paracoccidioidomycosis, candidiasis, chromomycosis, lobomycosis, and mycetoma with ketoconazole. Int J Dermatol. 1980;19:405–8.
20. Fischer M, Chrusciak Talhari A, Reinel D, Talhari S. [Sucessful treatment with clofazimine and itraconazole in a 46 year old patient after 32 years duration of disease]. Der Hautarzt; Zeitschrift fur Dermatologie, Venerologie, und verwandte Gebiete 2002;53:677–81.
21. Baruzzi RG, Rodrigues DA, Michalany NS, Salomao R. Squamous-cell carcinoma and lobomycosis (Jorge Lobo's disease). Int J Dermatol. 1989;28:183–5.
22. Hawksworth DL, Sutton BC, Ainsworth GC. Ainsworth & Bisby's dictionary of fungi. 7th ed. Kew: Commonwealth Mycological Institute; 1983.
23. Greer DL. Basidiomycetes as agents of human infections: a review. Mycopathologia. 1978;65:133–9.
24. Rihs JD, Padhye AA, Good CB. Brain abscess caused by *Schizophyllum commune*: an emerging basidiomycete pathogen. J Clin Microbiol. 1996;34:1628–32.
25. Restrepo A, Greer DL, Robledo M, Osorio O, Mondragon H. Ulceration of the palate caused by a basidiomycete *Schizophyllum commune*. Sabouraudia. 1973;11:201–4.
26. Catalano P, Lawson W, Bottone E, Lebenger J. Basidiomycetous (mushroom) infection of the maxillary sinus. Otolaryngol Head Neck Surg. 1990;102:183–5.
27. Clark S, Campbell CK, Sandison A, Choa DI. *Schizophyllum commune*: an unusual isolate from a patient with allergic fungal sinusitis. J Infect. 1996;32:147–50.
28. Kern ME, Uecker FA. Maxillary sinus infection caused by the homobasidio-mycetous fungus *Schizophyllum commune*. J Clin Microbiol. 1986;23:1001–5.
29. Rosenthal J, Katz R, DuBois DB, Morrissey A, Machicao A. Chronic maxillary sinusitis associated with the mushroom *Schizophyllum commune* in a patient with AIDS. Clin Infect Dis. 1992;14:46–8.
30. Sigler L, Estrada S, Montealegre NA, et al. Maxillary sinusitis caused by *Schizophyllum commune* and experience with treatment. J Med Vet Mycol. 1997;35:365–70.
31. Sigler L, Bartley JR, Parr DH, Morris AJ. Maxillary sinusitis caused by medusoid form of *Schizophyllum commune*. J Clin Microbiol. 1999;37:3395–8.
32. Roan JN, Hsieh HY, Tsai HW, et al. Pulmonary nodules caused by *Schizophyllum commune* after cardiac transplantation. J Infect. 2009;58:164–7.
33. Tullio V, Mandras N, Banche G, et al. *Schizophyllum commune*: an unusual of agent bronchopneumonia in an immunocompromised patient. Med Mycol. 2008;46:735–8.

34. Kamei K, Unno H, Nagao K, Kuriyama T, Nishimura K, Miyaji M. Allergic bronchopulmonary mycosis caused by the basidiomycetous fungus *Schizophyllum commune*. Clin Infect Dis. 1994;18:305–9.
35. Bulajic N, Cvijanovic V, Vukojevic J, Tomic D, Johnson E. *Schizophyllum commune* associated with bronchogenous cyst. Mycoses. 2006;49:343–5.
36. Speller DE, MacIver AG. Endocarditis caused by a *Coprinus* species: a fungus of the toadstool group. J Med Microbiol. 1971;4:370–4.
37. Surmont I, Van Aelst F, Verbanck J, De Hoog GS. A pulmonary infection caused by *Coprinus cinereus* (*Hormographiella aspergillata*) diagnosed after a neutropenic episode. Med Mycol. 2002;40:217–9.
38. Verweij PE, van Kasteren M, van de Nes J, de Hoog GS, de Pauw BE, Meis JF. Fatal pulmonary infection caused by the basidiomycete *Hormographiella aspergillata*. J Clin Microbiol. 1997;35:2675–8.
39. Lagrou K, Massonet C, Theunissen K, et al. Fatal pulmonary infection in a leukaemic patient caused by *Hormographiella aspergillata*. J Med Microbiol. 2005;54:685–8.
40. Teo LH, Tay YK. *Ustilago* species infection in humans. Br J Dermatol. 2006;155:1096–7.
41. Marlier S, De Jaureguiberry JP, Aguilon P, Carloz E, Duval JL, Jaubert D. Chronic sinusitis caused by *Schizophyllum commune* in AIDS. Presse Méd. 1993;22:1107.
42. Gonzalez GM, Sutton DA, Thompson E, Tijerina R, Rinaldi MG. In vitro activities of approved and investigational antifungal agents against 44 clinical isolates of basidiomycetous fungi. Antimicrob Agents Chemother. 2001;45:633–5.
43. England DM, Hochholzer L. Adiaspiromycosis: an unusual fungal infection of the lung. Report of 11 cases. Am J Surg Pathol. 1993;17:876–86.
44. Pfaller MA, Diekema DJ. Unusual fungal and pseudofungal infections of humans. J Clin Microbiol. 2005;43:1495–504.
45. Dot JM, Debourgogne A, Champigneulle J, et al. Molecular diagnosis of disseminated adiaspiromycosis due to *Emmonsia crescens*. J Clin Microbiol. 2009;47:1269–73.
46. Doby-Dubois M, Chevrel ML, Doby JM, Louvet M. 1st human case of adiaspiromycosis, caused by *Emmonsia crescens*, Emmons and Jellison, 1960. Bull Soc Pathol Exot Fil. 1964;57:240–4.
47. Echavarria E, Cano EL, Restrepo A. Disseminated adiaspiromycosis in a patient with AIDS. J Med Vet Mycol. 1993;31:91–7.
48. Kamalam A, Thambiah AS. Adiaspiromycosis of human skin caused by *Emmonsia crescens*. Sabouraudia. 1979;17:377–81.
49. Turner D, Burke M, Bashe E, Blinder S, Yust I. Pulmonary adiaspiromycosis in a patient with acquired immunodeficiency syndrome. Eur J Clin Microbiol. 1999;18:893–5.
50. Mendes MO, Moraes MA, Renoiner EI, et al. Acute conjunctivitis with episcleritis and anterior uveitis linked to adiaspiromycosis and freshwater sponges, Amazon region, Brazil, 2005. Emerg Infect Dis. 2009;15:633–9.
51. Stebbins WG, Krishtul A, Bottone EJ, Phelps R, Cohen S. Cutaneous adiaspiromycosis: a distinct dermatologic entity associated with *Chrysosporium* species. J Am Acad Dermatol. 2004;51:S185–9.
52. Peres LC, Figueiredo F, Peinado M, Soares FA. Fulminant disseminated pulmonary adiaspiromycosis in humans. Am J Trop Med Hyg. 1992;46:146–50.
53. Barbas Filho JV, Amato MB, Deheinzelin D, Saldiva PH, de Carvalho CR. Respiratory failure caused by adiaspiromycosis. Chest. 1990;97:1171–5.
54. Severo LC, Geyer GR, Camargo JJ, Porto NS. Adiaspiromycosis treated successfully with ketoconazole. J Med Vet Mycol. 1989;27:265–8.
55. Herr RA, Ajello L, Taylor JW, Arseculeratne SN, Mendoza L. Phylogenetic analysis of *Rhinosporidium seeberi's* 18 S small-subunit ribosomal DNA groups this pathogen among members of the protoctistan Mesomycetozoa clade. J Clin Microbiol. 1999;37:2750–4.
56. Fredricks DN, Jolley JA, Lepp PW, Kosek JC, Relman DA. *Rhinosporidium seeberi*: a human pathogen from a novel group of aquatic protistan parasites. Emerg Infect Dis. 2000;6:273–82.
57. Wallin LL, Coleman GD, Froeling J, Parker GA. Rhinosporidiosis in a domestic cat. Med Mycol. 2001;39:139–41.
58. Miller RI, Baylis R. Rhinosporidiosis in a dog native to the UK. Vet Rec. 2009;164:210.
59. Mohan H, Chander J, Dhir R, Singhal U. Rhinosporidiosis in India: a case report and review of literature. Mycoses. 1995;38:223–5.
60. Moses JD, Shanmugham A. Epidemiological survey of rhinosporidiosis in man – a sample survey in a high school located in a hyperendemic area. Indian Vet J. 1987;64:34–8.
61. Capoor MR, Khanna G, Rajni, et al. Rhinosporidiosis in Delhi, north India: case series from a non-endemic area and mini-review. Mycopathologia. 2009;168:89–94.
62. Owor R, Wamukota WM. Rhinosporidiosis in Uganda: a review of 51 cases. E Afr Med J. 1978;55:582–6.
63. Londero AT, Santos MN, Freitas CJ. Animal rhinosporidiosis in Brazil. Report of three additional cases. Mycopathologia. 1977;60:171–3.
64. van der Coer JM, Marres HA, Wielinga EW, Wong-Alcala LS. Rhinosporidiosis in Europe. J Laryngol Otol. 1992;106:440–3.
65. Seeber G. Un Nuevo esporozuario parasito del hombre: dos casos encontrades en polipos nasals. Thesis, Universidad nacional de Buenos Aires 1900.
66. Kennedy FA, Buggage RR, Ajello L. Rhinosporidiosis: a description of an unprecedented outbreak in captive swans (*Cygnus* spp.) and a proposal for revision of the ontogenic nomenclature of *Rhinosporidium seeberi*. J Med Vet Mycol. 1995;33:157–65.
67. Mahakrisnan A, Rajasekaram V, Pandian PJ. Disseminated cutaneous rhinosporidiosis treated with dapsone. Trop Geogr Med. 1981;33:189–92.
68. Qureshi F, Abdulmannan MS, Eltayeb AA, Qadri S, Al-Qahtani H, Gabr A. Rhinosporidiosis of the male urethra. Ann Saudi Med. 2004;24:299–300.
69. Amritanand R, Nithyananth M, Cherian VM, Venkatesh K, Shah A. Disseminated rhinosporidiosis destroying the talus: a case report. J Orthop Surg (Hong Kong). 2008;16:99–101.
70. Rajakannu M, Sri Vengadesh G, Pai D, Jagdish S. Disseminated rhinosporidiosis – an unusual presentation with pulmonary involvement. Int J Dermatol. 2006;45:297–8.
71. Roberson MC. Conjunctival rhinosporidiosis. Ann Ophthalmol. 1985;17:262–3.
72. Chaudhary SK, Joshi KR. Diagnosis of rhinosporidiosis by nasal smear examination. J Indian Med Assoc. 1986;84:274–6.
73. Firouz-Abadi A, Moghimi M, Azad Y. Rhinosporidiosis in Iran (Persia) – a study of seventy-four cases. Mycopathol Mycol Appl. 1971;44:249–60.
74. Job A, Venkateswaran S, Mathan M, Krishnaswami H, Raman R. Medical therapy of rhinosporidiosis with dapsone. J Laryngol Otol. 1993;107:809–12.
75. Ho MS, Tay BK. Disseminated rhinosporidiosis. Ann Acad Med Singapore. 1986;15:80–3.
76. Nair KK. Clinical trial of diaminodiphenylsulfone (DDS) in nasal and nasopharyngeal rhinosporidiosis. Laryngoscope. 1979;89:291–5.
77. Bosco S, Bagagili E, Araujo Jr JP, Candeias JM, et al. Human pythiosis, Brazil. Emerg Infect Dis. 2005;11:715–7.
78. Prasertwitayakij N, Louthrenoo W, Kasitanon N, Thamprasert K, Vanittanakon N. Human pythiosis, a rare cause of arteritis: case report and review of the literature. Semin Arthritis Rheum. 2003;33:204–14.
79. Rivierre C, Laprie C, Guiard-Marigny O, Bergeaud P, Berthelemy M, Guillot J. Pythiosis in Africa. Emerg Infect Dis. 2005;11:479–81.
80. de Cock AW, Mendoza L, Padhye AA, Ajello L, Kaufman L. *Pythium insidiosum* sp. nov., the etiologic agent of pythiosis. J Clin Microbiol. 1987;25:344–9.

81. Krajaejun T, Sathapatayavongs B, Pracharktam R, et al. Clinical and epidemiologic analyses of human pythiosis in Thailand. Clin Infect Dis. 2006;43:567–75.
82. Schurko AM, Mendoza L, de Cock AW, Bedard JE, Klassen GR. Development of a species-specific probe for *Pythium insidiosum* and the diagnosis of pythiosis. J Clin Microbiol. 2004;42:2411–8.
83. Mendoza L, Kaufman L, Standard PG. Immunodiffusion test for diagnosing and monitoring pythiosis in horses. J Clin Microbiol. 1986;23:813–6.
84. Schenep JL, Englis BK, Kaufman L, et al. Successful medical therapy for deeply invasive facial infection due to *Pythium insidiosum* in a child. Clin Infect Dis. 1998;27:1388–93.

Part VIII
Special Patient Populations

Fungal Infections in Neutropenic Patients

Juan C. Gea-Banacloche, Andreas H. Groll, and Thomas J. Walsh

Magnitude and Scope of the Problem

Invasive fungal infections (IFIs) continue to be a significant problem in neutropenic patients. They are common, difficult to diagnose, and associated with high mortality rates. Their frequency may be estimated by two types of studies: autopsy surveys and controlled trials of antifungal agents for empirical treatment of prolonged fever during neutropenia. Autopsy studies are surprisingly consistent over the years, and some of them are summarized in Table 1.

Bodey reviewed the records of all 454 patients with acute leukemia who died at the National Institutes of Health between 1954 and 1964 and found that 107 patients (24%) had a "major" fungal infection (excluding focal candidiasis) [1]. In a similar single-center review of 1,017 autopsies during a 15-year period (1989–2003) published 40 years later, investigators at the MD Anderson Cancer Center identified IFIs in 31% [3]. Other autopsy studies are consistent with this high frequency in leukemia [2, 6]. The proportions are much lower for patients with solid tumors (1–8%). The autopsy studies are also consistent on the fact that a large percentage (frequently the majority) of fungal infections went undiagnosed during life. The most important change over the years is that filamentous fungi (moulds), mainly invasive aspergillosis (IA), have become the most commonly identified IFI, replacing invasive candidiasis [3, 5, 7]. A report from Germany suggests other trends, including a possible decrease in undiagnosed infections in the most recent period analyzed, 2001–2005 (from 70% to 58%) [5].

These numbers must be interpreted with caution and should be considered the highest end of the estimate because of the selection bias inherent in autopsy studies and the various definitions used in the different series [8, 9]. A different estimate comes from the large trials of empirical antifungal therapy in neutropenic fever, which have documented relatively low frequencies of IFI either at the initiation of the antifungal agent (between 1.5% and 5.9%) [10, 11] or as breakthrough infections during treatment (between 2.6% and 5.5%) [10, 12, 13]. Given the limitations of diagnostic tools for the detection of IFIs, these studies may underestimate the true frequency of mycoses in neutropenic hosts.

This broad range of estimates reflects in part methodologic and definition issues [14, 15], but it also underscores the fact that not all neutropenic patients are at the same risk [16, 17]. The essential concepts are that IFIs are common and difficult to diagnose and that most of them are caused by *Aspergillus* and *Candida* species.

The relative proportions of pathogens have changed over the years. Recent autopsy studies show a preponderance of moulds over yeasts [3, 5, 7]. In the period 2001–2005 Donhuijsen et al. documented 17 cases of aspergillosis and 2 of candidiasis in 67 autopsies, in contrast with the period 1976–1980, when 10 cases of aspergillosis and 26 of candidiasis were noted in 335 autopsies [5]. Similarly, investigators at the MD Anderson Cancer Center documented 68 mould infections and 23 *Candida* infections in 268 autopsies in the period 1998–2003, compared with 89 and 62, respectively, in 466 autopsies performed between 1989 and 1993 [3]. The randomized controlled trials of empirical therapy show candidiasis as the most common baseline infection, and *Aspergillus* and *Candida* are the most common breakthrough fungal pathogens (Table 2) [12, 13, 18]; this has been confirmed also in case series from several institutions [19].

Studies of systemic prophylaxis (Table 3) show that *Candida albicans* has been almost completely eliminated and that aspergillosis is a more common breakthrough infection than non-*albicans Candida* species [20–23]. A few cases of IFI are caused by *Fusarium*, Zygomycetes, *Trichosporon,* and other fungi.

Most cases of candidiasis in neutropenic patients receiving fluconazole prophylaxis are now caused by non-*albicans Candida* species [24–26], particularly *C. glabrata* and *C. krusei* [27, 28]. These species are often more resistant and

J.C. Gea-Banacloche (✉)
Infectious Diseases Section, Experimental Transplantation and Immunology Branch, National Cancer Institute, National Institutes of Health, Bethesda, MD, USA
e-mail: banacloj@mail.nih.gov

C.A. Kauffman et al. (eds.), *Essentials of Clinical Mycology*,
DOI 10.1007/978-1-4419-6640-7_28, © Springer Science+Business Media, LLC 2011

Table 1 Selected autopsy studies of patients with hematological malignancies

	Bodey [1]	Bodey et al. [2]	Chamilos et al. [3]	Larbcharoensub et al. [4]	Donhuijsen et al. [5]
Setting	Single Research Center	12 Hospitals Canada, Japan and Europe	Single Cancer Center, US	Single Center Thailand	Single Center Germany
Years surveyed	1954–64	1980–1988	1989–2003	1997–2006	1976–2005
Patients	Acute leukemia	All malignancies	Hematologic malignancies	All autopsies	Hematologic malignancies
Number	454	4,096	1,017	1,652	1,591
Patients with IFI (%)	107 (24%)	455 (11.1%)	314 (31%)	155 (9.4%)	340 (21.4%)
Candida	71	265	113	50	122
Aspergillus	38	137	178	62	188
Other molds	6	52	36	5	
Mixed/other	40	24	63	38	
Leukemic patients with IFI	107/454 (24%)	157/633 (25%)	NA	NA	167/565 (29.6%)
Proportion of IFIs undiagnosed during life	75%	> 80%	75% (as proven or probable by EORTC-MSG[a])	36%	70% (1976–83) to 58% (1998–2005)

IFI invasive fungal infection, *NA* not available, *EORTC/MSG* European Organization for Research and Treatment of Cancer/Mycoses Study Group

[a]This 75% does not mean the fungal infections were not unsuspected; it just means that they did not meet EORTC/MSG criteria for probable or proven IFIs. This statistic may be more an illustration of the limitations of the criteria than of the current tendency to consider IFIs in neutropenic patients

Table 2 Baseline and breakthrough fungal infections documented in selected studies of empirical antifungal treatment for persistent fever during neutropenia

	Walsh et al. [18]		Walsh et al. [12]		Walsh et al. [13]		
	AmB-d	L-AmB	Vori	L-AmB	Caspo	L-AmB	Total
Number	344	343	415	422	556	539	2,619
Antifungal prophylaxis	ND	ND	222	250	313	304	
Total IFIs at baseline[a] (%)	11 (3%)	11 (3%)	13 (3.1%)	6 (1.4%)	27 (4.9%)	27 (5%)	95
Aspergillus			2	2	12	12	28
Candida	11	11	10	3	12	12	59
Zygomycetes			1		1	0	2
Other				1	2	3	6
Total breakthrough IFI (%)[b]	27 (7.8%)	11 (3.2%)	8 (1.6%)	21 (5%)	29 (5.2%)	24 (4.5%)	120 (4.6%)
Aspergillus	12	6	4	13	10	9	54
Candida	12	3	2	6	16	15	54
Zygomycetes	0	1	2	0	2	0	5
Other	3	1	0	2	2	1	9

AmB-d Amphotericin B deoxycholate, *L-AmB* liposomal amphotericin B, *Vori* voriconazole, *Caspo* caspofungin, *IFIs* invasive fungal infections

[a]Baseline infections were those present on or before day 1–2 of the study

[b]Breakthrough infections those identified on day 2–3 or later

Table 3 Breakthrough fungal infections documented in selected studies of systemic antifungal prophylaxis during neutropenia

	Winston et al. [20]		Van Burik et al. [21]		Marr et al. [22]		Cornely et al. [23]		
	Flu	Itra	Flu	Mica	Flu	Itra	Flu/Itra	Posa	Total
	67	71	457	425	148	151	298	304	1,921
Candida albicans	0	0	0	1	0	0	0	0	1
Non-albicans Candida	8	2	2	3	4	3	2	3	27
Aspergillus	8	3	7	1	17	8	20	2	66
Zygomycetes	0	1	0	1	1	0	2	0	5
Fusarium	1	0	2	1	1	0	0	0	5
Other	0	0	0	0	0	0	0	1	1
"Rescue" antifungal for suspected IFI	ND	ND	94	68	25	19	101	68	
Total IFI probable/proven	17	6	11	7	22	11	25	7	106

Flu = fluconazole, Itra = itraconazole, Mica = micafungin, Posa = posaconazole cause higher attributable mortality rates than *C. albicans* or *C. parapsilosis* [29].

Fungal infections are associated with a high mortality rate in neutropenic patients. Neutropenia as a risk factor for mortality in IFIs has been documented by retrospective series [30–33] and controlled trials [34]. In the case of candidiasis, the overall response rate decreases from 70% to approximately 50% in neutropenic patients in most randomized controlled trials [35, 36]. The therapeutic options for candidiasis and aspergillosis may result in successful outcomes, even in cases of prolonged neutropenia, but some infections, such as fusariosis and scedosporiosis, still have a very poor prognosis unless neutrophil recovery ensues [33, 37].

Deficits in Host Defenses Predisposing Neutropenic Patients to Invasive Fungal Infections

Protracted, profound myelosuppression has been recognized as the major risk factor for development of IFIs [38–41]. Other risk factors that should be considered [16] include the use of broad-spectrum antibacterial agents, corticosteroids, central venous catheters, the status of the patient's underlying disease, and the type of cytotoxic chemotherapy, especially agents which disrupt mucosal integrity [42] (Table 4).

Table 4

Host factors associated with increased development of invasive fungal infections in granulocytopenic patients
Protracted granulocytopenia
Corticosteroid therapy
Broad spectrum antibiotics
Relapsed neoplastic disease
Hematological neoplasias
Previous invasive pulmonary aspergillosis
Central venous catheters
Total body irradiation
Allogeneic bone marrow transplantation
T-cell depletion[a]
Graft versus host disease[a]
Host factors associated with possibly reduced development of invasive fungal infections in granulocytopenic patients
Solid tumors
Remission of neoplastic disease
Recovery from granulocytopenia related to
Spontaneous recovery
Recombinant hematopoietic cytokines[b]
Stem cell reconstitution[b]
Granulocyte transfusions[b]

[a]Additional host factors further compromising the allogeneic bone marrow transplant recipient

[b]Investigational for reducing development of invasive fungal infections

Candida colonization has been shown to be an important risk factor for the development of superficial candidiasis and subsequent invasive infection [43, 44], and broad-spectrum antibiotics increase the risk of fungal colonization [45]. Patients with hematologic malignancies, particularly acute myelogenous leukemia (AML), have a much higher frequency of opportunistic mycoses than do patients with solid tumors [46]. Patients with relapsed versus newly diagnosed neoplastic disease have an increased risk for infectious complications for several reasons, including diminished bone marrow reserve and need for more intensive chemotherapy, with subsequent increased mucosal disruption and opportunities for fungal colonization. The disruption of the mucosal barriers is an important factor in establishing disseminated candidiasis in animal models of granulocytopenia [47]. Similar findings have been observed in patients receiving cytarabine for acute leukemia [42]. Venous catheters represent another portal of entry into the bloodstream for yeast-like fungi.

Corticosteroid use increases the risk of invasive aspergillosis (IA), mainly through an inhibitory effect on phagocytosis [48]. The duration and dosage of glucocorticoids correlate strongly with the development of aspergillosis following allogeneic stem cell transplantation (HSCT) [49], Corticosteroids also result in defective cell-mediated immunity. Other agents that have immunosuppressive action have a less clear effect on fungal infections. As an example, fludarabine seems to be associated mainly with an increased incidence of cryptococcosis [50]. Radiation therapy also decreases cell-mediated immunity and contributes to the disruption of mucosal barriers.

Clinical Manifestations of Invasive Fungal Infections in the Neutropenic Host

The clinical manifestations of IFI in neutropenic patients are seldom specific, and early detection remains difficult. A Consensus Group of the European Organization for Research and Treatment of Cancer/Invasive Fungal Infections Cooperative Group and the National Institute of Allergy and Infectious Diseases Mycoses Study Group (EORTC/MSG) put forward [14] and revised [15] definitions of IFIs in patients with cancer and HSCT. IFIs are classified as proven, probable, and possible, based on a combination of host factors, clinical criteria (which include clinical manifestations and radiologic evidence), and mycologic criteria (which include direct microbiologic or pathologic evidence as well as indirect tests that detect fungal antigens or cell wall constituents). Even if these criteria are for clinical research and not to indicate treatment of individual patients, the concept is helpful and allows for a better understanding of the published evidence.

Invasive Candidiasis

Acute disseminated candidiasis is typically characterized by fever, with or without sepsis syndrome. The physical examination may reveal vitreal opacities related to *Candida* endophthalmitis, erythematous maculopapular cutaneous lesions, and myalgias [51] (Fig. 1). Chronic disseminated candidiasis (hepatosplenic candidiasis) characteristically presents as new fever after recovery from neutropenia, with alkaline phosphatase elevation and tenderness in the right or left upper quadrants [52]. Radiologic investigations are typically unrevealing in acute hematogenous candidiasis, but are frequently the key diagnostic test in chronic disseminated candidiasis, in which ultrasound, computed tomography (CT), and magnetic resonance imaging (MR) may reveal characteristic "target-like" lesions in liver, spleen, and kidneys [52–54] (Fig. 2).

Invasive Aspergillosis

The most common clinical presentation of IA in the neutropenic patient is persistent or recurrent fever [55, 56].

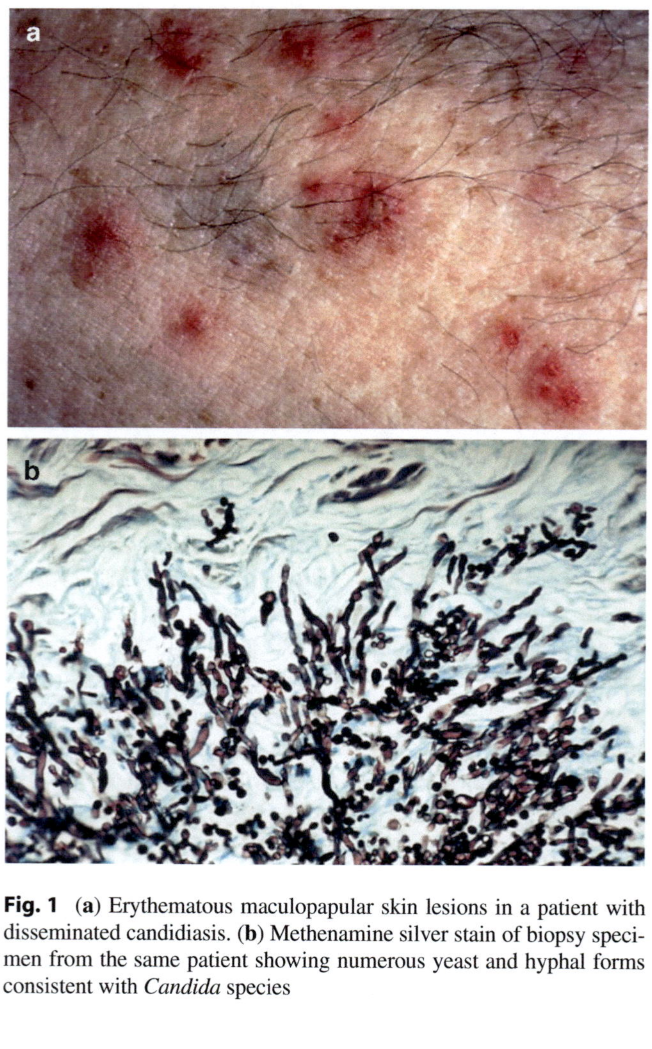

Fig. 1 (**a**) Erythematous maculopapular skin lesions in a patient with disseminated candidiasis. (**b**) Methenamine silver stain of biopsy specimen from the same patient showing numerous yeast and hyphal forms consistent with *Candida* species

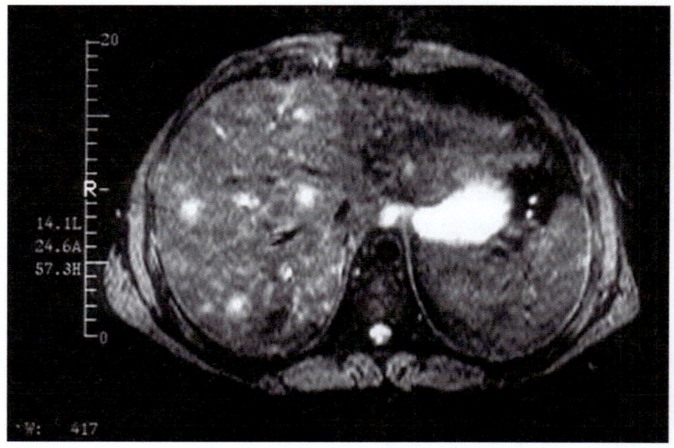

Fig. 2 Scan showing characteristic enhancing lesions in the liver and spleen in a patient with chronic disseminated candidiasis

The respiratory tract is the most common portal of entry and target of *Aspergillus* species. In neutropenic hosts, *Aspergillus* has a strong propensity for invasion of blood vessels resulting in vascular thrombosis, infarction, and tissue necrosis [57]. This process contributes to many of the clinical manifestations of pulmonary aspergillosis, including pleuritic pain, nonproductive cough, hemoptysis, pleural rub, and occasionally adventitious breath sounds [58, 59]. In the case of sinus involvement, signs and symptoms include fever, orbital swelling, facial pain, and nasal congestion [60]. Angioinvasion by the mould may cause cavernous sinus thrombosis. An ulcerated lesion on the hard palate or gingiva may be present [61].

Radiographic manifestations of invasive pulmonary aspergillosis include bronchopneumonia, lobar consolidation, segmental pneumonia, multiple nodular lesions resembling septic emboli, and cavitary lesions [62–66]. The chest radiograph may initially appear normal due to the poor inflammatory response. However, with early use of CT scanning it has been shown that the "halo sign" may be observed early in the majority of neutropenic patients with proven IA [63]. The halo sign consists of a delicate infiltrate at the edges of the denser consolidation and likely represents edema around the infarcted tissue [64, 65, 67, 68]. With initiation of antifungal therapy, this process may be stabilized or reversed [69]; after recovery from neutropenia, cavitation and appearance of a "crescent sign" may occur [63, 70, 71] (Fig. 3). Other early lesions visible on CT scan are peripheral or subpleural nodules contiguous with the pulmonary vascular tree. Early radiographic recognition of pulmonary lesions by CT contributes to more prompt initiation of appropriate antifungal therapy [65, 67, 72].

Dissemination involves characteristically the central nervous system (CNS) and the skin. CNS involvement may be clinically silent or present dramatically as an embolic stroke [73]. Imaging, preferably by MR scanning, is indicated when the diagnosis of aspergillosis is made, even in the absence of symptoms. The neuroradiologic findings are variable, as the

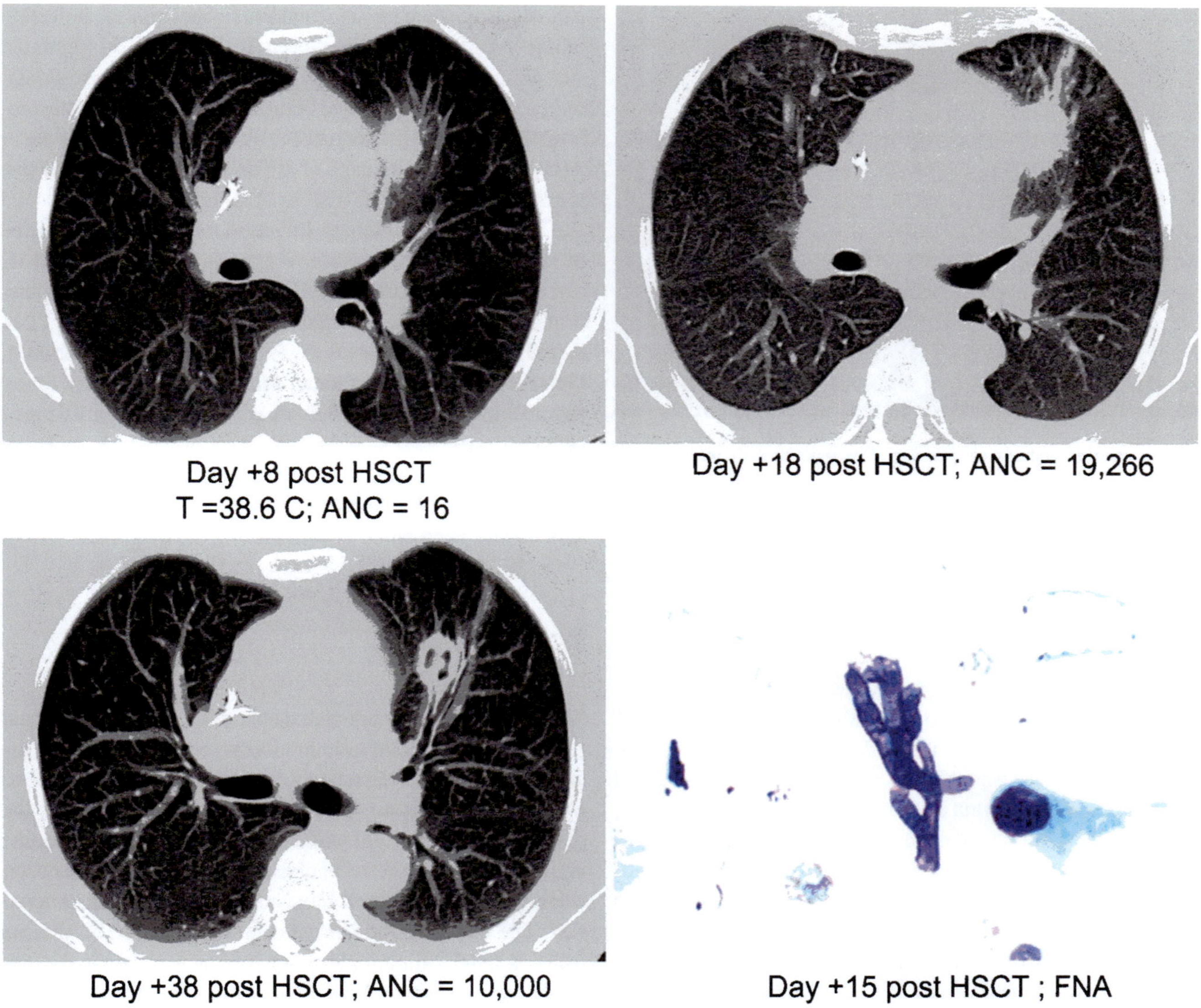

Fig. 3 Chest CT scan showing various manifestations of invasive aspergillosis in a patient who had received a hematopoietic stem cell transplant (*HSCT*) and was neutropenic. (**a**) Nodular mass with ground glass changes surrounding the nodule (halo sign) when the absolute neutrophil count (*ANC*) was extremely low; (**b**) enlarging mass as neutrophils recover; (**c**) cavitation as the immune response improves; (**d**) Smear of fine-needle aspirate obtained just before recovery of neutrophils showing septate hyphae with dichotomous branching consistent with *Aspergillus* species

pathologic lesions may be infarction, hemorrhage, or abscess [74–76]. The lesions may lack ring enhancement, particularly during neutropenia. Disseminated aspergillosis involving the skin is characterized by erythematous nodules with hemorrhagic infarctions. Septated hyphae with dichotomous branching are detected in the biopsy.

Fusariosis

Fusarium species (*Fusarium solani*, *Fusarium oxysporum*, *Fusarium moniliforme*, and *Fusarium chlamydosporum*) in granulocytopenic patients undergoing intensive antileukemic chemotherapy or HSCT have been recognized during the past 15 years to cause severe pulmonary, sinus, and disseminated infections [77–81]. The portals of entry of *Fusarium* species include lungs, sinuses, catheters, and skin, particularly periungual regions. *Fusarium* has become increasingly recognized as a cause of paronychia in neutropenic patients receiving broad-spectrum antibiotics. These portals of entry may lead to widespread dissemination, fungemia with positive blood cultures in approximately one-half of cases, and, occasionally, chronic hepatic infection upon recovery from neutropenia. On physical examination one may observe nodular cutaneous lesions as a reflection of disseminated infection [82] (Fig. 4). Biopsy of these lesions reveals hyaline branching septate hyphae that are not reliably distinguishable from those of *Aspergillus* and extensive necrosis surrounding the fungal elements [77].

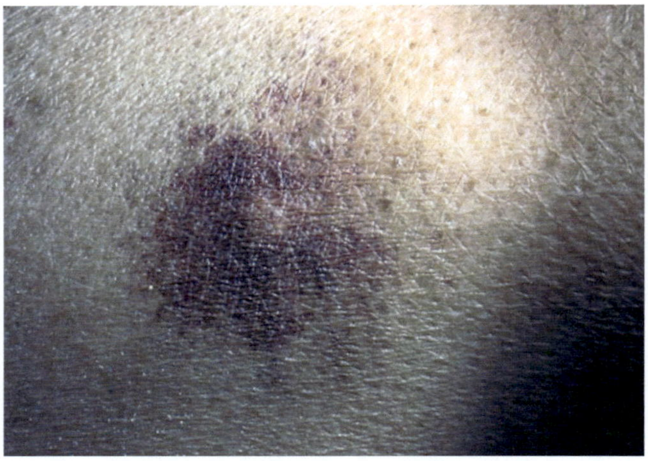

Fig. 4 Painful nodular skin lesion in a patient with disseminated fusariosis

Scedosporiosis

Scedosporium species causes pneumonia and disseminated infections in neutropenic and other compromised hosts [83–88]. Pneumonia due to *Scedosporium* species is clinically indistinguishable from that due to *Aspergillus* species. As with pulmonary aspergillosis, dissemination complicating *Scedosporium* pneumonia often involves the CNS [83, 89, 90] and may cause multiple cutaneous lesions. Diagnostic procedures and approaches, including thoracic CT scan, bronchoalveolar lavage (BAL), and lung biopsy are also similar to those for invasive pulmonary aspergillosis.

The organism in tissue and direct smears resembles the angular, septate, dichotomously branching hyphae of *Aspergillus* species. However, terminal annelloconidia may be observed histologically in some infected tissues. Definitive microbiologic diagnosis is established by culture, in which the organism may grow as the synanamorph *Scedosporium apiospermum* or as the teleomorph *Pseudallescheria boydii* with cleistothecia. *Scedosporium prolificans* in culture is characterized by distended phialides.

Zygomycosis (Mucormycosis)

This class of organisms, which has undergone recent nomenclature changes, is characterized by the presence of sparsely septated or nonseptated broad hyphae in tissue. Recent case series from Europe and the USA have reported the characteristics of the disease over the last decade [91–94], and a review of all documented cases has been published [95]. Rhinocerebral, pulmonary, and disseminated mucormycosis are the most frequently encountered conditions in immunocompromised patients. Rhinocerebral infection usually begins as an infection of the paranasal sinuses, especially maxillary and ethmoid sinuses, which progresses to invade the orbit, retro-orbital region, cavernous sinus, and brain. Angioinvasion with thrombosis causes ischemic necrosis. A black eschar on the palate or nasal mucosa and drainage of a black discharge from the eye are characteristic manifestations of infarction.

Diagnosis of pulmonary infection requires a high degree of suspicion and an aggressive approach [91–94, 96]. BAL can be performed in almost all patients. Brushings and transbronchial biopsies require an adequate platelet count. CT can define the extent of disease and guide fine-needle aspiration. Open lung biopsy by thoracoscopy in select cases or by thoracotomy is sometimes the only definitive diagnostic procedure for detection of pulmonary infection. Rarely, primary cutaneous disease may develop in a neutropenic patient [97], producing risk of subsequent dissemination. Biopsy of new skin lesions is essential to establishing the diagnosis.

Trichosporonosis

Trichosporon species are pathogenic yeasts which cause fatal disseminated infection in immunocompromised patients, particularly those with neutropenia, and mucosal disruption due to cytotoxic chemotherapy [98, 99]. The portals of entry are the gastrointestinal tract and vascular catheters; however, increasingly investigators are recognizing that aspiration may occur, leading to a *Trichosporon* bronchopneumonia and dissemination. The characteristic constellation of disseminated disease includes renal failure, pulmonary infiltrates, multiple cutaneous lesions, and characteristic chorioretinitis. This process can evolve into chronic hepatic trichosporonosis in patients who recover from neutropenia. Persistent fungemia despite administration of amphotericin B (AmB) is a clue to this infection.

Detection of Fungal Pathogens in the Neutropenic Host

Candidiasis

Direct Examination

Direct examination of a specimen provides information about the cellular composition of any inflammatory reaction, the relative amount of *Candida* species present, the distinctive morphologic features of the organism, such as the presence of blastoconidia (budding yeast forms), pseudohyphae, and hyphae, as well as the presence of other pathogens. Direct examination of urine may promptly identify *Candida* species as the cause of a urinary tract infection. The significance of candiduria depends greatly upon the immune status of the host and the presence or absence of specific risk factors for disseminated candidiasis [100, 101]. Febrile neutropenic patients with candiduria of any colony count from a correctly collected urine specimen should be considered as having a high probability for invasive candidiasis [102]. As yeast-like fungi other than *Candida* species may infect neutropenic patients, differentiation from other genera, especially *Cryptococcus, Trichosporon, Rhodotorula,* and *Malassezia* is important [103–105].

Detection of Fungemia

Detection of *Candida* species in the bloodstream must be considered to be significant until proven otherwise. Blood cultures growing *Candida* species from a vascular catheter are not considered mere catheter colonization; vascular catheters may be the target of fungemia from a distal site or the portal of entry of *Candida* species [106–108]. Negative peripheral blood cultures do not reliably exclude the diagnosis of disseminated candidiasis. Berenguer et al. addressed this question by determining the frequency with which lysis centrifugation blood cultures yielded *Candida* species in patients with autopsy-proven invasive candidiasis [109]. Blood cultures were positive in 7 of 9 patients with >3 organs infected in comparison with only 5 of 18 patients with 1 organ infected ($p=0.024$). This study demonstrated that there is a direct relation between the tissue burden of *Candida* and the frequency of detection of fungemia and that the lysis centrifugation system had a relatively low sensitivity for detecting fungemia in early deep candidiasis.

Depending on the method used, blood cultures should be incubated for 5–7 days when there is suspicion of fungemia [110, 111]. The automated blood culture systems have been shown to be equivalent to the lysis centrifugation technique in detection of candidemia [112, 113].

Immunodiagnostic and Molecular Methods

The limitations of clinical assessment and blood culture systems in early detection of invasive candidiasis warrant development of newer nonculture methods. Most of these methods should be considered investigational at this time, but assays for the detection of (1→3) beta-D-glucan (BG) are commercially available and have been approved by the FDA for the diagnosis of invasive fungal infections, including candidiasis. BG is a component of the cell wall of many fungi, including *Candida* spp., *Aspergillus* spp., *Fusarium* spp., *Trichosporon* spp., and others [114]. The organisms causing mucormycosis do not contain BG and cannot be detected by this assay, and *Cryptococcus* does not contain enough BG to be detected by this assay [115]. With the currently available FDA-approved test (Fungitell®), levels above 80 pg/mL are considered positive. A list of causes of false-positive BG tests is shown on Table 5.

Table 5 Known causes of false positive ß-D-glucan

Causes of false-positive β-D-glucan
Intravenous amoxicillin-clavulanic [116]
Surgical gauze [117]
Dialysis membranes (cellulose) [118]
Albumin [119]
Intravenous immunoglobulin [119, 120]
Coagulation factors (contamination with cellulose membranes) [119]
Some episodes of bacteremia: *Pseudomonas aeruginosa* [121], streptococcal bacteremia [122]

The first published studies of BG validated the assay and established cutoff values and showed a wide range for sensitivity (55–100%) and specificity (87–93%) [123–126]. These studies included a variety of patient populations and designs. A case series supported high sensitivity for invasive candidiasis, but raised the concern of high frequency of false-positive results in cases of bacteremia [122]. Subsequently a clinical trial in 190 neutropenic episodes in 96 patients with acute leukemia who were not receiving antifungal prophylaxis used intensive monitoring of BG and strict EORTC/MSG criteria to define probable and proven IFI to study the efficiency of the test when analyzed as a single value or as two consecutive values [127]. In this study, which used the Japanese BG assay, the investigators found that the best diagnostic performance of the test was achieved by using two consecutive values≥7 pg/mL as the diagnostic cutoff, which resulted in sensitivity of 63% (95% CI, 44–79%) and specificity of 96% (95% CI, 89–98%). There were no false-positive results caused by bacteremia. All "false-positives" were in patients with heavy fungal mucosal colonization, and most false-negatives occurred in patients receiving systemic antifungal agents [127]. Another study from a single center monitored 85 patients, 65 with EORTC/MSG proven or probable fungal infection and 20 nonneutropenic controls with solid tumors, during 12 weeks and compared BG with galactomannan [128]. In this case-control design, the monitoring was much less intensive, and the results showed the BG test had a sensitivity of approximately 60% and specificity of about 90% using the manufacturer's recommended cutoff of 80 pg/mL and two consecutive positive tests.

The published evidence does not allow for a definitive recommendation regarding the use of BG in neutropenic patients. At the present time, it seems most useful as a screening test to be obtained several times weekly in patients at risk rather than as an "ad hoc" diagnostic test in the neutropenic patient suspected of having an IFI.

Several different DNA-amplification systems are being developed for the diagnosis of *Candida* infections [129, 130].

In one of the most promising trials, McMullan et al. correctly identified eight of nine patients with *C. albicans* candidemia and two of two patients with *C. glabrata* infection by using a combination of three sets of nested real-time polymerase chain reaction (PCR), each set with primers specific for a few species of *Candida* [129]. Most notably, there were no false-positive results in 491 serum samples. The future role of this approach is difficult to predict, as the routine application of nested PCR has logistical difficulties [131], and it may be argued that the actual need is for a method that will be more sensitive than blood culture.

Aspergillosis

Microbiology and Direct Examination

The genus *Aspergillus* consists of more than 600 species, but only a few are pathogenic for humans [132]. The most common of these are *Aspergillus fumigatus* and *Aspergillus flavus*. Other species, such as *Aspergillus terreus*, *Aspergillus ustus*, and *Aspergillus nidulans,* are also known pulmonary pathogens in humans. *Aspergillus niger* is commonly isolated as a saprophyte, but is seldom proven to be a cause of IA in cancer patients.

Aspergillus species in tissue form angular dichotomously branching septate hyphae. This histopathologic pattern may be observed in infection due to *Aspergillus* species, *Pseudallescheria boydii*, *Fusarium* species, and several less common fungi. Culture is the only way to distinguish these invasive fungi. Because the antifungal susceptibility of these various genera varies, this distinction has therapeutic importance.

Aspergillus is an uncommon contaminant in most clinical microbiology laboratories. Early studies conducted by Aisner et al. found that positive nasal surveillance cultures of *A. flavus* during the midst of an outbreak of nosocomial aspergillosis in granulocytopenic patients correlated significantly with IA [133]. These findings have not been consistently corroborated in non-outbreak settings, and surveillance cultures are not routinely recommended. In contrast, isolation of *Aspergillus* species from respiratory secretions from febrile neutropenic patients with pulmonary infiltrates is strongly associated with IA. Among 108 consecutive patients from whom *Aspergillus* species were isolated, Yu et al. found that all 17 patients with granulocytopenia and/or leukemia who had lung tissue examined had IA [134], but IA was not found in nonimmunosuppressed patients or in nongranulocytopenic patients with solid tumors. Another retrospective study also underscored the significance of isolation of *Aspergillus* species from respiratory secretions in high-risk populations [135]. Thus, isolation of *Aspergillus* species from respiratory tract cultures of febrile neutropenic patients with pulmonary infiltrates should be considered evidence of IA.

Mucosal eschars may be observed by careful examination of the nasal septum and turbinates in patients with *Aspergillus* sinusitis. Biopsy and culture of these lesions may reveal hyphae. A sinus aspirate demonstrating hyphae may preclude the need for bronchoscopy. Although *Aspergillus* is the most common fungus isolated from the sinuses of immunocompromised patients, other fungi, including Zygomycetes, *Fusarium*, *Scedosporium*, *Curvularia,* and *Alternaria,* may be recovered.

BAL has been found to yield variable results in patients with tissue-proven IA, with sensitivity varying from 30% to 59% [136–138]. The combination of microbiologic culture with cytopathology increases the diagnostic yield [139]. The presence of *Aspergillus* species in BAL fluid in a febrile granulocytopenic patient with new pulmonary infiltrates is indicative of IA. However, the absence of hyphal elements or positive culture by no means excludes the diagnosis. In the case of very peripheral nodular lesions, a fine-needle biopsy may have a better yield, even if the morbidity is potentially higher [140–142]. If the foregoing methods do not yield a microbiologic diagnosis, then lung biopsy should be performed for histopathology and culture. Ideally the biopsy should include both the periphery as well as the central areas of abnormal lung because the distribution of organisms may vary.

Immunodiagnostic and Molecular Methods

The current definitions of invasive fungal infections in immunocompromised hosts now include *Aspergillus* galactomannan (GM) in the CSF, BAL fluid, or blood as one of the microbiologic criteria for probable and possible aspergillosis [15, 143–145]. The current FDA-approved, commercially available GM test (Platelia® Aspergillus, Bio-Rad Laboratories) is an enzyme immunoassay (EIA) that uses rat monoclonal antibodies, which recognize ß (1→5)–linked galactofuranose. The result is compared to a cutoff control and expressed as a GM index [146]. Some early studies used an index ≥ 1 as positive [147, 148], but it was subsequently demonstrated that an index ≥ 0.5 is more sensitive for detecting IA [149], and this value is used as a cutoff in the USA. Table 6 shows a list of known causes of false-positive GM results. The use of piperacillin-tazobactam and other beta-lactam antibiotics derived from *Penicillium* has been particularly well documented.

Several studies addressing the accuracy of the GM assay have been performed, using diverse settings and a variety of patient populations [168–171]. While initial reports suggested that the test lacked specificity in pediatric patients, more recent studies demonstrate a level of specificity and sensitivity in neutropenic children that is comparable to that of adult patients

Table 6 Known causes of false-positive galactomannan

Causes of false-positive galactomannan
Piperacillin-Tazobactam [150, 151]
Other beta-lactams [152]: ampicillin [153], amoxicillin-clavulanate [154, 155] – antibiotics that are fermentation products of *Penicillium*
Infant formula [156]
Enteral feeding with soybean protein [157]
Aspiration pneumonia [158]
PlasmaLyte (both IV and in bronchoalveolar lavage) [159, 160] or other gluconate-containing solutions [161]
Graft-versus-host disease [162]
Contamination with cardboard particles [163]
Other fungi (cross-reactive galactomannan): *Histoplasma* [164, 165], *Penicillium* spp. [166], *Geotrichum* spp. [167], *Neosartoria* spp. and possibly *Paecilomyces* spp., *Alternaria* spp., *Trichophyton* spp., *Botrytis* spp., *Wallemia* spp., *Cladosporium* spp., *Bifidobacterium* spp. [146].

with leukemia [172]. The best results during neutropenia have been reported by Maertens and colleagues, who retrospectively tested serum samples that had been collected daily or twice a week from 203 patients who had 239 episodes of neutropenia [173]. Thirty-five patients developed 38 episodes of IA (19 proven, 19 probable) using EORTC/MSG criteria [14] without considering the results of the GM assay. This design allowed the investigators to determine the performance of the test with different cutoff points – either as a single value or as two positive values. The optimal performance was found with a cutoff of the GM index ≥ 0.5 and a requirement for two abnormal results. This resulted in a sensitivity of 92% (84% for probable, 100% for proven) and a specificity of 97.5%. The GM frequently became positive a week before the diagnosis by conventional methods was made, although the sensitivity was higher the week of the diagnosis.

Determining the GM in BAL fluid may offer increased sensitivity, particularly in neutropenic patients [170, 174]; however, compared to serum, the experience is more limited and the optimization of the cutoff point for different patient populations has not been elucidated [175–177].

With increased experience in the use of GM, several points have become clear. The test is most useful as a screening test obtained at least twice weekly [178]. The sensitivity in clinical practice is lower than the optimal results of the clinical studies, and it may be less than 50% in some patient populations [128]. The sensitivity is much higher in profoundly neutropenic patients who have an absolute neutrophil count (ANC) <100 [179]. The GM may be useful as a surrogate marker of the response of the patient to treatment of IA [180]. The performance of the GM assay when it is used "ad hoc" as a diagnostic tool in immunocompromised patients with a clinical suspicion of IA is not known [146].

Regarding the use of the BG assay for the diagnosis of IA, it is unclear how it compares with GM. A case-control study from the MD Anderson Cancer Center suggests the two assays may offer similar sensitivity for IA [128]. Depending on the clinical setting, it may be advantageous to use only GM or both tests.

Molecular techniques for the diagnosis of IA have been studied for more than a decade [181] and are still considered investigational. The sensitivity and specificity vary widely [125, 182], and many questions remain regarding optimal specimen type, DNA extraction method, primer specificity, and PCR format. In some studies the PCR has performed worse than the GM [125], whereas in others the combination of both seems to be quite promising [183]. There is considerable interest in using molecular techniques in tissue samples to discern the etiologic agent. Rickerts et al. compared histopathology with culture and PCR, using two seminested polymerase chain reaction assays identifying *Aspergillus* species and Zygomycetes from 58 consecutive biopsies, and showed that PCR was superior to culture to identify the pathogen [184]. The etiologic diagnosis in the 27 patients with proven IFI increased from 63 to 96. When both histopathology and culture were negative (29 biopsies), the PCR was positive in two cases only.

Fusariosis

Fusarium species are frequently detected by automated blood culture detection systems or lysis centrifugation methods. *Fusarium* species initially grow on solid media with hyphae with phialides and microconidia. The typical plantain-shaped macroconidia (phragmospores) appear in more mature cultures. Consequently, initial culture reports from the laboratory may describe an *Acremonium* species, while subsequent reports are modified to *Fusarium* species. Thus, any culture report from blood or tissue growing *Acremonium* species from a neutropenic patient should be considered a possible early form of *Fusarium* species. Current diagnostic approaches depend upon bedside evaluation, diagnostic imaging, biopsy, and culture, but PCR methods also are being developed for detection of this lethal pathogen [185, 186]. *Fusarium* produces ß-D-glucan, and the BG test may be positive in cases of disseminated fusariosis.

Zygomycetes (Mucorales)

Examination by calcofluor staining or by KOH-digested sputum and cultures of respiratory tract secretions are frequently negative. If sputum examination and evaluation of BAL specimens are nondiagnostic, then more invasive diagnostic tests are warranted, including fine-needle aspirate and thoracoscopic or open lung biopsy, depending on local expertise and pace of the illness. Any suspicious cutaneous lesions should be biopsied. Organisms in tissue exhibit broad, 15- to 20-μm, irregular, usually non-septate, coenocytic hyphae with nondichotomous side branching.

These fungi are easily rendered nonviable if infected tissue is ground or homogenized in preparation for plating on culture media. The recovery rate may be enhanced if the tissue specimen is sliced into small pieces without grinding or homogenization. The Mucorales typically grow rapidly within 24–48 h. Recent advances in molecular detection in serum and BAL fluid may lead to improved diagnosis of this lethal infection [187].

Trichosporonosis

Cultures of blood, urine, and sputum may be persistently positive even with concomitant administration of AmB. *Trichosporon asahii* (previously *Trichosporon beigelii*) grows as a rugose or powdery yeast; microscopically, one can see blastoconidia, arthroconidia, hyphae, and occasionally pseudohyphae. *Trichosporon* species may germinate under conditions used for detecting *C. albicans*. Biopsies of cutaneous lesions generally reveal typical arthroconidia, blastoconidia, pseudohyphae, true hyphae, and vascular invasion. Trichosporon produces ß-D-glucan, and the BG test may be positive in cases of fungemia. The serum latex agglutination test for cryptococcal antigen may be positive due to shared antigens and resultant cross-reactivity between *Trichosporon* species and *C. neoformans*.

Prevention of Fungal Infections During Neutropenia

Established fungal infections have an extremely high mortality rate in persistently neutropenic patients and are difficult to diagnose early. This has resulted in the current practice of administering antifungal agents to patients who are at risk, even in the absence of proven infection. Ultimately, the goal is to prevent morbidity and mortality caused by fungal infections. Different terms have been used to characterize the administration of antifungal agents in the absence of documented fungal infections. The most commonly used are prophylaxis, empirical treatment, and preemptive treatment [188–191]. The administration of an antifungal agent to all patients undergoing conditioning chemotherapy is appropriately called prophylaxis, whereas the administration of an antifungal agent to a persistently febrile neutropenic patient is called empirical treatment. However, in both cases an antifungal agent is being given to many patients who do not need it in order to ensure that the patients who really need it do receive treatment.

As an example of the first case (prophylaxis), it has been shown that 10–15% of patients undergoing HSCT will develop invasive fungal infection when fluconazole prophylaxis is not given, as opposed to 3–5% of patients who do receive fluconazole [192, 193]. The use of an agent with very little toxicity, such as fluconazole, is easily justifiable in this setting, even if 85–90% of the patients would not have benefited from it. In the second case (empirical treatment), persistent fever during neutropenia acts as a marker for risk, identifying a group of patients in whom the frequency of fungal infection is much higher. A fungal infection is documented in only approximately 3–5% of these patients (but up to 10% in "high-risk" subgroups); however, the administration of a potentially toxic antifungal agent seems justified because of the extremely high mortality rate from these infections. Although many patients probably do not benefit from it, the use of empirical antifungal therapy has become accepted clinical practice [194].

The term "preemptive therapy" has been used to describe the administration of antifungal agents in persistently febrile neutropenic patients who have some other clinical evidence of fungal infection [195]. This represents an attempt to minimize exposure to a toxic antifungal therapy, and it lies somewhere between empirical treatment and treatment of documented infection. The important concept is that diverse approaches may be used to decrease the morbidity and mortality associated with fungal infections during neutropenia.

Prevention of Exposure: Environmental Control

Prevention of exposure is not possible for *Candida* infections but is feasible, at least partially, for *Aspergillus*. A review of nosocomial aspergillosis found that the most common sources of clusters and outbreaks were hospital construction and renovation and defective and contaminated ventilation systems [55]. Exposure of patients to *Aspergillus* conidia can be significantly decreased by the use of high-efficiency particulate air filtration (HEPA) filters and positive pressure rooms [196]. During an outbreak, IA developed in 50% of patients treated during a 4-month period of extensive renovation of the hematology ward and decreased to 0% after the installation of HEPA filters [197].

The risk of IA in HSCT recipients who were not in HEPA-filtered rooms was 5.6 times higher in a classic study from the Fred Hutchinson Medical Center [198]. Data from the International Bone Marrow Transplant Registry have confirmed that use of HEPA and/or laminar air flow (LAF) to prevent infections decreases transplant-related mortality rates and increases survival rates after allogeneic HSCT for leukemia [199].

Use of HEPA filters has become more common, but still some patients develop pulmonary aspergillosis and other mould infections while in the hospital. There is growing evidence that contamination of the water distribution system with *Aspergillus* [200] and other moulds, such as *Fusarium* [201], plays a role in the epidemiology of hospital-acquired fungal infection. There have been fatal infections with *Aspergillus terreus* from the soil of hospital plants [202]. This may be a rare event, but exposure to wet soil should be avoided during profound neutropenia.

Primary Prophylaxis of Invasive Fungal Infections

Patients with prolonged neutropenia secondary to chemotherapy have been shown to benefit from systemic antifungal prophylaxis with fluconazole, itraconazole, posaconazole, voriconazole, and micafungin. Topical treatment with nystatin, oral AmB, or clotrimazole troches decreases fungal colonization, but has not been shown to decrease the incidence of invasive disease.

Prophylaxis with Fluconazole

Candida is a common inhabitant of the human gastrointestinal tract. The majority of invasive *Candida* infections during neutropenia originate after mucosal colonization evolves into superficial infection. However, prevention of oropharyngeal candidiasis does not necessarily lead to prevention of deeply invasive candidiasis [203], and superficial candidiasis is not an appropriate end point in clinical trials.

Many studies of prophylaxis have found a relatively low incidence of IFI, and consequently they have been underpowered [204–207]. However, the studies of systemic agents for prophylaxis in populations at substantial risk, especially allogeneic HSCT recipients, have clearly shown a beneficial effect [192, 193]. In the study by Goodman et al., fluconazole 400 mg daily or placebo was initiated on day 1 of marrow-ablative chemotherapy to 356 HSCT recipients. Invasive candidiasis developed in 28 of 178 patients (15.7%) who received placebo and 5 of 179 (2.8%) who received fluconazole ($p<0.001$). This 13% reduction in absolute risk means only eight patients need to be treated to prevent one infection. There was a significant reduction in fungal infection–attributable mortality rates, but no difference in overall mortality rates. Fluconazole was associated with minimal adverse effects.

Another randomized, placebo-controlled trial of fluconazole in HSCT recipients showed a significant reduction in the number of fungal infections, 10 of 152 (7%) in fluconazole-treated patients compared with 26 of 148 (18%) in placebo-treated patients ($p=0.004$) and improved survival rates (31 deaths compared with 52 deaths in placebo recipients ($p = 0.004$)) [192]. Long-term follow-up of these patients has confirmed the benefit in survival rates [208]. In a multicenter study that included patients receiving intensive chemotherapy for acute leukemia or autologous HSCT, fluconazole prophylaxis, when compared with placebo, decreased superficial fungal infections, definite and probable invasive fungal infections (9 of 141 vs 32 of 133), and decreased deaths attributable to fungal infection (1 of 15 vs 6 of 15), respectively [209].

Rex et al. reported a retrospective analysis of the effect of systemic antifungal prophylaxis in 833 episodes of neutropenia in 322 patients treated for AML at the MD Anderson Medical Center between 1988 and 1992 [41]. Although retrospective, this comparison between episodes of neutropenia in which prophylaxis, typically fluconazole 400 mg daily or amphotericin B 40 mg daily, was given and episodes in which prophylaxis was not given, has the advantages of size and power that many prospective randomized trials lack. The results show statistically significant reductions in invasive fungal infection (5% vs 13%), empirical AmB use (26% vs 34%), and death within 30 days of the first neutropenic episode (23% vs 35%). As expected, the difference in invasive fungal infections was accounted for by a reduction in yeast infections (2% vs 8%), with no difference in the frequency of mould infections.

In summary, the beneficial effect of prophylaxis with systemic antifungal agents is demonstrable in high-risk patients, particularly allogeneic HSCT recipients and patients with AML, but difficult to demonstrate in lower-risk neutropenic patients. When the risk is low, most studies are underpowered. Not surprisingly, a meta-analysis shows that the use of azole or systemic AmB prophylaxis in oncology patients with severe neutropenia is associated with significant benefit regarding four main end points: decreased need for therapeutic doses of parenteral antifungal agents, decreased superficial fungal infection, decreased invasive fungal infection, and decreased fungal-related mortality [210]. The number of patients that require treatment to prevent one event for each one of these four end points are 10, 12, 22, and 52, respectively. Similar to a previous meta-analysis [211], there was no difference in overall mortality, and there was no effect on aspergillosis.

Prophylaxis with Itraconazole

Fluconazole has no activity against moulds. Therefore it is not expected to decrease the incidence of aspergillosis. Conversely, itraconazole has good activity against *Aspergillus* and many dematiaceous molds and maintains activity against yeasts. Several studies have compared itraconazole oral solution in a formulation with hydroxyprolyl-ß-cyclodextrin with placebo [212], itraconazole with oral AmB [213], and itraconazole with fluconazole, either in capsules [214] or as an oral solution [215]. Studies using the intravenous formulation of itraconazole, which is currently unavailable in most countries, as prophylaxis in allogeneic HSCT have been reported [20, 22].

Itraconazole oral solution (2.5 mg/kg twice daily) reduced the frequency of proven and suspected fungal infections compared to placebo in a randomized, double-blind, multicenter study of 405 patients with hematologic malignancies [212]. There was no difference in mortality rates. Itraconazole oral solution (2.5 mg/kg twice daily) was not statistically significantly better than oral AmB in another double-blind, double-placebo, randomized, multicenter trial that enrolled 557 patients [213], although trends favoring itraconazole were seen for proven IFI (3.6% vs 9.4%) and proven IA (1.8% vs 3.3%). Of note, the median plasma concentration of itraconazole during the first week was <0.5 μg/mL. Lower itraconazole levels have been associated with the occurrence of invasive fungal infections [216, 217]. Low levels of itraconazole may also have played some role in another study that compared itraconazole capsules (100 mg twice daily) with fluconazole capsules (50 mg twice daily) in 213 adult patients with hematologic malignancies [214] and found no difference in any of the measured clinical end points. The comparison of itraconazole oral solution (5 mg/kg daily) with fluconazole oral solution (100 mg daily) showed fewer proven systemic fungal infections (1 in 288 neutropenic episodes vs 4 in 293 neutropenic episodes) in the itraconazole-treated group. No cases of IA were documented in the itraconazole group versus 4 in the fluconazole group. There were also fewer deaths caused by fungal infection in the itraconazole group [215]. However, the oral solution of itraconazole caused significantly more toxicity than fluconazole, particularly nausea, vomiting, and diarrhea – most likely due to the cyclodextrin vehicle. The increased toxicity and poor tolerability of itraconazole also were factors in the studies comparing the IV formulation to fluconazole [20, 22].

Prophylaxis with Posaconazole

In a randomized controlled trial, posaconazole showed higher efficacy, including a survival advantage, than fluconazole or itraconazole as prophylaxis during neutropenia [23] (Table 3 summarizes the results). This multicenter study included more than 600 patients. The estimated number of patients needed to treat to prevent one death was only 15, making posaconazole the antifungal prophylaxis of choice when IA is a consideration, such as during prolonged neutropenia and when adequate absorption of the drug, currently available only as an oral formulation, is anticipated. It is questionable if the results of this study are specific for posaconazole or whether they serve as proof of principle that a well-tolerated azole with activity against *Aspergillus* will result in better outcomes than fluconazole during prolonged neutropenia [218].

Prophylaxis with Voriconazole

One randomized controlled trial compared voriconazole to fluconazole as antifungal prophylaxis in HSCT recipients [219]. Antifungal prophylaxis was administered for 100 days (not just during neutropenia) in the context of close monitoring with structured use of empirical antifungal therapy for suspected invasive fungal infection. The primary end point was fungal-free survival at 6 months. There was no overall difference between the two groups, but there was a trend toward fewer cases of aspergillosis in the voriconazole arm. In a second, very small, randomized controlled trial 25 patients with AML undergoing induction of remission were randomized to voriconazole ($n=10$) or placebo ($n = 15$) [220]. The study was stopped early because the use of placebo was considered unacceptable after the results of the posaconazole trial mentioned above were made public. There was a trend toward fewer pulmonary infiltrates (0 vs 5) and less hepatosplenic candidiasis (0 vs. 4) in the voriconazole arm compared with the placebo arm. Despite the lack of evidence from controlled trials, voriconazole is used frequently in clinical practice as prophylaxis for high-risk patients. Of particular concern with the use of voriconazole prophylaxis is the frequency of reports of breakthrough IFI with zygomycetes [221–224].

Prophylaxis with Echinocandins

Given that echinocandins have excellent activity against *Candida* and significant activity against *Aspergillus*, they constitute a very reasonable option for prophylaxis. In a randomized, controlled multicenter trial comparing micafungin with fluconazole, 882 patients who were to undergo HSCT were randomized to receive micafungin, 50 mg daily, or fluconazole, 400 mg daily. Both drugs prevented invasive candidiasis. However, micafungin had a greater impact on the prevention of IA during neutropenia (1 case vs 7, $p=0.07$) [21].

Prophylaxis with Amphotericin B

AmB has been used as prophylaxis orally to prevent superficial fungal infection; inhaled and intravenous amphotericin B deoxycholate (AmB-d) and lipid formulations of AmB have been used [213, 225–227]. A study of oral fluconazole versus high-dose oral AmB-d (2 g in four divided doses) in a large population of neutropenic patients described equivalent effects of both regimens in preventing invasive candidiasis [227]. Fluconazole, however, was better tolerated. In our opinion, the lack of patient compliance with oral AmB-d and the toxicity of prophylactic AmB-d preclude the use of this agent as a viable prophylactic compound.

Aerosolized AmB-d was not effective in the prevention of IA in a large prospective, randomized, multicenter trial [228]. In contrast, aerosolized liposomal amphotericin B (L-AmB) was superior to placebo in neutropenic patients (all subject were also receiving fluconazole prophylaxis) to prevent pulmonary aspergillosis [229]. This study should be considered more a proof of principle than a currently available approach.

Systemic, low-dose AmB-d has been used [230], but it has never shown more efficacy than fluconazole, and it has proven significantly more toxic. The use of lipid formulations of AmB has also been attempted. In a randomized, double-blind placebo-controlled study of L-AmB, 2 mg/kg three times weekly, the drug was well tolerated, but there was no significant reduction in proven or suspected IFI, in part due to the low-risk population that was studied [231]. There were no proven IFIs in patients on L-AmB and only three in the group that received placebo (3.4%). In an interim analysis of a prospective study, Uhlenbrock et al. found that antifungal prophylaxis with L-AmB, 1 mg/kg three times weekly, was no more effective than no prophylaxis [232].

Secondary Prophylaxis of Invasive Fungal Infections

A patient may be successfully treated for an IFI and still require further myelosuppressive chemotherapy or HSCT. The ultimate objective is to successfully treat the patient's neoplastic disease while preventing breakthrough fungal infection. In the case of aspergillosis, Karp et al. demonstrated that aggressive antifungal therapy during neutropenia induced by subsequent courses of chemotherapy prevented exacerbation or recurrence of IA in patients with acute leukemia [233]. Similar strategies have been used in HSCT [234–236]. Most patients have been treated with prophylactic antifungal agents – itraconazole [235], AmB, or voriconazole [237]. Surgical resection of remaining foci of disease prior to myeloablation has been used, but it is not always adequate [236, 238]. The largest published systematic study is a retrospective case series of 48 patients, 20 of whom had undergone surgical resection, for proven or probable IA prior to HSCT [239]. Sixteen patients (33%) had a relapse a median of 15 days after the transplant (range 0–120 days). Ten patients were receiving systemic antifungal therapy (8 AmB and 4 itraconazole) at the time of relapse. Better results have been noted with voriconazole [237].

The use of secondary antifungal prophylaxis is mandatory in the setting of IA for patients ongoing chemotherapy. We recommend voriconazole, based on the results of the prophylactic and therapeutic trials of this agent [12, 34], small series, and case reports [237, 240]. Surgical resection of an isolated pulmonary lesion may be highly beneficial, but is not mandatory.

Recommendations for Prophylaxis

Systemic antifungal prophylaxis is effective and should be used in groups at high risk. In the case of neutropenia, this applies to patients with acute leukemia, particularly AML, and HSCT recipients. We recommend the use of prophylaxis during induction or reinduction chemotherapy for AML or myelodysplastic syndrome and in HSCT, particularly when using a myeloablative regimen.

Fluconazole is the treatment of choice as long as the risk of IA is low, as in patients who have an anticipated short duration of neutropenia. Fluconazole has shown significant effectiveness in high-risk groups and is very well tolerated [192, 193]. The role of itraconazole in prophylaxis in neutropenic patients is unclear, given the problems with absorption, tolerability of the liquid form, and drug interactions. If the activity against *Aspergillus* is considered necessary, there is strong clinical evidence favoring posaconazole [23].

The efficacy of voriconazole against IA [34], its comparison with L-AmB in high-risk patients with persistent febrile neutropenia [18], and the availability of an intravenous form make it a very attractive option. However, voriconazole has only been properly studied as a prophylactic agent in allogeneic HSCT [219].

The echinocandins offer great promise as prophylactic compounds. They have excellent activity against fluconazole-susceptible and -resistant *Candida* species [241] and activity against *Aspergillus* [242] and *Pneumocystis* [243]. Micafungin can be used to prevent invasive candidiasis and possibly aspergillosis during the neutropenic phase of HSCT [21]. The role of these agents in antifungal prophylaxis in patients with leukemia remains undefined at this point.

Finally, no prophylaxis can be universally effective. In the same way that the use of fluconazole prophylaxis has resulted in increasing incidence of *C. glabrata* and *C. krusei* infection, it is inevitable that more resistant pathogens will break through the newer, broader-spectrum agents. The development of mould infections during prophylaxis with echinocandins, voriconazole, or posaconazole should suggest the possibility of zygomycosis [221], fusariosis [244], or scedosporiosis [245].

Empirical Antifungal Therapy

The use of empirical antifungal therapy in the presence of persistent or recurrent fever during neutropenia is the last step in an attempt to prevent morbidity and mortality secondary to fungal infection before a definitive diagnosis is established. It is understood that the majority of neutropenic patients with persistent fever do not have an occult fungal infection, but the proportion who do steadily increases with the duration of neutropenia [39]. At some point the risk of not administering effective antifungal therapy outweighs the risk associated with the toxicity of the drugs. Empirical treatment should then be started. The availability of newer, less toxic agents should alter this balance and allow earlier intervention.

The evidence supporting the empirical addition of antifungal agents in persistently febrile neutropenic patients is less than optimal but reflects the state of the art of antifungal therapy at the time. Two randomized studies compared antifungal therapy against no therapy in the setting of persistent fever during neutropenia [246, 247]. Both studies were completed when CT of the chest was used less frequently and before the wide use of fluconazole prophylaxis and hematopoietic growth factor support. Both studies are limited by a small sample size. In the study by Pizzo et al. 50 patients with persistent fever and neutropenia after 7 days of broad-spectrum antibiotics (cefazolin, carbenicillin, and gentamicin, the standard regimen at the time) were randomized to one of three treatments: discontinuing antibiotics and reevaluating, continuing the same regimen, or adding AmB-d, 0.5 mg/kg daily, until resolution of fever and neutropenia. Several results of this study deserve emphasis. Deep-seated fungal infections or esophageal candidiasis was documented in 1 of the 18 patients who received AmB-d and 7 of the 32 who did not. Two deaths caused by fungal infection occurred in the patients who did not receive AmB-d and one in the treated group. These differences were not statistically significant, but suggested a trend and led to a randomized trial by the EORTC.

The EORTC study randomized 132 patients to receive 0.6 mg/kg of AmB-d or continue just antibiotics after 3 days of neutropenic fever [247]. Six fungal infections were documented in the group receiving antibiotics alone and only one in the group that received AmB-d. The fungal-related deaths were 4 versus 0, respectively, in no therapy versus AmB-d arms ($p=0.05$). The greatest benefits accrued to those who had not received antifungal prophylaxis ($p = 0.04$), those who were severely neutropenic ($p = 0.06$), those with a clinically documented infection ($p = 0.03$), and those >15 years old ($p=0.06$). The EORTC authors concluded that early AmB-d in granulocytopenic patients with continued fever despite broad-spectrum antibiotics may be beneficial. Moreover, the authors further emphasized that this approach would be most beneficial for selected subgroups of persistently febrile neutropenic patients. This observation was prescient of subsequent studies that also have demonstrated the benefits in this approach in the highest-risk patients with prolonged neutropenia.

It is reasonable to question if these two studies constitute adequate proof that all neutropenic patients with persistent fever should receive antifungal therapy [248]. In fact, the idea of acknowledging the differences between different groups of patients is not new [16, 17]. We strongly believe that high-risk patients with prolonged neutropenia derive the greatest benefit from empirical antifungal therapy. The specific circumstances of each individual patient should be considered before starting antifungal therapy. The current Guidelines from the Infectious Disease Society of America [194] suggest 5–7 days of persistent fever as the time to start AmB.

The decision may be considerably simplified thanks to the use of newer agents with a much more favorable benefit-toxicity profile. Empirical antifungal therapy has been controversial because of the risk of AmB-related toxicity. In a retrospective analysis of 239 patients, Wingard et al. found that the creatinine level doubled in 53%, and 14.5% of the patients required dialysis [249]. If the newer drugs have much less toxicity with similar efficacy, the decision to use empirical therapy will be easier. Conversely, if a group of patients with significantly higher risk of developing a fungal infection can be identified, even potentially toxic interventions may be justified.

During the last decade several large studies have compared the use of AmB with alternative antifungal agents. These trials have included more than 3,500 patients, and have demonstrated that several antifungal agents can be used successfully during neutropenic fever. The clinician can choose depending on risk factors and toxicity. A summary of the three studies that have established the current state of the art is shown in Table 2.

Fluconazole Versus Amphotericin B: Only if the Risk of Mold Infection Is Negligible

Two multicenter randomized trials have compared fluconazole with AmB as empirical treatment of neutropenic fever. This approach does not make sense if the incidence of IA is high. The first study compared fluconazole, 6 mg/kg daily, with AmB-d, 0.8 mg/kg, and was stopped early after an interim analysis showed excess toxicity in the AmB-d group [250]. Importantly, patients with abnormal x-rays, a history of aspergillosis, or colonization with *Aspergillus* were not eligible, and patients could have received nonabsorbable antifungal prophylaxis before enrollment. There were no documented fungal infections in this trial, which makes it difficult to draw any conclusions, other than AmB-d is more toxic than fluconazole.

In the other open-label trial, neutropenic patients with persistent fever after 4 days of antibiotics were randomized to receive either fluconazole, 400 mg daily ($n=158$), or AmB-d, 0.5 mg/kg daily ($n = 159$) [11]. Patients were not eligible if they had been receiving systemic antifungal agents or if they were colonized with *Aspergillus*. This study used a composite end point that defined success if the patient was afebrile, had no clinical or microbiologic evidence of fungal infection, and did not require study termination due to lack of efficacy, drug toxicity, or death. Both regimens were similar in terms of the proportion of "satisfactory responses" – 68% versus 69%. The failures in the fluconazole group were typically related to persistent fever. In the AmB-d group, most failures were due to toxicity. Overall, 4% of the patients in each group developed new fungal infections during therapy, there were no differences in mortality, and toxicity was less in the fluconazole arm. The authors concluded that fluconazole may be appropriate empirical therapy in persistently febrile neutropenic patients at low risk for IA.

Lipid Formulations of Amphotericin B: At Least as Effective and Less Toxic

A double-blind, randomized controlled trial of amphotericin B colloidal dispersion (ABCD), 4 mg/kg daily, compared to AmB-d, 0.8 mg/kg daily, enrolled 213 patients with febrile neutropenia ≥ 3 days [251]. More than half the patients in the study were receiving cyclosporine or tacrolimus after an allogeneic HSCT. A successful treatment outcome included all of the following criteria: survival for 7 days after the last dose of the study drug, lack of suspected or documented IFI during the study and within 7 days of the last dose of the study drug, lack of study drug discontinuation because of adverse events, and lack of fever on the day of discontinuation of therapy. There were no differences in the therapeutic responses between both groups: 50% of the 98 ABCD recipients and 43.2% of the AmB-d recipients responded. The causes for discontinuation of the study drug were similar in both study arms. Although ABCD produced significantly less renal toxicity, it was associated with more frequent infusion-related toxicities, particularly hypoxemia. This study lacked the power to find a difference in frequency of breakthrough IFI.

The Mycoses Study Group compared L-AmB, 3 mg/kg daily, to AmB-d, 0.6 mg/kg daily, in a double-blind randomized trial that enrolled 689 patients [18]. This was a noninferiority study, where success was defined as a composite of five criteria: survival for 7 days after initiation of the study drug; resolution of fever during the period of neutropenia; successful treatment of any baseline fungal infection; absence of breakthrough fungal infections during administration of the study drug or within 7 days after the completion of treatment; and absence of premature discontinuation of the study drug because of toxicity or lack of efficacy. The study showed similar outcomes in both groups, 50% versus 49%, although there were significantly fewer proven IFI in patients receiving L-AmB – 11 (3.2%) versus 27 (7.8%), $p=0.009$. This difference was independent of risk category, age, and antifungal prophylaxis. There was a trend for improved overall survival rates in the L-AmB group, and infusion-related toxicity and nephrotoxicity were significantly less with L-AmB. This study unequivocally established L-AmB as an alternative to AmB-d in the empirical management of fever and neutropenia. Prentice et al. compared two different dosages of L-AmB, 1 mg/kg daily and 3 mg/kg daily, with AmB-d, 1 mg/kg daily, in 204 children and 134 adults with neutropenic fever. The primary end point was safety, and efficacy was only a secondary end point. Response was defined as a composite of defervescence for 3 consecutive days and until the end of the study, when recovery of neutropenia occurred, with no addition of another antifungal agent and no breakthrough fungal infection. Toxicity was clearly more frequent in the AmB-d group; a total of 24% of the patients doubled their serum creatinine, compared with 10% and 12% receiving the two dosages of L-AmB.

A multicenter, randomized double-blind study compared the safety of L-AmB, 3 mg/kg daily or 5 mg/kg daily, with ABLC, 5 mg/kg daily, in 244 patients [252]. The study drugs were initiated after ≥ 3 days of persistent neutropenic fever. The results of the study showed that L-AmB was significantly less toxic than ABLC, both in nephrotoxicity and in infusion-related reactions. The efficacy analysis showed no significant differences among the three study arms (33–42% efficacy). The reasons for failure were similar for both drugs; eight patients developed breakthrough fungal infections.

Itraconazole Versus Amphotericin B Deoxycholate: Of Historical Interest Only

An open-label, multicenter, randomized study powered to show equivalence enrolled 394 adult neutropenic patients with fever that persisted ≥ 3 days while receiving broad-spectrum antibiotics [10]. HSCT recipients were excluded. Other exclusion criteria included strong suspicion of fungal infections during previous episodes of neutropenia and current treatment with drugs known to interact with itraconazole. Itraconazole was administered intravenously at a dosage of 200 mg twice daily for the first 2 days, followed by 200 mg daily on days 3–14. Oral itraconazole solution could be substituted after day 7. AmB-d was given at a dose of 0.7–1.0 mg/kg daily. Most patients had received previous antifungal prophylaxis. The primary analysis used criteria similar to those of earlier studies. A favorable response (defervescence and recovery from neutropenia) was documented in 47% of the patients in the itraconazole group and

38% of the patients in the AmB-d group. In the AmB-d group, 38 patients failed because of intolerance to the drug; in the itraconazole group, 20 patients failed because fever persisted after the resolution of neutropenia and 19 because the fever required a change in the antifungal regimen.

Voriconazole Versus Liposomal Amphotericin B: Another Option

In this noninferiority trial, summarized in Table 2, 849 patients in 73 participating centers were randomized to receive either L-AmB or voriconazole after 96 h of fever and neutropenia [12]. Voriconazole was given at a dose of 6 mg/kg twice daily for 2 days, followed by 4 mg/kg twice daily; L-AmB was given at a dosage of 3 mg/kg daily. Patients were stratified according to risk, with allogeneic HSCT and chemotherapy for relapsed leukemia considered high risk. The end point of the study was success or failure defined according to the composite end point that had been validated in previous trials [10, 11, 18, 253]. The overall success rate was only 26% for voriconazole and 30.6% for those receiving L-AmB, much lower than in previous studies. This low success rate can be explained by the requirement of resolution of fever for 48 h prior to recovery from neutropenia as part of the composite end point. As the median time to recovery from neutropenia was only 5.4–5.5 days, there was very little time available to become and remain afebrile for 48 h. If defervescence is excluded from the composite end point, the success rate more than doubles to 82% in the voriconazole group and 86% in the L-AmB group. Although voriconazole narrowly failed to fulfill the criteria for noninferiority (the confidence interval for the difference was –10.6% to 1.6%, and the predefined lower limit for equivalence was 10%), there was a striking and significant difference favoring voriconazole in breakthrough fungal infections (8 vs 21, $p=0.02$). This difference was even more marked in the high-risk category: 2 of 143 (1.4%) versus 13 of 141 (9.2%). As in other open-label studies, many more patients discontinued voriconazole (22) than L-AmB (5) for persistent fever, which was never due to breakthrough fungal infections. There was no difference in the proportion of patients discontinuing the study drug because of adverse effects. This study showed that voriconazole is comparable to L-AmB in overall therapeutic success, and it is superior in reducing documented breakthrough fungal infections, particularly in high-risk neutropenic patients.

Caspofungin Versus Liposomal Amphotericin B: Yet Another Option

Using a noninferiority design and composite end point similar to the prior studies, Walsh et al. compared caspofungin with L-AmB in a multicenter, randomized double-blind clinical trial in 1,095 patients [13]. The results of the study, summarized in Table 2, determined caspofungin was as effective as L-AmB in all groups – high-risk, low-risk, on antifungal prophylaxis or not – and for each one of the individual components of the composite end point. The overall success rate was 33.9% for the caspofungin group and 33.7% for the L-AmB group. Caspofungin treated successfully the IFIs diagnosed at baseline 51.9% of the time, which compared favorably with the 25.9% achieved by L-AmB. Drug-related adverse events were less common with caspofungin, and overall survival was also statistically significantly better with caspofungin. This study clearly established that a much less toxic agent was noninferior to the standard of care for empirical therapy.

Recommendations for Empirical Therapy

Several antifungal agents have been shown in well-designed clinical trials to be adequate for the management of persistently febrile neutropenic patients. Fluconazole should generally not be used, except in lower-risk patients [254]. Lipid formulations of AmB, voriconazole, and caspofungin have emerged as viable alternatives to the standard AmB-d, with similar efficacy and much less toxicity. Each of these agents may be preferable under different circumstances. Lipid formulations of AmB are at least as effective as AmB-d [18, 252, 253]. It is possible that the initial high acquisition cost of L-AmB and other lipid formulations could be offset by the savings associated with the prevention of renal toxicity [255]. Caspofungin seems to be the safest alternative, is at least as effective as L-AmB, and has less potential for drug interactions than voriconazole. Its main downside is acquisition cost.

Voriconazole, despite failing the noninferiority requirement in the randomized trial that compared it with L-AmB, was significantly better at preventing breakthrough fungal infections, particularly in the high-risk group. It is less nephrotoxic than L-AmB, and the transient visual disturbances and hallucinations associated with it are usually manageable, but it has higher potential for drug interactions than caspofungin [256].

Preemptive Antifungal Therapy

The term preemptive antifungal therapy describes the administration of antifungal agents in persistently febrile neutropenic patients with some other clinical evidence of fungal infection [195]. The underlying rationale for this idea is that most neutropenic patients with persistent fever do not, in fact, have an IFI. Administering an antifungal may be life-saving for the relatively small fraction who are infected, but may result in unnecessary toxicity in a sizeable group. It would be desirable to narrow the group of patients who receive unneeded antifungal drugs, as long as no one with an early occult IFI goes untreated [188–190]. The new serologic and molecular tests for diagnosing IFI, together with the increased availability of CT imaging, have resulted in exploratory studies [257] and randomized controlled trials [258, 259] that test this approach.

It is appropriate to question if this idea still has merit in face of the antifungal agents currently available. In the trial of empirical therapy comparing L-AmB with AmB-d, 18.7% and 33% of the patients developed creatinine increases ≥2× the baseline, respectively [18]. However, in the voriconazole versus L-AmB trial, these proportions were 7% and 7.6% [12] and in the caspofungin versus L-AmB trial, 2.6% and 11.6% [13]. Preemptive therapy may be perfectly reasonable when one-third of the patients exposed to empirical therapy may develop significant nephrotoxicity [18], but not so reasonable if the risk is less than 3% [13].

In a "proof of principle" trial, Maertens and colleagues used daily monitoring with GM in 88 high-risk patients undergoing chemotherapy for AML, myelodysplastic syndrome, or myeloablative HSCT [257]. If the patients developed persistent fever, recrudescent fever, signs and symptoms of IFI, or two consecutive GM tests ≥0.5, high-resolution CT and bronchoscopy with BAL were performed. Antifungal treatment with L-AmB, 5 mg/kg daily, was triggered only when GM was positive or when suggestive CT findings were supported by a culture or microscopic evaluation positive for a mold. The investigators diagnosed 19 cases of IA (7 proven, 12 probable) [14]. Except for one case of mucormycosis, no cases of IFI went undiagnosed. The survival rate for patients with IA was 63.1% at 6 months. This study showed that it is possible to limit the number of patients receiving empirical antifungal treatment without missing IFIs, but did not address whether this approach was better than traditional empirical treatment.

More recently a multicenter, open-label, randomized noninferiority trial compared empirical treatment with preemptive antifungal therapy in 293 patients with prolonged neutropenia [259]. The antifungal of choice was AmB-d, 1 mg/kg daily, or L-AmB, 3 mg/kg daily, for patients with renal dysfunction. AmB was started in the preemptive arm in patients who had repeatedly positive GM assays and any of several signs or symptoms, including pneumonia, sinusitis, suggestive skin lesions, or unexplained CNS symptoms. Patients in the empirical treatment arm received AmB if they had persistent fever for more than 4 days or recurrent fever. The survival rate was 97.3% with empirical treatment and 95.1% with preemptive treatment. Despite the fact that this difference was within the prespecified noninferiority margin, the authors expressed some concerns. The frequency of IFIs was higher in the preemptive arm than in the empirical treatment arm (9.1% vs 2.7%), and in an exploratory analysis of the high-risk subgroup, in which most cases of aspergillosis occurred, inferiority could not be ruled out.

A slightly different approach was adopted by Hebart and colleagues, who randomized 403 allogeneic HSCT recipients to empirical treatment with L-AmB, 3 mg/kg daily, in case of persistent fever for ≥120 h or to a PCR-based treatment, in which L-AmB was initiated because of a positive PCR for *Candida* or *Aspergillus* OR persistent fever [258, 260]. The preemptive part of this approach is that L-AmB was supposed to decrease to 1 mg/kg daily after 3 days of treatment unless the condition of the patient deteriorated. The study resulted in more patients being treated in the PCR-based treatment arm (112 of 196 vs 76 of 207), but a slightly lower total dosage of L-AmB per patient. There was no difference in the number of IFIs, overall mortality, or mortality caused by fungal infection between the treatment arms.

Recommendations for Preemptive Therapy

We believe empirical treatment of persistent fever during neutropenia is a very safe approach with the currently available drugs. Preemptive treatment was an attractive idea when the only empirical option was AmB-d, which carried significant toxicity. Currently, the toxicity associated with caspofungin, voriconazole, and L-AmB is very low. It is concerning that efforts to limit administration of antifungal therapy may result in delayed or missed diagnoses of IFIs, and we consider the preemptive approach experimental at this time.

This in no way negates the importance of exhaustively looking for IFIs in neutropenic patients with persistent fever. On the contrary, determining the presence and nature of IFI has serious implications for the management of the patient. Aspergillosis, breakthrough candidemia and less common mold infections, such as mucormycosis and fusariosis, require different treatment. As an example, caspofungin is an effective drug for empirical management of persistent fever, but it is not the treatment of choice for any mould infection. Consequently, trying to establish the presence of an IFI is of paramount importance. We try to obtain a CT of the chest and sinuses in neutropenic patients with persistent fever, and pursue pulmonary abnormalities with bronchoscopy and BAL with the goal of obtaining cultures for bacterial, fungal, nocardial, and mycobacterial pathogens. We perform specific stains, including direct fluorescence assay for *Pneumocystis*, and also perform cytologic examination with silver and Fite stains. We measure GM in the BAL and early on consider obtaining tissue for specific diagnosis. With several options available, empirical management can be tailored to the specific situation of the patient.

Table 7 Pathogen-specific antifungal therapy in neutropenic patients

Pathogen	Treatment of choice	Alternative	Comments
Candida [261]			
Suspected candidemia	L-AmB 3–5 mg/kg daily or caspofungin (70 mg loading dose, then 50 mg daily), or voriconazole (6 mg/kg every 12 h for 1 day, then 3 mg/kg twice daily)	Fluconazole 800-mg IV (12 mg/kg) loading dose, then 400 mg (6 mg/kg) daily	Azoles should not be used for empirical therapy in patients who have received an azole for prophylaxis
Proven candidemia	An echinocandin (caspofungin, loading 70 mg, then 50 mg daily; micafungin, 100 mg daily; anidulafungin, loading 200 mg, then 100 mg daily) or L-AmB (3–5 mg/kg daily)	For patients who are less critically ill and who have no recent azole exposure Fluconazole 800 mg IV (12 mg/kg) loading dose, then 400 mg (6 mg/kg) IV daily	For *C. glabrata*, an echinocandin is preferred; for *C. parapsilosis*, fluconazole or AmBLF is preferred as initial therapy; for *C. krusei*, an echinocandin, AmBLF, or voriconazole is recommended Intravenous catheter removal should be considered
Chronic disseminated candidiasis	Fluconazole 400 mg (6 mg/kg) daily for clinically stable patients. L-AmB 3–5 mg/kg daily or AmB-d 0.5–0.7 mg/kg daily in acutely ill patients or patients with refractory disease	Anidulafungin (loading dose of 200 mg, then 100 mg daily), micafungin (100 mg daily), or caspofungin (loading dose of 70 mg, then 50 mg daily)	Therapy should be continued for weeks to months, until calcification occurs or lesions resolve. Patients who require ongoing chemotherapy or undergo HCT should continue to receive antifungal therapy throughout the period of high risk
Aspergillosis [262]	Voriconazole 6 mg/kg IV every 12 h for 1 day, followed by 4 mg/kg IV every 12 h	L-AmB 3–5 mg/kg/day, or ABLC 5 mg/kg/day, or caspofungin (loading dose of 70 mg, then 50 mg daily), or posaconazole 200 mg QID initially, then 400 mg BID PO after stabilization of disease [263]	Primary combination therapy is not routinely recommended based on lack of clinical data; addition of another agent or switch to another drug class for salvage therapy may be considered in individual patients. Posaconazole is only available by mouth and takes several days to achieve adequate tissue levels; it should not be used as single agent in the critically ill neutropenic patient
Zygomycosis [95]	L-AmB 5 mg/kg/day, or ABLC 5 mg/kg/day [264]	Posaconazole 200 mg QID initially, then 400 mg BID PO after stabilization of disease [265] New iron chelators (deferasirox, deferiprone) have been combined with antifungal agents [266, 267] and are investigational at this point [268, 269]	Many infections with zygomycetes require surgery. Primary combination therapy is not routinely recommended based on lack of clinical data; addition of caspofungin may be considered in individual patients based on theoretical considerations and anecdotal evidence. Posaconazole is only available by mouth and takes several days to achieve adequate tissue levels; it should not be used as single agent in the critically ill neutropenic patient
Fusariosis [33, 37, 270]	Voriconazole 6 mg/kg IV every 12 h for 1 day, followed by 4 mg/kg IV every 12 h	L-AmB 3–5 mg/kg/day, or ABLC 5 mg/kg/day [271] or posaconazole 200 mg QID initially, then 400 mg BID PO after stabilization of disease [272]	Consider combination antifungal treatment adding caspofungin [273]; consider granulocyte transfusions
Trichosporonosis [270]	Voriconazole 6 mg/kg IV every 12 h for 1 day, followed by 4 mg/kg IV every 12 h [274, 275]	Fluconazole 800 mg IV (12 mg/kg) loading dose, then 400 mg (6 mg/kg) IV daily [276] or L-AmB 3–5 mg/kg/day or ABLC (5 mg/kg/day)	No in vivo comparison between fluconazole and voriconazole has been carried out; voriconazole may have better activity in vitro. Amphotericin failures are common

Scedosporiosis [270]			
Scedosporium apiospermium (*Pseudallescheria boydii*)	Voriconazole 6 mg/kg IV every 12 h for 1 day, followed by 4 mg/kg IV every 12 h [277, 278]	L-AmB 3–5 mg/kg/day, or ABLC 5 mg/kg/day	
Scedosporium prolificans			Medical therapy of nonresectable disseminated disease seems to be ineffective. Consider augmentation of the immune response with interferon gamma or GM-CSF
Dematiaceous molds [270]	Voriconazole 6 mg/kg IV every 12 h for 1 day, followed by 4 mg/kg IV every 12 h	Posaconazole 200 mg QID initially, then 400 mg BID PO or Itraconazole (dose depends on the formulation) or L-AmB 3–5 mg/kg/day, or ABLC 5 mg/kg/day	Triazoles are considered more effective than amphotericin B formulations

QID: four times a day; BID: twice a day. All forms of amphotericin B and all echinocandins are administered intravenously (IV) only. Fluconazole and voriconazole are available in oral (PO) and IV formulations. We believe IV administration should be preferred for these immunocompromised patients. Posaconazole is only available PO.

L-AmB liposomal amphotericin B, *AmBLF* lipid formulation of amphotericin B, *ABLC* amphotericin B lipid complex

Treatment of Established Fungal Infections

The critical elements of successful management of the invasive fungal infections complicating neutropenia are (1) early diagnosis, (2) initiation of aggressive pharmacologic treatment, (3) reversal of immunosuppression, including recovery from neutropenia, discontinuation or reduction of immunosuppressive agents such as corticosteroids, and administration of cytokines or granulocyte transfusions, and (4) when feasible, surgical resection of lesions.

Pharmacologic Treatment

A full review of antifungal agents as well as the specific issues regarding each possible pathogen are beyond the scope of this chapter. The reader should consult the appropriate chapters elsewhere in this textbook. We will focus on a few selected topics that pertain specifically to neutropenic hosts (Table 7).

Candidiasis

Of the different clinical presentations of candidiasis, chronic disseminated candidiasis (hepatosplenic candidiasis) should be briefly discussed because it is a specific manifestation of candidiasis in neutropenic patients. Clinical manifestations characteristically appear when neutropenia resolves. Most cases are caused by *C. albicans*, but *C. tropicalis*, *C. glabrata,* and *C. krusei* have also been reported [279, 280]. Several agents have been reported to be effective, including AmB-d [53, 280–282], lipid formulations of AmB [283], fluconazole, and caspofungin [284–286]. Generally, fluconazole is the agent of choice if the patient is clinically stable [287]. Duration seems to be the most important variable related to successful treatment. In a recent series of 23 leukemic patients, the median duration of antifungal therapy was 112 days (range 42–175 days) [280]. Very rarely, splenectomy may be required [288]. Due to the chronicity of this infection, a dilemma often occurs between treating the underlying neoplastic disease and the fungal infection, because of concern that immunosuppression could lead to progression of candidiasis or breakthrough candidemia. However, cancer chemotherapy can proceed despite the presence of active infection, as long as continuous antifungal treatment and careful monitoring are performed [281, 285, 289]. For example, among 17 patients treated for chronic disseminated candidiasis, all but 2 were treated for their neoplastic process without progressive disease [281]. Premature discontinuation of antifungal therapy during cancer chemotherapy was the likely cause of progressive chronic disseminated candidiasis in these two patients.

Aspergillosis

Voriconazole should be considered the treatment of choice for IA in neutropenic patients. The strongest evidence comes from a multicenter, open-label, randomized, clinical trial [34]. The investigators compared voriconazole, 6 mg/kg twice daily on day 1 of treatment, followed by 4 mg/kg twice daily IV for at least 7 days, after which time patients could switch to oral voriconazole, 200 mg twice daily with intravenous AmB-d, 1.0–1.5 mg/kg daily. Patients with intolerance or no response to therapy could be switched to "other licensed antifungal therapy," including lipid formulations, and continue to be included in the analysis. Only patients with probable or definite IA were included. Among the 391 patients who were randomized, results were the same whether analyzed by intention-to-treat or by the modified intention-to-treat population, which included 144 patients in the voriconazole group and 133 in the AmB-d group. The proportion of neutropenic patients was 45% in both groups. Voriconazole proved superior to AmB overall (successful outcome 49.7% vs 27.8%) and in almost every subgroup analysis. In the neutropenic patients, the success rate was 50.8% for voriconazole and 31.7% for AmB. Voriconazole had better survival rate at 12 weeks: (70.8% vs 57.9%), as well as fewer adverse events. The results of this trial were in agreement with a previously published observational study that had shown a response rate of 48% [290], with in vitro data [291], and with observations in animal models [292, 293]. Although we now consider voriconazole the agent of choice against aspergillosis in neutropenic patients, it must be pointed out that the overall satisfactory response rate is only approximately 50%. New strategies are clearly needed for the treatment of this disease.

The disappointing 27.8% response rate of AmB demonstrated in the aforementioned randomized trial [34] is within the range previously reported for this compound [30]. Although lipid formulations of AmB are less nephrotoxic than conventional AmB-d, the value of these agents in improving the response rate or overall survival rate in neutropenic patients with IA is unclear. Lipid formulations have been shown to be at least as effective as AmB-d in pulmonary aspergillosis in persistently neutropenic rabbits [294, 295] and in clinical studies [296]. Lipid formulations also have been useful in many cases as salvage therapy [264] and are appropriate for neutropenic patients who are intolerant of or refractory to voriconazole.

Itraconazole has been used for pulmonary aspergillosis, with an acceptable response rate of 48.5% in 31 immunocompromised patients, 60% of whom were neutropenic [297]. However, the discontinuation of the intravenous formulation of itraconazole and the availability of voriconazole has all but eliminated itraconazole as a viable alternative in neutropenic patients.

Surgical Management

Surgical intervention is frequently a critical component of the management of invasive fungal infections, particularly during neutropenia. Acute invasive fungal rhinosinusitis during neutropenia should be considered a surgical emergency and treated aggressively with extensive debridement and appropriate antifungal agents [60, 298]. Blood vessel invasion by the mould causes vascular thrombosis, tissue ischemia, and infarction of adjacent tissue. Rhinocerebral zygomycosis usually begins as an infection of the maxillary and ethmoid sinuses. Involvement of the ethmoid sinus may progress to invade the orbit, retro-orbital region, cavernous sinus, and brain. A similar clinical picture may be caused by *Aspergillus*, particularly *A. flavus*, and by *Fusarium*. Because the zygomycetes are not susceptible to voriconazole, treatment of rhinosinusitis in neutropenic patients should include high-dose lipid formulation AmB pending definitive identification of the pathogen. Although posaconazole has demonstrated clinical activity against some genera of the family, this drug takes at least 5 days to achieve adequate tissue levels and should not be used as first line of therapy during an emergency.

In the case of pulmonary infection, surgery has been used for both diagnosis and therapy, and several series have reported excellent results when early resection of localized pulmonary fungal lesions is performed [67, 299–302]. The goal of early surgery is to reduce the burden of disease and to prevent life-threatening hemoptysis. The indications for surgery for pulmonary IA include resection of lesions threatening the great vessels, involvement of pericardium or other mediastinal structures, hemoptysis from a large cavitary lesion, intractable pleuritic pain, and invasion of ribs and other chest wall structures. Generally, surgery may be indicated in *Aspergillus* osteomyelitis, CNS aspergillosis, sinusitis (particularly involving the ethmoid sinus), and primary cutaneous ulcerative aspergillosis.

Massive hemoptysis typically occurs during the recovery phase after chemotherapy, when the neutropenia has resolved and the platelet count is rising [303–306], and it is often fatal. Panos and colleagues found that aspergillosis was the most common cause of fatal hemoptysis in patients with acute leukemia [304]. Caillot and colleagues performed emergency surgery to prevent massive hemorrhage when the CT showed a fungal lesion that appeared to be contiguous to the pulmonary artery or its branches [67, 299]. The presence of multiple lesions, thrombocytopenia, and neutropenia are not contraindications for surgery in this setting. The most common procedure is lobectomy, plus segmentectomy and angioplasty if required. These investigators have reported an improved prognosis for their patients over the years after the introduction of this approach; 16 of 19 patients (84%) were considered cured in one of their reports [299].

Other groups [300–302, 307] have reported their experience with surgical management of fungal infections during neutropenia. Although the series are retrospective and relatively small, several conclusions can be drawn. First, surgery can be performed in compromised patients with IA. Surgical complications, including bronchial dehiscence, pleural contamination, and prolonged chest tube drainage, are significant, but the perioperative mortality rate is only 11–14%, and the overall survival rate compares favorably with series based exclusively on medical management. Second, experience is essential for favorable outcomes, and third, there is no clear consensus on the indications for surgery. When evaluating the surgical series, which report cure and survival rates apparently better than average (69–84% cure rate), it is necessary to be aware that patients who undergo surgery are not representative of all patients with IA. In their analysis of the 87 cases of IA seen between 1982 and 1995 at the Royal Free Hospital in London, Yeghen et al. found that the mere presence of at least one lesion with imaging suggestive of aspergillosis was associated with a better prognosis, irrespective of surgery [308].

Granulocyte Transfusions

Granulocyte transfusions may be useful for the treatment of fungal infections in neutropenic patients under certain conditions. The effectiveness of granulocyte transfusions in bacterial and fungal infections in neutropenic animal models was shown decades ago [309–311]. Several studies in neutropenic patients with infection during treatment for acute leukemia seemed to support the use of this intervention, either prophylactically or therapeutically [312–317]. Subsequently, however, its use declined during the 1980s because of questionable overall efficacy [318, 319] and the occurrence of cases of severe toxicity, in particular acute respiratory distress syndrome [320], Wright et al. reported severe reactions with acute dyspnea, hypoxemia, and interstitial infiltrates in 14 of 22 courses of granulocyte transfusions when AmB-d was administered at the same time as the granulocytes, but only in 2 of 35 courses when AmB-d was not given [320]. It was hypothesized that the AmB-d caused aggregation of neutrophils and enhanced pulmonary leukostasis [321]; however, these severe pulmonary reactions were not confirmed by other investigators [322], and in retrospect seem to be explained by a combination of diverse causes, predominantly alloimmunization and infection [323]. These reactions have seldom been observed in the more recent reports of granulocyte transfusions, although most investigators recommend separating in time the administration of granulocytes and any form of AmB.

Several critical reviews and meta-analyses of the initial reports have been published [324–326], and they conclude that granulocyte transfusions have demonstrated efficacy in the treatment of uncontrolled bacterial infections during persistent neutropenia. The data on fungal infections are less conclusive, mainly because of a smaller number of patients treated, as well as the presence of confounding factors. The technical advances of the last 15 years, in particular the use of G-CSF to mobilize granulocytes and the use of continuous flow apheresis techniques for harvesting the cells, offer the promise of 2–10 times more neutrophils than were obtained with corticosteroids alone in the past [327–329], which could yield potentially higher efficacy.

Reflecting the renewed interest in granulocyte transfusions, several case series or phase I/II clinical trials of neutropenic patients treated with GCSF-mobilized granulocytes [330–334] and a randomized controlled trial [335] have been published in the last decade. As anticipated, the combination of G-CSF plus dexamethasone resulted in higher yields than either agent alone. The leukocyte concentrates used in these studies contained $\geq 10^{10}$ neutrophils. Transfused neutrophils have persisted in the circulation with sustained increases in the ANC for up to 24 h, and a cumulative effect of repeated transfusions on the ANC has been documented. The correlation between the administered dose and the increase in ANC has been poor, although in general doses $>2 \times 10^9$/kg have been associated with increments of the ANC $>2 \times 10^3$/μL [332].

There are several case reports in which granulocyte transfusions seem to have been life-saving during fungal infection, both in neutropenic patients [336–339] and in others with abnormal neutrophil function, such as chronic granulomatous disease [340]. The study by Dignani et al. of 15 neutropenic patients with refractory invasive fungal infection showed that 11 had favorable responses, probably due to the high neutrophil dose, which elicited a mean increase of the ANC in the recipients of 396/μL 24 h after the transfusion [330].

Granulocyte transfusions may be life saving when given to the appropriate hosts. At the NIH Clinical Center we have used them selectively. The general requirements include fungal infection unresponsive to optimal medical therapy, neutropenia that is bound to persist for more than 4 or 5 days, and reasonable chance of ultimate bone marrow function recovery. The only prophylactic indication we consider is for patients with previously documented invasive fungal infections who are to undergo profound, prolonged neutropenia. As a significant fraction of our neutropenic patients with fungal infection exhibit some degree of respiratory compromise, careful monitoring and adjustment of the rates and doses of granulocytes are warranted.

Recombinant Human Cytokines in the Management of Established Fungal Infections in Neutropenic Patients

The preceding discussion has emphasized the importance of neutrophil recovery to control invasive fungal infections in neutropenic patients. From this standpoint, it is logical to recommend the use of agents that have been shown in controlled trials to decrease the duration of neutropenia, even if their documented effect on clinically significant outcomes is unclear. The American Society for Clinical Oncology recently updated its recommendations for the use of hematopoietic colony-stimulating factors [341]. Although two meta-analyses suggest that the overall outcome of fever and neutropenia is not significantly changed by the use of colony-stimulating factors [342, 343], the consensus is that they should be considered for high-risk patients, including those with ANC <100/μL, uncontrolled primary disease, pneumonia, hypotension, sepsis syndrome, and invasive fungal infection. We would strongly recommend the administration of recombinant G-CSF or GM-CSF to persistently neutropenic patients who have a proven invasive fungal infection.

Both G-CSF and GM-CSF accelerate myelopoiesis and decrease the duration of neutropenia, but they are different cytokines with different targets and immunomodulatory effects. (For a review of the comparison and potential use as adjuvant therapy of fungal infections in nonneutropenic hosts, see the review by Root and Dale [344]). G-CSF, GM-CSF, and M-CSF have been shown to increase the fungicidal action of phagocytes against *Candida* and *Aspergillus* in a variety of experimental systems, both in vitro and ex vivo [345–347]. GM-CSF also prevents dexamethasone suppression of killing of *A. fumigatus* conidia by bronchoalveolar and peritoneal macrophages in mice [346, 348, 349]. Interferon gamma may be superior at enhancing the antifungal activity of phagocytes [345, 350].

There is some evidence that Th1 immune responses may be necessary for the optimal control of fungal infections [351, 352]. In this regard, immune interventions to polarize the immune response toward a Th1 type may be beneficial. Two of the main cytokines involved in this kind of response are IL-12 and interferon-gamma, and it has been shown in animal models that the administration of interferon-gamma had some protective effect in BALB/c mice challenged with *Aspergillus* conidia [353]. Evidence of a Th1/Th2 dysimmunoregulation in hepatosplenic candidiasis [354] and IA [355], characterized by increased circulating levels of IL-10, has been demonstrated in humans. These patterns of cytokine dysregulation provide a rationale for use of GM-CSF and interferon-gamma alone or in combination for adjunctive treatment of persistent or progressive invasive fungal infections.

References

1. Bodey GP. Fungal infections complicating acute leukemia. J Chronic Dis. 1966;19:667–87.
2. Bodey G, Bueltmann B, Duguid W, et al. Fungal infections in cancer patients: an international autopsy survey. Eur J Clin Microbiol Infect Dis. 1992;11:99–109.
3. Chamilos G, Luna M, Lewis RE, et al. Invasive fungal infections in patients with hematologic malignancies in a tertiary care cancer center: an autopsy study over a 15-year period (1989-2003). Haematologica. 2006;91:986–9.
4. Larbcharoensub N, Srisuma S, Ngernprasertsri T, et al. Invasive fungal infection in Ramathibodi hospital: a ten-year autopsy review. J Med Assoc Thai. 2007;90:2630–7.
5. Donhuijsen K, Petersen P, Schmid WK. Trend reversal in the frequency of mycoses in hematological neoplasias: autopsy results from 1976 to 2005. Dtsch Arztebl Int. 2008;105:501–6.
6. Jandrlic M, Kalenic S, Labar B, et al. An autopsy study of systemic fungal infections in patients with hematologic malignancies. Eur J Clin Microbiol Infect Dis. 1995;14:768–74.
7. Sinko J, Csomor J, Nikolova R, et al. Invasive fungal disease in allogeneic hematopoietic stem cell transplant recipients: an autopsy-driven survey. Transpl Infect Dis. 2008;10:106–9.
8. Krick JA, Remington JS. Opportunistic invasive fungal infections in patients with leukaemia lymphoma. Clin Haematol. 1976; 5:249–310.
9. Fraser DW, Ward JI, Ajello L, Plikaytis BD. Aspergillosis and other systemic mycoses. The growing problem. JAMA. 1979;242:1631–5.
10. Boogaerts M, Winston DJ, Bow EJ, et al. Intravenous and oral itraconazole versus intravenous amphotericin B deoxycholate as empirical antifungal therapy for persistent fever in neutropenic patients with cancer who are receiving broad-spectrum antibacterial therapy. A randomized, controlled trial. Ann Intern Med. 2001;135:412–22.
11. Winston DJ, Hathorn JW, Schuster MG, Schiller GJ, Territo MC. A multicenter, randomized trial of fluconazole versus amphotericin B for empiric antifungal therapy of febrile neutropenic patients with cancer. Am J Med. 2000;108:282–9.
12. Walsh TJ, Pappas P, Winston DJ, et al. Voriconazole compared with liposomal amphotericin B for empirical antifungal therapy in patients with neutropenia and persistent fever. N Engl J Med. 2002;346:225–34.
13. Walsh TJ, Teppler H, Donowitz GR, et al. Caspofungin versus liposomal amphotericin B for empirical antifungal therapy in patients with persistent fever and neutropenia. N Engl J Med. 2004;351:1391–402.
14. Ascioglu S, Rex JH, de Pauw B, et al. Defining opportunistic invasive fungal infections in immunocompromised patients with cancer and hematopoietic stem cell transplants: an international consensus. Clin Infect Dis. 2002;34:7–14.
15. De Pauw B, Walsh TJ, Donnelly JP, et al. Revised definitions of invasive fungal disease from the european organization for research and treatment of cancer/invasive fungal infections Cooperative Group and the National Institute of Allergy and Infectious Diseases Mycoses Study Group (EORTC/MSG) Consensus Group. Clin Infect Dis. 2008;46:1813–21.
16. Walsh TJ, Hiemenz J, Pizzo PA. Evolving risk factors for invasive fungal infections – all neutropenic patients are not the same. Clin Infect Dis. 1994;18:793–8.
17. Prentice HG, Kibbler CC, Prentice AG. Towards a targeted, risk-based, antifungal strategy in neutropenic patients. Br J Haematol. 2000;110:273–84.
18. Walsh TJ, Finberg RW, Arndt C, et al. Liposomal amphotericin B for empirical therapy in patients with persistent fever and neutropenia. N Engl J Med. 1999;340:764–71.
19. Martino R, Subira M, Rovira M, et al. Invasive fungal infections after allogeneic peripheral blood stem cell transplantation: incidence and risk factors in 395 patients. Br J Haematol. 2002;116:475–82.
20. Winston DJ, Maziarz RT, Chandrasekar PH, et al. Intravenous and oral itraconazole versus intravenous and oral fluconazole for long-term antifungal prophylaxis in allogeneic hematopoietic stem-cell transplant recipients. A multicenter, randomized trial. Ann Intern Med. 2003;138:705–13.
21. van Burik JA, Ratanatharathorn V, Stepan DE, et al. Micafungin versus fluconazole for prophylaxis against invasive fungal infections during neutropenia in patients undergoing hematopoietic stem cell transplantation. Clin Infect Dis. 2004;39:1407–16.
22. Marr KA, Crippa F, Leisenring W, et al. Itraconazole versus fluconazole for prevention of fungal infections in patients receiving allogeneic stem cell transplants. Blood. 2004;103:1527–33.
23. Cornely OA, Maertens J, Winston DJ, et al. Posaconazole vs. fluconazole or itraconazole prophylaxis in patients with neutropenia. N Engl J Med. 2007;356:348–59.
24. Abbas J, Bodey GP, Hanna HA, et al. *Candida krusei* fungemia. An escalating serious infection in immunocompromised patients. Arch Intern Med. 2000;160:2659–64.
25. Bodey GP, Mardani M, Hanna HA, et al. The epidemiology of *Candida glabrata* and *Candida albicans* fungemia in immunocompromised patients with cancer. Am J Med. 2002;112:380–5.
26. Pfaller MA, Diekema DJ, Gibbs DL, et al. Results from the ARTEMIS DISK Global Antifungal Surveillance study, 1997 to 2005: an 8.5-year analysis of susceptibilities of *Candida* species and other yeast species to fluconazole and voriconazole determined by CLSI standardized disk diffusion testing. J Clin Microbiol. 2007;45:1735–45.
27. Safdar A, van Rhee F, Henslee-Downey JP, Singhal S, Mehta J. *Candida glabrata* and *Candida krusei* fungemia after high-risk allogeneic marrow transplantation: no adverse effect of low-dose fluconazole prophylaxis on incidence and outcome. Bone Marrow Transplant. 2001;28:873–8.
28. Hachem R, Hanna H, Kontoyiannis D, Jiang Y, Raad I. The changing epidemiology of invasive candidiasis: *Candida glabrata* and *Candida krusei* as the leading causes of candidemia in hematologic malignancy. Cancer. 2008;112:2493–9.
29. Horn DL, Neofytos D, Anaissie EJ, et al. Epidemiology and outcomes of candidemia in 2019 patients: data from the prospective antifungal therapy alliance registry. Clin Infect Dis. 2009;48:1695–703.
30. Patterson TF, Kirkpatrick WR, White M, et al. Invasive aspergillosis. Disease spectrum, treatment practices, and outcomes. Medicine. 2000;79:250–60.
31. Marr KA, Carter RA, Crippa F, Wald A, Corey L. Epidemiology and outcome of mould infections in hematopoietic stem cell transplant recipients. Clin Infect Dis. 2002;34:909–17.
32. Upton A, Kirby KA, Carpenter P, Boeckh M, Marr KA. Invasive aspergillosis following hematopoietic cell transplantation: outcomes and prognostic factors associated with mortality. Clin Infect Dis. 2007;44:531–40.
33. Nucci M, Marr KA, Queiroz-Telles F, et al. *Fusarium* infection in hematopoietic stem cell transplant recipients. Clin Infect Dis. 2004;38:1237–42.
34. Herbrecht R, Denning DW, Patterson TF, et al. Voriconazole versus amphotericin B for primary therapy of invasive aspergillosis. N Engl J Med. 2002;347:408–15.
35. Mora-Duarte J, Betts R, Rotstein C, et al. Comparison of caspofungin and amphotericin B for invasive candidiasis. N Engl J Med. 2002;347:2020–9.

36. Kuse ER, Chetchotisakd P, da Cunha CA, et al. Micafungin versus liposomal amphotericin B for candidaemia and invasive candidosis: a phase III randomised double-blind trial. Lancet. 2007;369:1519–27.
37. Kontoyiannis DP, Bodey GP, Hanna H, et al. Outcome determinants of fusariosis in a tertiary care cancer center: the impact of neutrophil recovery. Leuk Lymphoma. 2004;45:139–41.
38. Bodey GP, Buckley M, Sathe YS, Freireich EJ. Quantitative relationships between circulating leukocytes and infection in patients with acute leukemia. Ann Intern Med. 1966;64:328–40.
39. Gerson SL, Talbot GH, Hurwitz S, Strom BL, Lusk EJ, Cassileth PA. Prolonged granulocytopenia: the major risk factor for invasive pulmonary aspergillosis in patients with acute leukemia. Ann Intern Med. 1984;100:345–51.
40. Uzun O, Ascioglu S, Anaissie EJ, Rex JH. Risk factors and predictors of outcome in patients with cancer and breakthrough candidemia. Clin Infect Dis. 2001;32:1713–7.
41. Rex JH, Anaissie EJ, Boutati E, Estey E, Kantarjian H. Systemic antifungal prophylaxis reduces invasive fungal in acute myelogenous leukemia: a retrospective review of 833 episodes of neutropenia in 322 adults. Leukemia. 2002;16:1197–9.
42. Bow EJ, Shore TB, Kilpatrick MG, Scott BA, Schacter B. Relationship of invasive fungal disease and high-dose cytarabine plus etoposide containing remission-induction regimens for acute myeloid leukemia. Blood. 1991;78(suppl):55A.
43. Schwartz RS, Mackintosh FR, Schrier SL, Greenberg PL. Multivariate analysis of factors associated with invasive fungal disease during remission induction therapy for acute myelogenous leukemia. Cancer. 1984;53:411–9.
44. Guiot HF, Fibbe WE, van't Wout JW. Risk factors for fungal infection in patients with malignant hematologic disorders: implications for empirical therapy and prophylaxis. Clin Infect Dis. 1994;18:525–32.
45. Gualtieri RJ, Donowitz GR, Kaiser DL, Hess CE, Sande MA. Double-blind randomized study of prophylactic trimethoprim/sulfamethoxazole in granulocytopenic patients with hematologic malignancies. Am J Med. 1983;74:934–40.
46. Denning DW, Marinus A, Cohen J, et al. An EORTC multicentre prospective survey of invasive aspergillosis in haematological patients: diagnosis and therapeutic outcome. EORTC Invasive Fungal Infections Cooperative Group. J Infect. 1998;37:173–80.
47. Walsh TJ, Pizzo PA. Experimental gastrointestinal and disseminated candidiasis in immunocompromised animals. Eur J Epidemiol. 1992;8:477–83.
48. Schaffner A, Schaffner T. Glucocorticoid-induced impairment of macrophage antimicrobial activity: mechanisms and dependence on the state of activation. Rev Infect Dis. 1987;9 Suppl 5:S620–9.
49. Ribaud P, Chastang C, Latge JP, et al. Survival and prognostic factors of invasive aspergillosis after allogeneic bone marrow transplantation. Clin Infect Dis. 1999;28:322–30.
50. Chim CS, Liang R, Wong SS, Yuen KY. Cryptococcal infection associated with fludarabine therapy. Am J Med. 2000;108:523–4.
51. Arena FP, Perlin M, Brahman H, Weiser B, Armstrong D. Fever, rash, and myalgias of dissseminated candidiasis during antifungal therapy. Arch Intern Med. 1981;141:1233.
52. Kontoyiannis DP, Luna MA, Samuels BI, Bodey GP. Hepatosplenic candidiasis. A manifestation of chronic disseminated candidiasis. Infect Dis Clin North Am. 2000;14:721–39.
53. Thaler M, Pastakia B, Shawker TH, O'Leary T, Pizzo PA. Hepatic candidiasis in cancer patients: the evolving picture of the syndrome. Ann Intern Med. 1988;108:88–100.
54. Sallah S, Semelka R, Kelekis N, Worawattanakul S, Sallah W. Diagnosis and monitoring response to treatment of hepatosplenic candidiasis in patients with acute leukemia using magnetic resonance imaging. Acta Haematol. 1998;100:77–81.
55. Walsh TJ, Dixon DM. Nosocomial aspergillosis: environmental microbiology, hospital epidemiology, diagnosis and treatment. Eur J Epidemiol. 1989;5:131–42.
56. Denning DW, Stevens DA. Antifungal and surgical treatment of invasive aspergillosis: review of 2, 121 published cases. Rev Infect Dis. 1990;12:1147–201.
57. Berenguer J, Allende MC, Lee JW, et al. Pathogenesis of pulmonary aspergillosis. Granulocytopenia versus cyclosporine and methylprednisolone-induced immunosuppression. Am J Respir Crit Care Med. 1995;152:1079–86.
58. Gerson SL, Talbot GH, Lusk E, Hurwitz S, Strom BL, Cassileth PA. Invasive pulmonary aspergillosis in adult acute leukemia: clinical clues to its diagnosis. J Clin Oncol. 1985;3:1109–16.
59. Gerson SL, Talbot GH, Hurwitz S, Lusk EJ, Strom BL, Cassileth PA. Discriminant scorecard for diagnosis of invasive pulmonary aspergillosis in patients with acute leukemia. Am J Med. 1985;79:57–64.
60. Drakos PE, Nagler A, Or R, et al. Invasive fungal sinusitis in patients undergoing bone marrow transplantation. Bone Marrow Transplant. 1993;12:203–8.
61. Talbot GH, Huang A, Provencher M. Invasive *aspergillus* rhinosinusitis in patients with acute leukemia. Rev Infect Dis. 1991;13:219–32.
62. Aquino SL, Kee ST, Warnock ML, Gamsu G. Pulmonary aspergillosis: imaging findings with pathologic correlation. AJR Am J Roentgenol. 1994;163:811–5.
63. Caillot D, Couaillier JF, Bernard A, et al. Increasing volume and changing characteristics of invasive pulmonary aspergillosis on sequential thoracic computed tomography scans in patients with neutropenia. J Clin Oncol. 2001;19:253–9.
64. Hruban RH, Meziane MA, Zerhouni EA, Wheeler PS, Dumler JS, Hutchins GM. Radiologic-pathologic correlation of the CT halo sign in invasive pulmonary aspergillosis. J Comput Assist Tomogr. 1987;11:534–6.
65. Kuhlman JE, Fishman EK, Siegelman SS. Invasive pulmonary aspergillosis in acute leukemia: characteristic findings on CT, the CT halo sign, and the role of CT in early diagnosis. Radiology. 1985;157:611–4.
66. Orr DP, Myerowitz RL, Dubois PJ. Patho-radiologic correlation of invasive pulmonary aspergillosis in the compromised host. Cancer. 1978;41:2028–39.
67. Caillot D, Casasnovas O, Bernard A, et al. Improved management of invasive pulmonary aspergillosis in neutropenic patients using early thoracic computed tomographic scan and surgery. J Clin Oncol. 1997;15:139–47.
68. Caillot D, Mannone L, Cuisenier B, Couaillier JF. Role of early diagnosis and aggressive surgery in the management of invasive pulmonary aspergillosis in neutropenic patients. Clin Microbiol Infect. 2001;7 Suppl 2:54–61.
69. Walsh TJ, Garrett K, Feurerstein E, et al. Therapeutic monitoring of experimental invasive pulmonary aspergillosis by ultrafast computerized tomography, a novel, noninvasive method for measuring responses to antifungal therapy. Antimicrob Agents Chemother. 1995;39:1065–9.
70. Curtis AM, Smith GJ, Ravin CE. Air crescent sign of invasive aspergillosis. Radiology. 1979;133:17–21.
71. Slevin ML, Knowles GK, Phillips MJ, Stansfeld AG, Lister TA. The air crescent sign of invasive pulmonary aspergillosis in acute leukaemia. Thorax. 1982;37:554–5.
72. Aisner J, Wiernik PH, Schimpff SC. Treatment of invasive aspergillosis: relation of early diagnosis and treatment to response. Ann Intern Med. 1977;86:539–43.
73. Walsh TJ, Hier DB, Caplan LR. Aspergillosis of the central nervous system: clinicopathological analysis of 17 patients. Ann Neurol. 1985;18:574–82.
74. Yamada K, Shrier DA, Rubio A, et al. Imaging findings in intracranial aspergillosis. Acad Radiol. 2002;9:163–71.
75. DeLone DR, Goldstein RA, Petermann G, et al. Disseminated aspergillosis involving the brain: distribution and imaging characteristics. AJNR Am J Neuroradiol. 1999;20:1597–604.

76. Dietrich U, Hettmann M, Maschke M, Doerfler A, Schwechheimer K, Forsting M. Cerebral aspergillosis: comparison of radiological and neuropathologic findings in patients with bone marrow transplantation. Eur Radiol. 2001;11:1242–9.
77. Anaissie E, Kantarjian H, Ro J, et al. The emerging role of *Fusarium* infections in patients with cancer. Medicine. 1988;67:77–83.
78. Anaissie E, Kantarjian H, Jones P, et al. *Fusarium*. A newly recognized fungal pathogen in immunosuppressed patients. Cancer. 1986;57:2141–5.
79. Boutati EI, Anaissie EJ. *Fusarium*, a significant emerging pathogen in patients with hematologic malignancy: ten years' experience at a cancer center and implications for management. Blood. 1997;90:999–1008.
80. Martino P, Gastaldi R, Raccah R, Girmenia C. Clinical patterns of *Fusarium* infections in immunocompromised patients. J Infect. 1994;28 Suppl 1:7–15.
81. Segal BH, Walsh TJ, Liu JM, Wilson JD, Kwon-Chung KJ. Invasive infection with *Fusarium chlamydosporum* in a patient with aplastic anemia. J Clin Microbiol. 1998;36:1772–6.
82. Nucci M, Anaissie E. Cutaneous infection by *Fusarium* species in healthy and immunocompromised hosts: implications for diagnosis and management. Clin Infect Dis. 2002;35:909–20.
83. Berenguer J, Rodriguez-Tudela JL, Richard C, et al. Deep infections caused by *Scedosporium prolificans*. A report on 16 cases in Spain and a review of the literature. *Scedosporium prolificans* Spanish Study Group. Medicine. 1997;76:256–65.
84. Travis LB, Roberts GD, Wilson WR. Clinical significance of *Pseudallescheria boydii*: a review of 10 years' experience. Mayo Clin Proc. 1985;60:531–7.
85. Walsh TJ, Peter J, McGough DA, Fothergill AW, Rinaldi MG, Pizzo PA. Activities of amphotericin B and antifungal azoles alone and in combination against *Pseudallescheria boydii*. Antimicrob Agents Chemother. 1995;39:1361–4.
86. Groll AH, Walsh TJ. Uncommon opportunistic fungi: new nosocomial threats. Clin Microbiol Infect. 2001;7 Suppl 2:8–24.
87. Jabado N, Casanova JL, Haddad E, et al. Invasive pulmonary infection due to *Scedosporium apiospermum* in two children with chronic granulomatous disease. Clin Infect Dis. 1998; 27:1437–41.
88. Walsh TJ, Groll AH. Emerging fungal pathogens: evolving challenges to immunocompromised patients for the twenty-first century. Transpl Infect Dis. 1999;1:247–61.
89. Yoo D, Lee WH, Kwon-Chung KJ. Brain abscesses due to *Pseudallescheria boydii* associated with primary non-Hodgkin's lymphoma of the central nervous system: a case report and literature review. Rev Infect Dis. 1985;7:272–7.
90. Nguyen BD. Pseudallescheriasis of the lung and central nervous system: multimodality imaging. AJR Am J Roentgenol. 2001;176:257–8.
91. Pagano L, Ricci P, Tonso A, et al. Mucormycosis in patients with haematological malignancies: a retrospective clinical study of 37 cases. GIMEMA Infection Program (Gruppo Italiano Malattie Ematologiche Maligne dell'Adulto). Br J Haematol. 1997;99:331–6.
92. Maertens J, Demuynck H, Verbeken EK, et al. Mucormycosis in allogeneic bone marrow transplant recipients: report of five cases and review of the role of iron overload in the pathogenesis. Bone Marrow Transplant. 1999;24:307–12.
93. Kontoyiannis DP, Wessel VC, Bodey GP, Rolston KV. Zygomycosis in the 1990s in a tertiary-care cancer center. Clin Infect Dis. 2000;30:851–6.
94. Herbrecht R, Letscher-Bru V, Bowden RA, et al. Treatment of 21 cases of invasive mucormycosis with amphotericin B colloidal dispersion. Eur J Clin Microbiol Infect Dis. 2001;20:460–6.
95. Roden MM, Zaoutis TE, Buchanan WL, et al. Epidemiology and outcome of zygomycosis: a review of 929 reported cases. Clin Infect Dis. 2005;41:634–53.
96. Sugar AM. Mucormycosis. Clin Infect Dis. 1992;14 Suppl 1:S126–9.
97. Wirth F, Perry R, Eskenazi A, Schwalbe R, Kao G. Cutaneous mucormycosis with subsequent visceral dissemination in a child with neutropenia: a case report and review of the pediatric literature. J Am Acad Dermatol. 1997;36:336–41.
98. Walsh TJ, Newman KR, Moody M, Wharton RC, Wade JC. Trichosporonosis in patients with neoplastic disease. Medicine. 1986;65:268–79.
99. Hoy J, Hsu KC, Rolston K, Hopfer RL, Luna M, Bodey GP. *Trichosporon beigelii* infection: a review. Rev Infect Dis. 1986;8:959–67.
100. Goldberg PK, Kozinn PJ, Wise GJ, Nouri N, Brooks RB. Incidence and significance of candiduria. JAMA. 1979;241:582–4.
101. Lundstrom T, Sobel J. Nosocomial candiduria: a review. Clin Infect Dis. 2001;32:1602–7.
102. Navarro EE, Almario JS, Schaufele RL, Bacher J, Walsh TJ. Quantitative urine cultures do not reliably detect renal candidiasis in rabbits. J Clin Microbiol. 1997;35:3292–7.
103. Samonis G, Anatoliotaki M, Apostolakou H, Maraki S, Mavroudis D, Georgoulias V. Transient fungemia due to *Rhodotorula rubra* in a cancer patient: case report and review of the literature. Infection. 2001;29:173–6.
104. Rusthoven JJ, Feld R, Tuffnell PG. Systemic infection by *Rhodotorula* spp in the immunocompromised host J Infect. 1984;8:241–6.
105. Dankner WM, Spector SA, Fierer J, Davis CE. *Malassezia* fungemia in neonates and adults: complication of hyperalimentation. Rev Infect Dis. 1987;9:743–53.
106. Lecciones JA, Lee JW, Navarro EE, et al. Vascular catheter-associated fungemia in patients with cancer: analysis of 155 episodes. Clin Infect Dis. 1992;14:875–83.
107. Nucci M, Anaissie E. Should vascular catheters be removed from all patients with candidemia? An evidence-based review. Clin Infect Dis. 2002;34:591–9.
108. Walsh TJ, Bustamente CI, Vlahov D, Standiford HC. Candidal suppurative peripheral thrombophlebitis: recognition, prevention, and management. Infect Control. 1986;7:16–22.
109. Berenguer J, Buck M, Witebsky F, Stock F, Pizzo PA, Walsh TJ. Lysis-centrifugation blood cultures in the detection of tissue-proven invasive candidiasis. Disseminated versus single-organ infection. Diagn Microbiol Infect Dis. 1993;17:103–9.
110. Masterson KC, McGowan Jr JE. Detection of positive blood cultures by the Bactec NR660. The clinical importance of five versus seven days of testing. Am J Clin Pathol. 1988;90:91–4.
111. Varettas K, Taylor PC, Mukerjee C. Determination of the optimum incubation period of continuously monitored blood cultures from patients with suspected endocarditis or fungaemia. Pathology. 2002;34:167–9.
112. Archibald LK, McDonald LC, Addison RM, et al. Comparison of BACTEC MYCO/F LYTIC and WAMPOLE ISOLATOR 10 (lysis-centrifugation) systems for detection of bacteremia, mycobacteremia, and fungemia in a developing country. J Clin Microbiol. 2000;38:2994–7.
113. Creger RJ, Weeman KE, Jacobs MR, et al. Lack of utility of the lysis-centrifugation blood culture method for detection of fungemia in immunocompromised cancer patients. J Clin Microbiol. 1998;36:290–3.
114. Yoshida M, Obayashi T, Iwama A, et al. Detection of plasma (1 –>3)-beta-D-glucan in patients with *Fusarium, Trichosporon, Saccharomyces* and *Acremonium* fungaemias. J Med Vet Mycol. 1997;35:371–4.
115. Obayashi T, Negishi K, Suzuki T, Funata N. Reappraisal of the serum (1–>3)-beta-D-glucan assay for the diagnosis of invasive fungal infections – a study based on autopsy cases from 6 years. Clin Infect Dis. 2008;46:1864–70.

116. Mennink-Kersten MA, Warris A, Verweij PE. 1, 3-beta-D-glucan in patients receiving intravenous amoxicillin-clavulanic acid. N Engl J Med. 2006;354:2834–5.
117. Kanamori H, Kanemitsu K, Miyasaka T, et al. Measurement of (1-3)-beta-D-glucan derived from different gauze types. Tohoku J Exp Med. 2009;217:117–21.
118. Kato A, Takita T, Furuhashi M, Takahashi T, Maruyama Y, Hishida A. Elevation of blood (1–>3)-beta-D-glucan concentrations in hemodialysis patients. Nephron. 2001;89:15–9.
119. Usami M, Ohata A, Horiuchi T, Nagasawa K, Wakabayashi T, Tanaka S. Positive (1–>3)-beta-D-glucan in blood components and release of (1–>3)-beta-D-glucan from depth-type membrane filters for blood processing. Transfusion. 2002;42:1189–95.
120. Ogawa M, Hori H, Niiguchi S, Azuma E, Komada Y. False-positive plasma (1–>3)-beta-D-glucan test following immunoglobulin product replacement in an adult bone marrow recipient. Int J Hematol. 2004;80:97–8.
121. Mennink-Kersten MA, Ruegebrink D, Verweij PE. *Pseudomonas aeruginosa* as a cause of 1, 3-beta-D-glucan assay reactivity. Clin Infect Dis. 2008;46:1930–1.
122. Pickering JW, Sant HW, Bowles CA, Roberts WL, Woods GL. Evaluation of a (1->3)-beta-D-glucan assay for diagnosis of invasive fungal infections. J Clin Microbiol. 2005;43:5957–62.
123. Odabasi Z, Mattiuzzi G, Estey E, et al. Beta-D-glucan as a diagnostic adjunct for invasive fungal infections: validation, cutoff development, and performance in patients with acute myelogenous leukemia and myelodysplastic syndrome. Clin Infect Dis. 2004;39:199–205. Epub 2004 Jun 28.
124. Ostrosky-Zeichner L, Alexander BD, Kett DH, et al. Multicenter clinical evaluation of the (1–>3) beta-D-glucan assay as an aid to diagnosis of fungal infections in humans. Clin Infect Dis. 2005;41:654–9.
125. Kawazu M, Kanda Y, Nannya Y, et al. Prospective comparison of the diagnostic potential of real-time PCR, double-sandwich enzyme-linked immunosorbent assay for galactomannan, and a (1–>3)-beta-D-glucan test in weekly screening for invasive aspergillosis in patients with hematological disorders. J Clin Microbiol. 2004;42:2733–41.
126. Pazos C, Ponton J, Del Palacio A. Contribution of (1->3)-beta-D-glucan chromogenic assay to diagnosis and therapeutic monitoring of invasive aspergillosis in neutropenic adult patients: a comparison with serial screening for circulating galactomannan. J Clin Microbiol. 2005;43:299–305.
127. Senn L, Robinson JO, Schmidt S, et al. 1, 3-Beta-D-glucan antigenemia for early diagnosis of invasive fungal infections in neutropenic patients with acute leukemia. Clin Infect Dis. 2008;46:878–85.
128. Hachem RY, Kontoyiannis DP, Chemaly RF, Jiang Y, Reitzel R, Raad I. Utility of galactomannan enzyme immunoassay and (1, 3) beta-D-glucan in diagnosis of invasive fungal infections: low sensitivity for *Aspergillus fumigatus* infection in hematologic malignancy patients. J Clin Microbiol. 2009;47:129–33.
129. McMullan R, Metwally L, Coyle PV, et al. A prospective clinical trial of a real-time polymerase chain reaction assay for the diagnosis of candidemia in nonneutropenic, critically ill adults. Clin Infect Dis. 2008;46:890–6.
130. White PL, Shetty A, Barnes RA. Detection of seven *Candida* species using the Light-Cycler system. J Med Microbiol. 2003;52:229–38.
131. Bennett J. Is real-time polymerase chain reaction ready for real use in detecting candidemia? Clin Infect Dis. 2008;46:897–8.
132. Rinaldi MG. Invasive aspergillosis. Rev Infect Dis. 1983;5:1061–77.
133. Aisner J, Murillo J, Schimpff SC, Steere AC. Invasive aspergillosis in acute leukemia: correlation with nose cultures and antibiotic use. Ann Intern Med. 1979;90:4–9.
134. Yu VL, Muder RR, Poorsattar A. Significance of isolation of *Aspergillus* from the respiratory tract in diagnosis of invasive pulmonary aspergillosis. Results from a three- year prospective study. Am J Med. 1986;81:249–54.
135. Treger TR, Visscher DW, Bartlett MS, Smith JW. Diagnosis of pulmonary infection caused by *Aspergillus*: usefulness of respiratory cultures. J Infect Dis. 1985;152:572–6.
136. Reichenberger F, Habicht J, Matt P, et al. Diagnostic yield of bronchoscopy in histologically proven invasive pulmonary aspergillosis. Bone Marrow Transplant. 1999;24:1195–9.
137. Verea-Hernando H, Martin-Egana MT, Montero-Martinez C, Fontan-Bueso J. Bronchoscopy findings in invasive pulmonary aspergillosis. Thorax. 1989;44:822–3.
138. Albelda SM, Talbot GH, Gerson SL, Miller WT, Cassileth PA. Role of fiberoptic bronchoscopy in the diagnosis of invasive pulmonary aspergillosis in patients with acute leukemia. Am J Med. 1984;76:1027–34.
139. Kahn FW, Jones JM, England DM. The role of bronchoalveolar lavage in the diagnosis of invasive pulmonary aspergillosis. Am J Clin Pathol. 1986;86:518–23.
140. Jantunen E, Piilonen A, Volin L, et al. Radiologically guided fine needle lung biopsies in the evaluation of focal pulmonary lesions in allogeneic stem cell transplant recipients. Bone Marrow Transplant. 2002;29:353–6.
141. Jantunen E, Piilonen A, Volin L, et al. Diagnostic aspects of invasive *Aspergillus* infections in allogeneic BMT recipients. Bone Marrow Transplant. 2000;25:867–71.
142. Tikkakoski T, Lohela P, Paivansalo M, Kerola T. Pleuro-pulmonary aspergillosis. US and US-guided biopsy as an aid to diagnosis. Acta Radiol. 1995;36:122–6.
143. Reiss E, Lehmann PF. Galactomannan antigenemia in invasive aspergillosis. Infect Immun. 1979;25:357–65.
144. Lehmann PF, Reiss E. Invasive aspergillosis: antiserum for circulating antigen produced after immunization with serum from infected rabbits. Infect Immun. 1978;20:570–2.
145. Dupont B, Huber M, Kim SJ, Bennett JE. Galactomannan antigenemia and antigenuria in aspergillosis: studies in patients and experimentally infected rabbits. J Infect Dis. 1987;155:1–11.
146. Wheat LJ, Walsh TJ. Diagnosis of invasive aspergillosis by galactomannan antigenemia detection using an enzyme immunoassay. Eur J Clin Microbiol Infect Dis. 2008;27:245–51.
147. Bretagne S, Marmorat-Khuong A, Kuentz M, Latge JP, Bart-Delabesse E, Cordonnier C. Serum *Aspergillus* galactomannan antigen testing by sandwich ELISA: practical use in neutropenic patients. J Infect. 1997;35:7–15.
148. Maertens J, Verhaegen J, Demuynck H, et al. Autopsy-controlled prospective evaluation of serial screening for circulating galactomannan by a sandwich enzyme-linked immunosorbent assay for hematological patients at risk for invasive aspergillosis. J Clin Microbiol. 1999;37:3223–8.
149. Maertens J, Theunissen K, Verbeken E, et al. Prospective clinical evaluation of lower cut-offs for galactomannan detection in adult neutropenic cancer patients and haematological stem cell transplant recipients. Br J Haematol. 2004;126:852–60.
150. Adam O, Auperin A, Wilquin F, Bourhis JH, Gachot B, Chachaty E. Treatment with piperacillin-tazobactam and false-positive *Aspergillus* galactomannan antigen test results for patients with hematological malignancies. Clin Infect Dis. 2004;38:917–20.
151. Viscoli C, Machetti M, Cappellano P, et al. False-positive galactomannan platelia *Aspergillus* test results for patients receiving piperacillin-tazobactam. Clin Infect Dis. 2004;38:913–6.
152. Aubry A, Porcher R, Bottero J, et al. Occurrence and kinetics of false-positive *Aspergillus* galactomannan test results following treatment with beta-lactam antibiotics in patients with hematological disorders. J Clin Microbiol. 2006;44:389–94.
153. Fortun J, Martin-Davila P, Alvarez ME, et al. False-positive results of *Aspergillus* galactomannan antigenemia in liver transplant recipients. Transplantation. 2009;87:256–60.
154. Maertens J, Theunissen K, Verhoef G, Van Eldere J. False-positive *Aspergillus* galactomannan antigen test results. Clin Infect Dis. 2004;39:289–90.

155. Mattei D, Rapezzi D, Mordini N, et al. False-positive *Aspergillus* galactomannan enzyme-linked immunosorbent assay results in vivo during amoxicillin-clavulanic acid treatment. J Clin Microbiol. 2004;42:5362–3.
156. Aceti A, Corvaglia L, Faldella G. Infant formulas thickened with carob bean gum causing false-positive galactomannan test reactivity. Pediatr Infect Dis J. 2008;27:769.
157. Murashige N, Kami M, Kishi Y, Fujisaki G, Tanosaki R. False-positive results of *Aspergillus* enzyme-linked immunosorbent assays for a patient with gastrointestinal graft-versus-host disease taking a nutrient containing soybean protein. Clin Infect Dis. 2005;40:333–4.
158. Tomita Y, Sugimoto M, Kawano O, Kohrogi H. High incidence of false-positive *Aspergillus* galactomannan test results in patients with aspiration pneumonia. J Am Geriatr Soc. 2009;57:935–6.
159. Hage CA, Reynolds JM, Durkin M, Wheat LJ, Knox KS. Plasmalyte as a cause of false-positive results for *Aspergillus* galactomannan in bronchoalveolar lavage fluid. J Clin Microbiol. 2007;45:676–7.
160. Racil Z, Kocmanova I, Lengerova M, Winterova J, Mayer J. Intravenous PLASMA-LYTE as a major cause of false-positive results of platelia *Aspergillus* test for galactomannan detection in serum. J Clin Microbiol. 2007;45:3141–2.
161. Surmont I, Stockman W. Gluconate-containing intravenous solutions: another cause of false-positive galactomannan assay reactivity. J Clin Microbiol. 2007;45:1373.
162. Asano-Mori Y, Kanda Y, Oshima K, et al. False-positive *Aspergillus* galactomannan antigenaemia after haematopoietic stem cell transplantation. J Antimicrob Chemother. 2008;61:411–6.
163. Girmenia C, Ballaro D, Martino P. Contamination by cardboard particles as a cause of false-positive results for *Aspergillus* galactomannan enzyme immunoassays. Clin Vaccine Immunol. 2007;14:929.
164. Jones O, Cleveland KO, Gelfand MS. A case of disseminated histoplasmosis following autologous stem cell transplantation for Hodgkin's lymphoma: an initial misdiagnosis with a false-positive serum galactomannan assay. Transpl Infect Dis. 2009;11:281–3.
165. Narreddy S, Chandrasekar PH. False-positive *Aspergillus galactomannan* (GM) assay in histoplasmosis. J Infect. 2008;56:80–1.
166. Huang YT, Hung CC, Liao CH, Sun HY, Chang SC, Chen YC. Detection of circulating galactomannan in serum samples for diagnosis of *Penicillium marneffei* infection and cryptococcosis among patients infected with human immunodeficiency virus. J Clin Microbiol. 2007;45:2858–62.
167. Giacchino M, Chiapello N, Bezzio S, et al. *Aspergillus* galactomannan enzyme-linked immunosorbent assay cross-reactivity caused by invasive Geotrichum capitatum. J Clin Microbiol. 2006;44:3432–4.
168. Maertens J, Verhaegen J, Lagrou K, Van Eldere J, Boogaerts M. Screening for circulating galactomannan as a noninvasive diagnostic tool for invasive aspergillosis in prolonged neutropenic patients and stem cell transplantation recipients: a prospective validation. Blood. 2001;97:1604–10.
169. Herbrecht R, Letscher-Bru V, Oprea C, et al. *Aspergillus* galactomannan detection in the diagnosis of invasive aspergillosis in cancer patients. J Clin Oncol. 2002;20:1898–906.
170. Becker MJ, Lugtenburg EJ, Cornelissen JJ, Van Der Schee C, Hoogsteden HC, De Marie S. Galactomannan detection in computerized tomography-based broncho-alveolar lavage fluid and serum in haematological patients at risk for invasive pulmonary aspergillosis. Br J Haematol. 2003;121:448–57.
171. Marr KA, Balajee SA, McLaughlin L, Tabouret M, Bentsen C, Walsh TJ. Detection of galactomannan antigenemia by enzyme immunoassay for the diagnosis of invasive aspergillosis: variables that affect performance. J Infect Dis. 2004;190:641–9.
172. Hayden R, Pounds S, Knapp K, et al. Galactomannan antigenemia in pediatric oncology patients with invasive aspergillosis. Pediatr Infect Dis J. 2008;27:815–9.
173. Maertens JA, Klont R, Masson C, et al. Optimization of the cutoff value for the *Aspergillus* double-sandwich enzyme immunoassay. Clin Infect Dis. 2007;44:1329–36.
174. Penack O, Rempf P, Graf B, Blau IW, Thiel E. *Aspergillus* galactomannan testing in patients with long-term neutropenia: implications for clinical management. Ann Oncol. 2008;19:984–9.
175. Nguyen MH, Jaber R, Leather HL, et al. Use of bronchoalveolar lavage to detect galactomannan for diagnosis of pulmonary aspergillosis among nonimmunocompromised hosts. J Clin Microbiol. 2007;45:2787–92.
176. Husain S, Paterson DL, Studer SM, et al. *Aspergillus* galactomannan antigen in the bronchoalveolar lavage fluid for the diagnosis of invasive aspergillosis in lung transplant recipients. Transplantation. 2007;83:1330–6.
177. Clancy CJ, Jaber RA, Leather HL, et al. Bronchoalveolar lavage galactomannan in diagnosis of invasive pulmonary aspergillosis among solid-organ transplant recipients. J Clin Microbiol. 2007;45:1759–65.
178. Pfeiffer CD, Fine JP, Safdar N. Diagnosis of invasive aspergillosis using a galactomannan assay: a meta-analysis. Clin Infect Dis. 2006;42:1417–727.
179. Cordonnier C, Botterel F, Ben Amor R, et al. Correlation between galactomannan antigen levels in serum and neutrophil counts in haematological patients with invasive aspergillosis. Clin Microbiol Infect. 2009;15:81–6.
180. Maertens J, Buve K, Theunissen K, et al. Galactomannan serves as a surrogate endpoint for outcome of pulmonary invasive aspergillosis in neutropenic hematology patients. Cancer. 2009;115:355–62.
181. Hope WW, Walsh TJ, Denning DW. Laboratory diagnosis of invasive aspergillosis. Lancet Infect Dis. 2005;5:609–22.
182. Buchheidt D, Hummel M, Schleiermacher D, et al. Prospective clinical evaluation of a LightCycler-mediated polymerase chain reaction assay, a nested-PCR assay and a galactomannan enzyme-linked immunosorbent assay for detection of invasive aspergillosis in neutropenic cancer patients and haematological stem cell transplant recipients. Br J Haematol. 2004;125:196–202.
183. Cuenca-Estrella M, Meije Y, Diaz-Pedroche C, et al. Value of serial quantification of fungal DNA by a real-time PCR-based technique for early diagnosis of invasive aspergillosis in patients with febrile neutropenia. J Clin Microbiol. 2009;47:379–84.
184. Rickerts V, Mousset S, Lambrecht E, et al. Comparison of histopathological analysis, culture, and polymerase chain reaction assays to detect invasive mold infections from biopsy specimens. Clin Infect Dis. 2007;44:1078–83.
185. Walsh TJ, Francesconi A, Kasai M, Chanock SJ. PCR and single-strand conformational polymorphism for recognition of medically important opportunistic fungi. J Clin Microbiol. 1995;33:3216–20.
186. Kappe R, Fauser C, Okeke CN, Maiwald M. Universal fungus-specific primer systems and group-specific hybridization oligonucleotides for 18 S rDNA. Mycoses. 1996;39:25–30.
187. Kasai M, Harrington SM, Francesconi A, et al. Detection of a molecular biomarker for zygomycetes by quantitative PCR assays of plasma, bronchoalveolar lavage, and lung tissue in a rabbit model of experimental pulmonary zygomycosis. J Clin Microbiol. 2008;46:3690–702.
188. Maertens J, Deeren D, Dierickx D, Theunissen K. Preemptive antifungal therapy: still a way to go. Curr Opin Infect Dis. 2006;19:551–6.
189. Segal BH, Almyroudis NG, Battiwalla M, et al. Prevention and early treatment of invasive fungal infection in patients with cancer and neutropenia and in stem cell transplant recipients in the era of newer broad-spectrum antifungal agents and diagnostic adjuncts. Clin Infect Dis. 2007;44:402–9.
190. Rieger CT, Ostermann H. Empiric vs. preemptive antifungal treatment: an appraisal of treatment strategies in haematological patients. Mycoses. 2008;51 Suppl 1:31–4.
191. Almyroudis NG, Segal BH. Prevention and treatment of invasive fungal diseases in neutropenic patients. Curr Opin Infect Dis. 2009;22:385–93.

192. Slavin MA, Osborne B, Adams R, et al. Efficacy and safety of fluconazole prophylaxis for fungal infections after marrow transplantation–a prospective, randomized, double-blind study. J Infect Dis. 1995;171:1545–52.
193. Goodman JL, Winston DJ, Greenfield RA, et al. A controlled trial of fluconazole to prevent fungal infections in patients undergoing bone marrow transplantation. N Engl J Med. 1992;326:845–51.
194. Hughes WT, Armstrong D, Bodey GP, et al. 2002 guidelines for the use of antimicrobial agents in neutropenic patients with cancer. Clin Infect Dis. 2002;34:730–51.
195. Walsh TJ, Lee JW. Prevention of invasive fungal infections in patients with neoplastic disease. Clin Infect Dis. 1993;17 Suppl 2:S468–80.
196. Rhame FS. Prevention of nosocomial aspergillosis. J Hosp Infect. 1991;18(Suppl A):466–72.
197. Oren I, Haddad N, Finkelstein R, Rowe JM. Invasive pulmonary aspergillosis in neutropenic patients during hospital construction: before and after chemoprophylaxis and institution of HEPA filters. Am J Hematol. 2001;66:257–62.
198. Wald A, Leisenring W, van Burik JA, Bowden RA. Epidemiology of *Aspergillus* infections in a large cohort of patients undergoing bone marrow transplantation. J Infect Dis. 1997;175:1459–66.
199. Passweg JR, Rowlings PA, Atkinson KA, et al. Influence of protective isolation on outcome of allogeneic bone marrow transplantation for leukemia. Bone Marrow Transplant. 1998;21:1231–8.
200. Anaissie EJ, Stratton SL, Dignani MC, et al. Cleaning patient shower facilities: a novel approach to reducing patient exposure to aerosolized *Aspergillus* species and other opportunistic molds. Clin Infect Dis. 2002;35:E86–8.
201. Anaissie EJ, Kuchar RT, Rex JH, et al. Fusariosis associated with pathogenic Fusarium species colonization of a hospital water system: a new paradigm for the epidemiology of opportunistic mold infections. Clin Infect Dis. 2001;33:1871–8.
202. Lass-Florl C, Rath P, Niederwieser D, et al. *Aspergillus terreus* infections in haematological malignancies: molecular epidemiology suggests association with in-hospital plants. J Hosp Infect. 2000;46:31–5.
203. Walsh TJ, Merz WG. Pathologic features in the human alimentary tract associated with invasiveness of *Candida tropicalis*. Am J Clin Pathol. 1986;85:498–502.
204. Winston DJ, Chandrasekar PH, Lazarus HM, et al. Fluconazole prophylaxis of fungal infections in patients with acute leukemia. Results of a randomized placebo-controlled, double-blind, multicenter trial. Ann Intern Med. 1993;118:495–503.
205. Schaffner A, Schaffner M. Effect of prophylactic fluconazole on the frequency of fungal infections, amphotericin B use, and health care costs in patients undergoing intensive chemotherapy for hematologic neoplasias. J Infect Dis. 1995;172:1035–41.
206. Chandrasekar PH, Gatny CM. Effect of fluconazole prophylaxis on fever and use of amphotericin in neutropenic cancer patients. Chemotherapy. 1994;40:136–43.
207. Kern W, Behre G, Rudolf T, et al. Failure of fluconazole prophylaxis to reduce mortality or the requirement of systemic amphotericin B therapy during treatment for refractory acute myeloid leukemia: results of a prospective randomized phase III study. Cancer. 1998;83:291–301.
208. Marr KA, Seidel K, Slavin MA, et al. Prolonged fluconazole prophylaxis is associated with persistent protection against candidiasis-related death in allogeneic marrow transplant recipients: long-term follow-up of a randomized, placebo-controlled trial. Blood. 2000;96:2055–61.
209. Rotstein C, Bow EJ, Laverdiere M, Ioannou S, Carr D, Moghaddam N. Randomized placebo-controlled trial of fluconazole prophylaxis for neutropenic cancer patients: benefit based on purpose and intensity of cytotoxic therapy. The Canadian Fluconazole Prophylaxis Study Group. Clin Infect Dis. 1999;28:331–40.
210. Bow EJ, Laverdiere M, Lussier N, Rotstein C, Cheang MS, Ioannou S. Antifungal prophylaxis for severely neutropenic chemotherapy recipients: a meta analysis of randomized-controlled clinical trials. Cancer. 2002;94:3230–46.
211. Gotzsche PC, Johansen HK. Meta-analysis of prophylactic or empirical antifungal treatment versus placebo or no treatment in patients with cancer complicated by neutropenia. BMJ. 1997;314:1238–44.
212. Menichetti F, Del Favero A, Martino P, et al. Itraconazole oral solution as prophylaxis for fungal infections in neutropenic patients with hematologic malignancies: a randomized, placebo-controlled, double-blind, multicenter trial. GIMEMA Infection Program. Gruppo Italiano Malattie Ematologiche dell' Adulto. Clin Infect Dis. 1999;28:250–5.
213. Harousseau JL, Dekker AW, Stamatoullas-Bastard A, et al. Itraconazole oral solution for primary prophylaxis of fungal infections in patients with hematological malignancy and profound neutropenia: a randomized, double-blind, double-placebo, multicenter trial comparing itraconazole and amphotericin B. Antimicrob Agents Chemother. 2000;44:1887–93.
214. Huijgens PC, Simoons-Smit AM, van Loenen AC, et al. Fluconazole versus itraconazole for the prevention of fungal infections in haemato-oncology. J Clin Pathol. 1999;52:376–80.
215. Morgenstern GR, Prentice AG, Prentice HG, Ropner JE, Schey SA, Warnock DW. A randomized controlled trial of itraconazole versus fluconazole for the prevention of fungal infections in patients with haematological malignancies. U.K. Multicentre Antifungal Prophylaxis Study Group. Br J Haematol. 1999;105:901–11.
216. Glasmacher A, Hahn C, Leutner C, et al. Breakthrough invasive fungal infections in neutropenic patients after prophylaxis with itraconazole. Mycoses. 1999;42:443–51.
217. Lamy T, Bernard M, Courtois A, et al. Prophylactic use of itraconazole for the prevention of invasive pulmonary aspergillosis in high risk neutropenic patients. Leuk Lymphoma. 1998;30:163–74.
218. De Pauw BE, Donnelly JP. Prophylaxis and aspergillosis–has the principle been proven? N Engl J Med. 2007;356:409–11.
219. Wingard JR, Carter SL, Walsh TJ, et al. Randomized, double-blind trial of fluconazole vs. voriconazole for the prevention of invasive fungal infection (IFI) after allogeneic hematological cell transplantation. Blood 2010; doi:10.1182/Blood-2010-02-268151.
220. Vehreschild JJ, Bohme A, Buchheidt D, et al. A double-blind trial on prophylactic voriconazole (VRC) or placebo during induction chemotherapy for acute myelogenous leukaemia (AML). J Infect. 2007;55:445–9.
221. van Well GT, van Groeningen I, Debets-Ossenkopp YJ, van Furth AM, Zwaan CM. Zygomycete infection following voriconazole prophylaxis. Lancet Infect Dis. 2005;5:594.
222. Lionakis MS, Kontoyiannis DP. Sinus zygomycosis in a patient receiving voriconazole prophylaxis. Br J Haematol. 2005;129:2.
223. Siwek GT, Dodgson KJ, de Magalhaes-Silverman M, et al. Invasive zygomycosis in hematopoietic stem cell transplant recipients receiving voriconazole prophylaxis. Clin Infect Dis. 2004;39:584–7.
224. Mattner F, Weissbrodt H, Strueber M. Two case reports: fatal *Absidia corymbifera* pulmonary tract infection in the first postoperative phase of a lung transplant patient receiving voriconazole prophylaxis, and transient bronchial *Absidia corymbifera* colonization in a lung transplant patient. Scand J Infect Dis. 2004;36:312–4.
225. Ezdinli EZ, O'Sullivan DD, Wasser LP, Kim U, Stutzman L. Oral amphotericin for candidiasis in patients with hematologic neoplasms. An autopsy study. JAMA. 1979;242:258–60.
226. Bodey GP. The effect of amphotericin B on the fungal flora in feces. Clin Pharmacol Ther. 1969;10:675–80.
227. Menichetti F, Del Favero A, Martino P, et al. Preventing fungal infection in neutropenic patients with acute leukemia: fluconazole compared with oral amphotericin B. The GIMEMA Infection Program. Ann Intern Med. 1994;120:913–8.

228. Schwartz S, Behre G, Heinemann V, et al. Aerosolized amphotericin B inhalations as prophylaxis of invasive *Aspergillus* infections during prolonged neutropenia: results of a prospective randomized multicenter trial. Blood. 1999;93:3654–61.
229. Rijnders BJ, Cornelissen JJ, Slobbe L, et al. Aerosolized liposomal amphotericin B for the prevention of invasive pulmonary aspergillosis during prolonged neutropenia: a randomized, placebo-controlled trial. Clin Infect Dis. 2008;46:1401–8.
230. Bodey GP, Anaissie EJ, Elting LS, Estey E, O'Brien S, Kantarjian H. Antifungal prophylaxis during remission induction therapy for acute leukemia fluconazole versus intravenous amphotericin B. Cancer. 1994;73:2099–106.
231. Kelsey SM, Goldman JM, McCann S, et al. Liposomal amphotericin (AmBisome) in the prophylaxis of fungal infections in neutropenic patients: a randomised, double-blind, placebo-controlled study. Bone Marrow Transplant. 1999;23:163–8.
232. Uhlenbrock S, Zimmermann M, Fegeler W, Jurgens H, Ritter J. Liposomal amphotericin B for prophylaxis of invasive fungal infections in high-risk paediatric patients with chemotherapy-related neutropenia: interim analysis of a prospective study. Mycoses. 2001;44:455–63.
233. Karp JE, Burch PA, Merz WG. An approach to intensive antileukemia therapy in patients with previous invasive aspergillosis. Am J Med. 1988;85:203–6.
234. Richard C, Romon I, Baro J, et al. Invasive pulmonary aspergillosis prior to BMT in acute leukemia patients does not predict a poor outcome. Bone Marrow Transplant. 1993;12:237–41.
235. Martino R, Nomdedeu J, Altes A, et al. Successful bone marrow transplantation in patients with previous invasive fungal infections: report of four cases. Bone Marrow Transplant. 1994;13:265–9.
236. Martino R, Lopez R, Sureda A, Brunet S, Domingo-Albos A. Risk of reactivation of a recent invasive fungal infection in patients with hematological malignancies undergoing further intensive chemo-radiotherapy. A single-center experience and review of the literature. Haematologica. 1997;82:297–304.
237. Cordonnier C, Maury S, Pautas C, et al. Secondary antifungal prophylaxis with voriconazole to adhere to scheduled treatment in leukemic patients and stem cell transplant recipients. Bone Marrow Transplant. 2004;33:943–8.
238. Michailov G, Laporte JP, Lesage S, et al. Autologous bone marrow transplantation is feasible in patients with a prior history of invasive pulmonary aspergillosis. Bone Marrow Transplant. 1996;17:569–72.
239. Offner F, Cordonnier C, Ljungman P, et al. Impact of previous aspergillosis on the outcome of bone marrow transplantation. Clin Infect Dis. 1998;26:1098–103.
240. Uriz J, de Andoin NG, Calvo C, et al. Secondary prophylaxis with voriconazole in a leukemic patient with pulmonary aspergillosis. Pediatr Infect Dis J. 2007;26:971–2.
241. Villanueva A, Arathoon EG, Gotuzzo E, Berman RS, DiNubile MJ, Sable CA. A randomized double-blind study of caspofungin versus amphotericin for the treatment of candidal esophagitis. Clin Infect Dis. 2001;33:1529–35.
242. Maertens J, Raad I, Petrikkos G, et al. Efficacy and safety of caspofungin for treatment of invasive aspergillosis in patients refractory to or intolerant of conventional antifungal therapy. Clin Infect Dis. 2004;39:1563–71.
243. Ito M, Nozu R, Kuramochi T, et al. Prophylactic effect of FK463, a novel antifungal lipopeptide, against Pneumocystis carinii infection in mice. Antimicrob Agents Chemother. 2000;44:2259–62.
244. Cudillo L, Girmenia C, Santilli S, et al. Breakthrough fusariosis in a patient with acute lymphoblastic leukemia receiving voriconazole prophylaxis. Clin Infect Dis. 2005;40:1212–3.
245. Tong SY, Peleg AY, Yoong J, Handke R, Szer J, Slavin M. Breakthrough Scedosporium prolificans infection while receiving voriconazole prophylaxis in an allogeneic stem cell transplant recipient. Transpl Infect Dis. 2007;9:241–3.
246. Pizzo PA, Robichaud KJ, Gill FA, Witebsky FG. Empiric antibiotic and antifungal therapy for cancer patients with prolonged fever and granulocytopenia. Am J Med. 1982;72:101–11.
247. EORTC International Antimicrobial Therapy Cooperative Group. Empiric antifungal therapy in febrile granulocytopenic patients. Am J Med. 1989;86:668–72.
248. Bennett J. Editorial response: choosing amphotericin B formulations-between a rock and a hard place. Clin Infect Dis. 2000;31:1164–5.
249. Wingard JR, Kubilis P, Lee L, et al. Clinical significance of nephrotoxicity in patients treated with amphotericin B for suspected or proven aspergillosis. Clin Infect Dis. 1999;29:1402–7.
250. Viscoli C, Castagnola E, Van Lint MT, et al. Fluconazole versus amphotericin B as empirical antifungal therapy of unexplained fever in granulocytopenic cancer patients: a pragmatic, multicentre, prospective and randomised clinical trial. Eur J Cancer. 1996;32A:814–20.
251. White MH, Anaissie EJ, Kusne S, et al. Amphotericin B colloidal dispersion vs. amphotericin B as therapy for invasive aspergillosis. Clin Infect Dis. 1997;24:635–42.
252. Wingard JR, White MH, Anaissie E, Raffalli J, Goodman J, Arrieta A. A randomized, double-blind comparative trial evaluating the safety of liposomal amphotericin B versus amphotericin B lipid complex in the empirical treatment of febrile neutropenia. L Amph/ABLC Collaborative Study Group. Clin Infect Dis. 2000;31:1155–63.
253. Prentice HG, Hann IM, Herbrecht R, et al. A randomized comparison of liposomal versus conventional amphotericin B for the treatment of pyrexia of unknown origin in neutropenic patients. Br J Haematol. 1997;98:711–8.
254. Bodey GP. Management of persistent fever in the neutropenic patient. Am J Med. 2000;108:343–5.
255. Cagnoni PJ, Walsh TJ, Prendergast MM, et al. Pharmacoeconomic analysis of liposomal amphotericin B versus conventional amphotericin B in the empirical treatment of persistently febrile neutropenic patients. J Clin Oncol. 2000;18:2476–83.
256. Zonios DI, Gea-Banacloche J, Childs R, Bennett JE. Hallucinations during voriconazole therapy. Clin Infect Dis. 2008;47:e7–10.
257. Maertens J, Theunissen K, Verhoef G, et al. Galactomannan and computed tomography-based preemptive antifungal therapy in neutropenic patients at high risk for invasive fungal infec tion: a prospective feasibility study. Clin Infect Dis. 2005;41: 1242–50.
258. Hebart H, Klingspor L, Klingebiel T, et al. A prospective randomized controlled trial comparing PCR-based and empirical treatment with liposomal amphotericin B in patients after allo-SCT. Bone Marrow Transplant. 2009;43:553–61.
259. Cordonnier C, Pautas C, Maury S, et al. Empirical versus preemptive antifungal therapy for high-risk, febrile, neutropenic patients: a randomized, controlled trial. Clin Infect Dis. 2009;48:1042–51.
260. Einsele H, Hebart H, Roller G, et al. Detection and identification of fungal pathogens in blood by using molecular probes. J Clin Microbiol. 1997;35:1353–60.
261. Pappas PG, Kauffman CA, Andes D, et al. Clinical practice guidelines for the management of candidiasis: 2009 update by the Infectious Diseases Society of America. Clin Infect Dis. 2009;48:503–35.
262. Walsh TJ, Anaissie EJ, Denning DW, et al. Treatment of aspergillosis: clinical practice guidelines of the Infectious Diseases Society of America. Clin Infect Dis. 2008;46:327–60.
263. Walsh TJ, Raad I, Patterson TF, et al. Treatment of invasive aspergillosis with posaconazole in patients who are refractory to or intolerant of conventional therapy: an externally controlled trial. Clin Infect Dis. 2007;44:2–12.
264. Walsh TJ, Hiemenz JW, Seibel NL, et al. Amphotericin B lipid complex for invasive fungal infections: analysis of safety and efficacy in 556 cases. Clin Infect Dis. 1998;26:1383–96.
265. van Burik JA, Hare RS, Solomon HF, Corrado ML, Kontoyiannis DP. Posaconazole is effective as salvage therapy in zygomycosis: a retrospective summary of 91 cases. Clin Infect Dis. 2006;42:e61–5.
266. Ibrahim AS, Edwards Jr JE, Fu Y, Spellberg B. Deferiprone iron chelation as a novel therapy for experimental mucormycosis. J Antimicrob Chemother. 2006;58:1070–3.

267. Spellberg B, Andes D, Perez M, et al. Safety and outcomes of open-label deferasirox iron chelation therapy for mucormycosis. Antimicrob Agents Chemother. 2009;53:3122–5.
268. Pagano L, Valentini CG, Caira M, Fianchi L. ZYGOMYCOSIS: current approaches to management of patients with haematological malignancies. Br J Haematol. 2009;146:597–606.
269. Rogers TR. Treatment of zygomycosis: current and new options. J Antimicrob Chemother. 2008;61 Suppl 1:i35–40.
270. Walsh TJ, Groll A, Hiemenz J, Fleming R, Roilides E, Anaissie E. Infections due to emerging and uncommon medically important fungal pathogens. Clin Microbiol Infect. 2004;10 Suppl 1:48–66.
271. Perfect JR. Treatment of non-Aspergillus moulds in immunocompromised patients, with amphotericin B lipid complex. Clin Infect Dis. 2005;40 Suppl 6:S401–8.
272. Raad II, Hachem RY, Herbrecht R, et al. Posaconazole as salvage treatment for invasive fusariosis in patients with underlying hematologic malignancy and other conditions. Clin Infect Dis. 2006;42:1398–403.
273. Lamaris GA, Lewis RE, Chamilos G, et al. Caspofungin-mediated beta-glucan unmasking and enhancement of human polymorphonuclear neutrophil activity against *Aspergillus* and non-*Aspergillus* hyphae. J Infect Dis. 2008;198:186–92.
274. Antachopoulos C, Papakonstantinou E, Dotis J, et al. Fungemia due to *Trichosporon asahii* in a neutropenic child refractory to amphotericin B: clearance with voriconazole. J Pediatr Hematol Oncol. 2005;27:283–5.
275. Falk R, Wolf DG, Shapiro M, Polacheck I. Multidrug-resistant *Trichosporon asahii* isolates are susceptible to voriconazole. J Clin Microbiol. 2003;41:911.
276. Walsh TJ, Lee JW, Melcher GP, et al. Experimental *Trichosporon* infection in persistently granulocytopenic rabbits: implications for pathogenesis, diagnosis, and treatment of an emerging opportunistic mycosis. J Infect Dis. 1992;166:121–33.
277. Walsh TJ, Lutsar I, Driscoll T, et al. Voriconazole in the treatment of aspergillosis, scedosporiosis, and other invasive fungal infections in children. Pediatr Infect Dis J. 2002;21:240–8.
278. Perfect JR, Marr KA, Walsh TJ, et al. Voriconazole treatment for less-common, emerging, or refractory fungal infections. Clin Infect Dis. 2003;36:1122–31.
279. Quintini G, Barbera V, Gambino R, Spadola V, Minardi V, Mariani G. Successful treatment of hepatosplenic candidiasis in an elderly patient with acute myeloid leukemia using liposomal daunorubicin and fluconazole. Haematologica. 2001;86:E18.
280. Sallah S, Semelka RC, Wehbie R, Sallah W, Nguyen NP, Vos P. Hepatosplenic candidiasis in patients with acute leukaemia. Br J Haematol. 1999;106:697–701.
281. Walsh TJ, Whitcomb PO, Revankar SG, Pizzo PA. Successful treatment of hepatosplenic candidiasis through repeated cycles of chemotherapy and neutropenia. Cancer. 1995;76:2357–62.
282. Pagano L, Mele L, Fianchi L, et al. Chronic disseminated candidiasis in patients with hematologic malignancies. Clinical features and outcome of 29 episodes. Haematologica. 2002;87:535–41.
283. Lopez-Berestein G, Bodey GP, Frankel LS, Mehta K. Treatment of hepatosplenic candidiasis with liposomal-amphotericin B. J Clin Oncol. 1987;5:310–7.
284. Kauffman CA, Bradley SF, Ross SC, Weber DR. Hepatosplenic candidiasis: successful treatment with fluconazole. Am J Med. 1991;91:137–41.
285. Anaissie E, Bodey GP, Kantarjian H, et al. Fluconazole therapy for chronic disseminated candidiasis in patients with leukemia and prior amphotericin B therapy. Am J Med. 1991;91:142–50.
286. Sora F, Chiusolo P, Piccirillo N, et al. Successful treatment with caspofungin of hepatosplenic candidiasis resistant to liposomal amphotericin B. Clin Infect Dis. 2002;35:1135–6.
287. Rex JH, Walsh TJ, Sobel JD, et al. Practice guidelines for the treatment of candidiasis. Infectious Diseases Society of America. Clin Infect Dis. 2000;30:662–78.
288. Ratip S, Odabasi Z, Karti S, et al. Clinical microbiological case: chronic disseminated candidiasis unresponsive to treatment. Clin Microbiol Infect. 2002;8:442–4.
289. Katayama K, Koizumi S, Yamagami M, et al. Successful peritransplant therapy in children with active hepatosplenic candidiasis. Int J Hematol. 1994;59:125–30.
290. Denning DW, Ribaud P, Milpied N, et al. Efficacy and safety of voriconazole in the treatment of acute invasive aspergillosis. Clin Infect Dis. 2002;34:563–71.
291. Espinel-Ingroff A, Boyle K, Sheehan DJ. In vitro antifungal activities of voriconazole and reference agents as determined by NCCLS methods: review of the literature. Mycopathologia. 2001;150:101–15.
292. Kirkpatrick WR, McAtee RK, Fothergill AW, Rinaldi MG, Patterson TF. Efficacy of voriconazole in a guinea pig model of disseminated invasive aspergillosis. Antimicrob Agents Chemother. 2000;44:2865–8.
293. Chandrasekar PH, Cutright J, Manavathu E. Efficacy of voriconazole against invasive pulmonary aspergillosis in a guinea-pig model. J Antimicrob Chemother. 2000;45:673–6.
294. Allende MC, Lee JW, Francis P, et al. Dose-dependent antifungal activity and nephrotoxicity of amphotericin B colloidal dispersion in experimental pulmonary aspergillosis. Antimicrob Agents Chemother. 1994;38:518–22.
295. Francis P, Lee JW, Hoffman A, et al. Efficacy of unilamellar liposomal amphotericin B in treatment of pulmonary aspergillosis in persistently granulocytopenic rabbits: the potential role of bronchoalveolar D-mannitol and serum galactomannan as markers of infection. J Infect Dis. 1994;169:356–68.
296. Leenders AC, Daenen S, Jansen RL, et al. Liposomal amphotericin B compared with amphotericin B deoxycholate in the treatment of documented and suspected neutropenia-associated invasive fungal infections. Br J Haematol. 1998;103:205–12.
297. Caillot D, Bassaris H, McGeer A, et al. Intravenous itraconazole followed by oral itraconazole in the treatment of invasive pulmonary aspergillosis in patients with hematologic malignancies, chronic granulomatous disease, or AIDS. Clin Infect Dis. 2001;33:e83–90.
298. Rizk SS, Kraus DH, Gerresheim G, Mudan S. Aggressive combination treatment for invasive fungal sinusitis in immunocompromised patients. Ear Nose Throat J. 2000;79:278–80. 82, 84-5.
299. Bernard A, Caillot D, Couaillier JF, Casasnovas O, Guy H, Favre JP. Surgical management of invasive pulmonary aspergillosis in neutropenic patients. Ann Thorac Surg. 1997;64:1441–7.
300. Pidhorecky I, Urschel J, Anderson T. Resection of invasive pulmonary aspergillosis in immunocompromised patients. Ann Surg Oncol. 2000;7:312–7.
301. Salerno CT, Ouyang DW, Pederson TS, et al. Surgical therapy for pulmonary aspergillosis in immunocompromised patients. Ann Thorac Surg. 1998;65:1415–9.
302. Reichenberger F, Habicht J, Kaim A, et al. Lung resection for invasive pulmonary aspergillosis in neutropenic patients with hematologic diseases. Am J Respir Crit Care Med. 1998;158:885–90.
303. Albelda SM, Talbot GH, Gerson SL, Miller WT, Cassileth PA. Pulmonary cavitation and massive hemoptysis in invasive pulmonary aspergillosis. Influence of bone marrow recovery in patients with acute leukemia. Am Rev Respir Dis. 1985;131:115–20.
304. Panos RJ, Barr LF, Walsh TJ, Silverman HJ. Factors associated with fatal hemoptysis in cancer patients. Chest. 1988;94:1008–13.
305. Pagano L, Ricci P, Nosari A, et al. Fatal haemoptysis in pulmonary filamentous mycosis: an underevaluated cause of death in patients with acute leukaemia in haematological complete remission. A retrospective study and review of the literature. Gimema Infection Program (Gruppo Italiano Malattie Ematologiche dell'Adulto). Br J Haematol. 1995;89:500–5.
306. Gorelik O, Cohen N, Shpirer I, et al. Fatal haemoptysis induced by invasive pulmonary aspergillosis in patients with acute leukaemia during bone marrow and clinical remission: report of two cases and review of the literature. J Infect. 2000;41:277–82.

307. Baron O, Guillaume B, Moreau P, et al. Aggressive surgical management in localized pulmonary mycotic and nonmycotic infections for neutropenic patients with acute leukemia: report of eighteen cases. J Thorac Cardiovasc Surg. 1998;115:63–8. discussion 8-9.
308. Yeghen T, Kibbler CC, Prentice HG, et al. Management of invasive pulmonary aspergillosis in hematology patients: a review of 87 consecutive cases at a single institution. Clin Infect Dis. 2000;31:859–68.
309. Ruthe RC, Andersen BR, Cunningham BL, Epstein RB. Efficacy of granulocyte transfusions in the control of systemic candidiasis in the leukopenic host. Blood. 1978;52:493–8.
310. Debelak KM, Epstein RB, Andersen BR. Granulocyte transfusions in leukopenic dogs: in vivo and in vitro function of granulocytes obtained by continuous-flow filtration leukopheresis. Blood. 1974;43:757–66.
311. Dale DC, Reynolds HY, Pennington JE, Elin RJ, Pitts TW, Graw RG. Experimental pneumonia due to *Pseudomonas* in dogs: controlled trial of granulocyte transfusion therapy. J Infect Dis. 1974;130(Suppl):S143–4.
312. Graw Jr RG, Herzig G, Perry S, Henderson ES. Normal granulocyte transfusion therapy: treatment of septicemia due to gram-negative bacteria. N Engl J Med. 1972;287:367–71.
313. Boggs DR. Transfusion of neutrophils as prevention or treatment of infection in patients with neutropenia. N Engl J Med. 1974;290:1055–62.
314. Higby DJ, Yates JW, Henderson ES, Holland JF. Filtration leukapheresis for granulocyte transfusion therapy. Clinical and laboratory studies. N Engl J Med. 1975;292:761–6.
315. Alavi JB, Root RK, Djerassi I, et al. A randomized clinical trial of granulocyte transfusions for infection in acute leukemia. N Engl J Med. 1977;296:706–11.
316. Herzig RH, Herzig GP, Graw Jr RG, Bull MI, Ray KK. Successful granulocyte transfusion therapy for gram-negative septicemia. A prospectively randomized controlled study. N Engl J Med. 1977; 296:701–5.
317. Clift RA, Sanders JE, Thomas ED, Williams B, Buckner CD. Granulocyte transfusions for the prevention of infection in patients receiving bone-marrow transplants. N Engl J Med. 1978;298: 1052–7.
318. Strauss RG, Connett JE, Gale RP, et al. A controlled trial of prophylactic granulocyte transfusions during initial induction chemotherapy for acute myelogenous leukemia. N Engl J Med. 1981;305:597–603.
319. Winston DJ, Ho WG, Gale RP. Therapeutic granulocyte transfusions for documented infections. A controlled trial in ninety-five infectious granulocytopenic episodes. Ann Intern Med. 1982;97:509–15.
320. Wright DG, Robichaud KJ, Pizzo PA, Deisseroth AB. Lethal pulmonary reactions associated with the combined use of amphotericin B and leukocyte transfusions. N Engl J Med. 1981;304:1185–9.
321. Berliner S, Weinberger M, Ben-Bassat M, et al. Amphotericin B causes aggregation of neutrophils and enhances pulmonary leukostasis. Am Rev Respir Dis. 1985;132:602–5.
322. Dana BW, Durie BG, White RF, Huestis DW. Concomitant administration of granulocyte transfusions and amphotericin B in neutropenic patients: absence of significant pulmonary toxicity. Blood. 1981;57:90–4.
323. Dutcher JP, Kendall J, Norris D, Schiffer C, Aisner J, Wiernik PH. Granulocyte transfusion therapy and amphotericin B: adverse reactions? Am J Hematol. 1989;31:102–8.
324. Engelhard D, Nagler A, Hardan I, et al. Antibody response to a two-dose regimen of influenza vaccine in allogeneic T cell-depleted and autologous BMT recipients. Bone Marrow Transplant. 1993;11:1–5.
325. Vamvakas EC, Pineda AA. Meta-analysis of clinical studies of the efficacy of granulocyte transfusions in the treatment of bacterial sepsis. J Clin Apher. 1996;11:1–9.
326. Vamvakas EC, Pineda AA. Determinants of the efficacy of prophylactic granulocyte transfusions: a meta-analysis. J Clin Apher. 1997;12:74–81.
327. Strauss RG. Neutrophil (granulocyte) transfusions in the new millennium. Transfusion. 1998;38:710–2.
328. Liles WC, Huang JE, Llewellyn C, SenGupta D, Price TH, Dale DC. A comparative trial of granulocyte-colony-stimulating factor and dexamethasone, separately and in combination, for the mobilization of neutrophils in the peripheral blood of normal volunteers. Transfusion. 1997;37:182–7.
329. Stroncek DF, Yau YY, Oblitas J, Leitman SF. Administration of G–CSF plus dexamethasone produces greater granulocyte concentrate yields while causing no more donor toxicity than G–CSF alone. Transfusion. 2001;41:1037–44.
330. Dignani MC, Anaissie EJ, Hester JP, et al. Treatment of neutropenia-related fungal infections with granulocyte colony-stimulating factor-elicited white blood cell transfusions: a pilot study. Leukemia. 1997;11:1621–30.
331. Peters C, Minkov M, Matthes-Martin S, et al. Leucocyte transfusions from rhG-CSF or prednisolone stimulated donors for treatment of severe infections in immunocompromised neutropenic patients. Br J Haematol. 1999;106:689–96.
332. Price TH, Bowden RA, Boeckh M, et al. Phase I/II trial of neutrophil transfusions from donors stimulated with G-CSF and dexamethasone for treatment of patients with infections in hematopoietic stem cell transplantation. Blood. 2000;95:3302–9.
333. Lee JJ, Chung IJ, Park MR, et al. Clinical efficacy of granulocyte transfusion therapy in patients with neutropenia-related infections. Leukemia. 2001;15:203–7.
334. Illerhaus G, Wirth K, Dwenger A, et al. Treatment and prophylaxis of severe infections in neutropenic patients by granulocyte transfusions. Ann Hematol. 2002;81:273–81.
335. Seidel MG, Peters C, Wacker A, et al. Randomized phase III study of granulocyte transfusions in neutropenic patients. Bone Marrow Transplant. 2008;42:679–84.
336. Helm TN, Longworth DL, Hall GS, Bolwell BJ, Fernandez B, Tomecki KJ. Case report and review of resolved fusariosis. J Am Acad Dermatol. 1990;23:393–8.
337. Catalano L, Fontana R, Scarpato N, Picardi M, Rocco S, Rotoli B. Combined treatment with amphotericin-B and granulocyte transfusion from G-CSF-stimulated donors in an aplastic patient with invasive aspergillosis undergoing bone marrow transplantation. Haematologica. 1997;82:71–2.
338. Barrios NJ, Kirkpatrick DV, Murciano A, Stine K, Van Dyke RB, Humbert JR. Successful treatment of disseminated *Fusarium* infection in an immunocompromised child. Am J Pediatr Hematol Oncol. 1990;12:319–24.
339. Samadi DS, Goldberg AN, Orlandi RR. Granulocyte transfusion in the management of fulminant invasive fungal rhinosinusitis. Am J Rhinol. 2001;15:263–5.
340. Bielorai B, Toren A, Wolach B, et al. Successful treatment of invasive aspergillosis in chronic granulomatous disease by granulocyte transfusions followed by peripheral blood stem cell transplantation. Bone Marrow Transplant. 2000;26:1025–8.
341. Smith TJ, Khatcheressian J, Lyman GH, et al. 2006 update of recommendations for the use of white blood cell growth factors: an evidence-based clinical practice guideline. J Clin Oncol. 2006;24:3187–205.
342. Berghmans T, Paesmans M, Lafitte JJ, et al. Therapeutic use of granulocyte and granulocyte-macrophage colony-stimulating factors in febrile neutropenic cancer patients. A systematic review of the literature with meta-analysis. Support Care Cancer. 2002;10:181–8.
343. Clark OA, Lyman GH, Castro AA, Clark LG, Djulbegovic B. Colony-stimulating factors for chemotherapy-induced febrile neutropenia: a meta-analysis of randomized controlled trials. J Clin Oncol. 2005;23:4198–214.

344. Root RK, Dale DC. Granulocyte colony-stimulating factor and granulocyte-macrophage colony-stimulating factor: comparisons and potential for use in the treatment of infections in nonneutropenic patients. J Infect Dis. 1999;179 Suppl 2:S342–52.
345. Roilides E, Holmes A, Blake C, Pizzo PA, Walsh TJ. Effects of granulocyte colony-stimulating factor and interferon-gamma on antifungal activity of human polymorphonuclear neutrophils against pseudohyphae of different medically important *Candida* species. J Leukoc Biol. 1995;57:651–6.
346. Roilides E, Sein T, Holmes A, et al. Effects of macrophage colony-stimulating factor on antifungal activity of mononuclear phagocytes against *Aspergillus fumigatus*. J Infect Dis. 1995;172: 1028–34.
347. Gaviria JM, van Burik JA, Dale DC, Root RK, Liles WC. Modulation of neutrophil-mediated activity against the pseudohyphal form of *Candida albicans* by granulocyte colony-stimulating factor (G-CSF) administered in vivo. J Infect Dis. 1999;179:1301–4.
348. Brummer E, Maqbool A, Stevens DA. Protection of peritoneal macrophages by granulocyte/macrophage colony-stimulating factor (GM-CSF) against dexamethasone suppression of killing of *Aspergillus*, and the effect of human GM-CSF. Microbes Infect. 2002;4:133–8.
349. Brummer E, Maqbool A, Stevens DA. In vivo GM-CSF prevents dexamethasone suppression of killing of *Aspergillus fumigatus* conidia by bronchoalveolar macrophages. J Leukoc Biol. 2001; 70:868–72.
350. Gaviria JM, van Burik JA, Dale DC, Root RK, Liles WC. Comparison of interferon-gamma, granulocyte colony-stimulating factor, and granulocyte-macrophage colony-stimulating factor for priming leukocyte-mediated hyphal damage of opportunistic fungal pathogens. J Infect Dis. 1999;179:1038–41.
351. Centeno-Lima S, Silveira H, Casimiro C, Aguiar P, do Rosari VE. Kinetics of cytokine expression in mice with invasive aspergillosis: lethal infection and protection. FEMS Immunol Med Microbiol. 2002;32:167–73.
352. Brieland JK, Jackson C, Menzel F, et al. Cytokine networking in lungs of immunocompetent mice in response to inhaled *Aspergillus fumigatus*. Infect Immun. 2001;69:1554–60.
353. Nagai H, Guo J, Choi H, Kurup V. Interferon-gamma and tumor necrosis factor-alpha protect mice from invasive aspergillosis. J Infect Dis. 1995;172:1554–60.
354. Roilides E, Sein T, Schaufele R, Chanock SJ, Walsh TJ. Increased serum concentrations of interleukin-10 in patients with hepatosplenic candidiasis. J Infect Dis. 1998;178:589–92.
355. Roilides E, Sein T, Roden M, Schaufele RL, Walsh TJ. Elevated serum concentrations of interleukin-10 in nonneutropenic patients with invasive aspergillosis. J Infect Dis. 2001;183: 518–20.

Fungal Infections in Stem Cell Transplant Recipients

Dionissios Neofytos and Kieren A. Marr

Since the first hematopoietic stem cell transplant (HSCT) was performed more than 50 years ago, significant progress has been attained in the field, with changes in conditioning regimens, stem cell sources, and outcomes. The preparative regimen for HSCT may be fully myeloablative or less aggressive (nonmyeloablative). Different sources of stem cells have been used, including bone marrow (BM), peripheral blood stem cells (PBSCs), and cord blood. Stem cells may originate from an identical twin (syngeneic), one's own self (autologous), and another donor (allogeneic). Allogeneic donors may be related (family members) or unrelated to the recipients, with match or mismatch in human leukocyte antigens (HLA). Finally, manipulation of grafts (e.g., T cell depletion, CD34+ selection) may be used to modulate outcomes such as graft-versus-host disease (GVHD) and relapsed malignancy. All these variables impact the risks, timing, and outcomes of opportunistic infections, including invasive fungal infections (IFIs). Historically, infections due to *Candida* species have been predominately encountered soon after HSCT (prior to engraftment), while invasive mould infections, mainly invasive aspergillosis (IA), occur both early and later (after engraftment). Damage of the gastrointestinal tract mucosa and neutropenia due to conditioning regimens – particularly those designed to be myeloablative – represent the main risks for IFIs prior to engraftment. Neutrophil and T cell impairment associated with delayed engraftment or GVHD and associated therapies are the main risks for IFIs later after a HSCT.

The incidence, epidemiology, and clinical outcomes of IFIs among HSCT recipients have changed over the last several decades as a result of changes in the host, preventive strategies, and antifungal therapies. While the frequency of invasive candidiasis has decreased since the early 1990s, increasing frequency of IA among HSCT recipients was noted during the 1990s [1–3]. In addition, IFIs due to moulds other than *Aspergillus*, namely the Zygomycetes and *Fusarium* species, have also been appreciated as a significant problem [4, 5]. The clinical presentation, dynamically changing epidemiology, and outcomes of the most frequently observed IFIs, namely candidiasis, aspergillosis, zygomycosis (also known as mucormycosis), and other moulds, will be discussed.

D. Neofytos (✉)
Transplant and Oncology, Infectious Diseases Program, Johns Hopkins University, Baltimore, MD, USA
e-mail: dneofyto1@jhmi.edu

Invasive Candidiasis

Clinical Presentation

The main risks for *Candida* infections post HSCT include skin and mucosal membrane damage due to the presence of central intravenous catheters and conditioning-related gastrointestinal mucositis, respectively. Neutropenia before engraftment is another significant factor impacting risks for invasive candidiasis, and this is affected by the preparative regimens, stem cell source, HSCT manipulation, which is longer with ablative conditioning, and use of cord blood. HSCT recipients with *Candida* infections most commonly present with candidemia, which can be accompanied by sepsis. Candidemia may be sustained despite administration of appropriate therapy and rapidly disseminate to involve other organs. A diffuse maculopapular skin rash may be observed. As skin lesions in HSCT recipients may represent a number of different entities, it is pertinent to rapidly identify these findings and proceed with the appropriate diagnostic procedure to obtain a diagnosis in a timely fashion.

Hepatosplenic candidiasis is the result of *Candida* species invasion into the portal vasculature and subsequent dissemination to the liver and spleen. Clinical presentation frequently occurs when neutropenia resolves and inflammation develops. Blood cultures are negative in the vast majority of cases, and the diagnosis is usually made based on clinical suspicion. Patients present with right upper quadrant pain and tenderness on physical examination and have abnormal liver enzymes. Computed tomography (CT) or magnetic resonance imaging (MRI) of the abdomen may reveal liver, spleen,

C.A. Kauffman et al. (eds.), *Essentials of Clinical Mycology*,
DOI 10.1007/978-1-4419-6640-7_29, © Springer Science+Business Media, LLC 2011

and/or kidney micronodular lesions. For a definitive diagnosis, biopsy of hepatic lesions is required, if feasible, which may reveal fungal forms consistent with *Candida* species. In clinical practice, diagnosis is frequently based on the presence of fever, abdominal pain, elevated alkaline phosphatase, and liver lesions on imaging. Notably, multiple other organisms (e.g., bacteria, filamentous fungi) may present similarly and should be appropriately ruled out. Finally, resolution of signs and symptoms may be late despite appropriate antifungal therapy.

Epidemiology

In the 1980s *Candida* species were appreciated to be the major fungal pathogen affecting HSCT recipients, with reported incidence rates between 11% and 18% [6–8]. This observation was followed by two large randomized, placebo-controlled trials testing primary antifungal prophylaxis with fluconazole after autologous and allogeneic HSCT [7, 9]. A significant decrease in IFIs, mainly due to *Candida* species, was observed in both studies. In one study, fluconazole administration was significantly associated with decreased overall mortality among allogeneic HSCT recipients [9, 10]. The above studies resulted in the widespread administration of fluconazole for antifungal prophylaxis in the early post-transplant period in the early 1990s and lower rates (4.7–7%) of invasive candidiasis among HSCT recipients [7–9, 11, 12]. Epidemiologic studies performed in European centers suggest that the incidence of candidiasis among allogeneic HSCT recipients has remained low (1–3%) since the 1980s [13–16] (Fig. 1). Differences in conditioning, transplant practices, and prophylactic strategies among different centers and countries may, in part, account for differences in epidemiology and outcomes.

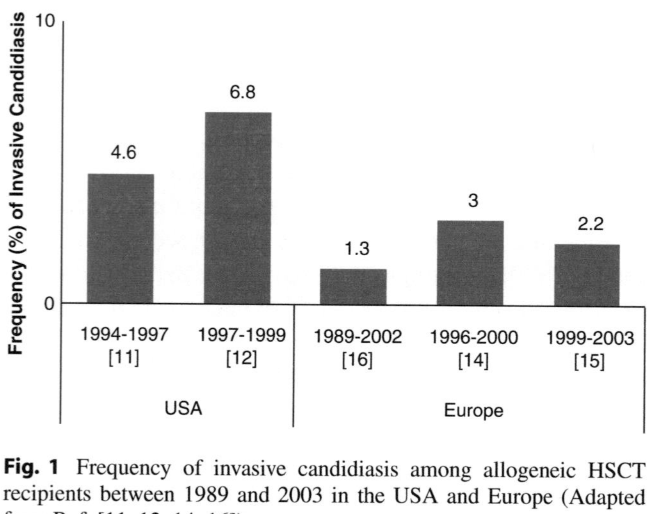

Fig. 1 Frequency of invasive candidiasis among allogeneic HSCT recipients between 1989 and 2003 in the USA and Europe (Adapted from Ref. [11, 12, 14–16])

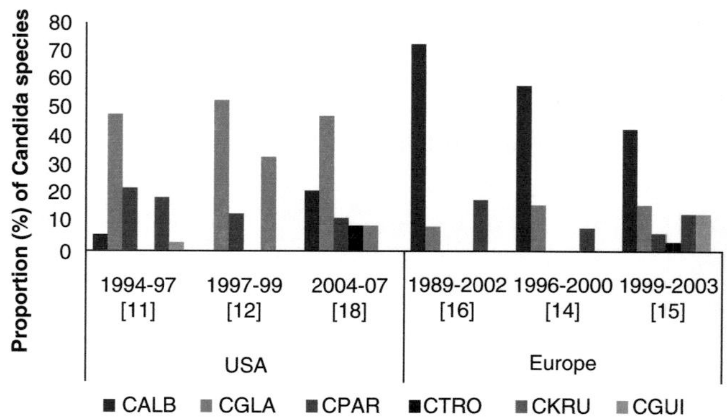

Fig. 2 Proportion of *Candida* species among HSCT recipients with invasive candidiasis between 1989 and 2007 in the USA and Europe (Adapted from Ref. [11, 12, 14–16, 18]). *CALB C. albicans, CGLA C. glabrata, CPAR C. parapsilosis, CTRO C. tropicalis, CKRU C. krusei, CGUI C. guilliermondii*

In early studies, *C. albicans* counted for >50% of episodes, followed by *C. tropicalis*; *C. glabrata* and *C. krusei* were less frequently identified [6]. However, the epidemiology of *Candida* species among HSCT recipients has changed; the proportion of invasive infection caused by potentially azole-resistant *Candida* species, such as *C. glabrata* and *C. krusei*, has increased since the early 1990s, perhaps as a result of the selective pressure from extensive use of fluconazole [11, 12, 15–19] (Fig. 2). Wingard et al. reported a sevenfold increase between 1989 and 1990 in the frequency of invasive candidiasis due to *C. krusei* in patients with leukemia and HSCT recipients that received fluconazole for prophylaxis compared with those who did not receive prophylaxis (p = 0.0002) [17]. The same group reported higher rates of infection due to *C. glabrata* among leukemic patients and HSCT recipients receiving fluconazole [20]. Recent prospectively collected data from a multicenter registry on HSCT recipients who had IFIs between 2004 and 2007 suggest that species other than *C. albicans* are the most common cause of invasive candidiasis, with *C. glabrata* most frequently isolated (43.5%) [19]. Finally, resistance developing among traditionally azole-susceptible *Candida* species can occur. In one study, 5.3% of *C. albicans* isolated were found to be resistant to fluconazole, which is consistent with other concurrent reports [11, 21, 22].

Invasive Mould Infections

Clinical Presentation

HSCT recipients are at risk for invasive mould infections by virtue of their underlying disease, complications, and administered therapies. The most frequently encountered moulds affecting HSCT recipients include *Aspergillus* species, *Fusarium* species, *Scedosporium* species, and the agents of mucormycosis. HSCT recipients are exposed to moulds through direct skin inoculation and gastrointestinal tract invasion, but the predominant exposure is via inhalation. Normally, macrophages identify and kill conidia in the alveoli before they germinate and form hyphae. Therapies for GVHD, including high-dose corticosteroids and other immunosuppressive agents, significantly affect neutrophil and T cell function, both pertinent for containing mould infections, preventing tissue invasion, and clearing pulmonary inflammation [23–26]. Risk factors for IA appear to differ based on the timing after transplant, with neutropenia and GVHD being the major driving forces before and after engraftment, respectively (Table 1). Recent data suggest that polymorphisms in different pattern recognition receptors (e.g., Toll-like receptors) and other genes, such as those regulating plasminogen, in HSCT donors and recipients may also affect the risks for IA following HSCT [27–29].

Invasive mould infections among HSCT recipients may present with local invasion of lung and sinuses or with dissemination to multiple sites. *Aspergillus* species are the most frequent cause, identified in more than 90% of pulmonary invasive mould disease, followed by other filamentous fungi, including *Fusarium* species, *Scedosporium* species, and the agents of mucormycosis [4, 5, 30]. Clinical and radiologic presentations of pulmonary syndromes due to different moulds are often similar. Patients present with fever, cough, dyspnea, hemoptysis, and pleuritic chest pain [5, 31]. A "halo sign" (nodular lesion surrounded by a halo representing alveolar hemorrhage) may be identified in up to 93% of patients with acute pulmonary IA [32–37]. Notably, the halo sign is not specific for IA, as other infections can present similarly, including those caused by other moulds and bacteria, such as *Pseudomonas* species [38–40]. Radiographic patterns may be variable, especially in non-neutropenic hosts [35, 36, 41]. Abnormalities may include small or large nodules, patchy, segmental, or wedge-shaped consolidations, peribronchial infiltrates, tree-in-bud distribution, and cavities [35, 36] (Fig. 3). Recent studies suggest that allogeneic HSCT recipients with IA in the setting of GVHD may present with variable radiographic findings, such as bronchopneumonia or focal infiltrates rather than isolated nodules [41]. Retrospective data suggest that presence of concomitant sinusitis, multiple (>10) pulmonary nodules, and pleural effusion may be predictive of pulmonary mucormycosis [42]. Because therapies differ, aggressive diagnostic workup, including bronchoscopy and testing for galactomannan,

Table 1 Risk factors associated with invasive aspergillosis among HSCT recipients

	Overall	Early (0–40 days)	Late (>40 days)
Host-related	Age >40 [1, 2, 4, 15]	Age >40 [1, 2]	Age >19 [1]
	CMV seropositivity [2, 26]		CMV seropositivity [2]
Underlying disease	Hematologic malignancy[a] [1, 2, 4]	Hematologic malignancy[a] [1, 2]	Hematologic malignancy[a] [1]
	Multiple myeloma [1]	Aplastic anemia [1, 2]	Multiple myeloma [2]
	Myelodysplastic syndrome [1, 2]	Myelodysplastic syndrome [1, 2]	
Transplant-related			
Conditioning	Total body irradiation [15]		
Donor–recipient	Mismatched donor [1, 2]	Mismatched donor [1]	Unrelated donor [1]
	Unrelated donor [2, 4, 15]		
	TLR4 donor polymorphism [26]		
	Plasminogen gene recipient polymorphism [27]		
Stem cell source/manipulation	Cord blood [2]	Cord blood [2]	T cell depletion [2]
	T cell depletion [2]		CD34 selection [2]
	CD34 selection [2]		
Transplant complications	Neutropenia [1, 2]		Neutropenia [1, 2]
	GVHD acute 2–4 [2]		Lymphopenia [2]
	Chronic extensive GVHD [2]		Acute GVHD grade 2–4 [1, 2]
			Corticosteroids [1]
Concomitant infections	CMV disease [2]	CMV disease [2]	CMV disease [2]
	Respiratory viral infection [2]		Respiratory viral infections [2]
Other factors		No laminar air room [1]	Present construction [1]
		Summer [1]	

CMV cytomegalovirus, *TLR* Toll-like receptors, *GVHD* graft-versus-host disease
[a]Other than chronic myelogenous leukemia, chronic phase and first remission
Only results found significant in multivariate analyses are included

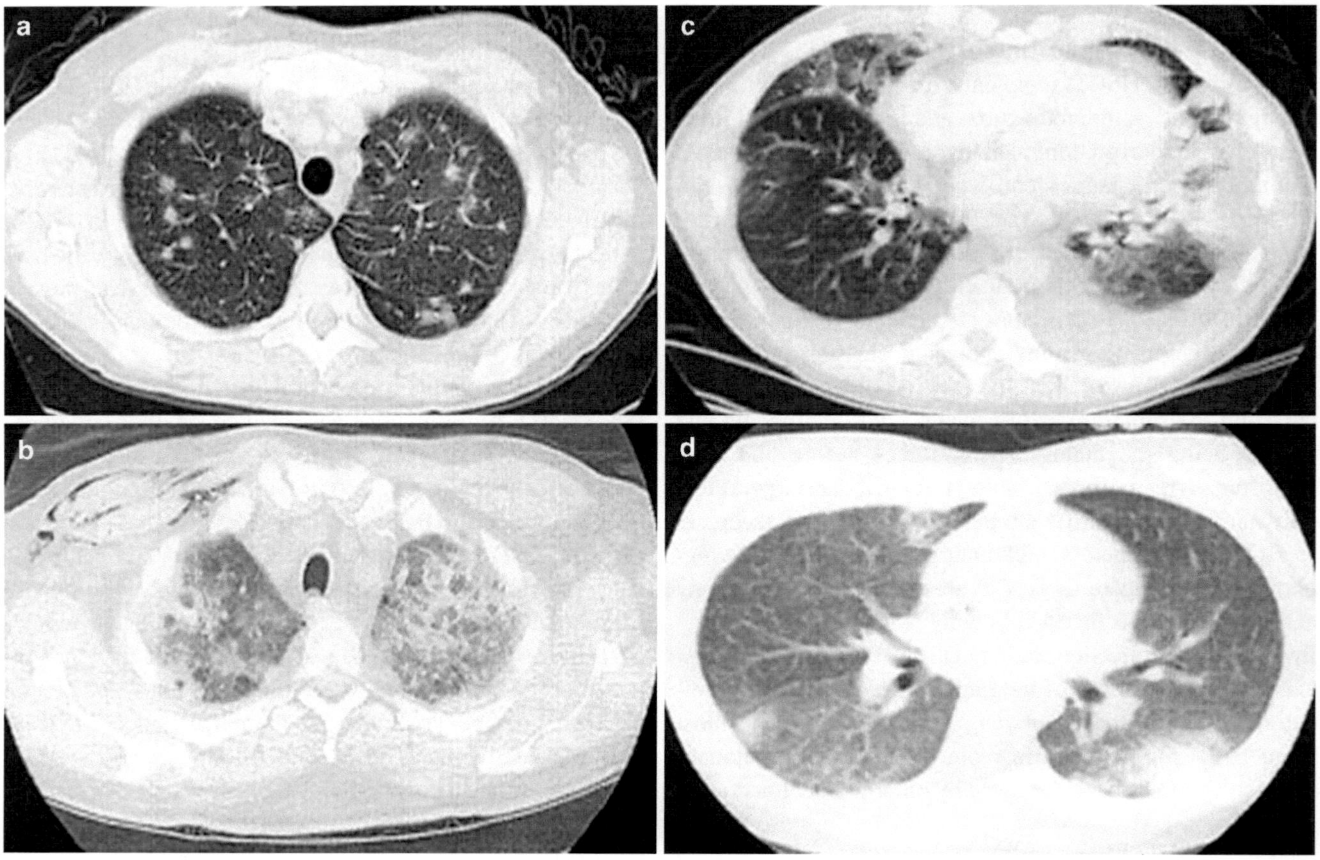

Fig. 3 Radiographic presentations of aspergillosis in allogeneic HSCT recipients. Appearance can vary from (**a**) isolated pulmonary lesions, to (**b**) cavitary lesions, to (**c** and **d**) infiltrates. Infiltrates are frequently pleural based (**c** and **d**), and ground glass changes can appear surrounding nodular lesions (**a**) or as an isolated finding (**d**)

should be promptly initiated to allow the accurate diagnosis of invasive mould infections and initiation of appropriate therapies.

Sinusitis is a common manifestation of invasive mould infections among HSCT recipients, with *Aspergillus* species and the Zygomycetes representing the major pathogens. Sinus disease can be very subtle and is occasionally found on routine sinus CT, but most patients present with facial tenderness, congestion, and fever. A CT scan showing sinus disease is not specific, as multiple different moulds and bacterial pathogens can cause sinusitis. Definitive diagnosis relies on biopsy and culture of the affected tissue, if feasible. These organisms may invade and spread into the orbits or brain causing significant necrosis of the palate, often presenting as a necrotic, black eschar. The absence of distinct lesions upon direct visualization of the sinuses should not exclude tissue biopsy.

Invasive mould infections among HSCT recipients can spread to other contiguous sites or rapidly disseminate to skin, leading to multiple papular to nodular necrotic lesions, and to other organs, including the lungs and brain [4, 43–48]. *Fusarium* species can sporulate in vivo and produce adventitious forms that disseminate and are able to grow in blood cultures [4, 49]. A classic presentation of fusariosis is that of disseminated papular-to-ulcerated skin lesions and blood cultures positive for a filamentous organism [48, 50]. Other filamentous organisms, predominately *S. prolificans*, can also be detected in blood cultures [45, 51].

Epidemiology

In the 1990s data from the Fred Hutchinson Cancer Research Center in Seattle, Washington, suggested that the incidence of IA among allogeneic HSCT recipients increased compared to the 1980s (11.2% vs 5.7%, respectively; $p = 0.02$) [1]. Multiple centers have since reported that the rates of IA among allogeneic HSCT recipients remained as high as 10% during the 1990s and early 2000s [2–4, 13, 14, 52–54]. All HSCT recipients are not equally affected by *Aspergillus* species. The incidence of IA differs based on factors predicting severity and duration of neutropenia and GVHD: (1) type of transplant (lower among autologous [0–5.3%] compared to allogeneic HSCT [10%]), (2) HLA match (higher in HLA mismatched and unrelated donors [10.5% vs matched related 7.3%]), and (3) graft manipulation (higher in T-cell-depleted

[4–16%] vs unmanipulated grafts [2.2–7%]) [2, 4, 15, 53–58]. In contrast, differences in the conditioning regimen do not seem to significantly affect the incidence of IA postallogeneic HSCT, with recipients of nonablative conditioning regimens exhibiting high risks during GVHD [57, 59–62].

Although less frequently encountered, the incidence of mucormycosis among HSCT recipients significantly increased from 0.25% (10 cases among 4,020 HSCT recipients) between 1989 and 1998 to 1.5% (13 of 834) from 2002 to 2004 in one center [30]. Similarly, other groups have reported a relative increase in the frequency of infections due to moulds other than IA among HSCT recipients since the 1990s (Fig. 3) [4, 15, 19, 30].

Despite the routine administration of prophylactic therapy and aggressive monitoring of HSCT recipients, almost one-third of IA cases are observed prior to engraftment, particularly among autologous HSCT recipients [3, 15, 19]. However, the majority of cases of other mould infections occur post engraftment, during periods of acute or chronic GVHD [3, 4, 19, 30, 48, 63, 64]. In one series, all cases of zygomycosis and fusariosis occurred after engraftment, with >50% diagnosed after day 100 [3].

A. fumigatus has been the most commonly isolated *Aspergillus* species in HSCT recipients with IA, ranging from 22.1 to 80.5% in different series (Fig. 4) [1, 4, 13–15, 19, 52]. The frequency of infections with *A. flavus*, *A. terreus*, and *A. niger* has varied in different studies, but these species are noted much less commonly than *A. fumigatus* [1, 4, 13–15, 19, 52, 57]. Clusters of cases of IA due to *A. ustus* or *A. calidoustus*, both potentially multi-drug-resistant pathogens, have been reported among HSCT recipients [65–67]. Recently infections caused by previously unrecognized species within the section *Fumigati,* specifically *A. lentulus, Neosartorya udagawae,* and *N. pseudofischeri*, have been reported in HSCT recipients from multiple centers [68–72]. These species include several that exhibit high resistance profiles to multiple antifungal agents, including voriconazole and amphotericin B, which raises questions regarding the potential clinical significance of antifungal resistance in cases with poor outcomes. In addition, *A. terreus* has been reported to be resistant to amphotericin B [73–75].

The above observations underscore the importance of establishing a microbiologic diagnosis for IA when feasible. Unfortunately, recent reports suggest that *Aspergillus* species remain either unknown or not identified in as many as 49–62% of cases (Fig. 4) [15, 19]. This may, in part, be related to the availability of noninvasive diagnostic tests such as CT scans and galactomannan assays that provide a possible or probable diagnosis without requiring an invasive procedure such as bronchoscopy and lung tissue biopsy. Although this may facilitate and, at times, expedite the diagnosis of IA, the emergence of new *Aspergillus* species with different susceptibility profiles and azole resistance among *Aspergillus* species should be taken into consideration when treating HSCT recipients with IA, particularly those that fail to respond to the administered therapies.

Prevention

Therapy of IFIs entails both preventive strategies as well as treatment of established infection. In HSCT recipients, prevention of infection is critical. It can be argued that the most important therapeutic advances in the supportive care of HSCT recipients within the last decade have occurred due to

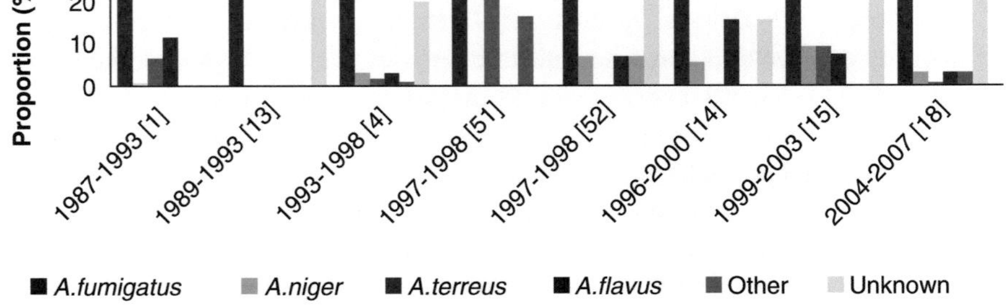

Fig. 4 Epidemiology of *Aspergillus* species between 1987 and 2007 among HSCT recipients with invasive aspergillosis (Adapted from Ref. [1, 4, 13–15, 18, 51, 52])

the effective measures to prevent gram-negative bacterial infections, CMV disease, and candidiasis. One multivariable analysis of outcomes among unrelated donor HSCT recipients with chronic myelogenous leukemia found that two important predictors of overall survival were receipt of ganciclovir for preventing CMV infection and fluconazole for preventing candidiasis [76].

Strategies to prevent fungal infections may rely on administration of antifungals "prophylactically" in high-risk patients, "empirically" in patients with fever during neutropenia, and "preemptively" in patients in whom a more specific indicator of fungal infection is detected. There are advantages and disadvantages to each of these strategies.

Prophylaxis

Prophylactic administration of azole antifungal drugs has become common practice in HSCT recipients. Several randomized trials performed in the early 1990s showed efficacy in preventing candidiasis [7, 9]. The first large randomized trial that compared fluconazole with placebo until neutrophil engraftment in both autologous and allogeneic HSCT recipients showed that fluconazole was associated with decreased fungal infections and fungal infection-related deaths, but there was no difference in overall survival [7]. A second trial compared fluconazole with placebo, both administered for a longer period of time during GVHD in allograft recipients [9]. The results of this trial, and a subsequent long-term follow-up study of the same randomized cohort, verified that fluconazole decreased infections, infection-related deaths, and the overall mortality rate of allograft recipients [9, 10]. Another study documented that the prophylactic use of fluconazole decreased the incidence of hepatosplenic candidiasis in HSCT recipients [77]. Optimal doses and duration of fluconazole administration continue to be a matter of debate.

Unfortunately, the successful prevention of fungal infections has been dampened due to the emergence of azole-resistant *Candida* species and moulds. Most reports suggest that liberal azole use is associated with selection of resistant *Candida* species, namely *C. glabrata* and *C. krusei* [11, 78, 79]. Perhaps more importantly, the incidence of IA has increased in many centers, with this organism surpassing yeasts as the cause of infection-related mortality. The estimated incidence of IA approximates 10–15% in most HSCT centers, with the majority of infections diagnosed late after engraftment – during GVHD [1, 53, 80]. Due to this shift in epidemiology, efforts turned toward establishing a preventive strategy that would encompass moulds as well as yeasts.

Several studies were performed to determine if itraconazole was better than placebo, amphotericin B, or fluconazole for preventing infection in neutropenic patients [81–83]. Although the results of these studies suggested promise regarding prevention of IA, the studies were not performed in high-risk HSCT recipients. Two trials that compared outcomes of HSCT patients who received either itraconazole or fluconazole for at least 100 days after transplant demonstrated the potential utility of itraconazole in preventing invasive mould infections; however, the rate of toxicities was high [84]. Two large studies have demonstrated utility of posaconazole in preventing IFI, especially those caused by moulds, in HSCT patients with GVHD and in patients who are neutropenic following therapy for acute myelocytic leukemia or myelodysplastic syndrome [85, 86]. Another large trial that compared outcomes of voriconazole to fluconazole in "standard risk" HSCT recipients has been completed, with numbers of IFI suggesting potential utility of the mould-active drug [87]. Finally, other methods of administering mould-active antifungals, such as inhaled lipid amphotericin B formulations, may provide utility in preventing IA, but this practice is not yet the standard of care [88].

Empirical and Preemptive Therapy

Another approach to prevention of IFIs is to administer antifungal agents to neutropenic patients with fever that persists despite antibiotics. This practice was established in the 1980s, with the performance of two randomized trials that compared outcomes of febrile neutropenic patients who received either no antifungal therapy or amphotericin B deoxycholate [89, 90]. Both trials showed that amphotericin B was associated with fewer fungal infections. Which antifungal is best for treating fever during neutropenia has been the subject of multiple studies performed subsequently. Most of these studies did not enroll enough HSCT patients to compare efficacy of preventing infection, especially in people already receiving some type of systemically absorbed antifungal drug as prophylaxis [91]. Evaluation of toxicity end points and composite variables showed efficacy, but fewer toxicities with empirical therapy with fluconazole, itraconazole, and lipid formulations of amphotericin B compared to amphotericin B deoxycholate [91, 92]. Whether the toxicity concerns are great enough to warrant the use of the more expensive formulations is a matter of continued debate. Expense has limited their widespread adoption in many large cancer centers. Mould-active triazole antifungal drugs, such as voriconazole and lipid amphotericin B formulations, may be appropriate for treatment of fever during neutropenia in HSCT recipients who have received fluconazole prophylactically [93, 94]. However, fever during neutropenia is not frequently caused by fungal infections in patients who are receiving prophylaxis. Recent studies have found that <5% of high-risk HSCT recipients who are febrile while receiving systemically absorbed antifungal prophylaxis actually had fungal infections as a cause of their fevers [94].

Preemptive is a term used to describe therapy administered early during the course of infection in some settings in an attempt to prevent the development of disease. For CMV, strategies using pp65 antigenemia and PCR to identify infection in HSCT recipients have been very successful at preventing CMV disease and attributable mortality [95]. The development of new diagnostic assays for fungal infections may allow for the similar development of preventive strategies. Early studies focused on the use of serial CT-scanning to initiate early antifungal therapy. Although one small study noted that screening with sensitive radiographic tests may lead to decreased *Aspergillus*-associated mortality compared to historic controls, the costs and inability to routinely screen for long durations after HSCT have limited the applicability of this approach [96]. Other studies have reported that screening with PCR or antigenemia assays may permit establishment of an earlier diagnosis of aspergillosis [97].

Recently, two large studies have evaluated, in a comparative fashion, the potential utility of preemptive therapy. In one, patients were randomized to "standard care" versus care augmented with PCR-based screening. Results did not demonstrate clear benefits in the PCR-based approach; more antifungals were used and there was no large difference in clinical outcomes [98]. Another study randomized neutropenic patients to receive either "standard care" with empirical therapy or an approach that utilized composite clinical and laboratory criteria, including galactomannan screening tests, to trigger the initiation of antifungal therapy [99]. In that study, there were trends to fewer IFIs, particularly those caused by *Candida* species, in the standard "empirical" therapy arm, suggesting that a preemptive approach driven by these clinical criteria may not be sufficient for early therapy in patients who are not receiving fluconazole as prophylactic therapy. While these studies have tremendous importance in providing first efforts for comparative evaluation of preemptive approaches, neither can be considered to provide definitive results, and more efforts are needed to optimize preventative strategies.

Other Methods

Aside from prophylactic or preemptive antifungal administration, other methods to prevent IFIs in HSCT recipients include avoiding exposure and minimizing the severity or duration of risk. *Aspergillus* and other moulds are most frequently acquired from the hospital or external environment, although a certain number of HSCT patients who develop disease early after transplant appear to have reactivation from a previously acquired infection. Efforts to minimize exposure to *Aspergillus* species during the periods of risk have focused on air filtration, either through laminar airflow or high-efficiency particulate air (HEPA) filtration. No randomized trials have been performed to measure the utility of these measures; however, several multivariable models to define risk factors for IA have shown that both may be useful to prevent infection early after transplant [1, 100, 101]. The important limitation to using containment practices is that they are only useful during the period of time during which they are employed. Many experienced clinicians have recently questioned the utility of laminar air flow at a time when disease is most frequently acquired outside of the hospital, late after transplant.

The environmental source of *Aspergillus* species has also been called into question with the results of several recent studies suggesting that moulds may be a common contaminant in hospital water supplies [102–106]. The findings of *Aspergillus* (including *A. fumigatus*) and *Fusarium* species in hospital water supplies, with high amounts of spores recovered in and around patient bathrooms, have led some clinicians to suggest that it may be prudent to avoid aerosolization of water through showering during the period of high risk. Other studies have reported outbreaks of hospital-acquired *A. terreus* infections from apparent association with vegetation (plants) within the hospital [107].

Although the exact environmental source of moulds is rarely determined, even during periods of outbreaks, most centers have instituted infection control practices that focus on air monitoring, patient avoidance of vegetation and food known to have high mould content, such as pepper, and patient avoidance of activities that are associated with aerosolization of conidia, including mowing the lawn, gardening, vacuuming, etc. More studies are necessary to determine whether other infection control practices can minimize infection late after HSCT.

It may also be possible to prevent infection by minimizing the severity and the duration of risks. Efforts to prevent fungal infections have focused on the roles of immune modulators to decrease neutropenia. Few placebo-controlled randomized studies employing hematopoietic growth factors or granulocyte infusions to prevent infection have been performed; however, the results of small randomized trials and risk factor analyses suggest that minimizing the period of neutropenia is associated with fewer *Candida* and *Aspergillus* infections [108]. Optimizing risk reduction during the GVHD period is important, and recent risk factor analyses have shown that factors other than neutropenia, namely corticosteroid exposure, viral (CMV) infections, and lymphopenia may be the strongest predictors of post-engraftment aspergillosis [2, 53]. Minimizing the use of corticosteroids for GVHD is prudent, when possible.

Treatment

For a long time, clinicians have balanced the need for establishing a microbial diagnosis of fungal infections with the desire to minimize complications associated with invasive procedures. Mould infections are especially difficult to diagnose with certainty without performance of some type of invasive procedure, such as bronchoalveolar lavage or lung biopsy. Although complications are rare subsequent to lavage, lung biopsy may elicit hemorrhage and infection in neutropenic, thrombocytopenic patients [109]. One may treat patients with suggestive radiographic lesions presumptively with antifungal agents; however, without a definitive diagnosis, there is a substantial risk of administering misdirected therapy. Establishing a microbial diagnosis has become especially important now that multiple effective antifungal drugs other than amphotericin B deoxycholate are available for use.

Treatment of Candidiasis

Therapy of infections caused by *Candida* depends on the causative species. While fluconazole has been shown to be equivalent to amphotericin B for treatment of candidemia in nonneutropenic patients, candidiasis in neutropenic patients and HSCT recipients is frequently caused by azole-resistant organisms, such as *C. glabrata* or *C. krusei* [1, 110, 111]. In these patients, even *C. albicans* may become resistant to fluconazole through continued exposure during prophylactic therapy [11, 78, 112]. For this reason, and because azole drugs, especially fluconazole and itraconazole, have not been evaluated extensively for therapy of invasive infection in severely immunosuppressed patients, standard therapy of bloodstream infection should include an amphotericin B formulation or an echinocandin. Therapy with lipid formulations of amphotericin B or one of the echinocandins is supported by the results of randomized trials, in which these agents – caspofungin, micafungin, and anidulafungin – were compared with amphotericin B, lipid formulations of amphotericin B, or fluconazole. Results of these studies suggest comparable efficacy, with potentially fewer toxicities associated with echinocandin therapy [113–116]. Duration of therapy for candidemia should continue for at least 2 weeks after the first negative blood culture in order to minimize the likelihood of metastatic sequelae, such as chorioretinitis and endocarditis [117].

Multiple antifungal drugs, including fluconazole, have been shown to be effective for the treatment of hepatosplenic candidiasis, as most infections are caused by susceptible *C. albicans*. Although no randomized studies have been performed to identify the best antifungal agent for treatment, most clinicians favor the use of an amphotericin B formulation as initial therapy, followed by maintenance therapy with an azole antifungal until resolution of lesions occurs [118]. Anecdotal success has been reported using echinocandin antifungals for therapy of hepatosplenic candidiasis as well, which is consistent with the distribution of these drugs to the liver [119]. The reader is referred to a detailed discussion of treatment of *Candida* infections in Chap. 11.

Treatment of Mould Infections

Historically, the only effective therapy for mould infections was amphotericin B. The introduction of new triazoles and echinocandins has now challenged this "gold standard," with evidence that alternative therapy may be indicated for non-*Aspergillus* mould infections and for treatment of infection that does not initially respond to amphotericin B formulations. No randomized studies have compared therapy with amphotericin B deoxycholate to lipid formulations of amphotericin B, although the latter formulations have fewer nephrotoxicities and infusion-related toxicities, both of which may occur at high frequency in HSCT recipients [94, 120]. Differentiating infections with *Aspergillus* species and other mould pathogens has become critical, as optimal therapy for each may differ. While amphotericin B remains the current therapy of choice for zygomycosis, several retrospective open-label studies suggest that the best outcomes result from therapy with high doses of lipid amphotericin B formulations in conjunction with aggressive surgical debridement of involved tissue and granulocyte stimulation or replacement [5, 121]. Emerging data indicate that optimal therapy for *Fusarium* species and *Scedosporium* species may be a mould-active triazole antifungal drug. Reports of outcomes using voriconazole and posaconazole have been encouraging, leading some experienced clinicians to suggest that these drugs should now be considered first-line therapy for these opportunistic filamentous mould infections.

The historic algorithm for treating IA has been to administer amphotericin B deoxycholate as initial (primary) therapy and then to switch to either a mould-active triazole, an echinocandin, or a lipid formulation of amphotericin B if the patient develops serious toxicities or fails to respond to initial therapy. Only one randomized, double-blind study has been performed to evaluate the use of a lipid formulation of amphotericin B as primary therapy for IA. In this study, amphotericin B colloidal dispersion (ABCD) at a dose of 6 mg/kg/day was equivalent in efficacy to amphotericin B deoxycholate, 1.0–1.5 mg/kg/day, but was associated with significantly less nephrotoxicity [122]. Despite the lack of data to support superior efficacy, the lipid formulations are favored by many clinicians because of their potential to deliver high doses of amphotericin B to target tissues without an increase in toxicities. A recent study that compared two doses of liposomal amphotericin B (3 mg/kg vs 10 mg/kg) did not demonstrate better outcomes with the higher dose, in which there were also more toxicities [123]. Salvage studies have shown that voriconazole, posaconazole, and caspofungin are associated with successful therapy when used as a second-line agent in approximately 40% of patients.

The algorithm for standard therapy for IA changed with trials that compared amphotericin B with voriconazole.

Although the response rates of aspergillosis in allogeneic HSCT recipients using amphotericin B formulations only approximated 10–15%, responses were noted in 26% of allogeneic HSCT patients who received voriconazole either as primary or secondary therapy [33, 124–126]. More convincing evidence that voriconazole may be an effective therapy comes from the randomized trial that compared voriconazole as primary therapy with the standard algorithm of amphotericin B followed by the investigator's choice of other licensed antifungal therapy. The results of this trial indicate that clinical outcomes and overall survival rates improve with voriconazole used as primary therapy [127].

In vitro and in vivo studies suggest that combination antifungal therapy, employing an echinocandin with either a mould-active triazole or an amphotericin B formulation for IA, may be more efficacious [128–131]. Retrospective data from the Fred Hutchinson Cancer Center showed that voriconazole combined with caspofungin as salvage treatment of IA in HSCT recipients, most of whom had received an allogeneic transplant, was associated with improved 3-month survival compared to voriconazole alone [132]. In multivariate model analyses, salvage therapy with the combination of voriconazole and caspofungin was associated with reduced mortality rates, compared with therapy with voriconazole (HR, 0.28; 95% CI, 0.28–0.92; $p = 0.01$), independent of other prognostic variables [132]. A prospective double-blind, randomized, multicenter, international study to address the efficacy of combination therapy of voriconazole with an echinocandin in HSCT recipients and high-risk hematologic malignancy patients is currently underway (Clinical Trials Gov: NCT00531479).

Recently, attention has turned toward the potential need for therapeutic drug monitoring to assure "good" levels of voriconazole. Studies have shown that approximately 20% of patients do not have measurable levels of the drug despite standard dosing, and if levels are too high, there may be a higher incidence of neurotoxicity and/or hepatotoxicity [133–135]. While the optimal algorithm for dosing and following up on voriconazole has yet to be defined, levels have to at least be considered, especially in patients who are not responding or who have demonstrated toxicities. Clinical studies evaluating the safety and efficacy of the various combinations, especially combining voriconazole with an echinocandin, are underway. Common practice is to continue antifungal therapy for the duration of time that the patient is receiving immunosuppressive drugs. Allogeneic HSCT recipients with pulmonary mould infections should receive prolonged antifungal therapy, at least as long as they are receiving high doses of corticosteroid therapy for GVHD. The cumulative dose and duration of corticosteroid exposure are closely associated with negative outcomes of antifungal therapy; consequently, every effort should be made to minimize exposure to corticosteroids [33].

Adjunctive Therapy

The utility of adjunctive therapy using immune modulating agents, such as hematopoietic growth factors or granulocyte transfusions, continues to be a matter of debate. No definitive randomized studies have been performed. Up to now, studies have only justified the safety of immunomodulating therapy, with anecdotes suggesting efficacy. Granulocyte colony-stimulating factor (G-CSF) and granulocyte-macrophage colony-stimulating factor (GM-CSF) are used frequently in patients who are neutropenic and have invasive fungal infections. Adjunctive immunotherapy may be especially important for treatment of mould infections characterized by a large circulating fungal burden and relative resistance to antifungal drugs, as with disseminated fusariosis. In addition, other reports emphasize that outcomes of therapy for zygomycosis improve with rapid resolution of neutropenia [5]. The potential utility of neutrophil transfusions as adjunctive therapy has been rejuvenated with the development of G-CSF-primed community donor transfusions [136]. Studies evaluating the safety and efficacy of such transfusions, and the use of interferon-gamma for adjunctive therapy of aspergillosis in neutropenic patients, are either ongoing or in development.

The role of surgical debridement of pulmonary fungal lesions is also a matter of debate, as no randomized studies have been performed, and noncontrolled studies are impacted by selection bias. Anecdotal reports and case series suggest that there is a definite role for surgical resection in patients who present with severe hemoptysis and fungal lesions abutting large vessels, and in patients in whom further myelosuppressive therapy is intended [137]. In many centers, patients who present pretransplant with isolated pulmonary fungal lesions undergo resection when possible. This practice is justified by the results of case series that suggest that recurrent fungal infection occurs less frequently in patients who have undergone surgical resection before myeloablative therapy. As mentioned above, surgical resection of infection caused by Zygomycetes appears to be strongly associated with successful therapy.

Clinical Outcomes

Clinical outcomes among HSCT recipients with invasive candidiasis remain poor, in part due to the underlying compromised immune status and organ function of these patients. Mortality rates ranged between 22% and 40% during the 1980–1990s [6, 8, 11]. In a US multicenter study performed between 2004 and 2007, the crude 12-week mortality rate among HSCT recipients with invasive candidiasis was found to be 48.9% [19]. Although less frequently encountered due to routine prophylaxis with fluconazole, invasive candidiasis appears to be a significant factor affecting outcomes among

HSCT recipients. More aggressive HSCT practices, such as performing high-risk transplants, might have resulted in sicker patients with worse prognoses due to their comorbidities and prolonged immunosuppressed state. Estimating the actual attributable mortality of invasive candidiasis in this population is difficult.

The reported 4–12-month mortality rates among HSCT recipients with IA have historically been as high as 90% [1, 2, 4, 33]. Recent data suggest that outcomes may be improving, with 12-week overall survival ranging from 44 to 64.5% [19, 138, 139]. Improved contemporary clinical outcomes may in part reflect improved diagnostic modalities leading to earlier recognition of IA and prompt initiation of antifungal treatment at an earlier stage. In fact, early diagnosis of pulmonary IA based on chest CT scan was associated with improved 12-week survival rate (71% vs 53%, $p < 0.01$) and treatment response (52% vs 29%, $p < 0.001$) [37]. The availability of potent and well-tolerated antifungal agents might have also allowed for earlier treatment initiation and improved outcomes. Different centers have reported an association between improved survival rates and voriconazole administration [138, 139]. In addition, transplant-related variables, such as nonmyeloablative conditioning and use of peripheral blood cells as a stem cell source, have been associated with improved survival rates [138, 139]. In contrast, predictors of mortality among HSCT recipients with IA have included younger age, HLA-mismatched donors, neutropenia, monocytopenia, abnormal renal and liver function, disseminated disease, presence of a pleural effusion, administration of corticosteroids, and uncontrolled GVHD [19, 139, 140].

While the clinical outcomes of IA appear to be improving, survival among HSCT recipients with mucormycosis and other mould infections remains poor, with reported mortality rates ranging between 64% and 100% [4, 19, 121]. Historically, HSCT recipients with an invasive infection due to *Fusarium* species have had poor outcomes, with survival rates ranging between 13% and 21% [4, 48, 141]. Similarly, infections with *Scedosporium* species have been associated with 30-day mortality rates reaching 100% [4]. The prolonged duration of profound immunosuppression of HSCT recipients, cumbersome and frequent late diagnosis of these infections, and limited treatment options likely contribute to the poor outcomes associated with mould infections.

References

1. Wald A, Leisenring W, van Burik JA, Bowden RA. Epidemiology of *Aspergillus* infections in a large cohort of patients undergoing bone marrow transplantation. J Infect Dis. 1997;175(6):1459–66.
2. Marr KA, Carter RA, Boeckh M, Martin P, Corey L. Invasive aspergillosis in allogeneic stem cell transplant recipients: changes in epidemiology and risk factors. Blood. 2002;100(13):4358–66.
3. Garcia-Vidal C, Upton A, Kirby KA, Marr KA. Epidemiology of invasive mould infections in allogeneic stem cell transplant recipients: biological risk factors for infection according to time after transplantation. Clin Infect Dis. 2008;47(8):1041–50.
4. Marr KA, Carter RA, Crippa F, Wald A, Corey L. Epidemiology and outcome of mould infections in hematopoietic stem cell transplant recipients. Clin Infect Dis. 2002;34(7):909–17.
5. Kontoyiannis DP, Wessel VC, Bodey GP, Rolston KV. Zygomycosis in the 1990s in a tertiary-care cancer center. Clin Infect Dis. 2000;30(6):851–6.
6. Goodrich JM, Reed EC, Mori M, et al. Clinical features and analysis of risk factors for invasive candidal infection after marrow transplantation. J Infect Dis. 1991;164(4):731–40.
7. Goodman JL, Winston DJ, Greenfield RA, et al. A controlled trial of fluconazole to prevent fungal infections in patients undergoing bone marrow transplantation. N Engl J Med. 1992;326(13):845–51.
8. Meyers JD. Fungal infections in bone marrow transplant patients. Semin Oncol. 1990;17(3 Suppl):10–3.
9. Slavin MA, Osborne B, Adams R, et al. Efficacy and safety of fluconazole prophylaxis for fungal infections after marrow transplantation-a prospective, randomized, double-blind study. J Infect Dis. 1995;171(6):1545–52.
10. Marr KA, Seidel K, Slavin MA, et al. Prolonged fluconazole prophylaxis is associated with persistent protection against candidiasis-related death in allogeneic marrow transplant recipients: long-term follow-up of a randomized, placebo-controlled trial. Blood. 2000;96(6):2055–61.
11. Marr KA, Seidel K, White TC, Bowden RA. Candidemia in allogeneic blood and marrow transplant recipients: evolution of risk factors after the adoption of prophylactic fluconazole. J Infect Dis. 2000;181(1):309–16.
12. Safdar A, van Rhee F, Henslee-Downey JP, Singhal S, Mehta J. *Candida glabrata* and *Candida krusei* fungemia after high-risk allogeneic marrow transplantation: no adverse effect of low-dose fluconazole prophylaxis on incidence and outcome. Bone Marrow Transplant. 2001;28(9):873–8.
13. Jantunen E, Ruutu P, Niskanen L, et al. Incidence and risk factors for invasive fungal infections in allogeneic BMT recipients. Bone Marrow Transplant. 1997;19(8):801–8.
14. Martino R, Subira M, Rovira M, et al. Invasive fungal infections after allogeneic peripheral blood stem cell transplantation: incidence and risk factors in 395 patients. Br J Haematol. 2002;116(2):475–82.
15. Pagano L, Caira M, Nosari A, et al. Fungal infections in recipients of hematopoietic stem cell transplants: results of the SEIFEM B-2004 study-Sorveglianza Epidemiologica Infezioni Fungine Nelle Emopatie Maligne. Clin Infect Dis. 2007;45(9):1161–70.
16. Jantunen E, Nihtinen A, Volin L, et al. Candidaemia in allogeneic stem cell transplant recipients: low risk without fluconazole prophylaxis. Bone Marrow Transplant. 2004;34(10):891–5.
17. Wingard JR, Merz WG, Rinaldi MG, Johnson TR, Karp JE, Saral R. Increase in *Candida krusei* infection among patients with bone marrow transplantation and neutropenia treated prophylactically with fluconazole. N Engl J Med. 1991;325(18):1274–7.
18. Persons DA, Laughlin M, Tanner D, Perfect J, Gockerman JP, Hathorn JW. Fluconazole and *Candida krusei* fungemia. N Engl J Med. 1991;325(18):1315.
19. Neofytos D, Horn D, Anaissie E, et al. Epidemiology and outcome of invasive fungal infection in adult hematopoietic stem cell transplant recipients: analysis of multicenter prospective antifungal therapy (PATH) alliance registry. Clin Infect Dis. 2009;48(3):265–73.
20. Wingard JR, Merz WG, Rinaldi MG, Miller CB, Karp JE, Saral R. Association of *Torulopsis glabrata* infections with fluconazole prophylaxis in neutropenic bone marrow transplant patients. Antimicrob Agents Chemother. 1993;37(9):1847–9.
21. Nolte FS, Parkinson T, Falconer DJ, et al. Isolation and characterization of fluconazole- and amphotericin B-resistant *Candida*

albicans from blood of two patients with leukemia. Antimicrob Agents Chemother. 1997;41(1):196–9.
22. Mori T, Matsumura M, Kanamaru Y, et al. Myelofibrosis complicated by infection due to *Candida albicans*: emergence of resistance to antifungal agents during therapy. Clin Infect Dis. 1997;25(6):1470–1.
23. Brummer E, Kamberi M, Stevens DA. Regulation by granulocyte-macrophage colony-stimulating factor and/or steroids given in vivo of proinflammatory cytokine and chemokine production by bronchoalveolar macrophages in response to *Aspergillus* conidia. J Infect Dis. 2003;187(4):705–9.
24. Grazziutti ML, Rex JH, Cowart RE, Anaissie EJ, Ford A, Savary CA. *Aspergillus fumigatus* conidia induce a Th1-type cytokine response. J Infect Dis. 1997;176(6):1579–83.
25. Hebart H, Bollinger C, Fisch P, et al. Analysis of T-cell responses to *Aspergillus fumigatus* antigens in healthy individuals and patients with hematologic malignancies. Blood. 2002;100(13):4521–8.
26. Philippe B, Ibrahim-Granet O, Prevost MC, et al. Killing of *Aspergillus fumigatus* by alveolar macrophages is mediated by reactive oxidant intermediates. Infect Immun. 2003;71(6):3034–42.
27. Bochud PY, Chien JW, Marr KA, et al. Toll-like receptor 4 polymorphisms and aspergillosis in stem-cell transplantation. N Engl J Med. 2008;359(17):1766–77.
28. Zaas AK, Liao G, Chien JW, et al. Plasminogen alleles influence susceptibility to invasive aspergillosis. PLoS Genet. 2008;4(6):e1000101.
29. Kesh S, Mensah NY, Peterlongo P, et al. TLR1 and TLR6 polymorphisms are associated with susceptibility to invasive aspergillosis after allogeneic stem cell transplantation. Ann NY Acad Sci. 2005;1062:95–103.
30. Kontoyiannis DP, Lionakis MS, Lewis RE, et al. Zygomycosis in a tertiary-care cancer center in the era of aspergillus-active antifungal therapy: a case-control observational study of 27 recent cases. J Infect Dis. 2005;191(8):1350–60.
31. Hachem R, Sumoza D, Hanna H, Girgawy E, Munsell M, Raad I. Clinical and radiologic predictors of invasive pulmonary aspergillosis in cancer patients: should the European Organization for Research and Treatment of Cancer/Mycosis Study Group (EORTC/MSG) criteria be revised? Cancer. 2006;106(7):1581–6.
32. Kuhlman JE, Fishman EK, Siegelman SS. Invasive pulmonary aspergillosis in acute leukemia: characteristic findings on CT, the CT halo sign, and the role of CT in early diagnosis. Radiology. 1985;157(3):611–4.
33. Ribaud P, Chastang C, Latge JP, et al. Survival and prognostic factors of invasive aspergillosis after allogeneic bone marrow transplantation. Clin Infect Dis. 1999;28(2):322–30.
34. Caillot D, Couaillier JF, Bernard A, et al. Increasing volume and changing characteristics of invasive pulmonary aspergillosis on sequential thoracic computed tomography scans in patients with neutropenia. J Clin Oncol. 2001;19(1):253–9.
35. Kami M, Kishi Y, Hamaki T, et al. The value of the chest computed tomography halo sign in the diagnosis of invasive pulmonary aspergillosis. An autopsy-based retrospective study of 48 patients. Mycoses. 2002;45(8):287–94.
36. Horger M, Hebart H, Einsele H, et al. Initial CT manifestations of invasive pulmonary aspergillosis in 45 non-HIV immunocompromised patients: association with patient outcome? Eur J Radiol. 2005;55(3):437–44.
37. Greene RE, Schlamm HT, Oestmann JW, et al. Imaging findings in acute invasive pulmonary aspergillosis: clinical significance of the halo sign. Clin Infect Dis. 2007;44(3):373–9.
38. Greene R. The radiological spectrum of pulmonary aspergillosis. Med Mycol. 2005;43 Suppl 1:S147–54.
39. Primack SL, Hartman TE, Lee KS, Muller NL. Pulmonary nodules and the CT halo sign. Radiology. 1994;190(2):513–5.
40. Lee YR, Choi YW, Lee KJ, Jeon SC, Park CK, Heo JN. CT halo sign: the spectrum of pulmonary diseases. Br J Radiol. 2005;78(933):862–5.
41. Kojima R, Tateishi U, Kami M, et al. Chest computed tomography of late invasive aspergillosis after allogeneic hematopoietic stem cell transplantation. Biol Blood Marrow Transplant. 2005;11(7):506–11.
42. Chamilos G, Marom EM, Lewis RE, Lionakis MS, Kontoyiannis DP. Predictors of pulmonary zygomycosis versus invasive pulmonary aspergillosis in patients with cancer. Clin Infect Dis. 2005;41(1):60–6.
43. Martino P, Gastaldi R, Raccah R, Girmenia C. Clinical patterns of *Fusarium* infections in immunocompromised patients. J Infect. 1994;28 Suppl 1:7–15.
44. Jahagirdar BN, Morrison VA. Emerging fungal pathogens in patients with hematologic malignancies and marrow/stem-cell transplant recipients. Semin Respir Infect. 2002;17(2):113–20.
45. Husain S, Munoz P, Forrest G, et al. Infections due to *Scedosporium apiospermum* and *Scedosporium prolificans* in transplant recipients: clinical characteristics and impact of antifungal agent therapy on outcome. Clin Infect Dis. 2005;40(1):89–99.
46. Garcia-Arata MI, Otero MJ, Zomeno M, de la Figuera MA, de las Cuevas MC, Lopez-Brea M. *Scedosporium apiospermum* pneumonia after autologous bone marrow transplantation. Eur J Clin Microbiol Infect Dis. 1996;15(7):600–3.
47. Safdar A, Papadopoulos EB, Young JW. Breakthrough *Scedosporium apiospermum* (*Pseudallescheria boydii*) brain abscess during therapy for invasive pulmonary aspergillosis following high-risk allogeneic hematopoietic stem cell transplantation. Scedosporiasis and recent advances in antifungal therapy. Transpl Infect Dis. 2002;4(4):212–7.
48. Nucci M, Marr KA, Queiroz-Telles F, et al. *Fusarium* infection in hematopoietic stem cell transplant recipients. Clin Infect Dis. 2004;38(9):1237–42.
49. Liu K, Howell DN, Perfect JR, Schell WA. Morphologic criteria for the preliminary identification of *Fusarium*, *Paecilomyces*, and *Acremonium* species by histopathology. Am J Clin Pathol. 1998;109(1):45–54.
50. Dignani MC, Anaissie E. Human fusariosis. Clin Microbiol Infect. 2004;10 Suppl 1:67–75.
51. Idigoras P, Perez-Trallero E, Pineiro L, et al. Disseminated infection and colonization by *Scedosporium prolificans*: a review of 18 cases, 1990–1999. Clin Infect Dis. 2001;32(11):E158–65.
52. Baddley JW, Stroud TP, Salzman D, Pappas PG. Invasive mould infections in allogeneic bone marrow transplant recipients. Clin Infect Dis. 2001;32(9):1319–24.
53. Grow WB, Moreb JS, Roque D, et al. Late onset of invasive *Aspergillus* infection in bone marrow transplant patients at a university hospital. Bone Marrow Transplant. 2002;29(1):15–9.
54. Cornet M, Fleury L, Maslo C, Bernard JF, Brucker G. Invasive aspergillosis surveillance network of the assistance Publique-Hopitaux de Paris. Epidemiology of invasive aspergillosis in France: a six-year multicentric survey in the greater Paris area. J Hosp Infect. 2002;51(4):288–96.
55. Jantunen E, Salonen J, Juvonen E, et al. Invasive fungal infections in autologous stem cell transplant recipients: a nation-wide study of 1188 transplanted patients. Eur J Haematol. 2004;73(3):174–8.
56. Mihu CN, King E, Yossepovitch O, et al. Risk factors and attributable mortality of late aspergillosis after T-cell depleted hematopoietic stem cell transplantation. Transpl Infect Dis. 2008;10(3):162–7.
57. Morgan J, Wannemuehler KA, Marr KA, et al. Incidence of invasive aspergillosis following hematopoietic stem cell and solid organ transplantation: interim results of a prospective multicenter surveillance program. Med Mycol. 2005;43 Suppl 1:S49–58.
58. van Burik JA, Carter SL, Freifeld AG, et al. Higher risk of cytomegalovirus and *Aspergillus* infections in recipients of T cell-depleted

unrelated bone marrow: analysis of infectious complications in patients treated with T cell depletion versus immunosuppressive therapy to prevent graft-versus-host disease. Biol Blood Marrow Transplant. 2007;13(12):1487–98.

59. Labbe AC, Su SH, Laverdiere M, et al. High incidence of invasive aspergillosis associated with intestinal graft-versus-host disease following nonmyeloablative transplantation. Biol Blood Marrow Transplant. 2007;13(10):1192–200.
60. Junghanss C, Marr KA, Carter RA, et al. Incidence and outcome of bacterial and fungal infections following nonmyeloablative compared with myeloablative allogeneic hematopoietic stem cell transplantation: a matched control study. Biol Blood Marrow Transplant. 2002;8(9):512–20.
61. Fukuda T, Boeckh M, Carter RA, et al. Risks and outcomes of invasive fungal infections in recipients of allogeneic hematopoietic stem cell transplants after nonmyeloablative conditioning. Blood. 2003;102(3):827–33.
62. Martino R, Caballero MD, Canals C, et al. Reduced-intensity conditioning reduces the risk of severe infections after allogeneic peripheral blood stem cell transplantation. Bone Marrow Transplant. 2001;28(4):341–7.
63. Imhof A, Balajee SA, Fredricks DN, Englund JA, Marr KA. Breakthrough fungal infections in stem cell transplant recipients receiving voriconazole. Clin Infect Dis. 2004;39(5):743–6.
64. Trifilio SM, Bennett CL, Yarnold PR, et al. Breakthrough zygomycosis after voriconazole administration among patients with hematologic malignancies who receive hematopoietic stem-cell transplants or intensive chemotherapy. Bone Marrow Transplant. 2007;39(7):425–9.
65. Pavie J, Lacroix C, Hermoso DG, et al. Breakthrough disseminated *Aspergillus ustus* infection in allogeneic hematopoietic stem cell transplant recipients receiving voriconazole or caspofungin prophylaxis. J Clin Microbiol. 2005;43(9):4902–4.
66. Panackal AA, Imhof A, Hanley EW, Marr KA. *Aspergillus ustus* infections among transplant recipients. Emerg Infect Dis. 2006;12(3):403–8.
67. Alastruey-Izquierdo A, Cuesta I, Houbraken J, Cuenca-Estrella M, Monzon A, Rodriguez-Tudela JL. In vitro activity of nine antifungal agents against clinical isolates of *Aspergillus calidoustus*. Med Mycol. 2010;48:97–102.
68. Balajee SA, Gribskov JL, Hanley E, Nickle D, Marr KA. *Aspergillus lentulus* sp. nov., a new sibling species of *A. fumigatus*. Eukaryot Cell. 2005;4(3):625–32.
69. Balajee SA, Nickle D, Varga J, Marr KA. Molecular studies reveal frequent misidentification of *Aspergillus fumigatus* by morphotyping. Eukaryot Cell. 2006;5(10):1705–12.
70. Chim CS, Ho PL, Yuen KY. Simultaneous *Aspergillus fischeri* and Herpes simplex pneumonia in a patient with multiple myeloma. Scand J Infect Dis. 1998;30(2):190–1.
71. Jarv H, Lehtmaa J, Summerbell RC, Hoekstra ES, Samson RA, Naaber P. Isolation of *Neosartorya pseudofischeri* from blood: first hint of pulmonary aspergillosis. J Clin Microbiol. 2004; 42(2):925–8.
72. Vinh DC, Shea YR, Sugui JA, et al. Invasive aspergillosis due to *Neosartorya udagawae*. Clin Infect Dis. 2009;49(1):102–11.
73. Lass-Florl C, Kofler G, Kropshofer G, et al. In-vitro testing of susceptibility to amphotericin B is a reliable predictor of clinical outcome in invasive aspergillosis. J Antimicrob Chemother. 1998;42(4):497–502.
74. Steinbach WJ, Stevens DA, Denning DW. Combination and sequential antifungal therapy for invasive aspergillosis: review of published in vitro and in vivo interactions and 6281 clinical cases from 1966 to 2001. Clin Infect Dis. 2003;37 Suppl 3:S188–224.
75. Rex JH, Pfaller MA, Walsh TJ, et al. Antifungal susceptibility testing: practical aspects and current challenges. Clin Microbiol Rev. 2001;14(4):643–58.
76. Hansen JA, Gooley TA, Martin PJ, Appelbaum F, Chancey TR, Clift RA, et al. Bone marrow transplants from unrelated donors for patients with chronic myeloid leukemia. N Engl J Med. 1998;338:962–8.
77. van Burik JH, Leisenring W, Myerson D, et al. The effect of prophylactic fluconazole on the clinical spectrum of fungal diseases in bone marrow transplant recipients with special attention to hepatic candidiasis. An autopsy study of 355 patients. Medicine (Baltimore). 1998;77(4):246–54.
78. Marr KA, White TC, van Burik JA, Bowden RA. Development of fluconazole resistance in *Candida albicans* causing disseminated infection in a patient undergoing marrow transplantation. Clin Infect Dis. 1997;25(4):908–10.
79. Bodey GP, Mardani M, Hanna HA, et al. The epidemiology of *Candida glabrata* and *Candida albicans* fungemia in immunocompromised patients with cancer. Am J Med. 2002;112(5): 380–5.
80. Williamson EC, Millar MR, Steward CG, et al. Infections in adults undergoing unrelated donor bone marrow transplantation. Br J Haematol. 1999;104(3):560–8.
81. Menichetti F, Del Favero A, Martino P, et al. Itraconazole oral solution as prophylaxis for fungal infections in neutropenic patients with hematologic malignancies: a randomized, placebo-controlled, double-blind, multicenter trial. GIMEMA infection program. Gruppo Italiano Malattie Ematologiche dell' Adulto. Clin Infect Dis. 1999;28(2):250–5.
82. Harousseau JL, Dekker AW, Stamatoullas-Bastard A, et al. Itraconazole oral solution for primary prophylaxis of fungal infections in patients with hematological malignancy and profound neutropenia: a randomized, double-blind, double-placebo, multicenter trial comparing itraconazole and amphotericin B. Antimicrob Agents Chemother. 2000;44(7):1887–93.
83. Morgenstern GR, Prentice AG, Prentice HG, Ropner JE, Schey SA, Warnock DW. A randomized controlled trial of itraconazole versus fluconazole for the prevention of fungal infections in patients with haematological malignancies. U.K. multicentre antifungal prophylaxis study group. Br J Haematol. 1999;105(4): 901–11.
84. Marr KA, Crippa F, Leisenring W, et al. Itraconazole versus fluconazole for prevention of fungal infections in patients receiving allogeneic stem cell transplants. Blood. 2004;103(4):1527–33.
85. Cornely OA, Maertens J, Winston DJ, et al. Posaconazole vs. fluconazole or itraconazole prophylaxis in patients with neutropenia. N Engl J Med. 2007;356(4):348–59.
86. Ullmann AJ, Lipton JH, Vesole DH, et al. Posaconazole or fluconazole for prophylaxis in severe graft-versus-host disease. N Engl J Med. 2007;356(4):335–47.
87. Wingard JR, Carter SL, Walsh TJ, et al. Randomized, double-blind trial of fluconazole vs. voriconazole for the prevention of invasive fungal infection (IFI) after allogeneic hemotopoietic cell transplantation. Blood 2010; doi: 10.1182/blood-2010–02-268151.
88. Rijnders BJ, Cornelissen JJ, Slobbe L, et al. Aerosolized liposomal amphotericin B for the prevention of invasive pulmonary aspergillosis during prolonged neutropenia: a randomized, placebo-controlled trial. Clin Infect Dis. 2008;46(9):1401–8.
89. Pizzo PA, Robichaud KJ, Gill FA, Witebsky FG. Empiric antibiotic and antifungal therapy for cancer patients with prolonged fever and granulocytopenia. Am J Med. 1982;72(1):101–11.
90. EORTC International Antimicrobial Therapy Cooperative Group. Empiric antifungal therapy in febrile granulocytopenic patients. Am J Med. 1989;86(6 Pt 1):668–72.
91. Marr KA. Empirical antifungal therapy-new options, new tradeoffs. N Engl J Med. 2002;346(4):278–80.
92. Walsh TJ, Hiemenz JW, Seibel NL, et al. Amphotericin B lipid complex for invasive fungal infections: analysis of safety and efficacy in 556 cases. Clin Infect Dis. 1998;26(6):1383–96.

93. Walsh TJ, Finberg RW, Arndt C, et al. Liposomal amphotericin B for empirical therapy in patients with persistent fever and neutropenia. National Institute of Allergy and Infectious Diseases Mycoses Study Group. N Engl J Med. 1999;340(10):764–71.
94. Walsh TJ, Pappas P, Winston DJ, et al. Voriconazole compared with liposomal amphotericin B for empirical antifungal therapy in patients with neutropenia and persistent fever. N Engl J Med. 2002;346(4):225–34.
95. Boeckh M. Current antiviral strategies for controlling cytomegalovirus in hematopoietic stem cell transplant recipients: prevention and therapy. Transpl Infect Dis. 1999;1(3):165–78.
96. Caillot D, Casasnovas O, Bernard A, et al. Improved management of invasive pulmonary aspergillosis in neutropenic patients using early thoracic computed tomographic scan and surgery. J Clin Oncol. 1997;15(1):139–47.
97. Walsh TJ, Chanock SJ. Diagnosis of invasive fungal infections: advances in nonculture systems. Curr Clin Top Infect Dis. 1998;18:101–53.
98. Hebart H, Loffler J, Reitze H, et al. Prospective screening by a panfungal polymerase chain reaction assay in patients at risk for fungal infections: implications for the management of febrile neutropenia. Br J Haematol. 2000;111(2):635–40.
99. Cordonnier C, Pautas C, Maury S, et al. Empirical versus preemptive antifungal therapy for high-risk, febrile, neutropenic patients: a randomized, controlled trial. Clin Infect Dis. 2009;48(8):1042–51.
100. Sherertz RJ, Belani A, Kramer BS, et al. Impact of air filtration on nosocomial *Aspergillus* infections. Unique risk of bone marrow transplant recipients. Am J Med. 1987;83(4):709–18.
101. Cornet M, Levy V, Fleury L, et al. Efficacy of prevention by high-efficiency particulate air filtration or laminar airflow against *Aspergillus* airborne contamination during hospital renovation. Infect Control Hosp Epidemiol. 1999;20(7):508–13.
102. Anaissie EJ, Costa SF. Nosocomial aspergillosis is waterborne. Clin Infect Dis. 2001;33(9):1546–8.
103. Anaissie EJ, Stratton SL, Dignani MC, et al. Pathogenic *Aspergillus* species recovered from a hospital water system: a 3-year prospective study. Clin Infect Dis. 2002;34(6):780–9.
104. Anaissie EJ, Kuchar RT, Rex JH, et al. Fusariosis associated with pathogenic *Fusarium* species colonization of a hospital water system: a new paradigm for the epidemiology of opportunistic mould infections. Clin Infect Dis. 2001;33(11):1871–8.
105. Warris A, Gaustad P, Meis JF, Voss A, Verweij PE, Abrahamsen TG. Recovery of filamentous fungi from water in a paediatric bone marrow transplantation unit. J Hosp Infect. 2001;47(2):143–8.
106. Warris A, Voss A, Abrahamsen TG, Verweij PE. Contamination of hospital water with *Aspergillus fumigatus* and other moulds. Clin Infect Dis. 2002;34(8):1159–60.
107. Lass-Florl C, Rath P, Niederwieser D, et al. *Aspergillus terreus* infections in haematological malignancies: molecular epidemiology suggests association with in-hospital plants. J Hosp Infect. 2000;46(1):31–5.
108. Wingard J. Growth factors and other immunomodulators. In: Bowden R, Ljungman P, Paya C, editors. Transplant Infections. Philadelphia: Lippincott-Raven; 1998. p. 367–78.
109. Hoffer FA, Gow K, Flynn PM, Davidoff A. Accuracy of percutaneous lung biopsy for invasive pulmonary aspergillosis. Pediatr Radiol. 2001;31(3):144–52.
110. Rex JH, Bennett JE, Sugar AM, et al. A randomized trial comparing fluconazole with amphotericin B for the treatment of candidemia in patients without neutropenia. Candidemia Study Group and the National Institute. N Engl J Med. 1994;331(20):1325–30.
111. Viscoli C, Castagnola E, Machetti M. Antifungal treatment in patients with cancer. J Intern Med Suppl. 1997;740:89–94.
112. Marr KA, Lyons CN, Ha K, Rustad TR, White TC. Inducible azole resistance associated with a heterogeneous phenotype in *Candida albicans*. Antimicrob Agents Chemother. 2001;45(1):52–9.
113. Mora-Duarte J, Betts R, Rotstein C, et al. Comparison of caspofungin and amphotericin B for invasive candidiasis. N Engl J Med. 2002;347(25):2020–9.
114. Kuse ER, Chetchotisakd P, da Cunha CA, et al. Micafungin versus liposomal amphotericin B for candidaemia and invasive candidosis: a phase III randomised double-blind trial. Lancet. 2007;369(9572): 1519–27.
115. Pappas PG, Rotstein CM, Betts RF, et al. Micafungin versus caspofungin for treatment of candidemia and other forms of invasive candidiasis. Clin Infect Dis. 2007;45(7):883–93.
116. Reboli AC, Rotstein C, Pappas PG, et al. Anidulafungin versus fluconazole for invasive candidiasis. N Engl J Med. 2007; 356(24):2472–82.
117. Pappas PG, Kauffman CA, Anies D, et al. Clinical practice guidelines for the management of candidiasis: 2009 update by the Infectious Diseases Society of America. Clin Infect Dis. 2009;48:503–35.
118. Kontoyiannis DP, Luna MA, Samuels BI, Bodey GP. Hepatosplenic candidiasis. A manifestation of chronic disseminated candidiasis. Infect Dis Clin North Am. 2000;14(3):721–39.
119. Groll AH, Walsh TJ. Caspofungin: pharmacology, safety and therapeutic potential in superficial and invasive fungal infections. Expert Opin Investig Drugs. 2001;10(8):1545–58.
120. Wingard JR, White MH, Anaissie E, et al. A randomized, double-blind comparative trial evaluating the safety of liposomal amphotericin B versus amphotericin B lipid complex in the empirical treatment of febrile neutropenia. L Amph/ABLC Collaborative Study Group. Clin Infect Dis. 2000;31(5):1155–63.
121. Herbrecht R, Letscher-Bru V, Bowden RA, et al. Treatment of 21 cases of invasive mucormycosis with amphotericin B colloidal dispersion. Eur J Clin Microbiol Infect Dis. 2001;20(7):460–6.
122. Bowden R, Chandrasekar P, White MH, et al. A double-blind, randomized, controlled trial of amphotericin B colloidal dispersion versus amphotericin B for treatment of invasive aspergillosis in immunocompromised patients. Clin Infect Dis. 2002;35(4): 359–66.
123. Cornely OA, Maertens J, Bresnik M, et al. Liposomal amphotericin B as initial therapy for invasive mould infection: a randomized trial comparing a high-loading dose regimen with standard dosing (AmBiLoad trial). Clin Infect Dis. 2007;44(10):1289–97.
124. Denning DW, Ribaud P, Milpied N, et al. Efficacy and safety of voriconazole in the treatment of acute invasive aspergillosis. Clin Infect Dis. 2002;34(5):563–71.
125. Patterson TF, Kirkpatrick WR, White M, et al. Invasive aspergillosis. Disease spectrum, treatment practices, and outcomes. Aspergillus study group. Medicine (Baltimore). 2000;79(4):250–60.
126. Lin SJ, Schranz J, Teutsch SM. Aspergillosis case-fatality rate: systematic review of the literature. Clin Infect Dis. 2001;32(3): 358–66.
127. Herbrecht R, Denning DW, Patterson TF, et al. Voriconazole versus amphotericin B for primary therapy of invasive aspergillosis. N Engl J Med. 2002;347(6):408–15.
128. Arikan S, Lozano-Chiu M, Paetznick V, Rex J. In vitro synergy of caspofungin and amphotericin B against *Aspergillus* and *Fusarium* spp. Antimicrob Agents Chemother. 2002;46:245–7.
129. Perea S, Gonzalez G, Fothergill AW, Kirkpatrick WR, Rinaldi MG, Patterson TF. In vitro interaction of caspofungin acetate with voriconazole against clinical isolates of *Aspergillus* spp. Antimicrob Agents Chemother. 2002;46:3039–41.
130. Kirkpatrick WR, Perea S, Coco BJ, Patterson TF. Efficacy of caspofungin alone and in combination with voriconazole in a Guinea pig model of invasive aspergillosis. Antimicrob Agents Chemother. 2002;46:2564–8.
131. Kontoyiannis DP, Hachem R, Lewis RE, et al. Efficacy and toxicity of caspofungin in combination with liposomal amphotericin B as primary or salvage treatment of invasive aspergillosis in patients with hematologic malignancies. Cancer. 2003;98:292–9.

132. Marr KA, Boeckh M, Carter RA, et al. Combination antifungal therapy for invasive aspergillosis. Clin Infect Dis. 2004;39: 797–802.
133. Trifilio S, Pennick G, Pi J, et al. Monitoring plasma voriconazole levels may be necessary to avoid subtherapeutic levels in hematopoietic stem cell transplant recipients. Cancer. 2007;109(8): 1532–5.
134. Trifilio S, Singhal S, Williams S, et al. Breakthrough fungal infections after allogeneic hematopoietic stem cell transplantation in patients on prophylactic voriconazole. Bone Marrow Transplant. 2007;40(5):451–6.
135. Pascual A, Calandra T, Bolay S, Buclin T, Bille J, Marchetti O. Voriconazole therapeutic drug monitoring in patients with invasive mycoses improves efficacy and safety outcomes. Clin Infect Dis. 2008;46(2):201–11.
136. Hubel K, Dale DC, Liles WC. Granulocyte transfusion therapy: update on potential clinical applications. Curr Opin Hematol. 2001;8(3):161–4.
137. Offner F, Cordonnier C, Ljungman P, et al. Impact of previous aspergillosis on the outcome of bone marrow transplantation. Clin Infect Dis. 1998;26(5):1098–103.
138. Nivoix Y, Velten M, Letscher-Bru V, et al. Factors associated with overall and attributable mortality in invasive aspergillosis. Clin Infect Dis. 2008;47(9):1176–84.
139. Upton A, Kirby KA, Carpenter P, Boeckh M, Marr KA. Invasive aspergillosis following hematopoietic cell transplantation: outcomes and prognostic factors associated with mortality. Clin Infect Dis. 2007;44(4):531–40.
140. Cordonnier C, Ribaud P, Herbrecht R, et al. Prognostic factors for death due to invasive aspergillosis after hematopoietic stem cell transplantation: a 1-year retrospective study of consecutive patients at French transplantation centers. Clin Infect Dis. 2006;42(7): 955–63.
141. Nucci M, Anaissie EJ, Queiroz-Telles F, et al. Outcome predictors of 84 patients with hematologic malignancies and *Fusarium* infection. Cancer. 2003;98(2):315–9.

Fungal Infections in Solid Organ Transplant Recipients

Peter G. Pappas

Organ transplantation is an effective life-sparing modality for thousands of patients with organ failure syndromes. In spite of important advances in surgical technique and immunosuppressive regimens that have made organ transplantation a safer procedure today when compared to previous decades, there remain substantial risks of infection and other complications related to these procedures. Among the infectious complications of organ transplantation, none is associated with a greater impact on morbidity and mortality than invasive fungal infections (IFI) [1–5]. Fungal infections in organ transplant recipients (OTRs) vary in frequency, etiology, and pathogenesis according to the type of organ transplant procedure. Variations in immunosuppressive regimens, surgical technique, infection control, and exposure history further complicate evaluation of these patients. Moreover, the incidence of IFIs among this group of patients varies considerably from center to center [6].

The clinician is faced with a number of diagnostic and therapeutic challenges in approaching a transplant recipient who has a possible IFI. First, there is a lack of sensitive and specific diagnostic assays that might lead to early intervention. Second, antifungal therapy is frequently associated with dose-limiting toxicity. Third, significant potential for drug–drug interactions exists between existing antifungal agents and immunosuppressive agents. Fourth, only limited data are available that facilitate early identification of patients who are at the highest risk for IFI within each transplant group. This chapter describes risk factors for developing IFIs among OTRs, reviews the specific fungal pathogens, and discusses an approach to the diagnosis, therapy, and prevention of these potentially devastating infections.

P.G. Pappas (✉)
Division of Infectious Diseases, University of Alabama at Birmingham School of Medicine, Birmingham, AL USA
e-mail: pappas@uab.edu

Determining the "Net State of Immunosuppression"

As advanced by Rubin [7] and Fishman [8], the concept of "net state of immunosuppression" is a useful, albeit vague, assessment of the overall risk of infection in the OTR. Quantitation of this risk in a reliable and reproducible manner is difficult. Assessing the net state of immunosuppression encompasses a number of host and environmental factors, each of which can impact host defense (Table 1). Included among these factors are dose, duration, and temporal sequence of specific immunosuppressive agents; underlying immune deficiency such as autoimmune disease and other functional immune deficits; integrity of the mucocutaneous barrier; anatomic abnormalities, such as devitalized tissue and fluid collections; neutropenia and lymphopenia; underlying metabolic conditions, such as renal insufficiency, malnutrition, diabetes mellitus, hepatic failure; and infection with immunomodulating viruses such as cytomegalovirus (CMV), Epstein-Barr virus (EBV), hepatitis B and C viruses, human herpes virus (HHV-6), and human immunodeficiency virus (HIV) [7, 8].

While this approach is a useful guide to the assessment of risk for infection in OTRs, it does not take into account specific risk factors related to different organ transplants and/or to variations in surgical technique, intraoperative time, and use of blood products. A gross estimate of overall immunologic impairment can be made, but it does not provide a specific means by which the physician might more accurately determine the risk of IFI.

Specific Factors Associated with Invasive Fungal Infection in Organ Transplant Recipients

The development of IFI following solid organ transplantation is influenced by a number of different variables. These include the type and timing of the organ transplant; the

C.A. Kauffman et al. (eds.), *Essentials of Clinical Mycology*,
DOI 10.1007/978-1-4419-6640-7_30, © Springer Science+Business Media, LLC 2011

Table 1 Factors influencing the net state of immunosuppression in solid organ transplant recipients (Adapted from [8])

Immunosuppressive therapy
Dose and duration of individual agents
Recent rejection episodes
Use of antithymocyte globulin, total nodal irritation
Underlying immune disorders
Autoimmune disease
Antibody deficiency, complement deficiency, and other functional immune defects
Integrity of mucocutaneous barrier
Devitalized tissue, undrained fluid collections, hematomas
Neutropenia, lymphopenia
Metabolic conditions
Acute or chronic renal failure
Hepatic failure
Malnutrition
Diabetes mellitus
Alcoholism
Metabolic acidosis
Chronic viral infections
BK virus
Cytomegalovirus
Epstein-Barr virus
Hepatitis B and C viruses
Human herpesvirus 6
Human immunodeficiency virus types 1 and 2
Human T cell lymphotrophic virus type 1

specific immunosuppressive regimen, including the timing and frequency of rejection episodes; donor-transmitted infections; comorbid conditions and coinfections in the recipient, especially viral infections; perioperative fungal colonization; and other factors, including previous exposure and recent epidemiology. Each of these variables is discussed below.

Type of Solid Organ Transplant

The risk of IFI depends on the organ transplanted. Moreover, distribution of causative organisms also varies with the type of transplant [1–6, 8, 9]. Some risk factors, such as retransplantation, prolonged ICU stay with mechanical ventilation, requirement for surgical reexploration, primary graft nonfunction, and active CMV infection, are common to all OTRs. Other risk factors are specific to the type of transplant, and may relate to the type of anastomosis, differences in intensity of immunosuppression, or other variables. The distribution of infection by type and proportion of individual IFI according to the type of transplant for the TRANSNET prospective surveillance study conducted from 2001 to 2006 is demonstrated in Table 2 [6].

Kidney

Kidney transplantation is associated with the least risk of IFI. The published cumulative incidence of IFI following renal transplantation varies between 2% and 14% [10–12], but the most recent data from the multicenter TRANSNET surveillance study suggests that the 12-month cumulative incidence for IFI is 1.3% [6]. The most common fungi causing infection in renal transplant recipients are *Candida* species, *Aspergillus* species, and *Cryptococcus neoformans* [6, 10–12]. In geographic regions in which *Histoplasma capsulatum* and *Coccidioides* species are endemic, these organisms can also be important pathogens in the posttransplant period [13–15]. The TRANSNET study and sporadic reports support a significant role for infections due to *Fusarium* species and other hyalohyphomycetes, the zygomycetes, *Trichosporon asahii* and other pathogenic yeasts, and the dematiaceous fungi [6, 16–19].

Candida infection may be mucocutaneous, urinary, or deeply invasive. Factors predisposing to urinary tract infection include bladder catheterization, structural abnormalities or disruption of urinary flow, corticosteroids, and diabetes mellitus. Asymptomatic urinary tract colonization with *Candida* species is particularly common in renal transplant recipients and can be associated with significant consequences. Renal parenchymal disease may result from ascending infection from the bladder [20]. Rarely, urinary tract colonization can be associated with the development of a ureteral fungus ball, leading to obstruction of urinary flow and threatening allograft survival. Nosocomial candidemia in renal transplant recipients is most commonly associated with recognized risk factors, such as indwelling venous catheters, that are related to infection among nontransplanted patients and can occasionally lead to secondary involvement of the allograft from hematogenous spread [20].

Risk factors for the development of invasive aspergillosis are less well established in renal transplant patients. Underlying diabetes mellitus, cadaveric allograft, increased corticosteroid usage, retransplantation, and recent CMV infection have been associated with invasive aspergillosis [21–23]. Involvement of the lungs or disseminated multiorgan disease is most common, but focal extrapulmonary disease, e.g., cerebral abscess [24, 25], endocarditis [26], tuboovarian abscess [27, 28], and focal prostatic or ureteral involvement, [29, 30], has been reported.

C. neoformans is the third most common invasive fungal pathogen reported among renal transplant recipients, occurring in as many as 2% of patients [6, 31, 32]. Zygomycoses, phaeohyphomycoses, and hyalohyphomycoses are much less commonly reported. Risk factors for the development of these infections are poorly defined, but most occur beyond 4–6 months posttransplantation and are often associated with chronic allograft rejection and intense immunosuppression [1–6, 10].

Table 2 Percent of invasive fungal infection cases stratified by organism/group, according to transplant type in the surveillance cohort [6]

IFI type	Kidney	Liver	Pancreas	Lung	Heart	Sm. bowel
Candidiasis	164 (49)[a]	255 (68)	97 (76)	56 (23)	48 (49)	19 (85)
Aspergillosis	47 (14)	42 (11)	6 (5)	109 (44)	23 (23)	0 (0)
Zygomycosis	8 (2)	9 (2)	0 (0)	8 (3)	3 (3)	0 (0)
Other moulds	10 (3.0)	9 (2.4)	4 (3.1)	49 (19.8)	7 (7.1)	0 (0)
Unspecified moulds	7 (2.1)	8 (2.1)	0 (0)	7 (2.8)	2 (2.0)	0 (0)
Cryptococcosis	49 (15)	24 (6)	6 (5)	6 (2)	10 (10)	1 (5)
Endemic mycoses	33 (10)	17 (5)	8 (6)	3 (1)	3 (3)	0 (0)
Pneumocystosis	5 (1)	0 (0)	1 (1)	4 (2)	3 (3)	0 (0)
Other yeast	6 (1.8)	9 (2.4)	5 (3.9)	0 (0)	0 (0)	1 (4.6)
Unspecified yeast	3 (0.9)	5 (1.3)	1 (0.8)	6 (2.4)	0 (0)	1 (4.6)
Total IFI cases	332	378	128	248	99	22

[a]Number in parentheses represent percent of total for each organ type

Pancreas and Kidney–Pancreas

Invasive fungal infections among pancreas and kidney–pancreas transplant recipients occur much more frequently than among renal transplant recipients. Historically, the cumulative incidence of IFIs in this group has ranged between 6% and 38% [1–5]; TRANSNET demonstrated a 4% incidence in this group [6]. Most of these infections are due to *Candida* species [1, 6, 33, 34], with a much smaller proportion secondary to cryptococcosis, aspergillosis., and non-*Aspergillus* moulds [6, 33, 35].

The increased risk of IFI in this group largely relates to surgical and technical issues. Specifically, the type of surgical anastomosis can be associated with local complications and *Candida* superinfection [34–37]. Bladder-drained pancreas transplants are associated with a much higher incidence of urinary tract infections due to all causes, but especially due to *Candida* species. In contrast, enterically drained pancreatic transplants are much more likely to develop enteric leaks leading to polymicrobial intraabdominal infections in which *Candida* is an important pathogen [37]. Some experts disagree as to which of these two anastomotic and drainage procedures leads to fewer postoperative fungal infections, as the published data vary according to center. As with other OTRs, the risk of IFI is significantly greater among patients with recent CMV infection, graft rejection or failure, surgical reoperation, higher dose immunosuppression (especially corticosteroids), and bacterial coinfection.

Liver

The risk of IFI among liver transplant recipients has traditionally been very high, with a cumulative incidence of up to 42% [38]. The incidence of IFI has declined in recent years [5, 9], and the TRANSNET study demonstrated a 12-month incidence of only 4.7% [6]. Improvements in surgical technique, immunosuppressive regimens, and improved patient selection have contributed to this decrease. The majority of IFIs in liver transplant recipients are caused by *Candida* species with the peak incidence in the first month posttransplant [5, 6]. Aspergillosis, cryptococcosis, and mucormycosis also are commonly recognized in this population [12, 39–46].

Risk factors for the development of IFI have been best defined in the liver transplant population. In the study by Collins and colleagues, several important and independent variables were related to increased risk of fungal infection in the posttransplant period [47]. These included baseline creatinine >3 mg/dL, operative time >11 h, retransplantation, active CMV infection, and an intraoperative requirement of >40 units of blood products. The risk of fungal infection was 1% without any risk factor, compared to 67% among patients with two or more of these risk factors [47]. In addition, choledochojejunostomy anastomosis and early colonization with a fungal pathogen were strongly associated with the development of IFI in this study. Others have identified similar trends among liver transplant recipients and have consistently related prolonged intraoperative time, requirement for a large number of blood products, CMV infection, and choledochojejunostomy anastomosis to an increased risk of developing IFI [48, 49].

Heart

There is a modest risk of IFI following heart transplantation. The reported rate of occurrence ranges from 4% to 35% [50, 51], although recent reports consistently demonstrate an overall rate <10% [52]. TRANSNET observed an incidence of 3.4% [6]. *Candida* species account for at least two-thirds of the fungal infections; invasive aspergillosis is somewhat more common in heart compared to liver and kidney transplant recipients for reasons probably related to the increased intensity of immunosuppression [52].

Invasive *Candida* infections among heart transplant recipients are usually limited to candidemia and its complications. In addition, preexisting colonization with *Candida* species of ventricular assist devices is an established risk factor for the subsequent development of invasive *Candida* infection

[53, 54]. Mediastinitis due to *Candida* is an uncommon postoperative complication. Active CMV infection, the use of antilymphocyte antibodies, and treatment for rejection are the most common risk factors associated with IFI in heart transplant recipients.

Lung and Heart-Lung

In most recent studies, the incidence of IFI in lung and heart-lung transplant recipients is among the highest of all OTRs [55–57]. The cumulative incidence among this group of transplant recipients from smaller studies ranged between 10% and 36%; the TRANSNET data demonstrated a 12-month incidence of 8.6% [6]. *Aspergillus* species have emerged as dominant pathogens in this population [55–59]. In the TRANSNET study, invasive aspergillosis accounted for 44% of IFIs among lung and heart-lung recipients [6].

Invasive aspergillosis occurs in between 3.3% and 16% of lung and heart-lung recipients in different studies [55–61]. The enhanced risk of developing invasive aspergillosis among lung transplant recipients probably relates to several factors: prior airway colonization with *Aspergillus* species [60]; CMV infection [61]; environmental exposure through routine daily activities; and hypogammoglobulinemia [62]. Smoking substances such as marijuana is an additional risk [63]. Furthermore, patients with single lung transplants appear to have a greater risk of invasive aspergillosis than double lung transplants, a risk that is likely due to colonization with *Aspergillus* species in the remaining native lung [59]. Interestingly, preexisting *Aspergillus* species and *Scedosporium* colonization among patients with cystic fibrosis is not associated with a significantly increased risk of IFI due to these organisms posttransplantation [64, 65]. In fact, among all lung transplant recipients, those with cystic fibrosis appear to be at somewhat less risk of invasive mould disease than other lung transplant recipients.

Candida infections complicating lung transplantation include candidemia, mycotic aneurysm involving the vascular anastomoses, mediastinal wound infection, and necrotizing bronchitis at the tracheal anastomotic site [51, 66–68].

Pneumocystis jiroveci pneumonia (PCP) can occur in all OTRs, but appears to be most common in lung and heart recipients [69]. *P. jiroveci* pneumonia has become uncommon owing to the widespread use of trimethoprim/sulfamethoxazole (TMP/SMX) prophylaxis.

Small Bowel

The highest risk of IFI following organ transplantation occurs among small bowel recipients, with an incidence ranging from a low of 11.6% in TRANSNET [6], to as high as 59% [70, 71]. In addition to risk factors common to other OTRs, intraoperative complications include small bowel anastomotic leaks as a unique risk factor associated with this type of transplantation. Not surprisingly, *Candida* species constitute the majority of fungal pathogens in small bowel transplant recipients, with *Aspergillus* and other moulds playing less of a role. Prospective data among small bowel transplant patients are limited given the relative rarity of this transplant procedure, which has largely been limited to children with congenital small bowel disorders and highly selected adult patients.

Timing of Invasive Fungal Infection Following Organ Transplantation

In spite of differences in frequency and distribution of pathogens among the various transplant groups, the timing of these infections following organ transplantation is similar. As such, the posttransplant period can be generally divided into three intervals when assessing the risk and type of IFI: 0–1 month, 1–6 months, and beyond 6 months posttransplant. Understanding the temporal relatedness of the posttransplant interval to the risk and type of IFI can be very useful to the clinician in formulating a diagnosis and guiding empiric therapy. It also highlights the differences in pathogenesis for IFI during these intervals [1, 6, 8, 9].

Infections in the first month posttransplant are dominated by *Candida* species and are usually related to technical and surgical issues in addition to traditional nosocomial risk factors. Thus, anastomotic leaks, early graft failure, reoperation, central venous catheter–associated fungemia, and catheter-associated urinary tract infections are common. In one study among liver transplant recipients, over 50% of IFIs occurred within the first 10 days posttransplant, almost all of them caused by *Candida* species [47]. In the absence of early graft failure, retransplantation, significant pretransplant immunosuppression, or other mitigating circumstances, mould infections, especially those due to *Aspergillus* species, are uncommon during this period. Donor-related infections, especially those due to *Candida* species and *Aspergillus* species, often present during this first interval, 0–1 months posttransplantation.

During the second interval, 1–6 months posttransplantation, the effects of intense immunosuppression become manifest as the impact of nosocomial and surgical-related infections diminish. This second phase is dominated by mould infections, especially aspergillosis, zygomycosis, scedosporiosis, and less common mould diseases. *P. jiroveci* pneumonia is also common during this period among patients not receiving TMP/SMX prophylaxis. The peak incidence of aspergillosis is between 1 and 4 months posttransplantation, but there continues to be small risk of invasive aspergillosis throughout the posttransplant period

[5, 6, 8, 22]. The development of IFI during this time interval often follows evidence of active disease with an immunomodulating virus, such as CMV, HHV-6, EBV, hepatitis B, or hepatitis C.

The interval beyond 6 months posttransplantation is generally considered to be the period during which IFI is least likely to occur. Nonetheless, especially among patients with chronic rejection, graft dysfunction, late CMV infection, and other transplant-associated viral infections, IFI do occur. The late posttransplant period is dominated by fungal infections due to *C. neoformans*, regionally endemic mycoses, and some of the more unusual pathogens, including the dematiaceous fungi [6, 19, 31, 72–74]. However, mould infections due to *Aspergillus* species and the agents of zygomycoses may occur at any time in the posttransplant period [6, 75].

Immunosuppressive Regimen

The most important factor affecting the risk of IFI after the first month of transplantation is the intensity and duration of immunosuppressive agents that prevent organ rejection. Immunosuppression is initiated at high levels in the immediate posttransplant period when the risk of graft rejection is greatest. Most OTRs currently receive either a cyclosporine- or tacrolimus-based immunosuppressive regimen, usually in combination with mycophenylate mofetil. A growing number of patients receive antithymocyte globulin (ATG), alemtuzumab, basiliximab, daclizumab, or other monoclonal antibodies in the immediate posttransplant period to decrease the risk of rejection and minimize the need for glucocorticosteroids [76]. Reduction in overall glucocorticosteroid exposure has significantly decreased the overall incidence of IFI among OTRs. In an uncomplicated posttransplant setting, these regimens are continued at higher doses in the early posttransplant period, and are gradually tapered to a chronic maintenance regimen within 6 months in the absence of significant rejection. Undoubtedly the approach to immunotherapy in OTRs will continue to evolve as safer and more effective agents are developed.

Cyclosporine and tacrolimus have not demonstrated any clear difference with respect to incidence of IFI [77]. Similarly, studies among renal transplant recipients comparing regimens utilizing mycophenolate mofetil or azathioprine have not demonstrated any significant difference in rate of IFIs [78]. Moreover, recent data suggest that use of the calcineurin inhibitors (cyclosporine and tacrolimus) has led to decreased rates and severity of IFI because of their modest in vitro antifungal activity [79]. Thus, the recent reduction in IFIs associated with the calcineurin inhibitors may not only relate to a glucocorticosteroid-sparing effect, but also to modest antifungal activity.

The timing and frequency of rejection episodes as they relate to intensification of immunosuppressive regimens are also important factors associated with IFIs in OTRs. Pulse-dose glucocorticosteroids are commonly administered in this setting, usually coupled with an overall intensification of immunosuppressive therapy. In addition, specific antilymphocyte therapy with ATG or monoclonal antibodies is often administered in this setting. These interventions are associated with higher rates of CMV reactivation, which leads to an increased risk of IFI [76].

Donor-Related Fungal Infections

The vast majority of donor-related transplant infections are viral in origin. Well-documented donor-related infections are CMV, EBV, hepatitis B, hepatitis C, and HIV. Donor-related fungal infections are much less common; often the source of the pathogen is suspected to be the donor, but convincing proof is lacking. Nonetheless, several well-documented cases of donor-transmitted fungal infections have been described, including cases of histoplasmosis [80, 81], coccidioidomycosis [82–84], cryptococcosis [68], candidiasis [85, 86], and aspergillosis [87]. A recent French study found that graft site candidiasis could be traced to donor transmission, and occurred in 1 per 1,000 renal transplant recipients [86].

Among donors from endemic areas for histoplasmosis and coccidioidomycosis, a suspicion for latent disease must be maintained. Donor transmission of these two pathogens, *H. capsulatum* and *C. immitis*, is uncommon, and it remains difficult to accurately discern the source of these pathogens with certainty. Donor-derived *Aspergillus* infection among lung transplant recipients, while theoretically common because of frequent airway colonization, is rarely demonstrated [87]. Similarly, donor-derived cryptococcosis is infrequently recognized.

Comorbid Illnesses

Underlying diseases in the host contribute to the "net state of immunosuppression," and no doubt influence the risk of IFI. Factors that have most commonly been associated with an increased risk include renal dysfunction and the need for peritoneal or hemodialysis, diabetes mellitus, neutropenia, malnutrition, mechanical ventilation, admission to an intensive care unit, and chronic immunosuppressive therapy pretransplant [7, 8]. The degree to which these factors individually influence risk is uncertain.

Several viral infections increase the risk of IFI in the transplant recipient. CMV is the most commonly recognized immunomodulating viral infection in this population. Ample evidence from large retrospective studies relate active CMV disease to increased risk of fungal infection in OTRs [47, 48, 61]. Additional data suggest that active hepatitis B and C, HHV-6, and HIV infection are important risk factors for posttransplantation IFI [8].

Specific Fungal Pathogens

Candida Species

Candida species are the commonest invasive fungal pathogens among OTRs. Virtually all of the more common *Candida* species, particularly *C. albicans*, *C. glabrata*, *C. tropicalis*, *C. parapsilosis*, *C. krusei*, *C. lusitaniae*, and *C. guilliermondii*, have been reported in this population. *Candida albicans* is the commonest species, followed by *Candida glabrata*, *C. tropicalis*, and *C. parapsilosis* [6]. In contrast to hematopoietic stem cell transplant recipients, *Candida krusei* is an uncommon pathogen in OTRs [6, 41, 66]. Reflecting a similar trend among nontransplant hospitalized patients, the broad use of prophylactic and empiric antifungal therapy, particularly with the azoles, has probably played an important role in the emergence of non-*albicans Candida* species in this population. Factors leading to candidemia are similar among OTRs and nontransplant patients, but the rate of complicated infection as evidenced by disseminated disease appears to be greater among OTRs than among nontransplanted patients [41]. Candidemia is the most common manifestation of invasive candidiasis in the transplant population, accounting for at least 60% of all episodes [6].

Intraabdominal infections secondary to *Candida* infections are significantly more common among liver, pancreas, and small bowel transplant recipients compared to other OTRs. These patients undergo disruption of the normal anatomy of the small bowel, common bile duct, and/or pancreatic duct with the potential for intraabdominal anastomotic leakage. Intraabdominal infectious complications frequently occur within the first month posttransplant and are often polymicrobial. Sternal wound infections among heart and heart-lung transplants due to *Candida* species have been reported, and can be associated with significant morbidity and mortality [67]. Among lung transplants, bronchial anastomotic infections secondary to *Candida* species have been reported [68].

Urinary tract infections due to *Candida* are common among OTRs owing to the need for bladder catheterization during the period of hospitalization, particularly in the immediate postoperative period. Candiduria can be a harbinger of complicated upper tract disease, but in a large prospective study of candiduria in renal transplant recipients, patients who received treatment with fluconazole did not have better outcomes than those who were not treated [88]. An unusual complication of *Candida* urinary tract infection in OTRs is the development of a ureteral fungus ball due to *Candida* species [89]. This complication is most often seen in renal transplant recipients, but it is also seen in other OTRs, and may clinically mimic fungus ball due to less common urinary pathogens such as *Aspergillus* species

A rare but important syndrome due to *Candida* species relates to vascular anastomotic infections. True "mycotic" aneurysms occurring at the site of the vascular anastomosis due to *Candida* species have been reported among pancreatic [90], renal [86, 91], and heart-lung transplant recipients [92]. Among renal transplant recipients this manifestation has been associated with donor origin of the organism [86]. These represent a very significant and highly lethal postoperative complication. Less common complications of *Candida* infection include septic arthritis, chronic meningitis, endocarditis, and rarely, pneumonia [93, 94].

Aspergillus

Invasive aspergillosis is reported among all transplant groups; however, lung transplant recipients seem to be particularly predisposed to infections with *Aspergillus* species. As many as 10% of lung transplant recipients will develop significant infection with *Aspergillus* and another 10% will develop *Aspergillus* colonization posttransplantation [21, 22]. Among non-lung OTRs, the overall risk of invasive aspergillosis is substantially less [6]. *Aspergillus fumigatus* is the most common causative species; however, infections due to *A. flavus*, *A. niger*, *A. terreus*, *A. nidulans*, *A. glaucus*, *A. ustus*, *A. versicolor*, and other less common species have been reported. Moreover, multiple species may be isolated from the same patient. Newer molecular techniques have provided the means of identifying several less common *Aspergillus* species, including *A.lentulus*, *A. calidoustus*, and *A. tubingensis* [95].

Aspergillus spores are ubiquitous in the environment, and infection usually begins as a result of inhalation, resulting in lower respiratory tract colonization. Disease may be confined to the lungs or may disseminate to virtually any organ, most commonly the skin, central nervous system, heart, and the endocrine glands, especially the thyroid. Disseminated disease is associated with a mortality rate of greater than 80% [96, 97]. Ulcerative tracheobronchitis due to *Aspergillus* is a well-described syndrome among lung transplant recipients that is characterized by superficial invasion of the tracheobronchial tree, typically at the site of an anastomosis, but it may occur anywhere within the proximal airway [98]. The disease has been reported among other transplant groups [99], but is distinctly uncommon outside of lung transplant recipients. Patients with this ulcerative tracheobronchitis may be asymptomatic or minimally symptomatic with chronic nonproductive cough. Bronchoscopy reveals single or multiple ulcerative lesions at the anastomotic site.

Aspergillus species frequently colonize the upper airways, making it difficult to distinguish between invasive disease and asymptomatic colonization. However, the detection of significant *Aspergillus* colonization in the upper airways is strongly predictive of invasive disease in most OTRs with a positive predictive value of at least 60% [60, 100–102]. Recently, the measurement of *Aspergillus* galactomannan by EIA in bronchoalveolar lavage fluid has proven to be a sensitive indicator of pulmonary invasive aspergillosis and should become an important component of the evaluation of patients with suspected disease [103].

Other manifestations of invasive aspergillosis in OTRs include sinusitis, thoracic empyema, and angioinvasion at virtually any site. *Aspergillus* has been reported as a cause of urinary tract fungus ball and prostatic abscess in renal and liver transplant recipients [28, 29]. Invasive aspergillosis may occur several years following transplantation, especially among patients undergoing intensification of immunosuppressive therapy or receiving higher-dose corticosteroids for allograft rejection [6, 22, 75]. Additional risk factors for invasive aspergillosis include CMV infection, renal failure, and early graft failure [22, 61].

The source of *Aspergillus* infection can be difficult to discern. Recent studies have suggested that nosocomial transmission occurs, although the frequency of this event is unclear [104]. Also, the recipients may serve as their own reservoirs for *Aspergillus*, especially those with single lung transplants [59]. Community-acquired infection occurs, but its relative importance compared to nosocomial acquisition and donor transmission remains unknown [87].

Cryptococcus

Cryptococcus is overall the third most common IFI in OTRs, and usually occurs relatively late in the posttransplant period [31]. In the TRANSNET study, the median time to development of cryptococcosis was 575 days posttransplantation [6]. Disease is usually due to *C. neoformans*, although disease due to *C. gattii*, *C. albidus*, and *C. laurentii* is reported. Manifestations of cryptococcal disease are similar among OTRs and HIV-infected individuals. Primary infection usually occurs following inhalation [105] although there are sporadic reports of direct primary cutaneous disease possibly resulting from direct inoculation [106, 107]. Most patients present with nonspecific respiratory symptoms, unexplained fever, or an asymptomatic nodule on chest roentgenogram. Asymptomatic infection with *C. neoformans* is common; thus, it is unclear how often extrapulmonary dissemination occurs in OTRs. The central nervous system (CNS) is the most common extrapulmonary site of cryptococcal disease in OTRs, followed by involvement of the skin and subcutaneous tissue, bones, and prostate. Necrotizing cellulitis is a common cutaneous manifestation in this population, and must be distinguished from cellulitis due to common bacterial and mycobacterial pathogens [108–110]. Based on data from TRANSNET and other studies, there seems to be little predilection for the type of organ transplant and the development of cryptococcosis [6]. Cryptococcemia is especially common in this group and is generally associated with a worse clinical outcome [111].

Recent experience among OTRs with cryptococcosis suggest that outcomes are at least as good as outcomes among patients who are otherwise normal hosts [45, 111]. This paradox is not well understood, but could relate to the intensity of patient follow-up after organ transplantation and the ability to make a diagnosis earlier in the course of infection. Corticosteroids may have an ameliorating effect early in the course of cryptococcosis, particularly when the CNS is involved. The calcineurin inhibitors, especially tacrolimus, possess not only modest in vitro antifungal activity, but also excellent CNS penetration, and may have a beneficial effect on the natural history and severity of CNS cryptococcosis in OTRs [79, 112]. Investigators also suggest that a relative increase in cutaneous expression of disease may be the result of poor antifungal activity of tacrolimus at lower temperatures found in cutaneous tissue [31].

Transplant-related immune reconstitution inflammatory syndrome (IRIS) has been best described among patients with cryptococcosis and relates to the rapid withdrawal of immunosuppressive therapy from patients with active infection. The clinical manifestation of IRIS is a paradoxical worsening of disease, relating to the rapid conversion from a TH2 to a TH1 host immunologic response [113–116].

Mucorales (Zygomycetes)

Mucormycosis or zygomycosis, has been reported in all OTRs. Disease has been reported due to several genera, most commonly *Rhizopus* species, *Mucor* species, *Cunninghamella bertholletiae*, and *Absidia* species. Risk factors for invasive disease include neutropenia, ketoacidosis, renal failure, and treatment of chronic rejection, especially with higher-dose steroids.

Clinical disease often involves the paranasal sinuses, leading to destructive lesions and CNS involvement by direct extension. The lungs are also a commonly involved site, although virtually any organ can be involved [42–44, 49, 117–119]. Multiple organ involvement consistent with hematogenous dissemination is reported, but is less common than that due to invasive aspergillosis, even though the pathogenesis of both disorders involves angioinvasion. *Conidiobolus coronatus*, an organism infecting patients living in tropical areas, has been reported as a cause of disseminated disease in a renal transplant recipient [120].

The typical clinical finding associated with mucormycosis is a necrotizing, locally invasive process. Necrotizing wound infections have been described [119], as has infection of a renal allograft [17]. In addition, localized gastrointestinal mucormycosis, characterized by giant gastric and/or colonic ulcers, has been reported [121–123].

Phaeohyphomycoses

The agents of phaeohyphomycosis consist of over 100 pigmented moulds (dematiaceous fungi), and a growing number of these species have been reported to cause disease among OTRs [19, 74]. The clinical spectrum of these infections includes invasive sinusitis, pneumonia, endophthalmitis, skin and musculoskeletal involvement, CNS disease, gastrointestinal involvement, and disseminated disease. Infections due to *Exophiala* species, *Dactylaria constricta*, *Alternaria* species, *Bipolaris spicifera*, *Curvularia* spp., *Cladophialophora bantiana*, *Colletotrichum crassipes*, *Phaeocremonium parasiticum*, and *Fonsecaea pedrosoi* have been reported [124–131]. In one review of disseminated phaeohyphomycosis in OTRs, only 16% of patients survived, even with therapy [19]. In another review, Singh and colleagues noted that cutaneous and synovial involvement was usually caused by *Exophiala* species, whereas systemic infections, including CNS involvement, were caused by less common organisms, such as *Ochroconis gallopavum* and *Cladophialophora bantiana* [74]. Phaeohyphomycosis is usually late-occurring, and specific risk factors for development have not been clearly delineated.

Endemic Fungi

Infections due to *C. immitis* and *H. capsulatum* are not uncommon among OTRs who have lived in endemic areas. The true incidence of these infections is unknown, but estimates range between 0.2% and 6% [72, 73, 132–139]. Endemic fungal infections tend to occur late in the post-transplantation period, with a median time of greater than 1 year posttransplant. In the TRANSNET cohort, infections with the endemic fungi occurred a median of 343 days following transplantation [6]. Transmission from the donor organ has been documented in several of these cases [81–83, 138], but a history of prior infection without evidence of active disease should not exclude potential donors or recipients. Nonetheless, the potential for donor-related transmission with these organisms remains a concern in endemic areas. Several recent reports clearly document donor-related *H. capsulatum* and *C. immitis* transmission to recipients residing in nonendemic areas for these organisms, underscoring the need to consider the donor as a potential source of infection in patients with undifferentiated fever [81–83].

Histoplasmosis is the most commonly reported endemic mycosis among OTRs. Most reports have involved renal transplant recipients, although disease has been described in liver, heart, and lung recipients [135–141]. Histoplasmosis in OTRs usually presents as disseminated disease, although focal involvement of the CNS, skin, renal papilla, and gastrointestinal tract has been described. In addition, cecal and ileal perforation associated with gastrointestinal histoplasmosis has been described.

Coccidioidomycosis following organ transplantation has been reported in up to 6% of OTRs living in the endemic desert areas in the southwestern USA [142]. Disease is due to either recent environmental exposure or to reactivation of a latent infection; there is less documentation of donor-related transmission. Clinical features of coccidioidomycosis in this population vary from pneumonia to disseminated disease involving skin, musculoskeletal structures, and the CNS [15, 132–134]. The majority of cases of posttransplant coccidioidomycosis have been reported among renal, heart, and liver transplant recipients.

Blastomycosis is distinctly uncommon among OTRs, even among patients residing in endemic areas [143–145]. There has been no evidence to suggest donor-related transmission of *B. dermatitidis* to date. Disease manifestations in this group tend to parallel those of the normal host; however, disseminated disease, including involvement of the CNS, is more commonly observed in OTRs. Overall, the mortality rate among OTRs and other immunocompromised hosts with blastomycosis has been significantly higher than among otherwise normal patients [145].

Sporotrichosis due to *Sporothrix schenckii* and *S. cyanensis* has been reported sporadically among OTRs [146]. There is no evidence to suggest donor-transmitted infections, and most cases have been reported in conjunction with recognized environmental exposure. Disease has been limited to the skin and subcutaneous tissue in most cases, although pulmonary and disseminated disease has been reported [147].

Other Fungi

Disease due to other pathogenic yeasts and moulds has been reported sporadically among OTRs. Fusariosis due to *F. solani*, *F. oxysporum*, *F. moniliforme*, and *F. sacchari* has been reported [16, 148, 149]. Infection due to *Fusarium* species is often associated with prolonged periods of neutropenia, although fusariosis can present among OTRs without neutropenia. Patients with fusariosis are frequently fungemic [150]. Localized infection involving the sinuses, lungs, skin, and soft tissue, as well as disseminated disease, are reported. Another ubiquitous hyalohyphomycete, *Paecilomyces lilacinus*, is a cause of cutaneous and sinus disease in OTRs [151–153].

Trichosporonosis due to *T. asahii*, a pathogenic yeast often associated with intravenous catheter-related infections, may cause disseminated disease in OTRs. In addition, funguria due to *T. asahii* has been reported among OTRs [18]. Fatal fungemia due to *Trichoderma harzianum* has also been observed [154].

Pneumocystis jiroveci

Infection due to *Pneumocystis jiroveci* is reported in all organ transplant recipients, although it is most commonly reported among lung and heart-lung transplant recipients [69]. The incidence of *Pneumocystis* pneumonia (PCP) is greatest within the first year after transplantation. Gordon and colleagues suggested an eight-fold higher incidence of PCP in the first year following transplant compared to the combined incidence in all subsequent years among OTRs at one institution [155].

For patients with PCP associated with transplantation, recent receipt of antithymocyte globulin, CMV infection, and therapy for organ rejection are considered important risk factors [69]. Extrapulmonary disease similar to that seen among patients with AIDS can occur. Antimicrobial prophylaxis with trimethoprim/sulfamethoxazole or sulfadoxine/pyrimethamine in the first 6–12 months posttransplantation is highly effective in preventing PCP [156]; dapsone, atovaquone, and inhaled pentamidine are reasonable alternatives to these agents.

Approach to Diagnosis

A diagnosis of IFI in OTRs is frequently challenging, relating in part to the relative paucity and nonspecificity of the signs and symptoms associated with IFI in immunocompromised patients in general and in OTRs, specifically. Thus, a high index of suspicion and an aggressive approach to diagnosis is warranted in clinically compatible situations. The recently revised EORTC/MSG criteria for the diagnosis of IFI [157] are based on the following criteria: (1) the isolation of a pathogenic organism from a properly obtained clinical specimen, associated with clinical or radiographic evidence of disease, (2) the demonstration of fungal organisms in cytologic or histopathologic studies, or (3) serologic detection of a specific antibody or fungal antigen from blood, serum, urine, cerebrospinal fluid, or bronchoalveolar lavage (BAL) fluid. These definitions are categorized as proven, probable, or possible based on the strength of the host, clinical, radiographic, and microbiologic criteria.

Culture of certain fungi from any site virtually always suggests disease, even in the absence of clinical signs and symptoms. Examples include *H. capsulatum*, *C. immitis*, *B. dermatitidis*, *S. schenckii*, and *P. brasiliensis*. Isolation of *C. neoformans* from specimens other than sputum is always indicative of invasive disease. In rare circumstances, isolation of *C. neoformans* from the sputum can represent colonization only, but the recovery of this organism from respiratory secretions in an OTR must always be accompanied by an aggressive diagnostic approach, including chest CT scan and/or bronchoscopy, directed at evaluating the possibility of parenchymal lung disease.

Isolation of *Candida* species from the blood, regardless of whether it was obtained from a peripheral site or an intravascular catheter, should always be considered a true infection, even in the absence of clinical signs and symptoms. Isolates of *Candida* from other normally sterile sources should similarly be regarded as indicative of invasive disease. *Candida* species isolated from drains, urinary catheters, sputum, and other nonsterile sites often represent colonization only, and must be interpreted in the clinical context of the individual patient. The main value of isolation of *Candida* from a nonsterile site is to help predict the future development of invasive candidiasis and guide empiric therapy in patients who are perceived to be at high risk.

Isolation of *Aspergillus* species from blood cultures is rare. By comparison, *Fusarium* species, *Scedosporium* species, *P. lilacinus*, and other rare moulds are frequently isolated from blood cultures among patients with disseminated disease. The isolation of a mould from other clinical specimens such as sputum, BAL fluid, or tissue biopsy are best interpreted with clinical, radiographic, and histopathologic correlation [57, 60, 100, 102].

Direct visualization of an organism on a histopathologic specimen is an indispensable means of establishing tissue invasion. The demonstration on biopsy of fungal elements invading tissue often distinguishes a proven from a possible or probable case of invasive mould disease in an immunocompromised patient. Special stains such as Gomori's methanamine silver, periodic acid–Schiff, and Fontana-Masson can help to demonstrate fungal organisms in tissue.

Several serologic tests have been used successfully in the early detection of fungal infections. Among the approved tests, detection of cryptococcal antigen in serum or cerebrospinal fluid remains the most reliable of these serologic assays, maintaining a high sensitivity and specificity.

The measurement of *Histoplasma* antigen in serum and urine has also been extremely useful in the diagnosis of histoplasmosis in immunocompromised patients. The urine *Histoplasma* antigen assay has a sensitivity of at least 90% among immunocompromised patients with disseminated disease. In addition, among AIDS patients with disseminated histoplasmosis, serial urine *Histoplasma* antigens have been utilized to follow response to therapy and to predict relapse. Among the other endemic fungi, reliable serologic testing is available for *C. immitis*. The detection of antibodies to *Coccidioides* is a sensitive and specific marker of coccidioidomycosis.

Serologic assays for detecting early evidence of invasive candidiasis and invasive aspergillosis are available [158, 159]. The serum 1–3 beta-D-glucan is approved as an adjunctive assay for the diagnosis of invasive candidiasis. The test is approved but not widely utilized due to cost and technical factors. The *Aspergillus* galactomannan EIA is approved for use in serum and BAL, but has proven to be less useful in OTRs than in patients with hematologic malignancies and in stem cell transplant recipients. Nonetheless, this assay is an important step forward in the earlier diagnosis of invasive aspergillosis.

Prophylactic Antifungal Therapy

Antifungal prophylaxis is widely practiced but inadequately studied in liver, pancreas, lung, and heart-lung transplant recipients. With the exception of liver transplant recipients, there are limited studies of targeted prophylaxis in OTRs. The largest study to date compared fluconazole 400 mg daily to placebo given for the first 70 days posttransplant among 212 liver transplant recipients in a randomized, double-blind study. In this study, 6% versus 23% of fluconazole and placebo recipients, respectively, developed IFI, but neither regimen demonstrated reduced mortality rates [160]. In a small, randomized, double-blind study of 86 liver transplant patients, 0% versus 16% (p, 0.01) of recipients of a lipid formulation of amphotericin B versus placebo, respectively, developed an IFI in the first month posttransplant [161].

In an observational study of 200 low-risk liver transplant recipients who did not receive antifungal prophylaxis, the incidence of IFI was 3.6% during the first 100 days posttransplant, suggesting that antifungal prophylaxis in a low-risk population is unnecessary [162]. A recently published study comparing 71 high-risk liver transplant recipients who received either fluconazole (400 mg/day) or liposomal amphotericin (2 mg/kg/day) as posttransplantation prophylaxis both given for 14 days, demonstrated a low incidence of IFI and no differences between the two arms [163].

Some authors have advocated targeted prophylaxis and/or preemptive therapy in selected clinical situations. These include early posttransplant pulmonary colonization with *Aspergillus* species, the discovery that removed focal pulmonary nodules contain *C. neoformans* or *H. capsulatum* without evidence of extrapulmonary disease, and asymptomatic candiduria in the renal transplant recipient [164].

Recent studies among lung transplant recipients have examined the use of inhaled amphotericin B preparations for primary prophylaxis of invasive fungal pneumonia and bronchitis. These uncontrolled studies demonstrate the safety of a nebulized lipid agent and amphotericin B deoxycholate and efficacy in preventing IFI in the early postoperative period [165, 166]. Aside from these studies, there are few data that address the best approach to antifungal prophylaxis in OTRs. As such, antifungal prophylaxis is largely practiced in a center-to-center approach based on local experience, epidemiology, and perceived risk of IFI.

References

1. Paya CV. Fungal infections in solid-organ transplantation. Clin Infect Dis. 1993;16:677–88.
2. Hibberd PL, Rubin RH. Clinic aspects of fungal infection in organ transplant recipients. Clin Infect Dis. 1994;19 Suppl 1:33–40.
3. Hadley S, Karchmer AW. Fungal infections in solid organ transplant recipients. Infect Dis Clin N Am. 1995;9:1045–74.
4. Dictar MO, Maiolo E, Alexander B, Jacob N, Veron MT. Mycoses in the transplanted patient. Med Mycol. 2000;38:251–8.
5. Silveira FP, Husain S. Fungal infections in solid organ transplantation. Med Mycol. 2007;45:305–20.
6. Pappas PG, Alexander BD, Andes DR, et al. Invasive fungal infections among organ transplant recipients in the United States: results of the Transplant-Associated Infection Surveillance Network (TRANSNET). Clin Infect Dis. 2010;50:1101–12.
7. Rubin RH. Infection in the organ transplant recipient. In: Rubin RH, Young LS, editors. Clinical approach to infections in the compromised host. 3rd ed. New York: Plenum; 1994. p. 629–705.
8. Fishman JA. Infection in solid-organ transplant recipients. N Eng J Med. 2007;357:2601–14.
9. Patel R, Paya CV. Infections in solid organ transplant recipients. Clin Microbiol Rev. 1997;10:86–124.
10. Patel R. Infections in recipients of kidney transplants. Infect Dis Clin N Am. 2001;15:901–51.
11. Abbott KC, Hypolite I, Poropatich RK, et al. Hospitalizations for fungal infections after renal transplantation in the United States. Transpl Infect Dis. 2001;3:203–11.
12. Singh N. Fungal infections in the recipients of solid organ transplantation. Infect Dis Clin N Am. 2003;17:113–34.
13. Cuellar-Rodriguez J, Avery RK, Lard M, et al. Histoplasmosis in solid organ transplant recipients: 10 years of experience at a large transplant center in an endemic area. Clin Infect Dis. 2009; 49:710–6.
14. Wheat LJ, Smith EJ, Sathapatayavongs B, et al. Histoplasmosis in renal allograft recipients: two large urban outbreaks. Arch Intern Med. 1983;143:703–7.
15. Blair JE. Coccidioidomycosis in patients who have undergone transplantation. Ann NY Acad Sci. 2007;1111:365–76.
16. Heinz T, Perfect J, Schell W, Ditter E, Ruff G, Serafin D. Soft tissue fungal infections: surgical management of 12 immunocompromised patients. Plast Reconstr Surg. 1996;97:1391–9.

17. Chkhotua A, Yussim A, Tovar A, et al. Mucormycosis of the renal allograft: case report and review of the literature. Transpl Int. 2001;14:438–41.
18. Lussier N, Laverdiere M, Delorme J, Weiss K, Dandavino R. *Trichosporon beigelii* funguria in renal transplant recipients. Clin Infect Dis. 2000;31:1299–301.
19. Revankar SG, Patterson JE, Sutton DA, Pullen R, Rinaldi MG. Disseminated phaeohyphomycosis: review of an emerging mycosis. Clin Infect Dis. 2002;34:467–76.
20. Nampoory MR, Khan ZU, Johny KV, et al. Invasive fungal infections in renal transplant recipients. J Infect. 1996;33:95–101.
21. Paterson DL, Singh N. Invasive aspergillosis in transplant recipients. Medicine (Baltimore). 1999;78:123–38.
22. Singh N, Paterson DL. *Aspergillus* infections in transplant recipients. Clin Microbiol Rev. 2005;18:44–69.
23. Patterson JE, Peters J, Calhoon JH, et al. Investigation and control of aspergillosis and other filamentous fungal infections in solid organ transplant recipients. Transpl Infect Dis. 2000;2:22–8.
24. Carlini A, Angelini D, Burrows L, DeQuirico G, Antonelli A. Cerebral aspergillosis: long term efficacy and safety of liposomal amphotericin B in kidney transplant. Nephrol Dial Transplant. 1998;13:2659–61.
25. Garcia A, Mazuecos A, Flayo A, et al. Isolated cerebral aspergillosis without a portal of entry-complete recovery after liposomal amphotericin B and surgical treatment. Nephrol Dial Transplant. 1998;9:2385–7.
26. Marin P, Garcia-Martos P, Carcia-Doncel A, et al. Endocarditis by *Aspergillus fumigatus* in a renal transplant. Mycopathologia. 1999;145:127–9.
27. Viertel A, Ditting T, Pistorius K, Geiger H, Scheuermann EH. Just-Nubling G. An unusual case of *Aspergillus* endocarditis in a kidney transplant recipient. Transplantation. 1999;68:1812–3.
28. Kim SW, Nah MY, Ueum CH, et al. Pelvic aspergillosis with tubo-ovarian abscess in a renal transplant recipient. J Infect. 2001;42:215–7.
29. Shirwany A, Sargent SJ, Dmochowski RR, Bronze MS. Urinary tract aspergillosis in a renal transplant recipient. Clin Infect Dis. 1998;27:1336.
30. Kaplan-Pavlovcic S, Masera A, Ovcak Z, Kmetec A. Prostatic aspergillosis in a renal transplant recipient. Nephrol Dial Transplant. 1999;14:1778–80.
31. Husain S, Wagener MM, Singh N. *Cryptococcus neoformans* infection in organ transplant recipients: variables influencing clinical characteristics and outcome. Emerg Infect Dis. 2001;7:1–14.
32. Singh N, Dromer F, Perfect JR, Lortholary O. Cryptococcosis in solid organ transplant recipients: current state of the science. Clin Infect Dis. 2008;47:1321–7.
33. Lumbreras C, Fernandez I, Velosa J, Munn S, Sterioff S, Paya CV. Infectious complications following pancreatic transplantation: incidence, microbiological and clinical characteristics, and outcome. Clin Infect Dis. 1995;20:514–20.
34. Benedetti E, Gruessner AC, Troppmann C, et al. Intra-abdominal fungal infections after pancreatic transplantation: incidence, treatment, and outcome. J Am Coll Surg. 1996;183:307–16.
35. Smets YF, van der Piji JW, van Dissel JT, Ringers FJ, de Fijter JW, Lemkes HH. Infectious disease complications of simultaneous pancreas kidney transplantation. Nephrol Dial Transplant. 1997;12:764–71.
36. Hesse UJ, Sutherland DER, Najarian JS, Simmons RL. Intra-abdominal infections in pancreas transplant recipients. Ann Surg. 1986;203:153–62.
37. Pirsch JD, Odorico JS, D'Alessandro AM, Knechtle SJ, Becker BN, Sollinger HW. Post-transplant infections in enteric versus bladder-drained simultaneous pancreas-kidney transplant recipients. Transplantation. 1998;66:1746–50.
38. Wajszczuk CP, Dummer JS, Ho M, et al. Fungal infections in liver transplant recipients. Transplantation. 1985;40:347–53.
39. Singh N, Pruett TL, Houston S, et al. Invasive aspergillosis in the recipients of liver retransplantation. Liver Transpl. 2006;12:1205–9.
40. Singh N, Avery RK, Munoz P, et al. Trends in risk profiles for and mortality associated with invasive aspergillosis among liver transplant recipients. Clin Infect Dis. 2003;36:46–52.
41. Husain S, Tollemar J, Dominguez EA, et al. Changes in the spectrum and risk factors for invasive candidiasis in liver transplant recipients: prospective, multicenter, case-controlled study. Transplantation. 2003;75:2023–9.
42. Stelzmueller I, Lass-Floerl C, Geltner C, et al. Zygomycosis and other rare filamentous fungal infections in solid organ transplant recipients. Transpl Int. 2008;21:534–46.
43. Sun HY, Singh N. Emerging importance of infections due to zygomycetes in organ transplant recipients. Int J Antimicrob Agents. 2008;32 Suppl 2:S115–8.
44. Sun HY, Aguado JM, Bonatti H, et al. Pulmonary zygomycosis in solid organ transplant recipients in the current era. Am J Transplant. 2009;9:2166–71.
45. Davis JA, Horn DL, Marr KA, Fishman JA. Central nervous system involvement in cryptococcal infection in individuals after solid organ transplantation or with AIDS. Transpl Infect Dis. 2009;11:432–7.
46. Sun HY, Wagener MM, Singh N. Cryptococcosis in solid-organ, hemtopoietic stem cell, and tissue transplant recipients: evidence-based evolving trends. Clin Infect Dis. 2009;48:1566–76.
47. Collins LA, Samore MH, Roberts MS, et al. Risk factors for invasive fungal infections complicating orthotopic liver transplantation. J Infect Dis. 1994;170:644–52.
48. Patel R, Portela D, Badley AD, et al. Risk factors of invasive *Candida* or non-*Candida* fungal infections after liver transplantation. Transplantation. 1996;62:926–34.
49. Singh N, Aguado JM, Bonatti H, et al. Zygomycosis in solid organ transplant recipients: a prospective, matched case-control study to assess risks for disease and outcome. J Infect Dis. 2009; 200:1002–11.
50. Waser M, Maggiorini M, Luthy A, et al. Infectious complications in 100 consecutive heart transplant recipients. Eur J Clin Microbiol Infect Dis. 1994;13:12–8.
51. Kramer MR, Marshal SE, Starnes VA, Gamberg P, Amitai Z, Theodore J. Infectious complications in heart-lung transplantation analysis of 200 episodes. Arch Intern Med. 1993; 153:2010–6.
52. Grossi P, Glaudio F, Fiocchi R, Dalla Gasperina D. Prevalence and outcome of invasive fungal infections in 1,963 thoracic organ transplant recipients. Transplantation. 2000;70:112–6.
53. Goldstein DJ, El-Amir NG, Ashton RC, et al. Fungal infections in left ventricular assist device recipients: incidence, prophylaxis, and treatment. ASAIO J. 1995;41:873–5.
54. Argenziano M, Catanese KA, Moazami N, et al. The influence of infection on survival and successful transplantation in patients with left ventricular assist devices. J Heart Lung Transplant. 1997;16:822–31.
55. Gordon SM, Avery RK. Aspergillosis in lung transplantation: incidence, risk factors, and prophylactic strategies. Transpl Infect Dis. 2001;3:161–7.
56. Singh N, Husain S. *Aspergillus* infections after lung transplantation: clinical differences in type of transplant and implications for management. J Heart Lung Transplant. 2003;22:258–66.
57. Mehrad B, Giusppe P, Martinez FJ, Clark T, Iannettoni MD, Lynch JP. Spectrum of *Aspergillus* infection in lung transplant recipients. Chest. 2001;119:169–75.
58. Yeldandi V, Laghi F, McCabe MA, et al. *Aspergillus* and lung transplantation. J Heart Lung Transplant. 1995;14:883–90.

59. Westney GE, Kesten S, de Hoyos A, Chapparro C, Winton T, Maurer JR. *Aspergillus* infection in single and double lung transplant recipients. Transplantation. 1996;61:915–9.
60. Cahill BC, Hibbs JR, Savik K, et al. *Aspergillus* airway colonization and invasive disease after lung transplantation. Chest. 1997;112:1160–4.
61. Husni RN, Gordon SM, Longworth DL, et al. Cytomegalovirus infection is a risk factor for invasive aspergillosis in lung transplant recipients. Clin Infect Dis. 1998;26:753–5.
62. Goldfarb NS, Avery RK, Goormastic M, et al. Hypogammaglobulinemia in lung transplant recipients. Transplantation. 2001;71:242–6.
63. Marks WH, Florence L, Lieberman J, et al. Successfully treated invasive pulmonary aspergillosis associated with smoking marijuana in a renal transplant recipient. Transplantation. 1996;61:1771–83.
64. Nunley DR, Ohori NP, Grgurich WF, et al. Pulmonary aspergillosis in cystic fibrosis lung transplant recipients. Chest. 1998;114:1321–9.
65. Cimon B, Carrere J, Vinatier JF, Chazalette JP, Chabasse D, Bouchara JP. Clinical significance to *Scedosporium apiospermum* in patients with cystic fibrosis. Eur J Clin Microbiol Infect Dis. 2000;19:53–6.
66. Horn DL, Neofytos D, Anaissie EJ, et al. Epidemiology and outcomes of candidemia in 2019 patients: data from the prospective antifungal therapy alliance registry. Clin Infect Dis. 2009;48:1695–703.
67. Dauber HJ, Paradis IL, Dummer JS. Infectious complications in pulmonary allograft recipients. Clin Chest Med. 1990;11:291–308.
68. Kanj SS, Welty-Wolf K, Madden J, et al. Fungal infections in lung and heart transplant recipients: report of 9 cases and review of the literature. Medicine (Baltimore). 1996;75:142–56.
69. Rodriguez M, Fishman JA. Prevention of infection due to *Pneumocystis* spp. in human immunodeficiency virus-negative immunocompromised patients. Clin Microbiol Rev. 2004;17:770–82.
70. Reyes J, Abu-Elmagd K, Tzakis A, et al. Infectious complications after human small bowel transplantation. Transplantation. 1992;24:1249–50.
71. Kusne S, Furukawa H, Abu-Elmagd K, et al. Infectious complications after small bowel transplantation in adults: an update. Transplant Proc. 1996;28:2761–2.
72. Freifeld AG, Iwen PC, Lesiak BL, Gilroy RK, Stevens RB, Kalil AC. Histoplasmosis in solid organ transplant recipients at a large Midwestern university transplant center. Transpl Infect Dis. 2005;7:109–15.
73. Peddi VR, Hariharan S, First MR. Disseminated histoplasmosis in renal allograft recipients. Clin Transplant. 1996;10:160–5.
74. Singh N, Chang FY, Gayowski T, Marino IR. Infections due to dematiaceous fungi in organ transplant recipients: case report and review. Clin Infect Dis. 1997;24:369–74.
75. Singh N, Limaye AP, Forrest G, et al. Late-onset invasive aspergillosis in organ transplant recipients in the current era. Med Mycol. 2006;44:445–9.
76. Issa NC, Fishman JA. Infectious complications of antilymphocyte therapies in solid organ transplantation. Clin Infect Dis. 2009;48:772–86.
77. The US Multicenter FK506 Liver Study Group. A comparison of tacrolimus (FK 506) and cyclosporine for immunosuppresion in liver transplantation. N Engl J Med. 1994;331:1110–5.
78. Bernabeu-Wittel M, Naranjo M, Cisneros JM, et al. Infections in renal transplant recipients receiving mycophenolate versus azathioprine-based immunosuppression. Eur J Clin Microbiol Infect Dis. 2002;21:173–80.
79. Kontoyiannis DP, Lewis RE, Alexander BD, et al. Calcineurin inhibitor agents interact synergistically with antifungal agents in vitro against *Cryptococcus neoformans* isolates: correlation with outcome in solid organ transplant recipients with cryptococcosis. Antimicrob Agents Chemother. 2008;52:735–8.
80. Wong SY, Allen DM. Transmission of disseminated histoplasmosis via cadaveric renal transplantation: case report. Clin Infect Dis. 1992;14:232–4.
81. Limaye AP, Connolly PA, Sagar M, et al. Transmission of *Histoplasma capsulatum* by organ transplantation. N Engl J Med. 2000;343:1163–6.
82. Wright P, Pappagianis D, Davis CA, et al. Transmission of *Coccidioides immitis* from donor organs: a description of two fatal cases of disseminated coccidioidomycosis. Clin Infect Dis. 2003;37:1265–9.
83. Brugière O, Forget E, Biondi G, et al. Coccidioidomycosis in a lung transplant recipient acquired from the donor graft in France. Transplantation. 2009;88:1319–20.
84. Tripathy U, Yung GL, Kriett JM, Thistlewaite PA, Kapelanski DP, Jamieson SW. Donor transfer of pulmonary coccidioidomycosis in lung transplantation. Ann Thoracic Surg. 2002;73:306–8.
85. Battaglia M, Ditonno P, Fiore T, De Ceglie G, Regina G, Selvaggi FP. True mycotic arteritis by *Candida albicans* in 2 kidney transplant recipients from the same donor. J Urol. 2000;163:1236–7.
86. Albano L, Bretagne S, Mamzer-Bruneel MF, et al. Evidence that graft-site candidiasis after kidney transplantation is acquired during organ recovery: a multicenter study in France. Clin Infect Dis. 2009;48:194–202.
87. Keating MR, Guerrero MA, Daly RC, Walker RC, Davies SF. Transmission of invasive aspergillosis from a subclinically infected donor to three different organ transplant recipients. Chest. 1996;109:1119–24.
88. Safdar N, Slattery WR, Knasinski V, et al. Predictors and outcomes of candiduria in renal transplant recipients. Clin Infect Dis. 2005;40:1413–21.
89. Gallis HA, Berman RA, Cate TR, Hamilton JD, Gunnels JC, Stickel DL. Fungal infections following renal transplantation. Arch Intern Med. 1975;135:1163–72.
90. Ciancio G, Burke GW, Viciana AL, et al. Destructive allograft fungal arteritis following simultaneous pancreas-kidney transplantation. Transplantation. 1996;61:1172–5.
91. Potti A, Danielson B, Sen K. "True" mycotic aneurysm of a renal artery allograft. Am J Kidney Dis. 1998;31:E3.
92. Dowling RD, Baladi N, Zenati M, et al. Disruption of the aortic anastomosis after heart-lung transplantation. Ann Thoracic Surg. 1990;49:118–22.
93. Ralph ED, Hussain Z. Chronic meningitis caused by *Candida albicans* in a liver transplant recipient: usefulness of the polymerase chain reaction for diagnosis and for monitoring treatment. Clin Infect Dis. 1996;23:191–2.
94. Choi IS, Kim SJ, Kim BY, et al. *Candida* polyarthritis in a renal transplant patient: case report of a patient successfully treated with amphotericin B. Transplant Proc. 2000;32:1963–4.
95. Balajee SA, Kano R, Baddley JW, et al. Molecular identification of *Aspergillus* species collected for the Transplant-Associated Infection Surveillance Network. J Clin Microbiol. 2009;47:3138–41.
96. Patterson TF, Kirkpatrick WR, White M, et al. Invasive aspergillosis: disease spectrum, treatment, practice, and outcomes. Medicine (Baltimore). 2000;79:250–60.
97. Lin SJ, Schranz J, Teutsch SM. Aspergillosis case-fatality rate: systemic review of the literature. Clin Infect Dis. 2001;32:658–66.
98. Kramer MR, Denning DW, Marshall SE, et al. Ulcerative tracheobronchitis after lung transplantation: a new form of invasive aspergillosis. Am Rev Respir Dis. 1991;144:552–8.
99. Sayiner A, Kursat S, Toz H, Duman S, Onal B, Tumbay E. Pseudomembranous necrotizing bronchial aspergillosis in a renal transplant recipient. Nephrol Dial Transplant. 1999;14:1784–5.
100. Horvath JA, Dummer S. The use of respiratory-tract cultures in the diagnosis of invasive pulmonary aspergillosis. Am J Med. 1996;100:171–8.

101. Brown RS, Lake JR, Katzman BA, et al. Incidence of significance of *Aspergillus* cultures following liver and kidney transplantation. Transplantation. 1996;61:666–9.
102. Perfect JR, Cox GM, Lee JY, et al. The impact of culture isolation of *Aspergillus* species: a hospital-based survey of aspergillosis. Clin Infect Dis. 2001;33:1824–33.
103. Husain S, Paterson DL, Studer SM, et al. *Aspergillus* galactomannan antigen in the bronchoalveolar lavage fluid for the diagnosis of invasive aspergillosis in lung transplant recipients. Transplantation. 2007;83:1330–6.
104. Patterson JE. Epidemiology of fungal infections in solid organ transplant patients. Transpl Infect Dis. 1999;1:229–36.
105. Kapoor A, Flechner SM, O'Malley K, Paolone D, File TM, Cutrona AF. Cryptococcal meningitis in renal transplant patients associated with environmental exposure. Transplant Infect Dis. 1999;1:213–7.
106. Hunger RE, Paredes BE, Quattroppani C, Krahenbuhl S, Braathen LR. Primary cutaneous cryptococcosis in a patient with systemic immunosuppression after liver transplantation. Dermatology. 2000;200:352–5.
107. Nosanchuk JD, Shoham S, Fries BC, Shapiro S, Levitz SM, Casadevall A. Evidence of zoonotic transmission of *Cryptococcus neoformans* from a pet cockatoo to an immunocompromised patient. Ann Intern Med. 2000;132:205–8.
108. Anderson DJ, Schmidt C, Goodman J, Pomeroy C. Cryptococcal disease presenting as cellulitis. Clin Infect Dis. 1992;14:666–72.
109. Baer S, Baddley JW, Gnann JW, Pappas PG. Cryptococcal disease presenting as necrotizing cellulitis in transplant recipients. Transpl Infect Dis. 2009;11:353–8.
110. Chandesris LF, MO PS, et al. Cellulitis revealing a cryptococcosis-related immune reconstitution inflammatory syndrome in a renal allograft recipient. Am J Transplant. 2007;7:2826–8.
111. Pappas PG, Perfect JR, Cloud GA, et al. Cryptococcosis in human immunodeficiency virus-negative patients in the era of effective azole therapy. Clin Infect Dis. 2001;33:690–9.
112. Singh N, Alexander BD, Lortholary O, et al. *Cryptococcus neoformans* in organ transplant recipients: impact of calcineurin-inhibitor agents on mortality. J Infect Dis. 2007;195:756–64.
113. Singh N, Perfect JR. Immune reconstitution syndrome associated with opportunistic mycoses. Lancet Infect Dis. 2007;7:395–401.
114. Singh N, Lortholary O, Alexander BD, et al. An immune reconstitution syndrome-like illness associated with *Cryptococcus neoformans* infection in organ transplant recipients. Clin Infect Dis. 2005;40:1756–61.
115. Singh N, Lortholary O, Alexander BD, et al. Allograft loss in renal transplant recipients with *Cryptococcus neoformans* associated immune reconstitution syndrome. Transplantation. 2005;80:1131–3.
116. Singh N, Lortholary O, Dromer F, et al. Central nervous system cryptococcis in solid organ transplant recipients: clinical relevance of abnormal neuroimaging findings. Transplantation. 2008;86:647–51.
117. Demirag A, Elkhammas EA, Henry ML, et al. Pulmonary *Rhizopus* infection in a diabetic renal transplant recipient. Clin Transplant. 2000;14:8–10.
118. Lee E, Vershvovsky Y, Miller F, Waltzer W, Suh H, Nord EP. Combined medical surgical therapy for pulmonary mucormycosis in a diabetic renal allograft recipient. Am J Kidney Dis. 2001;38:E37.
119. Jimenez C, Lumbreras C, Aguado JM, et al. Successful treatment of *Mucor* infection after liver or pancreas-kidney transplantation. Transplant. 2002;73:476–80.
120. Walker SD, Clark RV, King CT, Humphries JE, Lytle LS, Butkus DE. Fatal disseminated *Conidiobolus coronatus* infection in a renal transplant patient. Review. Am J Clin Pathol. 1992;98:559–64.
121. Sheu BS, Lee PC, Yang HB. A giant gastric ulcer caused by mucormycosis infection in a patient with renal transplantation. Endoscopy. 1998;30:S60–1.
122. Ju JH, Park HS, Shin MJ, et al. Successful treatment of massive lower gastrointestinal bleeding caused by mixed infection of cytomegalovirus and mucormycosis in a renal transplant recipient. Am J Nephrol. 2001;21:232–6.
123. Timmouth J, Baker J, Gardiner G. Gastrointestinal mucormycosis in a renal transplant patient. Can J Gastroenterol. 2001;15:269–71.
124. Gold WL, Vellend H, Salit IE, et al. Successful treatment of systemic and local infections due to *Exophiala* spp. Clin Infect Dis. 1994;19:339–41.
125. Salama AD, Rogers T, Lord GM, Lechler RI, Mason PD. Multiple *Cladosporium* brain abscesses in a renal transplant patient: aggressive management improves outcome. Transplantation. 1997; 63:160–2.
126. von Eiff C, Bettin D, Proctor RA, et al. *Phaeocremonium parasiticum* infective endocarditis following liver transplantation. Clin Infect Dis. 1997;25:1251–3.
127. Mesa A, Henao J, Gil M, Durango G. Phaeohyphomycosis in kidney transplant patients. Clin Transplant. 1999;13:273–6.
128. Malani PN, Bleicher JJ, Kauffman CA, Davenport DS. Disseminated *Dactylaria constricta* infection in a renal transplant recipient. Transpl Infect Dis. 2001;3:40–3.
129. Castro LG, da Silva Lacaz C, Guarro J, et al. Phaeohyphomycotic cyst caused by *Colletotrichum crassipes*. J Clin Microbiol. 2001;39:2321–4.
130. Magina S, Libosa C, Santos P, et al. Cutaneous alternariosis by *Alternaria chartarum* in a renal transplanted patient. Br J Dermatol. 2000;142:1261–2.
131. Halaby T, Boots H, Vermeulen A, et al. Phaeohyphomycosis caused by *Alternaria infectoria* in a renal transplant recipient. J Clin Microbiol. 2001;39:1952–5.
132. Blair JE. Coccidioidomycosis in liver transplantation. Liver Transplant. 2006;12:31–9.
133. Blair JE, Logan JL. Coccidioidomycosis in solid organ transplantation. Clin Infect Dis. 2001;33:1536–44.
134. Braddy CM, Heilman RL, Blair JE. Coccidioidomycosis after renal transplantation in an endemic area. Am J Transplant. 2006;6:340–5.
135. Marques SA, Hozumi S, Camargo RM, Carvalho MF, Marques ME. Histoplasmosis presenting as cellulitis 18 years after renal transplantation. Med Mycol. 2008;46:725–8.
136. McGuinn ML, Lawrence ME, Proia L, Segreti J. Progressive disseminated histoplasmosis presenting as cellulitis in a renal transplant recipient. Transplant Proc. 2005;37:4313–4.
137. Bacal F, Andrade AC, Migueletto BC, et al. Histoplasmosis as a late infectious complication following heart transplantation in a patient with Chagas' disease. Arquivos Brasileiors de Cardiologia. 2001;76:403–8.
138. Botterel F, Romand S, Saliba F, et al. A case of disseminated histoplasmosis likely due to infection from a liver allograft. Eur J Clin Microbiol Infect Dis. 1999;18:662–4.
139. Livas IC, Nechay PS, Nauseef WM. Clinical evidence of spinal and cerebral histoplasmosis twenty years after renal transplantation. Clin Infect Dis. 1995;20:692–5.
140. Zainudin BM, Kassim F, Annuar NM, Lim CS, Ghazali AK, Murad Z. Disseminated histoplasmosis presenting with ileal perforation in a renal transplant recipient. J Trop Med Hygiene. 1992;95:276–9.
141. Brett MT, Kwan JT, Bending MR. Caecal perforation in a renal transplant patient with disseminated histoplasmosis. J Clin Pathol. 1988;41:992–5.
142. Cohen IM, Galgini JN, Potter D, Ogden DA. Coccidioidomycosis in renal transplant replacement therapy. Arch Intern Med. 1982;142:489–94.
143. Serody JS, Mill MR, Detterbeck FC, Harris DT, Cohen MS. Blastomycosis in transplant recipients: report of a case and review. Clin Infect Dis. 1993;16:54–8.

144. Gauthier GM, Safdar N, Klein BS, Andes DR. Blastomycosis in solid organ transplant recipients. Transpl Infect Dis. 2007;9:310–7.
145. Pappas PG, Threlkeld MG, Bedsole GD, Cleveland KO, Gelfand MS, Dismukes WE. Blastomycosis in immunocompromised patients. Medicine (Baltimore). 1994;72:311–25.
146. Agarwal SK, Tiwari SC, Dash SC, et al. Urinary sporotrichosis in a renal allograft recipient. Nephron. 1994;66:485.
147. Gullberg RM, Quintanilla A, Levin ML, Williams J, Phair JP. Sporotrichosis: recurrent cutaneous, articular, and central nervous system infection in a renal transplant recipient. Rev Infect Dis. 1987;9:369–75.
148. Guarro J, Nucci M, Akiti T, Gene J, Barreiro MD, Goncalves RT. Fungemia due to *Fusarium sacchari* in an immunosuppressed patient. J Clin Microbiol. 2000;38:419–21.
149. Sampathkumar P, Paya CV. *Fusarium* infection after solid-organ transplantation. Clin Infect Dis. 2001;32:1237–40.
150. Boutati EI, Anaissie EJ. *Fusarium*, a significant emerging pathogen in patients with hematologic malignancy: ten years' experience at a cancer center and implications for management. Blood. 1997;90:999–1008.
151. Clark NM. *Paecilomyces lilacinus* infection in a heart transplant recipient and successful treatment with terbinafine. Clin Infect Dis. 1999;28:1169–70.
152. Blackwell W, Ahmed K, O'Docherty C, Hay RJ. Cutaneous hyalohyphomycosis caused by *Paecilomyces lilacinus* in a renal transplant patient. Br J Dermatol. 2000;143:873–5.
153. Hilmarsdottir I, Thorsteinsson SB, Asmundsson P, Bodvarsson M, Arnadottir M. Cutaneous infection caused by *Paecilomyces lilacinus* in a renal transplant patient: treatment with voriconazole. Scand J Infect Dis. 2000;32:331–2.
154. Guarro J, Antolin Ayala MI, Gene J, Gutierrez-Calzada J, Nieves-Diez C, Ortoneda M. Fatal case of *Trichoderma harzianum* infection in a renal transplant recipient. J Clin Microbiol. 1999;37:3751–5.
155. Gordon SM, LaRosa SP, Kalmadi S, et al. Should prophylaxis for *Pneumocystis carinii* pneumonia in solid organ transplant recipients ever be discontinued? Clin Infect Dis. 1999;28:240–6.
156. Torre-Cisneros J, De la Mata M, Pozo JC, et al. Randomized trial of weekly sulfadoxine/pyrimethamine versus daily low-dose trimethoprim-sulfamethoxazole for the prophylaxis of *Pneumocystis carinii* pneumonia after liver transplantation. Clin Infect Dis. 1999;29:771–4.
157. De Pauw B, Walsh TJ, Donnelly JP, et al. Revised definitions of the EORTC/MSG Consensus Group for invasive fungal diseases. Clin Infect Dis. 2008;46:1813–21.
158. Ostrosky-Zeichner L, Alexander BD, Kett DH, et al. Multicenter clinical evaluation of the (1,3) β-D glucan assay as an aid to diagnosis of fungal infections in humans. Clin Infect Dis. 2005;41:654–9.
159. Husain S, Kwak EJ, Obman A, et al. Prospective assessment of Platelia *Aspergillus* galactomannan antigen for the diagnosis of invasive aspergillosis in lung transplant recipients. Am J Transplant. 2004;4:796–802.
160. Winston DJ, Pakrasi A, Busuttil RW. Prophylactic fluconazole in liver transplant recipients: a randomized, double-blind, placebo-controlled trial. Ann Intern Med. 1999;131:729–37.
161. Tollemar J, Hockerstedt K, Ericzon BG, Jalanko H, Ringden O. Liposomal amphotericin B prevents invasive fungal infections in liver transplant recipients. Transplantation. 1995;59:45–50.
162. Pappas PG, Andes D, Schuster M, et al. Invasive fungal infections in low-risk liver transplant recipients: a multi-center prospective observational study. Am J Transplant. 2006;6:386–91.
163. Hadley S, Huckabee C, Pappas PG, et al. Outcomes of antifungal prophylaxis in high-risk liver transplant recipients. Transpl Infect Dis. 2009;11:40–8.
164. Marty FM, Rubin RH. The prevention of infection post-transplant: the role of prophylaxis, preemptive and empiric therapy. Transpl Int. 2006;19:2–11.
165. Palmer SM, Drew RH, Whitehouse JD, et al. Safety of aerosolized amphotericin B lipid complex in lung transplant recipients. Transplantation. 2001;72:545–8.
166. Monforte V, Roman A, Gavalda J, et al. Nebulized amphotericin B prophylaxis for *Aspergillus* infection in lung transplantation: study of risk factors. J Heart Lung Transplant. 2001;20:1274–81.

Fungal Infections Among Patients with AIDS

Olivier Lortholary and Bertrand Dupont

Fungal infections are the most frequent opportunistic diseases occurring during the course of HIV infection. Those mycoses that are usually controlled by cellular immunity are most commonly observed. However, in patients with AIDS, the immune deficit is complex and worsens with time in untreated patients, allowing mycotic diseases to develop [1–3]. *Pneumocystis jiroveci* and *Candida albicans*, which are responsible for mucosal candidiasis, and *Cryptococcus neoformans*, the most frequent cause of meningitis, are the three major fungal pathogens in patients with AIDS [4, 5]. In endemic areas, infections due to dimorphic fungi also represent an important group. *Histoplasma capsulatum*, *Coccidioides* species, and *Penicillium marneffei* are the most important endemic pathogens. In some AIDS patients, mycotic disease is often the consequence of reactivation several years after a primary infection [6].

The time of occurrence of opportunistic fungal infections parallels the intensity of the immune deficit. Fungal infections can be the initial sign of HIV infection, are a good marker of the severity of the immune deficit, and have prognostic value. Some fungal infections, such as oropharyngeal candidiasis, are relatively benign, but others, such as cryptococcal meningitis and invasive aspergillosis, are usually severe and have a poor prognosis. Since 1996 the use of highly active antiretroviral therapy (HAART) has markedly reduced the incidence and the severity of opportunistic fungal infections in patients living in countries that can afford the high costs of HAART. Several helpful reviews are devoted to fungal infections in patients with AIDS [6–8].

O. Lortholary (✉)
Infectious and Tropical Diseases Departement, Centre d' Infectiologie Necker-Pasteur, Université Paris Descartes, Hôpital Necker Enfants malades, Paris, France
e-mail: olivier.lortholary@nck.aphp.fr

Candidiasis

Mucosal candidiasis is the most prevalent infection in HIV-positive patients, and nearly all AIDS patients will develop some clinical manifestations of candidiasis during the course of their illness [9]. Among *Candida* species, *C. albicans* is almost exclusively responsible for clinical disease. Other species such as *Candida glabrata*, *Candida tropicalis*, *Candida krusei*, or *Candida parapsilosis* may be associated with *C. albicans* in culture; however these non-*albicans* species are often present in low number and their pathogenic role is doubtful and rarely proven. *Candida dubliniensis* may be mistaken for *C. albicans*; the former has been isolated from the oral cavity in patients suffering from recurrent episodes of infection [10]. Beside impairment of cellular immunity and of Th1 and Th2 type responses, a lack of integrity of host tissue and an alteration in equilibrium of the oral flora predispose to oropharyngeal candidiasis. Antimicrobial drugs given for a bacterial or a parasitic infection may represent an additional predisposing factor. An increase in colonization precedes infection. HIV-positive patients can be heavily colonized without clinical signs or symptoms.

Oropharyngeal Candidiasis

Oropharyngeal candidiasis is the most common disease and will occur in 90% of HIV-infected patients if they do not receive HAART. The lower the CD4 cell count, the higher the risk of developing thrush, although this disease can occur in patients with CD4 counts of 200–400 cells/μL. Thrush, or acute pseudomembranous candidiasis, is the most common clinical form and is characterized by the presence of white patches on an erythematous mucosa. Patches can become confluent, with white pseudomembranes generally spread throughout the oral cavity, involving the dorsal and ventral parts of the tongue, gums, cheeks, and hard and soft palate. The membranes are adherent to the underlying mucosa and can be removed by scraping, revealing a raw erythematous base.

C.A. Kauffman et al. (eds.), *Essentials of Clinical Mycology*,
DOI 10.1007/978-1-4419-6640-7_31, © Springer Science+Business Media, LLC 2011

Symptoms vary from patient to patient and may not be proportional to the intensity of the intraoral disease. Some patients are symptomless, while others will complain of a furrowed tongue, mouth pain, odynophagia, dysphagia, or burning mouth. Mycologic examination of wet preparations of specimens obtained by scraping or swabbing shows numerous blastospores and pseudohyphae with few polymorphonuclear leukocytes. Heavy growth of *Candida* species is obtained when culture is performed.

Patients who develop thrush should be tested for HIV infection. Presence of thrush allows classification of the patient as having symptomatic HIV disease. Other clinical forms of oropharyngeal candidiasis include atrophic erythematous candidiasis, which involves the tongue and/or palatal mucosa, is less frequent than thrush, possibly underdiagnosed, and can precede the appearance of typical thrush. Angular cheleitis is generally associated with thrush present on the adjacent buccal mucosa. A saburral tongue, also called "dirty tongue," may be difficult to differentiate from thrush, and mycologic sampling of the mouth is useless, as HIV-positive patients are often heavily colonized with *Candida*, even in the absence of disease. From a clinical viewpoint, thrush is rarely exclusively found on the tongue. Hairy leukoplakia, due to EBV and often associated with thrush, is characterized by white parallel vertical striae localized to both sides of the tongue.

Treatment of the first episode of oropharyngeal candidiasis should be with a topical antifungal agent that is formulated so as to allow prolonged contact with the affected mucosa. Topical medications should be given 4–6 times a day, administered apart from meals, held in the mouth for several minutes, and continued for 2–3 weeks. Suitable topical drugs include amphotericin B, nystatin, or clotrimazole troches. Numerous commercial formulations are available in different countries as suspensions, powders, oral gels, and tablets for chewing or sucking. In cases of relapsing or chronic candidiasis, topical treatment is less likely to be effective and may be refused by the patient. The treatment of choice is oral fluconazole, 100 mg daily for 7–14 days. The oral solution of itraconazole, 100–200 mg daily, is an effective alternative. In patients with an inadequate response, the daily dose of fluconazole or itraconazole can be raised. Chronic suppressive therapy with fluconazole is effective in the prevention of relapse, but emergence of azole resistance is a concern [11].

Esophageal Candidiasis

Esophageal candidiasis, typically observed in patients with more advanced immunosuppression, classifies the patient's condition as AIDS. Oral thrush is almost always present in patients with esophagitis, but this may not be true in patients treated with a topical oral agent. Esophagitis may be latent and discovered by an endoscopic examination performed for a nonspecific gastric disturbance. The most suggestive symptom of esophageal candidiasis is odynophagia. Some patients complain of nausea or vomiting and can have esophageal bleeding. Patients can have fever and, occasionally, posterior thoracic pain. Endoscopic examination of the esophagus reveals characteristic confluent white plaques adherent to the erythematous mucosa and sometimes covering the entire mucosal surface. A stratification of severity can be established based on extent of lesions, presence of ulcerations, and narrowing of the lumen. In a patient with oral thrush and retrosternal odynophagia, an endoscopic examination of the esophagus is not mandatory to prove the diagnosis of esophageal candidiasis. A trial of a systemic antifungal agent can be used as a diagnostic trial. However, if failure of systemic antifungal therapy occurs, endoscopic examination is needed to rule out azole resistance and other etiologies of ulcers, such as herpes simplex virus, cytomegalovirus, atypical mycobacterial infection, and idiopathic ulcers [12].

Systemic therapy is required to effectively treat esophageal candidiasis. Oral fluconazole 200–400 mg daily for 2–3 weeks is the drug of choice [11]. Itraconazole, voriconazole, and echinocandins are alternative therapies and are less toxic than amphotericin B. In cases of failure due to resistance to fluconazole, these therapies are usually effective [13, 14].

Other Candida Infections

Other forms of candidiasis in HIV-infected/AIDS patients are less frequent. Laryngitis should be suspected in a patient with thrush and hoarseness and is sometimes diagnosed during bronchoscopy. Symptomatic vulvovaginitis is much less frequent than thrush, and anal and penile candidiasis are uncommon. *Candida* intertrigo and paronychia are no more frequent than in HIV-negative persons. Invasive candidiasis in AIDS patients is rare. When candidemia does occur it is usually due to the presence of an infected intravenous catheter [15]. Candidemia is treated with either an echinocandin or fluconazole according to the specific *Candida* species and previous azole exposure [11, 16]. Anecdotal reports have been published describing cholecystitis, prostatitis, and osteoarticular infections due to *Candida* species in HIV-infected patients.

Refractory Mucosal Candidiasis

Oropharyngeal candidiasis and esophagitis have a tendency to recur in patients with a low CD4 count. Consequently, these patients are often treated with protracted or repeated courses of systemic antifungal agents. Cases refractory to fluconazole were reported in up to 15% of patients with advanced AIDS before the era of HAART. Low CD4 counts ≤50/μL, frequent courses of azole therapy, and prolonged treatment have been shown to predispose to clinical resistance [17, 18]. Higher minimum inhibitory concentrations (MIC) to fluconazole correlate with clinical failure [19, 20]. Clinical resistance has been reported in patients not previously exposed to fluconazole but who were sexual partners of patients who were receiving this antifungal agent and harboring *Candida* strains with a high MIC [21]. Molecular biology studies indicate that a majority of patients carry the same clone of *Candida* for many years [19]. Since the advent of HAART there has been a marked decrease in all forms of candidiasis in HIV-infected patients. Resistance of *Candida* to antifungal drugs among AIDS patients appears to be less common than in the 1990s.

Cryptococcosis

Cryptococcosis is caused by *Cryptococcus neoformans* var. *neoformans* and *Cryptococcus neoformans* var. *grubii. Cryptococcus gattii* has recently been given species status and is infrequently described in HIV-infected patients. Both varieties of *C. neoformans* are cosmopolitan and are found in soil and bird droppings, whereas *C. gatti* is found mostly in subtropical areas and the Pacific Northwest. Most laboratories do not differentiate between the two varieties in AIDS or non-AIDS patients [22], and the organism will be referred to simply as *C. neoformans* in this section.

The prevalence of exposure to *Cryptococcus* is high, with up to 80% of adults having been exposed, as evidenced by serology. HIV infection represents the most prevalent underlying disease in patients with cryptococcosis. Studies from the western world revealed HIV infection in 29% of patients; in 58% of these patients, cryptococcosis was an AIDS-defining illness [23]. The overall incidence of cryptococcosis has declined by 46% in France between 1997 and 2002 [23]. However, cryptococcosis is of increasing concern in Africa and Southeast Asia. It is encountered in 15–20% of AIDS patients in Africa and Cambodia [24, 25]. It is estimated that there are now one million new cases of cryptococcosis seen annually [26], and this disease has become the leading cause of meningitis in the world and the fourth most common cause of mortality related to infections. The male/female ratio is >2; this disease rarely affects children who are HIV-infected.

The portal of entry is pulmonary following environmental exposure. Pulmonary infection is mostly asymptomatic in immunocompetent individuals [5]. When cellular immunodeficiency occurs, yeasts multiply and fungemia occurs with subsequent occurrence of central nervous system (CNS) infection. A primary skin portal of entry has been described rarely [27]. Polysaccharide antigen is shed during growth of the organism, is associated with numerous immunomodulatory effects, and may be responsible for elevated cerebrospinal fluid (CSF) opening pressure without hydrocephalus. Cellular immunodeficiency is pivotal in the occurrence of extrapulmonary cryptococcosis. The median CD4 cell count at the time of diagnosis is 20/μL [28].

Clinical Manifestations

Meningoencephalitis is the classic presentation of cryptococcosis and accounts for 90% of the cases in HIV-infected patients. Neurologic symptoms are most often subacute but can also be acute, in which case there is a worse prognosis. Fever and headache are common, but meningeal symptoms are not consistently noted. Cranial nerve palsies, seizures, motor weakness, and obtundation can occur. Loss of visual acuity usually is a consequence of increased intracranial pressure.

In all cases of cryptococcal meningitis occurring in patients with AIDS, cerebral imaging, using CT or MRI scanning when available, should be performed [29]. Imaging is normal in 50% of cases; however, cortical atrophy, hydrocephalus, and nodules can be found in the others. MRI is more sensitive and can show T2 hyperintensity in the basal meninges and dilation of Virchow-Robin spaces. When performing lumbar puncture, measurement of CSF opening pressure is mandatory as increased pressure is found in 30–50% of AIDS patients with cryptococcal meningitis. The prognosis is highly associated with the magnitude of the increased intracranial pressure that is found.

Pneumonia is often symptomatic in AIDS patients, causing cough and dyspnea and, less commonly, chest pain and hemoptysis [30]. Other opportunistic pulmonary infections and extrapulmonary dissemination of *C. neoformans* are often found. Acute respiratory distress syndrome occurs and is associated with a worse prognosis. Chest radiographs and CT scans show interstitial infiltrates, nodules, pleural effusions, mediastinal lymphadenopathy, or cavitary lesions [31].

Cryptococcal skin involvement is often manifested by lesions resembling molluscum contagiosum, but other types of lesions, including papules, pustules, nodules, and cellulitis, are also found. Disseminated cryptococcosis should be suspected in febrile HIV-infected patients who present with skin lesions. Urinary tract involvement occurs commonly and is usually asymptomatic. The prostate can serve as a sanctuary for *C. neoformans* in patients who have had a response to treatment for meningitis.

Diagnosis

Microscopic examination of CSF allows a rapid diagnosis. Analysis with India ink preparation of the pellet obtained after centrifugation of the CSF allows the diagnosis of cryptococcal meningitis by showing encapsulated yeasts in more than 80% of HIV-infected patients. However, many laboratories no longer perform this assay and rely instead on the demonstration of cryptococcal antigen in the CSF. In tissues, the organisms are seen as yeasts that are circumscribed by an unstained halo corresponding to the capsule.

C. neoformans is readily grown in culture at 35–37°C on many types of culture media, with the exception of those containing cycloheximide. Growth is usually obtained in 2–7 days, but samples should be incubated at least 4 weeks. The positivity rate is improved by the collection of larger volumes of CSF. Blood cultures should be performed in all patients, and if possible the centrifugation/lysis technique should be used [32].

Cryptococcal antigen should be searched for in serum and CSF. Commercially available tests are sensitive (≥95%) and specific (≥95%), and false-positive results are rare. In developing areas, it has been shown that the detection of cryptococcal antigen in the serum of AIDS patients allows the early diagnosis of a large number of asymptomatic cases [25, 33]. A high serum antigen titer is associated with a higher mycologic failure rate. However, serum titers cannot be followed to determine the course of the infection as it has been shown that a lack of decrease is not predictive of a worse outcome.

Treatment

Antifungal agents used to treat cryptococcosis include amphotericin B, flucytosine, and fluconazole [32]. For initial therapy, the combination of amphotericin B and flucytosine has been shown to be superior to monotherapy, and flucytosine use is an independent predictor of early mycologic outcome [28, 34]. Amphotericin B in association with high-dose fluconazole, 800 mg daily, may also be an option [35], and the combination of high-dose fluconazole and flucytosine has also been validated.

The appropriate management of elevated CSF opening pressure strongly influences early mortality. Overall, mortality remains at 17% in France, although delayed mortality has been dramatically reduced with the availability of HAART [28]. Amphotericin B, 0.7 mg/kg daily, and flucytosine, 100 mg/kg daily, is the regimen of choice for induction therapy, when flucytosine is available, and should be given for a minimum of 14 days [32, 34, 36, 37]. If clinical outcome is favorable and CSF culture has become negative, therapy can be switched to oral fluconazole, 400 mg daily, for a duration of 8–10 weeks. Maintenance therapy with fluconazole, 200 mg daily, should be given until persistent immune restoration is obtained. If the patient has renal failure, liposomal amphotericin B, 3–5 mg/kg daily, can be used [38, 39]. Ideally, in order to avoid flucytosine hematologic toxicity, serum drug concentrations should be monitored; a peak flucytosine concentration <100 μg/mL is sought.

In patients who have an elevated CSF opening pressure (≥25 cm H_2O), repeated lumbar punctures should be performed every 1–3 days in order to withdraw CSF until the pressure returns to a normal value [32, 40]. In cases of persistently increased intracranial pressure, a ventriculoperitoneal shunt or a lumbar drain should be placed. Mannitol and acetazolamide have not been proven to be helpful for the management of raised intracranial pressure, and steroids have been reported to be deleterious based on a post hoc analysis of a large clinical trial [41].

For patients who have localized extrameningeal cryptococcosis, such as pulmonary infection in the absence of dissemination, fluconazole, 400 mg daily, can be given. However, with disseminated infection, the treatment is the same as that outlined for meningeal cryptococcosis [32].

In a patient who is noted to have an isolated positive serum cryptococcal antigen titer, an exhaustive workup should be performed to search for a site of infection, and if none is found and the patient has a CD4 count <200/μL, therapy with fluconazole should be initiated.

Before the availability of HAART, relapses were observed in 37–60% of patients in whom maintenance therapy with an azole was stopped. In the HAART era, several studies have clearly demonstrated that maintenance therapy can be safely withdrawn in patients who are on HAART and who have a CD4 cell count >100/μL and an undetectable viral load for at least 3 months [42–45].

Primary prophylaxis with fluconazole or itraconazole has been shown to reduce the incidence of cryptococcal disease without any impact on mortality. Prophylaxis is not recommended in developed countries that have relatively low rates of cryptococcosis. However, in developing countries, such as Thailand, where the prevalence of cryptococcosis is as high as 38% of all hospitalized patients, fluconazole, 400 mg weekly, has been found to be effective, and this regimen has now been adopted by several countries in Africa and Southeast Asia [46].

Pneumocystosis

This chapter does not address *Pneumocystis jiroveci* infections in AIDS patients. For a detailed discussion on this topic, see Chap. 26.

Dimorphic (Endemic) Fungal Infections

Among fungal infections due to dimorphic fungi, only three – histoplasmosis, coccidioidomycosis, and penicilliosis – are frequently found in AIDS patients [7, 47–49].

Histoplasmosis

Histoplasmosis due to *H. capsulatum* is endemic in the USA, the Caribbean, and Central and South America and occurs with much less frequency in Africa and Southeast Asia. In HIV-positive patients living in endemic areas in the midwestern USA, the incidence of histoplasmosis varies from 1% to 25% [48, 50]. Disease can be due to primary infection following an exposure event or to reactivation of a latent infection. Outside endemic areas, such as when histoplasmosis occurs in Europe, infection usually represents reactivation occurring several years after the primary infection [8, 49]. It is important to obtain a travel history, including trips to and former residence in geographic areas endemic for histoplasmosis, and to ask about activities, such as spelunking, cleaning old buildings, or disrupting soil. Histoplasmosis generally occurs in patients with CD4 counts <100 cells/μL and is an AIDS-defining illness in its disseminated form.

Clinical Manifestations

In AIDS patients, histoplasmosis is usually disseminated and presents with fever, weight loss, fatigue, and night sweats. Pneumonia is present in over half of the cases, and hepatomegaly, splenomegaly, and lymphadenopathy are common findings. Signs and symptoms of septic shock and respiratory failure are seen in about 10% of cases and are associated with a poor prognosis [51]. Central nervous system involvement, either meningitis or a space-occupying lesion, occurs in approximately 15% of patients [48]. Various cutaneous lesions are seen, including maculopapular rashes, pustules, papules, and ulcers, and mucosal ulcers are typical. Gastrointestinal involvement is fairly frequent, manifesting as fever, abdominal pain, anorexia, and weight loss. Mediastinal granuloma and chronic cavitary lung disease are unusual in this population.

Histoplasmosis due to *H. duboisii* does not occur frequently in AIDS patients. This form of histoplasmosis is seen exclusively among patients living in, or having traveled to, Central and West Africa and Madagascar. It is likely that histoplasmosis due to *H. duboisii* is underdiagnosed in the endemic area [52].

Diagnosis

Pancytopenia is common at presentation. Increases of serum lactic dehydrogenase and ferritin are commonly found but are nonspecific. The chest radiograph demonstrates patchy infiltrates or diffuse interstitial pneumonitis in more severe cases.

Microscopic examination of biopsy specimens or body fluid aspirates represents the fastest diagnostic approach, but the sensitivity varies. The greatest yield is from bone marrow, skin, and mucosal lesions. The classic 2–4 μm budding yeasts, visualized best by periodic acid–Schiff or methenamine silver stains, should be sought. The typical yeasts also can be seen in smears of buffy coat or blood. Material for culture for *H. capsulatum* should be obtained from blood, bone marrow, bronchoalveolar lavage fluid, and tissue samples.

Serodiagnostic tests by immunodiffusion or complement fixation are often negative but may be helpful when positive. *Histoplasma* antigen detection in blood, urine, or CSF is a specific and sensitive test among patients with disseminated disease. Antigenuria correlates well with response to therapy and is useful to detect relapsing histoplasmosis [53].

Treatment

Amphotericin B and itraconazole are effective against both *H. capsulatum* and *H. duboisii* [53]. Among patients with severe disease, including those with diffuse pneumonia, septic shock, or other life-threatening complications, initial treatment should be with liposomal amphotericin B, 3 mg/kg daily, or alternatively, amphotericin B, 0.7–1.0 mg/kg daily [53]. When patients have improved, generally after several weeks, the regimen can be switched to oral itraconazole, 200 mg twice daily for 12 months. Milder illness due to histoplasmosis can be treated initially with itraconazole, beginning with a loading dose of 200 mg thrice daily for 3 days, then giving 200 mg twice daily for 12 months [53]. Monitoring of serum itraconazole levels is mandatory in AIDS patients. Fluconazole is less effective than itraconazole, but can be given at a dosage of 400–800 mg daily if itraconazole is not tolerated. The role of newer azoles has not been established.

Maintenance therapy with itraconazole is necessary to avoid relapses in AIDS patients. Before 1996, relapse rates varied between 35% and 80%. In the HAART era, a prospective study has clearly documented that withdrawal of itraconazole is a safe strategy in patients who have been treated with itraconazole for at least 12 months, have at least two measurements of CD4 cell counts >150/μL in the preceding 6 months, and have received HAART for at least 6 months [54]. Maintenance therapy should be restarted when CD4 cells fall below 100/μL. Primary prophylaxis can be considered in areas in which the incidence of histoplasmosis is highest [55].

Coccidioidomycosis

Coccidioides immitis and *Coccidioides posadasii* are dimorphic fungi found in semi-arid areas in the southwestern USA, Mexico, and Central and South America, The disease is acquired by inhalation of arthroconidia present in the soil. The lung is the primary target organ. In highly endemic areas, such as Arizona, the annual rate of infection is as high as 27% among patients with AIDS compared with <4% in non-AIDS patients [56]. Disease can occur following reactivation or as a primary infection. Extrathoracic coccidioidomycosis involving sites other than the respiratory tract is an AIDS-defining illness. Risk factors for developing coccidioidomycosis in HIV-infected patients include African American race, the presence of oropharyngeal candidiasis (undoubtedly reflecting immune suppression), and lack of treatment with HAART [57].

Clinical Manifestations

The most common symptoms of coccidioidomycosis in AIDS patients are fever, cough, and weight loss. Chest radiography reveals a variety of abnormalities, including focal pulmonary alvelolar infiltrates, discrete nodules, hilar lymphadenopathy, and pleural effusions in more than 60% of patients. In 40% of those with radiographic findings, a diffuse reticulonodular infiltrate is present. Approximately 12% of patients develop meningitis. Lymphadenopathy, cutaneous lesions, and subcutaneous abscesses are common. Fungemia, thyroiditis, peritonitis, adrenal involvement, osteoarticular disease, and prostatic involvement also have been reported [56, 58, 59].

Diagnosis

The CD4 cell count is usually <200 cells/μL and often <50 cells/μL. Definitive diagnosis relies on visualization of the typical large spherules containing numerous endospores in clinical specimens and isolation of *Coccidioides* species in culture. *Coccidioides* are considered to be bioterrorism agents, and thus this organism cannot be handled in clinical microbiology laboratories. Serologic tests, including complement fixation and immunodiffusion, can be negative in as many as 25% of AIDS patients with active coccidioidal disease. Cerebrospinal fluid analysis typically shows leukocytic pleocytosis, decreased glucose, and increased protein values. Culture for *Coccidioides* species in CSF is often negative, but serology is positive and can establish the diagnosis of coccidioidal meningitis.

Treatment

The drug of choice for severe life-threatening coccidioidal infection, including diffuse reticulonodular lung involvement, is amphotericin B, 1 mg/kg daily, or a lipid formulation of amphotericin B, 3–5 mg/kg daily [60]. When the disease is controlled, generally after 2–3 weeks, switching to an oral triazole drug should be considered. Fluconazole 400 mg daily is a good alternative, particularly in patients with meningitis; itraconazole 400 mg daily has also given good results, especially in patients with skeletal disease [60, 61]. Fluconazole is the currently preferred treatment of coccidioidal meningitis [60]. Lifelong maintenance therapy with a triazole, either fluconazole 400 mg daily or itraconazole 400 mg daily, is necessary to avoid relapse in AIDS patients [62].

Penicilliosis

Penicillium marneffei is a dimorphic fungus present in soil in Southeast Asia, including northern Thailand, south China, Laos, Cambodia, and Vietnam. A few cases of penicilliosis have also been reported from Hong Kong, India, and Indonesia. A probable autochthonous case was reported in Africa. *Penicillium marneffei* is associated with several species of bamboo rats; however, contact with soil seems the most important risk factor regarding exposure to this fungus. In northern Thailand, penicilliosis has become the third most common AIDS-defining opportunistic disease, following tuberculosis and cryptococcosis [47, 63, 64]. Penicilliosis probably occurs as a silent primary infection and only becomes clinically apparent following reactivation years later when cellular immunity is profoundly depressed due to advanced HIV disease [65].

Clinical Manifestations

The portal of entry is the lung in most reported cases. As with histoplasmosis, disseminated penicilliosis is very common at presentation, and CD4 counts are uniformly very low, usually below 50 cells/μL. In one study of 92 patients with disseminated penicilliosis seen at Chiang Mai University Hospital in Thailand, 86 (93%) were HIV infected [47]. The mean duration of illness before patients presented for care in this study was 4 weeks (range 1 day to 3 years). Most patients were young men. The clinical characteristics of these patients included fever (93%), anemia (78%), pronounced weight loss (76%), skin lesions (68%), generalized lymphadenopathy (58%), hepatomegaly (51%), cough (49%), diarrhea (31%), splenomegaly (16%), and jaundice (8%). Skin lesions, especially a generalized papular rash, are very suggestive of the diagnosis of penicilliosis in patients at risk. Some of the papules with central umbilication mimic lesions caused by molluscum contagiosum. Subcutaneous nodules, acne-like lesions, and folliculitis may also be present. Genital ulcers and palatal papules also have been reported. Chest radiography is abnormal in almost 30% of patients with disseminated penicilliosis. Diffuse reticulonodular opacities and localized alveolar opacities are most common, and diffuse alveolar infiltrates and pleural effusion are less common [63, 64].

Diagnosis

Imported cases of penicilliosis are generally diagnosed earlier in the course of disease. Fever, with or without pancytopenia, skin, and/or lung lesions could also suggest a diagnosis of leishmaniasis or disseminated histoplasmosis. For any HIV-positive patient, a history of living in or previous travel to Southeast Asia is the first clue suggesting a diagnosis of penicilliosis [8, 49].

In the Chiang Mai series, diagnosis of penicilliosis was made by culture of the fungus from blood (76%), skin lesions (90%), bone marrow aspirate (100%), and sputum [47]. At 25°C, the organism grows as a mould within several days. The organism has a symmetric or asymmetric biverticillium structure and produces a distinctive red pigment that diffuses into the culture medium. The organism grows as a yeast when incubated at 35–37°C. The galactomannan test for detection of *Aspergillus* antigen cross-reacts with *P. marneffei*; however, the diseases are clinically different and direct examination of culture easily distinguishes between the two organisms. A presumptive diagnosis of penicilliosis can be made by examination of sputum or from biopsy material from bone marrow, skin, or lymph node. The typical oval or elongated, nonbudding *P. marneffei* yeasts that are 8–13 μm in length, with a characteristic septation, should be sought.

Treatment

Itraconazole and amphotericin B are the mainstays of therapy for penicilliosis in all patients, regardless of their immune status. A combination regimen of induction treatment with amphotericin B 0.6 mg/kg daily for approximately 2 weeks, followed by consolidation treatment with itraconazole 400 mg daily for 10 weeks, has been reported to be effective in 95% of patients [66]. This regimen clears fungal cultures more rapidly than a course of itraconazole alone. Voriconazole has also been shown to be effective. Suppressive therapy with itraconazole, 200 mg daily, is recommended for all patients with persistent immunocompromise [67]. In geographic areas in which *P. marneffei* is endemic, primary prophylaxis with itraconazole 200 mg daily is recommended [68].

Paracoccidioidomycosis

Paracoccidioidomycosis is not commonly reported in AIDS patients, a fact that remains unexplained. In a review of 27 cases, paracoccidioidomycosis occurred mainly in patients with advanced AIDS who were not receiving prophylaxis with trimethoprim-sulfamethoxazole for *P. jiroveci* [69]. In areas endemic for *Paracoccidioides brasiliensis*, HIV positivity has been limited mostly to larger towns, and paracoccidioidomycosis is generally seen more in rural areas. Almost all reported cases of AIDS-associated paracoccidioidomycosis have occurred in Brazil, with only one case reported from Venezuela. In the series reported by Goldani and Sugar, the overall male-to-female ratio was 3.5:1, which is lower than the sex ratio of 13:1 observed in the HIV-negative population [69, 70]. Reactivation of latent disease probably accounts for most cases, but among patients living in rural areas, primary infection cannot be excluded [70]. Most of the reported patients had advanced AIDS with CD4 cell counts well below 200/μL.

In most AIDS patients with paracoccidioidomycosis, the disease is widely disseminated. About two-thirds of patients have lung involvement with severe cough and dyspnea. Chest radiography is usually nonspecific, revealing diffuse interstitial infiltrates in most patients. Approximately 50% of patients have skin lesions that include a diffuse maculopapular rash, nodules, or ulcerative lesions. Adenopathy is present in approximately one-third of patients. Prolonged fever, weight loss, hepatomegaly, and splenomegaly are common. Meningitis is rare.

The diagnosis of paracoccidioidomycosis is usually made by direct microscopic examination and culture of clinical specimens, most commonly skin and lymph nodes. Biopsy material shows the characteristic large yeast with multiple buds around its border. Cultures of blood, bone marrow, and sputum may also be positive. Antibody detection is positive in a small number of patients. An assay for *P. brasiliensis* antigen and PCR for *P. brasiliensis* DNA are promising diagnostic tools in these patients.

Therapeutic options include trimethoprim-sulfamethoxazole, amphotericin B, ketoconazole, and itraconazole as primary treatment. Lifelong maintenance therapy with trimethoprim-sulfamethoxazole or itraconazole is recommended [71].

Blastomycosis

Blastomycosis is uncommon among HIV-infected patients [72]. Over 30 cases of blastomycosis have been reported in patients with AIDS, and most had CD4 cell counts well below 200/μL. Reactivation disease can occur as evidenced among patients who have been out of the endemic area for several years when they develop blastomycosis. Localized pleuropulmonary disease and disseminated infection have been seen in AIDS patients. Disseminated disease is associated with a high early mortality.

Amphotericin B is considered the initial treatment of choice for patients with severe disease and for all immunosuppressed patients [73]. For patients who are improved after 2–4 weeks of therapy with amphotericin B, it is reasonable to switch to oral itraconazole, 200 mg twice daily, and to maintain chronic suppressive therapy with itraconazole indefinitely in those patients who remain severely immunosuppressed [72, 73].

Sporotrichosis

Sporotrichosis usually manifests as a localized lymphocutaneous disease in the immunocompetent host. Disseminated disease occurs most frequently in severely immunocompromised individuals. In a review of 16 cases of disseminated sporotrichosis among HIV-infected patients, all patients presented with diffuse ulcerative skin lesions [74]. Other sites of disease included the CNS, joints, eyes, spleen, and bone marrow. *Sporothrix schenckii* fungemia was noted in two patients. Fifteen of the 16 patients were men. The mean CD4 cell count was 73/μL. Six of these patients died despite therapy. A second series of cases of sporotrichosis in AIDS patients has recently been reported [75].

Examination of tissue biopsies or material aspirated from skin lesions usually leads to the diagnosis when the typical cigar-shaped yeast forms are seen. However, the organism may be hard to discern. Culture of tissue or body fluids at 25°C reveals the mould form of *S. schenckii*.

The optimal therapy for disseminated sporotrichosis in HIV-positive patients has not been determined. Amphotericin B for the most severe cases followed by itraconazole appears to be the most reasonable approach to therapy. Itraconazole should be considered for long-term maintenance therapy among those patients who remain immunosuppressed [76].

Other Opportunistic Moulds and Yeasts

Aspergillosis

Invasive aspergillosis has been reported among patients with advanced HIV disease, especially in patients with CD4 cell counts <50/μL [77–79]. The classic risk factors for invasive aspergillosis, namely, neutropenia and corticosteroid therapy, are absent in many of the reported *Aspergillus* infections in persons with AIDS.

The lungs are the most common site of infection. In a study of 33 AIDS patients with invasive aspergillosis, most of whom had pulmonary disease, fever, cough, and dyspnea were the predominant symptoms, and chest pain and hemoptysis were noted less frequently [79]. On chest radiographs, nodular lesions and cavitary infiltrates are common and suggestive of aspergillosis; bilateral interstitial infiltrates are also noted. Invasive necrotizing tracheobronchitis, manifested by acute dyspnea and wheezing, is a clinical form of aspergillosis also seen in AIDS patients. Bronchoscopy reveals necrotic ulceration of the trachea with pseudomembranes [80]. Obstructing bronchial aspergillosis with chest pain, hemoptysis, and dyspnea may precede necrotizing tracheobronchitis [77]. A majority of patients have a history of prior pulmonary infection; preexisting cystic pulmonary lesions and bullae may represent risk factors for invasive pulmonary aspergillosis among patients with AIDS. Disseminated aspergillosis can occur and often involves the CNS and myocardium. *Aspergillus* endocarditis and sinusitis also have been reported among patients with AIDS.

There is a good correlation between a positive bronchoalveolar lavage culture for *Aspergillus* and histologically proven diagnosis in immunocompromised patients, including AIDS patients. The *Aspergillus* species most often implicated in disease are *A. fumigatus*, *Aspergillus flavus*, *Aspergillus niger*, and *Aspergillus terreus*. Detection of galactomannan antigen in serum or bronchoalveolar lavage fluid and/or PCR for *Aspergillus* may help to establish the diagnosis of invasive disease.

Although not specifically studied for AIDS patients, voriconazole has now become the recommended therapy for invasive aspergillosis in all patient groups, including AIDS patients [81]. Drug interactions with protease inhibitors and non-nucleoside reverse transcriptase inhibitors have to be carefully monitored when azole agents are used. An alternative therapy is a lipid formulation of amphotericin B. The prognosis of invasive aspergillosis in AIDS patients is poor, with a mean survival of 2–4 months despite antifungal treatment. This opportunistic infection is very unusual among patients receiving and responding to HAART.

Other Moulds

Zygomycosis, or mucormycosis, is usually encountered among AIDS patients with other risk factors, including diabetic ketoacidosis, neutropenia, hemodialysis, and intravenous drug use. Isolated renal infection has been described [82–84]. Rhinocerebral disease and brain abscesses, cutaneous infections, osteoarticular infections, and an unusual presentation with pharyngeal ulcerations have all been reported in AIDS patients [85–90]. The causative organisms of zygomycosis in AIDS patients have included *Absidia corymbifera*, *Cunninghamella bertholletiae*, and *Rhizopus oryzae*.

Scedosporium apiospermum (*Pseudallescheria boydii*) infections in patients with AIDS include pneumonia, renal infection, endocarditis, meningitis, brain abscess, and sinusitis [2, 91–95]. *Scedosporium prolificans* was responsible for a case of cutaneous and pulmonary disease [2]. Other uncommon moulds causing infections among AIDS patients include invasive alternariosis [96], disseminated and pulmonary adiaspiromycosis [97, 98], disseminated cutaneous *Emmonsia pasteuriana* infection [99], invasive *Fusarium* infections [100–102], and infections due to *Schizophyllum commune*, *Scytalidium dimidiatum*, and *Lecythophora hoffmannii* [103, 104].

Other Yeast-Like Fungi

Several cases of infection due to *Saccharomyces cerevisiae* in AIDS patients have been reported [2, 3, 105], and catheter-associated fungemia due to *Rhodotorula rubra* has been noted [106]. Three cases caused by *Trichosporon* species have been reported in AIDS patients, including two with central venous catheter–associated fungemia and one with peritonitis and a peritoneal catheter. Outcome was favorable in each case with antifungal treatment and removal of the catheter [107–109].

Impact of Antiretroviral Therapy on Fungal Infections

Antiretroviral therapy has had a major impact on the natural course of opportunistic infections in AIDS patients. Therapy has led to a marked decrease in the number of infections and has made it possible to stop primary prophylaxis for fungal infections and suppressive therapy of established fungal infections [110, 111]. The routine use of HAART has resulted in dramatic declines in morbidity and mortality among HIV-infected patients with advanced immune dysfunction [111]. In effectively treated patients, the incidence of opportunistic infections has decreased 50–70%. HAART has had an especially important impact on the incidence of *P. jiroveci* pneumonia, *Mycobacterium avium* complex disease, cytomegalovirus infection, mucosal candidiasis, cryptococcosis, dimorphic fungal infections, and invasive aspergillosis. Additionally, suppressive therapy for mucosal candidiasis, histoplasmosis, and cryptococcosis are no longer needed when immune reconstitution occurs with HAART [112]. Clinical resistance to fluconazole in patients with mucosal candidiasis has almost disappeared in patients responding to HAART.

A successful response to HAART is characterized by a marked reduction in viral load and a subsequent increase in CD4 cell count. However, the partial restoration of cell-mediated immunity and possibly other immune effectors may facilitate the development of an inflammatory reaction at the site of previous infection, which can mimic reactivation of the opportunistic disease [113]. Immune reconstitution inflammatory syndrome (IRIS) has been reported in AIDS patients with cryptococcosis and histoplasmosis [114–121]. The symptoms and signs of IRIS raise the diagnostic challenge for the clinician to decide whether the patient is experiencing a relapse of the initial infection, a new infection, or IRIS. The issue of timing of the initiation of HAART following initial treatment of an acute opportunistic infection is still not clarified. In cases of IRIS, treatment with anti-inflammatory agents, including corticosteroids, may be effective without necessitating a change in HAART or the anti-infective treatment.

In a prospective study of 101 AIDS patients who had cryptococcal meningitis, IRIS developed in 13% [120]. Risk factors for development of IRIS that were noted in various studies include early initiation of HAART after the diagnosis of cryptococcosis, high CSF antigen titer, fungemia, low CD4 cell count, and high viral load. IRIS can present as aseptic meningitis with increased intracranial pressure. Other manifestations include necrotic lymphadenopathy, necrotizing pneumonia, and cerebral or medullary abscesses. Although guidelines recommend starting HAART shortly after the occurrence of an opportunistic infection, some recommend waiting until CSF cultures have become negative [62]. In cases of IRIS reported during the course of histoplasmosis in AIDS patients, uveitis, liver abscesses, arthritis, and necrotizing lymphadenopathy have been reported.

References

1. Spellberg B, Edwards Jr JE. Type 1/Type 2 immunity in infectious diseases. Clin Infect Dis. 2001;32:76–102.
2. Cunliffe NA, Denning DW. Uncommon invasive mycoses in AIDS. AIDS. 1995;9:411–20.
3. Perfect JR, Schell WA, Rinaldi MG. Uncommon invasive fungal pathogens in the acquired immunodeficiency syndrome. J Med Vet Mycol. 1993;31:175–9.
4. Catherinot E, Lanternier F, Bougnoux ME, Lecuit M, Couderc LJ, Lortholary O. *Pneumocystis jiroveci* pneumonia. Infect Dis Clin North Am. 2010;24(1):107–38.
5. Mitchell TG, Perfect JR. Cryptococcosis in the era of AIDS – 100 years after the discovery of *Cryptococcus neoformans*. Clin Microbiol Rev. 1995;8:515–48.
6. Wheat J. Endemic mycoses in AIDS: a clinical review. Clin Microbiol Rev. 1995;8:146–59.
7. Ampel NM. Emerging disease issues and fungal pathogens associated with HIV infection. Emerg Infect Dis. 1996;2:109–16.
8. Dupont B, Crewe Brown HH, Westermann K, et al. Mycoses in AIDS. Med Mycol. 2000;38:259–67.

9. Klein RS, Harris CA, et al. Oral candidiasis in high risk patients as the initial manifestation of the acquired immunodeficiency syndrome. N Engl J Med. 1984;311:354–8.
10. Sullivan D, Coleman D. *Candida dubliniensis*: characteristics and identification. J Clin Microbiol. 1998;36:329–34.
11. Pappas PG, Kauffman CA, Andes D, et al. Clinical practice guidelines for the management of candidiasis: 2009 update by the Infectious Diseases Society of America. Clin Infect Dis. 2009;48:503–35.
12. Wilcox CM. Esophageal disease in the acquired immunodeficiency syndrome: etiology, diagnosis, and management. Am J Med. 1992;92:412–21.
13. Villanueva A, Arathoon EG, Gotuzzo E, Berman RS, DiNubile MJ, Sable CA. A randomized double-blind study of caspofungin versus amphotericin B for the treatment of candidal esophagitis. Clin Infect Dis. 2001;33:1529–35.
14. Ally R, Schürmann, Kreisel W, et al. A randomized, double-blind, double dummy, multicenter trial of voriconazole and fluconazole in the treatment of esophageal candidiasis in immunocompromised patients. Clin Infect Dis. 2001;33:1447–54.
15. Launay O, Lortholary O, Bourges C, Jarrousse B, Bentata M, Guillevin L. Candidemia: a nosocomial complication in adults with late-stage AIDS. Clin Infect Dis. 1998;26:1134–41.
16. Charlier C, Hart E, Lefort A, et al. Fluconazole for the management of invasive candidiasis: where do we stand after 15 years? J Antimicrob Chemother. 2006;57:384–410.
17. Maenza JR, Keruly JC, Moore RD, Chaisson RE, Merz WG, Gallant JE. Risk factors for fluconazole-resistant candidiasis in human immunodeficiency virus-infected patients. J Infect Dis. 1996;173:219–25.
18. Walmsley S, King S, McGeer A, Ye Y, Richardson S. Oropharyngeal candidiasis in patients with human immunodeficiency virus: correlation of clinical outcome with in vitro resistance, serum azole levels, and immunosuppression. Clin Infect Dis. 2001;32: 1554–61.
19. Redding S, Smith J, Farinacci G, et al. Resistance of *Candida albicans* to fluconazole during treatment of oropharyngeal candidiasis in a patient with AIDS: documentation by in vitro susceptibility testing and DNA subtype analysis. Clin Infect Dis. 1994;18:240–2.
20. Revankar SG, Dib OP, Kirkpatrick WR, et al. Clinical evaluation and microbiology of oropharyngeal infection due to fluconazole-resistant *Candida* in human immunodeficiency virus-infected patients. Clin Infect Dis. 1998;26:960–3.
21. Dromer F, Improvisi L, Dupont B, Eliaszewicz M, Pialoux G, Fournier S. Oral transmission of *Candida albicans* isolates between partners in HIV-infected couples could contribute to dissemination of fluconazole-resistant isolates. AIDS. 1997;11:1095–101.
22. Kwon-Chung KJ, Varma A, Howard DH. Ecology of *Cryptococcus neoformans* and prevalence of its two varieties in AIDS and non-AIDS associated cryptococcosis. In: Vanden Bossche H, MacKenzie DWR, Cauwenbergh G, Van Cutsem J, Drouhet E, Dupont B, editors. Mycoses in AIDS patients. New York: Plenum Press; 1990. p. 103–13.
23. Dromer F, Mathoulin-Pélissier S, Fontanet A, et al. Epidemiology of HIV-associated cryptococcosis in France (1985–2001): comparison of the pre- and post-HAART eras. AIDS. 2004;18:555–62.
24. Jarvis JN, Dromer F, Harrison TS, Lortholary O. Managing cryptococcosis in the immunocompromised host. Curr Opin Infect Dis. 2008;21:596–603.
25. Micol R, Lortholary O, Sar B, et al. Prevalence, determinants of positivity, and clinical utility of cryptococcal antigenemia in Cambodian HIV-infected patients. J Acquir Immune Defic Syndr. 2007;45:555–9.
26. Park BJ, Wannemuehler KA, Marston BJ, Govender N, Pappas PG, Chiller TM. Estimation of the current global burden of cryptococcal meningitis among persons living with HIV/AIDS. AIDS. 2009;23:525–30.
27. Neuville S, Dromer F, Morin O, et al. Primary cutaneous cryptococcosis: a distinct clinical entity. Clin Infect Dis. 2003;6:337–44.
28. Dromer F, Mathoulin-Pélissier S, Launay O, Lortholary O. French Cryptococcosis Study Group. Determinants of disease presentation and outcome during cryptococcosis: the CryptoA/D study. PLoS Med. 2007;4:e21.
29. Charlier C, Dromer F, Lévêque C, et al. Cryptococcal neuroradiological lesions correlate with severity during cryptococcal meningoencephalitis in HIV-positive patients in the HAART era. PLoS ONE. 2008;3:e1950.
30. Cameron ML, Bartlett JA, Gallis HA, Waskin HA. Manifestations of pulmonary cryptococcosis in patients with acquired immunodeficiency syndrome. Rev Infect Dis. 1990;12:768–77.
31. Meyohas MC, Roux P, Bollens D, et al. Pulmonary cryptococcosis: localized and disseminated infections in 27 patients with AIDS. Clin Infect Dis. 1995;21:628–33.
32. Perfect JR, Dismukes WE, Dromer F, et al. Clinical practice guidelines for the management of cryptococcal disease: 2010 Update by the Infectious Disease Society of America. Clin Infect Dis. 2010;50:291–322.
33. Jarvis JN, Lawn SD, Vogt M, Bangani N, Wood R, Harrison TS. Screening for cryptococcal antigenemia in patients accessing an antiretroviral treatment program in South Africa. Clin Infect Dis. 2009;48:856–62.
34. van der Horst CM, Saag MS, Cloud GA, et al. Treatment of cryptococcal meningitis associated with the acquired immunodeficiency syndrome. N Engl J Med. 1997;337:15–21.
35. Pappas PG, Chetchotisakd P, Larsen RA, et al. A phase II randomized trial of amphotericin B alone or combined with fluconazole in the treatment of HIV-associated cryptococcal meningitis. Clin Infect Dis. 2009;48:1775–83.
36. Dromer F, Bernede-Bauduin C, Guillemot D, Lortholary O. French Cryptococcosis Study Group. Major role for amphotericin B-flucytosine combination in severe cryptococcosis. PLoS One. 2008;3:e2870.
37. Saag MS, Powderly WG, Cloud GA, et al. Comparison of amphotericin B with fluconazole in the treatment of acute AIDS-associated cryptococcal meningitis. N Engl J Med. 1992;326:83–9.
38. Coker RJ, Viviani M, Gazzard BG, et al. Treatment of cryptococcosis with liposomal amphotericin B (AmBisome) in 23 patients with AIDS. AIDS. 1993;7:829–35.
39. Leenders AC, Reiss P, Portegies P, et al. Liposomal amphotericin B (AmBisome) compared with amphotericin B followed by oral fluconazole in the treatment of AIDS-associated cryptococcal meningitis. AIDS. 1997;11:1463–71.
40. Liliang P-C, Liang C-L, Chang W-N, Lu K, Lu C-H. Use of ventriculoperitoneal shunts to treat uncontrollable intracranial hypertension in patients who have cryptococcal meningitis without hydrocephalus. Clin Infect Dis. 2002;34:e64–8.
41. Graybill JR, Sobel J, Saag M, et al. Diagnosis and management of increased intracranial pressure in patients with AIDS and cryptococcal meningitis. Clin Infect Dis. 2000;30:47–54.
42. Aberg JA, Price RW, Heeren DM, Bredt B. A pilot study of the discontinuation of antifungal therapy for disseminated cryptococcal disease in patients with acquired immunodeficiency syndrome, following immunologic response to antiretroviral therapy. J Infect Dis. 2002;185:1179–82.
43. Mussini C, Pezzotti P, Miró JM, et al. Discontinuation of maintenance therapy for cryptococcal meningitis in patients with AIDS treated with highly active antiretroviral therapy: an international observational study. Clin Infect Dis. 2004;38:565–71.
44. Lortholary O, Poizat G, Zeller V, et al. Long-term outcome of AIDS-associated cryptococcosis in the era of combination antiretroviral therapy. AIDS. 2006;20:2183–91.
45. Vibhagool A, Sungkanuparph S, Mootsikapun P, et al. Discontinuation of secondary prophylaxis for cryptococcal meningitis in human immunodeficiency virus-infected patients treated with highly active

antiretroviral therapy: a prospective, multicenter, randomized study. Clin Infect Dis. 2003;36:1329–31.
46. Chetchotisakd P, Sungkanuparph S, Thinkhamrop B, Mootsikapun P, Boonyaprawit P. A multicentre, randomized, double-blind, placebo-controlled trial of primary cryptococcal meningitis prophylaxis in HIV-infected patients with severe immune deficiency. HIV Med. 2004;5:140–3.
47. Supparatpinyo K, Khamwan C, Baosoung V, Nelson KE, Sirisanthana T. Disseminated *Penicillium marneffei* infection in Southeast Asia. Lancet. 1994;334:110–3.
48. Wheat LJ, Connolly-Stringfield PA, Baker RL, et al. Disseminated histoplasmosis in the acquired immune deficiency syndrome: clinical findings, diagnosis and treatment, and review of the literature. Medicine (Baltimore). 1990;69:361–74.
49. Warnock DW, Dupont B, Kauffman CA, Sirisanthana T. Imported mycoses in Europe. Med Mycol. 1998;36:87–94.
50. McKinsey D, Spiegel RA, Hutwagner L, et al. Prospective study of histoplasmosis patients infected with human immunodeficiency virus: incidence, risk factors, and pathophysiology. Clin Infect Dis. 1997;24:1195–203.
51. Wheat J, Chetchotisakd P, Williams B, Connolly P, Shutt K, Hajjeh R. Factors associated with severe manifestations of histoplasmosis in AIDS. Clin Infect Dis. 2000;30:877–81.
52. Loulergue P, Bastides F, Baudouin V, et al. Literature review and case histories of *Histoplasma capsulatum* var. *duboisii* infections in HIV-infected patients. Emerg Infect Dis. 2007;13:1647–52.
53. Wheat LJ, Freifeld AG, Kleiman MB, et al. Clinical practice guidelines for the management of patients with histoplasmosis: 2007 update by the Infectious Diseases Society of America. Clin Infect Dis. 2007;45:807–25.
54. Goldman M, Zackin R, Fichtenbaum CJ, et al. Safety of discontinuation of maintenance therapy for disseminated histoplasmosis after immunologic response to antiretroviral therapy. Clin Infect Dis. 2004;38:1485–9.
55. McKinsey DS, Wheat LJ, Cloud GA, et al. Itraconazole prophylaxis for fungal infections in patients with advanced human immunodeficiency virus infection: randomized, placebo-controlled, double-blind study. Clin Infect Dis. 1999;28:1049–56.
56. Bronnimann DA, Adam RD, Galgiani JN, et al. Coccidioidomycosis in the acquired immunodeficiency syndrome. Ann Intern Med. 1987;106:372–9.
57. Woods CW, McRill C, Plikaytis BD, et al. Coccidioidomycosis in human immunodeficiency virus-infected persons in Arizona, 1994–1997: incidence, risk factors, and prevention. J Infect Dis. 2000;181:1428–34.
58. Fish DG, Ampel NM, Galgiani JN, et al. *Coccidioides immitis* in patients with human immunodeficiency virus infections: a review of 77 patients. Medicine (Baltimore). 1990;69:384–91.
59. Galgiani JN, Ampel NM. *Coccidioides immitis* in patients with human immunodeficiency virus infections. Semin Respir Infect. 1990;5:151–4.
60. Galgiani JN, Ampel NM, Blair JE, et al. Coccidioidomycosis. Clin Infect Dis. 2005;41:1217–23.
61. Galgiani JN, Catanzaro A, Cloud GA, et al. Comparison of oral fluconazole and itraconazole for progressive non-meningeal coccidioidomycosis. Ann Intern Med. 2000;133:676–86.
62. Kaplan JE, Benson C, Holmes KK, Brooks JT, Pau A, Masur H. Guidelines for the prevention and treatment of opportunistic infections in HIV-infected adults and adolescents. MMWR. 2009;58(RR-11):1–166.
63. Deng Z, Ribas JL, Gibson DW, Connor DH. Infection caused by *Penicillium marneffei* in China and Southeast Asia: review of eighteen published cases and report of four more Chinese cases. Rev Infect Dis. 1998;10:640–52.
64. Drouhet E. Penicilliosis due to *Penicillium marneffei*: a new emerging systemic mycosis in AIDS patients travelling or living in Southeast Asia. Review of 44 cases reported in HIV infected patients during the last 5 years compared to 44 cases of non-AIDS patients reported over 20 years. J Mycol Med. 1993;4:195–224.
65. Sobottka I, Albrecht H, Mack D, et al. Systemic *Penicillium marneffei* infection in a German AIDS patient. Eur J Clin Microbiol Infect Dis. 1996;15:256–69.
66. Sirisanthana T, Supparatpinyo K, Periens T, Nelson KE. Amphotericin B and itraconazole for treatment of disseminated *Penicillium marneffei* infection in human immunodeficiency virus-infected patients. Clin Infect Dis. 1998;26:1107–10.
67. Supparatpinyo K, Perriens J, Nelson KE, Srisanthana T. A controlled trial of itraconazole to prevent relapse of *Penicillium marneffei* infection in patients infected with the human immunodeficiency virus. N Engl J Med. 1998;339:1739–43.
68. Chariyalertsak S, Supparatpinyo K, Sirisanthana T, Nelson KE. A controlled trial of itraconazole as primary prophylaxis for systemic fungal infections in patients with advanced human immunodeficiency virus infection in Thailand. Clin Infect Dis. 2002;34:277–84.
69. Goldani LZ, Sugar AM. Paracoccidioidomycosis in AIDS: an overview. Clin Infect Dis. 1995;21:1275–81.
70. Benard G, Duarte AJS. Paracoccidioidomycosis: a model for evaluation of the effects of human immunodeficiency virus infection on the natural history of endemic tropical diseases. Clin Infect Dis. 2000;31:1032–9.
71. Paniago AM, de Freitas AC, Aguiar ES, et al. Paracoccidioidomycosis in patients with human immunodeficiency virus: review of 12 cases observed in an endemic region in Brazil. J Infect. 2005;51:248–52.
72. Pappas PG, Pottage JC, Powderly WG, et al. Blastomycosis in patients with the acquired immunodeficiency syndrome. Ann Intern Med. 1992;116:847–53.
73. Chapman SW, Dismukes WE, Proia LA, et al. Clinical practice guidelines for the management of blastomycosis: 2008 update by the Infectious Diseases Society of America. Clin Infect Dis. 2008;46:1801–12.
74. Al-Tawfiq JA, Wools KK. Disseminated sporotrichosis and *Sporothrix schenckii* fungemia as the initial presentation of human immunodeficiency virus infection. Clin Infect Dis. 1998;26:1403–6.
75. Rocha MM, Dassin T, Lira R, Lima EL, Severo LC, Londero AT. Sporotrichosis in patients with AIDS: report of case and review. Rev Iber Micol. 2001;18:133–6.
76. Kauffman CA, Bustamante B, Chapman SW, Pappas PG. Clinical practice guidelines for the management of sporotrichosis: 2007 update by the Infectious Diseases Society of America. Clin Infect Dis. 2007;45:1255–65.
77. Denning DW, Follansbee SE, Scolaro M, Norris S, Edelstein H, Stevens DA. Pulmonary aspergillosis in the acquired immunodeficiency syndrome. N Engl J Med. 1991;324:654–62.
78. Khoo S, Denning DW. *Aspergillus* infection in the acquired immune deficiency syndrome. Clin Infect Dis. 1994;19:541–8.
79. Lortholary O, Meyohas MC, Dupont B, et al. Invasive aspergillosis in patients with acquired immunodeficiency syndrome: report of 33 cases. Am J Med. 1993;95:177–87.
80. Kemper CA, Hostetler JS, Follansbee S, et al. Ulcerative and plaque-like tracheobronchitis due to infection with *Aspergillus* in patients with AIDS. Clin Infect Dis. 1993;17:344–52.
81. Walsh TJ, Anaissie EJ, Denning DW, et al. Treatment of aspergillosis: clinical practice guidelines of the Infectious Diseases Society of America. Clin Infect Dis. 2008;46:327–60.
82. Smith AG, Bustamante CI, Gilmor GD. Zygomycosis (absidiomycosis) in an AIDS patient. Mycopathologia. 1989;105:7–10.
83. Vesa J, Bielsa O, Arango O, Liado C, Gelabert A. Massive renal infarction due to mycormycosis in an AIDS patient. Infection. 1992;20:234–6.
84. Santos J, Espigado P, Romero C, Andreu J, Rivero A, Pineda JA. Isolated renal mucormycosis in two AIDS patients. Eur J Clin Microbiol Infect Dis. 1994;13:430–2.

85. Micozzi MS, Wetli CV. Intravenous amphetamine abuse, primary cerebral mucormycosis, and acquired immunodeficiency. J Forensic Sci. 1985;30:504–10.
86. Cuadrado LM, Guerrero A, Garcia Asenjo JAL, Martin F, Palau E, Urra DG. Cerebral mucormycosis in two cases of acquired immunodeficiency syndrome. Arch Neurol. 1998;45:109–11.
87. Blatt SP, Lucey DR, De Hoff D, Zellmer RB. Rhinocerebral zygomycosis in a patient with AIDS. J Infect Dis. 1991;164:215–6.
88. Hopwood V, Hicks DA, Thomas S, Evans EGV. Primary cutaneous zygomycosis due to *Absidia corymbifera* in a patient with AIDS. J Med Vet Mycol. 1992;30:399–402.
89. Mostaza JM, Barbado FJ, Fernandez-Martin J, Pena-Yanez J, Vasquez-Rodriguez JJ. Cutaneoarticular mucormycosis due to *Cunninghamella bertholletiae* in a patient with AIDS. Rev Infect Dis. 1989;11:316–8.
90. Chavanet P, Lefranc T, Bonnin A, Waldner A, Portier H. Unusual cause of pharyngeal ulcerations in AIDS. Lancet. 1990;336:383–4.
91. Rollot F, Blanche P, Richaud-Thiriez B, et al. Pneumonia due to *Scedosporium apiospermum* in a patient with HIV infection. Scand J Infect Dis. 2000;32:439.
92. Raffanti SP, Fyfe B, Carreiro S, Sharp SE, Hyma BA, Ratzan KR. Native valve endocarditis due to *Pseudallescheria boydii* in a patient with AIDS: case report and review. Rev Infect Dis. 1990;12:993–6.
93. Montero A, Cohen JE, Fernandez MA, Mazzolini G, Gomez R, Perugini J. Cerebral pseudallescheriasis due to *Pseudallescheria boydii* as the first manifestation in AIDS. Clin Infect Dis. 1998;26:1476–7.
94. Eckburg PB, Zolopa AR, Montoya JG. Invasive fungal sinusitis due to *Scedosporium apiospermum* in a patient with AIDS. Clin Infect Dis. 1999;29:212–3.
95. Scherr GR, Evans SG, Kiyabu MT, Klatt EC. *Pseudallescheria boydii* infection in the acquired immunodeficiency syndrome. Arch Pathol Lab Med. 1992;116:535–6.
96. Wiest PM, Wiese K, Jacobs MR, et al. *Alternaria* infection in a patient with acquired immunodeficiency syndrome: case report and review of invasive *Alternaria* infections. Rev Infect Dis. 1987;9:799–803.
97. Turner D, Burke M, Bashe E, Blinder S, Yust I. Pulmonary adiaspiromycosis in a patient with acquired immunodeficiency syndrome. Eur J Clin Microbiol Infect Dis. 1999;18:893–5.
98. Echavarria E, Cano EL, Restrepo A. Disseminated adiaspiromycosis in a patient with AIDS. J Med Vet Mycol. 1993;31:91–7.
99. Gori S, Drouhet E, Gueho E, et al. Cutaneous disseminated mycosis in a patient with AIDS due to a new dimorphic fungus. J Mycol Med. 1998;8:57–63.
100. Bossi P, Mortier E, Michon C, et al. Sinusite à *Fusarium solani* chez un patient atteint de SIDA. J Mycol Med. 1995;5:56–7.
101. Del Palacio-Hernanz A, Casado VA, Lopez FP, Quiros HO, Palancar MP. Infeccion oportunista pulmonar por *Fusarium moniliforme* en paciente con SIDA. Rev Iber Micol. 1989;6:144–7.
102. Paugam A, Baixench MT, Frank N, et al. Localized oral *Fusarium* in an AIDS patient with malignant lymphoma. J Infect. 1999;39:153–4.
103. Marriott DJE, Wong KH, Aznar E, Harkness JL, Cooper DA, Muir D. *Scytalidium dimidiatum* and *Lecythophora hoffmannii*: unusual causes of fungal infections in a patient with AIDS. J Clin Microbiol. 1997;35:2949–52.
104. Rosenthal J, Katz R, Dubois DB, Morrissey A, Machicao A. Chronic maxillary sinusitis associated with the mushroom *Schizophyllum commune* in a patient with AIDS. Clin Infect Dis. 1992;14:46–8.
105. Al-Tawfik OW, Papasian CJ, Dixon AY, Potter LM. *Saccharomyces cerevisiae* pneumonia in a patient with acquired immune deficiency syndrome. J Clin Microbiol. 1989;27:1689–91.
106. Lui AY, Turett GS, Karter DL, Bellman PC, Kislak JW. Amphotericin B lipid complex therapy in AIDS patient with *Rhodotorula rubra* fungemia. Clin Infect Dis. 1998;27:892–3.
107. Barchiesi F, Morbiducci V, Ancarani F, Arzeni D, Scalise G. *Trichosporon beigelii* fungaemia in an AIDS patient. AIDS. 1993;7:139–40.
108. Leaf HL, Simberkoff MS. Invasive trichosporonosis in a patient with acquired immunodeficiency syndrome. J Infect Dis. 1989;160:356–7.
109. Parsonnet J. *Trichosporon beigelii* peritonitis. South Med J. 1989;82:1062–3.
110. Detels R, Tarwater P, Phair JP, Margolick J, Riddler SA, Munoz A. Effectiveness of potent antiretroviral therapies on the incidence of opportunistic infections before and after AIDS diagnosis. AIDS. 2001;15:347–55.
111. Palella Jr FJ, Delaney KM, Moorman AC, et al. Declining morbidity and mortality among patients with advanced human immunodeficiency virus infection. N Engl J Med. 1998;338:853–60.
112. Soriano V, Dona C, Rodriguez-Rosado R, Barreiro P, Gonzalez-Lahoz J. Discontinuation of secondary prophylaxis for opportunistic infections in HIV-infected patients receiving highly active antiretroviral therapy. AIDS. 2000;14:383–6.
113. Sempowski GD, Haynes BF. Immune reconstitution in patients with HIV infection. Ann Rev Med. 2002;53:269–84.
114. Blanche PH, Gombert B, Ginsburg CH, et al. HIV combination therapy: immune restitution causing cryptococcal lymphadenitis dramatically improved by anti-inflammatory therapy. Scand J Infect Dis. 1998;30:615–6.
115. De Simonne JA, Roger J, Pomerantz A, Babinchak TJ. Inflammatory reactions in HIV1-infected persons after initiation of active antiretroviral therapy. Ann Intern Med. 2000;133:447–54.
116. Cheng VCC, Yuen K-Y, Chan W-M, Wong SSY, Ma ESK, Chan RMT. Immunorestitution disease involving the innate and adaptive response. Clin Infect Dis. 2000;30:882–92.
117. Lortholary O, Fontanet A, Mémain N, et al. Incidence and risk factors of immune reconstitution inflammatory syndrome complicating HIV-associated cryptococcosis in France. AIDS. 2005;19:1043–9.
118. Breton G, Adle-Biassette H, Therby A, et al. Immune reconstitution inflammatory syndrome in HIV-infected patients with disseminated histoplasmosis. AIDS. 2006;20:119–21.
119. Shelburne SA, Darcourt J, White Jr AC, et al. The role of immune reconstitution inflammatory syndrome in AIDS-related *Cryptococcus neoformans* disease in the era of highly active antiretroviral therapy. Clin Infect Dis. 2005;40:1049–52.
120. Sungkanuparph S, Filler SG, Chetchotisakd P, et al. Cryptococcal immune reconstitution inflammatory syndrome after antiretroviral therapy in AIDS patients with cryptococcal meningitis: a prospective multicenter study. Clin Infect Dis. 2009;49:931–4.
121. Woods ML, MacGinly R, Eisen DP, Allworth AM. HIV combination therapy: partial immune restitution unmasking latent cryptococcal infection. AIDS. 1998;12:1491–4.

Index

C.A. Kauffman et al. (eds.), *Essentials of Clinical Mycology*,
DOI 10.1007/978-1-4419-6640-7, © Springer Science+Business Media, LLC 2011

R

MIX
Papier aus verantwortungsvollen Quellen
Paper from responsible sources
FSC® C105338

If you have any concerns about our products,
you can contact us on
ProductSafety@springernature.com

In case Publisher is established outside the EU,
the EU authorized representative is:
Springer Nature Customer Service Center GmbH
Europaplatz 3, 69115 Heidelberg, Germany

Printed by Libri Plureos GmbH
in Hamburg, Germany